Core Curriculum fo.
Lactation
Consultant
Practice

International
Lactation
Consultant
Association

**THIRD
EDITION**

EDITED BY

Rebecca Mannel, BS, IBCLC, FILCA
Lactation Center Coordinator and Clinical Instructor
OU Medical Center and OU Health Sciences Center
Oklahoma City, Oklahoma

Patricia J. Martens, IBCLC, PhD, FILCA
Director, Manitoba Centre for Health Policy
Professor, Department of Community Health Sciences
Faculty of Medicine
University of Manitoba
Winnipeg, Manitoba, Canada

Marsha Walker, RN, IBCLC
Executive Director, National Alliance for Breastfeeding Advocacy
Research, Education, and Legal Branch
Weston, Massachusetts

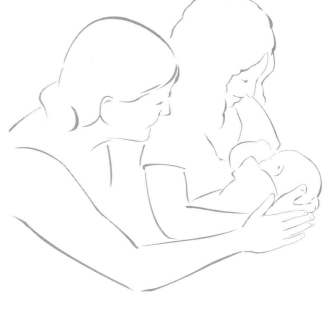

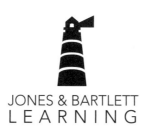

JONES & BARTLETT
L E A R N I N G

World Headquarters
Jones & Bartlett Learning
5 Wall Street
Burlington, MA 01803
978-443-5000
info@jblearning.com
www.jblearning.com

Jones & Bartlett Learning books and products are available through most bookstores and online booksellers. To contact Jones & Bartlett Learning directly, call 800-832-0034, fax 978-443-8000, or visit our website, www.jblearning.com.

Substantial discounts on bulk quantities of Jones & Bartlett Learning publications are available to corporations, professional associations, and other qualified organizations. For details and specific discount information, contact the special sales department at Jones & Bartlett Learning via the above contact information or send an email to specialsales@jblearning.com.

Production Credits

Publisher: Kevin Sullivan
Acquisitions Editor: Amanda Harvey
Editorial Assistant: Sara Bempkins
Associate Production Editor: Sara Fowles
Marketing Communications Manager: Katie Hennessy
V.P., Manufacturing and Inventory Control:
  Therese Connell

Composition: Jason Miranda, Spoke & Wheel
Cover Design and Illustration: Scott Moden
Printing and Binding: Edwards Brothers Malloy
Cover Printing: Edwards Brothers Malloy

Library of Congress Cataloging-in-Publication Data
Core curriculum for lactation consultant practice / [edited by] Rebecca Mannel,
Patricia J. Martens, Marsha Walker.
— 3rd ed.
p ; cm. Includes bibliographical references and index.
ISBN 978-0-7637-9879-6 (pbk.)
I. Mannel, Rebecca. II. Martens, Patricia J. III. Walker, Marsha.
[DNLM: 1. Breast Feeding. 2. Lactation. 3. Mothers—education. WS 125]
649.33—dc23
                                    2012011789
6048

Printed in the United States of America
16   10 9 8 7

CONTENTS

PART IV Nutrition and Biochemistry   **317**

SECTION III BREASTFEEDING MANAGEMENT **473**

PART V Breastfeeding Technique   **475**

Appendices

ACKNOWLEDGMENTS

This *Third Edition* of ILCA's *Core Curriculum for Lactation Consultant Practice* has truly been a collaborative undertaking. Our editorial team wishes to extend our sincere gratitude to all of the chapter authors whose diligence and expertise enabled the association to update the information in this text and to add new chapters. A special thanks also goes to the ILCA office team of Ashley Lehman and Natalie Sroka, for their invaluable assistance and support. This third edition could not have materialized without their team effort. We also wish to acknowledge the Jones & Bartlett Learning staff for their patience and support and the ILCA board of directors for their vision and action to ensure that this revision took place.

On a personal note, we wish to thank our families for their encouragement and support. A project of this magnitude takes a great deal of time away from your family. Thank you to our husbands, Robert Mannel, Gary Martens, and Hap Walker, for keeping our families intact and functioning! Last, we acknowledge all of our hardworking peers in lactation who keep us motivated to continue to strengthen our profession through publications such as the *Core Curriculum*.

Rebecca Mannel
Patricia J. Martens
Marsha Walker

PREFACE

With the vast amount of information available about breastfeeding and human lactation, it is challenging to reflect key concepts in a single core text. As the editors of the *Core Curriculum for Lactation Consultant Practice, Third Edition*, we envision this as a practical, succinct, and user-friendly resource for lactation consultants and other healthcare providers. The authors who participated in the creation of this resource provide a wealth of knowledge and expertise, resulting in information being available in one convenient location.

First and foremost, this text is designed to be used as a resource for practicing lactation consultants as well as for development of educational programs. The core curriculum content, along with its hundreds of citations, represents the knowledge base required to practice the profession of lactation consulting. In addition to its use as a valuable reference, it can be a source for staff development training, orientation of new staff, and as a resource when designing a curriculum for aspiring lactation consultants. Because this book will be utilized by a wide variety of healthcare providers, the editors chose the American Psychological Association style of referencing.

This text can also serve as a guide for aspiring lactation consultants as they study for the certification exam administered by the International Board of Lactation Consultant Examiners (IBLCE). Its content is patterned after the exam blueprint and encompasses all required topic areas. Use of this guide can help exam candidates assess their level of knowledge, experience, and expertise to develop an effective study plan. A unique feature of the book is a mapping plan that cross references topics found in the IBLCE exam blueprint with relevant information found in particular chapters. This information allows users to easily locate topics of specific interest in a quick reference format. Used in conjunction with lactation textbooks, the reader will find this core curriculum invaluable in devising an effective study plan.

We hope that this text is helpful to all who use it and that ultimately it benefits all the mothers, babies, and families with whom we interact in our lactation consultant roles.

Rebecca Mannel, BS, IBCLC, FILCA
Lactation Center Coordinator and Clinical Instructor
OU Medical Center and OU Health Sciences Center
Oklahoma City, Oklahoma

Patricia J. Martens, IBCLC, PhD, FILCA
Director, Manitoba Centre for Health Policy
Professor, Department of Community Health Sciences, Faculty of Medicine
University of Manitoba
Winnipeg, Manitoba, Canada

Marsha Walker, RN, IBCLC
Executive Director, National Alliance for Breastfeeding Advocacy
Research, Education, and Legal Branch
Weston, Massachusetts

CONTRIBUTORS

Teresa E. Baker, MD
Associate Professor
Department of OB/GYN
Texas Tech University School of Medicine
Amarillo, Texas

Jennifer Bañuelos, MAS
Human Lactation Center
Department of Nutrition
University of California
Davis, California

Priscilla G. Bornmann, JD
McKinley & Bornmann, PLC
Alexandria, Virginia

Elizabeth C. Brooks, JD, IBCLC, FILCA
Private Practice IBCLC
Wyndmoor, Pennsylvania

Karin Cadwell, PhD, FAAN, IBCLC
The Healthy Children Project
East Sandwich, Massachusetts

Cathy Carothers, BLA, IBCLC, FILCA
Codirector
Every Mother, Inc.
Greenville, Mississippi

Lisa M. Cleveland, PhD, RN, IBCLC
Assistant Professor, Family Nursing
University of Texas Health Science Center,
    School of Nursing
San Antonio, Texas

Suzanne Cox, AM, IBCLC, FILCA
Private Practice Lactation Consultants
Tasmania, Australia

Melissa Cross, RN, IBCLC
Saint Luke's Hospital
Kansas City, Missouri

Marie Davis, RN, IBCLC
Kaiser Permanente Riverside, Retired
Riverside, California

Catherine Watson Genna, BS, IBCLC
Private Practice Lactation Consultant
Woodhaven, New York

Sara L. Gill, PhD, RN, IBCLC
Associate Professor, Family & Community
    Health Systems
The University of Texas Health Science Center
    San Antonio School of Nursing
San Antonio, Texas

Jennifer Goldbronn, RD, MAS
Human Lactation Center
Department of Nutrition
University of California
Davis, California

M. Karen Kerkoff Gromada, MSN, IBCLC, FILCA
Lead Lactation Consultant Educator
TriHealth Hospitals
Cincinnati, Ohio

Thomas W. Hale, RPh, PhD
Professor of Pediatrics
Director, InfantRisk Center
Director, Clinical Research Unit
Texas Tech University School of Medicine
Amarillo, Texas

Susan W. Hatcher, RN, BSN, IBCLC
Private Practice Lactation Consultant
Director, HealthSource for Women
Chesapeake, Virginia

Joy Heads, RM, MHPEd, IBCLC
Lactation Consultant
Royal Hospital for Women
South Eastern Sydney Illawarra Area Health
    Service
New South Wales, Australia

M. Jane Heinig, PhD, IBCLC
Human Lactation Center
Department of Nutrition
University of California
Davis, California

Kay Hoover, MEd, IBCLC, FILCA
Pennsylvania State University
University Park, Pennsylvania

Maeve Howett, PhD, APRN, IBCLC
Nell Hodgson Woodruff School of Nursing,
    Emory University
Atlanta, Georgia

Vergie I. Hughes, MS, IBCLC, FILCA
Inova Learning Network
Fairfax, Virginia

Roberto Mario Silveira Issler, MD, PhD, IBCLC
Assistant Teacher
Pediatric Department, Faculdade de Medicina,
    Universidade Federal do Rio Grande do Sul
Porto Alegre, Brazil

Frances Jones, RN, MSN, IBCLC
Program Coordinator, Lactation Service & BC
    Women's Milk Bank
Children's and Women's Health Centre of
    British Columbia
Vancouver, British Columbia

Kathleen Kendall-Tackett, PhD, IBCLC, FAPA
Family Research Laboratory
University of New Hampshire
Durham, New Hampshire

Marion ("Lou") Lamb, RN, MS, IBCLC
Lactation Education Resources
Charlottesville, Virginia

Mary Grace Lanese, BSN, RN, IBCLC
Saint Luke's Hospital
Kansas City, Missouri

Judith Lauwers, BA, IBCLC, FILCA
Education Coordinator
International Lactation Consultant Association
Chalfont, Pennsylvania

Rachelle Lessen, MS, RD, IBCLC
Lactation Consultant and Pediatric Nutritionist
The Children's Hospital of Philadelphia
Philadelphia, Pennsylvania

Rebecca Mannel, BS, IBCLC, FILCA
Lactation Center Coordinator and Clinical
    Instructor
OU Medical Center and OU Health Sciences
    Center
Oklahoma City, Oklahoma

Lisa Marasco, MA, IBCLC, FILCA
Santa Barbara County Public Health
    Department
Nutrition Services/WIC
Santa Barbara, California

Patricia J. Martens, IBCLC, PhD, FILCA
Director, Manitoba Centre for Health Policy
Professor, Department of Community Health
    Sciences
Faculty of Medicine
University of Manitoba
Winnipeg, Manitoba, Canada

Nancy Mohrbacher, IBCLC, FILCA
Coauthor, *The Breastfeeding Answer Book*
Arlington Heights, Illinois

Chris Mulford, BA, BSN
Formerly: Chair of the Workplace Committee
    for the United State Breastfeeding Committee
Coordinator for Women and Work Task Force
    for the World Alliance for Breastfeeding
    Action
Swarthmore, Pennsylvania

Frank J. Nice, RPh, DPA, CPHP
National Institutes of Health
Bethesda, Maryland

Sallie Page-Goertz, MN, CPNP, IBCLC
Clinical Assistant Professor
Pediatrics
Kansas University School of Medicine
Kansas City, Kansas

Judith Rogers, OTR/L
Pregnancy and Parenting Equipment Specialist
Through the Looking Glass (National Resource
    Center for Parents with Disabilities)
Berkeley, California

Carol A. Ryan, MSN, IBCLC, FILCA
Georgetown University Hospital
Washington, D.C.

Michelle Scott, MA, RD/LD, IBCLC
Wellspring Nutrition and Lactation Services
Mason, New Hampshire

Noreen Siebenaler, MSN, RN, IBCLC
Lactation Consultant, Clinical Nurse Consultant
Adventist Health Central Valley Network
Adventist Medical Center
Selma, California

Angela Smith, RM, BA, IBCLC
Post Natal Nursing Unit Manager KGV
Royal Prince Alfred Hospital
Sydney, Australia

Linda J. Smith, MPH, IBCLC, FILCA
Director
Bright Future Lactation Resource Centre Ltd
Dayton, Ohio

Amy Spangler, MN, RN, IBCLC
President
Amy's Babies
Atlanta, Georgia

Elizabeth K. Stehel, MD, FAAP, IBCLC
Associate Professor, Department of Pediatrics
University of Texas Southwestern Medical Center
Dallas, Texas

Virginia Thorley, PhD, IBCLC, FILCA
Private Practice Lactation Consultant
Queensland, Australia

Mary Rose Tully, MPH, IBCLC
Formerly: Center for Infant/Young Child
    Feeding/Care
Maternal Child Health, School of Public Health
University of North Carolina
Chapel Hill, North Carolina

Cynthia Turner-Maffei, MA, IBCLC
Faculty
Healthy Children Project, Inc.
East Sandwich, Massachusetts

Marsha Walker, RN, IBCLC
Executive Director, National Alliance for
    Breastfeeding Advocacy
Research, Education, and Legal Branch
Weston, Massachusetts

Barbara Wilson-Clay, BSEd, IBCLC, FILCA
Private Practice Lactation Consultant
Manchaca, Texas

MAP OF THE
CORE CURRICULUM CHAPTERS

The following table is a "road map" of the objectives and standards in the IBLCE Exam cross-referenced to coverage of that topic in this book. Use it as a guide to explore each discipline in depth according to the perspective provided in relevant chapters.

Discipline	Chapters
A. Maternal and infant ANATOMY Includes: breast and nipple structure and development; blood, lymph, innervation, mammary tissue; infant oral anatomy and reflexes; assessment; anatomical variations.	15, 16, 17, 18, 27, 28, 29, 32, 39, 42
B. Maternal and infant normal PHYSIOLOGY and ENDOCRINOLOGY Includes: hormones; lactogenesis; endocrine/autocrine control of milk supply; induced lactation; fertility; infant hepatic, pancreatic and renal function; metabolism; effect of complementary feeds; digestion and gastrointestinal tract; voiding and stooling patterns.	15, 17, 18, 20, 28, 29, 30, 31, 32, 33, 35, 39, 40, 41, 42
C. Maternal and infant normal NUTRITION and BIOCHEMISTRY Includes: breastmilk synthesis and composition; milk components, function, and effect on baby; comparison with other products/milks; feeding patterns and intake over time; variations of maternal diet; ritual and traditional foods; introduction of solids.	5, 17, 19, 20, 21, 22, 24, 28, 29, 30, 31, 33, 42
D. Maternal and infant IMMUNOLOGY and INFECTIOUS DISEASE Includes: antibodies and other immune factors; cross-infection; bacteria and viruses in milk; allergies and food sensitivity; long-term protective factors.	19, 20, 23, 24, 29, 36, 41, Appendix B

(continues)

Discipline	Chapters
D. Maternal and infant IMMUNOLOGY and INFECTIOUS DISEASE Includes: antibodies and other immune factors; cross-infection; bacteria and viruses in milk; allergies and food sensitivity; long-term protective factors.	19, 20, 23, 24, 29, 36, 41, Appendix B
E. Maternal and infant PATHOLOGY Includes: acute/chronic abnormalities and diseases (both local and systemic); breast and nipple problems and pathology; endocrine pathology; mother/child physical and neurological disabilities; congenital abnormalities; oral pathology; neuro-logical immaturity; failure to thrive; hyperbilirubinemia and hypoglycemia; impact of pathology on breastfeeding.	16, 18, 24, 27, 29, 30, 31, 32, 33, 37, 38, 39, 40, 42, 43
F. Maternal and infant PHARMACOLOGY and TOXICOLOGY Includes: environmental contaminants; maternal use of medi-cation, over-the-counter preparations: effects of social or rec-reational drugs on the infant, on milk composition, and on lactation; galactagogues/suppressants; effects of medications used in labor; contraceptives; complementary therapies.	1, 25, 26, 35, 37, 39, 40, 41, 43
G. PSYCHOLOGY, SOCIOLOGY, and ANTHROPOLOGY Includes: counseling and adult education skills; grief, post-natal depression and psychosis; effect of socioeconomic, lifestyle, and employment issues on breastfeeding; maternal-infant relationship; maternal role adaptation; parenting skills; sleep patterns; cultural beliefs and practices; family; support systems; domestic violence; mothers with special needs, such as adolescents and migrants.	1, 3, 4, 5, 6, 7, 8, 9, 27, 28, 29, 30, 31, 32, 33, 35, 37, 38, 40
H. GROWTH PARAMETERS and DEVELOPMENTAL MILESTONES Includes: fetal and preterm growth; breastfed and artificially fed growth patterns; recognition of normal and delayed physi-cal, psychological, and cognitive developmental markers; breastfeeding behaviors to 12 months and beyond; weaning.	18, 20, 24, 28, 29, 30, 31, 38, 43
I. INTERPRETATION OF RESEARCH Includes: skills required to critically appraise and interpret research literature, lactation consultant educational material, and consumer literature; understanding terminology used in research and basic statistics; reading tables and graphs; sur-veys and data collection.	1, 11, 12, 14

Discipline	Chapters
J. ETHICAL AND LEGAL ISSUES Includes: IBLCE Code of Professional Conduct; ILCA Standards of Practice; practicing within scope of practice; referrals and interdisciplinary relationships; confidentiality; medical-legal responsibilities; charting and report writing skills; record keeping; informed consent; battery; maternal-infant neglect and abuse; conflict of interest; ethics of equipment rental and sales.	1, 7, 11, 12, 13, 14, 28, 32, 39, Appendix A
K. BREASTFEEDING EQUIPMENT AND TECHNOLOGY Includes: identification of breastfeeding devices and equipment, their appropriate use, and technical expertise to use them properly; handling and storing human milk, including human milk banking protocols.	1, 7, 29, 30, 32, 33, 34, 36, 38, Appendix B
L. TECHNIQUES Includes: breastfeeding techniques, positioning, and latch; assessing milk transfer; breastfeeding management; normal feeding patterns; milk expression.	7, 18, 28, 29, 30, 31, 32, 33, 35, 37, 38, 39
M. PUBLIC HEALTH Includes: breastfeeding promotion and community education; working with groups with low breastfeeding rates; creating and implementing clinical protocols; international tools and documents; International Code; Baby-Friendly Hospital Initiative implementation; prevalence, surveys and data collection for research purposes.	1, 2, 7, 8, 9, 10, 11, 12, 14, 30, 32, 37, Appendix A

Chronological Periods	Chapters
• Preconception	20, 21, 25, 26, 38, 41
• Prenatal	7, 18, 19, 20, 21, 23, 24, 25, 26, 30, 38, 41
• Labor and Birth (Perinatal)	5, 6, 18, 20, 21, 23, 24, 28, 30, 31, 33, 37, 38
• Prematurity	18, 20, 21, 23, 24, 25, 29, 30, 33, 40
• 0–2 Days	5, 6, 8, 18, 20, 21, 22, 23, 24, 25, 26, 28, 30, 31, 32, 33, 34, 37, 38, 39, 40, 41
• 3–14 Days	5, 6, 7, 8, 18, 20, 21, 22, 23, 24, 25, 26, 30, 31, 32, 33, 34, 37, 38, 39, 40, 41, 42, 43
• 15–28 Days	5, 6, 7, 8, 20, 21, 22, 23, 24, 25, 26, 30, 31, 32, 33, 37, 38, 39, 40, 41, 42, 43
• 1–3 Months	5, 6, 7, 8, 20, 21, 22, 23, 24, 25, 26, 30, 31, 32, 35, 38, 39, 40, 41, 43
• 4–6 Months	5, 6, 7, 8, 20, 21, 22, 23, 24, 25, 26, 30, 31, 32, 35, 38, 39, 41, 43
• 7–12 Months	5, 6, 7, 8, 20, 21, 22, 23, 24, 25, 26, 30, 31, 32, 35, 38, 39, 41
• 12 Months and Older	8, 20, 21, 23, 24, 30, 31, 32, 35, 39
• General Principles	2, 3, 4, 5, 6, 8, 9, 10, 11, 16, 19, 20, 21, 23, 30, 31, 34, 36, 38

IN MEMORIAM

In memory of two highly respected, much loved members of our profession and fellow authors of the Core Curriculum.

CHRIS MULFORD, RN, BSN, IBCLC
PENNSYLVANIA, USA

MARY ROSE TULLY, MPH, IBCLC
NORTH CAROLINA, USA

Section I

*Profession of
Lactation Consulting*

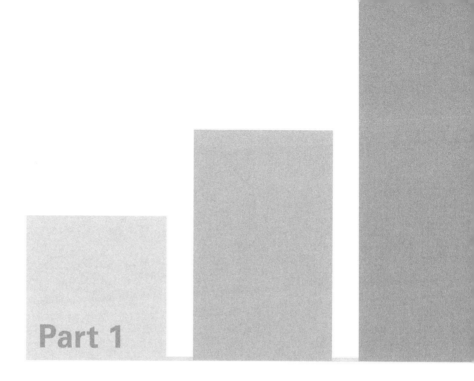

Part 1

Promotion and Support

CHAPTER 1
The IBLCE Code of Professional Conduct for IBCLCs

Elizabeth C. Brooks, JD, IBCLC, FILCA; Elizabeth K. Stehel, MD, FAAP, IBCLC; and Rebecca Mannel, BS, IBCLC, FILCA

OBJECTIVES

- Define the purpose of the Code of Professional Conduct for International Board Certified Lactation Consultants (IBCLCs) from the International Board of Lactation Consultant Examiners (IBLCE).[1]
- Discuss the Preamble, Definitions and Interpretations, and each principle of the IBLCE Code of Professional Conduct for IBCLCs, as they relate to lactation consultant practice.
- Describe when and how to report violations of the IBLCE Code of Professional Conduct for IBCLCs.

INTRODUCTION

The only internationally certified healthcare provider with expertise in breastfeeding and human lactation is the International Board Certified Lactation Consultant (IBCLC). The IBCLC earns the credential by successful completion of lactation-specific education, clinical practice, and the certification exam administered by the International Board of Lactation Consultant Examiners (IBLCE, 2011a). IBLCE has sole international authority to offer the IBCLC certification examination and confer the IBCLC credential through accreditation conferred by an independent organization, the National Commission for Certifying Agencies (NCCA). NCCA is based in the United States and operates under the aegis of the Institute for Credentialing Excellence (ICE), formerly known as the National Organization for Competency Assurance (Institute for Credentialing Excellence [ICE], 2011).

(continues)

---

[1] *IBCLC*© and *IBLCE*© are registered certification and service marks of the International Board of Lactation Consultant Examiners. For the readability of this chapter, the symbol is not repeated with each use of these terms. IBLCE has granted permission to ILCA to reproduce the CPC in this chapter. Contents of this chapter represent the views of the authors as individual IBCLCs.

The goal of any certification board is to establish that "the certification of specialized skill-sets affirms a knowledge and experience base for practitioners in a particular field, their employers, and the public at large" (ICE, 2009, para. 1). The "mission of NCCA is to help ensure the health, welfare, and safety of the public through the accreditation of certification programs that assess professional competence" (NCCA, 2007, p. 10). Thus, the IBLCE certification process (which includes education, clinical training, and examination) measures the skill of IBCLCs, who will use that expertise in their clinical and educational duties. A corollary concept is that there must be a "formal, published process for the enforcement of standards governing the professional behavior (i.e., ethics) of certificants" (NCCA, 2007, p. 22). This disciplinary process helps IBLCE ensure the public is protected against IBCLCs who do not practice using the requisite professional skills.

IBCLC certification is voluntarily sought, obtained, and maintained. The IBCLC credential is a conditional privilege that is revocable for cause. The purpose of the IBLCE Code of Professional Conduct (CPC) for IBCLCs is to provide guidance to the IBCLC in professional practice and conduct. The practitioner who chooses to earn IBCLC certification is bound by the professional behaviors described in the IBLCE Code of Professional Conduct for IBCLCs (IBLCE, 2011b), including consent to be governed by IBLCE Disciplinary Procedures (IBLCE, 2011c).[2]

History of the IBLCE Code of Professional Conduct

The IBLCE Code of Professional Conduct became effective November 1, 2011, and is a revision of the earlier IBLCE Code of Ethics (COE). The original COE was first enacted March 1, 1997, when the profession was about 10 years old (Scott, 1996). The COE applied to all IBCLCs who were "personally accountable for [their] practice and, in the exercise of professional accountability," were required to adhere to the enumerated principles (COE, 2003, para. 3, as cited in Scott & Calandro, 2008). The inaugural COE had 23 principles (Scott, 1996); a 24th principle relating to the *International Code of Marketing of Breast-milk Substitutes* was added in 1999 (IBLCE, 1999) and a 25th principle pertaining to intellectual property rights was made effective in 2004 (Scott et al., 2008).

Comparison of Code of Professional Conduct with Superseded Code of Ethics

IBCLCs certified through October 31, 2011, will have learned, and practiced under, the professional standards outlined in the COE. From November 1, 2011, onward, all current IBCLCs and all initial or recertification candidates are required to practice under the CPC. It is important for all IBCLCs to understand the CPC and how it affects their practice because

---

[2] The IBLCE Disciplinary Procedures were revised November 1, 2011. The IBLCE Disciplinary Procedures detail how one files a complaint against an IBCLC with IBLCE and the process that ensues to review and adjudicate the matter.

IBCLCs are bound to abide by the CPC. Most of the concepts from the old COE were retained and are a part of the new CPC. IBLCE changed the name because "professional conduct encompasses ethical behavior, and is a broader and stronger term" (IBLCE, 2011d, p. 1).

The IBLCE Code of Professional Conduct for IBCLCs

The following descriptions elaborate on each element of the CPC. Significant changes from the original COE, where pertinent, are explained. Interpretations of each principle and practice-guiding tips for the IBCLC are offered.

Introduction

The International Board of Lactation Consultant Examiners (IBLCE©) is the global authority that certifies practitioners in lactation and breastfeeding care.

IBLCE was founded to protect the health, welfare and safety of the public by providing the internationally recognized measure of knowledge in lactation and breastfeeding care through the IBLCE exam. Successful candidates become International Board Certified Lactation Consultants (IBCLCs).

A crucial part of an IBCLC's duty to protect mothers and children is adherence to the principles and aim of the *International Code of Marketing of Breast-milk Substitutes* and subsequent relevant World Health Organization resolutions. (IBLCE, 2011b, p. 1)

Interpretation

The first two introductory paragraphs of the CPC tell the reader about IBLCE: what it is, why it was founded, and whom it certifies. IBCLCs must pass the international certification exam in breastfeeding and human lactation, which is administered by one entity, the International Board of Lactation Consultant Examiners. IBLCE was founded precisely to administer the examination and award the IBCLC credential. This certification process is designed to protect the public by measuring the knowledge of IBCLCs, who will provide clinical care and education in breastfeeding and human lactation.

The third introductory paragraph of the CPC outlines IBCLC requirements related to the *International Code of Marketing of Breast-milk Substitutes,* often referred to as the *International Code.*

The *International Code* today is composed of the original language as passed in 1981, along with several subsequently adopted resolutions that have offered interpretation or expanded explanation of sections of the *International Code.* Full citation of the *International Code* is *International Code of Marketing of Breast-milk Substitutes* and all subsequent relevant World Health Assembly resolutions (World Health Organization [WHO], 2011).

It is important for IBCLCs to understand the principles of the *International Code,* which predates the profession of lactation consultation and was "perhaps the most significant international consumer protection standard of modern time" when passed in 1981 (Baumslaug et al., 1995, p. 164). It is a model for countries to use to create public health policy within their borders that seeks to support and promote breastfeeding. It asks governments to pass legislation to support the aims of the *International Code* and to provide sanctions against inappropriate and unethical marketing of breastmilk substitute products covered under its scope. Those products are infant formula, bottles, teats/bottle nipples, and other foods marketed to replace breastmilk for children (International Code Documentation Centre, 2006).

Anyone may choose to support the *International Code's* objectives on an individual level, regardless of governmental support or legislative status. If there are to be enforcement or sanctions elements, however, governments first must enact appropriate laws or regulations within their countries. Unfortunately, worldwide governmental support has not yet occurred (International Baby Food Action Network [IBFAN], 2011). IBCLCs are "health workers" under the *International Code*. Health workers and healthcare institutions are to have limited interactions with the marketers of the *International Code*–covered products to reduce inappropriate commercial influence on the provision of health care to breastfeeding families. Note that the *International Code* allows the covered products to be sold and purchased. Also, any IBCLC (or other health worker) is allowed to discuss any covered product with any mother, in a clinical or educational setting. The *International Code* is designed to prohibit inappropriate *marketing* of the products within its scope.

IBLCE has jurisdiction over IBCLCs worldwide and because governmental adoption of the *International Code* varies around the globe IBLCE's ability to enforce violations of the *International Code* also varies.

Practice-Guiding Tips

1. As an organization, IBLCE supports the *International Code,* stating that it "views the *WHO Code* as a practice-guiding document and encourages IBCLCs to adhere to the same irrespective of legal enforceability in many jurisdictions" (E. Stehel, personal communication, November 10, 2011). Any IBCLC who endeavors to practice ethically should follow the guidelines for health workers under the *International Code.*

2. The International Baby Food Action Network (IBFAN) and the International Code Document Centre (ICDC) are recognized international experts in interpreting and encouraging adoption of the *International Code* in countries around the world. They offer descriptions for health workers (such as IBCLCs) to support the aims of the *International Code* (IBFAN & ICDC, 2009). The International Lactation Consultant Association (ILCA) has also developed a concise overview of the *International Code,* which is provided in **Table 1-1.**

> **Preamble**
>
> IBLCE endorses the broad human rights principles articulated in numerous international documents affirming that every human being has the right to the highest attainable standard of health. Moreover, IBLCE considers that every mother and every child has the right to breastfeed. Thus, IBLCE encourages IBCLCs to uphold the highest standards of ethical conduct as outlined in the:
> - United Nations Convention on the Rights of the Child (UN, 1989)
> - United Nations Convention on the Elimination of All Forms of Discrimination Against Women (Article 12) (UN, 1979)
> - Council of Medical Specialty Societies Code for Interactions with Companies (CMSS, 2011)

To guide their professional practice, it is in the best interest of all IBCLCs and the public they serve that there is a Code of Professional Conduct which:

- Informs both IBCLCs and the public of the ***minimum*** standards of acceptable conduct;
- Exemplifies the commitment expected of all holders of the IBCLC credential;
- Provides IBCLCs with a framework for carrying out their essential duties;
- Serves as a basis for decisions regarding alleged misconduct. (IBLCE, 2011b, p. 1) (emphasis in original)

Interpretation

The first paragraph of the Preamble of the CPC embraces several documents. Two are United Nations Conventions (position statements) about human rights standards. They provide authority for protecting a child's right to good health and a woman's right to appropriate health care and nutrition during pregnancy and lactation. Promoting and protecting breast-feeding are seen as integral to optimal infant and young child feeding (the child's human

Table 1-1 Summary: International Code of Marketing of Breast-milk Substitutes

---

1. **Aim**: The Code aims to protect and promote breastfeeding by ensuring appropriate marketing and distribution of breastmilk substitutes.

2. **Scope**: The Code applies to breastmilk substitutes, when marketed or otherwise represented as a partial or total replacement for breastmilk. These breastmilk substitutes can include food and beverages such as:

   - infant formula
   - other milk products
   - cereals for infants
   - vegetable mixes
   - baby teas and juices
   - follow-up milks.

   The Code also applies to feeding bottles and teats. Some countries have expanded the scope of the Code to include foods or liquids used as breastmilk substitutes and pacifiers.

3. **Advertising**: No advertising of above products to the public.

4. **Samples**: No free samples to mothers, their families, or health workers.

5. **Healthcare facilities**: No promotion of products, i.e., no product displays, posters, or distribution of promotional materials. No use of mothercraft nurses or similar company-paid personnel.

6. **Health workers**: No gifts or samples to health workers. Product information must be factual and scientific.

7. **Supplies**: No free or low-cost supplies of breastmilk substitutes to any part of the healthcare system.

8. **Information**: Information and educational materials must explain the benefits of breastfeeding, the health hazards associated with bottle-feeding, and the costs of using infant formula.

9. **Labels**: Product labels must clearly state the superiority of breastfeeding, the need for the advice of a health worker and a warning about health hazards. No pictures of infants, or other pictures or text idealising the use of infant formula.

10. **Products**: Unsuitable products, such as sweetened condensed milk, should not be promoted for babies. All products should be of a high quality (Codex Alimentarius standards), have expiration dates, and take account of the climatic and storage conditions of the country where they are used.

Source: Reprinted with permission from ILCA. Original text courtesy of International Code Documentation Centre/IBFAN Penang, Malaysia.

right) provided by the mother (her human right) (United Nations General Assembly, 1979; WHO, 2006). The third document from the Council of Medical Specialty Societies (CMSS) is a model, voluntary code to guide professional healthcare societies in programs, policies, and advocacy positions to avoid commercial influences from pharmaceutical and medical device manufacturers (Council of Medical Specialty Societies [CMSS], 2011). IBLCE has endorsed the CMSS Code along with other international organizations to ensure IBLCE's "interaction with companies will be for the benefit of patients and members and for the improvement of care" (CMSS, 2011, p. 4).

The second paragraph of the Preamble sets up the basic framework: The CPC is the authoritative document from IBLCE describing *minimum* standards of professional conduct (as the original emphasizes); the expectation is that IBCLCs will follow these guidelines in the conduct of their duties. The CPC is the basis used to evaluate complaints of misconduct.

Practice-Guiding Tips

1. The CPC is the document describing the IBCLC's authority and responsibilities.
2. The CPC serves to inform all IBCLCs, and the families they work with, of the *minimum* standards that IBCLCs must meet in their professional practice. Any IBCLC is thus free to and should practice in a manner that sets a higher bar of ethical conduct (for example, abiding by the health worker elements of the *International Code of Marketing of Breast-milk Substitutes* regardless of legislative status in the IBCLC's country).
3. The CPC requires that IBCLCs consent to adjudication of any complaints against them under the disciplinary procedures established and enforced by IBLCE. Additionally, any complaints filed against an IBCLC must contain an allegation that an element of the CPC has been violated.

Definitions and Interpretations

1. For purposes of this document, the Code of Professional Conduct for IBCLCs will be referred to as the "CPC."
2. IBCLCs will comply fully with the IBLCE Disciplinary Procedures. (IBLCE, 2011b, p. 1)

Interpretation

This section is new to the CPC, although elements of the terms described were contained in the earlier COE as principles unto themselves. Those elements requiring comment are examined here.

An IBCLC agrees to be subject to the authority and jurisdiction of the IBLCE Ethics and Discipline Committee should a complaint be filed alleging failure to adhere to a principle of the CPC.

Practice-Guiding Tips

1. The IBCLC has agreed, by voluntarily becoming an IBCLC, to be subject to the jurisdiction of the IBLCE Ethics and Discipline Committee, which reviews and adjudicates complaints.

2. Any IBCLC against whom a complaint has been filed will be notified of the complaint in writing by IBLCE. It would be prudent for the IBCLC to contact his or her professional liability insurer and/or legal counsel for guidance on responding to the complaint.

    3. For the purposes of the CPC, "due diligence" refers to the obligation imposed on IBCLCs to adhere to a standard of reasonable care while performing any acts that could foreseeably harm others. (IBLCE, 2011b, p. 2)

    and

    6. "Misfeasance" describes an act that is legal but performed improperly, while "malfeasance" describes a wrongful act. (IBLCE, 2011b, p. 2)

Interpretation

The terms *due diligence*, *misfeasance*, and *malfeasance* are best discussed together because they all spring from legal concepts. *Due diligence* describes the broad, overarching principle that a healthcare provider (such as an IBCLC) who has a specialized skill (expertise in breastfeeding and human lactation) must take reasonable care not to harm someone (a patient/client, or the public). *Misfeasance* means doing something that a person has the legal right to do, but doing it improperly. *Malfeasance* means doing something that is illegal.

A hypothetical example can explain these concepts. A mother hires an IBCLC to consult with her on suspected oversupply of milk with her second baby, now 7 days of age. She had recurrent bouts of plugged ducts and mastitis with her first baby and is alarmed at how much milk she is producing. The IBCLC should provide a thorough lactation assessment of this mother and baby. She should devise a care plan that takes into account the baby's age and feeding pattern, mother's lactation history, current stage of lactogenesis, and milk production. She should also be available for follow-up to adjust the care plan as the mother's supply calibrates to baby's needs. Failing to use due diligence by competently providing all elements of the lactation consultation (assessment, care plan, and follow-up) could result in the harm of plugged ducts, mastitis, and even abscess or premature weaning. The IBCLC could be accused of misfeasance if she gave improper or incomplete oral instructions on techniques or frequency of milk removal to address plugged ducts, or instructions on how to ensure adequate milk intake by the infant. Malfeasance occurs if the IBCLC does something egregious, or illegal, such as fabricating information in the chart or the report sent to the primary healthcare provider to cover up a mistake.

Practice-Guiding Tips

The IBCLC should be familiar with all IBCLC practice-guiding documents. They outline the knowledge base and clinical expertise IBCLCs should possess, the scope of practice for lactation consultation, best practice parameters, and minimum conduct expectations. They describe for the IBCLC the elements of day-to-day practice, which require reasonable care, diligently exercised. The practice-guiding documents are as follows:

1. IBLCE Code of Professional Conduct for IBCLCs (IBLCE, 2011b)

2. IBLCE Scope of Practice for IBCLCs (IBLCE, 2008)

3. IBLCE Clinical Competencies for the Practice of IBCLCs (IBLCE, 2010a)

4. International Lactation Consultant Association (ILCA) Standards of Practice for IBCLCs (International Lactation Consultant Association [ILCA], 2006)

5. *International Code of Marketing of Breast-milk Substitutes* and all subsequent relevant World Health Assembly resolutions (International Code Documentation Centre [ICDC], 2006)

4. The term "intellectual property" (Principle 2.5) refers to copyrights (which apply to printed or electronic documents, manuscripts, photographs, slides and illustrations), trademarks, service and certification marks, and patents. (IBLCE, 2011b, p. 2)

Interpretation

Intellectual property rights are an area of law involving ownership and protections for authors, artists, and inventors. This definition makes it clear that IBLCE requires IBCLCs to respect intellectual property in all formats.

5. The exception to the statement "refrain from revealing any information" (Principle 3.1) means that, to the extent required, IBCLCs may disclose such information to:
   (a) comply with a law, court or administrative order, or this CPC;
   (b) protect the client, in consultation with appropriate individuals or entities in a position to take suitable action, when the IBCLC reasonably believes that a client is unable to act adequately in her own and her child's best interest and there is thus risk of harm;
   (c) establish a claim or defense on behalf of the IBCLC and the client, or a defense against a criminal charge or civil claim against the IBCLC based upon conduct in which the client was involved; or
   (d) respond to allegations in any proceeding concerning the services the IBCLC has provided to the client. (IBLCE, 2011b, p. 2)

Interpretation

As healthcare providers, IBCLCs have an obligation to maintain the confidentiality of their clients' and patients' information. The notion of protecting privacy is a fundamental tenet in health care. It arises from the premise that healthcare providers can more effectively advise and treat those in their care if they have accurate information about the patient. The patient is more likely to reveal personal information if he or she is assured the details will not be freely shared with others. Sharing otherwise-private information is allowed only in specific situations: under court or administrative order, if the client or her child is at risk of harm, or if needed to defend an IBCLC's conduct.

Practice-Guiding Tips

1. IBCLCs must assume and practice as though all information about the consultation with the client/patient is strictly confidential. They should permit confidential information to be revealed only when authorized in writing by the client or when required. IBCLCs must follow the procedures of their place of work (e.g., documentation requirements at the healthcare institution) and appropriate laws and regulations of their geopolitical region (e.g., the Health Insurance Portability and Accountability Act of 1996, in the United States [HIPAA, 2002]).

2. IBCLCs must avoid careless practices (e.g., leaving charts out or discussing a case in public) that allow others to learn details about a consultation with a client and violate privacy.

Code of Professional Conduct Principles

The CPC consists of eight principles, which require every IBCLC to:
1. Provide services that protect, promote and support breastfeeding
2. Act with due diligence
3. Preserve the confidentiality of clients
4. Report accurately and completely to other members of the healthcare team
5. Exercise independent judgment and avoid conflicts of interest
6. Maintain personal integrity
7. Uphold the professional standards expected of an IBCLC
8. Comply with the IBLCE Disciplinary Procedures
IBCLCs are personally accountable for acting consistently with the CPC to safeguard the interests of clients and justify public trust. (IBLCE, 2011b, p. 2)

Interpretation

The CPC is a *mandatory* practice-guiding document and every IBCLC is *required* to practice in accordance with its principles. The CPC is designed to ensure the safety of clients/patients and justify public trust in IBCLCs. Principles 1 through 6 address professional behavior in the clinical context. Principle 7 focuses on how the IBCLC comports him- or herself as a member of the profession. Principle 8 relates to the Disciplinary Procedures. The word *shall* in each principle reminds the IBCLC that these are mandatory obligations of competent, ethical practice.

Principle 1: Provide services that protect, promote and support breast-feeding. Every IBCLC shall:

>1.1 Fulfill professional commitments by working with mothers to meet their breastfeeding goals. (IBLCE, 2011b. p. 2)

Interpretation

This principle reminds the IBCLC that mothers have different lactation goals and might seek a lactation consultation with an IBCLC for many reasons.

Practice-Guiding Tips

The IBCLC should provide information and support to help mothers formulate and achieve their breastfeeding goals. Mothers need to know the risks and benefits of any decision regarding breastfeeding and human lactation. IBCLCs, the healthcare specialists in this area, are ideally suited to provide a mother information so that she can make fully informed decisions and to offer assistance to reach her goal.

>1.2 Provide care to meet clients' individual needs that is culturally appropriate and informed by the best available evidence. (IBLCE, 2011b, p. 2)

Interpretation

Principle 1.2 embraces the concept of evidence-based practice, where clinical decisions in health care are "based on the best research evidence available, clinical knowledge and expertise of the practitioner, and in consultation with the individual receiving care" (Riordan et al., 2010, p. 767). This is especially important because IBCLCs work with mothers all over the world. Social, cultural, religious, political, familial, and personal beliefs about breastfeeding vary widely. The IBCLC should provide information and support in a manner that is respectful of the personal beliefs of the mother.

Practice-Guiding Tips

1. Open-ended inquiries into mothers' concerns and customs or beliefs associated with breastfeeding provide an opportunity for the IBCLC to explore matters of importance to each mother and address her concerns in a sensitive manner.
2. Providing evidence-based care means IBCLCs should be aware of and evaluate research that affects human lactation. If research does not exist, expert opinion should guide practice. Where such technical or medical information does not exist and the IBCLC has clinical experience relevant to the issue at hand, the mother should be so informed.

>1.3 Supply sufficient and accurate information to enable clients to make informed decisions. (IBLCE, 2011b, p. 2)

Interpretation

The essence of informed decision making is that the IBCLC fills in gaps in a mother's knowledge so that she can make an educated decision.

Practice-Guiding Tips

It is the obligation of the IBCLC to provide the mother with information relevant to the issues at hand, taking into account all the present circumstances. Principles of adult education should guide teaching. Learning style should be considered and material presented at an appropriate pace, in a setting and format designed to maximize maternal understanding. A distraught or exhausted mother might not be able to absorb large amounts of new information. Does this mother have access to more than one IBCLC visit? If so, the IBCLC should evaluate which matters are critical for immediate discussion, and which can be discussed at subsequent visits. The IBCLC should offer suggestions of where and how the mother can get follow-up support in person or by phone and provide written materials about the care plan.

> 1.4 Convey accurate, complete and objective information about commercial products (see Principle [5.1]). (IBLCE, 2011b, p. 2)

Interpretation

The IBCLC may find that a consultation with a mother will involve discussion of the mother's use of a commercial product. It could be a medical device, such as a breast pump, or equipment for supplemental feedings. The IBCLC may discuss commercial products and still be *International Code* compliant. Information should be tailored to the clinical setting and be unbiased.

Practice-Guiding Tips

1. IBCLCs whose practice settings offer retail services along with clinical consultation (e.g., renting breast pumps or selling bras) must be careful to segregate commercial from clinical recommendations. For example, a mother might be advised to use a rental or hospital-grade breast pump for the clinical objective of building or preserving milk supply. The clinical necessity of the recommendation, including risks and benefits, should be explained. The IBCLC who offers this product as part of her retail operation should offer the mother several options of where to obtain the equipment and ensure that the recommendation is being made for clinical reasons, not to secure a sale.

2. A thorough lactation consultation involves consideration of all causes and corrections of breastfeeding issues, and use of purchased products should not be promoted over other solutions. For example, if the mother is seeking to build her milk supply, the baby might do the best job (by more frequent breastfeeding). If the mother and baby must be separated, hand expression might be the most efficient and effective means for the mother to express her breastmilk.

> 1.5 Present information without personal bias. (IBLCE, 2011b, p. 3)

Interpretation

The IBCLC should provide objective, unbiased information. All relevant information should be presented, including different recommendations (with an explanation of why the suggestions differ). Conflicting evidence should be acknowledged and discussed without bias, and a lactation care plan that meets the client's needs should be developed.

Practice-Guiding Tips

IBCLCs should provide objective, unbiased information with courtesy, respect, and in the spirit of collegiality.

The second Principle of the CPC applies to day-to-day practice.

> **Principle 2: Act with due diligence. Every IBCLC shall:**
>
> 2.1 Operate within the limits of the scope of practice. (IBLCE, 2011b, p. 3)

Interpretation

The IBLCE Scope of Practice for IBCLCs (SOP) (IBLCE, 2008) is a mandatory practice-guiding document describing the boundaries within which the IBCLC may practice. It applies to all IBCLCs around the world, regardless of their geographic or practice setting. It defines the IBCLC's areas of skill and expertise and the circumstances under which such expertise may be shared with the public (e.g., assisting breastfeeding mothers or providing evidence-based information to healthcare team members).

Practice-Guiding Tips

1. An IBCLC needs only the IBCLC certification to practice as an IBCLC; it is a stand-alone credential and profession. Nonetheless, many IBCLCs have first earned a degree or credential in another field (e.g., speech pathology, midwifery, doctor of medicine, registered dietitian, registered nurse). If the IBCLC has additional training, his or her scope of practice might encompass a wider range of clinical competencies. For example, an IBCLC who is also a registered nurse (RN) has a scope of practice including clinical competency to give an injection. An IBCLC does not. Those who hold more than one credential must be clear as to which clinical role they have in relation to the breastfeeding mother. The SOP defines those practices in which any IBCLC may engage.

2. The SOP clearly defines the IBCLC's role as a member of the healthcare team. Also helpful in describing the range and boundaries of IBCLC expertise is the ILCA *Position Paper on the Role and Impact of the IBCLC* (ILCA, 2011).

> 2.2 Collaborate with other members of the healthcare team to provide unified and comprehensive care. (IBLCE, 2011b, p. 3)

Practice-Guiding Tips

IBCLCs must work with other members of the healthcare team taking care of mother and baby so that lactation care can be aligned with and part of the overall care plan.

2.3 Be responsible and accountable for personal conduct and practice. (IBLCE, 2011b, p. 3)

Interpretation

The IBCLC should take responsibility for personal behavior and clinical practice regardless of practice setting.

Practice-Guiding Tips

1. IBCLCs are responsible for ensuring personal conduct is professional at all times.
2. Keeping current on research and continuing education on breastfeeding and human lactation is a means by which the IBCLC shows accountability for personal practice.
3. IBCLCs should learn how to identify and evaluate the medical literature. Published research involving human lactation is expanding rapidly; the IBCLC might need to explain results that seem contrary to the clinical experience or teaching of other healthcare providers.
4. Improve clinical and hands-on skills by training with or observing other IBCLCs. The ready availability of teaching videos and webinars on the Internet allow any IBCLC, anywhere, to observe face-to-face care. Asking a coworker or supervisor to perform chart reviews or to observe consultations is another way IBCLCs can improve clinical skills as is participating in quality improvement projects.
5. IBCLCs, as healthcare providers who assess breastfeeding dyads and draft care plans to address lactation issues, should carry professional liability (malpractice) insurance, regardless of their work setting or geopolitical location. Those who serve in dual professional roles (e.g., labor and delivery nurses who sometimes work as dedicated IBCLCs at the same institution) should be certain that their professional liability insurance covers all types of clinical work. Those who work in more than one position (e.g., hospital-based dietitian with a separate job as private practice IBCLC) must be certain that insurance covers activities in each role.

2.4 Obey all applicable laws, including those regulating the activities of lactation consultants. (IBLCE, 2011b, p. 3)

Interpretation

The IBCLC must obey laws governing practice by IBCLCs or similar allied healthcare providers if no laws specific to IBCLCs exist. The IBCLC must also adhere to the rules and policies in place at the work setting.

Practice-Guiding Tips

1. Because the profession of lactation consulting is less than 30 years old, there are not specific laws or regulations in all geopolitical jurisdictions of the world delineating an IBCLC's legal responsibilities. However, IBCLCs are allied healthcare providers, so any statutory or regulatory language defining responsibilities of such professionals can guide the IBCLC.

2. The IBCLC must follow whatever policies and procedures are in place at the work setting as a condition of employment.

> 2.5 Respect intellectual property rights. (IBLCE, 2011b, p. 3)

Interpretation

The IBCLC is required to respect intellectual property rights, a vast area of the law governing copyrights, trademarks and service marks, and patents. Laws to enforce and support creators and inventors who have rights in intellectual property are fairly uniform around the world. Copyright law is the intellectual property law IBCLCs might encounter most often in professional practice.

Practice-Guiding Tips

1. Materials do *not* have to show a copyright mark (©) to have copyright protection under the law. Mere creation vests in the originator an immediate copyright, including the right to decide who else may reproduce, show, or adapt the material. Thus, the IBCLC may *not* use materials created or developed by others (handouts, letters, articles, slides, presentations, photographs, drawings, graphs, etc.) unless there is specific permission granted first. This is true even if the IBCLC has no plans to sell the material, and even if the IBCLC plans to credit the originator (U.S. Copyright Office, Library of Congress, 2008).

2. IBCLCs who are preparing scholarly works (position papers, book chapters, or articles for publication in a professional journal or text) may cite sources, without prior permission, under the traditional conventions of academic and professional writing. When giving educational presentations that discuss another's work, the original author should be credited.

3. The Internet has greatly increased accessibility to material, but it has not diminished the requirement to respect copyright. An IBCLC may share a link to an article or abstract but should not provide access to a full article unless first given permission by the author and/or publisher.

4. Seeking permission to use another person's materials can be as simple as sending an email message to the originator. The IBCLC can describe the material that is sought for reuse and the conditions under which it will be shown and credited. IBCLCs should retain proof of the permission sought, and granted, to defend any challenge to use.

Principle 3: Preserve the confidentiality of clients. Every IBCLC shall:

3.1 Refrain from revealing any information acquired in the course of the professional relationship, except to another member of a client's healthcare team, or to other persons or entities for which the client has granted express permission, except only as provided in the Definitions and Interpretations to the CPC. (IBLCE, 2011b, p. 3)

Interpretation

The IBCLC will not reveal information about a lactation consultation unless the client/patient permits it or it is required as part of a court or legal proceeding.

Note that an IBCLC should, pursuant to Principle 2.2, collaborate with other members of the healthcare team, so the family receives "unified and comprehensive care" (IBLCE, 2011b, p. 3). CPC Principle 3.1 requires IBCLCs to maintain confidentiality and "refrain from revealing any information . . . except to another member of a client's healthcare team" (IBLCE, 2011b, p. 3). Principle 4.1, however, specifies that the mother *does* have to specifically agree to the sharing of her information with other healthcare providers (HCPs). Typically, consent is given on admission to a hospital or to receive care in an outpatient setting. Additional consent might be required to share information outside that healthcare team. Regardless of local regulations, optimal communication requires disclosing to the mother with whom and under what circumstances her or her baby's information might be shared.

Practice-Guiding Tips

1. Before commencing any lactation consultation, the IBCLC should be certain that the mother agrees (a) to be seen and (b) to have information about her situation shared, as circumstances warrant, with her own or her baby's HCP. For example, if a mother is hospitalized during delivery, she customarily agrees, upon admission, to the sharing of private health information. In this setting, the IBCLC may share information obtained during the consult with both the mother's and the infant's healthcare team. If the infant has a cleft palate and a specialist consults during the birth hospitalization, information can be shared either verbally or in written format when the specialist accesses the medical record. If the infant will be referred to a subspecialist at a separate children's hospital, then consent is required to share information outside the admitting institution.

2. Consent to be seen and consent to share clinical information with other members of the healthcare team are fairly standard forms routinely required of patients/clients. Those forms also traditionally spell out the caregiver's responsibility to keep the patient/client's information confidential. In a hospital or clinic setting, such paperwork is customarily handled during admission or at the first appointment. IBCLCs in private practice or public health who are the first to see a mother upon referral from another HCP may need to build a chart from the bottom up (including a record of consents and precautions taken to protect confidentiality).

3. Some laws impose further privacy-protecting requirements on the IBCLC who practices within that jurisdiction. For example, Health Insurance Portability and Accountability Act (HIPAA) regulations in the United States require that mothers be given a Notice of Privacy Practices by the HCP describing how her confidential information is protected (HIPAA, 2002).

4. IBCLCs working in clinical settings should follow their institution's policies on confidentiality (e.g., refrain from using information that can identify the mother if speaking in public areas about a case, log off computers when not in use, protect computer password information).

5. Prior permission is not required from the mother for the IBCLC to discuss her case *in anonymous fashion* with colleagues who are not part of the healthcare team. The IBCLC must be cognizant to avoid using bits of information that may unwittingly identify the mother. For example, the IBCLC who practices in a sparsely populated, remote area may find that saying "I worked with a mother of triplets" allows others to quickly detect the patient's identity, whereas the same description might not compromise privacy if used by the IBCLC in a large urban hospital setting.

6. Particular care should be taken to avoid use of client/patient identification clues when sharing case studies on websites or at conferences. IBCLCs must not share details that have even a remote chance of specifically identifying the mother and baby unless the mother has first consented.

> 3.2 Refrain from photographing, recording, or taping (audio or video) a mother or her child for any purpose unless the mother has given advance written consent on her behalf and that of her child. (IBLCE, 2011b, p. 3)

Interpretation

Written consent must be obtained from a mother before the IBCLC may photograph or record her or her child.

Practice-Guiding Tips

1. The IBCLC might consider adding a section to the consent-to-consult forms signed by the mother in which the mother grants permission for photographs and recordings to be taken and used. The consent form should be signed and dated and should include a description of uses permitted such as teaching, publication, or examination.

2. The IBCLC should consider whether additional requirements or consents are imposed by her employer for the making and use of photographs or recordings. Some institutions require the institution's own permission forms to be used and guidelines followed.

3. The IBCLC should not avoid taking and using images; rather, simply keep a supply of consent forms available.

4. Unauthorized use of a clinical image may subject the practitioner to liability beyond the CPC, such as a lawsuit for invasion of privacy or loss clinical privileges if institutional policies are not followed.

Principle 4: Report accurately and completely to other members of the healthcare team. Every IBCLC shall: (IBLCE, 2011b, p. 3)

Interpretation

This principle describes the IBCLC's responsibility to share information about the lactation consultation with other members of the family's healthcare team.

Practice-Guiding Tips

1. The method used to keep other members of the healthcare team apprised of the IBCLC's consultation varies by work setting and geographical custom. Electronic and paper medical records, if accessible by the other HCPs, suffice. Private practitioners may mail, email, or fax reports (taking care to protect confidentiality in the mode of communication). When the mother's or infant's clinical condition is critical, a phone call is indicated. The IBCLC should interpret situations conservatively and send a report to ensure that the primary HCPs are aware of lactation issues.

2. The custom has developed in some regions (i.e., Australia and Great Britain, where many IBCLCs came to the field from midwifery) to contact other HCPs only when lactation care goes beyond the routine.

3. Information shared with the HCPs need not be overly detailed or elaborate. IBCLCs can include at a minimum the IBCLC's name and contact information, identifying information for the mother and baby (name, gender, date of birth), basic clinical data (infant's weight at birth and at consult), date and reasons for the lactation consultation, the IBCLC's assessment, and care plan. Whenever there is *any* cause for concern for the health of the mother or baby, the IBCLC should initiate a phone or in-person conversation with the mother's or baby's primary HCP.

> 4.1 Receive a client's consent, before initiating a consultation, to share clinical information with other members of the client's healthcare team. (IBLCE, 2011b, p. 3)

Interpretation

IBCLCs must get consent from the mother to share information with the healthcare team before beginning a consultation. See also Principle 3.1.

Practice-Guiding Tips

1. Before commencing any lactation consultation, IBCLCs should be certain that the mother agrees (a) to be seen and (b) to have information about her situation shared, as circumstances warrant, with her own or her baby's HCP.

2. The IBCLC should take care that the transmission of private health information does not accidently allow outsiders to read the details of the consult or learn the mother's or baby's identification.

3. In certain circumstances, the mother may have legitimate reasons not to have her identifying information sent to an HCP. For example, if she and her children are at risk and under protection from domestic abuse or threats, the mother will not want a report with her address and phone number included in a report to the pediatrician if the baby's father can (in his own right) access the pediatric file. The IBCLC should endeavor to speak to the HCP by phone or in person to verbally describe the lactation assessment and care plan. The IBCLC also describes in the mother's lactation charting the reasons for the verbal report.

> 4.2 Inform an appropriate person or authority if it appears that the health or safety of a client or a colleague is at risk, consistent with Principle 3. (IBLCE, 2011b, p. 3)

Interpretation

When the health and safety of *either* the mother, baby, *or* a coworker is at risk or appears to be at risk, the IBCLC should *inform* the involved parties, and/or if appropriate, supervisors and authorities.

Practice-Guiding Tips

1. An IBCLC has a responsibility for the safety of mothers and children and to the profession of lactation consulting. An IBCLC who is practicing under conditions where health, safety, or professional decision making is compromised or at risk cannot provide competent, ethical care. When other IBCLCs become aware of, or suspect, such professional liabilities in a colleague, they should consider addressing their concerns with the colleague in question. They should also share these concerns with the lactation consultant's supervisor or administrator to trigger appropriate remedial and mitigating measures.

2. An IBCLC might be unable to professionally and ethically perform his or her duties for any number of reasons: substance abuse, mental or physical illness (such as depression, or a newly diagnosed disease), personal family crises detracting from concentration, and so forth. Any member of the profession who is aware that a colleague cannot meet his or her professional responsibilities should seek the guidance and assistance of appropriate authorities.

3. In many countries, an IBCLC is legally required to report any suspicion of child abuse to appropriate authorities.

4. In cases of suspected domestic abuse, the IBCLC should document the suspected abuse, directly ask the mother about her safety, and direct the mother to appropriate community resources (Isaac et al., 2001). If child abuse is also suspected, then the IBCLC should report to appropriate authorities as required by the law of the region in which he or she practices.

Principle 5: Exercise independent judgment and avoid conflicts of interest. Every IBCLC shall: (IBLCE, 2011b, p. 3)

This principle describes the IBCLC's responsibility to use independent clinical judgment in providing lactation care and to avoid conflicts of interest that can blur the motives of the IBCLC's clinical assessment.

> 5.1 Disclose any actual or apparent conflict of interest, including a financial interest in relevant goods or services, or in organizations which provide relevant goods or services. (IBLCE, 2011b, p. 3)

Interpretation

Full and advance disclosure of relationships that constitute real or perceived conflicts of interest coupled with a consent-to-consult process is important to maintain public trust in IBCLCs' professional practice. Generally speaking, a conflict of interest arises when the IBCLC is perceived as being more concerned about his or her own interests than those of the client. An example is the IBCLC who is employed by a company that manufactures or distributes products covered by the *International Code*. To avoid eroding public trust in the IBCLC and profession, the IBCLC should disclose this conflict of interest to the client.

Practice-Guiding Tips

1. An IBCLC who works in a hospital or birth center and who also has a private practice or retail operation as a second venture does not—by virtue of this two-job arrangement alone—have a conflict of interest. A conflict of interest arises only when the IBCLC in one job is seen to steer clients to herself in the second job. To avoid this, referral choices or lists of community resources should include all the available options.

2. An IBCLC should disclose any stipend, honorarium, sponsorship, or grant received from any organization or commercial entity in the course of professional work. For example, if the IBCLC speaks at a conference and her honorarium was paid by the manufacturer of maternity clothing, this fact should be openly disclosed to the conference attendees. Similarly, any research that is funded by a commercial interest should be disclosed when the findings are discussed, written, and reported. The IBCLC should avoid entering into any business arrangement in which her professional recommendations are dictated by anything other than best professional judgment.

> 5.2 Ensure that commercial considerations do not influence professional judgment. (IBLCE, 2011b, p. 3)

Interpretation

Principle 5.2 requires the IBCLC to demonstrate professional behavior motivated by a desire to provide evidence-based information and care to a breastfeeding family, and not by personal financial gain.

Practice-Guiding Tips

1. An IBCLC can, and should, talk about the use of breastfeeding equipment and supplies with a mother when clinically indicated. Their brand names, prices, advantages,
   and disadvantages must all be discussed so that the mother can make a fully informed
   decision about the care plan that will work best for her, given her circumstances. The
   IBCLC should be certain the mother is aware that this discussion of products is a necessary element in devising her care plan, and not because the IBCLC has a financial
   interest in the outcome of the consultation.

2. The mother can choose to purchase equipment from the IBCLC; it may well be that
   convenience, price, or availability make that the best decision for the mother. She
   should, however, make that decision from the standpoint of a well-informed consumer,
   and not because of insufficient information or pressure from the IBCLC.

> 5.3 Withdraw voluntarily from professional practice if the IBCLC has a physical
> or mental disability that could be detrimental to clients. (IBLCE, 2011b, p. 4)

Interpretation

Any IBCLC with a disability that prevents competent and ethical practice and that could
result in harm to the mother or baby should withdraw voluntarily from professional practice.

Practice-Guiding Tips

1. IBLCE does not discriminate on the basis of disability.

2. IBCLCs should be aware of personal disability and should not practice if that disability prevents competent and ethical practice. The level of withdrawal is determined by
   the disability. As an example, a temporary psychological disability might be managed
   by temporary cessation of clinical practice. The IBCLC could resume clinical practice
   when the condition resolves or is under control. A medical disability that prevents active
   clinical care might require withdrawal from clinical practice while teaching, research,
   and leadership might continue unaffected.

3. Some disabilities are so extensive that the IBCLC credential must be forfeited.
   "Voluntary surrender of the credential will cause [IBLCE] to look favorably upon
   resumption of its use once the disability has been ameliorated" (Scott et al., 2008, p. 14).

4. The responsibility for safe practice rests first with the individual. If the individual fails
   to recognize unsafe practices, IBCLC colleagues should approach the IBCLC or appropriate authorities to remedy the situation.

Principle 6: Maintain personal integrity. Every IBCLC shall:
(IBLCE, 2011b, p. 4)

This principle governs the personal integrity of the IBCLC.

> 6.1 Behave honestly and fairly as a health professional. (IBLCE, 2011b, p. 4)

Interpretation

This principle describes the notion that IBCLCs must be just and honest in their professional practice.

Practice-Guiding Tips

1. IBCLCs should abide by their word and use best efforts to serve patients/clients who come under their care. If an IBCLC promises a mother follow-up care, the IBCLC must make certain it happens or make other arrangements. If resources or information have been promised to an HCP, the IBCLC must make certain to follow through. IBCLCs should provide evidence-based information so that the mother can make a fully informed decision about lactation care for herself and her family and should support the mother's decision even if the IBCLC might have chosen a different course of action.

2. A fair fee should be charged for services rendered, in keeping with community standards and regulations for reimbursement.

3. IBCLCs should spend focused and caring time with each client/patient in his or her care. Accurate assessment of a feed necessarily requires the IBCLC to be there at the start, middle, and finish of the baby's time at breast. Any necessary equipment must be demonstrated. These professional behaviors ensure that the client/patient gets the lactation support needed.

> 6.2 Withdraw voluntarily from professional practice if the IBCLC has engaged in substance abuse that could affect the IBCLC's practice. (IBLCE, 2011b, p. 4)

Interpretation

Principle 6.2 requires the IBCLC who is impaired by addiction or substance abuse to withdraw from professional practice. IBCLCs are required to obey the laws in the country in which they live and abstain from illegal drug use. When use of legal substances such as alcohol or prescription drugs turns into addiction or abuse, the IBCLC's ability to practice competently could be compromised, placing the public in danger. The IBCLC should withdraw from practice until the addiction or abuse has been successfully treated. When the addiction is under control, the IBCLC can resume practice.

Practice-Guiding Tips

Colleagues might need to help an IBCLC realize that he or she is breaching the CPC because substance abuse or addiction can impair professional judgment.

6.3 Treat all clients equitably without regard to age, ethnicity, national origin, marital status, religion, or sexual orientation. (IBLCE, 2011b, p. 4)

Interpretation

The IBCLC should treat all families fairly and equally, harboring no ill will or prejudice based on the characteristics or circumstances of the client/patient.

Practice-Guiding Tips

1. The IBCLC must give the same skilled level of care to all mothers, no matter the personal beliefs or biases of the IBCLC. The IBCLC is obligated to learn about unfamiliar traditions and customs to understand the mother's goals and needs.

2. If the IBCLC realizes that personal beliefs make it difficult to provide competent, dispassionate care, he or she should make every effort to refer the mother to another colleague. The personal reasons prompting the transfer of care need not be shared with the mother. A general statement such as, "It is not possible right now for me to provide the lactation consultation services you require, but I will find a colleague who can see you" suffices.

Principle 7: Uphold the professional standards expected of an IBCLC. Every IBCLC shall: (IBLCE, 2011b, p. 4)

The seventh Principle describes the professional standards an IBCLC is expected to uphold.

7.1 Operate within the framework defined by the CPC. (IBLCE, 2011b, p. 4)

Interpretation

Principle 7.1 means that every IBCLC is expected to use professional behaviors that conform with those described in the CPC.

Practice-Guiding Tips

Every IBCLC should have a copy of the CPC. IBCLCs should review the CPC periodically (perhaps annually and at least at certification and recertification) to ensure clinical practice complies with the CPC.

7.2 Provide only accurate information to the public and colleagues concerning lactation consultant services offered. (IBLCE, 2011b, p. 4)

Interpretation

Any advertising or marketing of IBCLC services should accurately and honestly describe what a lactation consultation involves: how fees, payment, or reimbursement are handled; the IBCLC's obligation to share concerns with other HCPs; the protection of private health information; the mother's role in devising and implementing a care plan; how follow-up is arranged.

Practice-Guiding Tips

1. It is impossible for the IBCLC to guarantee a particular breastfeeding outcome. The variables in any lactation situation are simply too many. The IBCLC can promise to provide evidence-based information and support and to deliver professional services in a responsive, efficient, and ethical manner. The IBCLC should strive to help every client/patient achieve her breastfeeding goal and the best possible health outcome.

2. It is ethical and desirable for IBCLC services to be marketed. Private practitioners can distribute brochures and business cards. Hospitals can advertise that they have IBCLCs dedicated to providing care to breastfeeding mothers. Physician offices can inform patients that IBCLCs on staff are available for pre- and postnatal consultations. It is important that members of the medical community and the public know how and where to access IBCLC services in the community.

3. The *International Code* applies to unethical marketing of covered products, not IBCLC services, and does not prevent IBCLCs from marketing their services.

> 7.3 Permit use of the IBCLC's name for the purpose of certifying that lactation consultant services have been rendered only when the IBCLC provided those services. (IBLCE, 2011b, p. 4)

Interpretation

If a mother expects that she will be seen or requests to be seen by an IBCLC, then an IBCLC should perform the consultation. If a patient/client is billed for a consultation with an IBCLC, an IBCLC should have seen the patient/client.

Practice-Guiding Tips

1. An IBCLC may work with or supervise other breastfeeding helpers. Indeed, mother-to-mother counselors are the backbone of most community-based breastfeeding support programs around the world. The patient/client must always have a clear understanding of who is consulting and the limitations in the care a non-IBCLC can provide. The mother should not be led to think that an uncredentialed person is an IBCLC. In a similar vein, HCPs or third-party reimbursement agencies should be informed that the dyad was seen by an IBCLC only if that was the case.

2. IBCLCs may serve as mentors and help train and educate those who are fulfilling requirements to become an IBCLC. As time progresses, those students operate with diminishing direct supervision. These clinical training arrangements are an acceptable and ethical means to educate trainees. The mother should always be informed that part of her consult is being spent with a student with oversight provided by the responsible IBCLC. Note that the supervising IBCLC always must be aware of, confirm, and agree with whatever assessments and care plans the student devises. The mother thus always has an IBCLC directly involved in and ultimately accountable for the consult.

7.4 Use the acronyms "IBCLC" and "RLC" or the titles "International Board Certified Lactation Consultant" and "Registered Lactation Consultant" only when certification is current and in the manner in which IBLCE authorizes their use. (IBLCE, 2011b, p. 4)

Interpretation

The terms *IBCLC, RLC, International Board Certified Lactation Consultant*, and *Registered Lactation Consultant* are registered certification and service marks of IBLCE (IBLCE, 2011a). IBLCE thus controls the manner in which *IBCLC* or its variants may be used when describing professional qualifications. Note that only currently certified IBCLCs may use such a designation.

Practice-Guiding Tips

1. Aspiring IBCLCs, formerly certified IBCLCs whose certification has lapsed, or retired IBCLCs may *not* use the abbreviations *IBCLC, RLC*, or descriptors *International Board Certified Lactation Consultant* or *Registered Lactation Consultant.*
2. Continuing to represent oneself as an IBCLC when such certification has lapsed, or allowing oneself to be so described by others, is a breach not only of the CPC but of the trademark protections afforded to IBLCE for the registered acronyms and phrases.
3. Use of terms such as *IBCLC candidate* or *student IBCLC* are potentially misleading to the public. The student is advised to use a generic descriptor such as *student lactation consultant.*

Principle 8: Comply with the IBLCE Disciplinary Procedures. Every IBCLC shall: (IBLCE, 2011b, p. 4)

This principle governs the disciplinary procedures that are intended to enforce the CPC and to protect the health, safety, and welfare of the public. For details about how to report a violation of the CPC and current forms, refer to the IBLCE International Office website: www.iblce.org.

8.1 Comply fully with the IBLCE Ethics & Discipline process. (IBLCE, 2011b, p. 4)

Interpretation

The IBCLC must submit to the jurisdiction of IBLCE and the disciplinary procedures established to enforce the CPC as a condition of IBCLC certification (IBLCE, 2011c; E. Stehel, personal communication, November 10, 2011). The CPC is enforced through the IBLCE Ethics and Discipline Committee, composed of a subset of members of the board of directors for IBLCE and other experts in the lactation field.

Practice-Guiding Tips

The IBCLC is advised to become familiar with both the CPC (IBLCE, 2011b) and the IBLCE Disciplinary Procedures (IBLCE, 2011c). The Disciplinary Procedures underwent substantive revision and became effective November 1, 2011. The reasons for the changes were many:

- To ensure current procedures harmonize with the current CPC
- To ensure the procedures allow IBLCE to protect the public
- To ensure that IBCLCs against whom a complaint has been filed continue to be treated justly while the complaint is being investigated

> 8.2 Agree that a violation of this CPC includes any matter in which:
>
> > 8.2.1 The IBCLC is convicted of a crime under applicable law, where dishonesty, gross neglect or wrongful conduct in relation to the practice of lactation consulting is a core issue. (IBLCE, 2011b, p. 4)

Interpretation

An IBCLC might be a defendant in a criminal court proceeding involving some aspect of his or her work as an IBCLC. If the IBCLC is accused and found guilty of a crime that includes any one of the following:

- Dishonesty (e.g., lying)
- Gross negligence (the IBCLC's conscious and voluntary disregard for reasonable care led to injury)
- Wrongful conduct (the IBCLC's actions led to injury)

then the IBCLC will be found also to have violated the CPC.

Practice-Guiding Tips

The criminal charges must involve some aspect of the IBCLC's professional work or responsibilities to be considered a CPC violation.

> > 8.2.2 The IBCLC is disciplined by a state, province or other level of government and at least one of the grounds for discipline is the same as, or substantially equivalent to, this CPC's principle. (IBLCE, 2011b, p. 4)

Interpretation

Any disciplinary action against an IBCLC that involves professional practice covered under the CPC is also a violation of the CPC. IBCLCs should evaluate their practice arrangements and behavior to ensure that they provide professional and ethical practice, protect the public, and minimize the risk of violations of the CPC and disciplinary complaints.

8.2.3 A competent court, licensing board, certifying board or governmental authority determines that the IBCLC has committed an act of misfeasance or malfeasance directly related to the practice of lactation consulting. (IBLCE, 2011b, p. 4)

Interpretation

Principle 8.2.3 describes a proceeding where a certificant is examined about his or her professional activities as an IBCLC. If the IBCLC is found, in the course of professional practice, to have committed the intentional torts of misfeasance or malfeasance (see the section titled "Definitions and Interpretations" earlier in this text), then a violation of the CPC has occurred. An example of this type of proceeding is a case heard by a licensing agency, in those jurisdictions where an IBCLC is required to have a license to practice as an allied healthcare provider. Or the IBCLC may work in a special jurisdictional region, subject to the laws and procedures established for that location (e.g., military bases and facilities, or lands reserved by treaty or law to the control of certain peoples).

Practice-Guiding Tips

IBCLCs must practice ethically at all times and comply with the CPC and any local or national regulations that apply generally to healthcare providers and specifically to lactation consultants.

Conclusion

The IBLCE Code of Professional Conduct outlines the standard of professional, ethical conduct for IBCLCs credentialed by IBLCE. All IBCLCs should be familiar with each of the CPC principles and their subsections. The IBCLC whose practice fails to conform with the CPC may be subject to disciplinary action by IBLCE, under enforcement authority granted to the IBLCE Ethics and Discipline Committee. Sanctions can vary, ranging from private reprimand to forfeiture of certification and public censure (IBLCE, 2010c). IBLCE reports 47 complaints filed through 2011 (IBLCE, 2012), disposed of as follows: no probable cause = 19; complaint dismissed = 10; complaint withdrawn = 2; private reprimand = 9; public reprimand = 2; suspension = 1; certification surrendered = 2; revocation = 2. For complaints ultimately dismissed as without cause, the accused IBCLC is subjected to worry and concern during the disciplinary process. Proactively using excellent communication skills can help IBCLCs avoid the mixed messages that can result in the filing of a complaint. To comply with the requirements of the IBLCE Code of Professional Conduct, the IBCLC must provide evidence-based care, offer compassionate and undivided attention to the mother, and understand her concerns and goals so that the IBCLC and mother can fashion an appropriate care plan together. In this way, the IBCLC provides ethical and professional care.

References

Baumslag, N., & Michels, D. (1995). *Milk, money and madness: The culture and politics of breastfeeding.* Westport, CT: Bergin & Garvey.

Council of Medical Specialty Societies. (2011, March). *Code for interactions with companies* (Model policy). Retrieved from http://www.cmss.org/uploadedFiles/Site/CMSS_Policies/CMSS%20 Code%20for%20Interactions%20with%20Companies%20Approved%20Revised%20Version%20 3-19-11CLEAN.pdf

Health Information Portability and Accountability Act of 1996, P. L. No. 104-191, 45 C.F.R. § 160 & 164 (2002).

Institute for Credentialing Excellence. (2009). What is certification? Retrieved from http://www. credentialingexcellence.org/GeneralInformation/WhatisCertification/tabid/63/Default.aspx

Institute for Credentialing Excellence. (2011). Accredited certification programs. Retrieved from http://www.credentialingexcellence.org/NCCAAccreditation/AccreditedCertificationPrograms/ tabid/120/Default.aspx

International Baby Food Action Network. (2011, May). State of the Code by country. Retrieved from http://www.ibfan.org/code_watch-reports.html

International Baby Food Action Network & International Code Documentation Centre. (2009). *Code essentials 3: Responsibilities of health workers under the International Code of Marketing of Breast-milk Substitutes and subsequent WHA resolutions.* Penang, Malaysia: IBFAN.

International Board of Lactation Consultant Examiners. (1999, April 22). *Code of ethics* [Archival document]. Retrieved from International Board of Lactation Consultant Examiners website: http://web.archive.org/web/*/http://iblce.org

International Board of Lactation Consultant Examiners. (2008, March 8). *Scope of practice for International Board certified lactation consultants.* Retrieved from http://www.iblce.org/upload/dow nloads/ScopeOfPractice.pdf

International Board of Lactation Consultant Examiners. (2010a, December 6). *Clinical competencies for the practice of IBCLCs.* Retrieved from http://www.iblce.org/upload/downloads/ClinicalComp etencies.pdf

International Board of Lactation Consultant Examiners. (2010b, September 26). *IBLCE disciplinary procedures.* Formerly available at http://www.iblce.org/upload/downloads/IBLCEDisciplinaryPro cedures.pdf

International Board of Lactation Consultant Examiners. (2010c, April 22). *Sanctions imposed against IBCLCs.* Retrieved from http://iblce.org/upload/downloads/SanctionsList.pdf

International Board of Lactation Consultant Examiners. (2011a). Certification. Retrieved from http://iblce.org/certification

International Board of Lactation Consultant Examiners. (2011b, November 2). *Code of professional conduct for IBCLCs.* Retrieved from http://iblce.org/upload/downloads/CodeOfProfessionalCon duct.pdf

International Board of Lactation Consultant Examiners. (2011c, September 24). *Disciplinary procedures for the code of professional conduct for IBCLCs for the International Board of Lactation Consultant Examiners (IBLCE).* Retrieved from http://www.iblce.org/upload/downloads/IBLCE DisciplinaryProcedures.pdf

International Board of Lactation Consultant Examiners. (2011d, October 31). *Frequently asked questions (FAQs) regarding the code of professional conduct for IBCLC.* Retrieved from http://iblce.org/ upload/downloads/CodeOfConductFAQs.pdf

International Board of Lactation Consultant Examiners. (2012, April 24). Code *of professional conduct for IBCLCs (CPC)*. Webinar presented live, taped for later website access, www.iblce.org.

International Code Documentation Centre. (2006). *International Code of Marketing of Breast-milk Substitutes and relevant WHA resolutions*. Penang, Malaysia: IBFAN Penang. (Original work published 2005)

International Lactation Consultant Association. (2006). *Standards of practice for International Board certified lactation consultants*. Retrieved from http://www.ilca.org/files/resources/Standards-of-Practice-web.pdf

International Lactation Consultant Association. (2011, June). *Position paper on the role and impact of the IBCLC* (Monograph). Retrieved from http://www.ilca.org/files/resources/ilca_ publications/Role%20%20Impact%20of%20the%20IBCLC-webFINAL_08-15-11.pdf

Isaac, N., & Enos, V. P. (2001, September). *Documenting domestic violence: How health care providers can help victims* (Research in Brief). Washington, DC: National Institute of Justice, U.S. Department of Justice. Retrieved from https://www.ncjrs.gov/pdffiles1/nij/188564.pdf

National Commission for Certifying Agencies. (2007, December). *Standards for the accreditation of certification programs*. Retrieved from http://www.credentialingexcellence.org/portals/0/ STANDARDS%20-%20Updated%20January%202010.pdf

Riordan, J., & Wambach, K. (2010). *Breastfeeding and human lactation* (4th ed.). Sudbury, MA: Jones and Bartlett.

Scott, J., & Calandro, A. (2008). The code of ethics for International Board certified lactation consultants: Ethical practice. In R. Mannel, P. Martens, & M. Walker (Eds.), *Core curriculum for lactation consultant practice* (2nd ed., pp. 5–18). Sudbury, MA: Jones and Bartlett.

Scott, J. W. (1996, December). Code of ethics for International Board certified lactation consultants. *Journal of Human Lactation, 12*(4), 344–347. doi:10.1177/089033449601200449

United Nations General Assembly. (1979 [resolution passed], December 18). *Convention on the elimination of all forms of discrimination against women*. Retrieved from http://www.hrweb.org/ legal/cdw.html

U.S. Copyright Office, Library of Congress. (2008, July). *Circular 1: Copyright basics*. Retrieved from http://www.copyright.gov/circs/circ01.pdf

World Health Organization. (2006). *The International Code of Marketing of Breast-milk Substitutes: Frequently asked questions* [Brochure]. Retrieved from http://whqlibdoc.who.int/publications/ 2008/9789241594295_eng.pdf

World Health Organization. (2011). World Health Assembly. Retrieved from http://www.who.int/m ediacentre/events/governance/wha/en/index.html

IBLCE
International Board of Lactation Consultant Examiners

Code of Professional Conduct for IBCLCs

Effective: November 1, 2011

Supersedes: December 1, 2004 Code of Ethics for IBCLCs

The International Board of Lactation Consultant Examiners® (IBLCE®) is the global authority that certifies practitioners in lactation and breastfeeding care.

IBLCE was founded to protect the health, welfare and safety of the public by providing the internationally recognized measure of knowledge in lactation and breastfeeding care through the IBLCE exam. Successful candidates become International Board Certified Lactation Consultants (IBCLCs).

A crucial part of an IBCLC's duty to protect mothers and children is adherence to the principles and aim of the _International Code of Marketing of Breast-milk Substitutes_ and subsequent relevant World Health Assembly's resolutions.

Preamble

IBLCE endorses the broad human rights principles articulated in numerous international documents affirming that every human being has the right to the highest attainable standard of health. Moreover, IBLCE considers that every mother and every child has the right to breastfeed. Thus, IBLCE encourages IBCLCs to uphold the highest standards of ethical conduct as outlined in:

- United Nations Convention on the Rights of the Child
- United Nations Convention on the Elimination of All Forms of Discrimination Against Women (Article 12)
- Council of Medical Specialty Societies _Code for Interactions with Companies_
- To guide their professional practice, it is in the best interest of all IBCLCs and the public they serve that there is a Code of Professional Conduct which:
- Informs both IBCLCs and the public of the **minimum** standards of acceptable conduct;
- Exemplifies the commitment expected of all holders of the IBCLC credential;
- Provides IBCLCs with a framework for carrying out their essential duties;
- Serves as a basis for decisions regarding alleged misconduct.

Definitions and Interpretations

1. For the purposes of this document, the Code of Professional Conduct for IBCLCs will be referred to as the "CPC."

2. IBCLCs will comply fully with the *IBLCE Disciplinary Procedures.*

3. For the purposes of the CPC, "due diligence" refers to the obligation imposed on IBCLCs to adhere to a standard of reasonable care while performing any acts that could foreseeably harm others.

4. The term "intellectual property" (Principle 2.5) refers to copyrights (which apply to printed or electronic documents, manuscripts, photographs, slides, and illustrations), trademarks, service and certification marks, and patents.

5. The exception to the statement "refrain from revealing any information" (Principle 3.1) means that, to the extent required, IBCLCs may disclose such information to:
   (a) comply with a law, court or administrative order, or this CPC;

   (b) protect the client, in consultation with appropriate individuals or entities in a position to take suitable action, when the IBCLC reasonably believes that a client is unable to act adequately in her own and her child's best interest and there is thus risk of harm;

   (c) establish a claim or defense on behalf of the IBCLC and the client, or a defense against a criminal charge or civil claim against the IBCLC based upon conduct in which the client was involved; or

   (d) respond to allegations in any proceeding concerning the services the IBCLC has provided to the client.

6. "Misfeasance" describes an act that is legal but performed improperly, while "malfeasance" describes a wrongful act.

Code of Professional Conduct Principles

The CPC consists of eight principles, which require every IBCLC to:

1. Provide services that protect, promote and support breastfeeding
2. Act with due diligence
3. Preserve the confidentiality of clients
4. Report accurately and completely to other members of the healthcare team
5. Exercise independent judgment and avoid conflicts of interest
6. Maintain personal integrity
7. Uphold the professional standards expected of an IBCLC
8. Comply with the IBLCE Disciplinary Procedures

IBCLCs are personally accountable for acting consistently with the CPC to safeguard the interests of clients and justify public trust.

Principle 1: Provide services that protect, promote and support breastfeeding

Every IBCLC shall:

1.1 Fulfill professional commitments by working with mothers to meet their breastfeeding goals.

1.2 Provide care to meet clients' individual needs that is culturally appropriate and informed by the best available evidence.

1.3 Supply sufficient and accurate information to enable clients to make informed decisions.

1.4 Convey accurate, complete and objective information about commercial products (see Principle 7.1).

1.5 Present information without personal bias.

Principle 2: Act with due diligence

Every IBCLC shall:

2.1 Operate within the limits of the scope of practice.

2.2 Collaborate with other members of the healthcare team to provide unified and comprehensive care.

2.3 Be responsible and accountable for personal conduct and practice.

2.4 Obey all applicable laws, including those regulating the activities of lactation consultants.

2.5 Respect intellectual property rights.

Principle 3: Preserve the confidentiality of clients

Every IBCLC shall:

3.1 Refrain from revealing any information acquired in the course of the professional relationship, except to another member of a client's healthcare team or to other persons or entities for which the client has granted express permission, except only as provided in the Definitions and Interpretations to the CPC.

3.2 Refrain from photographing, recording or taping (audio or video) a mother or her child for any purpose unless the mother has given advance written consent on her behalf and that of her child.

Principle 4: Report accurately and completely to other members of the healthcare team

Every IBCLC shall:

4.1 Receive a client's consent, before initiating a consultation, to share clinical information with other members of the client's healthcare team.

4.2 Inform an appropriate person or authority if it appears that the health or safety of a client or a colleague is at risk, consistent with Principle 3.

Principle 5: Exercise independent judgment and avoid conflicts of interest

Every IBCLC shall:

5.1 Disclose any actual or apparent conflict of interest, including a financial interest in relevant goods or services, or in organizations which provide relevant goods or services.

5.2 Ensure that commercial considerations do not influence professional judgment.

5.3 Withdraw voluntarily from professional practice if the IBCLC has a physical or mental disability that could be detrimental to clients.

Principle 6: Maintain personal integrity

Every IBCLC shall:

6.1 Behave honestly and fairly as a health professional.

6.2 Withdraw voluntarily from professional practice if the IBCLC has engaged in substance abuse that could affect the IBCLC's practice.

6.3 Treat all clients equitably without regard to age, ethnicity, national origin, marital status, religion, or sexual orientation.

Principle 7: Uphold the professional standards expected of an IBCLC

Every IBCLC shall:

7.1 Operate within the framework defined by the CPC.

7.2 Provide only accurate information to the public and colleagues concerning lactation consultant services offered.

7.3 Permit use of the IBCLC's name for the purpose of certifying that lactation consultant services have been rendered only when the IBCLC provided those services.

7.4 Use the acronyms "IBCLC" and "RLC" or the titles "International Board Certified Lactation Consultant" and "Registered Lactation Consultant" only when certification is current and in the manner in which IBLCE authorizes their use.

Principle 8: Comply with the IBLCE Disciplinary Procedures

Every IBCLC shall:

8.1 Comply fully with the IBLCE Ethics & Discipline process.

8.2 Agree that a violation of this CPC includes any matter in which:

    8.2.1 the IBCLC is convicted of a crime under applicable law, where dishonesty, gross negligence or wrongful conduct in relation to the practice of lactation consulting is a core issue;

    8.2.2 the IBCLC is disciplined by a state, province or other level of government and at least one of the grounds for discipline is the same as, or substantially equivalent to, this CPC's principle;

    8.2.3 a competent court, licensing board, certifying board or governmental authority determines that the IBCLC has committed an act of misfeasance or malfeasance directly related to the practice of lactation consulting.

CHAPTER 2
International Initiatives to Promote, Protect, and Support Breastfeeding

Karin Cadwell, PhD, FAAN, IBCLC

OBJECTIVE

- Discuss international statements and documents that are used as tools to protect, promote, and support breastfeeding.

INTRODUCTION

In 1979, alarmed over the unnecessary deaths related to the industry-created bottle-feeding culture, two agencies of the United Nations, the World Health Organization (WHO) and the United Nations Children's Fund (UNICEF), held an international meeting concerning infant and young child feeding. The ultimate result was the creation of the *International Code of Marketing of Breast-milk Substitutes*. The *International Code of Marketing* and subsequent resolutions have been approved in the World Health Assembly. This document and others strive to replace the commercial barriers to breastfeeding with protection for a health-related behavior that is in danger of extinction. In addition, WHO and UNICEF produced the *Ten Steps to Successful Breastfeeding*, which became the core of the Baby-Friendly Hospital Initiative (BFHI).

In 2002, WHO and UNICEF jointly endorsed the Global Strategy for Infant and Young Child Feeding, which builds on these and other successful policies and programs of the past. There is an enormous amount of work yet to be done. Even with international policies

> no more than 35% of infants worldwide are exclusively breastfed during the first four months of life; complementary feeding frequently begins too early or too late, and foods are often nutritionally inadequate and unsafe. Malnourished children who survive are more frequently sick and suffer the life-long consequences of impaired development. Rising incidences of overweight and obesity in children are also a matter of serious concern. Because poor feeding practices are a major threat to social and economic development, they are among the most serious obstacles to attaining and maintaining health that face this age group. (World Health Organization [WHO], 2003, p. 5)

I. The Global Strategy for Infant and Young Child Feeding

A. In 2002, WHO and UNICEF jointly endorsed the Global Strategy for Infant and Young Child Feeding. This publication renewed the commitment of these organizations to continuing joint efforts including the Baby-Friendly Hospital Initiative (BFHI), the *International Code of Marketing of Breast-milk Substitutes*, and the Innocenti Declaration on the Protection, Promotion, and Support of Breastfeeding. The Global Strategy urges countries to "formulate, implement, monitor and evaluate a comprehensive national policy on infant and young child feeding" and includes "ensuring sufficient maternity leave to promote exclusive breastfeeding" (WHO, 2003).

B. According to the Global Strategy, appropriate infant and young child feeding practices include:

1. Exclusive breastfeeding for 6 months.
2. Timely initiation of nutritionally adequate and safe complementary foods while continuing breastfeeding up to 2 years or beyond.
3. Appropriate feeding of infants and young children living in especially difficult circumstances (low-birth-weight infants, infants of mothers who are positive for human immunodeficiency virus [HIV], infants in emergency situations, malnourished infants, etc.).

C. The strategy calls for action in the following areas:

1. "All governments should develop and implement a comprehensive policy on infant and young child feeding, in the context of national policies for nutrition, child and reproductive health, and poverty reduction. . . .
2. "All mothers should have access to skilled support to initiate and sustain exclusive breastfeeding for six months, and ensure the timely introduction of adequate and safe complementary foods with continued breastfeeding up to two years or beyond. . . .
3. "Health care workers should be empowered to provide effective feeding counseling, and their services should be extended in the community by trained lay or peer counselors. . . .
4. "Governments should review progress in national implementation of the International Code of Marketing of Breast-milk Substitutes, and consider new legislation or additional measures as needed to protect families from adverse commercial influences. . . .
5. "Governments should enact imaginative legislation protecting the breastfeeding rights of working women and establishing means for its enforcement in accordance with international labor standards" (WHO, 2003).

The strategy specifies not only responsibilities of governments, but also of international organizations, nongovernmental organizations (NGOs), and other concerned parties. It engages all relevant stakeholders and provides a framework for accelerated action, linking relevant intervention areas and using resources available in a variety of sectors.

II. ***The International Code of Marketing of Breast-milk Substitutes*** **According to the World Health Assembly (WHA)** *International Code of Marketing of Breast-Milk Substitutes* **and subsequent resolutions**

 A. Manufacturers of breastmilk substitutes, feeding bottles, and teats have cleverly communicated to mothers doubts and pressures about "not enough milk."
 B. WHO and UNICEF drafted the *International Code of Marketing of Breast-milk Substitutes*, which was adopted by the WHA in May 1981. An international recommendation, the code is put into effect at the national level. The International Baby Food Action Network (IBFAN) periodically publishes information on which countries have taken some action to implement the international code and the percentage of the world's population who lives in countries where laws are in place that broadly incorporate its main provisions.
 C. The IBFAN set up the International Code Documentation Centre (ICDC) with the task of keeping track of code compliance both by governments and by companies. IBFAN's work also includes the following initiatives:
    1. Networking with partners around the world in a spirit of solidarity for mutual support and empowerment
    2. Advocacy for the international code and resolutions in national and international measures
    3. Capacity building and code training courses for NGOs, consumers, and policymakers in all parts of the world
    4. Monitoring the state of implementation of and compliance with the international code and resolutions
    5. Awareness-raising through publications, the media, and grassroots outreach
    6. Coordinating manufacturer campaigns (such as the Nestlé boycott)
    7. Policy development on food standards, maternity legislation, emergency relief, and human immunodeficiency virus (HIV)
 D. Further resolutions have clarified and strengthened the code, including a statement that member states "ensure that there are no donations of free or subsidized supplies of breast milk substitutes and other products" covered by the code (World Health Organization Division of Nutrition, 1997). This resolution forbids healthcare facilities to accept free or low-cost supplies.
 E. The 1996 WHA resolution urges member states to "ensure that complementary foods are not marketed for or used in ways that undermine exclusive and sustained breastfeeding."
 F. The scope of the code applies to the marketing and practices related to the following items:
    1. Breastmilk substitutes, including infant formula; other milk products, foods, and beverages, including bottle-fed complementary foods, when marketed or otherwise represented to be suitable, with or without modification, for use as a partial or total replacement of breastmilk
    2. Feeding bottles and teats
    3. The quality, availability, and information concerning the use of products mentioned previously

G. The code stipulates how products covered by the code can be promoted to the public and the healthcare system:
  1. There is to be no advertising or other form of promotion (such as free samples or gifts of articles or utensils) to the general public of products within the scope of the code. There should be no promotion to healthcare workers as a means of indirect promotion to the public.
  2. Governments are responsible to "ensure that objective and consistent information is provided on infant and young child feeding" (World Health Organization Division of Nutrition, 1997).
H. There is a gray area between providing information and promotion that manufacturers may easily cross and that casts doubt on a woman's ability to breastfeed.
 I. Labeling is also covered under the code. Labels should offer information about the appropriate use of the product in a way that does not discourage breastfeeding. The label should be clear and understandable, using appropriate language, with no pictures of infants. Some countries also require the age recommended for introduction of particular infant foods to be included on the label, as well as place restraints on using certain health claims (such as the use of the word *hypoallergenic*).
 J. Definitions of terms used in the code:
  1. *Breastmilk substitute* means any food being marketed or otherwise represented as a partial or total replacement for breastmilk, whether or not suitable for that purpose.
  2. *Infant formula* means a breastmilk substitute formulated industrially in accordance with applicable Codex Alimentarius standards to satisfy the normal nutritional requirements of infants between 4 and 6 months of age and adapted to their physiologic characteristics. Infant formula can also be prepared at home, in which case it is described as *home prepared*.
  3. *Complementary food* means any food, whether manufactured or locally prepared, that is suitable as a complement to breastmilk or to infant formula when either becomes insufficient to satisfy the nutritional requirements of the infant. Such food is also commonly called *weaning food* or *breastmilk supplement*.

III. Relevant Parts of World Health Assembly Resolutions

A. WHA 39.28: "Any food or drink given before complementary feeding is nutritionally required may interfere with the initiation or maintenance of breastfeeding and therefore should neither be promoted nor encouraged for use by infants during this period; the practice being introduced in some countries of providing infants with specially formulated milks (so-called follow-up milks) is not necessary" (World Health Assembly [WHA], 1986).
B. WHA 47.5: Member states are urged to "foster appropriate complementary feeding from the age of about six months" (WHA, 1994).
C. WHA 49.15: Member states are urged to "ensure that complementary foods are not marketed for or used in ways that undermine exclusive and sustained breastfeeding" (WHA, 1996).

D. At the 58th World Health Assembly (May 2005), results of the joint Food and Agriculture Organization (FAO)/WHO expert meeting on *Enterobacter sakazakii* (now *Cronobacter sakazakii*) and other microorganisms in powdered infant formula, which had been held in 2004, were brought forward. The expert meeting concluded that intrinsic contamination of powdered infant formula with *E. sakazakii* (now *C. sakazakii*) and Salmonella had been a cause of infection and illness, including severe disease in infants, particularly preterm, low-birth-weight, or immuno-compromised infants, and could lead to serious developmental sequelae and death. There was recognition of the need for parents and caregivers to be fully informed of evidence-based public health risks of intrinsic contamination of powdered infant formula, the potential for introduced contamination, and the need for safe preparation, handling, and storage of prepared infant formula. The WHA urged member states to the following action:

1. "To continue to protect, promote and support exclusive breastfeeding for six months as a global public health recommendation, taking into account the findings of the WHO Expert Consultation on optimal duration of exclusive breastfeeding, and to provide for continued breastfeeding up to two years of age or beyond, by implementing fully the WHO global strategy on infant and young-child feeding that encourages the formulation of a comprehensive national policy, including where appropriate a legal framework to promote maternity leave and a supportive environment for six months' exclusive breastfeeding, a detailed plan of action to implement, monitor and evaluate the policy, and allocation of adequate resources for this process...

2. "To ensure that nutrition and health claims are not permitted for breast-milk substitutes, except where specifically provided for in national legislation...

3. "To ensure that clinicians and other health-care personnel, community health workers and families, parents and other caregivers, particularly of infants at high risk, are provided with enough information and training by health-care providers, in a timely manner on the preparation, use and handling of powdered infant formula in order to minimize health hazards; are informed that powdered infant formula may contain pathogenic microorganisms and must be prepared and used appropriately; and, where applicable, that this information is conveyed through an explicit warning on packaging...

4. "To ensure that financial support and other incentives for programs and health professionals working in infant and young-child health do not create conflicts of interest...

5. "To ensure that research on infant and young-child feeding, which may form the basis for public policies, always contains a declaration relating to conflicts of interest and is subject to independent peer review...

6. "To work closely with relevant entities, including manufacturers, to continue to reduce the concentration and prevalence of pathogens, including *Cronobacter sakazakii*, in powdered infant formula...

7. "To continue to ensure that manufacturers adhere to Codex Alimentarius or national food standards and regulations...

8. "To ensure policy coherence at national levels by stimulating collaboration between health authorities, food regulators and food standard-setting bodies...

9. "To participate actively and constructively in the work of the Codex Alimentarius Commission...

10. "To ensure that all national agencies involved in defining national positions on public health issues for use in all relevant international forums, including the Codex Alimentarius Commission, have a common and consistent understanding of health policies adopted by the Health Assembly, and to promote these policies" (WHO/FAO, 2008).

E. Continued support for the BFHI in the 63rd (2010) World Health Assembly resolutions:

> In the pre-operative paragraph: "Mindful of the fact that implementation of the global strategy for infant and young child feeding and its operational targets requires strong political commitment and a comprehensive approach, including strengthening of health systems and communities with particular emphasis on the Baby-friendly Hospital Initiative, and careful monitoring of the effectiveness of the interventions used;...

>> URGES Member States: "to strengthen and expedite the sustainable implementation of the global strategy for infant and young child feeding including emphasis on giving effect to the aim and principles of the International Code of Marketing of Breast-milk Substitutes, and the implementation of the Baby-friendly Hospital Initiative;...

>> REQUESTS the Director-General: "to support Member States, on request, in expanding their nutritional interventions related to the double burden of malnutrition, monitoring and evaluating impact, strengthening or establishing effective nutrition surveillance systems, and implementing the WHO Child Growth Standards, and the Baby-friendly Hospital Initiative." (WHO, 2010)

IV. The Baby-Friendly Hospital Initiative

A. The BFHI was designed to rid hospitals of their dependence on breastmilk substitutes and to encourage maternity services to be supportive of breastfeeding.

B. Launched by WHO and UNICEF in June 1991 at a meeting of the International Pediatric Association in Ankara, Turkey, the global initiative is aimed at promoting the adoption of the *Ten Steps to Successful Breastfeeding* (described later) in hospitals worldwide.

C. The BFHI is designed to remove hospital barriers to breastfeeding by creating a supportive environment with trained and knowledgeable healthcare workers.

D. The 10 steps to successful breastfeeding are as follows:

1. Have a written breastfeeding policy that is routinely communicated to all healthcare staff.

2. Train all healthcare staff in skills necessary to implement this policy.

3. Inform all pregnant women about the benefits and management of breastfeeding.

4. Help mothers initiate breastfeeding within a half hour (1 hour in the United States) of birth.

    5. Show mothers how to breastfeed and how to maintain lactation even if they should be separated from their infants.

    6. Give newborn infants no food or drink other than breastmilk unless medically indicated.

    7. Practice rooming-in: Enable mothers and infants to remain together 24 hours a day.

    8. Encourage breastfeeding on demand.

    9. Give no artificial teats or pacifiers (also called dummies or soothers) to breast-feeding infants.

    10. Foster the establishment of breastfeeding support groups and refer mothers to them upon discharge from the hospital or clinic.

E. The 2009 revision of the BFHI materials by WHO updates and expands the program to increase the integration of the BFHI with the *Global Strategy for Infant and Young Child Feeding*. The revision includes the expectation that staff have received the necessary training to provide support and education for mothers who are not breastfeeding in addition to breastfeeding mothers to ensure that all mothers get the feeding support they need.

    1. In addition, the 2009 revision includes encouragement to reexamine labor and delivery practices that enhance the infant's start in life and optimize breastfeeding in the postpartum period.

    2. Information on HIV and the childbearing family has also been integrated into BFHI training for countries when appropriate.

    3. Although all 10 steps have been examined and updated, the training and assessment related to step 4 has been most noticeably reworked from the original to reflect new research and understanding. Step 4 is now interpreted as follows: Babies should be placed skin-to-skin with their mother soon (immediately) after birth and remain there without interruption until the baby finds his or her way to the breast and completes the first breastfeeding. It is expected that this will take an hour or more. The role of the staff is to understand the normal progress of the baby to latch and begin breastfeeding when ready and to provide a safe, knowledgeable, and helpful environment for the first breastfeeding to take place unless there are justifiable reasons for this not to occur. Mothers who are not planning to breastfeed or for whom breastfeeding is contraindicated should hold their baby skin-to-skin for at least an hour immediately after birth.

V. The FAO/WHO International Conference on Nutrition

A. The FAO/WHO International Conference on Nutrition was held in Rome, Italy, in December 1992. Signatories adopted the World Declaration on Nutrition and the Plan of Action for Nutrition. Article 19 of the World Declaration on Nutrition pledges "to reduce substantially within this decade social and other impediments to optimal breastfeeding" (Food and Agriculture Organization of the United Nations & World Health Organization, 1992).

B. The plan of action endorses breastfeeding under sections on preventing and managing infectious diseases and preventing and controlling specific micronutrient deficiencies. The plan of action also calls for the promotion of breastfeeding by governments by providing maximum support for women to breastfeed.

VI. The Innocenti Declaration

A. In August 1990 in Florence, Italy, the Innocenti Declaration was adopted at a meeting sponsored jointly by UNICEF, WHO, the United States Agency for International Development, and the Swedish International Development Authority. The Innocenti Declaration called for concrete actions for governments to take by 1995.

B. Attainment of Innocenti goals requires, in many countries, the reinforcement of a "breastfeeding culture" and the vigorous defense against incursions of a "bottle-feeding culture."

C. Operational targets: By the year 1995, all national governments should have taken the following actions:

   1. Appointed a national breastfeeding coordinator of appropriate authority and established a multisector national breastfeeding committee composed of representatives from relevant governmental departments, nongovernmental organizations, and health professional associations.

   2. Ensured that every facility providing maternity services fully practices all 10 of the *Ten Steps to Successful Breastfeeding* set out in the joint WHO/UNICEF statement, *Protecting, Promoting and Supporting Breast-feeding: The Special Role of Maternity Services* (WHO, 1989).

   3. Taken action to implement the principles and aim of all articles of the *International Code of Marketing of Breast-milk Substitutes* and subsequent relevant WHA resolutions in their entirety.

   4. Enacted imaginative legislation protecting the breastfeeding rights of working women and established means for its enforcement.

D. All international organizations were called upon by the Innocenti Declaration to do the following:

   1. Draw up action strategies for protecting, promoting, and supporting breastfeeding, including global monitoring of the evaluation of their strategies.

   2. Support national situation analyses and surveys and the development of national goals and targets for action.

   3. Encourage and support national authorities in planning, implementing, monitoring, and evaluating their breastfeeding policies.

E. The Innocenti Declaration was adopted by the World Summit for Children in September 1990 and by the 45th World Health Assembly in May 1992 in Resolution WHA 45.34.

VII. Innocenti + 15

A. The targets of the 1990 Innocenti Declaration and the 2002 Global Strategy for Infant and Young Child Feeding remain the foundation for action. Although remarkable progress has been made, much more needs to be done.

B. Innocenti + 15 issued this call for action so that all parties:

   1. "Empower women in their own right, and as mothers and providers of breastfeeding support and information to other women.

   2. "Support breastfeeding as the norm for feeding infants and young children.

3. "Highlight the risks of artificial feeding and the implications for health and development throughout the life course.
4. "Ensure the health and nutritional status of women throughout all stages of life.
5. "Protect breastfeeding in emergencies, including by supporting uninterrupted breastfeeding and appropriate complementary feeding, and avoiding general distribution of breast-milk substitutes.
6. "Implement the HIV and Infant Feeding—Framework for Priority Action, including protecting, promoting and supporting breastfeeding for the general population while providing counseling and support for HIV-positive women." (*Innocenti Declaration 2005: On Infant and Young Child Feeding*, 2005)

C. All governments were called on to:

1. "Establish or strengthen national infant and young child feeding and breast-feeding authorities, coordinating committees and oversight groups that are free from commercial influence and other conflicts of interest.
2. "Revitalize the Baby-Friendly Hospital Initiative (BFHI), maintaining the global criteria as the minimum requirement for all facilities, expanding the initiative's application to include maternity, neonatal, and child health services and community-based support for lactating women and caregivers of young children.
3. "Implement all provisions of the *International Code of Marketing of Breast-Milk Substitutes* and subsequent relevant World Health Assembly resolutions in their entirety as a minimum requirement, and establish sustainable enforcement mechanisms to prevent and/or address noncompliance.
4. "Adopt maternity protection legislation and other measures that facilitate 6 months of exclusive breastfeeding for women employed in all sectors, with urgent attention to the nonformal sector.
5. "Ensure that appropriate guidelines and skill acquisition regarding infant and young child feeding are included in both preservice and in-service training of all healthcare staff, to enable them to implement infant and young child feeding policies and to provide a high standard of breastfeeding management and counseling to support mothers to practice optimal breastfeeding and complementary feeding.
6. "Ensure that all mothers are aware of their rights and have access to support, information, and counseling on breastfeeding and complementary feeding from health workers and peer groups.
7. "Establish sustainable systems for monitoring infant and young child feeding patterns and trends and use this information for advocacy and programming.
8. "Encourage the media to provide positive images of optimal infant and young child feeding, to support breastfeeding as the norm, and to participate in social mobilization activities such as World Breastfeeding Week.
9. "Take measures to protect populations, especially pregnant and breastfeeding mothers, from environmental contaminants and chemical residues.
10. "Identify and allocate sufficient resources to fully implement actions called for in the Global Strategy for Infant and Young Child Feeding.

11. "Monitor progress in appropriate infant and young child feeding practices and report periodically, including as provided in the Convention on the Rights of the Child." (*Innocenti Declaration 2005*, 2005)

D. All manufacturers and distributors of products within the scope of the international code were called on to do the following:
1. "Ensure full compliance with all provisions of the International Code and subsequent relevant World Health Assembly resolutions in all countries, independently of any other measures taken to implement the Code.
2. "Ensure that all processed foods for infants and young children meet applicable Codex Alimentarius standards." (*Innocenti Declaration 2005*, 2005)

VIII. The International Baby Food Action Network

A. The International Baby Food Action Network (IBFAN) was created at the WHO/UNICEF Meeting on Infant and Young Child Feeding, which took place in Geneva, Switzerland, in October 1979.

B. By the end of the meeting, representatives from six of the NGOs attending decided to form the IBFAN.

C. One of IBFAN's objectives is to monitor the marketing practices of the industry around the world and to share and publicize the information gathered.

D. The group also states that "there should be an international code of marketing of infant formula and other products used as breast milk substitutes" (WHO/UNICEF meeting on infant and young child feeding, 1980).

E. IBFAN has also set up the ICDC with the task of keeping track of code compliance both by governments and by companies.

IX. WHO Global Data Bank on Breastfeeding

A. The WHO Global Data Bank on Breastfeeding is maintained in the Nutrition Unit of WHO in Geneva. Information from national and regional surveys and studies that deals specifically with breastfeeding prevalence and duration is pooled.

B. Reports are prepared on breastfeeding trends in countries for which data are available. Every effort is made to achieve worldwide coverage.

X. *Pontificiae Academiae Scientiarum Documenta* 28

A. The Pontifical Academy of Sciences and the Royal Society held a Working Group on Breastfeeding: Science and Society on May 11–13, 1995, at the Vatican.

B. The meeting was part of an overall study on population and resources.

C. Pope Pius XII had urged Catholic mothers to nourish their children themselves. Pope John Paul II emphasized that "mothers need time, information and support in order to breastfeed; no one can substitute for the mother in this natural activity" (Pontifical Academy of Sciences 1995).

XI. *Protection, Promotion and Support of Breastfeeding in Europe: A Blueprint for Action*

This document was developed and written by participants of the project Promotion of Breastfeeding in Europe. Under six headings, the document intends that its application will achieve a Europe-wide improvement in breastfeeding practices and rates (initiation, exclusivity, and duration); more parents who are confident, empowered, and satisfied with their breastfeeding experience; and healthcare workers with improved skills and greater job satisfaction (EU Project on Promotion of Breastfeeding in Europe, 2004).

XII. Acceptable Medical Reasons for Use of Breastmilk Substitutes

The original (1992) list of acceptable medical reasons for supplementation of babies with breastmilk substitutes was part of the package of tools created to support the Baby-Friendly Hospital Initiative. The new 2009 document had been circulated and reviewed for several years before being published as both a standalone document and as part of the revision of the BFHI. After acknowledging the multiple positive health reasons for breastfeeding that accrue to mother and baby, the document addresses conditions of the infant or mother that may justify the permanent or temporary cessation of breastfeeding (World Health Organization & UNICEF, 2009a).

References

EU Project on Promotion of Breastfeeding in Europe. (2004). *Protection, promotion and support of breastfeeding in Europe: A blueprint for action*. Luxembourg: European Commission, Directorate Public Health and Risk Assessment. Retrieved from http://www.iblce-europe.org/Download/Blueprint/Blueprint%20English.pdf

Food and Agriculture Organization of the United Nations & World Health Organization. (1992). *World declaration and plan of action for nutrition*. International Conference for Nutrition. Rome, Italy: Author. Retrieved from http://whqlibdoc.who.int/hq/1992/a34303.pdf

Innocenti declaration on the protection, promotion, and support of breastfeeding. (1990). Presented at the Breastfeeding in the 1990s: A Global Initiative meeting, Florence, Italy.

Innocenti Declaration 2005: On infant and young child feeding. (2005). Retrieved from http://innocenti15.net/declaration.pdf.pdf

Pontificia Academia Scientiarum. (1996). *Breastfeeding: Science and society*. Citta Del Vaticano: Author.

The Pontifical Academy of Sciences (1995) *Pontificiae Academiae Scientiarum Documenta* 28 Report of the Working Group on Breastfeeding: Science and Society May 11–13, 1995.

Sokol, E. J. (2005). *The code handbook: A guide to implementing the international code of marketing of breast-milk substitutes* (2nd ed.). Penang, Malaysia: International Code Documentation Centre.

WHO/UNICEF meeting on infant and young child feeding. (1980). *Journal of Midwifery and Women's Health*, *25*, 31–38. doi:10.1016/0091-2182(80)90051-8

World Alliance for Breastfeeding Action. (2005). Celebrating Innocenti: 1990–2005. Retrieved from http://innocenti15.net/

World Health Assembly. (1986, May 16). Resolution 39.28. Retrieved from http://www.ibfanafrica.org.sz/index.php/wha-resolutions/24-wha-resolution-3928-1986?format=pdf

World Health Assembly. (1994). Resolution 47.4. Retrieved from http://www.ibfan.org/issue-international_code-full-475.html

World Health Assembly. (1996). Resolution 49.15. Retrieved from http://www.ibfan.org/issue-international_code-full-4915.html

World Health Organization. (1989). *Protecting, promoting and supporting breast-feeding: The special role of maternity services*. Geneva, Switzerland: Author.

World Health Organization. (2003). *Global strategy for infant and young child feeding*. Geneva, Switzerland: Author.

World Health Organization Division of Nutrition. (1997). *The international code of marketing of breast-milk substitutes: A common review and evaluation framework (CREF)*. Geneva, Switzerland: Author.

World Health Organization & UNICEF. (2009a). Acceptable medical reasons for use of breast-milk substitutes. Retrieved from http://whqlibdoc.who.int/hq/2009/WHO_FCH_CAH_09.01_eng.pdf

World Health Organization & UNICEF. (2009b). Section 1: Background and implementation. In *Baby-Friendly Hospital Initiative: Revised, Updated and Expanded for Integrated Care*. Retrieved from http://whqlibdoc.who.int/publications/2009/9789241594967_eng.pdf

World Health Organization (2010) Sixty-Third World Health Assembly. Resolutions and Decisions. Accessed December 31, 2011 from http://www.who.int/nutrition/topics/WHA63.23_iycn_en.pdf

World Health Organization and the Food and Agriculture Organization of the United Nations. (2008) *Enterobacter sakazakii (Cronobacter* spp.) Meeting Report. Accessed December 31, 2011. http://www.fao.org/ag/agn/agns/jemra/Sakazaki_FUF_report.pdf

Suggested Reading

Armstrong, H. C., & Sokol, E. (1994). *The international code of marketing of breast-milk substitutes: What it means for mothers and babies world-wide*. Raleigh, NC: International Lactation Consultant Association.

Cadwell, K., & Turner-Maffei, C. (2009). *Implementing continuity of care in breastfeeding*. Sudbury, MA: Jones and Bartlett.

Chetley, A., & Allain, A. (1998). *Protecting infant health: A health worker's guide to the International Code of Marketing of Breastmilk Substitutes* (9th ed.). Geneva, Switzerland: International Baby Food Action Network.

Infant Feeding Action Coalition (INFACT) Canada. http://www.infactcanada.ca/

Innocenti declaration on the protection, promotion, and support of breastfeeding. (1990). Presented at the Breastfeeding in the 1990s: A Global Initiative meeting, Florence, Italy.

International Baby Food Action Network. http://ibfan.org/

International Baby Food Action Network. (1998). *Complying with the code? A manufacturers' and distributors' guide to the code*. Penang, Malaysia: Author.

International Baby Food Action Network. (2004). *Breaking the rules: Stretching the rules 2004. Evidence of violations of the international code of marketing of breastmilk substitutes and subsequent resolutions*. Geneva, Switzerland: Author. Retrieved from http://www.ibfan.org/art/302-2.pdf

International Labour Organization. (2000). Convention on maternity protection. Retrieved from http://www.ilo.org/ilolex/cgi-lex/convde.pl?C183

International Lactation Consultant Association (ILCA). http://www.ilca.org/i4a/pages/index.cfm?pageid=1

The Joint Commission. (2010). *Specifications manual for Joint Commission national quality core measures (2010A2): Exclusive breast milk feeding*. http://manual.jointcommission.org/releases/TJC2010A/MIF0170.html

The Joint Commission. (2010). *Specifications manual for Joint Commission national quality core measures (2010A2): Reasons for not exclusively feeding breast milk.* Retrieved from http://manual.jointcommission.org/releases/TJC2010A/DataElem0274.html

Office of the United Nations High Commissioner for Human Rights. (1966). International covenant on economic, social, and cultural rights. Retrieved from http://www2.ohchr.org/english/law/cescr.htm

Office of the United Nations High Commissioner for Human Rights. (1989). Convention on the rights of the child. Retrieved from http://www2.ohchr.org/english/law/crc.htm

Richter, J. (1998). *Engineering of consent: Uncovering corporate PR.* Dorset, England: Corner House.

Salisbury, L., & Blackwell, A. G. (1981). *Petition to alleviate domestic infant formula misuse and provide informed infant feeding choice.* San Francisco, CA: Public Advocates.

Sethi, S. P. (1994). *Multinational corporations and the impact of public advocacy on corporate strategy: Nestlé and the infant formula controversy.* Norwell, MA: Kluwer Academic Publishers.

Shuber, S. (1998). *The international code of marketing of breast-milk substitutes: An international measure to protect and promote breastfeeding.* Cambridge, MA: Kluwer Law International.

Sokol, E. J. (2005). *The code handbook: A guide to implementing the International Code of Marketing of Breast-milk Substitutes* (2nd ed.). Penang, Malaysia: International Code Documentation Center/ IBFAN.

United Nations Division for the Advancement of Women. (2009). Convention on the elimination of all forms of discrimination against women. Retrieved from http://www.un.org/womenwatch/daw/cedaw/

U.S. Department of Health and Human Services. (2010). 2020 topics and objectives: Maternal, infant, and child health. In *Healthy People 2020.* Washington, DC: Public Health Service. Retrieved from http://www.healthypeople.gov/2020/topicsobjectives2020/objectiveslist.aspx?topicid=26

World Alliance for Breastfeeding Action. http://www.waba.org.my/

World Alliance for Breastfeeding Action. (1994). Protect breastfeeding: Making the code work. Retrieved from http://worldbreastfeedingweek.net/webpages/1994.html

World Alliance for Breastfeeding Action. (2006). Code watch: 25 year of protecting breastfeeding. Retrieved from http://worldbreastfeedingweek.net/webpages/2006.html

World Breastfeeding Week. http://worldbreastfeedingweek.org/

World Health Organization. (2010, May). *World Health Assembly Journal.* Retrieved from http://apps. who.int/gb/ebwha/pdf_files/WHA63/A63_J3-en.pdf

World Health Organization. (2003). *Global strategy for infant and young child feeding.* Geneva, Switzerland: Author. Retrieved from http://www.who.int/nutrition/topics/global_strategy/en/index.html

World Health Organization & UNICEF. (2009). Section 2: Strengthening and sustaining the baby-friendly hospital initiative: A course for decision-makers. In *Baby-friendly hospital initiative: Revised, updated and expanded for integrated care.* Retrieved from http://whqlibdoc.who.int/publications/2009/9789241594974_eng.pdf

World Health Organization and the Food and Agriculture Organization of the United Nations. (2008) *Enterobacter sakazakii (Cronobacter* spp.) Meeting Report. Accessed December 31, 2011. http://www.fao.org/ag/agn/agns/jemra/Sakazaki_FUF_report.pdf

CHAPTER 3
Communication and Counseling Skills

Judith Lauwers, BA, IBCLC, FILCA

OBJECTIVES

- Identify principles of adult learning that lead to the empowerment of mothers.
- Describe the relative importance of the three components of communication and how to strengthen the message that is sent.
- Describe the counseling process and strategies for meeting the mother's needs for emotional support, understanding, and action.
- Discuss the relative roles of the consultant and the mother in guiding and leading counseling methods and the appropriate use of each method.
- Demonstrate a variety of guiding skills that will elicit information from and provide support to the mother.
- Implement effective problem solving and follow-up within the context of consulting.
- Recognize the needs of grieving parents and strategies for providing support.

INTRODUCTION

Effective counseling skills and communication techniques are essential tools of the lactation consultant. Use of these skills provides mothers with the support and teaching that will help them develop confidence in their mothering and breastfeeding. The degree to which mothers are helped by support and advice from a lactation consultant is determined in large part by the lactation consultant's attitude and approach. Adult learners need to perceive themselves as having control over their outcomes. Therefore, an approach that establishes a partnership between the mother and lactation consultant fosters the mother's learning and growth. This approach also increases the likelihood of the mother complying with her lactation consultant's advice.

New mothers and those who are breastfeeding for the first time are vulnerable to messages and impressions that compromise their self-confidence. An awareness of effective body language and voice tone assists the lactation consultant in creating an atmosphere in which the mother feels empowered and self-confident. Choice of positive words and phrases also contributes to an effective learning climate. Providing emotional support to mothers is pivotal to helping them feel confident and empowered in their breastfeeding. Learning how to listen attentively and respond with sensitivity

(continues)

and validation increase the mother's sense of value and control. It is important that the lactation consultant gather sufficient information and insights during a consultation before engaging in problem solving. Use of the counseling skills presented in this chapter optimizes the lactation consultant's effectiveness with mothers and contributes to meaningful interactions. They can be considered tools in the lactation consultant's toolbox to be pulled out as each situation warrants.

I. Principles of Adult Learning

A. The adult learner expects frankness and honesty.
  1. Healthcare providers have a responsibility to give parents the information they need to make informed decisions (Northouse, 1985).
  2. Educating parents empowers them to become informed healthcare consumers and to make responsible choices.
  3. Trust parents to learn about the health consequences of not breastfeeding and to make an informed decision about infant feeding.
      a. The fear of creating guilt if a mother chooses not to breastfeed should not be allowed to compromise the parents' right to evidence-based facts.
      b. Women experience lack of breastfeeding as a loss regardless of whether the choice not to breastfeed is by decision or imposed (Labbok, 2008).
B. The adult learner is an active participant in the learning process (Knowles, 1980).
  1. Planning is done mutually with self-direction, self-reliance, and risk taking encouraged.
  2. The mother develops problem-solving skills, takes ownership for the plan, and is responsible for the outcome.
  3. The mother evaluates her own learning and takes necessary action.
  4. A hands-off approach puts the mother in control and contributes to her personal growth (Law et al., 2007).
C. Learning climate influences the learning outcome.
  1. Personal knowledge and a flexible environment are the best predictors of women's satisfaction with decision making about healthcare issues (Wittmann-Price, 2006).
  2. Creating a positive impression enhances learning.
      a. Display self-confidence, an ability to relate to people, a sense of humor, enthusiasm, and informality.
      b. Respect the learner and be willing to be flexible and to adapt.
      c. Be neat, clean, and wear tasteful attire.
      d. Maintain positive body language, frequent eye contact, a strong voice, and carefully pronounced words.
      e. Maintain a strong knowledge base and demonstrate a desire to share knowledge.

D. A multisensory approach enhances the learning process.
  1. Engaging multiple senses can help visual, auditory, and kinesthetic learning to take place (Russell, 2006).
  2. Integrating appropriate and culturally sensitive humor with learning promotes critical thinking and emotional intelligence (Chabeli, 2008; Ziv, 1983).
    a. Humor reduces tension and anxiety and increases productivity.
    b. Humor stimulates divergent thinking and increases the mother's willingness to look at a situation in a new way.
    c. Humor stimulates and integrates the right and left hemispheres of the brain so that learning is at its highest level.
E. Every adult learning encounter is individualized to accommodate the particular mother and baby.
  1. Recognize the abilities of every mother and baby and let them set the pace.
  2. Respect the mother's background and tap into it.
  3. Assess the mother's learning needs and her readiness to learn before engaging in problem solving.
    a. Capitalize on the "teachable moment" that will maximize her ability to learn and process information.
    b. Consider the mother's physical comfort, confidence level, emotional state, and the health of the mother and baby in determining the teachable moment.
    c. Use the mother's language style and imagery, and match her intensity and sense of humor.
  4. Make sure every intervention is focused and justified.
  5. Tailor suggestions and actions to the mother's responses and provide appropriate written materials.
F. Learning outcome depends on the level of learning that takes place.
  1. Sharing information verbally is the lowest level of learning (tell me and I may remember).
    a. Verbal instruction is appropriate when visual or interactive reinforcement is not needed.
    b. Example: discussion of contraception or nutrition.
  2. Combining visual reinforcement with verbal instruction increases the level of learning (show me and I may understand).
    a. This is appropriate when interactive reinforcement is not needed.
    b. Example: use of a cloth breast to demonstrate latch-on.
  3. Engaging the learner to participate actively in the learning process produces the highest level of learning (involve me and I may master).
    a. The combination of verbal and visual reinforcement demonstrates whether the mother has mastered the technique being taught.
    b. Example: demonstration of the use of a breast pump with the mother giving a return demonstration.

II. Components of Communication

A. Communication is the delivery and the reception of a message.

B. The human brain is hard wired to process stories better than scientific data (Green et al., 2002).

    1. A mother's decisions can be biased by anecdotal messages from her friends or from the Internet.

    2. Mothers may ignore statistical data in favor of stories they hear from their environment.

    3. Stories are more vivid and easier to process than hard data and are useful in professional communications. Evidence-based storytelling makes use of an anecdote that relates to research-based practices.

C. Three factors that determine how a message is received are the spoken message, tone of voice, and body language (DeVito, 1989).

D. The words the speaker uses account for about 7% of the message received.

    1. Select words and phrases that correct inappropriate practices without compromising the mother's self-confidence or implying the mother is doing or saying something wrong.

       a. The conjunction *but* negates the first half of a thought and can be replaced with the word *and* as in, "You are holding your baby in a good position, (but) and if you turn him slightly, you will find that he can get an even better latch."

       b. The verb *should* implies judgment and can be avoided by rephrasing. Instead of, "You should feed your baby whenever he wants," rephrase to, "When you feed your baby whenever he wants, you will be meeting his needs."

    2. Avoid medical jargon and use words that are on the mother's intellectual level.

    3. If the mother's native language is different from yours, make sure she understands you and consider whether she needs a translator.

    4. Avoid negative terminology and imagery that undermine the mother's self-confidence, including words that imply success or failure, adequacy or inadequacy.

    5. Avoid sending mixed messages to ensure that your words create the desired effect.

    6. Supplement verbal messages with demonstrations, visual aids, and written instructions to strengthen understanding.

E. Voice tone accounts for about 38% of the message received.

    1. Manner of speech can create a warm, friendly, humorous atmosphere.

    2. Use a moderate volume (not too loud or too low).

    3. Use a moderate rate of speech (not too fast or too slow).

    4. Use a moderate pitch, and guard against your voice becoming higher pitched when you are angry or excited.

F. Body language accounts for about 55% of the message received.

    1. Body language is based on the behavioral patterns of nonverbal communication and includes all body movements (Fast, 1970).

       a. It ranges from a very deliberate to an unconscious movement or posture.

       b. It may vary culturally or cut across cultural barriers and needs to reflect the client population.

    2. Women rely on visual communication cues such as facial expressions and eye contact to determine whether they are accepted (Brizendine, 2006).

        a. A smile adds to a warm and inviting atmosphere, puts mothers at ease, and elicits a smile from the mother.

        b. Eye contact conveys a desire to communicate and establishes a warm, caring, and inviting climate.

           i. Eye contact serves as a powerful tool for influencing others.

           ii. Failure to establish eye contact sends a negative message in most cultures; try to maintain eye contact at least 85% of the time when culturally appropriate.

    3. A relaxed and comfortable posture creates a warm and inviting climate.

        a. Sit or stand squarely with both feet flat on the floor.

        b. Rest the arms at one's side, or on one's knees when sitting.

        c. Open body posture shows an openness to communicate on a meaningful level; crossing the arms or legs conveys disinterest and emotional distance.

        d. Combining open posture with leaning forward further conveys interest in engaging the mother.

    4. Altitude and distance can either enhance or detract from a message.

        a. Establish a comfortable position—not too far away or too close—using the mother's reactions as a guide. Standing or sitting too close invades another's personal space (comfort zone). Standing or sitting too far away conveys a message of being too busy or uninterested.

        b. Height in relation to another person conveys who possesses the greatest importance or control. A position equal to or below the mother puts her in control and leads to greater self-reliance and empowerment.

    5. Touch can convey warmth, caring, and encouragement.

        a. It must come at the right moment and in the right context.

        b. Ask permission before touching the mother's breasts or her baby.

    6. Learn to read the body language of mothers.

        a. Facial expression changes to reflect any emotion that is felt (Coon et al., 2008).

        b. Observe and respond to the mother's reactions and body language.

        c. Be alert for nonverbal messages the mother sends and watch for signs of physical discomfort.

III. The Counseling Process

    A. Personality and attitude are important to the counseling process.

        1. Knowledge of people's attitudes provides insight into understanding and predicting their behavior.

        2. Personal experience and other sources of information can change attitude.

        3. A warm and caring attitude shows genuine concern and empathy.

           a. Openness to disclosing feelings and thoughts encourages trust and openness in the mother when done appropriately.

      b. Acknowledging the mother's individuality and worth, without judgment, gives the mother freedom to be herself.

      c. Clear, accurate communication reduces confusion and frustration.

      d. Flexibility helps the counselor respond appropriately to the mother at different stages in the counseling process.

  4. Ineffective communication skills may transmit an attitude of disinterest or emotional distance.

  5. A noncommittal attitude about breastfeeding by healthcare workers has the potential to unintentionally promote the use of artificial baby milk.

B. Effective counseling fulfills the mother's need for emotional support.

  1. Education and support enhance self-perception and empower mothers to reach their goals (Betzold et al., 2007).

  2. Empowering a mother with confidence extends her duration of breastfeeding (O'Brien et al., 2008).

  3. Help the mother arrive at a state where she can take in information and solve problems.

      a. Provide a sense of security that encourages her to verbalize feelings and anxieties.

      b. Praise her actions and validate her feelings, emotions, and concerns.

      c. Listen to what she is *not* saying; look for her underlying message.

      d. Send the message that you genuinely care about her well-being and concerns.

C. Effective counseling increases understanding and self-efficacy.

  1. Interventions aimed at improving mothers' self-efficacy with breastfeeding result in longer and more exclusive breastfeeding (Nichols et al., 2009; Sisk et al., 2006).

  2. Giving a mother tools and support to identify and solve problems can improve breastfeeding self-efficacy (Kang et al., 2008).

      a. She understands herself and her feelings to clearly define and understand the problem and its cause.

      b. She understands her options in resolving problems.

      c. She makes informed choices and assumes responsibility for her actions.

      d. She feels empowered to actively work on solutions.

D. Parents progress through stages as they acquire the parental role, and some mothers may respond better to a more direct counseling approach in the early stages. (See Chapter 4, "The Parental Role.")

E. The counseling process can be hindered when the mother has physical discomfort.

  1. The mother may be too uncomfortable to listen and learn.

  2. Help her relieve discomfort before proceeding with educating and problem solving.

IV. Methods of Counseling

A. Counseling involves three distinct methods: guiding, leading, and follow-up (Brammer, 1973).

B. The process of guiding helps you genuinely listen to the mother and empathize with her through understanding her feelings, goals, and other factors that influence her actions.

   1. Begin with guiding and continue to use it throughout the contact.

   2. The guiding process provides emotional support to the mother.

     a. It transmits a message of acceptance and concern.

     b. It encourages her to express her ideas and concerns openly.

     c. It helps her hear what you are saying.

   3. The guiding process is characterized by limited direction from the counselor.

     a. The mother is encouraged to do most of the talking.

     b. You listen most of the time to gather necessary information and insights.

     c. Careful listening helps you hear what the mother is *not* saying.

C. The leading method requires a more active role by the counselor in directing the conversation.

   1. It helps you and the mother see the situation more clearly.

   2. It helps the mother who is unable to solve a problem.

   3. It helps define options that will lead to a plan of action.

   4. It enables you and the mother to form a problem-solving partnership.

D. Follow-up is essential to the counseling process.

   1. It determines how and when to plan the next contact.

   2. It identifies what preparation is needed for the next contact.

   3. It analyzes the efficacy of the contact.

   4. It indicates whether your suggestions have been useful.

   5. It identifies the mother's need for further support or assistance.

   6. It lets the mother know how concerned you are in helping her.

V. Skills in the Guiding Method

A. Counseling skills in the guiding method encourage the mother to continue talking freely and promote her active participation in the discussion.

B. Listening skills reinforce what is said, clarify the mother's statements, show acceptance of her situation, and encourage her to arrive at solutions.

   1. Attending is the lowest level of listening.

     a. You listen passively to indicate that you are paying attention.

     b. Examples of attending include eye contact, open posture, calm gestures, a silent pause, or saying, *Yes* or *Mmm*.

   2. Active listening, also called reflective listening, paraphrases what you believe the mother meant.

     a. Shows acceptance of the mother's viewpoint.

     b. Encourages a response from the mother.

     c. Clarifies the message so that the mother can reflect on it.

    3. Empathetic listening goes beyond merely reflecting words.
       a. You listen with the intent to understand emotionally and intellectually.
       b. You rephrase both the content and the feeling of what she said.
       c. It helps the mother know whether she sent the intended message.

C. Facilitating skills actively encourage the mother to give more information and define her situation better.
    1. They focus on specific concerns and pinpoint issues and feelings to explore.
    2. Clarifying helps to make a point clear, as in, "Do you mean that your nipples hurt only when…"
    3. Asking open-ended questions is a useful skill for gathering information.
       a. It is a question that cannot be answered by a simple "yes" or "no."
       b. The question begins with who, what, when, where, why, how, how much, or how often.
       c. Instead of asking, "Does your baby nurse often enough?" ask, "How many times does she nurse in 24 hours?"
    4. Interpreting takes active listening one step further to empathetic listening.
       a. You interpret what was said rather than merely restating it.
       b. It enables the mother to process your interpretation and to agree or disagree.
       c. It describes the emotion that is being expressed, as in, "You're worried that your baby is not getting enough milk."
    5. Focusing pursues a topic that is helpful to explore or condenses several points.
       a. Selects one particular point to repeat.
       b. Useful when the mother gets into an unrelated topic.
       c. Example: "Tell me more about…"
    6. Summarizing highlights and reinforces important information.
       a. Restates the plan of action.
       b. Reassures the mother that you are tuned into her.
       c. Helps you know that you understood the mother.
       d. Most effective when done by the mother, as in, "We talked about several things to try; which will work best for you?"

D. Influencing skills instill a positive outlook in the mother and encourage her to continue to seek help.
    1. Reassuring helps a mother see that her situation is normal and assures her that her situation will improve, as in, "Your breasts will feel more comfortable after the initial fullness goes down."
    2. Building hope helps the mother see how her feelings relate to her situation.
       a. Encourages her to talk about her feelings.
       b. Helps relieve tension.
       c. Encourages her to take positive action.
       d. Example: "I'm glad your mother plans to join us. She may be more supportive when she has a better understanding of breastfeeding."

3. Identifying strengths helps the mother focus on her positive qualities and those of her baby.
   a. Counteracts negative factors.
   b. Encourages the mother to persevere.
   c. Encourages the mother to develop and rely on her own resources.
   d. Helps her to recall enjoyable memories.
   e. Example: You did that really well!

VI. Skills in the Leading Method

A. Skills in the leading method place more responsibility for the direction of the discussion on the counselor.
B. The goal is to understand a problem and develop a plan of action.
   1. It is used when the mother is unable to solve a problem.
   2. It provides additional resources to lead the mother toward a solution.
   3. Gather enough information so that your problem solving is not premature or incorrect.
   4. Take time to gain the mother's trust and clarify the situation before problem solving.
   5. Give parents proper information at the appropriate time.
C. Informing explains how something functions and the reasons behind it.
   1. Correct misconceptions or mismanagement with sensitivity.
   2. Suggest appropriate resources to help them grow as parents.
   3. Provide anticipatory guidance at times when retention will be high and decision making will occur.
   4. Encourage initial learning before delivery so that postpartum teaching can focus on reinforcement.
   5. Example: When your baby suckles, it stimulates the nerve endings, and in turn signals milk production. Therefore,...
D. Problem solving is accomplished by forming a partnership between the mother and counselor.
   1. Form your first hunch (a hunch refers to an idea or a hypothesis) based on information and impressions you gained.
   2. Look for additional factors that will confirm the hunch.
   3. Test the hunch by suggesting what the problem might be.
   4. If the mother rejects the hunch, explore alternative hunches with the use of guiding skills to gain further insights and information.
   5. When the hunch is confirmed, develop a plan of action with the mother.
   6. Use a nonassertive approach to encourage the mother to be active in problem solving.
   7. Limit suggestions to two or three actions to avoid overwhelming the mother.
   8. Ask the mother to summarize the plan to demonstrate her understanding.
   9. Set a time limit on the actions to be taken, and follow up to learn whether the plan worked or whether further suggestions are needed.

VII. Skills in Follow-Up

A. Follow-up is an ongoing process and should be done after every contact. The urgency of the situation will determine how soon and how frequent follow-up is necessary.

B. Evaluating the session.
   1. Determine how effective the contact was and whether the mother's needs were met.
   2. Assess the use of appropriate counseling skills.
   3. Evaluate the information and advice given to the mother.
   4. Evaluate the method of documentation.

C. Arranging the next contact.
   1. Let the mother know what follow-up to expect, when the contact will occur, and who will initiate it.
   2. Determine any additional information or assistance that is needed.
   3. Leave the door open for the mother to contact you when needed.
   4. Make appropriate referrals to other healthcare professionals and community resources.
   5. Arrange frequent contact during the early weeks postpartum, either personally or through referral to a support group.

D. Researching outside sources.
   1. Accessing information and resources helps you grow as a lactation consultant and provides further input and a fresh outlook on a problem.
   2. Seek support and advice from colleagues.

E. Renewing the counseling process.
   1. The counseling process begins anew with each successive contact.
   2. Begin with guiding skills and progress to leading skills and further follow-up as needed.

VIII. Counseling a Mother Who Is Grieving

A. Parents who lose a baby progress through several stages of grief before their loss is resolved (**Figure 3-1**).
   1. They need time and privacy with their family immediately after the loss to begin the grieving process.
   2. Talking about her feelings helps the mother through the grief process.
   3. Resolution could take as long as 2 years, depending on the amount of support and understanding the parents receive.
   4. Mothers who had been nursing or expressing milk for their babies can be further comforted in knowing they gave their babies the best possible care.
   5. Donating milk that may help save another baby's life can be a part of the mother's emotional healing.
   6. Talking with other parents who have had similar experiences can help their perspective.
   7. Counseling is available through local clergy and social service organizations.

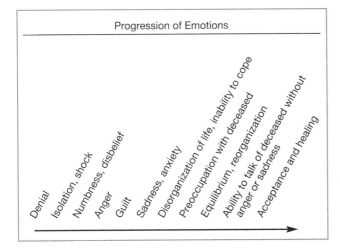

Progression of Emotions

Denial — Isolation, shock — Numbness, disbelief — Anger — Guilt — Sadness, anxiety — Disorganization of life, inability to cope — Preoccupation with deceased — Equilibrium, reorganization — Ability to talk of deceased without anger or sadness — Acceptance and healing

Figure 3-1
Sequence of the Grief Process

Source: Lauwers, J., & Swisher. A. (2010). *Counseling the nursing mother: A lactation consultant's guide (5th ed.).* Sudbury, MA: Jones & Bartlett Learning.

B. Appropriate counseling techniques, insight into the mother's emotions, and sincere empathy help you approach the situation confident in your ability to comfort the mother.
1. Reflect back to the mother how you imagine she must feel, as in, "You must be heartbroken," or, "I can't imagine the loss you feel."
2. Acknowledge her baby's importance by asking his name and using it during conversations.
3. Let her know you will be glad to listen, while assuring her that you do not want to invade her privacy.
4. Help parents assert their rights to hold or see their baby after he dies, take pictures, and keep the identification bracelet as mementos.
5. You may wish to attend the funeral if you have cared for the mother and baby.
C. Parents of high-risk infants may experience a similar grief process.
1. They may avoid contact with other parents who have healthy babies.
2. They may avoid involvement with their baby to protect themselves from becoming attached to a baby they may lose.
3. Such feelings usually subside after they accept their baby's condition.
4. Parents also grieve when it is necessary to transfer their infant to another facility.
5. Encourage parents to seek support, both in the hospital and within their community.

References

Betzold, C.M., Laughlin, K.M. & Shi, C. (2007). A family practice breastfeeding education pilot program: An observational, descriptive study. *International Breastfeeding Journal*, *2*(4).

Brammer, L. M. (1973). *The helping relationship*. Upper Saddle River, NJ: Prentice Hall.

Brizendine, L. (2006). *The female brain*. New York, NY: Morgan Road Books/Random House.

Chabeli, M. (2008). Humor: A pedagogical tool to promote learning. *Curationis*, *31*(3), 51–59.

Coon, D., & Mitterer, J. (2008). *Brain and behavior*. In *Psychology: A Journey*. Belmont, CA: Thomson Higher Education.

DeVito, J. A. (1989). *The interpersonal communication book* (5th ed.). New York, NY: Harper & Row.

Fast, J. (1970). *Body language*. New York, NY: Pocket Books.

Green, M. C., Strange, J. J., & Brock, T. C. (2002). *Narrative impact: Social and cognitive foundations*. Mahwah, NJ: Lawrence Erlbaum.

Kang, J. S., Choi, S. Y., & Ryu, E. J. (2008). Effects of a breastfeeding empowerment programme on Korean breastfeeding mothers: A quasi-experimental study. *International Journal of Nursing Studies*, *45*(1), 14–23.

Knowles, M. (1980). *The modern practice of adult education from pedagogy to andragogy*. Chicago, IL: Follett Publishing.

Labbok, M. (2008). Exploration of guilt among mothers who do not breastfeed: The physician's role. *Journal of Human Lactation*, *24*(1), 80–84.

Law, S., Dunn,O., & Wallace, L. (2007). Breastfeeding best start study: Training midwives in a "hands off" positioning and attachment intervention. *Maternal and Child Nutrition*, *3*(3), 194–205.

Nichols, J., Schutte, N., & Brown, R. (2009). The impact of a self-efficacy intervention on short-term breast-feeding outcomes. *Health Education and Behavior*, *36*, 250–258.

Northouse, P. G. (1985). *Health communication: A handbook for health professionals*. Englewood Cliffs, NJ: Prentice Hall.

O'Brien, M., Buikstra, E. & Hegney, D. (2008). The influence of psychological factors on breastfeeding duration. *Journal of Advanced Nursing*, *63*(4), 397–408.

Russell, S. (2006). An overview of adult-learning processes. *Urologic Nursing*, *26*(5), 349–352, 370.

Sisk, P. M., Lovelady, C.A., & Dillard, R.G. (2006). Lactation counseling for mothers of very low birth weight infants: Effect on maternal anxiety and infant intake of human milk. *Pediatrics*, *117*(1), e67–e75.

Wittmann-Price, R. A. (2006). Exploring the subconcepts of the Wittmann-Price theory of emancipated decision-making in women's health care. *Journal of Nursing Scholarship*, *38*(4), 377–382.

Ziv, A. (1983). The influence of humorous atmosphere on divergent thinking. *Contemporary Educational Psychology*, *9*, 413–421.

Suggested Reading

Ellis, D., Livingstone, V. H., & Hewat, R. J. (1993). Assisting the breastfeeding mother: A problem-solving process. *Journal of Human Lactation*, *9*, 89–93.

Fletcher, D., & Harris, H. (2000). The implementation of the HOT program at the Royal Women's Hospital. *Breastfeeding Review*, *8*, 19–23.

Isselman, M., Deubner, L. S., & Hartman, M. (1993). A nutrition counseling workshop: Integrating counseling psychology into nutrition practice. *Journal of the American Dietetic Association*, *93*, 324–326.

Lauwers, J., & Swisher, A. (2010). *Counseling the nursing mother: A lactation consultant's guide* (5th ed.). Sudbury, MA: Jones and Bartlett.

CHAPTER 4
The Parental Role

Revised by Judith Lauwers, BA, IBCLC, FILCA

OBJECTIVES

- Describe parents' role in the healthcare system.
- Identify factors in parent–infant bonding and attachment.
- Describe the common emotions of new parents and recognize signs of inadequate coping.
- Recognize signs of a history of sexual abuse.
- Discuss postpartum sexual adjustments and family planning options.
- Describe breastfeeding in the context of a major life change and alternative family styles.
- Identify support systems for mothers.

INTRODUCTION

Parenting roles and family relationships are influenced by social, cultural, and historical factors. Parents share many of the same goals across cultures but differ in how they approach meeting them. Some cultures place a strong emphasis on family and group identity. Others value individuality and independence. Childrearing attitudes and recommendations have changed over the years, as have the roles of men and women. Mothers and fathers often are challenged with balancing multiple roles while promoting the optimal development of their children. Articles and books contain conflicting information and advice that can be confusing for both parents and children. Parents who are in nuclear families have lost the modeling and influence of the extended family in their learning and practicing for the parental role. Any number of family configurations can be found, from the traditional married man and woman with the man as the major breadwinner to blended families through divorce and remarriage, to single mothers with children. Families living in poverty face significant parenting challenges and barriers. As hospital stays shorten, families are geographically spread out, and economic factors force women into employment after short maternity leaves, so educational needs for new parents have burgeoned. The lactation consultant is in a unique position both to assist with breastfeeding and offer valuable support to new families.

I. Parents' Roles in the Healthcare System

A. Parents who are active and informed healthcare consumers are responsible decision makers regarding their care and the care of their baby.

B. Encourage parents to:

1. Express concerns and preferences in a courteous manner.

2. Reinforce positive aspects of their care.

3. Carry through on an agreed plan of care and accept the consequences of their actions.

4. Allow reports and follow-up to their physicians for coordination of care.

II. Acquiring the Parental Role

A. Anticipatory guidance and active involvement in the pregnancy and birth enhance parental role acquisition (Freed et al., 1992; Gamble et al., 1992; Jordan et al., 1990).

1. Becoming a parent is a stressful experience (Randall et al., 2009).

a. Parents experience greater declines in marital satisfaction compared to non-parents (Lawrence et al., 2007).

b. Couples with higher levels of social support in pregnancy report significantly lower levels of distress 6 weeks postnatally (Castle et al., 2008).

c. Family transitions provide opportunities to strengthen marriage (Schulz et al., 2006).

d. Change in the relationship often results in a more closely united relationship (Fägerskiöld, 2008).

2. The term *maternal role attainment*, first described by Rubin (1967a, 1967b), describes the phases of taking in, taking hold, and letting go as characteristic of the behavior of new mothers.

a. Breastfeeding is part of a woman's transition to motherhood (Marshall et al., 2007).

b. Helping women cope with pressures of early mothering can increase breastfeeding duration (O'Brien et al., 2009).

c. Good maternal care is essential for a mother's psychological health (Barett, 2006).

3. Fathers report progressing from being overwhelmed to being masters of the new situation, to a new completeness in life (Premberg et al., 2008).

4. New parents often turn to the Internet for information and interaction (Plantin et al., 2009).

B. Stages of parental role acquisition (Bocar et al., 1987)

1. *Anticipatory:* The anticipatory stage occurs before delivery and is a time when parents begin learning about their new roles. They read, talk with their own parents, ask questions of other family members and parents, and attend classes.

2. *Formal:* The formal stage begins after delivery. Parents create the "perfect parent" image or an idealized version of parenting. They are interested in mastering practical child care skills. They may lack self-confidence and become

easily overwhelmed and confused by conflicting information. New parents need concrete demonstrations and suggestions as well as acknowledgment that they are the experts on their own baby. Once they develop confidence in their ability to meet their baby's basic needs, they progress to the informal stage.

    3. *Informal:* During the informal stage, parents begin interacting with their peers and have other informal interactions. They begin to relax the more rigid rules and directions used to acquire the caretaking behaviors.

    4. *Personal:* The personal stage is when parents modify their practices and evolve their own unique parenting styles.

C. Parents who follow rigid "baby training" programs that prescribe scheduled feedings, limited contact, and specified sleep periods find it difficult to move beyond the formal stage of parenting.

    1. Upwardly mobile, career-minded professionals are drawn to such programs.

    2. There are concerns about the psychological outcome of children left to "cry it out" (Aney, 1998). Some infants demonstrate detachment, depression, eating issues, and self-stimulating and self-soothing behaviors (Webb, 2003; Williams, 1998, 1999).

    3. Low milk supply, low infant weight gain, or the baby rejecting the breast may result (Aney, 1998; Moody, 2002).

    4. These babies are at risk for attachment problems; babies who are left to "cry it out" might sleep through the night after abandoning hope of being parented in the evening and might experience despair.

    5. With reflective listening, you can be accepting of parents without endorsing their practices. A nonjudgmental approach creates a climate where parents can question their approach and be open to alternatives.

III. Attachment and Bonding

A. Infant-to-parent attachment

    1. Attachment is viewed as a behavioral system (Bowlby, 1969).

      a. Infant attachment or signaling behaviors such as cooing, smiling, and crying initiate and maintain contact between the mother and infant.

      b. A secure attachment helps the infant develop a sense of security that was described by Erikson (1950) as basic trust.

      c. The first 6 months of life are considered a sensitive period when the infant develops a trusting relationship with the caregiver.

      d. Parents should watch their baby and respond to approach behaviors and feeding cues.

      e. Keeping mothers and babies together and avoiding unnecessary separations enhance bonding and attachment.

    2. Ainsworth et al. (1978) described three general patterns of infant-to-parent attachment: avoidant, ambivalent, and secure.

      a. Avoidant infants show little distress during separation, treat a stranger the same way as the mother, and avoid proximity or interaction with the mother during a reunion after separation.

     b. Ambivalent infants resist contact with a stranger and might be angry or resistant to the mother upon reunion following a separation; once contact with the mother is initiated, the infant seeks to maintain it.

     c. Securely attached infants seek proximity and contact with the mother (especially during reunions) and also explore the environment.

  3. Parental sensitivity and responsiveness may be key indicators of a parent's attachment to his or her infant and can affect the infant's subsequent attachment to the parent (Graham, 1993).

     a. Mothers who are sensitive and responsive to the infant's needs during the early months and who promptly meet the infant's needs foster the development of secure attachment relationships.

     b. Mothers who fail to respond to their infants or respond inappropriately foster the development of avoidant or ambivalent attachments.

  4. Secure infant-to-parent attachments at age 12 to 18 months are related to the child's adaptive problem-solving ability at 2 years of age and to social competence at age 3 years.

B. Parent-to-infant attachment

  1. Parents begin to form attachments to the baby in utero, and their interaction during the early weeks is a get-acquainted process.

  2. Parental, situational, and infant factors are related to the development of a parent's attachment to the infant.

     a. Early contact and bonding behaviors have been suggested as being important during the early hours following birth; Klaus et al. (1982) describe a sensitive period following birth as being important in establishing attachment; although humans are capable of adaptation and growth in this area, the concept might be of special importance to mothers who are at risk of developing maladaptive parent–child relationships.

     b. Attachment behaviors of all women are enhanced by avoiding epidurals and other birth interventions and keeping mothers and babies together in a rooming-in environment; this may be especially relevant to low-income or indigent women.

     c. If there are discrepancies between what parents had fantasized their baby would be like and the reality of their child, parents might be delayed in their attachment progress.

  3. The temperament of an infant has a great effect on parental feelings of competence and interactions.

     a. Compatibility can have an effect on parenting behaviors.

     b. Infants who are difficult to console or whose needs are difficult to meet might have parents who feel it is a challenge to develop high-quality interactions.

     c. When parents perceive their efforts as successful in meeting the needs of their infants, they perceive themselves as competent and effective caregivers.

4. Father's interaction with baby
   a. Father-to-infant attachment is enhanced by the father being actively involved in the pregnancy and birth and having extended contact with his infant during the newborn period (Sears et al., 2003).
   b. Fathers have unique ways of interacting with their infants, frequently called engrossment in the early period.
   c. Fathers learn their role through society's definitions, experience with their own fathers, and pressure from family members and other men.
   d. The father often feels as though he has lost his mate because she seems immersed in the care of the baby.
   e. Fathers experience a hormonal response to their babies' cries, with a rise in prolactin and testosterone levels (Delahunty et al., 2007; Fleming et al., 2002).
   f. Fathers benefit from learning about infant cues and responsiveness to recognize what is normal and how to interact with their young infants (Delight et al., 1991).

IV. Emotional Adjustments Postpartum

A. Maternal postpartum mood changes are usually mild and self-limiting.
   1. There is disagreement in the literature as to whether postpartum psychological complications are unique to the postpartum period or are symptoms of an underlying disorder that is triggered by childbirth.
   2. Possible causes include hormonal adjustments, chemical imbalances, a genetic predisposition, poor ego development, low self-esteem, poor interpersonal relationships, and the perception of the inability to meet others' needs.
B. "Baby blues"
   1. As many as 50% to 80% of postpartum women experience a period of emotional distress beginning 2 to 3 days after delivery.
   2. Baby blues are characterized by feelings of ambivalence, tearfulness, sadness, insomnia, anxiety, irritability, poor concentration, and lack of self-confidence.
   3. Baby blues are more common in women with their first baby. A disappointing birth experience, poor nutrition, and a fussy baby increase feelings of sadness.
   4. Emotional support, practical help, realistic expectations, and interaction with other new mothers can minimize baby blues.
   5. If the baby blues last more than 2 weeks, these feelings indicate that the mother may be depressed (Kendall-Tackett, 2005). See Chapter 6, "Maternal Mental Health and Breastfeeding."
   6. The average rate of depression among new fathers is 10%, twice the rate in the general population of men (Paulson et al., 2006).
      a. Fathers report lack of support networks and having no one to turn to other than their partner and work colleagues (Deave et al., 2008).
      b. Paternal depression, like maternal depression, adversely affects infant learning (Kaplan et al., 2007).

V. Postpartum Sexual Adjustments

A. Sexuality and intercourse

1. Many physicians recommend waiting to resume sexual relations until after the 6-week checkup; not all couples will need to wait for that period, however.
2. Adjustments in routine
   a. Having a baby interferes with freedom and sexual spontaneity, and some fathers may resent the attention the baby receives.
   b. Some women might feel tired, "touched out," or too overwhelmed to concentrate on sexual needs.
   c. Nursing the baby immediately before bedtime and taking advantage of moments alone during naptime can provide the parents with an opportunity for intimacy.
   d. Other forms of intimacy and variations in techniques or routines can be explored during this time.
3. Physical adjustments
   a. Kegel exercises help with general toning and facilitate entrance in intercourse.
   b. Vaginal dryness caused by hormonal changes may cause some physical discomfort when first resuming sexual intercourse. The mother can relieve her discomfort with an artificial lubricant.
   c. Some women find that their breasts are very sensitive to touch or not sensitive at all.
   d. Adjustments in positioning can help alleviate physical discomfort caused by a painful incision or full breasts.
   e. Oxytocin released during orgasm may cause the breasts to leak. Feeding the baby or expressing milk beforehand reduces leakage during lovemaking.
   f. Experiencing increased sensuality when breastfeeding is a result of oxytocin release and is a normal response for many women.

B. Amenorrhea and ovulation

1. During the immediate postpartum period and for varying lengths of time thereafter, the breastfeeding mother experiences amenorrhea or the absence of the menses.
   a. Return of menses depends on factors such as exclusive breastfeeding, nighttime breastfeeding, short intervals between breastfeedings, and duration of feeds; the average time to menses for women following these practices is around 14 months (Kippley, 1987; Kippley et al., 1972).
      i. The return of menses in a breastfeeding mother occurs at 3 months for 9% to 30% of mothers, and at 6 months for 19% to 53% of mothers.
      ii. Some women do not resume their cycles until after weaning has occurred.
   b. Some women experience scanty show before their true cycles resume.
   c. The menstrual cycle absence can be followed by anovulatory cycles (absent egg release).

    d. Menstruation causes no significant changes in the composition of the mother's milk but may change the taste of her milk and cause the baby to be fussy or refuse to nurse.

  2. Suppression of ovulation is associated with levels of growth hormone, luteinizing hormone, follicle-stimulating hormone, and estrogen (McNeilly, 1993).

  3. Lactation can delay the return of fertility during the postpartum period (Radwan et al., 2009; Subhani et al., 2008; Aryal, 2006).

  4. The most important factor in suppression of ovulation during lactation is the early establishment of frequent and strong suckling by the baby (Academy of Breastfeeding Medicine Protocol Committee [ABM], 2006; McNeilly, 1993; Tay et al., 1996).

  5. Factors in the length of amenorrhea and infertility include the following:

    a. Breastfeeding frequency and short intervals between feedings (Gray et al., 1993)

    b. Duration of feedings (Diaz et al., 1991; Gellen, 1992; McNeilly et al., 1994; Vestermark et al., 1994)

    c. Nighttime feedings (Vestermark et al., 1994)

    d. Absence of supplemental foods in the baby's diet (Diaz et al., 1992)

  6. Women can become pregnant while they are breastfeeding and have a number of family planning options.

VI. Contraception

  A. Natural family planning methods rely on fertility awareness to prevent or space pregnancies. These methods include calendar, basal body temperature, cervical mucus, and symptothermal.

  B. Lactational amenorrhea method (LAM) offers pregnancy protection during the first 6 months postpartum (Kennedy et al., 1998; Labbok et al., 1997).

    1. Only 1.5% of unintended pregnancies occur when all three prerequisites of LAM are present (Shaaban et al., 2008).

      a. The mother's menses have not yet returned.

      b. The baby is breastfed around the clock and receives no other foods or pacifiers.

      c. The baby is younger than 6 months of age.

    2. If any one of these conditions is not met, backup contraception is needed.

    3. In one study, more than 61% of breastfeeding mothers with unintended pregnancies failed to use contraception because they believed breastfeeding would prevent pregnancy (Tilley et al., 2009).

  C. Hormonal contraceptives (Academy of Breastfeeding Medicine [ABM], 2006)

    1. Generally, breastfeeding women should use nonestrogen contraceptive methods.

      a. Those that contain both estrogen and progesterone appear to cause the most difficulty in lactating women, especially in the early postpartum period before lactation is well established.

      b. Estrogen can lower milk production and can pass into the milk (Kelsey, 1996; Koetsawang, 1987; World Health Organization [WHO], 2004).

2. Oral contraceptives have been in use for more than 40 years. Two types are on the market today: a combined estrogen/progestin pill and a progestin-only formulation.
   a. Breastfeeding women usually use the progestin-only pill in the early phase of breastfeeding (the first 6 months).
   b. Progestin-only oral contraceptives do not appear to interfere with milk production, and therefore are acceptable during lactation (Bjarnadottir et al., 2001; Dunson et al., 1993; Kelsey, 1996; Speroff, 1992–1993). However, mothers should delay use of progesterone injectables until lactation is well established (Academy of Breastfeeding Medicine Protocol Committee, 2006).
3. Intrauterine devices (IUDs) prevent a fertilized egg from implanting (Williams, 2003).
   a. The nonhormonal IUD does not seem to have any effect on lactation (Koetsawang, 1987).
   b. The progesterone-releasing IUD has been associated with a slight decrease in milk volume (Kelsey, 1996).
   c. Women are at a higher risk of expulsion of the IUD during the early breastfeeding period because of the uterine contractions caused by suckling.
4. The vaginal ring is a hormone-releasing ring a woman can self-insert. Effectiveness, milk production, and infant growth with a progesterone-releasing ring are similar to those of IUD use (Sivin et al., 1997).
5. An etonogestrel implant (Implanon) is a flexible, plastic progestin implant that is inserted surgically under the skin of the upper arm.
   a. It slowly releases progesterone for up to 3 years.
   b. Some women continue to ovulate and some discontinue because of unpleasant side effects.
6. Depo-Provera is a progestin injection given every 3 months, with infertility lasting up to 1 year.
   a. When administered immediately postpartum, an impaired milk supply may result, though one clinical study showed no impact on lactation (Danli et al., 2000).
   b. Mothers should delay use of Depo-Provera for 6 weeks until lactation is well established.
7. The "patch" delivers estrogen and progesterone through the skin into the bloodstream and is about as effective as combination oral contraceptives.
8. Spermicidals prevent pregnancy by destroying sperm before it can reach and fertilize an egg. Vaginal spermicides are 69% to 89% effective and are used after the cervix has closed. There are no side effects or contraindications while breastfeeding.

D. Barrier methods
  1. Condoms have about a 14% failure rate (Williams, 2003).
     a. A male condom is a thin latex or silicone sheath that covers the male penis. The male condom combined with spermicidal foam is an effective contraceptive.
     b. A female condom is a thin polyurethane sheath with soft rings that fit over the cervix and part of the perineum and labia during intercourse. The female condom does not require fitting by a healthcare professional.
  2. A diaphragm must be refitted after each pregnancy.
  3. A cervical cap is placed over the cervix.
E. Sterilization
  1. Bilateral tubal ligation ties the fallopian tubes in the woman. There is no evidence that it hampers milk production.
  2. Vasectomy severs the vas deferens in the man, the main duct through which sperm travel during ejaculation.

VII. Siblings and Breastfeeding

A. Each child needs time and understanding to prepare for and adjust to the arrival of a new sibling. Planning time each day where the mother's total attention is devoted to the older sibling helps the adjustment.
B. Tandem nursing (breastfeeding of two or more children of different ages)
  1. The new baby takes precedence over the toddler, with access to both breasts before the toddler nurses.
  2. If a mother wishes to wean the older sibling, she can wean in a gradual manner by substituting activities for nursings, and feeding the new baby when the older child is either not present or is occupied with other things.
  3. Some mothers reserve time each day for the older sibling to nurse to provide special time together.
C. Accommodating a sibling during feedings
  1. Mothers can nurse where there is ample room to read a book or play simple games. Using the football hold frees the mother's hand for cuddling the older child.
  2. A child who has previously weaned might show renewed interest in breastfeeding when he or she sees the new baby at the breast. This renewed interest in breastfeeding is usually temporary. The sibling may simply be curious about the taste of the milk, so expressing some into a cup may satisfy this curiosity.

VIII. Family Lifestyle

A. The mother's ability to adapt her lifestyle to motherhood depends on her emotional well-being, her physical recovery, her maturity, and the support she receives from family and friends.
B. Women in the United States with unwanted pregnancies are less likely to initiate or continue breastfeeding than are women with intended pregnancies (Taylor et al., 2002).

C. Single mothers
1. In the United States, 34% of births in 2002 were to unmarried women (Centers for Disease Control and Prevention [CDC], 2003).
2. A woman may have sole responsibility of her baby because of a choice to remain single, separation or divorce, the death of the spouse, or a situation that requires the baby's father to be away from home for extended periods.
   a. She may live alone, with a partner or roommate, or with family members.
   b. She may have multiple responsibilities of work, school, household chores, and parenting.
   c. She may have little privacy or support for what she is doing.
   d. Emotional stress and demands for dealing with divorce, separation, or loss of a spouse may result in missed feedings and lowered milk production.
   e. Single mothers who are divorced or in the process of divorcing may have custody or visitation issues that affect separations and breastfeeding.
3. The lactation consultant's role is to be familiar with community resources for single mothers and to find ways to meet the mother's and baby's needs while preserving breastfeeding.
D. Adolescent mothers
1. Many pregnant teenagers elect to keep their babies, and about 17% go on to have a second child within 3 years (Ventura et al., 2001).
2. Teens have a higher incidence of preterm, low-birth-weight infants, stillbirths, and neonatal death than do postadolescent mothers (March of Dimes/National Foundation, 2002).
3. Adolescents are physically and psychologically capable of breastfeeding.
4. Breastfeeding rates are lower for teen mothers than for adults, partly because of lack of knowledge (Dewan et al., 2002).
   a. They typically choose to breastfeed because it is good for the baby and because of the closeness of the relationship.
   b. Some choose to breastfeed because it gives them some control over the situation.
   c. Those who have a dependent relationship with their mothers are less likely to breastfeed.
5. Teens who are the most likely to breastfeed
   a. Older teens who are exposed to other breastfeeding mothers and/or prenatal breastfeeding education
   b. Older teens who are married and no longer in school during their pregnancy (Lizarraga et al., 1992)
   c. Teens who see other women breastfeed and who were breastfed as babies (Leffler, 2000)
6. Adolescent mothers want to be treated as adults.
   a. They respond poorly to lecturing, advice-giving, mandates, and patronizing discussions or actions.

     b. They respond best to sincere, consistent, and honest support.

     c. They respond best to interactive learning and the right to refuse to participate if they feel threatened.

     d. They learn best in an environment that is nonjudgmental, fun, and supportive of their decisions.

  7. An adolescent mother faces unique challenges.

     a. Poor nutrition and inadequate prenatal care

     b. A mother who opposes breastfeeding or creates a power struggle

     c. Difficulty seeing beyond her own needs

     d. Unresolved issues about her sexuality and concerns about modesty

     e. Resentment toward the baby and parenting because they interfere with her social life

     f. The need to return to school within as little as 2 weeks after delivery and to plan breastfeeding or milk expression around breaks and classes

  8. Adolescent mothers need a strong information and support system.

     a. An adolescent mother needs a trusting relationship with her mother, grandmother, partner, or pregnancy coordinator (Dykes et al., 2003).

     b. Other family members, especially the teen's mother, might need information about breastfeeding and can be provided with ideas for supporting it.

     c. Peer counselors are a valuable addition to the support for teen mothers.

     d. One prenatal program resulted in 97.6% wanting to breastfeed and 82.8% breastfeeding at discharge (Greenwood et al., 2002).

     e. Staff in the hospital can encourage adolescent mothers to room-in with their baby, invite interaction between the mother and baby, and treat the mother in an adult manner, giving options and including her in decision making.

     f. Teachers may need help in understanding that breastfeeding is not being used as an excuse to miss classes.

E. Co-sleeping

  1. *Co-sleeping* refers to the infant sleeping in close social and/or physical contact with a committed caregiver.

     a. Parent–child co-sleeping provides physical protection for the infant against cold and extends the duration of breastfeeding (McKenna, 1986; McKenna et al., 1993).

     b. Parents should be educated about risks and benefits of co-sleeping and unsafe co-sleeping practices and make their own informed decision (Academy of Breastfeeding Medicine Protocol Committee, 2006).

     c. The American Academy of Pediatrics (AAP) recommends that mothers and infants sleep in proximity to each other to facilitate breastfeeding (American Academy of Pediatrics Task Force on Sudden Infant Death Syndrome [AAP], 2005; Blair et al., 1999).

  2. *Bedsharing* refers to the infant sharing a bed with a committed caregiver.

     a. Bedsharing is controversial because of concern for the baby's safety (AAP, 2005).

  b. Bedsharing between parents and their babies is widely practiced (McCoy et al., 2004; Willinger et al., 2003). The baby should not share a bed with anyone other than a parent.

  c. Parents need to know safe bedsharing practices (Jenni et al., 2005; McKenna et al., 2005).

  d. Smothering is strongly linked to alcohol and drug use by bed partners.

  e. No research has yet shown a risk to the baby from a sober, nonsmoking, breastfeeding mother on a safe surface.

  f. Recommendations about bedsharing are different for the sober, nonsmoking, breastfeeding mother on a safe surface with her infant (see Sections E4 to E6).

3. Bedsharing may have potential health benefits for babies.

  a. Incidence of sudden infant death syndrome is decreasing at the same time as bedsharing is increasing (Arnestad et al., 2001).

  b. Increased sensory contact and close proximity with the mother have potential for behavioral and physiologic changes in the infant (Ball, 2003).

  c. Bedsharing breastfeeding mothers have heightened sensitivity and responsivity to their infants.

  d. Bedsharing breastfeeding mothers and infants have increased interactions and arousals, face-to-face body orientations, increased breastfeeding, increased heart rate, increased infant body temperatures, increased movements and awakenings, and less deep sleep (Goto et al., 1999).

4. Bedsharing safely requires a safe environment (Blair et al., 1999; Fleming et al., 1996; Hauck et al., 2003; Kemp et al., 2000; Nakamura et al., 1999).

5. Potentially unsafe practices related to bedsharing/co-sleeping (ABM, 2006; AAP, 2005) include the following:

  a. Environmental smoke exposure and maternal smoking

  b. Sharing sofas, couches, or daybeds with infants

  c. Sharing waterbeds or the use of soft bedding materials

  d. Sharing beds with adjacent spaces that could trap an infant

  e. Placement of the infant in the adult bed in the prone or side position

  f. The use of alcohol or mind-altering drugs by the adult(s) who is bedsharing

6. Safe sleep environments (ABM, 2006; AAP, 2005)

  a. Place babies in the supine position for sleep.

  b. Use a firm, flat surface and avoid waterbeds, couches, sofas, pillows, soft materials, or loose bedding.

  c. Use only a thin blanket to cover the infant.

  d. Ensure that the head will not be covered. In a cold room, the infant could be kept in an infant sleeper to maintain warmth.

  e. Avoid the use of quilts, duvets, comforters, pillows, and stuffed animals in the infant's sleep environment.

  f. Never put an infant down to sleep on a pillow or adjacent to a pillow.

  g. Never leave an infant alone on an adult bed.

h. Ensure that there are no spaces between the mattress and headboard, walls, and other surfaces, which may entrap the infant and lead to suffocation. Placement of a firm mattress directly on the floor away from walls may be a safe alternative.

IX. Support Systems for Mothers

A. Mothers who have a strong support system for breastfeeding have better outcomes (Ekstrom et al., 2003; Rose et al., 2004; Sikorski et al., 2003).

1. There is a correlation between low parental confidence and a high perception of milk insufficiency (McCarter-Spaulding et al., 2001).
2. Enhancing a mother's self-efficacy and increasing her confidence in her ability to breastfeed help her persevere if she encounters difficulties (Blythe et al., 2002).
3. A mother's self-esteem increases with a positive breastfeeding experience (Locklin et al., 1993).
4. Interventions need to shift from education to enhancing the mother's confidence regarding breastfeeding (Ertem et al., 2001).

B. Mother-to-mother support groups are a valuable resource.

1. They reinforce women's traditional patterns of seeking and receiving advice from relatives and friends.
2. They educate women about options and help them make informed choices.
3. Open communication and cooperation with the medical community and breastfeeding professionals empower mothers to make informed decisions.
4. They provide anticipatory guidance to help mothers learn what to expect, avoid potential problems, and resolve issues before they become obstacles.

C. Opposition to breastfeeding often manifests as subtle undermining of the mother's efforts.

1. Questions and comments that prompt mothers to explain and defend their decision to breastfeed can undermine a mother's confidence and cause her to doubt her decision or her capability to breastfeed.
   a. A mother who is confident about her decision to breastfeed is less likely to yield to the opinions or rude remarks of a stranger.
   b. Objections from people close to the mother are more difficult to cope with.
   c. Developing friendships and relationships with people who are supportive of breastfeeding or who are breastfeeding mothers themselves may help her become more confident with breastfeeding (Dykes et al., 2003).
2. Employers who have had previous experience with breastfeeding employees often react more positively (Dunn et al., 2004).
   a. See Chapter 7, "Breastfeeding and Maternal Employment."
3. Physician lack of support is difficult for a mother. A checklist may help parents determine whether their physician truly supports breastfeeding (Newman et al., 2000).
4. In many cultures, the baby's grandmother has a pivotal role in a mother's breastfeeding experience (Ekstrom et al., 2003).

a. Some grandparents perceive breastfeeding as contributing to lack of sleep and a crying baby.
b. Many health and breastfeeding organizations have information geared directly to grandparents (Texas Department of Health, Bureau of Nutrition Services, 2002).

5. Opposition from the baby's father is especially difficult.

a. A father's opposition weighs greatly on the decision to initiate or continue breastfeeding (Chang et al., 2003; Kong et al., 2004; Rose et al., 2004).
b. As a man's role changes from mate to father, it may be difficult for him to regard the woman's breasts as something other than sexual.
c. Opposition may stem from concern for the well-being of the mother and baby; educating the father can address misconceptions.
d. Networking with families of older nursing babies and children enables the father to meet other breastfeeding families and find the practice more acceptable.
e. Lactation consultants must avoid placing themselves in the middle of a conflict between a mother and an unsupportive partner. If you suspect domestic violence, provide hotline numbers and local community resources and report the suspected abuse to legal authorities.

References

Academy of Breastfeeding Medicine Protocol Committee. (2006). ABM clinical protocol #13: Contraception during breastfeeding. *Breastfeeding Medicine, 1*(1), 43–51. Retrieved from http://www.bfmed.org/Media/Files/Protocols/Protocol_13.pdf

Academy of Breastfeeding Medicine Protocol Committee. (2008). ABM clinical protocol #6: Guideline on co-sleeping and breastfeeding. *Breastfeeding Medicine, 3*(1), 38–43. Retrieved from http://www.bfmed.org/Media/Files/Protocols/Protocol_6.pdf

Ainsworth, M. D. S., Blehar, M. C., Waters, E., & Wall, S. (1978). *Patterns of attachment—psychological study of the strange situation.* Hillsdale, NJ: Lawrence Erlbaum.

American Academy of Pediatrics Task Force on Sudden Infant Death Syndrome. (2005, November). The changing concept of sudden infant death syndrome: Diagnostic coding shifts, controversies regarding sleeping environment, and new variables to consider in reducing risk. *Pediatrics, 116*(5), 1245–1255.

Aney, M. (1998). Babywise linked to dehydration, failure to thrive. *AAP News, 14*(4), 21.

Arnestad, A. M., Andersen, A., Vege, Å., & Rognum, T. O. (2001). Changes in the epidemiological pattern of sudden infant death syndrome in southeast Norway, 1984–1998: Implications for future prevention and research. *Archives of Disease in Childhood, 85,* 108–115.

Ball, H. L. (2003). Breastfeeding, bed-sharing and infant sleep. *Birth, 30,* 181–188.

Barett, H. (2006). Parents and children: Facts and fallacies about attachment theory. *Journal of Family Health Care, 16*(1), 3-4.

Bar-Yam, N. B., & Darby, L. (1997). Fathers and breastfeeding: A review of the literature. *Journal of Human Lactation, 13,* 45–50.

Bjarnadottir, R., Gottfredsdottir, H., Siqurdardottir, K., et al. (2001). Comparative study of the effects of a progestogen-only pill containing desogestrel and an intrauterine contraceptive device in lactating women. *BJOG, 108,* 1174–1180.

Blair, P.S., Fleming, P. J., Smith, I. J., et al. (1999). Babies sleeping with parents: Case-control study of factors influencing the risk of the sudden infant death syndrome. *British Medical Journal, 319,* 1457–1462.

Blythe, R., Creedy, D., & Dennis, C. (2002). Effect of maternal confidence on breastfeeding duration: An application of breastfeeding self-efficacy theory. *Birth, 29*(4), 278–284.

Bocar, D. L., & Moore, K. (1987). *Acquiring the parental role: A theoretical perspective.* In *Lactation Consultant Series.* Franklin Park, IL: La Leche League International.

Bowlby, J. (1969). *Attachment. Attachment and loss,* vol. 1. New York, NY: Basic Books.

Bridges, C., Frank, D. & Curtin, J. (1997). Employer attitudes toward breastfeeding in the workplace. *Journal of Human Lactation, 13,* 215–219.

Castle, H., Slade P., & Barranco-Wadlow M. (2008). Attitudes to emotional expression, social support and postnatal adjustment in new parents. *Journal of Reproductive and Infant Psychology, 26*(3), 180–194.

Centers for Disease Control and Prevention. (2003). Births: Final data for 2002. *National Vital Statistics Report, 52*(10).

Chang, J. H., & Chan, W. T. (2003). Analysis of factors associated with initiation and duration of breast-feeding: A study in Taitung Taiwan. *Acta Paediatrica Taiwan, 44*(1), 29–34.

Danli, S., Qingxiang, S., & Guowei, S. (2000). A multicentered clinical trial of the long-acting injectable contraceptive Depo Provera in Chinese women. *Contraception, 62,* 15–18.

Deave, T., & Johnson, D. (2008). Transition to parenthood: The needs of parents in pregnancy and early parenthood. *BMC Pregnancy and Childbirth, 8,* 30.

Delahunty, K., McKay, D., & Noseworthy, D. (2007). Prolactin responses to infant cues in men and women: Effects of parental experience and recent infant contact. *Hormones and Behavior, 51*(2), 213–220.

Delight, E., Goodall, J., & Jones, P. W. (1991). What do parents expect antenatally and do babies teach them? *Archives of Disease in Childhood, 66,* 1309–1314.

Dennis, C., & McQueen, K. (2009). The relationship between infant-feeding outcomes and postpartum depression: A qualitative systematic review. *Pediatrics, 123*(4), e736–751.

Dewan, N., Wood, L., Maxwell, S., et al. (2002). Breast-feeding knowledge and attitudes of teenage mothers in Liverpool. *Journal of Human Nutrition and Dietetics, 15,* 33–37.

Diaz, S., Cardenas, H., Brandeis, A., et al. (1991). Early difference in the endocrine profile of long and short lactational amenorrhea. *Journal of Clinical Endocrinology and Metabolism, 72,* 196–201.

Diaz, S., Cardenas, H., Brandeis, A., et al. (1992). Relative contributions of anovulation and luteal phase defect to the reduced pregnancy rate of breastfeeding women. *Fertility and Sterility, 58,* 498–503.

Doucet, S., Dennis, C., & Letourneau, N. (2009). Differentiation and clinical implications of postpartum depression and postpartum psychosis. *Journal of Obstetric, Gynecologic, and Neonatal Nursing, 38*(3), 269–279.

Dunn, B., Zavela K., & Cline A. (2004). Breastfeeding practices in Colorado businesses. *Journal of Human Lactation, 20*(2), 170–177.

Dunson, T. R., McLaurin, V. L., Grubb, G. S., & Rosman, A. W. (1993). A multicenter clinical trial of a progestin-only oral contraceptive in lactating women. *Contraception, 47,* 23–35.

Dykes, F., Moran, V. H., Burt, S., & Edwards, J. (2003). Adolescent mothers and breastfeeding: Experiences and support needs: An exploratory study. *Journal of Human Lactation, 19,* 391–401.

Ekstrom, A., Widstrom, A. M., & Nissen, E. (2003). Breastfeeding support from partners and grandmothers: Perceptions of Swedish women. *Birth, 30,* 261–266.

Erikson, E. H. (1950). *Childhood and society.* New York, NY: W.W. Norton.

Ertem, I., Votto, N., & Leventhal, J. (2001). The timing and predictors of the early termination of breastfeeding. *Pediatrics, 107*(3), 543–548.

Fägerskiöld, A. (2008). A change in life as experienced by first-time fathers. *Scandinavian Journal of Caring Science, 22*(1), 64-71.

Fleming, A., Corter, C., Stallings, J., & Steiner, M. (2002). Testosterone and prolactin are associated with emotional responses to infant cries in new fathers. *Hormones and Behavior, 42*, 399–413.

Fleming, P. J., Blair, P. S., Bacon, C. , et al. (1996). Environment of infants during sleep and risk of the sudden infant death syndrome: Results of 1993–5 case-control study for confidential inquiry into stillbirths and deaths in infancy. *British Medical Journal, 313*, 191–195.

Freed, G., Fraley, J. K., & Schanler, R. J. (1992). Attitudes of expectant fathers regarding breastfeeding. *Pediatrics, 90*, 224–227.

Gamble, D., & Morse, J. (1992). Fathers of breastfed infants: Postponing and types of involvement. *Journal of Obstetric, Gynecologic, and Neonatal Nursing, 22*, 358–365.

Gellen, J. (1992). The feasibility of suppressing ovarian activity following the end of amenorrhea by increasing the frequency of suckling. *International Journal of Gynecology and Obstetrics, 39*, 321–325.

Goto, K., Miririan, M., Adams, M., et al. (1999). More awakenings and heart rate variability during sleep in preterm infants. *Pediatrics, 10*, 603–609.

Graham, M. (1993). Parental sensitivity to infant cues: Similarities and differences between mothers and fathers. *Journal of Pediatric Nursing, 8*, 376–384.

Gray, R., Apelo, R., Campbell, O., et al. (1993). The return of ovarian function during lactation: Results of studies from the US and the Philippines. In R. Gray, H. Leridon, & A. Spira (Eds.), *Biomedical and demographic determinants of reproduction* (pp. 428–445). Oxford, England: Colorado Press.

Greenwood, K., & Littlejohn, P. (2002). Breastfeeding intentions and outcomes of adolescent mothers in the Starting Out program. *Breastfeeding Review, 10*, 19–23.

Hasselmann, M. (2008). Symptoms of postpartum depression and early interruption of exclusive breastfeeding in the first two months of life. *Cadernos de Saúde Pública, 24*(Suppl. 2), S341–352.

Hauck, F. R., Herman, S. M., Donovan, M., et al. (2003). Sleep environment and the risk of sudden infant death syndrome in an urban population: The Chicago Infant Mortality Study. *Pediatrics, 111*, 1207–1214.

Jenni, O., Fuhrer, H., Iglowstein, I., et al. (2005). A longitudinal study of bed sharing and sleep problems among Swiss children in the first 10 years of life. *Pediatrics, 115*(Suppl.), 233–240.

Jolley, S., Elmore, S., & Barnard, K. (2007). Dysregulation of the hypothalamic-pituitary-adrenal axis in postpartum depression. *Biological Research for Nursing, 8*(3), 210–222.

Jordan, P., & Wall, V. (1990). Breastfeeding and fathers: Illuminating the darker side. *Birth, 17*, 210–213.

Kaplan, P., Sliter, J., & Burgess, A. (2007). Infant-directed speech produced by fathers with symptoms of depression: Effects on infant associative learning in a conditioned-attention paradigm. *Infant Behavior and Development, 30*(4), 535–545.

Kelsey, J. (1996). Hormonal contraception and lactation. *Journal of Human Lactation, 12*, 315–318.

Kemp, J. S., Unger, B., Wilkins, D., et al. (2000). Unsafe sleep practices and an analysis of bedsharing among infants dying suddenly and unexpectedly: Results of a four-year, population-based, death-scene investigation study of sudden infant death syndrome and related deaths. *Pediatrics, 106*, 341–349.

Kendall-Tackett, K. (2005). *The hidden feelings of motherhood: Coping with stress, depression and burnout* (2nd ed.). Amarillo, TX: Pharmasoft Publishing.

Kennedy, K. I., Kotelchuck, M., Visness, C. M., et al. (1998). Users' understanding of the lactational amenorrhea method and the occurrence of pregnancy. *Journal of Human Lactation, 14*, 209–218.

Kippley, S. (1986). Breastfeeding survey results similar to 1971 study. *CCL News, 13*, 10.

Kippley, S. (1987). Breastfeeding survey results similar to 1971 study. *CCL News, 13*, 5.

Kippley, S., & Kippley, J. F. (1972). The relation between breastfeeding and amenorrhea. *Journal of Obstetric, Gynecologic, and Neonatal Nursing, 1*, 15–21.

Klaus, M. H., & Kennell, J. H. (1982). *Parent–infant bonding* (2nd ed.). St. Louis, MO: Mosby.

Koetsawang, S. (1987). The effects of contraceptive methods on the quality and quantity of breast milk. *International Journal of Gynaecology and Obstetrics, 25*(Suppl.), 115–127.

Kong, S., & Lee, D. (2004). Factors influencing decision to breastfeed. *Journal of Advanced Nursing, 46*(4), 369–379.

Labbok, M. H., Hight Laukaran, V., Peterson, A. E., et al. (1997). Multicentre study of the lactational amenorrhea method (LAM). I. Efficacy, duration and implications for clinical application. *Contraception, 55*, 327–336.

Lawrence, E., Nylen, K. & Cobb, R. (2007). Prenatal expectations and marital satisfaction over the transition to parenthood. *Journal of Family Psychology, 21*(2), 155–164.

Leffler, D. (2000). U.S. high school age girls may be receptive to breastfeeding promotion. *Journal of Human Lactation, 16*, 36–40.

Lizarraga, J., Maehr, J., & Wingard, D. (1992). Psychosocial and economic factors associated with infant feeding intentions of adolescent mothers. *Journal of Adolescent Health, 13*, 676–681.

Locklin, M., & Naber, S. (1993). Does breastfeeding empower women? Insights from a select group of educated, low-income, minority women. *Birth, 20*, 30–35.

March of Dimes/National Foundation. (2002). *Facts you should know about teen pregnancy.* White Plains, NY: March of Dimes.

Marshall, J. L., Godfrey, M., & Renfrew, M. J. (2007). Being a "good mother": Managing breastfeeding and merging identities. *Social Science and Medicine, 65*(10), 2147–2159.

McCarter-Spaulding, D., & Kerarney, M. (2001). Parenting self-efficacy and perception of insufficient breast milk. *Journal of Obstetric, Gynecologic, and Neonatal Nursing, 30*(5), 515–522.

McCoy, R. C., Corwin, M. J., Willinger, M., et al. (2004). Frequency of bed sharing and its relationship to breastfeeding. *Journal of Deviant Behavior in Pediatrics, 25*, 141–149.

McKenna, J. J. (1986). An anthropological perspective on the sudden infant death syndrome (SIDS): The role of parental breathing cues and speech breathing adaptations. *Medical Anthropology, 10*, 9–92.

McKenna, J. J., & McDade, T. (2005). Why babies should never sleep alone: A review of the co-sleeping controversy in relation to SIDS, bedsharing and breast feeding. *Paediatric Respiratory Reviews, 6*, 134–152.

McKenna, J. J., Thoman, E. B., Anders, T. F., et al. (1993). Infant–parent co-sleeping in an evolutionary perspective: Implications for understanding infant sleep development and the sudden infant death syndrome. *Sleep, 16*, 263–282.

McNeilly, A. (1993). Lactational amenorrhea. *Endocrinology Metabolism Clinics of North America, 22*, 59–73.

McNeilly, A., Tay, C. C., & Glasier, A. (1994). Physiological mechanisms underlying lactational amenorrhea. *Annals of the New York Academy of Science, 709*, 145–155.

Moody, L. (2002). Case studies of moms who had problems using Babywise or Preparation for Parenting. Retrieved from www.angelfire.com/md2/moodyfamily/casestudies.html

Nakamura, S., Wond, M., & Danello, M. A. (1999). Review of the hazards associated with children placed in adult beds. *Archives of Pediatric Adolescent Medicine, 153*, 1019–1023.

Newman, J., & Pitman, T. (2000). *The ultimate breastfeeding book of answers.* Roseville, CA: Prima Pub.

O'Brien, M. L., Buikstra, E., & Fallon, T. (2009). Strategies for success: A toolbox of coping strategies used by breastfeeding women. *Journal of Clinical Nursing, 18*(11), 1574–1582.

Otsuka, K., Dennis, C., & Tatsuoka, H. (2008). The relationship between breastfeeding self-efficacy and perceived insufficient milk among Japanese mothers. *Journal of Obstetric, Gynecologic, and Neonatal Nursing, 37*(5), 546–555.

Paulson, J. F., Dauber, S. & Leiferman, J. A. (2006). Individual and combined effects of postpartum depression in mothers and fathers on parenting behavior. *Pediatrics, 118*, 659–668.

Plantin, L., & Daneback, K. (2009). Parenthood, information and support on the Internet. A literature review of research on parents and professionals online. *BMC Family Practice, 10*, 34.

Premberg, A., Hellström, A. & Berg, M. (2008). Experiences of the first year as father. *Scandinavian Journal of Caring Science, 22*(1), 56–63.

Radwan, H., Mussaiger, A. & Hachem, F. (2009). Breast-feeding and lactational amenorrhea in the United Arab Emirates. *Journal of Pediatric Nursing, 24*(1), 62–68.

Randall, A., & Bodenmann, G. (2009). The role of stress on close relationships and marital satisfaction. *Clinical Psychology Review, 29*(2), 105–115.

Rose, V., Warrington, V., & Linder, R. (2004). Factors influencing infant feeding method in an urban community. *Journal of the National Medical Association, 96*(3), 325–331.

Rubin, R. (1967a). Attainment of the maternal role: Part 1, Processes. *Nursing Research, 16*, 237–245.

Rubin, R. (1967b). Attainment of the maternal role. Part II, Models and referents. *Nursing Research, 16*, 342–346.

Schulz, M., Cowan, C., & Cowan, P. (2006). Promoting healthy beginnings: A randomized controlled trial of a preventive intervention to preserve marital quality during the transition to parenthood. *Journal of Consulting and Clinical Psychology, 74*(1), 20–31.

Sears, W., & Gotsch, G. (2003). *Becoming a father* (2nd ed.). Schaumburg, IL: La Leche League International.

Shaaban, O., & Glasier, A. (2008). Pregnancy during breastfeeding in rural Egypt. *Contraception, 77*(5), 350–354.

Sikorski, J., Renfrew, M. J., Pindoria, S., & Wade, A. (2003). Support for breastfeeding mothers: A systematic review. *Paediatric and Perinatal Epidemiology, 17*, 407–417.

Sivin, I., Diaz, S., Croxatto, H. B., et al. (1997). Contraceptives for lactating women: A comparative trial of a progesterone-releasing vaginal ring and the copper T 380A IUD. *Contraception, 55*, 225–232.

Speroff, L. (1992–1993). Postpartum contraception: Issues and choices. *Dialogues in Contraception, 3*, 1–3, 67.

Subhani, A., Gill, G., & Islam, A. (2008). Duration of lactational amenorrhoea: A hospital based survey in district Abbottabad. *Journal of Ayub Medical College Abbottabad, 20*(1), 122–124.

Tay, C., Glasier, A. F., & McNeilly, A. S. (1996). Twenty-four hour patterns of prolactin secretion during lactation and the relationship to suckling and the resumption of fertility in breast-feeding women. *Human Reproduction, 11*, 950–955.

Taylor, J., & Cabral, H. (2002). Are women with an unintended pregnancy less likely to breastfeed? *Journal of Family Practice, 51*(5), 431–436.

Texas Department of Health, Bureau of Nutrition Services. (2002). *Just for grandparents.* No. 13-06-11288. Austin, TX: Author.

Tilley, I., et al. (2009). Breastfeeding and contraception use among women with unplanned pregnancies less than 2 years after delivery. *International Journal of Gynaecology and Obstetrics*, *105*(2), 127–130.

Valdimarsdóttir, U., Hultman, C., & Harlow, B. (2009). Psychotic illness in first-time mothers with no previous psychiatric hospitalizations: A population-based study. *PLoS Medicine*, *6*(2), e13.

Ventura, S. J., Mathews, T. J., & Hamilton, B. E. (2001, September 25). Births to teenagers in the United States, 1940–2000. *National Vital Statistics Reports, 49*(10), 1–24. Retrieved from http://www.cdc.gov/nchs/data/nvsr/nvsr49/nvsr49_10.pdf

Vestermark, V., Hoqdall, C. K., Plenov, G., & Birch, M. (1994). Postpartum amenorrhoea and breastfeeding in a Danish sample. *Journal of Biosocial Science, 26*, 1–7.

Webb, C. (2003, July). Is the Babywise method right for you? What you should know about Babywise and Growing Kids God's Way. http://www.tulsakids.com.

Williams, M. (2003, August 1). *Epigee birth control guide*. Retrieved from http://www.epigee.org/guide/birth_control_guide.html

Williams, N. (1998). Counseling challenges: Helping mothers handle conflicting information. *Leaven, 34*(2), 19–20.

Williams, N. (1999, July 5). *Dancing with differences: Helping mothers handle conflicting information, including scheduled feeding and sleep training*. Presented at the La Leche League International 1999 Conference, Orlando, FL.

Willinger, M., et al. (2003). Trends in infant bed sharing in the United States, 1993–2000. *Archives of Pediatric and Adolescent Medicine, 157*, 43–49.

World Health Organization. (2004). *Medical eligibility criteria for contraceptive use* (3rd ed.). Geneva, Switzerland: Author.

CHAPTER 5
Normal Infant Behavior

M. Jane Heinig, PhD, IBCLC; Jennifer Goldbronn, MAS, RD; and Jennifer Bañuelos, MAS

OBJECTIVES

- Explain how infant behavior may influence infant-feeding practices.
- Describe the six infant states.
- Differentiate infant cues.
- List reasons why infants may cry.
- Describe infant sleep patterns.

INTRODUCTION

In many areas of the world, the majority of women initiate breastfeeding, but duration and exclusivity remain low (Agboado et al., 2010; Al-Hreashy et al., 2008; Antoniou et al., 2005; Butler et al., 2004; Cattaneo et al., 2005; Chalmers et al., 2009; Chan et al., 2000; Cramton et al., 2009; Dashti et al., 2010; Gartner et al., 2005; Gill, 2009; Hauck et al., 2011; Lanting et al., 2005; Ryan et al., 2002; Ryan et al., 2006; Walker, 2007). Although many factors influence women's infant-feeding decisions, perceived insufficient milk is reported to be one of the most common reasons for supplementing or weaning healthy breastfed infants (Bunik et al., 2010; Colin et al., 2002; Gatti, 2008; Lewallen et al., 2006; Sacco et al., 2006). Despite education about clinical indicators of sufficient milk supply, mothers of healthy, thriving infants may be convinced that their infants are not satisfied by breastmilk alone because of their infants' behaviors (such as crying and waking) (Donath et al., 2005; Grummer-Strawn et al., 2008; Heinig et al., 2006; Jacknowitz et al., 2007). Given how frequently women report that their infants are not satisfied by their breastmilk (Baeck et al., 2007; Black et al., 2001; Gross et al., 2010; Hiscock, 2006; Hodges et al., 2008), lactation consultants can be better prepared to promote and support exclusive breastfeeding if they are familiar with normal infant behavior. Lactation consultants can use education about normal baby behavior to help parents develop realistic expectations about parenting of newborns and prevent unnecessary weaning.

I. The Six Infant Behavioral "States"

An infant state is indicated by a group of behaviors that occur together, including degree and nature of body movement, eye movement, respirations, and responsiveness (Nugent et al., 2007). Understanding infants' states and how and why they move through these states can help lactation consultants to engage parents who are seeking answers to questions about their infants' behavior and development.

A. There are six defined infant behavioral states.

1. *Crying infants* have jerky movements, facial color changes, muscle tension, and rapid breathing. Newborns do not shed tears; infants' tear ducts typically are blocked until infants are between 2 and 4 months of age. Crying infants initially may be unresponsive to caregiver efforts to calm them. Caregivers need to be reassured that calming crying infants takes time (Hiscock, 2006).

2. Infants in an *active alert* state have moderate to frequent body and facial movements, irregular breathing, and open eyes. They are sometimes fussy and sensitive to stimuli in the environment. The active alert state is common before feeding (Nugent et al., 2007).

3. Infants in a *quiet alert* state have little body movement; their eyes are open and they have steady, regular breathing. Infants in quiet alert are highly responsive and this is the best state for interaction and play with caregivers. Maintenance of this state is challenging for young infants and, consequently, they may tire quickly (Nugent et al., 2007).

4. *Drowsy infants* have variable body movement, irregular breathing, glazed eyes, and delayed reaction time. They may open and close their eyes. Typically, drowsy infants have limited interest in interaction (Nugent et al., 2007).

5. *Active sleep* is characterized by rapid eye movement, body and facial twitches, and irregular breathing. Infants dream during active sleep, and while dreaming, they are easily awakened (Peirano et al., 2003).

6. *Quiet sleep* results in very little body or facial movement except occasional bursts of sucking. Infants in quiet sleep may startle with movement or loud noises but typically do not wake. Respirations are regular and the baby's body is relaxed. Infants in deep sleep may be difficult to wake (Peirano et al., 2003).

B. Infants gain increasing ability to regulate their behavioral states over the first few months of life.

1. Newborns are challenged by a limited ability to shut out environmental stimuli (called habituation). Although some infants are born with more capacity to self-regulate their states, young infants' states are less predictable than those of older infants (Barnard, 2010).

2. As soon as they are able, infants may use a variety of self-soothing behaviors including bringing their hands to mouths, sucking, and providing cues to caregivers. However, the fact that infants attempt to console themselves does not imply that the infants should be left to cry. Rather, parents should allow infants' efforts to self-soothe but step in quickly with consoling behaviors as soon as it is clear that the baby's self-soothing behaviors are not effective (Barnard, 2010).

3. Caregiver actions can assist infants' efforts to regulate and change behavioral states (Barnard, 2010).

    a. Infants will wake up when exposed to a variety of stimuli. Termed "variety to waken" by Barnard, parents can be taught to use different positions, touch, or sounds to awaken a sleepy infant. This process can take a significant amount of time in a very sleepy baby, particularly those who are sleepy as a result of stress during birth or exposure to medications.

    b. Alternatively, infants who are overstimulated or distressed respond well to sustained, low-level, repetitive stimulation. Termed "repetition to soothe" by Barnard, interventions such as stroking, rocking, or speaking softly to infants using the same repeated words or phrases may be used to calm infants. It may take several minutes to calm a crying infant who is very upset or very young.

II. Infant Communication

A. Infants use simple cues to communicate their needs to caregivers.

1. Infants use "engagement cues" to communicate their desire to interact, play, or feed. Examples of these cues include open eyes; looking intently at the caregiver's face; following objects, voices, and faces with their eyes; relaxed face; smooth body movements; smiling; and feeding cues (White et al., 2002).

2. Infants use "disengagement cues" to communicate when they want a change in activity, circumstances, or environment. For example, infants often give disengagement cues such as turning or arching away when they are overwhelmed by an interaction. Other examples of disengagement cues include pushing away, crying, stiff hands and arms, grimacing, yawning, or falling asleep (White et al., 2002).

3. Infants use multiple cues at the same time to indicate important needs such as hunger or satiation.

    a. When an infant is hungry he may clench his fingers and fists over his chest and tummy, flex his arms and legs, show mouthing or rooting, quicken his breathing, and make sucking noises and motions (Rochat et al., 1997).

    b. When a healthy thriving infant is full, he may extend his arms and legs, turn or push away from the breast, arch his back, slow (decrease) or stop sucking, or fall asleep (Pridham et al., 1989). If these behaviors are seen early in a feed or in an infant who is gaining poorly, further evaluation of milk transfer is necessary.

4. Infant cues are nonspecific; parents may need to investigate the reasons behind the cues to determine how best to meet the baby's needs. When cues are not addressed promptly, infants may escalate the cue to obtain or redirect caregiver attention (Nugent et al., 2007). For example, overstimulated infants may first turn their faces away from interactions with excited siblings. If the child continues to engage the infant, the infant may "escalate" the cue by twisting away, arching away, or starting to cry.

B. Crying is an important means for infants to communicate their needs.

    1. Crying is a common and normal part of infancy. Infants use crying as a powerful means to communicate their distress (Evanoo, 2007) and to drive caregiver activity (Crockenberg, 1981; Kurth et al., 2010). There is enormous variation in crying behavior from baby to baby and even day to day within babies. Therefore, it is not possible to determine the amount or duration of "normal crying" during infancy (Evanoo, 2007).

    2. Infants cry for many reasons, though caregivers may believe that infants cry predominantly because of hunger (Heinig et al., 2006). This belief may result in weaning from the breast if mothers believe that crying indicates that their infant is "not satisfied" by breastmilk (Jacknowitz et al., 2007).

    3. Infants cry when they are uncomfortable (e.g., if they have a wet or dirty diaper, they are too hot or too cold, need to be burped, or are sick or hungry). They may also cry when they need a change in their environment (e.g., when they are overstimulated by too much noise or too many new faces). Crying infants also may need quiet time, to be close to their parents, or a break from stimulation. If parents respond quickly and effectively to infant cues, crying may be minimized (Barnard, 2010; Evanoo, 2007).

    4. Excessive crying has been referred to as "colic" in the past. However, the classification of crying as "excessive" is highly subjective and related to parents' cultural norms, their own expectations of how infants should behave, and the characteristics of the infant (Evanoo, 2007; Leavitt, 2001). Researchers in the field currently use *persistent* or *problem* crying to describe daily inconsolable crying (Douglas et al., 2010; Hiscock, 2006; Keefe et al., 2006).

    5. Persistent crying occurs in approximately 20% of infants and is rarely associated with an organic cause (Hiscock, 2006). Persistent crying is one of the most frequent reasons why parents seek medical care and, in extreme cases, may be associated with dysfunctional patterns of interactions with caregivers, maternal depression, and child abuse (Evanoo, 2007; Kurth et al., 2010). Although gastrointestinal distress is most often ascribed by caregivers as the cause of persistent crying, objective evidence does not support this association in the majority of cases. Multiple biopsychosocial factors are likely to be involved (Evanoo, 2007).

    6. Repetitive sustained stimuli may be used to reduce crying (Barnard, 2010). When infants continue to cry despite parents' efforts to address the immediate issue (such as a wet diaper or hunger), using "repetition to soothe" such as rocking, singing, or stroking may reduce the infant's level of stimulation and calm the infant (Barnard, 2010). A more extensive intervention called REST (regulation, entrainment, structure, touch) has been associated with reduced daily crying and parental stress during the early infancy period (Keefe et al., 2006). For a chart on REST, go to www.jblearning.com/corecurriculum.

III. Infant Sleep

A. Researchers have described two primary sleep states: active sleep (also called light sleep) and quiet sleep (also called deep sleep).

   1. Active sleep

     a. Dreaming occurs during active sleep, resulting in rapid eye movement beneath infants' eyelids, body and facial twitches, and irregular breathing (Barnard, 2010; Heraghty et al., 2008).

     b. During active sleep, blood flow to the brain is increased and neural cells are stimulated, contributing to brain growth and development (Peirano et al., 2003).

     c. Infants are easily awakened during active sleep periods (Peirano et al., 2003; Rosen, 2008). The ability to awaken easily is considered important for babies' health and safety, given that an inability to rouse may be associated with sudden unexpected infant death (SUID) (American Academy of Pediatrics, 2005).

   2. Quiet sleep

     a. During quiet sleep, infants exhibit little body or facial movement other than short bursts of sucking and startle responses. Their breathing is regular (Heraghty et al., 2008) and they are more difficult to rouse than infants in light sleep (Rosen, 2008).

     b. During quiet sleep, most infants sleep deeply and can resist environmental stimuli. This is a restorative state, important for accruing the energy required for interaction and feeding when the infant awakens (Nugent et al., 2007). Quiet sleep also plays a role in memory development (Graven et al., 2008).

B. Infant Sleep Patterns

   1. Infant sleep cycles differ from those of adults and change as infants get older. More information about the relationship between infant feeding and sleep patterns is presented in a later section.

     a. Adult sleep cycles are 90 minutes in length whereas infant sleep cycles are about 60 minutes long (Heraghty et al., 2008).

     b. Newborns fall asleep into active sleep, and after about 20 to 30 minutes, they cycle into quiet sleep (Peirano et al., 2003). Adults, on the other hand, initially fall asleep into quiet sleep (Coons et al., 1984; Peirano et al., 2003).

     c. Newborns sleep on average 16–17 hours, and older infants about 13–14 hours, per 24-hour period (Rosen, 2008). However, studies show wide variations in total amount of infant sleep. Newborns spend about an equal amount of time in active sleep and quiet sleep, in about 50- to 60-minute cycles (Peirano et al., 2003). Initially, newborns may wake with each cycle, or every 1 to 2 hours.

     d. Sleep patterns change as infants get older. Between 12 and 16 weeks, infants begin sleep in quiet sleep, as adults do, and night waking decreases (Heraghty et al., 2008). Sleep states are more consistent and percentage of total sleep spent in quiet sleep increases from 50% in newborns to 75% at 6 months of age (Heraghty et al., 2008; Hoppenbrouwers et al.,1988; Peirano et al., 2003).

2. Infants' longest stretch of sleep increases with age.
   a. By 2 to 6 weeks of age, infants are able to sleep 2 to 4 hours at one time. At approximately 6 to 8 weeks of age, an infant's sleep becomes more concentrated during the nighttime because he or she is more awake during the day (Coons et al., 1984; Jenni et al., 2006; Peirano et al., 2003).
   b. By 3 months of age, sleep–wake periods consolidate and circadian rhythms follow the light/dark cycle as circadian-driven hormones, such as cortisol and melatonin, become endogenously produced (Jenni et al., 2006; Peirano et al., 2003). Infants are able to sleep about 4 hours at one time, and typically the longest stretch is during the nighttime (Coons et al., 1984; Goodlin-Jones et al., 2001).
   c. By 6 months of age, babies may be capable of sleeping up to 6 hours at one time (Coons & Guilleminault, 1984; Goodlin-Jones et al., 2001). A 2004 study shows that by 6 months, 90% of infants "slept regularly through the night" (defined as sleeping 6 hours without waking but not necessarily every night) (Adams et al., 2004). Sleeping and waking patterns may change again among older infants, but description of these changes is beyond the scope of this chapter.
3. There are several benefits of periodic waking for both infants and their mothers.
   a. Night waking may be essential to infants' health (Horne, Parslow, Ferens, Watts, & Adamson, 2004). An infant's ability to arouse during sleep is important to signal parents that the infant has an unmet need such as hunger, discomfort, or temperature control. As infants get older, they typically require less adult intervention at night as they develop the ability to self-soothe upon awakening (Goodlin-Jones et al., 2001).
   b. Very young infants who have long periods of quiet sleep are at greater risk for SUID, possibly because arousal thresholds increase with time spent in quiet sleep (Horne et al., 2004).
   c. Night waking is also beneficial for mothers. Night waking and night feeds help build and maintain mothers' breastmilk supply, reduce risk of hormone-related cancers (Heinig et al., 1997), and delay menstruation (Heinig et al., 1994).
4. Several factors may influence infants' abilities to maintain sleep states. Infants with unexplained frequent waking should be referred to the appropriate medical professional.
   a. The following infant-related conditions may affect infants' abilities to maintain sleep states.
      i. In infants with physical immaturity, such as prematurity, a lack of brain maturation influences infant sleep states and patterns. Premature infants sleep more total hours than term infants do, but they wake more often and have shorter sustained bouts of sleep. Preterm infants are more likely than term infants to have limited ability to control and maintain active and quiet sleep states (Barnard, 2010; Trachtenbarg et al., 1998).

      ii. Ineffective or poor feeding may result in lower intakes and shorter intervals between feeds. Feeding assessment should be considered when parents report excessive infant waking. Also, infants need to be in an alert state to feed effectively. Lack of alertness during feedings can lead to difficulty with the infants' coordination of sucking, swallowing, and breathing needed to feed effectively (Barnard, 2010).

     iii. Discomfort caused by symptoms of common illness, such as congestion or pain from an ear infection, or minor injuries may cause an infant to wake more often than expected. Sleep disturbance may continue until the illness or injury is resolved (Sadeh et al., 1993; Tirosh et al., 1993).

  b. The following external factors also influence infant sleep states.

     i. The increase in stimulation from having a television on or other interruptions in the room where the infant sleeps may cause increased arousals, especially during active sleep phases. Some infants are more sensitive to lights and sounds. These infants must expend needed energy trying to shut out external stimuli during sleep (Nugent et al., 2007).

     ii. Caffeine intake of breastfeeding mothers can disrupt infant sleep. Transfer of caffeine to breastmilk is low, but caffeine accumulates in the infant because of the infant's limited ability to metabolize it. Six to eight cups of caffeinated beverages per day have been linked to infant hyperactivity and short sleep duration (Lawrence et al., 2010).

C. Effects of feeding on sleep

  1. Studies of the effects of type of feeding on infant sleep show mixed results.

    a. Whether breastfed or formula-fed infants wake more often is controversial and studies have yielded mixed results. Many studies of infant sleep include only small numbers of infants and have inconsistent definitions of "nighttime," which varied in one recent review of the literature from 5 to 12 hours (Rosen, 2008).

     i. Infant feeding may influence the pattern of infants' sleep cycles. Breastfed infants have more active sleep and thus would be more likely to wake up if they were uncomfortable or needed parental assistance. Horne et al. (2004) reported that breastfed infants were more likely to wake in active sleep than formula-fed infants at 2–3 months of age.

     ii. Assessments of sleep duration have yielded mixed results. Doan et al. (2007) reported that mothers who exclusively breastfed slept 45–47 minutes longer at night than those who supplemented with formula. Lee (2000) reported that breastfed infants, between the ages of 2 weeks and 4 months, showed longer total sleep but shorter stretches of sleep than that of formula-fed infants. In addition, formula-fed infants cried more frequently in the evenings and at night, suggesting increased awakenings needing parental assistance (Lee, 2000). Ball (2003) reported awakenings in breastfed infants at 1 and 3 months of age remained consistent whereas formula-fed infants' awakenings dropped at 3 months of age.

iii. Other researchers have reported no significant difference among maternal reports of total infant sleep (Macknin et al., 1989; Quillin, 1997) or night awakenings (Alley et al., 1986; Anders et al., 1992) by feeding method. Furthermore, no difference was found among formula-fed and breastfed infants in "sleep period length" at 2–4 weeks, 2–3 months, and 5–6 months in a study using polysomnography rather than maternal report (Horne et al., 2004).

2. Mothers may assume adding cereal to feedings will increase infant sleep; however, the research does not support this belief.

a. Two-thirds of the mothers (44 breastfeeding and 33 formula-feeding) in a small study thought that adding cereal to their infants' feeding would increase their sleep duration. However, the intervention showed no significant difference in sleep duration, number of night wakings (midnight–5 a.m.), or minutes awake during the nighttime (midnight–5 a.m.) among infants fed rice cereal at night compared to control (no cereal at night) (Keane, 1988).

b. Feeding cereal before bedtime does not increase likelihood of an infant sleeping through the night (Crocetti et al., 2004). Another study indicates that cereal added to bottles of formula or human milk did not influence sleep patterns. At 7 weeks of age, infants not given cereal were actually more likely to sleep 8 hours at night (Macknin et al., 1989).

References

Adams, S. M., Jones, D. R., Esmail, A., & Mitchell, E. A. (2004). What affects the age of first sleeping through the night? *Journal of Paediatrics and Child Health*, *40*, 96–101.

Agboado, G., Michel, E., Jackson, E., & Verma, A. (2010). Factors associated with breastfeeding cessation in nursing mothers in a peer support programme in Eastern Lancashire. *BMC Pediatrics*, *10*, 3.

Al-Hreashy, F. A., Tamim, H. M., Al-Baz, N., Al-Kharji, N. H., Al-Amer, A., Al-Ajmi, H., & Eldemerdash, A. A. (2008). Patterns of breastfeeding practice during the first 6 months of life in Saudi Arabia. *Saudi Medical Journal*, *29*, 427–431.

Alley, J. M., & Rogers, C. S. (1986). Sleep patterns of breast-fed and nonbreast-fed infants. *Pediatric Nursing*, *12*, 349–351.

American Academy of Pediatrics. (2005). The changing concept of sudden infant death syndrome: Diagnostic coding shifts, controversies regarding the sleeping environment, and new variables to consider in reducing risk. *Pediatrics*, *116*, 1245–1255.

Anders, T. F., Halpern, L. F., & Hua, J. (1992). Sleeping through the night: A developmental perspective. *Pediatrics*, *90*, 554–560.

Antoniou, E., Daglas, M., Iatrakis, G., Kourounis, G., & Greatsas, G. (2005). Factors associated with initiation and duration of breastfeeding in Greece. *Clinical and Experimental Obstetrics and Gynecology*, *32*, 37–40.

Baeck, H. E., & de Souza, M. N. (2007). Longitudinal study of the fundamental frequency of hunger cries along the first 6 months of healthy babies. *Journal of Voice*, *21*, 551–559.

Ball, H. L. (2003). Breastfeeding, bed-sharing, and infant sleep. *Birth*, *30*, 181–188.

Barnard, K. E. (2010). Keys to developing early parent–child relationships. In B. M. Lester & J. D. Sparrow (Eds.), *Nurturing children and families* (pp. 53–63). Malden, MA: Blackwell Publishing.

Black, M. M., Siegel, E. H., Abel, Y., & Bentley, M. E. (2001). Home and videotape intervention delays early complementary feeding among adolescent mothers. *Pediatrics, 107,* E67.

Bunik, M., Shobe, P., O'Connor, M. E., Beaty, B., Langendoerfer, S., Crane, L., & Kempe, A. (2010). Are 2 weeks of daily breastfeeding support insufficient to overcome the influences of formula? *Academic Pediatrics, 10,* 21–28.

Butler, S., Williams, M., Tukuitonga, C., & Paterson, J. (2004). Factors associated with not breastfeeding exclusively among mothers of a cohort of Pacific infants in New Zealand. *Journal of the New Zealand Medical Association, 117,* U908.

Cattaneo, A., Yngve, A., Koletzko, B., & Guzman, L. R. (2005). Protection, promotion and support of breast-feeding in Europe: Current situation. *Public Health Nutrition, 8,* 39–46.

Chalmers, B., Levitt, C., Heaman, M., O'Brien, B., Sauve, R., & Kaczorowski, J. (2009). Breastfeeding rates and hospital breastfeeding practices in Canada: A national survey of women. *Birth, 36,* 122–132.

Chan, S. M., Nelson, E. A., Leung, S. S., & Li, C. Y. (2000). Breastfeeding failure in a longitudinal post-partum maternal nutrition study in Hong Kong. *Journal of Paediatrics and Child Health, 36,* 466–471.

Colin, W. B., & Scott, J. A. (2002). Breastfeeding: Reasons for starting, reasons for stopping and problems along the way. *Breastfeeding Review, 10,* 13–19.

Coons, S., & Guilleminault, C. (1984). Development of consolidated sleep and wakeful periods in relation to the day/night cycle in infancy. *Developmental Medicine and Child Neurology, 26,* 169–176.

Cramton, R., Zain-Ul-Abideen, M., & Whalen, B. (2009). Optimizing successful breastfeeding in the newborn. *Current Opinion in Pediatrics, 21,* 386–396.

Crocetti, M., Dudas, R., & Krugman, S. (2004). Parental beliefs and practices regarding early introduction of solid foods to their children. *Clinical Pediatrics (Philadelphia), 43,* 541–547.

Crockenberg, S. B. (1981). Infant irritability, mother responsiveness, and social support influences on the security of infant-mother attachment. *Child Development, 52,* 857–865.

Dashti, M., Scott, J. A., Edwards, C. A., & Al-Sughayer, M. (2010). Determinants of breastfeeding initiation among mothers in Kuwait. *International Breastfeeding Journal, 5,* 7.

Doan, T., Gardiner, A., Gay, C. L., & Lee, K. A. (2007). Breast-feeding increases sleep duration of new parents. *Journal of Perinatal and Neonatal Nursing, 21,* 200–206.

Donath, S. M., & Amir, L. H. (2005). Breastfeeding and the introduction of solids in Australian infants: Data from the 2001 National Health Survey. *Australian and New Zealand Journal of Public Health, 29,* 171–175.

Douglas, P. S., & Hiscock, H. (2010). The unsettled baby: Crying out for an integrated, multidisciplinary primary care approach. *Medical Journal of Australia, 193,* 533–536.

Evanoo, G. (2007). Infant crying: A clinical conundrum. *Journal of Pediatric Health Care, 21,* 333–338.

Gartner, L. M., Morton, J., Lawrence, R. A., Naylor, A. J., O'Hare, D., Schanler, R. J., & Eidelman, A. I. (2005). Breastfeeding and the use of human milk. *Pediatrics, 115,* 496–506.

Gatti, L. (2008). Maternal perceptions of insufficient milk supply in breastfeeding. *Journal of Nursing Scholarship, 40,* 355–363.

Gill, S. L. (2009). Breastfeeding by Hispanic women. *Journal of Obstetric, Gynecologic, and Neonatal Nursing, 38,* 244–252.

Goodlin-Jones, B. L., Burnham, M. M., Gaylor, E. E., & Anders, T. F. (2001). Night waking, sleep-wake organization, and self-soothing in the first year of life. *Journal of Deviant Behavior in Pediatrics, 22*, 226–233.

Graven, S. N., & Browne, J. V. (2008). Sleep and brain development: The critical role of sleep in fetal and early neonatal brain development. *Newborn and Infant Nursing Reviews, 8*, 173–179.

Gross, R. S., Fierman, A. H., Mendelsohn, A. L., Chiasson, M. A., Rosenberg, T. J., Scheinmann, R., & Messito, M. J. (2010). Maternal perceptions of infant hunger, satiety, and pressuring feeding styles in an urban Latina WIC population. *Academic Pediatrics, 10*, 29–35.

Grummer-Strawn, L. M., Scanlon, K. S., & Fein, S. B. (2008). Infant feeding and feeding transitions during the first year of life. *Pediatrics, 122*(Suppl. 2), S36–S42.

Hauck, Y. L., Fenwick, J, Dhaliwal, S. S., & Butt, J. (2011). A Western Australian survey of breastfeeding initiation, prevalence and early cessation patterns. *Maternal and Child Health Journal, 15*, 260–268.

Heinig, M. J., & Dewey, K. G. (1997). Health effects of breast feeding for mothers: A critical review. *Nutrition Research Reviews, 10*, 35–56.

Heinig, M. J., Follett, J. R., Ishii, K. D., Kavanagh-Prochaska, K., Cohen, R., & Panchula, J. (2006). Barriers to compliance with infant-feeding recommendations among low-income women. *Journal of Human Lactation, 22*, 27–38.

Heinig, M. J., Nommsen-Rivers, L. A., Peerson, J. M., & Dewey, K. G. (1994). Factors related to duration of postpartum amenorrhoea among USA women with prolonged lactation. *Journal of Biosocial Science, 26*, 517–527.

Heraghty, J. L., Hilliard, T. N., Henderson, A. J., & Fleming, P. J. (2008). The physiology of sleep in infants. *Archives of Disease in Childhood, 93*, 982–985.

Hiscock, H. (2006). The crying baby. *Australian Family Physician, 35*, 680–684.

Hodges, E. A., Hughes, S. O., Hopkinson, J., & Fisher, J. O. (2008). Maternal decisions about the initiation and termination of infant feeding. *Appetite, 50*, 333–339.

Hoppenbrouwers, T., Hodgman, J., Arakawa, K., Geidel, S. A., & Sterman, M. B. (1998). Sleep and waking states in infancy: Normative studies. *Sleep, 11*, 387–401.

Horne, R. S., Parslow, P. M., Ferens, D., Watts, A. M., & Adamson, T. M. (2004). Comparison of evoked arousability in breast and formula fed infants. *Archives of Disease in Childhood, 89*, 22–25.

Jacknowitz, A., Novillo, D., & Tiehen, L. (2007). Special Supplemental Nutrition Program for Women, Infants, and Children and infant feeding practices. *Pediatrics, 119*, 281–289.

Jenni, O. G., & LeBourgeois, M. K. (2006). Understanding sleep–wake behavior and sleep disorders in children: The value of a model. *Current Opinions in Psychiatry, 19*, 282–287.

Keane, V. (1988). Do solids help baby sleep through the night? *American Journal of Diseases of Children, 142*, 404–405.

Keefe, M. R., Kajrlsen, K. A., Lobo, M. L., Kotzer, A. M., & Dudley, W. N. (2006). Reducing parenting stress in families with irritable infants. *Nursing Research, 55*, 198–205.

Kurth, E., Spichiger, E., Cignacco, E., Kennedy, H. P., Glanzmann, R., Schmid, M., Staehelin, K., Schindler, C., & Stutz, E. Z. (2010). Predictors of crying problems in the early postpartum period. *Journal of Obstetric, Gynecologic, and Neonatal Nursing, 39*, 250–262.

Lanting, C. I., Van Wouwe, J. P., & Reijneveld, S. A. (2005). Infant milk feeding practices in the Netherlands and associated factors. *Acta Paediatrica, 94*, 935–942.

Lawrence, R. A., & Lawrence, R. M. (2010). *Breastfeeding: A guide for the medical professional.* Maryland Heights, MO: Elsevier Mosby.

Leavitt, L. A. (2001). Infant crying: Expectations and parental response. In R. G. Barr, I. St. James-Roberts, & M. R. Keefe (Eds.), *New evidence on unexplained early infant crying: Its origins, nature, and management* (pp. 43–50). Langhorne, PA: Johnson and Johnson Pediatric Institute.

Lee, K. (2000). Crying and behavior pattern in breast- and formula-fed infants. *Early Human Development, 58*, 133–140.

Lewallen, L. P., Dick, M. J., Flowers, J., Powell, W., Zickefoose, K. T., Wall, Y. G., & Price, Z. M. (2006). Breastfeeding support and early cessation. *Journal of Obstetric, Gynecologic, and Neonatal Nursing, 35*, 166–172.

Macknin, M. L., Medendorp, S. V., & Maier, M. C. (1989). Infant sleep and bedtime cereal. *American Journal of Diseases of Children, 143*, 1066–1068.

Nugent, J., Keefer, C., Minear, S., Johnson, L., & Blanchard, Y. (2007). *Understanding newborn behavior and early relationships: The newborn behavioral observations (NBO) system handbook.* Baltimore, MD: Paul H. Brookes.

Peirano, P., Algarin, C., & Uauy, R. (2003). Sleep-wake states and their regulatory mechanisms throughout early human development. *Journal of Pediatrics, 143*, S70–79.

Pridham, K. F., Knight, C. B., & Stephenson, G. R. (1989). Mothers' working models of infant feeding: Description and influencing factors. *Journal of Advanced Nursing, 14*, 1051–1061.

Quillin, S. I. (1997). Infant and mother sleep patterns during 4th postpartum week. *Issues in Comprehensive Pediatric Nursing, 20*, 115–123.

Rochat, A., & Hespos, S. J. (1997). Differential rooting response by neonates: Evidence for an early sense of self. *Early Devopment and Parenting, 6*, 105–112.

Rosen, L. A. (2008). Infant sleep and feeding. *Journal of Obstetric, Gynecologic, and Neonatal Nursing, 37*, 706–714.

Ryan, A. S., Wenjun, Z., & Acosta, A. (2002). Breastfeeding continues to increase into the new millennium. *Pediatrics, 110*, 1103–1109.

Ryan, A. S., & Zhou, W. (2006). Lower breastfeeding rates persist among the Special Supplemental Nutrition Program for Women, Infants, and Children participants, 1978–2003. *Pediatrics, 117*, 1136–1146.

Sacco, L. M., Caulfield, L. E., Gittelsohn, J., & Martinez, H. (2006). The conceptualization of perceived insufficient milk among Mexican mothers. *Journal of Human Lactation, 22*, 277–286.

Sadeh, A., & Anders, T. (1993). Infant sleep problems: Origins, assessment, interventions. *Infant Mental Health Journal, 14*, 17–34.

Tirosh, E., Scher, A., Sadeh, A., Jaffe, M., Rubin, A., & Lavie, P. (1993). The effects of illness on sleep behaviour in infants. *European Journal of Pediatrics, 152*, 15–17.

Trachtenbarg, D. E., & Golemon, T. B. (1998). Care of the premature infant: Part I. Monitoring growth and development. *American Family Physician, 57*, 2123–2130.

van Sleuwen, B. E., L'Hoir, M. P., Engelberts, A. C., Busschers, W. B., Westers, P., Blom, M. A., Schulpen, T. W., & Kuis, W. (2006). Comparison of behavior modification with and without swaddling as interventions for excessive crying. *Journal of Pediatrics, 149*, 512–517.

Walker, M. (2007). International breastfeeding initiatives and their relevance to the current state of breastfeeding in the United States. *Journal of Midwifery and Women's Health, 52*, 549–555.

White, C., Simon, M., & Bryan, A. (2002). Using evidence to educate birthing center nursing staff about infant states, cues, and behaviors. *MCN: The American Journal of Maternal/Child Nursing, 27*, 294–298.

CHAPTER 6
Maternal Mental Health and Breastfeeding

Kathleen Kendall-Tackett, PhD, IBCLC, FAPA

OBJECTIVES

- Recognize the symptoms of depression and other mood disorders in new mothers.
- Describe the role of stress in the etiology of depression.
- Describe how breastfeeding protects maternal mental health.
- Recognize that breastfeeding problems increase the risk of depression and need to be addressed promptly.
- Recognize that depressed mothers are at higher risk for breastfeeding cessation.
- Provide information to mothers on treatment options for depression that are compatible with breastfeeding.

INTRODUCTION

A mother's mental health can have a dramatic influence on her well-being in the first postpartum year. Depression, anxiety disorders, posttraumatic stress disorder (PTSD), and other conditions can lead to breastfeeding cessation and have a negative impact on both mother and baby (Kendall-Tackett, 2010a). Breastfeeding protects maternal mental health (Dennis et al., 2009; Groer, 2005; Kendall-Tackett, 2010a; Kendall-Tackett et al., 2011,), but breastfeeding problems can increase the risk of depression (Amir et al., 1996).

When breastfeeding mothers are depressed, breastfeeding protects their babies from the potentially harmful effects of their mothers' depression (Jones et al., 2004). Breastfeeding mothers are significantly less likely to abuse and neglect their children (Strathearn et al., 2009), and breastfeeding also protects children's mental health throughout childhood (Oddy et al., 2009).

I. Postpartum Depression

A. Overview

1. Postpartum depression is relatively common, affecting 15% to 25% of new mothers (Centers for Disease Control and Prevention, 2008; Kendall-Tackett, 2010a), but rates vary widely in the United States and around the world.

2. Some populations have considerably higher rates of depression, such as low-income mothers (McKee et al., 2001); some U.S. ethnic minorities, such as Native Americans and African Americans; women with a history of sexual abuse or assault (Fergusson et al., 2008; Kendall-Tackett, 2010a); women with bipolar disorder (Freeman et al., 2002); and women with active eating disorders (Morgan et al., 2006). But in cultures where there are social structures, such as a distinct postpartum period and care for the new mother, rates of postpartum depression and other conditions can be quite low (Stern et al., 1983).

3. Symptoms of depression include moods of sadness, anhedonia (inability to experience pleasure in normally pleasurable activities), sleep difficulties unrelated to infant care, fatigue, inability to concentrate, hopelessness, and thoughts of death. For a diagnosis of major depressive disorder these symptoms must be present for at least 2 weeks.

4. Depression also may manifest as somatic complaints or severe fatigue. In many cultures, these symptoms are more socially acceptable than depression is. Another possible indication of depression is increased use of healthcare services for the mother or her baby.

5. The number of minutes that it takes for mothers to fall asleep is an important predictor of depression and is a nonintrusive way to ask about it. If it takes mothers more than 25 minutes to fall asleep, they are at high risk for depression (Goyal et al., 2007; Posmontier, 2008).

6. "Baby blues" are often mild and self-limiting. But many believe that the blues are an early manifestation of depression and therefore should not be ignored. (See Chapter 4.)

7. Only one treatment for depression is contraindicated for breastfeeding mothers (the monoamine oxidase inhibitors [MAOI] class of antidepressants). All other treatments for depression are compatible with breastfeeding (Hale, 2010; Kendall-Tackett, 2008, 2010a).

B. Inflammation in depression

1. Researchers in the field of psychoneuroimmunology (PNI) have found that inflammation is involved in the pathogenesis of depression (Kendall-Tackett, 2010a; Maes, 2001).

2. All types of physical and psychological stress increase the risk of depression in nonpostpartum samples, and also in new mothers. The types of stressors vary from mother to mother. But the underlying physiologic mechanism in response to these stressors is the same: an upregulation of the stress response, including the increase in proinflammatory cytokines (Kendall-Tackett, 2007b).

3. Puerperal women are especially vulnerable because their inflammation levels rise significantly during the last trimester of pregnancy—a time when they are also at high risk for depression. Moreover, common experiences of new motherhood, such as sleep disturbance, postpartum pain, and psychological trauma, also increase inflammation (Kendall-Tackett, 2007b, 2010a).

4. The human stress response: To understand the role of inflammation in depression, it is helpful to first review the normal physiologic response to stress. When faced with a threat, human bodies have a number of interdependent mechanisms in place designed to preserve our lives (Corwin et al., 2008; Kendall-Tackett, 2007b, 2010a; Maes, 2001).

   a. The sympathetic nervous system responds by releasing catecholamines (norepinephrine, epinephrine, and dopamine).

   b. The hypothalamic-pituitary-adrenal (HPA) axis also responds: The hypothalamus releases corticotrophin releasing hormone (CRH), the pituitary releases adrenocorticotropin hormone (ACTH), and the adrenal cortex releases cortisol, a glucocorticoid.

   c. The immune system responds by increasing production of proinflammatory cytokines, which increase systemic inflammation. Cytokines are proteins that regulate immune response. Proinflammatory cytokines help the body heal wounds and fight infection by stimulating an inflammatory response. These inflammatory molecules are measured in the plasma. In depressed people, inflammation is increased, including high levels of proinflammatory cytokines and acute-phase proteins, such as C-reactive protein (CRP), which are a physiologic response to chronic distress. Levels of inflammation can be 40% to 50% higher in depressed people than in their nondepressed counterparts (Pace et al., 2007).

      i. The proinflammatory cytokines that researchers identified most consistently as being elevated in depression are interleukin-1β (IL-1), interleukin-6 (IL-6), and tumor necrosis factor (TNF).

   d. Breastfeeding specifically downregulates the stress response and lowers ACTH and cortisol (Heinrichs et al., 2001) and inflammation (Williams et al., 2006), and this is likely one way that breastfeeding decreases the risk for depression. This downregulation is thought to have survival advantage as it directs the mother toward milk production, conservation of energy, and attachment to her baby (Groer et al., 2002).

C. Stressors that can increase inflammation and depression risk can be physical or psychological. The stress response is the same whether the stressors are physical or psychological. Three stressors—sleep disturbance, pain, and trauma—are particularly relevant to new mothers.

   1. Sleep disturbances

      a. The relationship between sleep disturbance and depression is bidirectional. Sleep disturbances can cause depression, and depression causes sleep disturbances (Posmontier, 2008).

    b. Fatigue and sleep problems are often overlooked or minimized because they are so common in new mothers. But fatigue is often of great concern to mothers.

    c. Even short periods of disrupted sleep can wreak havoc on physical health. Sleep disturbances increase inflammatory responses and, if chronic, increase the risk of chronic diseases, such as heart disease and metabolic syndrome (McEwen, 2003; Suarez et al., 2010).

    d. Breastfeeding protects maternal mental health by improving sleep quality and quantity. In a number of recent studies, exclusively breastfeeding mothers get more sleep than their mixed- or exclusively formula-feeding counterparts (Doan et al., 2007; Dorheim, Bondevik et al., 2009; Gay et al., 2004; Kendall-Tackett et al., 2011; Quillin et al., 2004).

    e. One study of 2,870 mothers found that disturbed sleep increased risk for postpartum depression, and that "not exclusively breastfeeding" was a risk factor for both (Dorheim et al., 2009).

    f. Breastfeeding mothers also get more of deeper slow-wave sleep (SWS) (Blyton et al., 2002). In a study of 31 women, breastfeeding mothers got an average of 182 minutes of SWS. Women in the nonpostpartum control group had an average of 86 minutes. Slow-wave sleep is an important marker of sleep quality, and those with a lower percentage of slow-wave sleep report more daytime fatigue.

    g. If a breastfeeding mother is very fatigued, physical causes, such as anemia, hypothyroidism, or low-grade infection, should be tested for and ruled out. Mothers may also need help in mobilizing their support network so that they can get more rest. Supplementing will likely decrease the amount of sleep that a mother is getting (Doan et al., 2007).

2. Pain

    a. Postpartum pain can also trigger postpartum depression and should be addressed promptly. In a study of 1,288 new mothers, severity of postpartum pain predicted postpartum depression. Acute pain increased depression risk by three times (Eisenach et al., 2008).

    b. Nipple pain is one common type of postpartum pain. In two studies, more than half of the new mothers reported nipple pain at 5 weeks (McGovern et al., 2006) and 2 months postpartum (Ansara et al., 2005), and this can also cause postpartum depression. In a study from Australia, 38% of mothers with nipple pain had postpartum depression compared with 14% of women who did not. When the nipple pain resolved, the maternal mood states returned to normal (Amir et al., 1996).

    c. Pain and inflammation are mutually upregulatory: Pain increases inflammation and inflammation increases pain (Beilin et al., 2003).

    d. People with major depression or posttraumatic stress disorder are also more likely to experience pain (Geracioti et al., 2006).

3. Psychological trauma
   a. Psychological trauma increases the risk for depression (Buist et al., 2001; Rohde et al., 2008).
   b. It also increases inflammation. In the Dunedin Multidisciplinary Health and Development Study, a birth cohort study from Dunedin, New Zealand, childhood maltreatment was related to increased inflammation (C-reactive protein) 20 years later. There was a dose-response effect: The more severe the abuse, the higher the level of inflammation (Danese et al., 2007). At the 32-year assessment, those who experienced childhood adversities (low socio-economic status, maltreatment, or social isolation) had higher rates of major depression, systemic inflammation, and at least three metabolic risk markers (Danese et al., 2009).
   c. With regard to new mothers, the most common types of psychological trauma are adverse childhood experiences and trauma related to their birth experiences.
   d. Adverse childhood experiences (ACEs)
      i. ACEs include childhood physical and sexual abuse, emotional abuse, neglect, witnessing domestic violence between parents or a parent and his or her partner, parental mental illness, substance abuse, or criminal activity (Anda et al., 2006; Chapman et al., 2004).
      ii. These types of experiences are common. In one large, middle-class U.S. sample, 51% had experienced at least one type of ACE (Felitti et al., 1998). Samples with higher risk populations may have even higher rates.
      iii. Childhood adversities are related to a number of chronic health conditions in adults, including cardiovascular disease, metabolic syndrome, and diabetes (Batten et al., 2004; Kendall-Tackett, 2007a, 2007e; Shonkoff et al., 2009).
      iv. Childhood adversities are also related to sleep disturbances (Kendall-Tackett, 2007a) and chronic pain syndromes (Sachs-Ericsson et al., 2007).
      v. ACEs can affect mothers postpartum, most notably by increasing the risk of depression and PTSD. This risk seems especially elevated in mothers who are sexual abuse or sexual assault survivors (Milgrom et al., 2008).
      vi. Women who have these types of experiences may have higher rates of intention to breastfeed and breastfeeding initiation rates (Kendall-Tackett, 2010a). Data from the Survey of Mothers' Sleep and Fatigue, a sample of 6,410 new mothers from 59 countries, including 994 sexual assault survivors, found no significant difference in breastfeeding rates between sexual assault survivors and women who were not (Kendall-Tackett et al., submitted for publication).
      vii. Practitioners may need to work with mothers who are abuse survivors to modify breastfeeding so that it is more comfortable. But practitioners should not assume that a woman with a history of sexual abuse or assault does not want to breastfeed; it may be a very important goal for her.

Depending on the mother's experience, some strategies that may make breastfeeding easier include using distraction while breastfeeding, avoiding nighttime feedings, reducing the amount of skin-to-skin contact, and pumping milk and using a bottle. Be flexible and help the mother find a way that works best for her.

e. Negative birth experiences

   i. Birth experiences can also cause psychological trauma. One review study found that 1.5% to 6% of women met the full criteria of PTSD following birth (Beck, 2004). In comparison, 7.5% of residents of lower Manhattan in New York City met the full criteria for PTSD following the 9/11 terrorist attacks (Galea et al., 2003).

   ii. Objective aspects of birth (e.g., cesarean vs. vaginal) account for only some reactions. Mothers who have cesarean births are at somewhat increased risk of having a negative reaction, but that is not always true. Subjective aspects of birth, such as the following, are more likely to lead to a woman's negative assessment of her birth:

   • Did she believe that giving birth was dangerous to herself or her baby?
   • Did she feel in control of either the medical situation or herself during labor?
   • Did she feel supported during labor and birth? (Kendall-Tackett, 2010a)

   iii. Mothers are more vulnerable to PTSD if they have had prior episodes of depression or PTSD, are abuse survivors (which increases the risk of both PTSD and depression), had prior episodes of loss (including childbearing loss), or were depressed during pregnancy (Kendall-Tackett, 2007c, 2007d).

   iv. Infant illness, preterm birth, and disability also can cause depression in mothers, particularly if the babies are at high risk (Kersting et al., 2005; Kersting et al., 2004; van Pampus et al., 2004). However, this reaction is often delayed and may not manifest until the babies are out of danger, or even several months after they are discharged.

   v. A highly stressful birth may delay lactogenesis II (Grajeda et al., 2002).

D. Treatment options: A variety of treatment options that are effective for mild, moderate, and severe depression is available. All but one of these modalities (MAOI antidepressants) are compatible with breastfeeding, and most can be safely combined. All effective treatments for depression are anti-inflammatory (Kendall-Tackett, 2008, 2010a; Maes et al., 2009).

1. Omega-3 fatty acids

   a. The long-chain omega-3 fatty acids EPA and DHA have been used successfully both to prevent and treat depression. Both of these are found in fatty fish. Populations who have high rates of fish consumption have lower rates of several types of mental illness, including postpartum depression (Hibbeln, 2002; Kendall-Tackett, 2008, 2010b).

   b. EPA is the omega-3 that treats depression because it specifically lowers
      proinflammatory cytokines and downregulates the stress response (Kiecolt-
      Glaser et al., 2007; Rees et al., 2005). EPA/DHA has been used by itself
      or has been combined with medications. When used with medications,
      EPA/DHA enhances the effectiveness of the medications. The American
      Psychiatric Association recognizes EPA as a promising treatment for mood
      disorders (Freeman et al., 2006).
   c. Even in relatively large doses, EPA and DHA are safe for pregnant and breast-
      feeding women and provide a number of other health benefits for women,
      including lowering their risk of heart disease and making them less vulnerable
      to stress (Dunstan et al., 2004; Grandjean et al., 2001).
   d. ALA, the omega-3 in flaxseed and other plant sources, such as walnuts and
      canola oil, does not prevent or treat depression. ALA is not harmful and can
      be helpful in other ways. But it is metabolically too far removed from EPA
      to aid in lessening depression.
2. Bright light therapy
   a. Bright light is another effective treatment for depression. It has also been
      used to treat depression in pregnant and breastfeeding women, although the
      sample sizes are still small (Oren et al., 2002).
   b. An illumination level of 10,000 lux for 30 to 40 minutes is the most com-
      monly used dosage. Regular home lighting is not sufficiently bright to alle-
      viate depression. Light therapy first thing in the morning is more effective
      than light therapy later in the day (Terman et al., 2005).
3. Exercise
   a. Exercise is as effective as medications for even major depression (Babyak
      et al., 2000; Blumenthal et al., 2007).
   b. Exercise lowers inflammation. Overall fitness level lowers the inflammatory
      response to stress (Emery et al., 2005; Kiecolt-Glaser et al., 2010).
   c. Exercise at a moderate level is safe during pregnancy or breastfeeding (Su
      et al., 2007).
4. Psychotherapy
   a. Two types of psychotherapy are effective for depression in pregnant and breast-
      feeding women: cognitive-behavioral therapy and interpersonal psychotherapy.
   b. Cognitive therapy's premise is that depression is caused by distortions in
      people's beliefs about themselves and the world. By addressing these beliefs,
      depression diminishes. It is as effective as medications for treating depres-
      sion and other conditions (Rupke et al., 2006).
   c. Interpersonal psychotherapy (IPT) specifically addresses women's key rela-
      tionships and the support they receive from those relationships. It teaches
      mothers to identify sources of support and increase the amount of support
      they receive from existing relationships. It has been used with many high-
      risk mothers both to prevent and treat depression during pregnancy and
      postpartum (Zlotnick et al., 2006).

5. St. John's wort
   a. The herbal antidepressant St. John's wort is the most widely prescribed anti-depressant in the world, and it is highly effective in treating depression. Its standard uses are for mild-to-moderate depression, but it has been used for major depression as well.
   b. When researchers have compared St. John's wort to Zoloft (sertraline) and Paxil (paroxetine), St. John's wort was as effective as medications and patients reported fewer side effects (Anghelescu et al., 2006; Van Gurp et al., 2002).
   c. It is compatible with breastfeeding (Hale, 2010).
   d. Used by itself, St. John's wort has an excellent safety record. But it does interact with several classes of medications, so it should not be combined with antidepressants, birth control pills, cyclosporins, and several other classes of medications (Kendall-Tackett, 2008; Schultz, 2006).
6. Antidepressants
   a. Most antidepressants are compatible with breastfeeding, but some medications are better than others in terms of amount of exposure the infant receives (Hale et al., 2010; Weissman et al., 2004).
   b. Tricyclic and selective serotonin reuptake inhibitors are compatible with breastfeeding (Kendall-Tackett et al., 2010).
   c. Monoamine oxidase inhibitors (MAOIs) are contraindicated for breastfeeding mothers (Hale, 2010).

II. Other Conditions

Several conditions can occur alone or co-occur with postpartum depression.
   A. Posttraumatic stress disorder
      1. Women may experience PTSD as a result of a prior trauma-producing event (e.g., childhood abuse, rape or assault, car accident, natural disaster) or as a result of the birth itself.
      2. A key aspect of what makes a traumatic event harmful is whether the mother believed that either her or a loved one's life was in danger. In terms of the mother's reaction, her perception is what counts. For birth, it does not matter if the mother's perception of risk is not medically "true." If she believes that she or her baby might have died, then she is likely to have a reaction.
      3. To meet full criteria for PTSD, women must have symptoms in three domains: reexperiencing, avoidance, and hyperarousal. Even when someone does not meet the full criteria, however, that person may still have troublesome symptoms. For example, emotional numbness after a traumatic birth may make it difficult initially for a mother to bond with her baby. Intrusive thoughts, nightmares, and chronic hyperarousal may compromise the quality of a mother's sleep, further impairing her mental health (Kendall-Tackett, 2010a).

B. General anxiety disorder (GAD)
   1. GAD is the most prevalent anxiety disorder, occurring in 7% to 8.2% of mothers in the first year. A further 15% to 20% of women are subsyndromal.
   2. Symptoms include uncontrollable and excessive worry, restlessness, fatigue, difficulties concentrating, irritability, muscle tension, and sleep disturbance (Wenzel, 2011).
   3. Depression and anxiety often co-occur and the relationship between depression and anxiety is bidirectional (Skouteris et al., 2009).
C. Bipolar disorder
   1. Bipolar disorder can manifest for the first time in the postpartum period.
   2. Postpartum bipolar disorder is tricky to diagnose because it almost always manifests as major depression. When the depression is treated, often with the selective serotonin reuptake inhibitor (SSRI) class of antidepressants, these medications can trigger a manic episode (Beck, 2006).
   3. Postpartum bipolar disorder can occur with or without psychosis and tends to run in families.
   4. Patients with bipolar disorder often have comorbid depression (Freeman, et al., 2002).
D. Eating disorders
   1. Eating disorders can occur during pregnancy and during the postpartum period.
   2. Active eating disorders during pregnancy increase the rate of postpartum depression (Morgan et al., 2006).
E. Obsessive-compulsive disorder (OCD)
   1. OCD is characterized by recurrent obsessions, which include unwelcome thoughts, ideas, doubts, and marked distress that people try to suppress or ignore. These lead to compulsions, which includes repetitive behaviors that the person feels driven to perform with the intent of reducing distress (Wenzel, 2011).
   2. In community samples of postpartum women, incidence of OCD ranges from 0.6% to 1.3%, with 17% to 31% indicating that it started in pregnancy (Wenzel, 2011).
   3. OCD can manifest as repetitive thoughts of infant harm. Generally speaking, these thoughts do not lead to an increased risk that the mother will harm her baby. In fact, she often goes to extreme measures to keep anything from happening to her baby (Abramowitz et al., 2002).
   4. OCD and co-occurring depression are treated with SSRIs (Kendall-Tackett, 2010a).

Internet Resources

Association for Behavioral and Cognitive Therapies (ABCT): *www.abct.org*
Breastfeeding Made Simple: www.breastfeedingmadesimple.com
   Information for mothers on postpartum depression, trauma, and treatment options
International Society for Interpersonal Psychotherapy: www.interpersonalpsychotherapy.org
National Alliance on Mental Illness: www.nami.org
National Association of Cognitive-Behavioral Therapists: www.nacbt.org

Postpartum Support International: www.postpartum.net

Resources and information for those who may be experiencing prenatal or postnatal mood or anxiety disorders

Uppity Science Chick: http://uppitysciencechick.com

Information on depression, sexual abuse, breastfeeding, and other women's issues is presented in articles, video clips, and other educational materials written by Kathleen Kendall-Tackett, PhD, IBCLC, FAPA; use and reprints are free with acknowledgment of source

U.S. Pharmacopeia: www.usp.org

Includes information about specific brands of fish oil products

References

Abramowitz, J. S., Schwartz, S. A., Moore, K., Carmin, C., Wiegartz, P. S., & Purdon, C. (2002). Obsessive-compulsive symptoms in pregnancy and the puerperium: A review of the literature. *Anxiety Disorders, 87,* 49–74.

Amir, L. H., Dennerstein, L., Garland, S. M., Fisher, J., & Farish, S. J. (1996). Psychological aspects of nipple pain in lactating women. *Journal of Psychosomatic Obstetrics and Gynecology, 17,* 53–58.

Anda, R. F., Felitti, V. J., Bremner, J. D., et al. (2006). The enduring effects of abuse and related adverse experiences in childhood. A convergence of evidence from neurobiology and epidemiology. *European Archives of Psychiatry and Clinical Neuroscience, 256*(3), 174–186. doi:10.1007/s00406-005-0624-4

Anghelescu, I. G., Kohnen, R., Szegedi, A., Klement, S., & Kieser, M. (2006). Comparison of *Hypericum* extract WS 5570 and paroxetine in ongoing treatment after recovery from an episode of moderate to severe depression: Results from a randomized multicenter study. *Pharmacopsychiatry, 39,* 213–219.

Ansara, D., Cohen, M. M., Gallop, R., Kung, R., Kung, R., & Schei, B. (2005). Predictors of women's physical health problems after childbirth. *Journal of Psychosomatic Obstetrics and Gynecology, 26,* 115–125.

Babyak, M., Blumenthal, J. A., Herman, S., et al. (2000). Exercise treatment for major depression: Maintenance of therapeutic benefit at 10 months. *Psychosomatic Medicine, 62,* 633–638.

Batten, S. V., Aslan, M., Maciejewski, P. K., & Mazure, C. M. (2004). Childhood maltreatment as a risk factor for adult cardiovascular disease and depression. *Journal of Clinical Psychiatry, 65,* 249–254.

Beck, C. T. (2004). Posttraumatic stress disorder due to childbirth. *Nursing Research, 53,* 216–224.

Beck, C. T. (2006). Postpartum depression: It isn't just the blues. *American Journal of Nursing, 106*(5), 40–50.

Beilin, B., Shavit, Y., Trabekin, E., Mordashev, B., Mayburd, E., Zeidel, A., & Bessler, H. (2003). The effects of postoperative pain management on immune response to surgery. *Anesthesia & Analgesia, 97,* 822–827.

Blumenthal, J. A., Babyak, M. A., Doraiswamy, P. M., Watkins, L., Hoffman, B. M., & Barbour, K. A., et al. (2007). Exercise and pharmacotherapy in the treatment of major depressive disorder. *Psychosomatic Medicine, 69,* 587–596.

Blyton, D. M., Sullivan, C. E., & Edwards, N. (2002). Lactation is associated with an increase in slow-wave sleep in women. *Journal of Sleep Research, 11*(4), 297–303.

Buist, A., & Janson, H. (2001). Childhood sexual abuse, parenting, and postpartum depression: A 3-year follow-up study. *Child Abuse and Neglect, 25,* 909–921.

Centers for Disease Control and Prevention. (2008). Prevalence of self-reported postpartum depressive symptoms—17 states, 2004-5. *Morbidity & Mortality Weekly Report, 57*(14), 361-366.

Chapman, D. P., Whitfield, C. L., Felitti, V. J., Dube, S. R., Edwards, V. J., & Anda, R. F. (2004). Adverse childhood experiences and the risk of depressive disorders in adulthood. *Journal of Affective Disorders, 82*(2), 217–225. doi:S016503270400028X [pii] 10.1016/j.jad.2003.12.013

Corwin, E. J., & Pajer, K. (2008). The psychoneuroimmunology of postpartum depression. *Journal of Women's Health, 17*(9), 1529–1534.

Danese, A., Moffitt, T. E., Harrington, H., et al., (2009). Adverse childhood experiences and adult risk factors for age-related disease: Depression, inflammation, and clustering of metabolic risk markers. *Archives of Pediatric and Adolescent Medicine, 163*(12), 1135–1143. doi:163/12/1135 [pii] 10.1001/archpediatrics.2009.214

Danese, A., Pariante, C. M., Caspi, A., Taylor, A., & Poulton, R. (2007). Childhood maltreatment predicts adult inflammation in a life-course study. *Proceedings of the National Academy of Sciences of the United States of America, 104*(4), 1319–1324. doi:0610362104 [pii] 10.1073/pnas.0610362104

Dennis, C.-L., & McQueen, K. (2009). The relationship between infant-feeding outcomes and postpartum depression: A qualitative systematic review. *Pediatrics, 123*, e736–e751.

Doan, T., Gardiner, A., Gay, C. L., & Lee, K. A. (2007). Breastfeeding increases sleep duration of new parents. *Journal of Perinatal and Neonatal Nursing, 21*(3), 200–206.

Dorheim, S. K., Bondevik, G. T., Eberhard-Gran, M., & Bjorvatn, B. (2009). Sleep and depression in postpartum women: A population-based study. *Sleep, 32*(7), 847–855.

Dunstan, J. A., Roper, J., Mitoulas, L., Hartmann, P. E., Simmer, K., & Prescott, S. L. (2004). The effect of supplementation with fish oil during pregnancy on breast milk immunoglobulin A, soluble CD14, cytokine levels and fatty acid composition. *Clinical and Experimental Allergy, 34*, 1237–1242.

Eisenach, J. C., Pan, P. H., Smiley, R., Lavand'homme, P., Landau, R., & Houle, T. T. (2008). Severity of acute pain after childbirth, but not type of delivery, predicts persistent pain and postpartum depression. *Pain, 140*, 87–94.

Emery, C. F., Kiecolt-Glaser, J. K., Glaser, R., Malarky, W. B., & Frid, D. J. (2005). Exercise accelerates wound healing among healthy older adults: A preliminary investigation. *Journals of Gerontology: Medical Sciences, 60A*, 1432–1436.

Felitti, V. J., Anda, R. F., Nordenberg, D., et al. (1998). Relationship of childhood abuse and household dysfunction to many of the leading causes of death in adults. The Adverse Childhood Experiences (ACE) Study. *American Journal of Preventive Medicine, 14*(4), 245–258. doi:S0749379798000178 [pii]

Fergusson, D. M., Boden, J. M., & Horwood, L. J. (2008). Exposure to childhood sexual and physical abuse and adjustment in early adulthood. *Child Abuse and Neglect, 32*, 607–619.

Freeman, M. P., Hibbeln, J. R., Wisner, K. L., et al. (2006). Omega-3 fatty acids: Evidence basis for treatment and future research in psychiatry. *Journal of Clinical Psychiatry, 67*, 1954–1967.

Freeman, M. P., Smith, K. W., Freeman, S. A., McElroy, S. L., Kmetz, G. F., Wright, R., & Keck, P. E., Jr. (2002). The impact of reproductive events on the course of bipolar disorder in women. *Journal of Clinical Psychiatry, 63*, 284–287.

Galea, S., Vlahov, D., Resnick, H., et al. (2003). Trends of probable post-traumatic stress disorder in New York City after the September 11 terrorist attacks. *American Journal of Epidemiology, 158*, 514–524.

Gay, C. L., Lee, K. A., & Lee, S.-Y. (2004). Sleep patterns and fatigue in new mothers and fathers. *Biological Nursing Research, 5*(4), 311–318.

Geracioti, T. D. J., Carpenter, L. L., Owens, M. J., et al. (2006). Elevated cerebrospinal fluid substance P concentrations in posttraumatic stress disorder and major depression. *American Journal of Psychiatry, 63,* 637–643.

Goyal, D., Gay, C. L., & Lee, K. A. (2007). Patterns of sleep disruption and depressive symptoms in new mothers. *Journal of Perinatal and Neonatal Nursing, 21*(2), 123–129.

Grajeda, R., & Perez-Escamilla, R. (2002). Stress during labor and delivery is associated with delayed onset of lactation among urban Guatemalan women. *Journal of Nutrition, 132,* 3055–3060.

Grandjean, P., Bjerve, K.S., Weihe, P., & Steuerwald, U. (2001). Birthweight in a fishing community: Significance of essential fatty acids and marine food contaminants. *International Journal of Epidemiology, 30,* 1272–1278.

Groer, M. W. (2005). Differences between exclusive breastfeeders, formula-feeders, and controls: A study of stress, mood, and endocrine variables. *Biological Nursing Research, 7*(2), 106–117.

Groer, M. W., Davis, M. W., & Hemphill, J. (2002). Postpartum stress: Current concepts and the possible protective role of breastfeeding. *Journal of Obstetric, Gynecologic, and Neonatal Nursing, 31*(4), 411–417.

Hale, T. W. (2010). *Medications and mothers' milk* (14th ed.). Amarillo, TX: Hale Publishing.

Hale, T. W., Kendall-Tackett, K. A., Cong, Z., Votta, R., & McCurdy, F. (2010). Discontinuation syndrome in newborns whose mothers took antidepressants while pregnant or breastfeeding. *Breastfeeding Medicine, 5, 283-288.*

Heinrichs, M., Meinlschmidt, G., Neumann, I., Wagner, S., Kirschbaum, C., Ehlert, U., & Hellhammer, D. H. (2001). Effects of suckling on hypothalamic-pituitary-adrenal axis responses to psychosocial stress in postpartum lactating women. *Journal of Clinical Endocrinology and Metabolism, 86,* 4798–4804.

Hibbeln, J. R. (2002). Seafood consumption, the DHA content of mothers' milk and prevalence rates of postpartum depression: A cross-national, ecological analysis. *Journal of Affective Disorders, 69,* 15–29.

Jones, N. A., McFall, B. A., & Diego, M. A. (2004). Patterns of brain electrical activity in infants of depressed mothers who breastfeed and bottle feed: The mediating role of infant temperament. *Biological Psychology, 67,* 103–124.

Kendall-Tackett, K. A. (2007a). Cardiovascular disease and metabolic syndrome as sequelae of violence against women: A psychoneuroimmunology approach. *Trauma, Violence and Abuse, 8,* 117–126.

Kendall-Tackett, K. A. (2007b). A new paradigm for depression in new mothers: The central role of inflammation and how breastfeeding and anti-inflammatory treatments protect maternal mental health. *International Breastfeeding Journal, 2,* 6. Retrieved from http://www.internationalbreastfeedingjournal.com/content/2/1/6

Kendall-Tackett, K. A. (2007c). The psychological impact of birth experience: An underreported source of trauma in the lives of women. *Trauma Psychology, 2*(3), 9–11.

Kendall-Tackett, K. A. (2007d). Violence against women and the perinatal period: The impact of lifetime violence and abuse on pregnancy, postpartum and breastfeeding. *Trauma, Violence and Abuse, 8*(3), 344–353.

Kendall-Tackett, K. A. (2007e). Why trauma makes people sick: Inflammation, heart disease, and diabetes in trauma survivors. *Trauma Psychology, 2*(1), 9–12.

Kendall-Tackett, K. A. (2008). *Non-pharmacologic treatments for depression in new mothers.* Amarillo, TX: Hale Publishing.

Kendall-Tackett, K. A. (2010a). *Depression in new mothers: Causes, consequences and treatment options* (2nd ed.). London, England: Routledge.

Kendall-Tackett, K. A. (2010b). Long-chain omega-3 fatty acids and women's mental health in the perinatal period. *Journal of Midwifery and Women's Health*, *55*(6), 561–567.

Kendall-Tackett, K. A., Cong, Z., & Hale, T. W. (2011a). Effect of breastfeeding and formula-feeding on sleep duration and rates of depression. *Clinical Lactation*, *2*(2), 22-26.

Kendall-Tackett, K.A., Cong, Z., & Hale, T.W. (2011b). *Breastfeeding rates among sexual assault survivors.* Submitted for publication.

Kendall-Tackett, K. A., & Hale, T. W. (2010). The use of antidepressants in pregnant and breastfeeding women: A review of recent studies. *Journal of Human Lactation*, *26*(2), 187–196.

Kersting, A., Dorsch, M., Kreulich, C., Reutemann, M., Ohrmann, P., Baez, E., & Arolt, V. (2005). Trauma and grief 2–7 years after termination of pregnancy because of fetal anomalies—A pilot study. *Journal of Psychosomatic Obstetrics and Gynecology*, *26*(1), 9–14.

Kersting, A., Dorsch, M., Wesselman, U., et al. (2004). Maternal posttraumatic stress response after the birth of a very low-birth-weight infant. *Journal of Psychosomatic Research*, *57*, 473–476.

Kiecolt-Glaser, J. K., Belury, M. A., Porter, K., Beversdoft, D., Lemeshow, S., & Glaser, R. (2007). Depressive symptoms, omega-6: Omega-3 fatty acids, and inflammation in older adults. *Psychosomatic Medicine*, *69*, 217–224.

Kiecolt-Glaser, J. K., Christian, L., Preston, H., Houts, C., Malarkey, W. B., Emery, C. F., & Glaser, R. (2010). Stress, inflammation, and yoga practice. *Psychosomatic Medicine*, *72*(2), 113–121.

Maes, M. (2001). Psychological stress and the inflammatory response system. *Clinical Science*, *101*, 193–194.

Maes, M., Yirmyia, R., Noraberg, J., et al. (2009). The inflammatory and neurodegenerative hypothesis of depression: Leads for future research and new drug developments in depression. *Metabolic Brain Disease*, *24*, 27–53.

McEwen, B. S. (2003). Mood disorders and allostatic load. *Biological Psychiatry*, *54*, 200–207.

McGovern, P., Dowd, B. E., Gjerdingen, D., et al. (2006). Postpartum health of employed mothers 5 weeks after childbirth. *Annals of Family Medicine*, *4*(2), 159–167.

McKee, M. D., Cunningham, M., Jankowski, K. R., & Zayas, L. (2001). Health-related functional status in pregnancy: Relationship to depression and social support in a multi-ethnic population. *Obstetrics and Gynecology*, *97*, 988–993.

Milgrom, J., Gemmill, A. W., Bilszta, J. L., et al. (2008). Antenatal risk factors for postnatal depression: A large prospective study. *Journal of Affective Disorders*, *108*(1–2), 147–157.

Morgan, J. F., Lacey, J. H., & Chung, E. (2006). Risk of postnatal depression, miscarriage, and preterm birth in bulimia nervosa: Retrospective contolled study. *Psychosomatic Medicine*, *68*, 487–492.

Oddy, W. H., Kendall, G. E., Li, J., et al. (2009). The long-term effects of breastfeeding on child and adolescent mental health: A pregnancy cohort study followed for 14 years. *Journal of Pediatrics*, *156*(4), 568–574.

Oren, D. A., Wisner, K. L., Spinelli, M., Epperson, C. N., Peindl, K. S., Terman, J. S., & Terman, M. (2002). An open trial of morning light therapy for treatment of antepartum depression. *American Journal of Psychiatry*, *159*, 666–669.

Pace, T. W., Hu, F., & Miller, A. H. (2007). Cytokine-effects on glucocorticoid receptor function: Relevance to glucocorticoid resistance and the pathophysiology and treatment of major depression. *Brain, Behavior and Immunity*, *21*(1), 9–19. doi:S0889-1591(06)00297-2 [pii] 10.1016/j.bbi.2006.08.009

Posmontier, B. (2008). Sleep quality in women with and without postpartum depression. *Journal of Obstetric, Gynecologic and Neonatal Nursing*, *37*(6), 722–737.

Quillin, S. I. M., & Glenn, L. L. (2004). Interaction between feeding method and co-sleeping on maternal-newborn sleep. *Journal of Obstetric, Gynecologic, and Neonatal Nursing, 33*(5), 580–588.

Rees, A.-M., Austin, M.-P., & Parker, G. (2005). Role of omega-3 fatty acids as a treatment for depression in the perinatal period. *Australia & New Zealand Journal of Psychiatry, 39*, 274–280.

Rohde, P., Ichikawa, L., Simon, G. E., Ludman, E. J., Linde, J. A., Jeffery, R. W., & Operskalski, B. H. (2008). Associations of child sexual and physical abuse with obesity and depression in middle-aged women. *Child Abuse and Neglect, 32*(9), 878–887.

Rupke, S. J., Blecke, D., & Renfrow, M. (2006). Cognitive therapy for depression. *American Family Physician, 73*, 83–86.

Sachs-Ericsson, N., Kendall-Tackett, K. A., & Hernandez, A. (2007). Childhood abuse, chronic pain, and depression in the National Comorbidity Survey. *Child Abuse and Neglect, 31*, 531–547.

Schultz, V. (2006). Safety of St. John's wort extract compared to synthetic antidepressants. *Phytomedicine, 13*, 199–204.

Shonkoff, J. P., Boyce, W. T., & McEwen, B. S. (2009). Neuroscience, molecular biology, and the childhood roots of health disparities: Building a new framework for health promotion and disease prevention. *Journal of the American Medical Association, 301*(21), 2252–2259. doi:301/21/2252 [pii] 10.1001/jama.2009.754

Skouteris, H., Wertheim, E. H., Rallis, S., Milgrom, J., & Paxton, S. J. (2009). Depression and anxiety through pregnancy and the early postpartum: An examination of prospective relationships. *Journal of Affective Disorders, 113*, 303–308.

Stern, G., & Kruckman, L. (1983). Multi-disciplinary perspectives on postpartum depression: An anthropological critique. *Social Science and Medicine, 17*, 1027–1041.

Strathearn, L., Mamun, A. A., Najman, J. M., & O'Callaghan, M. J. (2009). Does breastfeeding protect against substantiated child abuse and neglect? A 15-year cohort study. *Pediatrics, 123*(2), 483–493. doi:123/2/483 [pii] 10.1542/peds.2007-3546

Su, D., Zhao, Y., Binna, C., Scott, J., & Oddy, W. (2007). Breastfeeding mothers can exercise: Results of a cohort study. *Public Health Nutrition, 10*, 1089–1093.

Suarez, E. C., & Goforth, H. (2010). Sleep and inflammation: A potential link to chronic diseases. In K. A. Kendall-Tackett (Ed.), *The psychoneuroimmunology of chronic disease* (pp. 53–75). Washington, DC: American Psychological Association.

Terman, M., & Terman, J. S. (2005). Light therapy for seasonal and nonseasonal depression: Efficacy, protocol, safety, and side effects. *CNS Spectrums, 10*, 647–663.

Van Gurp, G., Meterissian, G. B., Haiek, L. N., McCusker, J., & Bellavance, F. (2002). St. John's wort or sertraline?: Randomized controlled trial in primary care. *Canadian Family Physician, 48*, 905–912.

van Pampus, M. G., Wolf, H., Weijmar Schultz, W. C. M., Neeleman, J., & Aarnoudse, J. G. (2004). Posttraumatic stress disorder following preeclampsia and HELLP syndrome. *Journal of Psychosomatic Obstetrics and Gynecology, 25*, 183–187.

Wei, G., Greaver, L. B., Marson, S. M., Herndon, C. H., Rogers, J., & Corporation, R. H. (2008). Postpartum depression: Racial differences and ethnic disparities in a tri-racial and bi-ethnic population. *Maternal Child Health Journal. 12*(6), 699–707.

Weissman, A. M., Levy, B. T., Hartz, A. J., Bentler, S., Donohue, M., Ellingrod, V. L., & Wisner, K. L. (2004). Pooled analysis of antidepressant levels in lactating mothers, breast milk, and nursing infants. *American Journal of Psychiatry, 161*(6), 1066–1078.

Wenzel, A. (2011). *Anxiety in childbearing women: Diagnosis and treatment.* Washington, DC: American Psychological Association.

Williams, M. J. A., Williams, S. M., & Poulton, R. (2006). Breastfeeding is related to C-reactive protein concentration in adult women. *Journal of Epidemiology and Community Health, 60*, 146–148.

Zlotnick, C., Miller, I. W., Pearlstein, T., Howard, M., & Sweeney, P. (2006). A preventive intervention for pregnant women on public assistance at risk for postpartum depression. *American Journal of Psychiatry, 163*, 1443–1445.

Suggested Reading

Humphrey, S. (2003) *Nursing mothers' herbal*. Minneapolis: Fairview Press.

The Complete German Commission E Monographs available online and for purchase from the American Botanical Council, www.herbalgram.org.

Kendall-Tackett, K.A. (2010). *Depression in new mothers, 2nd Edition*. London: Routledge.

Kendall-Tackett, K.A. (2008). *Non-pharmacologic treatments for depression in new mothers*. Amarillo, TX: Hale Publishing.

Wenzel, A. (2011). *Anxiety in childbearing women: Diagnosis and treatment*. Washington, DC: American Psychological Association.

CHAPTER 7
Breastfeeding and Maternal Employment

Cathy Carothers, BLA, IBCLC, FILCA, and Chris Mulford, BA, BSN

OBJECTIVES

- Identify the competing demands of work on a breastfeeding mother's time and energy and offer strategies for enlisting family, friends, and community to reduce those demands.
- Identify ways that employment affects breastfeeding initiation, intensity (or exclusivity), and duration.
- Discuss occupational hazards in the workplace in relation to breastfeeding.
- List benefits to employers, mothers, infants, and the community when breastfeeding is continued after the mother returns to her outside employment.
- Identify common barriers to sustaining lactation that affect employers and mothers.
- Describe basic workplace requirements to support the lactating employee.
- Identify strategies for motivating employers to establish lactation support for employees.
- Review counseling and strategies for mothers.
- Identify information that should be discussed with child care providers.
- Explain the key components of maternity protection policies and the lactation consultant's role as a community advocate.

INTRODUCTION

Worldwide approximately 60% of women of childbearing age are in the workforce (International Labor Organization [ILO], 2007), but *every* mother is a working mother. When a woman gives birth, her baby's care and feeding are added to her existing workload, which may already include unpaid carework for her family, home, and community; income-generating employment; unpaid work in a family business; and/or subsistence farming. Her paying job(s) may be in the formal economy—working either for the government (public sector) or in business (private sector)—or in the informal economy (such as handcrafts, street vending, domestic service, sweatshops, illegal activities, and many kinds of small-scale self-employment). It has been estimated that 25% of the world's workforce is in the informal economy, which in some nations

(continues)

employs more than 80% of workers (Maternity Protection Coalition, 2008). People who work in the informal economy often work just as hard or harder than do those in formal employment, but they lack the "safety net" that is provided by labor laws and the solidarity that comes with organization by trade unions.

Much of women's paid and unpaid work competes with breastfeeding for their time and energy. Lactation consultants help clients assess these competing demands and suggest ways either to modify the work demands to free up resources for breastfeeding or to modify breastfeeding to fit in with the mother's work. Lactation consultants also educate the community and advocate for policies that protect and support breastfeeding in the context of women's work.

Work often requires mother–baby separation with all the challenges that separation poses for breastfeeding mothers and babies. A wide range of proven strategies can help maintain the breastfeeding relationship, including (1) do the work and simultaneously care for the baby (multitasking); (2) arrange alternate child care at or near the workplace, taking breaks from work to feed the baby; and (3) arrange alternate child care for the whole workday; express milk at the workplace to store for later feedings; the caregiver feeds expressed milk to the baby (International Lactation Consultant Association [ILCA], 2007). A mother following the latter strategy whose baby takes complementary foods or infant formula for some of the missed feedings may feel less pressure to sustain full lactation. Some babies adapt to separation by "reverse cycle feeding"—sleeping more when mother is away and breastfeeding more when she is present.

The lactation consultant assists the employed mother to reach her goals for breastfeeding through anticipatory guidance so that the mother can plan a course of action to support her working and mothering goals. This counseling occurs during the prenatal period and continues in the early postpartum days and after the mother resumes her work. To assist the mother effectively, the lactation consultant must understand the physiology of lactation to help the mother establish and maintain adequate milk production. The lactation consultant must also be familiar with methods of milk expression, including hand expression and the use of breast pumps. He or she must be able to counsel on the use of alternate feeding devices, safe storage and handling of human milk, and coping methods for dealing with the challenges of working as a breastfeeding mother. The lactation consultant must be able to address employer barriers to providing worksite lactation support that enables women to meet their breastfeeding goals. In addition, the lactation consultant should understand the key components of maternity protection, including job protection, nondiscrimination, nursing breaks, and paid maternity leave/parental leave.

I. Competing Demands

A. Childbearing and child rearing take place within the context of a woman's life. The amount of time and energy she can devote to these activities varies with her age, her socioeconomic and health status, and the multiple roles that her family and her community expect her to fill, in addition to her goals for herself as a worker and mother.

B. The demands of "nonmother" work can be significant, including work weeks of 80 to 100 hours for a Western physician in training as a house officer or medical resident or the 5 hours per day that a woman in an African village may spend gathering firewood and carrying water.

C. Breastfeeding lends itself to multitasking. Mothers commonly combine breastfeeding with other activities such as eating, resting, sleeping, doing household chores, computer and telephone use, and minding older children.

D. Breastfeeding is an economic activity that provides food, health protection, and care for infants and young children. Other economic opportunities, such as a chance to work for pay, may raise the relative value of a mother's time and influence her decision to use alternative foods for her baby (Smith et al., 1998).

E. Household tasks can be done by other people, leaving time and energy for the mother to devote to breastfeeding. U.S. couples in which fathers routinely did a larger share of household tasks had lower risk of early breastfeeding cessation (Sullivan et al., 2004).

F. Support for breastfeeding can come from a variety of sources. A male-focused breastfeeding promotion program raised rates of breastfeeding by the partners of male employees in one U.S. corporate lactation program (Cohen et al., 2002).

G. Community support for breastfeeding varies among cultures. In many cultures, there is a traditional "lying-in period," typically about 40 days of rest after birth, in which other women assume the new mother's normal workload. The period of compulsory postpartum maternity leave in some European countries is a modern version of this practice.

H. Community programs such as the Baby-Friendly Community Initiative in the Gambia can build general and specific community support for mothers of young children, including a redistribution of their workload (Semega-Janneh, 1998).

I. Anticipatory guidance for women planning to breastfeed should include an assessment of their expected workload of family care, household tasks, and community volunteer work as well as any plans for paid employment.

II. Impact of Employment on Breastfeeding Initiation, Exclusivity, and Duration

A. Employment among women and mothers is common. Rates vary around the world, from 40 employed women per 100 employed men in the Middle East and North Africa to 91 women per 100 men in transitional economies such as the former Soviet states of eastern Europe and third world countries (ILO, 2004).

B. Women have a higher share in the number of working poor in the world. Sixty percent of the 550 million working poor worldwide are women, and they are typically employed in jobs characterized by low wages, little or no job security, and fewer human rights or autonomy over their work life situation (ILO, 2004).

C. Increased numbers of women are joining the migrant workforce, and women constitute more than 50% of migrant workers in Asia and Latin America (United Nations Women, n.d.).

D. New mothers return to work exceptionally early in the United States. One-third are back at work within 3 months of birth whereas only 5% of Swedish, German, and U.K. mothers take such a short period of leave (Berger et al., 2005). Two-thirds of U.S. mothers are back on the job by 6 months (United States Breastfeeding Committee, 2002).

E. Effects of employment on breastfeeding initiation
   1. Some studies show that intention to work can affect breastfeeding initiation. Women planning to work part time have been found to be more likely to initiate breastfeeding than are women planning to work full time (Fein et al., 1998; Mandal et al., 2010; Scott et al., 2001).

F. Effects on breastfeeding exclusivity
   1. Twelve percent of a group of Italian mothers cited return to work as a reason to use formula (Romero et al., 2006).
   2. Ghanaian women living near a large city considered exclusive breastfeeding incompatible with hawking goods in a market because they had no suitable place at work to feed their babies (Otoo et al., 2009).
   3. A study in Yolo County, northern California, found that 38% of women working full time were almost exclusively breastfeeding at 6 months compared to 62% of women who worked part time (Dabritz et al., 2009).

G. Effects on duration
   1. Type of occupation affects breastfeeding duration. Women classified as professional, administrative, or managerial are likely to breastfeed longer than are women employed in low-wage jobs or jobs requiring lower skills (Galtry, 1997; Hanson et al., 2003).
   2. The number of hours worked affects duration. The more hours a week a mother is on the job, the shorter the duration of breastfeeding (see **Table 7-1**) (Fein et al., 1998).
   3. Compared with breastfeeding mothers who were not employed, returning to work within 12 weeks and working more than 34 hours a week were associated with a significantly shorter duration of breastfeeding (Mandal et al., 2010).
   4. Intention and actual breastfeeding practices can improve duration rates of breastfeeding. Women who breastfeed exclusively during the first postpartum month and intend to breastfeed fully or partially are more likely to breastfeed longer than 6 months after returning to work (Piper et al., 1996).

Table 7-1 Breastfeeding duration relative to hours worked per week

Hours Worked Per Week	Not Working	20 hours	20–34 hours	35 hours
Average Duration of Breastfeeding	25.1 weeks	24.4 weeks	22.5 weeks	16.5 weeks

5. Returning to work within 12 weeks postpartum is related to the greatest decrease in breastfeeding duration (Galtry, 2003; Gielen et al., 1991; Taveras, 2003).

H. Other factors can affect breastfeeding outcomes.

1. High-wage job settings may offer better family benefits and more flexibility of work schedules (Fairness Initiative on Low-Wage Work, n.d.).

2. Different employment sectors may have different levels of legal protection. Iranian maternity protection laws exceed ILO standards but apply only to government workers (Olang et al., 2009). Malaysian workers in the public sector have 2 months of maternity leave, and those in the private sector get 3 months (Amin et al., 2011).

3. Even where employed mothers enjoy a high level of legal protection, other factors—sociocultural, economic, healthcare practices—can adversely affect breastfeeding outcomes, as in a group of Italian mothers, 95% of whom initiated breastfeeding but dropped to 35% breastfeeding at 6 months (9% exclusive) despite exemplary maternity leave and nursing breaks laws (Chapin, 2001; Romero et al., 2006).

III. Occupational Hazards and the Breastfeeding Woman

A. It is undeniably true that the presence of environmental contaminants has exposed human populations to elevated levels of toxins and carcinogens, some of which appear in human milk. This fact argues more for the reduction of such exposure than against breastfeeding. The long-term effects of toxic exposure via human milk are not yet known. Analysis of milk after accidental exposure to PCBs, DDE, and heptachlor has not demonstrated that the infants were harmed by breastfeeding, although level of exposure might be a mitigating factor (Condon, 2005; Kurinij et al., 1989). (For further detail, see Chapter 26, "Lactation Toxicology.")

B. It is prudent for pregnant and lactating women to avoid exposure to radiation, hazardous chemicals, volatile organics, smoke, and other hazardous materials. If a pregnant or lactating woman is exposed to these substances on the job, she should voice her concerns to the occupational health authority at her workplace, her trade union, and/or her government. Strategies to reduce exposure include use of protective devices and clothing, reassignment to workplace tasks that avoid toxic exposures, or temporary "precautionary" leave without loss of pay.

C. Protective clothing, masks, goggles, and air filters are strategies for pregnant or lactating women who work around toxic materials. Clothing should be changed and hands washed before handling the baby.

D. Women face a dilemma, however, when actions taken to protect their capacity for healthy reproduction limit their choice of jobs or put them at a competitive disadvantage for promotion or better-paying jobs.

E. Women may also be exposed to harmful substances when doing unpaid family care work. For instance, smoke from burning solid fuel (wood, animal dung, crop residues, charcoal) for cooking and heating kills more than 1.6 million people, primarily women and children, every year (Warwick et al., 2004).

F. Occupational exposures typically involve trace metals, solvents, and halogenated hydrocarbons (Lindberg, 1996).

G. Welders, painters, artists, ceramic workers, and workers who handle weapons must beware of lead exposure.

H. Household or agricultural herbicides and pesticides should not be directly handled or inhaled.

I. Healthcare workers should practice universal precautions (see Appendix B), especially given the potential for exposure to human immunodeficiency virus and hepatitis C.

J. Accidental exposure to toxins (such as hazardous chemicals or lead exposure) or potential infection (which can include exposure to viruses, bacteria, or bodily fluids) should be reported to the mother's healthcare provider. Although milk or blood can be tested, such testing may be expensive, the process may be lengthy, and the results may not be useful in deciding what to do. In most cases, women are advised to continue breastfeeding because the risk of not breastfeeding may be greater than a potential risk of exposure to toxins. Ultimately, the mother must weigh the risks and benefits of continued breastfeeding, interrupted breastfeeding, or weaning, in consultation with her physician.

IV. Supporting Breastfeeding Is a "Win-Win-Win" for Employers, Mothers, and Babies

A. For mothers, continuing to breastfeed results in
   1. Optimal outcomes for her baby's health, growth, and development (Agency for Healthcare Research and Quality, 2007)
   2. Significant reduction in numerous acute infections and chronic diseases in infants (American Academy of Pediatrics [AAP], 2005)
   3. Continued emotional bonding with baby
   4. Fewer missed days of work because her baby is healthier (Cohen et al., 1995)
   5. Lower healthcare costs (Ball et al., 1999)
   6. Saving the energy, time, and cost to purchase, store, and prepare infant formula
   7. Benefits of oxytocin released during breastfeeding and milk expression with increased feelings of relaxation and sense of well-being
   8. Strong sense of "reconnection" when mother and child are reunited following separation at work (Roche-Paull, 2010)

B. For employers, support for breastfeeding results in
   1. Fewer employee absences to care for a sick baby and shorter absences when employees do miss work, compared with women who do not breastfeed (Cohen et al., 1995).
   2. Lower costs for employers who provide health care (Ball & Wright, 1999; Cohen et al., 1995). An analysis of overall healthcare costs in the United States found that if 90% of women breastfed exclusively for 6 months as recommended by the American Academy of Pediatrics, the country could save $13 billion in healthcare costs (Bartick et al., 2010).
   3. Reduced turnover rates and improved employee loyalty to the company (Galtry, 1997; Lyness et al., 1999; Ortiz et al., 2004).

       4. Higher job satisfaction (Galtry, 1997).

       5. Community recognition as a "family-friendly business."

  C. For the community, workplace support for breastfeeding results in

       1. Longer duration of breastfeeding, with accompanying health and economic benefits (Bar-Yam, 1998; Cohen et al., 1994; Whaley et al., 2002)

V. Identified Barriers to Sustaining Lactation After Mothers Return to Work (U.S. Department of Health and Human Services [USDHHS], 2003)

  A. Barriers for women

       1. Real or perceived low milk supply (Arlotti et al., 1998; Lewallen et al., 2006; McLeod et al., 2002; Zinn, 2000)

       2. Lack of accommodations in the workplace to express milk (Corbett-Dick et al., 1997)

       3. Lack of time to express milk with resultant diminishing milk supply (Arthur et al., 2003)

       4. Fatigue, stress, and exhaustion (Frank, 1998; Nichols et al., 2004; Wambach, 1998)

       5. Feeling overwhelmed with demands of fulfilling job requirements and meeting the needs of their child (Hochschild et al., 2003)

       6. Child care concerns and reliance on family for help with children (Best Start Social Marketing, 1996; Corbett-Dick et al., 1997)

       7. Concerns over employers' and colleagues' support (Corbett-Dick et al., 1997; Frank, 1998)

  B. Employers' barriers to providing support

       1. Lack of awareness of the numbers of women breastfeeding or the ways breastfeeding can decrease employee absenteeism and lower healthcare costs to the company (Bridges et al., 1997; Chow et al., 2011; Libbus et al., 2002)

       2. Infrequent requests for breastfeeding accommodations (Chow et al., 2011)

       3. Belief that breastfeeding employees will be too fatigued and therefore less productive on the job (Brown et al., 2001; Chow et al., 2011)

       4. Belief that breastfeeding or milk expression in the workplace will interfere with an employee's productivity (Libbus et al., 2002)

       5. Lack of space to accommodate a lactation room and lack of time for employees to express milk (Brown et al., 2001; Chow et al., 2011)

       6. Liability concerns (Brown et al., 2001)

       7. Belief that breastfeeding is a personal decision and not the employer's responsibility (Dunn et al., 2004)

       8. Concerns that other employees will complain or resent covering for a coworker who takes time for nursing breaks (Brown et al., 2001) (Exposure to coworkers who are expressing milk at work may actually improve acceptance [Suyes, Abrahams, & Labbok, 2008].)

       9. Lack of knowledge of how to set up a lactation support program (Brown et al., 2001)

     10. Prioritizing other employee benefit programs ahead of lactation support (Tuttle & Slavit, 2009)

VI. Components of a Successful Lactation Support Program (USDHHS, 2003)

A. Space to breastfeed or express milk

    1. A place to express milk comfortably and in privacy assists with milk ejection and enables mothers to express milk more effectively.

    2. Options for private breastfeeding areas include the following:

        a. Converting small unused spaces such as large closets, offices, or other small rooms

        b. Creating space within a women's lounge

        c. Installing walls, partitions, or dividers in corners or areas of rooms

        d. Creating multiuser stations within a single room divided by partitions or curtains

    3. Requirements for the room: central area that is easy to access, private (preferably with a lock), nearby access to running water, electrical outlet, comfortable chair, table or flat surface, well lit, ventilated and heated/air conditioned.

    4. Optional: multiuser breast pump, telephone, parenting literature, soft lighting, storage space, foot stool, breastfeeding artwork.

    5. Use of a high-quality bilateral electric breast pump can facilitate quick milk expression (Corbett-Dick et al., 1997). Options include the following:

        a. Employer provides a hospital-grade multiuser pump and attachment kits.

        b. Employer provides a hospital-grade multiuser pump and each employee purchases a kit.

        c. Employer provides or subsidizes a portable electric breast pump for each employee.

        d. The employee provides her own equipment.

    6. A secure place to store milk is necessary. Options include the following:

        a. Employer provides a small refrigerator in the milk expression room.

        b. Employee provides an insulated container with cooler packs.

        c. Refrigerators shared with nonlactating coworkers may not be a good option because of the risk that someone may tamper with the milk.

B. Time to express milk (Wyatt, 2002)

    1. Established lunch and morning/afternoon breaks are usually sufficient for milk expression during a standard 8-hour workday (Slusser et al., 2004).

    2. Milk expression needs vary according to the baby's age and needs.

        a. A mother of a baby younger than 4 months old may need three 20-minute milk expression breaks during a standard 8-hour work period.

        b. A mother of a 6-month-old may need to express milk only two times per workday because her baby is likely to be starting solid foods.

        c. Mothers of babies older than 12 months may need to express milk only once or twice during the workday.

        d. Needs of infants may fluctuate (ex: during growth spurts), requiring mothers to breastfeed or express milk more often.

C. Education
   1. Standard information about the company lactation program is often included as part of new employee orientation, in employee benefits materials, wellness or work–life program initiatives, company newsletter, and posters/flyers posted in the workplace.
   2. Identify pregnant employees and provide information. Options include information packets and lunchtime prenatal classes and support groups led by a lactation consultant.
   3. Back-to-work consults for new mothers with a lactation consultant to tailor a milk expression schedule to fit her job situation.
   4. Resource center with books, videos, and materials on ways to maintain lactation after returning to work.
   5. Promotion of the program to supervisors and colleagues through flyers, newsletters, e-mail listservs, and staff meeting presentations.
D. Support (Whaley et al., 2002; Wyatt, 2002)
   1. Support from the employer is highly valued among breastfeeding women. This often begins with a policy at the workplace that addresses needs of breastfeeding employees and can include such components as providing flexible time and a private space to breastfeed or express milk, providing for consultations with a lactation consultant, and addressing responsibilities of the employee, supervisors, and colleagues. Although not all employers believe a policy is necessary and could actually limit flexibility with individuals' needs, others believe it can ensure consistent accommodations for employees within companies (Chow et al., 2011).
   2. Access to other breastfeeding employees enhances confidence and helps women reach their own goals for breastfeeding.

VII. Counseling Mothers (Angeletti, 2009; Page, 2008)

A. During the prenatal period:
   1. Help women understand reasons to breastfeed and continue after returning to work.
   2. Provide practical strategies, encouragement, and support for breastfeeding (Meek, 2001).
   3. Help women understand reasons to express milk while separated from the baby, including the following:
      a. Protecting the baby from illnesses and allergies
      b. Providing comfort for the mother
      c. Preventing engorgement, mastitis, and leaking
      d. Maintaining milk production.
      e. Sustaining the breastfeeding relationship (Win et al., 2006)
   4. Offer support and solutions to help her reach her goals for infant feeding. For instance, some mothers choose not to express milk at work or are unable to express because of worksite constraints. They need strategies for staying comfortable when they are separated from their babies.

5. Refer the mother to community breastfeeding classes and support groups.

6. Develop a plan for combining employment with breastfeeding, including the following:

   a. Timing her return to work with the maximum leave possible. The ILO standard for paid maternity leave is 14 weeks, and 18 weeks is recommended.

   b. Explore work options that enable her to spend as much time as possible with her baby. These can include job sharing (Vanek et al., 2001); part-time employment (Hills-Bonczyk et al., 1993; Ryan et al., 2002); gradual phaseback (part time before full time); or working at home/telecommuting (see **Table 7-2**).

7. Prepare her to speak with her supervisor about nursing break options, including time and flexibility needed, possibilities for access to the baby, and milk expression and milk storage locations.

8. Develop realistic milk expression schedules. Mothers with job constraints that do not allow lengthy milk expression sessions can be encouraged to pump even for shorter durations to relieve overfulness, with a longer milk expression break during a meal period.

9. Discuss strategies for managing potential schedule variations, such as interruptions or unexpected overtime.

10. Explore options for direct breastfeeding and milk expression during the workday, including bringing baby to work (Moquin, 2008), having baby brought to the mother during breaks, going to the child care center to feed the baby during breaks, using breaks to express milk. Women who breastfeed directly during the workday, with or without additional milk expression breaks, may sustain lactation the longest (Fein et al., 2008).

11. Advise about selection of breast pump equipment and milk storage. (See Chapter 33, "Milk Expression, Storage, and Handling.")

12. Explore child care options with providers who support her decision to breastfeed. Encourage the mother to seek providers close to her workplace to facilitate feeding baby either during the work period or immediately before and after work. (See Section IX, which follows.)

B. Before the mother returns to work, the lactation consultant can help her by sharing information to assist the mother to do the following (see **Table 7-3**):

1. Successfully establish breastfeeding immediately after birth, during postpartum recovery, and through the early weeks. This includes

   a. Develop an abundant milk supply. The most frequent reason for weaning is real or perceived insufficient milk supply (Bourgoin et al., 1997).

   b. Frequent breastfeeds/removal of milk during lactogenesis II increases development of prolactin receptors that affect long-term milk supply (Cox et al., 1996).

2. Address coping strategies, including dealing with fatigue and stress, eating nutritious meals, establishing good breastfeeding patterns, and having others do household chores to spare her energy (Sullivan et al., 2004).

Table 7-2 Descriptions of flexible work programs and their benefits for new mothers and employers.

Benefit	Definition	Advantages for New Mothers	Advantages for Employers
Earned time	Sick leave, vacation time, and personal days are grouped into one set of paid days off. Workers take these days at their own discretion.	Mothers do not have to justify time off to their supervisors. Often, earned time accrues over several years, giving new mothers substantial paid leave after childbirth.	Promotes loyalty because workers feel trusted and valued. Workers often willing to work extra time as need arises because their needs were met when they arose.
Part-time	Workers work less than 35–40 hours/week. Benefits are usually prorated to hours worked.	Gives new mothers more time at home. Often includes flexibility of which hours are worked.	Retains workers with valuable experience and training. Saves recruiting and training new workers.
Job sharing	Two workers each work part time and share the responsibilities and benefits of one job.	Gives mothers more time at home while keeping the same job.	Retrains workers with valuable experience and training. Saves recruiting and training new workers.
Phase back	Workers return from leave to full-time work load gradually over several weeks or months.	Longer return to work adjustment period for mother and baby. More time with infant, when breastfeeding is being established.	Retains workers with experience. Promotes loyalty and dedication of workers.
Flex-time	Workers arrange to work hours to suit their schedules, i.e., 7 AM–3 PM, or 10 AM–6 PM	Can work with spouse's schedule to require less paid child care. Can arrange hours around best times of day to be with baby. Shorter commutes in less traffic.	Workplace covered for more hours/day. Workers better able to focus when schedules suit their needs.
Compressed work week	Workers work more hours on fewer days, i.e., 7 AM–7 PM, 3 days/week.	Allows new mothers full days at home with their babies.	Workers better able to focus when schedules suit their needs. Retains workers with experience and training.
Telecommuting	Workers work all or part of their jobs from home.	Can work around baby's schedule. Less commuting time. Less work clothing and travel expenses.	Retains workers with experience and training. Saves office and parking space.
On-site or near-site day care	Day care provided on or near site, often sponsored by the company.	Can visit baby for nursing etc. during the work day. Commuting time is with baby.	Promotes loyalty among workers. Workers better able to focus when baby is accessible.

Source: Reprinted by permission: Bar-Yam N. Workplace lactation support, part 1: A return to work breastfeeding assessment tool. *J Hum Lact*. 1998;14:249–254.

Table 7-3 Return-to-work breastfeeding assessment worksheet.

	Yes	No	Notes
Type of Job			
1. What is the client's job?			
2. Does she have her own office?			
3. Does she keep her own calendar/control her own time?			
4. Does the client's job involve travel out of town or out of her office?			
5. Are most of her colleagues men or women?*			
Space			
Bathrooms are not acceptable breastfeeding/pumping spaces!			
1. Is there designated private breastfeeding/pumping space (Nursing Mothers' Room/NMR) in the workplace?			
2. Does the space have a sink, a chair, and electrical outlets?			
3. Are pumps available there?			
4. Where is the space in relation to the client's workspace?			
5. How long does it take to get from the workspace to the NMR?			
6. Where will the client store her milk?			
7. If there is no designated space, where will the mother pump?			
8. Can she use the same space every day?			
9. Are there electrical outlets there?			
10. Where is the nearest sink?			
Time			
Pumping should not come at the expense of the mother's lunch!			
1. How old will the baby be upon return to work?			
2. How often will the client be pumping/breastfeeding when she first returns to work?			
3. When will the client pump?			
4. What type of pump will she use? Is there a double pump?			
5. How many parts on the pump must be cleaned out with each use?			
6. Can breaks be taken reliably at the same time every day?			
7. If there is on-site or near-site day care, can the mother go to the baby to nurse?			
Support			
1. What at work knows that the client plans to breastfeed/pump at work?			
2. Does the supervisor need to be informed or consulted?			
3. If so, what are his/her feedings about the client's plan?			
4. Are there other new mothers at work (at the same workplace or colleagues at other workplaces) who are nursing or planning to nurse at work?			
5. Are there mothers at work who have done so in the past?			

	Yes	No	Notes
Support (cont'd)			
6. What are her partner's feelings about the mother's plan to nurse and work?			
7. Do day care providers know how to handle breast milk?			
8. How do they feel about it?			
9. Will on-site or near-site providers call the mother to nurse, if she requests it?			
Gatekeepers			
1. If there is no lactation support program, who can help the client find time and space to pump/breastfeed?			
2. Who is responsible for signing up spare offices/conference rooms?			
3. Who keeps the calendar, answers the phone, greets visitors?			
Supervisor			
1. Must the supervisor be consulted regarding making time and/or space available to pump/breastfeed?			
2. What is the relationship between the client and her supervisor?			
3. Has the client addressed this issue with her supervisor?			
4. If so, what was the response?			
5. If not, what are her concerns about doing so?			
Breastfeeding-Friendly Benefits			
1. Are there any policies in the workplace regarding nursing mothers?			
2. Are there any policies regarding flexibility for new mothers returning to work?			
3. Does the client have access to any of the following programs?			
a. earned time e. flex-time			
b. part-time f. compressed work week			
c. job sharing g. telecommuting			
d. phase back h. on-site or near-site day care			
4. If so, has the client thought about taking advantage of one or more of them!			
5. What is the procedure for doing so?			
6. If not, with whom would the client speak to try to arrange one or more of these programs?			
a. supervisor d. Employee Relations Officer			
b. Human Resources Officer e. Other (specify)			
c. Benefits Officer			

Note: Space for answers is not displayed to scale.

*In some workplaces, men are more understanding and supportive than women and sometimes it is the reverse, but it is good information to have.

Source: Reprinted by permission: Bar-Yam N. Workplace lactation support, part 1: A return-to-work breastfeeding assessment tool. *J Hum Lact*. 1998;14:249–254.

3. Provide anticipatory guidance to assist in prevention of engorgement, mastitis, and maintaining milk supply once she is separated from her baby.
4. Offer realistic expectations for early pumping attempts.
   a. It is normal not to express much milk at first (around 15 ml is common with the first few pumping sessions after 3–4 days postpartum).
   b. With practice, she will learn to trigger the milk ejection reflex with hand expression, massage, and/or pumping.
   c. Sessions of 12 to 15 minutes are generally sufficient to obtain milk for practice feeds and to begin storing milk in the freezer.
   d. Label milk with baby's name and date of expression, and freeze for later use.
5. Help the mother determine the amount of milk her baby will need while the two are apart.
   a. The amount needed depends on many factors, including whether she is exclusively breastfeeding, age of her baby, and the number of hours she is separated from her baby.
   b. Typically, as babies grow, they take less milk as they begin to eat solid foods.
6. A mother who has access to a freezer can begin expressing milk around 2 to 4 weeks postpartum and store it for use when she returns to work. The earlier the mother returns to work, the more frequently she will need to express milk when she is away from her baby.
7. Strategies to facilitate milk expression are included in another discussion (Chapter 30, "Milk Expression, Storage, and Handling").
8. Provide general guidelines on safe storage of human milk (see Chapter 33). Note that guidelines are generally more liberal for storage of milk for healthy infants than for hospitalized infants.
9. Provide strategies for introducing expressed milk to the baby.
   a. Milk can be offered to help the baby become accustomed to being fed by the method that the child care provider will use.
   b. Small volumes can serve to familiarize baby with alternative feeding methods and might be less stressful.
   c. Offer expressed milk when baby is not overly hungry; it is difficult for babies to learn new tasks when they are uncomfortable.
   d. Feedings can often be tolerated better by someone other than the mother.
   e. Waiting too long to introduce a bottle can cause problems with bottle refusal (Fein et al., 1998).
   f. Many mothers choose to use a cup for giving expressed milk to baby.
10. Discuss realistic expectations about her first days back on the job.
    a. Suggest that she return to work on a part-time basis or a partial workweek schedule to shorten the first week away from the baby.
11. Identify community sources for support to boost her confidence in her ability to combine breastfeeding and employment.

C. After the mother returns to work, the lactation consultant can provide information.

   1. Address lactation challenges brought on by separation from her baby (such as engorgement, leaking, and concerns about milk supply).

   2. Adapt the strategies for milk expression and storage to fit the unique work and child care situation she faces.

   3. Dealing with baby's changing feeding patterns:

     a. Many babies sleep long hours when mother is gone as a way of coping with the separation. This "reverse-cycle feeding" means baby wants to be held and nursed a lot when mother is with the baby.

     b. Mothers can view nursing times as a way to rest and cuddle with baby after being apart. Mothers need support from family members to decrease competition from other family work, such as demands from an older child.

     c. When mother and baby are separated during the day, night feedings become more important. Advise the mother not to expect her baby to sleep for long periods.

   4. Listen and validate mothers' feelings on returning to work.

VIII. Assisting Employers with Providing Lactation Support

A. Frame the topic of lactation support as a business conversation, making a business case to get the employer's attention. The U.S. Department of Health and Human Service, Health Resources and Services Administration's Maternal and Child Health Bureau (2008) has published a resource tool kit called *The Business Case for Breastfeeding* to provide that "business case."

B. The lactation consultant is a valuable resource for employers who can help them explore solutions for supporting breastfeeding employees.

C. Provide information and professional materials for employers that explain the business case for breastfeeding and simple steps for establishing a lactation support program (Centers for Disease Control and Prevention, n.d.).

D. Provide information about national, regional, provincial, or state laws related to working and breastfeeding. For example, the United States has enacted a federal law requiring employers to provide breastfeeding employees with the flexible time and private space to express milk during the work period (U.S. Department of Labor, 2011).

E. Offer to serve on a company task force to explore strategies for supporting breastfeeding employees.

F. Provide individual technical assistance to employers who want to establish a worksite lactation program. In some cases, the lactation consultant might be employed by the company to establish a corporate lactation program or to offer assistance to employees.

G. Provide resources for breastfeeding employees at the worksite, and be available for one-on-one assistance to address breastfeeding concerns.

H. Encourage programs in the community to recognize worksites that provide support to breastfeeding employees. For example, in the United States, many state breastfeeding coalitions such as in Washington, Rhode Island, Oklahoma, and Texas have well-developed recognition programs. These programs range from honoring the most outstanding business of the year (for example, Washington) to recognizing any business that meets established criteria (for example, Texas Mother-Friendly Worksite Program). Oklahoma and Rhode Island have established a tiered recognition program to encourage businesses to continue improving lactation support services for breastfeeding women.

IX. Child Care Providers (Roche-Paull, 2010, Chap. 11)

A. Background. A caregiver who supports breastfeeding can make the difference between sustaining breastfeeding and stopping early. Mothers should seek care providers with a positive attitude and who have prior experience with breastfed babies or are willing to learn.

B. Clear communication between parent and caregiver is crucial. They must exchange information daily about baby's feedings, output, and general comfort level.

C. Mothers should discuss their preferences for care, such as paced bottle feeding and ample body contact (holding and carrying), with the caregiver (Kassing, 2002).

D. Infants in child care have higher rates of diarrhea and upper respiratory infections; breastfeeding helps lower the rate of illnesses (Cohen et al., 1995).

E. Addressing child care providers' concerns about handling human milk:

1. Milk is not classified by the U.S. Occupational Safety and Health Administration as requiring "universal precautions" for handling (Kearny et al., 1991; see Appendix B).

2. If caregivers express concerns about handling milk, mothers can prepackage milk for individual feedings using solid, labeled containers.

3. Empty, used bottles are put in a bag for the mother to clean so that the caregiver never handles the milk, only the bottles.

F. See Chapter 31 (Sections VI, VII, VIII, and XIII) in Roche-Paull(2010) for further information about feeding devices and methods.

X. The Lactation Consultant's Role as an Advocate for Working Mothers

A. The lactation consultant is in a pivotal role within the community for encouraging policies and programs to support working mothers with breastfeeding. A lactation consultant must know the maternity protection laws of the city, state/province, and nation, which workers they apply to, how the laws are implemented and monitored, and how an individual worker can exercise her rights under the law.

B. Background. Maternity protection as defined by the International Labor Organization (ILO) includes seven key concepts: *scope* (who is covered by the law); *leave* (maternity leave, paternity leave, parental leave, family and medical leave—who gets it, for how long, whether it is paid, when it can be taken, whether it is optional or compulsory); *benefits* (medical care for pregnancy, birth, and recovery, income replacement during leave, who pays for benefits—public insurance/social security, the employer, both, or neither); *health protection* (women are protected from workplace risks during pregnancy and lactation, have the right to return to their job or an equivalent job when the risk period is over, and can take time from work for medical care during pregnancy); *job protection and nondiscrimination* (employed mothers are placed in the same job or an equivalent job when returning after leave, and they are treated the same on the job as men and women without children; *nursing breaks* (women have the right to one or more paid breaks or a daily reduction of hours of work for breastfeeding or expressing milk during the workday). The ILO also recommends *breastfeeding facilities* (a clean, private place at or near the workplace where a woman can breastfeed her baby or express milk, plus secure storage for the milk). National law in many countries requires employers to provide a *crèche* at or near the workplace if they have more than a minimum number of female workers.

C. Laws and programs that affect employed mothers may be implemented by various government agencies, such as those that cover labor, business and industry, employment, poverty alleviation, economic development, gender, or women's affairs.

D. Be aware that legal protection alone does not guarantee optimal infant feeding. Italy's breastfeeding rates are modest despite excellent national maternity protection laws (Chapin, 2001).

E. Advocacy for better laws can be conducted at local, state/provincial, national, regional, and international levels. Be strategic in choosing where to act.

F. Meet with your legislative representatives to discuss breastfeeding policy issues in your area.

G. Join with coalitions that advocate on behalf of workers and/or families. Educate them about breastfeeding issues while you learn from them about the broader work-related issues such as maternity leave and family leave.

H. Community education. Offer to speak at community business and service organization meetings, meetings of trade unions that employ many women (such as nurses, domestic workers, hospitality and retail workers, or teachers), or at employer organizations that meet regularly. Set up displays at job fairs or health fairs in the community to provide information on the importance of combining breastfeeding and employment.

I. Provide prenatal education about breastfeeding at lunchtime seminars with pregnant workers at selected worksites. Offer to facilitate a working mothers' support group meeting at worksites in the community that meets during lunch or in the evenings.

J. Begin a coalition, or ask the existing community breastfeeding coalition, to conduct outreach with local worksites. Provide companies with information about supporting breastfeeding and available resources in the community.

K. Alert the media about advancements in breastfeeding support in community worksites. Publicity helps women view continued breastfeeding as the social norm, provides positive public relations to employers, and encourages other worksites to follow their lead.

References

Agency for Healthcare Research and Quality. (2007). *Breastfeeding and maternal and infant health outcomes in developed countries.* Washington, DC: Author. Retrieved from http://www.ahrq.gov/downloads/pub/evidence/pdf/brfout/brfout.pdf

American Academy of Pediatrics. (2005). Policy statement on breastfeeding and the use of human milk. *Pediatrics, 115*, 496–506. Retrieved from http://aappolicy.aappublications.org/cgi/content/full/pediatrics;115/2/496

Amin, R., Said, Z., Sutan, R., Shah, S., Darus, A., & Shamsuddin, K. (2011). Work related determinants of breastfeeding discontinuation among employed mothers in Malaysia. *International Breastfeeding Journal, 6*(4). Retrieved from http://www.internationalbreastfeedingjournal.com/content/6/1/4

Angeletti, M. A. (2009). Breastfeeding mothers returning to work: Possibilities for information, anticipatory guidance and support from US health care professionals. *Journal of Human Lactation, 25*(2), 226–232.

Arlotti, J., Cottrell, B., Lee, S., & Curtin, J. (1998). Breastfeeding among low-income women with and without peer support. *Journal of Community Health Nursing, 5*, 163–178.

Arthur, C., Saenz, R. B., & Replogle, W. H. (2003). The employment-related breastfeeding decisions of physician mothers. *Journal of the Mississippi State Medical Association, 44*, 383–387.

Ball, T., & Wright, A. (1999). Health care costs of formula-feeding in the first year of life. *Pediatrics, 103*, 871–876.

Bartick, M., & Reinhold, A. (2010). The burden of suboptimal breastfeeding in the United States: A pediatric cost analysis. *Pediatrics, 125*, e1048–e1056.

Bar-Yam, N. (1998). Workplace lactation support, part 1: A return-to-work breastfeeding assessment tool. *Journal of Human Lactation, 14*, 249–254.

Berger, L. M., Hill, J., & Waldfogel, J. (2005). Maternity leave, early maternal employment and child health and development in the US. *Economic Journal, 115*, F29–F47.

Best Start Social Marketing. (1996). *Research brief: USDA WIC National Breastfeeding Loving Support Campaign.* Tampa, FL: Author.

Bocar, D. (1997). Combining breastfeeding and employment: Increasing success. *Journal of Perinatal and Neonatal Nursing, 11*, 23–43.

Bourgoin, G., Lahaie, N., Rheaume, B., et al. (1997). Factors influencing the duration of breastfeeding in the Sudbury region. *Canadian Journal of Public Health, 88*, 238–241.

Bridges, C., Frank, D., & Curtin, J. (1997). Employer attitudes toward breastfeeding in the workplace. *Journal of Human Lactation, 13*(3), 215–219.

Brown, C., Poag, S., & Kasprzycki, C. (2001). Exploring large employers' and small employers' knowledge, attitudes, and practices on breastfeeding support in the workplace. *Journal of Human Lactation, 17*, 39–46.

Centers for Disease Control and Prevention. Healthier Worksite Initiative. Retrieved from http://www.cdc.gov/nccdphp/dnpao/hwi/toolkits/lactation/index.htm

Chapin, E. M. (2001). The state of the Innocenti Declaration targets in Italy. *Journal of Human Lactation, 17*(3), 202–206.

Chow, T., Fulmer I., & Olson, B. (2011). Perspectives of managers toward workplace breastfeeding support in the State of Michigan. *Journal of Human Lactation, 27*, 138–146.

Cohen, R., Lange, L., & Slusser, W. (2002). A description of a male-focused breastfeeding promotion corporate lactation program. *Journal of Human Lactation, 18*(1), 61–65.

Cohen, R., & Mrtek, M. B. (1994). The impact of two corporate lactation programs on the incidence and duration of breastfeeding by employed mothers. *American Journal of Health Promotion, 8,* 436–441.

Cohen, R., Mrtek, M., & Mrtek, R. G. (1995). Comparison of maternal absenteeism and infant illness rates among breast-feeding and formula-feeding women in two corporations. *American Journal of Health Promotion, 10,* 148–153.

Condon, M. (2005). Breast is best, but it could be better: What is in breast milk that should not be? *Pediatric Nursing, 31*(4), 333–338.

Corbett-Dick, P., & Bezek, S. K. (1997). Breastfeeding promotion for the employed mother. *Journal of Pediatric Health Care, 11,* 12–19.

Cox, D. B., Owens, R. A., & Hartmann, P. E. (1996). Blood and milk prolactin and the rate of milk synthesis in women. *Experimental Physiology, 81,* 1007–1020.

Dabritz, H. A., Hinton, B. G., & Babb, J. (2009). Evaluation of lactation support in the workplace or school environment on 6-month breastfeeding outcomes in Yolo County, California. *Journal of Human Lactation, 25*(2), 182–193.

Dunn, B. F., Zavela, K. J., Cline, A. D., & Cost, P. A. (2004). Breastfeeding practices in Colorado businesses. *Journal of Human Lactation, 20*(2), 217–218.

Fairness Initiative on Low-Wage Work. (n.d.). The story of low wage work. Retrieved from http://www.lowwagework.org/story

Faught, L. (1994, September/October). Lactation programs benefit the family and the cooperation. *Journal of Compensation and Benefits,* 44–47.

Fein, S. B., Mandal, B., & Roe, B. E. (2008). Success of strategies for combining employment and breastfeeding. *Pediatrics, 122*(Suppl. 2), S562.

Fein, S. B., & Roe, B. (1998). The effect of work status on initiation and duration of breastfeeding. *American Journal of Public Health, 88,* 1042–1046.

Frank, E. (1998). Breastfeeding and maternal employment: Two rights don't make a wrong. *Lancet, 352,* 1083–1085.

Galtry, J. (1997). Lactation and the labor market: Breastfeeding, labor market changes, and public policy in the United States. *Health Care for Women International, 18,* 467–480.

Galtry, J. (2003). The impact on breastfeeding of labour market policy and practice in Ireland, Sweden, and the USA. *Social Science and Medicine, 57,* 167–177.

Gielen, A. C., Faden, R. R., O'Campo, P., et al. (1991). Maternal employment during the early postpartum period: Effects on initiation and continuation of breastfeeding. *Pediatrics, 87,* 298–305.

Hanson, M., Hellerstedt, W. L., Desvarieux, M., & Duval, S. J. (2003). Correlates of breast-feeding in a rural population. *American Journal of Health Behavior, 27,* 432–444.

Hills-Bonczyk, S. G., Avery, M. D., Savik, K., et al. (1993). Women's experiences with combining breastfeeding and employment. *Journal of Nurse Midwifery, 38,* 257–266.

Hochschild, A., & Machung, A. (2003). *The second shift.* New York, NY: Penguin Books.

International Labour Organization. (2004). *Global employment trends for women 2004.* Geneva, Switzerland: ILO. Retrieved from http://www.ilo.org/empelm/pubs/WCMS_114289/lang--en/index.htm

International Labour Organization. (2007). Women in the workplace: New ILO report highlights how action in the world of work can help reduce maternal deaths. Retrieved from http://www.ilo.org/global/about-the-ilo/press-and-media-centre/insight/WCMS_084620/lang--en/index.htm

International Lactation Consultant Association. (2007). *Position paper on breastfeeding and work.* Retrieved from http://www.ilca.org/files/resources/ilca_publications/BreasfeedingandWorkPP.pdf

Kassing, D. (2002). Bottle-feeding as a tool to reinforce breastfeeding. *Journal of Human Lactation, 18*(1), 56–60.

Katcher, A., & Lanese, M. (1985). Breastfeeding by employed mothers: A reasonable accommodation in the workplace. *Pediatrics, 75,* 644–647.

Kearny, M., & Cronenwett, L. (1991). Breastfeeding and employment. *Journal of Obstetric, Gynecologic, and Neonatal Nursing, 20,* 471–480.

Kurinij, N., Shiono, P., Ezrine, S., & Rhoades, G. (1989). Does maternal employment affect breastfeeding? *American Journal of Public Health, 79,* 1247–1250.

Lewallen, L. P., Dick, M. J., Flowers, J., et al. (2006). Breastfeeding support and early cessation. *Journal of Obstetric, Gynecologic, and Neonatal Nursing, 35,* 166–172.

Libbus, M., & Bullock, L. (2002). Breastfeeding and employment: An assessment of employer attitudes. *Journal of Human Lactation, 18,* 247–251.

Lindberg, L. D. (1996). Trends in the relationship between breastfeeding and postpartum employment in the United States. *Social Biology, 43,* 191–202.

Lyness, K., Thompson, C., Francesco, A., & Judiesch, M. (1999). Work and pregnancy: Individual and organizational factors influencing organizational commitment, timing of maternity leave, and return to work. *Sex Roles, 41,* 485–508.

Mandal, B., Roe, B., & Fein, S. (2010). The differential effects of full-time and part-time work status on breastfeeding. *Health Policy, 97*(1), 79–86.

Maternity Protection Coalition. (2008). *Maternity protection campaign kit, section 9: How to support women in the informal economy to combine their productive and reproductive roles.* Retrieved from http://www.waba.org.my/whatwedo/womenandwork/pdf/09.pdf

McLeod, D., Pullon, S., & Cookson, T. (2002). Factors influencing continuation of breastfeeding in a cohort of women. *Journal of Human Lactation, 18,* 335–343.

Meek, J. Y. (2001). Breastfeeding in the workplace. *Pediatric Clinics of North America, 48,* 461–474.

Moquin, C. (2008). *Babies at work: Bringing new life to the workplace.* Framingham, MA: Author. Retrieved from http://www.parentingatwork.org/help.html

Nichols, M., & Roux, G. (2004). Maternal perspectives on postpartum return to the workplace. *Journal of Obstetrical, Gynecological and Neonatal Nursing, 33*(4), 463–471.

Olang, B., Farivar, K., Heidarzadeh, A., Strandvik, B., & Yngve, A.

(please note spelling changes on Farivar and Strandvik) (2009). Breastfeeding in Iran: Prevalence, duration and current recommendations. *International Breastfeeding Journal, 4*(8). Retrieved from http://www.internationalbreastfeedingjournal.com/content/4/1/8

Ortiz, J., McGilligan, K., & Kelly, P. (2004). Duration of breast milk expression among working mothers enrolled in an employer-sponsored lactation program. *Pediatric Nursing, 30,* 111–119.

Otoo, G., Lartey, A., & Perez-Escamilla, R. (2009). Perceived incentives and barriers to exclusive breastfeeding among periurban Ghanian women. *Journal of Human Lactation, 25*(1), 34–41.

Page, D. (2008). Breastfeeding and returning to work… working out the details. *Journal of Human Lactation, 24,* 85.

Piper, B., & Parks, P. L. (1996). Predicting the duration of lactation: Evidence from a national survey. *Birth, 23,* 7–12.

Roche-Paull, R. (2010). *Breastfeeding in combat boots: A survival guide to successful breastfeeding while serving in the military.* Amarillo, TX: Hale Publishing.

Roe, B., Whittington, L. A., Fein, S. B., & Teisl, M. E. (1999). Is there competition between breastfeeding and maternal employment? *Demography, 36*, 157–171.

Romero, S. Q., Bernal, R., Barbiero, C., Passamonte, R., & Cattaneo, A. (2006). A rapid ethnographic study of breastfeeding in the north and south of Italy. *International Breastfeeding Journal, 1*, 14.

Ryan A, Wenjun…costa A. (2002). Breastfeeding continues to increase into the new millennium. *Pediatrics, 110*, 1103–1109.

Scott, J., Landers, M., Huges, R., & Binns, C. (2001). Factors associated with breastfeeding at discharge and duration of breastfeeding. *Journal of Paediatrics and Child Health, 37*, 254–261.

Semega-Janneh, I. J. (1998). Chapter 9: The second Abraham Horwitz lecture, 1998. Breastfeeding: From biology to policy. Retrieved from http://www.unsystem.org/scn/archives/npp17/ch11.htm

Slusser, W. M., Lange, L., Eickson, V., et al. (2004). Breast milk expression in the workplace: A look at frequency and time. *Journal of Human Lactation, 20*, 164–169.

Smith, J., & Elwood, M. (2006). *Where does a mother's day go? Preliminary estimates from the Australian Time Use Survey of New Mothers.* Canberra Australia: Australian Centre for Economic Research on Health, the Australian National University.

Smith, J. P., Ingham, L. H., & Dunstone, M. D. (1998, May). *The economic value of breastfeeding in Australia* (NCEPH Working Paper #40). Canberra, Australia: National Centre for Epidemiology and Population Health.

Sullivan, M. L., Leathers, S. J., & Kelley, M. A. (2004). Family characteristics associated with duration of breastfeeding during early infancy among primiparas. *Journal of Human Lactation, 20*(2), 196–205.

Suyes, K., Abrahams, S. W., & Labbok, M. H. (2008). Breastfeeding in the workplace: Other employees' attitudes towards services for lactating mothers. *International Breastfeeding Journal, 3*, 25.

Taveras, E., Capra, A., Braveman, P., Jensvold, N., Escobar, G., & Lieu, T. (2003). Clinician support and psychosocial risk factors associated with breastfeeding discontinuation. *Pediatrics, 112*, 108–115.

Tuttle, C. R., & Slavit, W. I. (2009). Establishing the business case for breastfeeding. *Breastfeeding Medicine, 4*(Suppl. 1), S59–62.

United Nations Women. Women migrant workers. Retrieved at http://www.unifem.org/gender_issues/women_poverty_economics/women_migrant_workers.php

United States Breastfeeding Committee. (2002). *Workplace breastfeeding support* [issue paper]. Raleigh, NC: Author. Retrieved from http://www.usbreastfeeding.org/LinkClick.aspx?link=Publications%2fWorkplace-2002-USBC.pdf&tabid=70&mid=388

U.S. Department of Health and Human Services, Health Resources and Services Administration, Maternal and Child Health Bureau. (2003). *Research brief: Using loving support to develop breastfeeding-friendly worksites support kit.* Rockville, MD: Author.

U.S. Department of Health and Human Services. Health Resources and Services Administration, Maternal and Child Health Bureau. (2008). *The business case for breastfeeding.* Rockville, MD: Author.

U.S. Department of Labor, Wage and Hour Division. (2011). Break time for nursing mothers. Retrieved from http://www.dol.gov/whd/nursingmothers/

Vanek, E. P., & Vanek, J. A. (2001). Job sharing as an employment alternative in group medical practice. *Medical Group Management Journal, 48*, 20–24.

Wambach, K. (1998). Maternal fatigue in breastfeeding primiparae during the first nine weeks postpartum. *Journal of Human Lactation, 14*, 219–229.

Warwick, H., & Doig, A. (2004). *Smoke—the killer in the kitchen: Indoor air pollution in developing countries*. London, England: ITDG Publishing. http://practicalaction.org/docs/smoke/itdg%20 smoke%20report.pdf

Whaley, S., Meehan, K., Lange, L., et al. (2002). Predictors of breastfeeding duration for employees of the Special Supplemental Nutrition Program for Women, Infants, and Children (WIC). *American Dietetic Association, 102*, 1290–1293.

Win, N. N., Binns, C. W., Zhao, Y., Scott, J. A., & Oddy, W. H. (2006). Breastfeeding duration in mothers who express breast milk: A cohort study. *International Breastfeeding Journal, 1*, 28.

Wyatt, S. (2002). Challenges of the working breastfeeding mother. Workplace solutions. *American Association of Occupational Health Nurses, 50*(2), 61–66.

Zinn, B. (2000). Supporting the employed breastfeeding mother. *Journal of Midwifery and Women's Health, 145*, 216–226.

Suggested Reading

Auerbach, K. (1990). Assisting the employed breastfeeding mother. *Journal of Nurse Midwifery, 35*, 26–34.

Bar-Yam, N. (1998). Workplace lactation support, part II: Working with the workplace. *Journal of Human Lactation, 14*, 321–325.

Lauwers, J., & Swisher, A. (2005). When breastfeeding is interrupted. In J. Lauwers & A. Swisher (Eds.), *Counseling the nursing mother* (Chap. 24, pp. 485–495). Sudbury, MA: Jones and Bartlett.

Maternity Protection Coalition. (2008). *Maternity protection campaign kit, section 9: How to support women in the informal economy to combine their productive and reproductive roles*. Retrieved from http://www.waba.org.my/whatwedo/womenandwork/pdf/09.pdf

Nichols, L. (2001). Then comes the baby in the baby carriage: The economic resource use of new mothers. *Abstracts International, 61*, 2925-A.

Petersen, D. J., & Boller, H. R. (2004). Employers' duty to accommodate breast-feeding, working mothers. *Employee Relations Law Journal, 30*, 80–88.

U.S. Department of Health and Human Services. Health Resources and Services Administration, Maternal and Child Health Bureau. (2008). *The Business case for Breastfeeding*. Rockville, MD.

Walker, M. (2005). Physical, medical, emotional, and environmental challenges to the breastfeeding mother. In M. Walker (Ed.), *Breastfeeding management for the clinician* (Chap. 9). Sudbury, MA: Jones and Bartlett.

Wambach, K., & Rojjanasrirat, W. (2005). Maternal employment and breastfeeding. In J. Riordan (Ed.), *Breastfeeding and human lactation* (Chap. 17). Sudbury, MA: Jones and Bartlett.

CHAPTER 8
Caring for Vulnerable Populations

Cynthia Turner-Maffei, MA, IBCLC

OBJECTIVES

- Describe cultural competency vis-à-vis breastfeeding.
- Identify two strategies that have been successful in promoting breastfeeding in vulnerable populations.
- Demonstrate awareness of the rationale for special concerns regarding breastfeeding and vulnerable populations.

INTRODUCTION

Lactation consultants strive to promote, support, and protect breastfeeding among all families. The benefits of breastfeeding are particularly advantageous for families living in vulnerable situations. Disparities and inequities in access to healthcare services, including breastfeeding care, abound within vulnerable populations as a result of financial, language, geographic, and cultural barriers. Special emphasis must be placed on meeting the needs of those who are less able to access breastfeeding education and support. Lactation consultants should endeavor to develop cultural competency to address these barriers. Lactation care providers must work with health systems and other key stakeholders to improve access to lactation and health care for all members of society. Lactation consultants should be aware of the need to protect, promote, and support appropriate infant feeding during disaster situations, whether related to natural events, political conflicts, terrorism, environmental disasters, and other events, and should work with their communities to recognize and support the unique resource of human milk in these situations.

I. Issues of Vulnerable Populations Regarding Breastfeeding

A. Low-income families

1. In some nations, women from low-income families are less likely to breast-feed. In other nations, the reverse is true. Data collected by UNICEF (2011) demonstrate that in South Asia, women of the highest income category are the most likely to initiate breastfeeding, while the reverse is true in East Asia and the Pacific, and North Africa and the Middle East, where women of the lowest income category are the most likely to breastfeed.

2. Infant formula is often beyond the economic reach of low-income families. As an expensive commodity, formula may have a greater perceived value than breast-milk. The ability to purchase formula is a status symbol in some communities.

3. Where the *International Code of Marketing of Breast-milk Substitutes* (World Health Organization [WHO], 1981) is unimplemented, or is incompletely implemented, low-income women may be at greater risk of changing practice because of messages received. For example, women who received samples or gifts of infant formula from healthcare providers and/or health systems have been shown to have more difficulty achieving their own exclusive breastfeed-ing intention (Declerq et al., 2009), as well as are at increased risk of cessation of breastfeeding within the first 2 weeks and early introduction of solid foods (Howard et al., 2000).

4. The ease of integrating breastfeeding and employment ranges widely. Women working full time outside the home have an increased risk of early cessation of breastfeeding and a shorter duration of exclusive breastfeeding (Dearden et al., 2002; Ryan et al., 2006). Women working in low-wage positions may have more difficulty getting approval for breaks for breastfeeding or milk expression.

5. Low-income populations often have limited access to healthcare services, including lactation care. Where lactation care is available largely on a fee-for-service basis, such help may be beyond the financial means of many families.

B. Minority families

1. Traditions, beliefs, and values surrounding breastfeeding vary widely among the world's cultures. The identity of the individual with the greatest influence regarding the parents' infant feeding choice varies from culture to culture.

   a. Some cultures value external authority figures, including healthcare provid-ers, as influential in decisions such as infant feeding.

   b. In other cultures, grandmothers, fathers, peers, and/or other community members may have the greatest authority. Mothers want and need support of these individuals, but their advice may not be in line with current man-agement of breastfeeding (Grassley et al., 2008).

   c. Authority-based breastfeeding promotion programs have the potential to be counterproductive if not carefully designed.

2. Many nations have collected data regarding racial/ethnic differences in breast-feeding and have divergent findings. Kelly et al. (2006) reported that the high-est breastfeeding rates occur among black and Asian women in the United

Kingdom, which they contrasted with the lowest rates in the United States recorded among non-Hispanic black mothers. Promotion strategies developed for one specific community may not apply to another.

3. Minority families may experience inequities in access to care on the basis of language as well as other factors. If the healthcare system does not embrace multicultural health beliefs and practices, individuals may be less likely to seek help from the system.

4. Workplace accommodations may also be an issue for women from minority cultures.

C. Immigrant families

1. Immigrant families may assume different breastfeeding patterns than were practiced in their homeland (Homer et al., 2002; Singh et al., 2007).

2. These changes in breastfeeding patterns may reflect immigrant women's assimilation of the infant feeding norms of their new nation. In some industrialized countries, breastfeeding is relatively invisible, practiced largely in private homes, whereas bottlefeedingis the visible cultural norm. One study found that although recent immigrants to the United States were more likely to breastfeed than native-born women, their likelihood of breastfeeding declined 4% with every year lived in the United States (Gibson-Davis et al., 2006).

3. Foreign workers may have less access to workplace accommodations for breastfeeding/expressing milk, which may shorten breastfeeding duration (Mohd Amin et al., 2011).

4. Other factors that may influence breastfeeding include the following:
   a. Degree of cultural acceptability of breastfeeding
   b. Availability, affordability, and visibility of breastmilk substitutes
   c. Presence or absence of support provided by larger family networks
   d. Access to lactation care and services

D. Families experiencing disasters and emergencies

1. Emergency situations such as natural disasters including floods, tsunamis, earthquakes, political conflicts, and environmental disasters appear to be increasing in incidence. Emergencies result in displacement of large numbers of people and food insecurity. The World Health Organization and UNICEF (2003) reported that refugees and internally displaced persons alone numbered 40 million worldwide, including 5.5 million children under the age of 5 years. The number and magnitude of such crises require a concerted approach regarding appropriate infant and young child feeding.

2. Families have an urgent need for infant feeding support during these crises. The resultant trauma, lack of access to safe water and food, insufficient medical care, violence, and displacement can have a long-lasting, unspoken effect on all aspects of daily life, including infant feeding.

3. Breastfeeding makes an unparalleled contribution to the health of children living in emergency situations. Research from Guinea-Bissau demonstrates that weaned children suffered a sixfold higher mortality than those who continued to breastfeed during the first 3 months of war (Jakobsen et al., 2003).

4. The visibility and accessibility of donated formula and powdered milk, along with general lack of awareness of women's abilities to continue to lactate and to relactate in emergency situations, can be deterrents to continued breastfeeding.

II. Helpful Approaches in Caring for Vulnerable Populations

A. Cultural competency.

1. Cultural competency is a key skill for lactation consultants. Cultural competence has been defined as follows:

> Cultural and linguistic competence is a set of congruent behaviors, attitudes, and policies that come together in a system, agency, or among professionals that enables effective work in cross-cultural situations. "Culture" refers to integrated patterns of human behavior that include the language, thoughts, communications, actions, customs, beliefs, values, and institutions of racial, ethnic, religious, or social groups. "Competence" implies having the capacity to function effectively as an individual and an organization within the context of the cultural beliefs, behaviors, and needs presented by consumers and their communities. (Office on Minority Health, 2001; adapted from Cross, 1989)

2. A survey of cultural competency of health professionals working with lactating women in a large U.S. city found that 77% did not achieve a score of cultural competence (Noble et al., 2009).

3. The first step toward developing cultural competency is for each provider to undertake self-assessment. Care is enhanced when each care provider identifies and endeavors to remain conscious of his or her own cultural values and biases.

4. Care providers and their clients might have divergent beliefs about issues such as the etiology of problems, appropriate care plans, and so on.

    a. Exploring the client's viewpoint is a key strategy for arriving at mutually acceptable care plans.

        i. The lactation consultant can ask respectful questions so as to begin to determine whether a mother's cultural traditions are helpful, harmless, or harmful to the breastfeeding relationship (Riordan, 2010).

        ii. Involve the father, grandmother, and others as appropriate in the counseling session. The identity of the most influential person in a woman's feeding decision varies among cultures. Some identified individuals are the mother's relatives (particularly the mother's mother), peers, partners, and healthcare providers (Narayanan et al., 2005; Susin et al., 2005).

        iii. Several sources have identified general medical beliefs and values of different cultures. Such information can provide a framework for initial exploration with clients (Kleinman, 2008; Office of Minority Health, n.d.).

        iv. Although it is possible to generalize about the experience of many groups of people, it is impossible to predict the meaning of an experience for any individual. Truly culturally competent care makes no assumptions about the experience, practices, or viewpoints of others.

    b. Cultural beliefs and practices such as avoiding breastfeeding during the colostral phase have an impact on breastfeeding (Hizel et al., 2006). The practice of feeding an infant other foods (including formula) during the first days of life might lead healthcare workers to assume incorrectly that a mother has chosen not to breastfeed. Failing to explore the meaning of the practice closes the door to mutual understanding.

    i. New educational media and strategies should be designed, tested, and evaluated based on input from members of the target community. Messages must be crafted to resonate with cultural ideas and values (Chen, 2010).

B. Strategies for individual education/counseling encounters

  1. Establish an environment of trust and respect.

    a. Distrust of health workers is a continuing concern in research among disenfranchised populations (Cricco-Lizza, 2007). Seek to build a trusting relationship with the mother and family (Sheppard et al., 2004). Cricco-Lizza (2007) suggests strategies to generate trust in a research setting, which have resonance for lactation care. These strategies include respectful entry into the field (taking time to establish the connection); recognizing and decreasing differences in power (acknowledging and addressing power imbalances); sensitivity to time and timing (acknowledging that there are other priorities in the client's life); and adopting a relational approach (seeking continuity in the relationship).

    b. Ask respectful, open-ended questions.

    c. Inquire about and practice sensitivity to different customs regarding eye contact, body language, touching the mother and the baby.

    d. Be aware that many mothers report that they dislike hands-on breastfeeding help (**Figure 8-1**) (Hannula et al., 2008; Weimers et al., 2006). These studies identify that women prefer a hands-off helping approach (**Figure 8-2**), in which the lactation care provider uses words, pictures, or a doll to guide the mother in changing the way in which she holds her baby and her breast.

  2. Seek to understand the unique perspective of each woman.

    a. Invite each woman to express her knowledge and concerns.

    b. A series of questions designed for this purpose (Kleinman, 2008, p. 106) can be helpful in elaborating a woman's understanding and cultural knowledge of the situation.

    c. Without such knowledge, the care provider might unwittingly provide information that violates a client's belief structure.

  3. Include partners and family members in encounters as is possible and propriate. Fathers are often not included in breastfeeding counseling, but research indicates that involving fathers can improve outcomes (Engebretsen et al., 2010; Pisacane et al., 2005; Susin et al., 2008). Grandmothers often play a key support role but may need updating on current breastfeeding management (Grassley & Eschiti, 2008; Susin et al., 2005; Narayanan et al., 2005).

  4. Acknowledge any expressed concerns. This type of active listening response tells the client that the counselor is listening to and values the client's viewpoint.

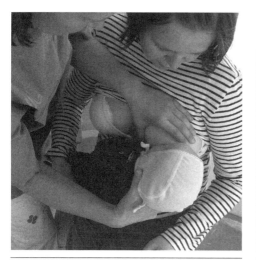

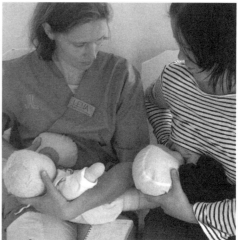

Figure 8-1 Hands-On Helping Method
Source: Courtesy of Lena Weimers, IBCLC

Figure 8-2 Hands-Off Helping
Source: Courtesy of Lena Weimers, IBCLC

5. Offer understanding and carefully targeted educational messages (Bryant et al., 1992).

6. Develop action plans together with the client, making sure to gather the client's feedback regarding suggested action plans.

   a. After proposing an action plan, ask for the client's feedback. For example, ask the client questions such as "Would you be willing to undertake such a plan?" "Do you have the resources needed to implement the plan?" and "What questions do you have about the plan as suggested?"

   b. Explore whether there are any specific concerns about proposed action plans. For example, the goal of treatment of the postpartum woman in the humoral health practices of many of the world's cultures is to keep the woman warm, eating, drinking, and surrounding herself with substances classified as "hot" and to avoid those that are associated with cold. Foods or practices that make the woman and baby safe in the postpartum period may conflict with best breastfeeding management practices (Fishman et al., 1988). For example, a woman practicing humoral health may perceive her lactation care provider's suggestion to apply ice to her engorged breasts as contradictory to her cultural practices.

7. Develop careful follow-up plans.

   a. Integrate breastfeeding follow-up with other services (such as pediatric follow-up) to the extent possible.

   b. Identify whether the woman is expected to contact the consultant or vice versa.

   c. Many clients move frequently and do not have regular access to a telephone. Establish backup communication plans.

8. Know that women who have familial or financial problems might require special attention and extra counseling sessions so that they can be helped to identify how to achieve and sustain exclusive breastfeeding (MacGregor et al., 2010).

9. If the lactation care provider cannot communicate effectively in the same language as the family being served, provisions should be made for the use of an interpreter. Children should not be depended on to convey medical information between mothers and healthcare providers. Provide written materials in the mother's native language at an easy reading level. Pictorially based materials are helpful for those who may not be able to read the language they speak.

10. Consider implementing breastfeeding peer counseling programs.
    a. Peer counseling programs have been identified among the most effective strategies for breastfeeding promotion and preservation (Agrasada et al., 2005; Haider et al., 2002; Leite et al., 2005; Martens, 2002).
    b. Women who have had successful breastfeeding experiences and who are members of the target community are recruited and trained to counsel and support pregnant and parenting mothers.
    c. Peer counseling programs are often low-cost methods of providing breastfeeding help. Further, they may have the effect of disseminating breastfeeding knowledge into communities that may be underserved by the existing health system structure, such as adolescents, migrant workers, and others.

11. Develop other social support strategies to provide a network of support.
    a. Many mothers consider social support more valuable than health system–based support (McInnes et al., 2008).
    b. Other models for social support have been described, including community-based breastfeeding support groups (Hoddinott et al., 2006); breastfeeding apprenticeships in which pregnant women visit with breastfeeding mothers in their neighborhood (Hoddinott et al., 1999); and grandmother support activities (Illinois State Breastfeeding Task Force, n.d.).

III. Improving Support for Vulnerable Populations in the Healthcare System

A. Integrate breastfeeding support into comprehensive medical care.
   1. Several researchers have shown that providing continuous lactation care within the framework of comprehensive prenatal, postpartum, and pediatric care is most effective in increasing incidence (Li et al., 2004), duration (Labarere et al., 2005), and exclusivity (Labarere et al., 2005) of breastfeeding.
   2. Encourage breastfeeding training for all healthcare providers interacting with breastfeeding families.
   3. Increase awareness of community breastfeeding support systems and services among healthcare providers.

B. Develop cultural competency programs within healthcare systems and among healthcare providers.

1. Identify individuals within the target community who are willing to serve as "cultural brokers" (Fadiman, 1998) to provide cultural interpretation when needed for lactation consultants and other members of the healthcare team.
2. Encourage cultural assessment to identify the major values, health beliefs, and practices of target populations (Tripp-Reimer et al., 1984).
3. Encourage systems and providers to study the impact of healthcare practices (for example, distribution of formula samples) on breastfeeding outcomes.
4. Explore barriers to breastfeeding through interviews with community members, and use this information to design new programs and strategies (Riordan et al., 2001).

C. Offer education regarding the identification of breastfeeding as the safest infant feeding method in all situations, including emergencies.

IV. Improving Support for Vulnerable Populations During Emergencies

A. Lactation consultants are encouraged to work with local disaster relief groups to increase knowledge of the role of exclusive breastfeeding and appropriate complementary feeding in protecting optimal child health. Lactation consultants may be called on to build the knowledge and skill of relief workers.

B. Lactation consultants should familiarize themselves with resources such as those offered by the IFE Core Group (2007a, 2007b, 2010) and the position statements of the International Lactation Consultant Association (ILCA, n.d.), the World Alliance for Breastfeeding Action (WABA, 2009), Wellstart International (2005), and other appropriate governmental and nongovernmental organizations regarding this topic.

C. Seek to educate the public about the possible negative effects of formula donation and the need to establish careful handling of infant formula during emergencies (IBFAN-ICDC, 2009).

Summary

Through self-assessment, cultural awareness, respectful counseling, and developed skill, lactation consultants can help vulnerable families have satisfying breastfeeding experiences. Just as breastfeeding is an empowering and satisfying experience for many women and their families, working with families who are in vulnerable situations provides lactation consultants many opportunities for professional growth and fulfillment.

References

Agrasada, G. V., Gustafsson, J., Kylberg, E., & Ewald, U. (2005). Postnatal peer counselling on exclusive breastfeeding of low-birthweight infants: A randomized, controlled trial. *Acta Paediatrica (Oslo, Norway: 1992)*, *94*(8), 1109–1115.

Akter, S., & Rahman, M. M. (2010). Duration of breastfeeding and its correlates in Bangladesh. *Journal of Health, Population, and Nutrition*, *28*(6), 595–601.

Bryant, C. A., Coreil, J., D'Angelo, S. L., Bailey, D. F., & Lazarov, M. (1992). A strategy for promoting breastfeeding among economically disadvantaged women and adolescents. *NAACOG's Clinical Issues in Perinatal and Women's Health Nursing*, *3*(4), 723–730.

Chen, W. (2010). Understanding the cultural context of Chinese mothers' perceptions of breastfeeding and infant health in Canada. *Journal of Clinical Nursing*, *19*(7–8), 1021–1029.

Cricco-Lizza, R. (2007). Ethnography and the generation of trust in breastfeeding disparities research. *Applied Nursing Research: ANR*, *20*(4), 200–204.

Dearden, K. A., Quan, L. N., Do, M., Marsh, D. R., Pachón, H., Schroeder, D. G., & Lang, T. T. (2002). Work outside the home is the primary barrier to exclusive breastfeeding in rural Viet Nam: Insights from mothers who exclusively breastfed and worked. *Food and Nutrition Bulletin*, *23*(4 Suppl.), 101–108.

Declercq, E., Labbok, M. H., Sakala, C., & O'Hara, M. (2009). Hospital practices and women's likelihood of fulfilling their intention to exclusively breastfeed. *American Journal of Public Health*, *99*(5), 929–935.

Engebretsen, I. M., Moland, K. M., Nankunda, J., Karamagi, C. A., Tylleskär, T., & Tumwine, J. K. (2010). Gendered perceptions on infant feeding in Eastern Uganda: Continued need for exclusive breastfeeding support. *International Breastfeeding Journal*, *5*, 13.

Fadiman, A. (1998). *The spirit catches you and you fall down: A Hmong child, her American doctors, and the collision of two cultures*. New York, NY: Farrar Straus and Giroux.

Fishman, C., Evans, R., & Jenks, E. (1988). Warm bodies, cool milk: Conflicts in post partum food choice for Indochinese women in California. *Social Science & Medicine*, 26(11), 1125–1132.

Gibson-Davis, C. M., & Brooks-Gunn, J. (2006). Couples' immigration status and ethnicity as determinants of breastfeeding. *American Journal of Public Health*, *96*(4), 641–646.

Grassley, J., & Eschiti, V. (2008). Grandmother breastfeeding support: What do mothers need and want? *Birth (Berkeley, Calif.)*, *35*(4), 329–335.

Haider, R., Kabir, I., Huttly, S. R. A., & Ashworth, A. (2002). Training peer counselors to promote and support exclusive breastfeeding in Bangladesh. *Journal of Human Lactation*, *18*(1), 7–12.

Hannula, L., Kaunonen, M., & Tarkka, M. (2008). A systematic review of professional support interventions for breastfeeding. *Journal of Clinical Nursing*, *17*(9), 1132–1143.

Hizel, S., Ceyhun, G., Tanzer, F., & Sanli, C. (2006). Traditional beliefs as forgotten influencing factors on breast-feeding performance in Turkey. *Saudi Medical Journal*, *27*(4), 511–518.

Hoddinott, P., Lee, A. J., & Pill, R. (2006). Effectiveness of a breastfeeding peer coaching intervention in rural Scotland. *Birth*, *33*(1), 27–36.

Hoddinott, P., & Pill, R. (1999). Qualitative study of decisions about infant feeding among women in east end of London. *BMJ (Clinical Research Ed.)*, *318*(7175), 30–34.

Homer, C. S. E., Sheehan, A., & Cooke, M. (2002). Initial infant feeding decisions and duration of breastfeeding in women from English, Arabic and Chinese-speaking backgrounds in Australia. *Breastfeeding Review*, *10*(2), 27–32.

Howard, C., Howard, F., Lawrence, R., Andresen, E., DeBlieck, E., & Weitzman, M. (2000). Office prenatal formula advertising and its effect on breast-feeding patterns. *Obstetrics and Gynecology, 95*(2), 296–303.

IBFAN-ICDC. (2009, May). *ICDC Focus: The code and infant feeding in emergencies.* Penang, Malaysia: Author.

IFE Core Group. (2007a). *Infant and young child feeding in emergencies: Operational guidance for emergency relief staff and programme managers, version 2.1.* Oxford, England: Emergency Nutrition Network. Retrieved from http://www.ennonline.net/pool/files/ife/ops-guidance-2-1-english-010307-with-addendum.pdf

IFE Core Group. (2007b). *Protecting babies in emergencies: The role of the public.* Oxford, England: Emergency Nutrition Network. Retrieved from http://www.ennonline.net/pool/files/generalpublic/ife-guide.pdf

IFE Core Group. (2010). *IFE orientation package.* Oxford, England: Emergency Nutrition Network. Retrieved from http://www.ennonline.net/ife/orientation

Illinois State Breastfeeding Task Force. (n.d.). *Grandmothers' tea toolkit.* Retrieved from http://www.nal.usda.gov/wicworks/Sharing_Center/gallery/wic_fam3.htm#

International Lactation Consultant Association. (n.d.). *Position on infant feeding in emergencies.* Retrieved from http://www.ilca.org/files/resources/ilca_publications/InfantFeeding-EmergPP.pdf

Jakobsen, M., Sodemann, M., Nylén, G., Balé, C., Nielsen, J., Lisse, I., & Aaby, P. (2003). Breastfeeding status as a predictor of mortality among refugee children in an emergency situation in Guinea-Bissau. *Tropical Medicine & International Health: TM & IH, 8*(11), 992–996.

Kelly, Y. J., Watt, R. G., & Nazroo, J. Y. (2006). Racial/ethnic differences in breastfeeding initiation and continuation in the United Kingdom and comparison with findings in the United States. *Pediatrics, 118*(5), e1428–e1435.

Kleinman, A. (2008). *Patients and healers in the context of culture: An exploration of the borderland between anthropology, medicine and psychiatry* (12th ed.). Berkeley, CA: University of California Press.

Labarere, J., Gelbert-Baudino, N., Ayral, A., et al. (2005). Efficacy of breastfeeding support provided by trained clinicians during an early, routine, preventive visit: A prospective, randomized, open trial of 226 mother–infant pairs. *Pediatrics, 115*(2), e139–146.

Leite, A. J. M., Puccini, R. F., Atalah, A. N., Alves Da Cunha, A. L., & Machado, M. T. (2005). Effectiveness of home-based peer counselling to promote breastfeeding in the northeast of Brazil: A randomized clinical trial. *Acta Paediatrica (Oslo, Norway: 1992), 94*(6), 741–746.

Li, L., Zhang, M., Scott, J. A., & Binns, C. W. (2004). Factors associated with the initiation and duration of breastfeeding by Chinese mothers in Perth, Western Australia. *Journal of Human Lactation, 20*(2), 188–195.

MacGregor, E., & Hughes, M. (2010). Breastfeeding experiences of mothers from disadvantaged groups: A review. *Community Practitioner: The Journal of the Community Practitioners' and Health Visitors' Association, 83*(7), 30–33.

Martens, P. J. (2002). Increasing breastfeeding initiation and duration at a community level: An evaluation of Sagkeeng First Nation's community health nurse and peer counselor programs. *Journal of Human Lactation, 18*(3), 236–246.

McInnes, R. J., & Chambers, J. A. (2008). Supporting breastfeeding mothers: Qualitative synthesis. *Journal of Advanced Nursing, 62*(4), 407–427.

Mohd Amin, R., Mohd Said, Z., Sutan, R., Shah, S. A., Darus, A., & Shamsuddin, K. (2011). Work related determinants of breastfeeding discontinuation among employed mothers in Malaysia. *International Breastfeeding Journal, 6*(1), 4.

Narayanan, I., Dutta, A. K., Philips, E., & Ansari, Z. (2005). Attitudes, practices, and socio-cultural factors related to breastfeeding: Pointers for intervention programmes. In S. A. Atkinson et al. (Eds.), *Breastfeeding, nutrition, infection and infant growth in developed and emerging countries*. St. John's, Canada: ARTS Biomedical Publishers and Distributors.

Noble, L. M., Noble, A., & Hand, I. L. (2009). Cultural competence of healthcare professionals caring for breastfeeding mothers in urban areas. *Breastfeeding Medicine, 4*(4), 221–224.

Office on Minority Health, U.S. Department of Health and Human Services. (n.d.). *Think cultural health*. Washington, DC: Author. Retrieved from https://www.thinkculturalhealth.hhs.gov

Office on Minority Health, U.S. Department of Health and Human Services, O.P.S. (2001). *National standards for culturally and linguistically appropriate services in health care, executive summary*. Washington, DC: Author. Retrieved from http://minorityhealth.hhs.gov/assets/pdf/checked/executive.pdf

Pisacane, A., Continisio, G. I., Aldinucci, M., D'Amora, S., & Continisio, P. (2005). A controlled trial of the father's role in breastfeeding promotion. *Pediatrics, 116*(4), e494–e498.

Riordan, J. (2010). *Breastfeeding and human lactation* (4th ed.). Sudbury, MA: Jones and Bartlett.

Riordan, J., & Gill-Hopple, K. (2001). Breastfeeding care in multicultural populations. *Journal of Obstetric, Gynecologic, and Neonatal Nursing, 30*(2), 216–223.

Ryan, A. S., Zhou, W., & Arensberg, M. B. (2006). The effect of employment status on breastfeeding in the United States. *Women's Health Issues, 16*(5), 243–251.

Sheppard, V. B., Zambrana, R. E., & O'Malley, A. S. (2004). Providing health care to low-income women: A matter of trust. *Family Practice, 21*(5), 484–491.

Singh, G. K., Kogan, M. D., & Dee, D. L. (2007). Nativity/immigrant status, race/ethnicity, and socioeconomic determinants of breastfeeding initiation and duration in the United States, 2003. *Pediatrics, 119*(Suppl. 1), S38–46.

Susin, L. R. O., & Giugliani, E. R. J. (2008). Inclusion of fathers in an intervention to promote breastfeeding: Impact on breastfeeding rates. *Journal of Human Lactation, 24*(4), 386–392.

Susin, L. R. O., Giugliani, E. R. J., & Kummer, S. C. (2005). [Influence of grandmothers on breastfeeding practices]. *Revista De Saúde Pública, 39*(2), 141–147.

Tripp-Reimer, T., Brink, P. J., & Saunders, J. M. (1984). Cultural assessment: Content and process. *Nursing Outlook, 32*(2), 78–82.

UNICEF. (2011). *ChildInfo: Statistics by area/child nutrition*. Retrieved from http://www.childinfo.org/breastfeeding_status.html

Weimers, L., Svensson, K., Dumas, L., Navér, L., & Wahlberg, V. (2006). Hands-on approach during breastfeeding support in a neonatal intensive care unit: A qualitative study of Swedish mothers' experiences. *International Breastfeeding Journal, 1*, 20.

Wellstart International. (2005). *Infant and young child feeding in emergency situations*. Blue Jay, CA: Author. Retrieved from http://www.wellstart.org/Infant_feeding_emergency.pdf

World Alliance for Breastfeeding Action. (2009). *Breastfeeding—a vital emergency response: Are you ready?* Penang, Malaysia: Author.

World Health Organization. (1981). *International code of marketing of breast-milk substitutes*. Geneva, Switzerland: Author. retrieved from http://whqlibdoc.who.int/publications/9241541601.pdf

World Health Organization & UNICEF. (2003). *Global strategy for infant and young child feeding*. Geneva, Switzerland: WHO.

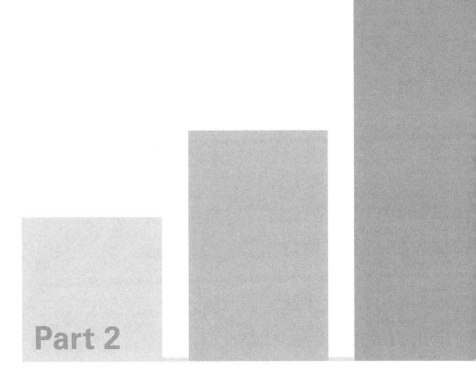

Part 2

Professional Development

CHAPTER 9
The IBCLC as Change Agent

Judith Lauwers, BA, IBCLC, FILCA

> *Never doubt that a small group of thoughtful, committed citizens*
> *can change the world. Indeed, it is the only thing that ever has.*
>
> —MARGARET MEAD

OBJECTIVES

- Use assertiveness and an understanding of culture and perception to promote change in breastfeeding practices and promotion.
- Recognize resistance as a natural part of change and use strategies to overcome it.
- Use strategies to work with conflict and with difficult people.
- Research and evaluate the need for change and implement a plan.
- Capitalize on personalities and group dynamics in the change process.
- Understand strategies in breastfeeding promotion that reflect women's attitudes and demographics.
- Use strategies to promote breastfeeding within the healthcare system throughout prenatal, postpartum, and post discharge.

INTRODUCTION

Healthcare professionals are in an ideal position to plan and implement changes to benefit mothers and babies. Inappropriate hospital practices increase the risk of weaning by 6 weeks 13-fold (DiGirolamo et al., 2008). Recognizing the need for change is the first step in the process of planned change. Unfortunately, not everyone shares equal enthusiasm for making dramatic changes in breastfeeding policies and practices. There is a descending scale of resistance to change, with the most resistant person arguing that there is no problem and thus no change needed. People who are most likely to embrace change acknowledge a problem exists and enthusiastically help to bring about the desired outcome. Demonstrating assertiveness and effective leadership and helping others embrace change can help return breastfeeding to the cultural norm (Mannel, 2007, 2008a, 2008b, 2008c, 2008d). The success of breastfeeding promotion depends on countless small changes enacted one person at a time, hospital by hospital, and country by country.

I. Assertive Behavior

A. Lactation consultants often practice within a hierarchical, male-dominated health-care setting (Manojlovich, 2007).

1. Women may worry that assertiveness will be perceived as aggressive behavior.

2. Powerlessness can lead to passive-aggressive behavior, frustration, and burnout.

B. Increasing assertiveness.

1. Embrace assertive behavior as a strong asset.

2. Analyze and emulate assertive behavior in others: what they say and how they say it.

3. Analyze how you respond in situations that call for assertiveness.

   a. Do others listen when you have something important to say?

   b. Are you able to convince others to comply with your wishes?

   c. Were there times when you came across as aggressive?

   d. Consider your language and nonverbal messages; what worked and what could you have done differently?

4. Practice assertiveness in interactions with family, friends, and coworkers.

   a. Visualize yourself being assertive.

   b. Approach an easy challenge with assertiveness.

   c. If results are not optimal, examine why and what you can do differently.

   d. Remain positive and adjust your approach with the next challenge.

II. Role of Culture and Perception

A. Cultural beliefs evolve from our paradigm, the way we perceive the world.

1. Cultural context involves the mother's family, support system, and birth environment.

2. Consider hospital culture and traditions regarding infant feeding (Mulford, 1995, 2008).

B. Perceptions of infant feeding create challenges in breastfeeding promotion.

1. Perceptions are influenced by our paradigm. **Figure 9-1** illustrates both a young aristocratic lady and an old woman.

2. You cannot persuade others to change their perceptions and beliefs; change must happen internally and at a comfortable pace.

III. Resistance to Change

A. Resistance is a natural part of the change process.

1. Change can create tension and stress.

2. Unless handled effectively, a changed practice risks being undermined or sabotaged.

3. Change could result in employee turnover, political battles, and a drain on resources.

4. Hospitals face financial issues when discontinuing "free" formula (Merewood et al., 2000; Walker, 2007a, 2007b) and implementing some of the

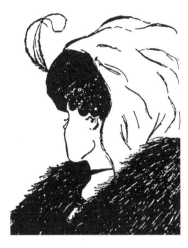

Figure 9-1 Both a young aristocratic lady and an old woman can be seen in this illustration.

Baby-Friendly Hospital Initiative (BFHI) policies. One study to date shows no significant difference in cost of care between BFHI-certified hospitals and those that are not certified (DelliFraine et al., 2011).

B. There are seven stages of resistance to change, adapted from materials developed by SARAR International and published by World Neighbors in Action (Anand, 2005).

1. *There is no problem.* I know human milk is good for babies, but artificial baby milk is perfectly safe.

2. *I recognize there is a problem, but it's not my responsibility.* I accept that breastfeeding is superior, but I can't get involved.

3. *I accept there is a problem, but I doubt anyone's ability to change it.* We have a problem, but formula companies are too influential.

4. *I accept there is a problem, but I'm afraid to get involved.* If I make too many waves, I might lose my job.

5. *We believe we can do something about it, and I will begin to look for solutions.* I will get involved, but I'm still unsure it will make a difference.

6. *We know we can do it and obstacles will not stop us.* Working together we can change things.

7. *We did it! Now we want to share our results with others.* We finally have policies and procedures that promote breastfeeding, and our staff is following the guidelines.

C. Change occurs when individuals reach the stage of group effort.

1. Each person enters the process of change at varying stages.

2. Members need time and patience to progress at their own rate.

3. The greatest resister may become a staunch advocate when able to progress through the necessary stages.

4. Some individuals may never change their opinions or beliefs.

5. Patience and flexibility help establish consensus for moving forward.

D. Reasons for resistance to change.
1. How people greet a change depends on the degree to which they feel they are in control of it.
   a. Some may worry about losing self-efficacy or power.
   b. Change is exciting when it is done by us and is threatening when it is done to us; empower others with legitimate choices.
2. Some people may feel uncertain about where a proposed change will lead.
   a. Share what is happening and avoid springing decisions without preparation.
   b. Divide big changes into several small steps over an extended period.
3. Some people simply want things to remain the same.
   a. They must question familiar habits and reprogram daily routines.
   b. Minimize the number of changes and leave as many routines unchanged as possible.
4. Some people feel embarrassed and self-conscious because of past actions.
   a. Help them appreciate that past actions were based on what was considered appropriate at the time.
   b. Thank them for their willingness to change to meet present needs and encourage them to view the change positively.
5. Some worry about their ability to be effective after the change.
   a. New ways often demand a new set of competencies.
   b. Provide sufficient training, positive reinforcement, and opportunity to practice new skills without judgment.
6. The change may interrupt other plans or projects and intrude on people's personal time.
   a. The change requires more energy, time, and mental preoccupation.
   b. Validate the concerns and give support and recognition for the extra effort.
   c. Introduce changes with flexibility, and be sensitive to the effect the process has on others.
7. Unresolved past grievances may surface.
   a. Undercurrents of professional jealousy or resentments may obstruct your efforts.
   b. Addressing past issues clears the air to focus on present issues.
8. The change may create winners and losers, resulting in people losing status or power.
   a. Create a supportive climate in which to let go of the past.
   b. Be sensitive to the loss of routines, comforts, traditions, and relationships.
   c. Avoid any pretense or false promises.
9. See **Table 9-1** for sample responses to resistance to the *Ten Steps to Successful Breastfeeding*.

Table 9-1 Responses to Arguments Against the Ten Steps to Successful Breastfeeding

Step 1 Have a written breastfeeding policy that is routinely communicated to all healthcare staff.

Stage of Resistance	Argument
There is no problem	We've had a policy for years. It's working well enough.
	We've been functioning well enough without one.
It's not my responsibility	I have too much to do already.
	I wouldn't know where to even begin writing a policy.
No one can do it	Even if we had a policy, no one would follow it.
	Mothers aren't motivated enough to breastfeed, so why bother.
I can't get involved	There are too many on the staff opposed to it.
	I wouldn't be able to get support from the supervisor or manager.
Let's begin	I can explore policies in other hospitals.
	I can contact ILCA to locate resources.
We can do it	Let's bring people together from all departments to work on it.
	Let's survey our patients to learn how satisfied they are.
We did it!	We accomplished our goal!

Step 2 Train all healthcare staff in skills necessary to implement this policy.

Stage of Resistance	Argument
There is no problem	We have IBCLCs, so we don't need to train the rest of the staff.
	Our nurses know what they need to know about breastfeeding.
It's not my responsibility	I don't have time to train everyone.
	I wouldn't know where to even begin with training.
No one can do it	The staff would never agree to 18 hours of training.
	We don't have enough money or time to train the entire staff.
I can't get involved	Staff would resent my suggesting that they need the training.
	I wouldn't be able to get support from the supervisor/manager.
Let's begin	I can explore how other hospitals do their training.
	I will take an extensive course in lactation.
We can do it	Let's survey staff to find out what they know about breastfeeding.
	Let's form a committee with people from several departments.
We did it!	We accomplished our goal!

Step 3 Inform all pregnant women about the benefits and management of breastfeeding.

Stage of Resistance	Argument
There is no problem	We have IBCLCs, so we don't need to train the rest of the staff.
	Our nurses know what they need to know about breastfeeding.
It's not my responsibility	Mothers learn what they need to know in their childbirth classes.
	It's the mother's responsibility to read and seek information.

(continues)

Table 9-1 Responses to Arguments Against the Ten Steps to Successful Breastfeeding (cont'd)

Step 3 (continued)	
No one can do it	We realize we need to, but we don't have the resources.
	If women want to bottle feed, it's our responsibility to help them.
I can't get involved	I don't have time to do prenatal teaching with everything else.
	I wouldn't be able to get support from the supervisor/manager.
Let's begin	I can explore breastfeeding initiation rates in other hospitals.
	I can make a questionnaire to screen mothers with difficulties.
We can do it	Let's survey our patients to find out how satisfied they are.
	Let's explore what we can improve in the labor and delivery department.
We did it!	We accomplished our goal!

Step 4 Help mothers initiate breastfeeding within a half-hour of birth.	
Stage of Resistance	**Argument**
There is no problem	We start breastfeeding as soon as the mother gets to her room.
	Most babies are too sleepy to breastfeed right away.
It's not my responsibility	If she breastfeeds after delivery, relatives will have to wait to see the baby.
	Babies get too cold in the delivery room.
No one can do it	The labor and delivery staff would never support such a policy.
	There are too many procedures that need to be done at that time.
I can't get involved	The staff is getting tired of all my suggestions about breastfeeding.
	I'm not very good at persuading people.
Let's begin	I can find someone in labor and delivery who will be receptive to change.
	I can teach the staff about the importance of early initiation of breastfeeding.
We can do it	Let's try it on a short-term trial basis and then evaluate it.
	We can find ways to keep babies warm.
We did it!	We accomplished our goal!

Step 5 Show mothers how to breastfeed and how to maintain lactation, even if they should be separated from their infants.	
Stage of Resistance	**Argument**
There is no problem	Breastfeeding is a natural instinct; we don't need to teach it.
	There are plenty of support groups who will help them.
It's not my responsibility	If the baby is in the NICU, those nurses are responsible for it.
	I can't possibly see every breastfeeding mother.
No one can do it	We don't have enough staff to spend the time required for this.
	A lot of our staff don't believe in pushing breastfeeding.
I can't get involved	I wouldn't get support from my supervisor for the time it will take.
	Staff won't spend so much time with breastfeeding mothers.

Step 5 (continued)

Let's begin	I can encourage staff to accompany me on rounds.
	I can propose telephone follow-up for breastfeeding mothers.
We can do it	Let's survey our patients about what would have helped them.
	Let's explore a program to mentor staff in breastfeeding.
We did it!	We accomplished our goal!

Step 6 Give newborn infants no food or drink other than breastmilk, unless medically indicated.

Stage of Resistance	Argument
There is no problem	We never do anything unless it is medically indicated.
	I am legally responsible to see that the baby is not dehydrated.
It's not my responsibility	I can't influence physician policies.
	Purchase of formula is an administrative decision, not mine.
No one can do it	Administration will never agree to begin purchasing formula.
	Formula companies will withdraw other funding if we make this change.
I can't get involved	I would not be able to get support from the supervisor/manager.
	What about jaundice? This could be dangerous.
Let's begin	I can explore how other hospitals have begun purchasing formula.
	I can teach staff the importance of exclusive breastfeeding.
We can do it	Let's review reasons we have been giving formula and water.
	Let's invite some mothers in to discuss how they managed.
We did it!	We accomplished our goal!

Step 7 Practice rooming-in—allow mothers and infants to remain together—24 hours a day.

Stage of Resistance	Argument
There is no problem	We have better security if babies are kept in the nursery.
	Babies could choke if they stay in the mother's room.
It's not my responsibility	Mothers are tired after laboring and delivering.
	That is an administrative decision.
No one can do it	If babies stay with their mothers, nursery staff will lose their jobs.
	Mothers do not want to keep their babies in the room.
I can't get involved	I will never get support from administration.
	The pediatricians will not examine babies in the mothers' rooms.
Let's begin	I can explore rooming-in policies at other hospitals.
	I can teach staff the importance of keeping babies with mothers.
We can do it	Let's invite pediatricians to meet with the breastfeeding committee.
	Let's record how much time babies spend away from their mothers.
We did it!	We accomplished our goal!

(continues)

Table 9-1 Responses to Arguments Against the Ten Steps to Successful Breastfeeding (cont'd)

Step 8 Encourage breastfeeding on demand.

Stage of Resistance	Argument
There is no problem	It is more efficient having scheduled feeding times. Babies need to get on a schedule as early as possible.
It's not my responsibility	I can do it with the mothers I see, but I can't see all of them. The babies must be fed at least two times on every shift.
No one can do it	Staff routines would be disrupted too much. It would be too hard to monitor babies for hypoglycemia without a schedule.
I can't get involved	Staff routines would be disrupted too much. This would be much too confusing.
Let's begin	I can teach staff the importance of the mother and baby setting the pace. I can help staff learn to recognize and teach feeding cues.
We can do it	Let's keep statistics to see if schedules make a difference. Let's try it for 6 months to see how it works.
We did it!	We accomplished our goal!

Step 9 Give no artificial teats or pacifiers (also called dummies or soothers) to breastfeeding infants.

Stage of Resistance	Argument
There is no problem	We have to test to see if the baby can suck and swallow. Babies have strong sucking needs and need pacifiers to keep calm.
It's not my responsibility	If parents want them, it is not my position to discourage it. Everyone uses pacifiers, so what's the big deal?
No one can do it	I'm the only one in the hospital who considers this to be a problem. Pacifiers are a part of our culture, just like baby bottles.
I can't get involved	The staff will think it takes too long to feed with a cup or spoon. There is nothing to document the use of cups for feeding babies.
Let's begin	I can teach staff about sucking preference and confusion. I can teach the staff how to cup feed a baby.
We can do it	Let's review why we give formula and water. Let's teach mothers to put the baby to breast rather than give a pacifier.
We did it!	We accomplished our goal!

Step 10 Foster the establishment of breastfeeding support groups and refer mothers to them on discharge from the hospital or clinic.

Stage of Resistance	Argument
There is no problem	We have the information at the desk if the patient requests it. Women in those groups make mothers feel guilty if they wean early.
It's not my responsibility	It is the mother's responsibility to seek help. The physician will refer her if there is a problem.

Step 10 (continued)	
No one can do it	We don't have enough resources to start a support group here. The counselors do not always give sound advice and information.
I can't get involved	If I do this, I'll have to do it on my own time. I don't have time to keep updating the referral list.
Let's begin	I can visit community support groups and foster a strong link. I can offer to train mother-to-mother support counselors.
We can do it	Let's give a name and telephone number to breastfeeding mothers. Let's explore an outpatient clinic and/or support group.
We did it!	We accomplished our goal!

Source: Lauwers, J., & Swisher, A. (2010). *Counseling the nursing mother: A lactation consultant's guide* (5th ed.). Sudbury, MA: Jones and Bartlett. Printed with permission.

IV. Conflict Resolution

    A. Introducing change results in a certain degree of conflict.

        1. Avoiding or dismissing conflict can lead to further conflict (Dana, 2000; Mayer, 2000).

        2. Exposing conflict allows honest, frank, and positive relationships to develop.

        3. Conflict can make people more receptive to finding creative solutions.

        4. Through conflict people learn to understand others and recognize the value of working together.

        5. People work to satisfy their own personal needs, and you must meet their needs as well as your own.

    B. Avoid confronting conflict in public or in the presence of others who are uninvolved.

    C. Remain focused on the solution rather than on individual problems.

    D. Find ways group members can join together to work through conflicts.

    E. Reflect emotions back through active listening to recognize and validate them.

    F. Identify common goals to set the stage for debating strategies for moving forward.

    G. Find outcomes with mutual benefit to set a tone of cooperation and problem solving.

V. Coping with Difficult People

    A. You cannot directly change the way a person responds to you.

    B. Finding a more effective way to communicate and present yourself can indirectly influence how others will respond.

        1. Give recognition and praise for accomplishments, and avoid placing blame.

        2. Write down what you plan to say.

        3. Use body language that shows a desire to interact and communicate in a meaningful way.

        4. Give your undivided attention and avoid distractions.

        5. Recycle the other person's message to make sure you understood it, and pause for a response before continuing to speak.

C. Some difficult people are aggressive to the point of being hostile.
  1. They have a strong sense of what others should do and how they should do it.
    a. They can be abrasive, abrupt, intimidating, and relentless.
    b. Their goal is to prove that you are wrong and they are right.
  2. An angry person cannot stay overtly angry for long if you remain calm.
    a. Listen attentively, look the person directly in the eye, and be ready to interrupt him or her.
    b. If the person interrupts you, hold your ground and insist on finishing.
  3. If sabotaged, expose the difficult person's undermining or that person will continue to breed discontent.
    a. Ask the person for ideas on positive, realistic solutions.
    b. Show that you respect that person's opinion and be prepared and accurate in your interactions with him or her.
    c. Try to engage others in the group for their input and support.
    d. Sitting directly next to the person reduces the potential for conflict.
  4. A leader who maintains a good sense of humor inspires tremendous loyalty and enthusiasm (Yerkes, 2001).

VI. The Art of Persuasion

A. A confident attitude and communication help persuade others.
B. Use the TALKING acronym for persuasion from Benjamin Franklin (Humes, 1992):
  1. **T**iming—choose the right moment.
  2. **A**ppreciation—learn to appreciate the other person's problems and concerns.
  3. **L**istening—Learn to listen well enough to find out what you need and how best to sell it to the other person.
  4. **K**nowledge—Learn where the other person is coming from and how to get them where you want to go.
  5. **I**ntegrity—Never misrepresent your fundamental beliefs or motives.
  6. **N**eed—Show others they are uniquely qualified to give you what you want.
  7. **G**iving—Learn the value of giving.

VII. The Process of Change

A. The first step in change is to gather information and supporting research.
  1. Gather breastfeeding rates and patient satisfaction data.
  2. Compare your findings with national, regional, or local statistics.
  3. Evaluate current policies and practices.
B. Target areas where improvements are needed.
  1. Prepare detailed rationale for each change.
  2. Write down anticipated arguments and possible responses to each one.
  3. Identify alternative approaches and methods in case you experience obstacles.
  4. Identify the people who will be most effective in proposing and instituting the particular change.

5. Identify who each change will affect and involve representatives from all affected areas in the process.

C. Define goals, objectives (short term, intermediate, and long term), strategies, and a timeline for planning and implementing the change.

1. Consider the anticipated level of difficulty in convincing others to support each change.
   a. Start with a change likely to garner the most support.
   b. Leave the toughest hurdles until you have several of the less difficult changes in place.
2. Monitor responses to learn whether any unanticipated problems arise.
3. Address staff education required and how the change will be communicated.
4. Link the change to the overall organizational structure and standardize it.

VIII. Group Dynamics in the Change Process

A. Composition of a breastfeeding committee influences its success.

1. Having enough members will enable meetings to be held when some are absent.
2. Including allies, those you expect will resist, and those who seem to be neutral helps to get buy-in and avoid sabotage.
3. The greatest resisters can become avid supporters when they understand the issues.
4. A quality improvement representative helps focus efforts (Cadwell, 1997).
5. Include representation from all areas the change will affect.

B. Having a range of personalities among members enhances group dynamics.

1. Six basic personality types prevalent among North Americans contribute positively (Kahler, 2008).
   a. Feelers (30%) are compassionate and react quickly to the feelings of others—they respond to assurances that they are valued.
   b. Thinkers (25%) are logical and organized—they want you to get to the point.
   c. Funsters/rebels (20%) are creative, spontaneous, and playful—they dislike rigid schedules.
   d. Believers/persisters (10%) are conscientious, observant, and dedicated—they have difficulty accepting criticism.
   e. Dreamers (10%) are imaginative—they like solitude and quiet surroundings.
   f. Doers/promoters (5%) are persuasive, charming, action oriented, firm, and direct.

C. An effective team leader requires empathy and encouraging the best from others.

1. Ask members to identify problems and how and where to start making changes.
2. Know when to keep quiet, sit back, and let the discussion flow.
3. Learn about the needs of each member before proposing solutions.
4. Help others meet the basic needs they have through their work.
   a. They want work that is interesting and challenging.
   b. They want appreciation expressed for their efforts.
   c. They want to be involved in and important to the overall scheme—with job security, reasonable pay, and opportunities for career growth and advancement.

IX. Change in the Context of Breastfeeding Promotion

A. The goal of breastfeeding promotion is to return breastfeeding to a natural activity and to normalize it within the cultures of mothers and families.

1. Breastfeeding promotion is a form of social marketing.

2. Effective marketing converts people's needs and wants into opportunities (Kotler et al., 2008).

3. Social marketing seeks to influence behavior and benefit society (Weinreich, 2006).

B. Understanding women's attitudes toward pregnancy and breastfeeding can lead to new strategies for promoting and maintaining breastfeeding (Sandes et al., 2007).

1. Messages need to reach mothers on multiple levels, in all aspects of their private and public lives (Mulford, 2008).

2. Strategies need to go beyond socioeconomic or demographic characteristics (Fonseca-Becker et al., 2006) to include generational traits and peer influence.

3. Promotion among working women needs to be geared toward the mother, her social network, and the entire community (Johnston et al., 2007) as well as mother–infant attachment and maternal sensitivity (Yoon et al., 2008).

4. Promotion efforts need to address trends among women living within resource-poor settings (Sibeko et al., 2005).

5. Strategies need to reflect an understanding of a woman's cultural heritage.

C. Insufficient staffing, lack of continuity, ineffective guidelines, and lack of commitment interfere with implementing breastfeeding-friendly practices (Bulhosa et al., 2007).

1. Increasing women's breastfeeding empowerment and efficacy in clinical settings is an effective promotional strategy (Kang et al., 2008).

   a. Most women make their infant feeding decision before delivery, yet little promotion of breastfeeding occurs in most prenatal practice settings (Dusdieker et al., 2006).

   b. Breastfeeding promotion should be incorporated into pediatric outpatient settings with specially trained pediatric staff (Böse-O'Reilly et al., 2008).

   c. Hospital policies and practices have a role and responsibility in the promotion and duration of breastfeeding (Manganaro et al., 2009).

   d. Promotion strategies need to remove barriers during labor, delivery, recovery, and postpartum (Komara et al., 2007).

2. Healthcare professionals need to develop trusting relationships, continuity of care, and clear, consistent education and support (Cricco-Lizza, 2006).

   a. Despite reporting favorable attitudes, many physicians fail to support breastfeeding mothers (Taveras et al., 2004).

   b. Providers' culture and attitudes, not their knowledge, most influence their efforts in breastfeeding promotion and support (Szucs et al., 2009).

   c. New strategies that focus on the attitudes and culture of physicians may help to enhance their promotion and support of breastfeeding (Barclay, 2008).

   d. Pediatric nurses have an important role in supporting breastfeeding (Hunt, 2006), as do midwives and dietitians.

e. There is a positive correlation between the services of lactation consultants and breastfeeding duration (Memmott et al., 2006; Thurman et al., 2008).

D. Combining prenatal and postnatal interventions has a larger effect on increasing breastfeeding duration than either pre- or postnatal interventions alone (Hannula et al., 2008).

1. Combining interventions with peer support or peer counseling increases short-term breastfeeding rates (Chung et al., 2008b).

2. Promotion efforts need to be developmentally appropriate, especially among adolescent mothers (Feldman-Winter et al., 2007).

3. Culturally and linguistically sensitive breastfeeding promotion and postpartum support services are needed (Sutton et al., 2007).

X. Role of Education in Promotion and Change

A. Breastfeeding education has a significant effect on increasing initiation rates (Dyson et al., 2005).

1. Educational programs are the single most effective intervention on initiation and short-term duration of breastfeeding (Guise et al., 2003).

2. Education within a context of risks and benefits helps inform mothers and promotes their commitment to exercise their right to breastfeed (Knaak, 2006).

3. Risk-based messages encourage social and institutional change but should not risk failing to recognize and respond to mothers' perceived barriers (Heinig, 2009).

4. Including fathers in education programs increases exclusive breastfeeding (Susin et al., 2008).

B. Caregivers' promotion efforts require adequate knowledge, skills, and attitude.

1. They need to learn about breastfeeding early in their medical training and be surrounded by a culture in which breastfeeding is the norm (Feldman-Winter et al., 2008).

2. Residency programs need to focus on medical rationale, techniques, and problem solving; expectations, beliefs, and an acceptance of data that demonstrate the health benefits of breastfeeding; and building confidence in providing effective counseling and support (American Academy of Family Physicians, 2007; Saenz, 2000).

3. The approach should facilitate personal reflection and critical engagement with sociopolitical issues (Dykes, 2006).

XI. Community Breastfeeding Promotion

A. Education and promotional strategies need to be targeted at the general public and health workers in maternity units (Chung et al., 2008a).

1. Communities need well-defined policies and strategies, financial resources, and strong political will to deliver effective promotional efforts at the community level (Bhandari et al., 2008).

2. A social and cultural change of the whole community toward breastfeeding increases breastfeeding rates (Mordini et al., 2009).

B. Promotion of breastfeeding at the government level increases the incidence and duration of breastfeeding (Merewood et al., 2004; Mitra et al., 2003).

C. Lobbying by lactation activists can be an effective way to change public policy (Wilson-Clay et al., 2005).

References

American Academy of Family Physicians. (2007). *Breastfeeding, family physicians supporting (position paper)*. Leawood, KS: Author. Retrieved from http://www.aafp.org/online/en/home/policy/policies/b/breastfeedingpositionpaper.html

American Academy of Family Physicians. (2008). Breastfeeding (policy statement). Retrieved from http://www.aafp.org/online/en/home/policy/policies/b/breastfeedingpolicy.html

Anand, R. K. (2005, February 7). *Transforming health colleagues into breastfeeding advocates* (WABA Activity Sheet No. 3). Penang, Malaysia: World Alliance for Breastfeeding Action.

Barclay, L. (2008). Pediatrician promotion of breast-feeding among their patients has declined. *Archives of Pediatric and Adolescent Medicine, 162*, 1142–1149.

Bhandari, N., et al. (2008). Mainstreaming nutrition into maternal and child health programmes: Scaling up of exclusive breast-feeding. *Maternal and Child Nutrition, 4*(1), 5–23.

Böse-O'Reilly, S., Wermuth, I., & Hellmann, J. (2008). Promotion of breast feeding in paediatric outpatient settings [in German]. *Gesundheitswesen, 70*(Suppl. 1), S34–S36.

Bulhosa, M. S., Lunardi, V., & Lunardi Filho, W. (2007). Promotion of breastfeeding by the nursing staff of a children-friendly hospital [in Portuguese]. *Revista Gaúcha de Enfermagem, 28*(1), 89–97.

Cadwell, K. (1997). Using the quality improvement process to affect breastfeeding protocols in United States hospitals. *Journal of Human Lactation, 13*, 5–9.

Chung, W., Kim, H. & Nam, C. (2008a). Breast-feeding in South Korea: Factors influencing its initiation and duration. *Public Health and Nutrition, 11*(3), 225–229.

Chung, M., Raman. G., & Trikalinos, T. (2008b). Interventions in primary care to promote breastfeeding: An evidence review for the U.S. Preventive Services Task Force. *Annals of Internal Medicine, 149*(8), 565–582.

Cricco-Lizza, R. (2006). Black non-Hispanic mothers' perceptions about the promotion of infant-feeding methods by nurses and physicians. *Journal of Obstetric, Gynecologic, and Neonatal Nursing, 35*(2), 173–1780.

Dana, D. (2000). *Conflict resolution*. New York, NY: McGraw-Hill.

DelliFraine, J., Langabeer, J., 2nd, Williams, J. F., Gong, A. K., Delgado, R. I., & Gill, S. L. (2011). Cost comparison of baby friendly and non-baby friendly hospitals in the United States. *Pediatrics, 127*(4), e989–994.

DiGirolamo, A. M., Grummer-Strawn, L. M., & Fein, S. B. (2008). Effect of maternity care practices on breastfeeding. *Pediatrics, 122*(Suppl. 2), S43–S49.

Dusdieker, L. B., Dungy, C.I. & Losch, M. E. (2006). Prenatal office practices regarding infant feeding choices. *Clinical Pediatrics, 45*(9), 841–845.

Dykes, F. (2006). The education of health practitioners supporting breastfeeding women: Time for critical reflection. *Maternal and Child Nutrition, 2*(4), 204–216.

Dyson, L., McCormick, F., & Renfrew, M. (2005). Interventions for promoting the initiation of breastfeeding. *Cochrane Database of Systematic Reviews, 2*, CD001688. doi:10.1002/14651858.CD001688.pub2

Feldman-Winter, L., & Shaikh, U. (2007). Optimizing breastfeeding promotion and support in adolescent mothers. *Journal of Human Lactation, 23*(4), 362–367.

Feldman-Winter, L. B., Schanler, R. J., & O'Connor, K. G. (2008). Pediatricians and the promotion and support of breastfeeding. *Archives of Pediatric and Adolescent Medicine, 162*(12), 1142–1149.

Fonseca-Becker, F., & Valente, T. W. (2006). Promoting breastfeeding in Bolivia: Do social networks add to the predictive value of traditional socioeconomic characteristics? *Journal of Health, Population, and Nutrition, 24*(1), 71–80.

Guise, J. M., Palda, V., & Westhoff, C. (2003). The effectiveness of primary care-based interventions to promote breastfeeding: Systematic evidence review and meta-analysis for the US Preventive Services Task Force. *Annals of Family Medicine, 1*(2), 70–78.

Hannula, L., Kaunonen, M. & Tarkka. (2008). A systematic review of professional support interventions for breastfeeding. *Journal of Clinical Nursing, 17*(9), 1132–1143.

Heinig, M. J. (2009). Are there risks to using risk-based messages to promote breastfeeding? *Journal of Human Lactation, 25*(1), 7–8.

Humes, J. C. (1992, June 15). Life lessons from Ben Franklin. *Bottom Line/Personal.*

Hunt, F. (2006). Breast feeding and society. *Paediatric Nursing, 18*(8), 24–26.

Johnston, M. L., & Esposito, N. (2007). Barriers and facilitators for breast-feeding among working women in the United States. *Journal of Obstetric, Gynecologic, and Neonatal Nursing, 36*(1), 9–20.

Kahler, T. (2008). *The process therapy model: The six personality types with adaptations.* Little Rock, AR: Taibi Kahler Associates.

Kang, J. S., Choi, S. Y., & Ryu, E. J. (2008). Effects of a breastfeeding empowerment programme on Korean breastfeeding mothers: A quasi-experimental study. *International Journal of Nursing Studies, 45*(1), 14–23.

Knaak, S. J. (2006). The problem with breastfeeding discourse. *Canadian Journal of Public Health, 97,* 412–414.

Komara, C., Simpson, D., & Teasdale, C. (2007). Intervening to promote early initiation of breastfeeding in the LDR. *MCN American Journal of Maternal and Child Nursing, 32*(2), 117–121.

Kotler, P., & Keller, K. (2008). *Marketing management* (13th ed.). Upper Saddle River, NJ: Prentice Hall.

Manganaro, R., Marseglia, L., & Mamì, C. (2009). Effects of hospital policies and practices on initiation and duration of breastfeeding. *Child: Care, Health, and Development, 35*(1), 106–111.

Mannel, R. (2007). Developing leadership. *Journal of Human Lactation, 23,* 229. doi:10.1177/0890334407304190

Mannel, R. (2008a). Essential leadership skills, part I: Defining vision. *Journal of Human Lactation, 24,* 11. doi:10.1177/0890334407313343

Mannel, R. (2008b). Essential leadership skills, part II: Build a team. *Journal of Human Lactation, 24,* 133. doi:10.1177/0890334408317556

Mannel, R. (2008c). Essential leadership skills, part III: Fostering change through collaboration. *Journal of Human Lactation, 24,* 244. doi:10.1177/0890334408320380

Mannel, R. (2008d). Essential leadership skills, part IV: Mentoring future leaders. *Journal of Human Lactation, 24,* 367. doi:10.1177/0890334408324468

Manojlovich, M. (2007). Power and empowerment in nursing: Looking backward to inform the future. *Online Journal of Issues in Nursing, 12*(1), 1. Retrieved from http://www.nursingworld.org/MainMenuCategories/ANAMarketplace/ANAPeriodicals/OJIN/TableofContents/Volume122007/No1Jan07/LookingBackwardtoInformtheFuture.aspx

Mayer, B. (2000). *The dynamics of conflict resolution: A practitioner's guide.* San Francisco, CA: Jossey-Bass.

Memmott, M. M., & Bonuck, K. A. (2006). Mother's reactions to a skills-based breastfeeding promotion intervention. *Maternal and Child Nutrition, 2*(1), 40–50.

Merewood, A., & Heinig, J. (2004). Efforts to promote breastfeeding in the United States: Development of a national breastfeeding awareness campaign. *Journal of Human Lactation, 20*(2), 140–145.

Merewood, A., & Philipp, B. (2000). Becoming baby-friendly: Overcoming the issue of accepting free formula. *Journal of Human Lactation, 16*(4), 279–282.

Mitra, A., Khoury, A. J., & Carothers, C. (2003). Evaluation of a comprehensive loving support program among state Women, Infants, and Children (WIC) program breast-feeding coordinators. *Southern Medical Journal, 96*(2), 168–171.

Mordini, B., Bortoli, E., & Pagano, R. (2009). Correlations between welfare initiatives and breastfeeding rates: A 10-year follow-up study. *Acta Paediatrica, 98*(1), 80–85.

Mulford, C. (1995). Swimming upstream: Breastfeeding care in a non-breastfeeding culture. *Journal of Obstetric, Gynecologic, and Neonatal Nursing, 24*(5), 464–474.

Mulford, C. (2008). Is breastfeeding really invisible, or did the health care system just choose not to notice it? *International Breastfeeding Journal, 3*, 13.

Saenz, R. (2000). A lactation management rotation for family medicine residents. *Journal of Human Lactation, 16*(4), 342–345.

Sandes, A. R., Nascimento, C., & Figueira, J. (2007). Breastfeeding: Prevalence and determinant factors [in Portuguese]. *Acta Médica Portuguesa, 20*(3), 193–200.

Sibeko, L., Dhansay, M. A., & Charlton, K. E. (2005). Beliefs, attitudes, and practices of breastfeeding mothers from a periurban community in South Africa. *Journal of Human Lactation, 21*(1), 31–38.

Susin, L. R., & Giugliani, E. R. (2008). Inclusion of fathers in an intervention to promote breastfeeding: Impact on breastfeeding rates. *Journal of Human Lactation, 24*(4), 386–392.

Sutton, J., He, M., & Despard, C. (2007). Barriers to breastfeeding in a Vietnamese community: A qualitative exploration. *Canadian Journal of Dietetic Practice and Research, 68*(4), 195–200.

Szucs, K. A., Miracle, D. J. & Rosenman, M. B. (2009). Breastfeeding knowledge, attitudes, and practices among providers in a medical home. *Breastfeeding Medicine, 4*(1), 31–42.

Taveras, E., Li, R., & Grummer-Strawn, L. (2004). Opinions and practices of clinicians associated with continuation of exclusive breastfeeding. *Pediatrics, 113*(4), e283–e290.

Thurman, S. E., & Allen, P. J. (2008). Integrating lactation consultants into primary health care services: Are lactation consultants affecting breastfeeding success? *Pediatric Nursing, 34*(5), 419–425.

Walker, M. (2007a). International breastfeeding initiatives and their relevance to the current state of breastfeeding in the United States. *Journal of Midwifery and Women's Health, 52*(6), 549–555.

Walker, M. (2007b). *Still selling out mothers and babies: Marketing of breast milk substitutes in the USA.* Weston, MA: NABA REAL.

Weinreich, N. (2006). What is social marketing? Retrieved from http://www.social-marketing.com/Whatis.html

Wilson-Clay, B., Rourke, J. W., & Bolduc, M. B. (2005). Learning to lobby for pro-breastfeeding legislation: The story of a Texas bill to create a breastfeeding-friendly physician designation. *Journal of Human Lactation, 21*(2), 191–198.

Yerkes, L. (2001). *Fun works: Creating places where people love to work.* San Francisco, CA: Berrett-Koehler.

Yoon, J., & Park, Y. (2008). Effects of a breast feeding promotion program for working women [in Korean]. *Journal of Korean Academy of Nursing, 38*(6), 843–852.

CHAPTER 10
Education and Mentoring

Karin Cadwell, PhD, FAAN, IBCLC

OBJECTIVE

- List resources for professional education and change in lactation.

INTRODUCTION

Almost all national and international statements regarding lactation call for change to improve education for healthcare providers and lactation management based on evidence. Changing current practice is a slow process that needs a well-thought-out plan. This chapter proposes the use of reflection, mentoring, and evidence-based practice as the foundation to make change.

I. Blueprint for Policymakers to Promote, Protect, and Support Breastfeeding (UNICEF)

A. Establish national breastfeeding committees.

B. Promote the Baby-Friendly Hospital Initiative.

C. Implement and enforce the *International Code of Marketing of Breast-milk Substitutes*.

D. Establish maternity protection.

E. Train medical personnel and health workers.

F. Support exclusive and sustained breastfeeding throughout the community.

G. Provide resources for support groups.

H. Promote breastfeeding campaigns.

I. Integrate breastfeeding messages into child health activities.

J. Improve women's social and economic status.

II. Policy

Policy has been shown to have an independent effect on changing outcome (Rosenberg et al., 2008). Evidence-based breastfeeding policies have been published, including the following:

A. *Sample Hospital Breastfeeding Policy for Newborns* (American Academy of Pediatrics, 2009)

B. Sample breastfeeding policy (U.K. Baby Friendly Initiative)

C. Clinical Protocol #7: Model Breastfeeding Policy (Academy of Breastfeeding Medicine, 2010)

D. *Clinical Guidelines for the Establishment of Exclusive Breastfeeding* (International Lactation Consultant Association, 2005)

E. *Altering Hospital Maternity Culture: Current Evidence to the Ten Steps for Successful Breastfeeding* (Cox, 2010)

F. *Continuity of Care in Breastfeeding: Best Practices in the Maternity Setting* (Cadwell et al., 2009)

G. *Breastfeeding Management for the Clinician: Using the Evidence*, second edition (Walker, 2009)

H. The Academy of Breastfeeding Medicine has as a central goal the development of evidence-based clinical protocols for managing common medical problems that may affect breastfeeding success. These protocols can be found at www.bfmed.org.

III. Practice Paradigms

Evidence-based and reflective practice paradigms are emerging models for examination of the validity of policies and practices.

A. These paradigms offer tools to address the tension between folklore and medicine by authority and between observed experience and authority.

B. Evidence-based practice might level the field by providing a forum for interdisciplinary discussion.

C. A hierarchy of evidence has been accepted in medical research literature (Guyatt et al., 1995).

1. Systematic reviews and meta-analyses

2. Randomized controlled trials

3. Cohort studies

4. Case-control studies

5. Cross-sectional surveys

6. Case reports

D. Reflective practice.

1. Emerges from 20th-century educators such as Dewey (1933) and Schön (1983) who encouraged practitioners and educators to develop their practice after conscious reflection of their experiences.

2. Asserts that integration of theory and practice happens on the level of the individual practitioner. A concern is that without conscious reflection, practitioners become habituated into routines that do not benefit themselves, the population they serve, or their organization.

3. Learning is lifelong. Experienced practitioners have opportunities to learn from everyday experiences as they transform information into knowledge. Knowledge accumulates, and the reflective practitioner can adapt to new situations and eventually can invent new strategies.

4. Applied to systems, reflective practice results in "learning organizations," which Schön et al. (1996) expanded from the model of the reflective practitioner.

E. Planning for change.
   1. Form a multidisciplinary practice committee.
   2. Develop a philosophy of care.
   3. Gather information.
      a. Explore the basis for current practice.
      b. Explore standards and guidelines from professional organizations.
      c. Review standards from regulatory agencies.
      d. Examine policies and procedures.
      e. Search the published literature.
      f. Grade the literature by using the following framework:
         i. Rituals versus rationales: Define current practices as rituals (for example, "We have always done it this way") or rationales (based on scientific principles, standards of care, and evidence).
         ii. Evaluate using current protocols.
         iii. Develop best practices for the breastfeeding family.
F. Evaluate current practice.
   1. No published standards or guidelines for care, but research support (for example, cup feeding for preterm infants)
   2. No published standards or guidelines for care and poor research support (for example, cabbage leaves for engorgement)
   3. Published standards and guidelines for care and literature support (for example, unrestricted breastfeeding times and frequency)
G. Benefits of evidence-based and reflective care.
   1. Practices are defensible during budget cuts and restrictions.
   2. Promotion of multidisciplinary collaboration.
   3. Assurance of patient safety.
   4. Reduction of liability.
H. Successful implementation of research into practice is a function of the interplay of three core elements:
   1. Level and nature of the evidence
   2. Context or environment into which the research is to be placed
   3. Method or way in which the process is facilitated (Rycroft-Malone et al., 2004)

IV. Three Levels of Objectives for Lactation Management Education (Naylor et al., 1994)

A. Level I: Awareness
   1. Target group: Medical students (preservice education).
   2. Example objective: Discuss, in general terms, findings from the basic and social sciences of lactation.
      a. Describe the general benefits of breastfeeding for the infant.

    B. Level II: Generalist
        1. Target group: Pediatricians, obstetric-gynecology physicians and residents, family medicine residents, and advanced practice nurses.
        2. Example objective: Apply the findings from the basic and social sciences to breastfeeding and lactation issues.
           a. Describe the unique properties of human milk for human infants.
           b. Describe the advantages of preterm milk for the preterm infant.
    C. Level III: Specialist
        1. Target group: Advanced/independent study, fellowships.
        2. Example objective: Critique the findings from the basic and social sciences and evaluate their applicability to clinical management issues.
           a. Discuss in detail the components of human milk and their functions.
           b. Describe in detail the suitability of preterm human milk for the preterm infant.

V. Education

The World Health Organization (WHO) and UNICEF have developed education specific to the field of breastfeeding and human lactation as the *Baby-Friendly Hospital Initiative: Revised, Updated and Expanded for Integrated Care* (2009). Four sections are available to the public as downloads from the Internet. Section 5 is available only to the national Baby-Friendly Hospital Initiative (BFHI) authority.
    A. BFHI Section 1: Background and implementation
    B. BFHI Section 2: Strengthening and sustaining the Baby-Friendly Hospital Initiative: A course for decision makers
    C. BFHI Section 3: Breastfeeding promotion and support in a baby-friendly hospital, a 20-hour course for maternity staff

VI. Components of Professional Knowledge According to Schein (1973)

    A. An underlying discipline or basic science component upon which the practice rests or from which it is developed
    B. An applied science or "engineering" component from which many of the day-to-day diagnostic procedures and problem solutions are derived
    C. A skills and attitudinal component that concerns the actual performance of services to the client using the underlying basic and applied knowledge

VII. Mentoring for Professional Development

    A. The concept of mentoring was first described by Homer in *The Odyssey*. Mentoring has advantages for the mentor and the person being mentored. The mentor (guide) benefits through the formalization of his or her reflective and evidence-based practice through transparent processing, reasoning, and problem solving of patient/client interactions. The person being mentored (referred to as "partner," "protégé," or "mentee") has the opportunity to experience personal advice and expertise from a professional colleague. Benner (2000) describes the process of professional growth in the book *From Novice to Expert*.

B. Ideally, mentoring occurs within a realistic environment in which there are challenges and the mentor can support the partner, demystify the consulting experience, and offer constructive criticism as well as positive feedback.

C. The person being mentored manages the work of the relationship. A sample contract may be found in the Appendix.

D. The European Mentoring and Coaching Council (2004) defines integrity and professionalism related to mentoring in its code of ethics.

E. Parsloe et al. (2000) describe a mentoring model for clinical practice:
1. Establish the aims of the mentoring.
2. Encourage self-management and self-direction.
3. Provide ongoing support.
4. Assist in evaluation.

F. Bayley et al. (2004) describe mentoring as a transformative process and suggest the individuals looking for a mentor seek out one who has the following characteristics:
1. Has a track record
2. Is committed to his or her own personal and professional development
3. Has the time and energy to fulfill the mentoring contract
4. Is flexible about developing the relationship
5. Is respected and trustworthy

G. International Board of Lactation Consultant Examiners (IBLCE) has developed specific mentoring guidelines to qualify as a candidate for Pathway 3. According to IBLCE (2011):
1. Pathway 3 clinical practice must be directly supervised.
2. Direct supervision is defined as a gradual, three-phase process that
   a. Begins with observation of the mentor at work
   b. Moves to clinical practice experience under the direct observation of the mentor (i.e., the mentor must be in the room with the applicant) until the skill is mastered
   c. Culminates with independent practice by the applicant with the mentor physically nearby to assist if needed

H. According to IBLCE (2011), mentors must
1. Be a currently certified International Board Certified Lactation Consultant (IBCLC) in good standing who has recertified at least once
2. Complete and submit a *Pathway 3 Mentor Agreement Form* accompanied by a CV or résumé
3. Provide a period of time during which the Pathway 3 applicant observes the mentor's practice before allowing the applicant to provide hands-on care to breastfeeding families
4. Directly supervise the applicant's clinical practice and determine the degree to which the applicant has mastered the clinical skills being practiced before permitting the applicant to practice independently

5. Log the clinical practice hours that the applicant has accumulated under the mentor's direct supervision by completing and signing a *Pathway 3 Time Sheet*
6. Assign additional learning activities, reading, and/or written assignments to the applicant, as needed
7. Provide a reference for the Pathway 3 applicant, upon request

VIII. Accreditation and Approval Review Committee

The Accreditation and Approval Review Committee (LEAARC) on Education in Human Lactation and Breastfeeding is jointly sponsored by the International Lactation Consultant Association (ILCA) and the International Board of Lactation Consultant Examiners (IBLCE). AARC's mission is to recognize educational programs that meet the minimum standards of quality to prepare individuals to enter the lactation consultant profession.

   A. LEAARC serves as a review committee for the Commission on Accreditation of Allied Health Education Programs (CAAHEP).
   B. LEAARC offers recognition to lactation programs in the form of AARC Approval or CAAHEP Accreditation.
   C. All programs recognized by LEAARC must have a recertified IBCLC as primary faculty.
   D. LEAARC makes recommendations for CAAHEP accreditation of academic lactation programs that meet LEAARC standards.
   E. CAAHEP-accredited programs must be taught through a postsecondary academic institution and meet the curriculum criteria contained in the LEAARC standards.
   F. LEAARC approval is available to free-standing lactation courses and academic programs that do not meet CAAHEP accreditation requirements.

References

Academy of Breastfeeding Medicine. (2010). Clinical protocol #7: Model breastfeeding policy. *Breastfeeding Medicine, 5*(4), 173–177.

American Academy of Pediatrics. (2009). *Sample hospital breastfeeding policy for newborns.* Retrieved from http://www.aapnj.org/uploadfiles/documents/f48.pdf

Bayley, H., Chambers, R., & Donovan, C. (2004). *The good mentoring toolkit for healthcare.* San Francisco, CA: Radcliffe Publishing.

Benner, P. (2000). *From novice to expert: Excellence and power in clinical nursing practice.* Upper Saddle River, NJ: Prentice Hall.

Cadwell, K., & Turner-Maffei, C. (2009). *Continuity of care in breastfeeding: Best practices in the maternity setting.* Sudbury, MA: Jones and Bartlett.

Cox, S. (2010). *Clinics in human lactation: Altering hospital maternity culture: Current evidence for the Ten Steps to Successful Breastfeeding* (Vol. 5). Amarillo, TX: Hale Publishing.

Dewey, J. (1933). *How we think. A restatement of the relation of reflective thinking to the educative process* (Rev. ed.). Boston, MA: D. C. Heath.

European Mentoring and Coaching Council. (2004). Code of ethics. Retrieved from http://www.emccouncil.org/src/ultimo/models/Download/4.pdf

Greenhalgh, T. (2006). *How to read a paper: The basics of evidence based medicine* (3rd ed.). London, England: BMJ Publishing Group.

Guyatt, G. H., Sackett, D. L., Sinclair, J. C., et al. (1995). User's guides to the medical literature IX. A method for grading health care recommendations. *Journal of the American Medical Association, 274*, 1800–1804.

International Board of Lactation Consultant Examiners. (2011). Pathways. Retrieved from http://www.americas.iblce.org/pathways

International Lactation Consultant Association. (2005). *Clinical guidelines for the establishment of exclusive breastfeeding*. Raleigh, NC: Author.

Naylor, A. J., Creer, A. E., Woodward-Lopez, G., & Dixon, S. (1994). Lactation management education for physicians. *Seminars in Perinatology, 18*, 525–531.

Parsloe, E., & Wray, W. (2000). *Coaching and mentoring—practical methods to improve learning*. London, England: Kogan Page.

Rosenberg, K. D., Stull, J. D., Adler, M. R., et al. (2008). Impact of hospital policies on breastfeeding outcomes. *Breastfeeding Medicine, 3*, 110–116.

Rycroft-Malone, J., Harvey, G., Seers, K., et al. (2004). An exploration of the factors that influence the implementation of evidence into practice. *Journal of Clinical Nursing, 13*, 913–924.

Schein, E. (1973). *Professional education*. New York, NY: McGraw-Hill.

Schön, D. (1983). *The reflective practitioner: How professionals think in action*. London, England: Temple Smith.

Schön, D., & Argyris, C. (1996). *Organizational learning II: Theory, method and practice*. Reading, MA: Addison Wesley.

Sinclair, J. C., Bracken M. B., & Horbar J. D. (1997). Introduction to neonatal systematic reviews. *Pediatrics, 100*, 892–895.

UNICEF. (1999). *Breastfeeding: Foundation for a healthy future*. New York, NY: Author.

Walker, M. (2009). *Breastfeeding management for the clinician: Using the evidence* (2nd ed.). Sudbury, MA: Jones and Bartlett.

World Health Organization. (1998). *Evidence for the Ten Steps to Successful Breastfeeding*. Geneva, Switzerland: Author.

World Health Organization. (2003). *Global strategy on infant and young child feeding*. Geneva, Switzerland: Author.

World Health Organization & UNICEF. (2009). *The baby-friendly hospital initiative: Revised, updated and expanded for integrated care*. Retrieved from http://www.who.int/nutrition/publications/infantfeeding/9789241594950/en/index.html

Suggested Reading

Lactation Education Accreditation and Approval Review Committee (LEAARC). http://www.aarclactation.org/

International Board of Lactation Consultant Examiners Pathway 3 information: http://www.americas.iblce.org/upload/Pathway%203%20Guide.pdf

U.K. Baby Friendly Initiative sample breastfeeding policy: http://www.unicef.org.uk/Documents/Baby_Friendly/Guidance/4/sample_maternity_policy.pdf?epslanguage=en

Sample Mentor–Partner Agreement

This agreement may serve as a template for Lactation Care Providers who want to enter into a mentor/partner relationship on their own. (Most institutions and agencies have standard agreements used in all mentor relationships.) It is recommended that an agreement always be used in order to formally ensure that both parties are considering concrete action items when making their arrangement.

A Mentor-Partner Arrangement is

- A relational process for developing an understanding of professional roles and responsibilities
- A relationship with a seasoned Lactation Care Provider who knows and understands the care setting culture and norms and knows how to navigate within the structure of the setting
- A relationship that can help the mentor and the partner develop additional professional relationships within and outside of the service delivery setting.

The Mentor Helps the Partner

- Create a vision for what can be accomplished in the care setting by role modeling the principles of evidence based practice
- Clarify and set goals for the partnership
- Shift perspectives to new possibilities through encouraging self reflection and accepting constructive criticism graciously
- Develop strategies and suggest resources for learning and role assumption
- Be accountable for the experience they say they want and what they say they will do
- Recognize and utilize the protégé's existing experience and knowledge

The Partner Takes Responsibility to

- Respect the mentor's availability and time
- Be receptive to constructive criticism, information, and feedback
- Set realistic expectations with the mentor
- Keep notes of the meetings and use self-reflection to maximize the experience
- Before the initial meeting, the mentor and partner should each consider what they would like to accomplish in the relationship.

Things to Consider

- Compatible professional values and use of the principles of evidence-based practice
- Compatible hours/schedule
- Mutual expectations of the relationship
- The shared ability to develop a relationship founded in trust and openness
- The gap between where the partner is professionally and where the partner wants to be professionally

Mentor/Partner Agreement

Mentor Name:

Affiliation:

Contact Information:

Goal(s)/Steps/Strategies

Example: Goal	**Example: Strategies**
Fulfill the clinical requirements to qualify for the IBLCE exam by _____ (year).	1. Create/discuss list of ways to achieve competent delivery of care to breastfeeding mothers and their babies.
	2. Identify practitioners I can observe and be observed by in the clinical setting.
Step:	Strategies:
Date:	
Step:	Strategies:
Date:	
Step:	Strategies:
Date:	

Duration of Agreement and Frequency of Meetings

Start Date:	**End Date**:

Frequency:

Signatures

We agree that mentoring conversations will be conducted within the following guidelines:
- Conversations will focus on results that we want to achieve professionally
- Conversations will be confidential
- Each participant agrees to maintain mutual dignity and respect
- We will be self-reflective and give and accept constructive criticism with dignity and respect
- We can opt out

Partner: Date:

Mentor: Date:

CHAPTER 11
Interpretation of Statistics and Quantitative Research Design

Patricia J. Martens, IBCLC, PhD, FILCA

OBJECTIVES

- Describe basic statistical concepts and how these relate to an understanding of quantitative research and its application to clinical practice.
- Describe basic epidemiologic concepts and how these relate to an understanding of research and its clinical application.
- Describe basic data collection tools and how to critique them.
- Describe a framework for critiquing quantitative research.

INTRODUCTION

This chapter focuses on understanding the basics of quantitative research, which is research based on numerical data collection and analysis. Many studies use only a numerical approach, such as a study on the average breastmilk intake of full-term babies at different points in time, or a study on initiation and duration rates of breastfeeding. Quantitative research is considered "generalizable" in the sense that it is expected to give you an idea of what is a typical result, how variable you could expect the result to be, and what you would estimate the population value to be based on the results of a sample of people from that population. Some people refer to quantitative research as "wide and thin" (in contrast to qualitative research being "narrow and deep"), meaning that you get a broad idea of a numerical value for a large population from the findings of your research, or an idea of which treatment works "better" from a number viewpoint, but you also might miss the subtleties of the qualitative information about why you see what you do or the rich context of the findings. Many people advocate for a mixed methods approach that combines the strengths of both quantitative and qualitative research into a single study.

PART 1 BASIC STATISTICAL CONCEPTS

I. Four Types of Quantitative Data

The type of quantitative data makes a difference as to the type of statistical test to use.

  A. Two types of categorical data
  1. *Nominal*: Distinctive named categories, but having no implied order
       a. Example: Eye color.
  2. *Ordinal*: Distinctive categories, but having an implied order
       a. Example: Satisfaction rating scale with categories of very unsatisfied, unsatisfied, neutral, satisfied, very satisfied (Likert scale)
  B. Two types of continuous data
  1. *Interval*: Data that are continuous, where the interval between numbers has real meaning but the numbers do not have a "true zero," that is, if you double the number, the true quantity doesn't double
       a. Example: Celsius temperature, where each degree of temperature has a constant interval. From $15°C$ to $16°C$ is the same interval change as from $30°C$ to $31°C$, but a change from $15°C$ to $30°C$ really doesn't double the amount of heat.
  2. *Ratio*: Data that are continuous and also have a "true zero" so that the ratio is meaningful
       a. Example: Pulse rate of 120 beats per minute is really double a pulse rate of 60 beats per minute.

II. Measures of Central Tendency: Mean, Median, and Mode, and When to Use Each One

Mean, median, and mode are ways to give a picture of the typical result in a data set.

  A. Mean: Arithmetic average
  1. Sum of all of the data, divided by N (where N is the total number of data points)
       a. Example: Five babies have birth weights of 2,500, 3,000, 3,500, 3,500, and 4,500 g, so the mean is the sum divided by the number of data points, or 17,000 g ÷ 5 = 3,400 g.
  2. Used for continuous data (ratio, interval)
  B. Median
  1. Halfway point of the dataset, where half of the data points are located above and half below the middle point (or if there is an even number of data points, the median is half way between the two middle points)
  2. Used for continuous and ordinal data
  3. Especially useful for *skewed* data (defined later)
  C. Mode
  1. Most frequently occurring number of the dataset
  2. Used for continuous, ordinal, and nominal data

D. Example: For a dataset of birth weights (in grams) for five newborns at 2,500, 3,000, 3,500, 3,500, and 4,500 g, the mean is 17,000 g ÷ 5 = 3,400 g; the *median* is the halfway point (third value in ascending order) = 3,500 g; and the *mode* is the most frequently occurring value = 3,500 g.

III. Measuring the Variability for Continuous Data: Range, Variance, and Standard Deviation (SD) and How to Interpret These Measures

A. Range
   1. Difference between the highest and lowest values
   2. Easy to calculate, but uses only the most extreme values to describe the dataset
B. Variance
   1. Calculated by taking every data point's distance from the mean, squaring that difference, adding these together, and dividing the sum by $(n - 1)$, that is, one less than the sample size
   2. Uses all data points, but the variance is in *squared units*, and as such is not easy to understand practically
C. Standard deviation (SD)
   1. The square root of the variance (see III-B above)
   2. Useful to describe normally distributed continuous datasets because 95% of the data should be within ±2 SD (read as "plus or minus two standard deviations") from the mean (the following section explains SD)
D. Example: For a dataset of birth weights (in grams) for five newborns at 2,500, 3,000, 3,500, 3,500, and 4,500 g, the *range* is 4,500 – 2,500, or 2,000 g; the *variance* is 550,000 grams squared (g^2); and the SD is 742 g.

IV. The Importance of a Normal Distribution for Continuous Data

A. Characteristics of a normally distributed continuous dataset
   1. Shows a specific pattern; the most frequently occurring number (mode) is the halfway point (median), which is also the arithmetic average (mean). The farther away the data are from the mean, the rarer it is to see those data points.
   2. Approximately 68% (around two-thirds) of the data fall within ±1 SD from the mean, and 95% of the data fall within ±2 SD from the mean.
B. Using a histogram to graph continuous data
   1. Group data into equal intervals (often 8 to 14 intervals) and count how many data points fit in each interval. Then, graph these data.
   2. Normally distributed data show a histogram shape that is high in the middle, very symmetrical, and where the mean, median, and mode values are similar.
   3. Skewed data result in a histogram shape that has a long "tail" either to the left (negatively skewed, lots of low numbers) or to the right (positively skewed, lots of high numbers). The mean, median, and mode values are not the same, and often the median is a better measure of the "typical" value than the mean is.
   4. Bimodal data show a histogram with two "peaks," meaning that there may be two very different groups within the dataset.

C. Example: **Figure 11-1** is a sample dataset of newborn birth weights (N = 812 newborns), with the mean = 3,624 g, SD = 464 g, median = 3,605 g, and mode = 3,595 g. It exhibits a pattern close to a perfect normal distribution.

1. The largest number of babies (n = ~275 babies) fit into the grouping from around 3,450 to 3,800 g, and very few babies (≤ 20) fit into each of the groupings from approximately 2,300 to 2,600 g, and from 4,600 to 5,000 g. (Note: There is an overlay of a perfect normal distribution shape.)

2. The mean, median, and mode values are similar and appear in the middle of the histogram where it peaks.

3. There is no *skewness*, that is, no tail at the low or high end.

4. In a perfect normal distribution, 68% of the data are within ±1 SD of the mean (that is, 3,624 ±464 g, or from 3,160 to 4,088 g), and 95% are within ±2 SD of the mean (from 2,696 to 4,552 g). In this dataset, 73% of the data are within ±1 SD, and 95% are within ±2 SD, close to the perfect normal distribution.

5. In the perfect normal distribution, you would have 2.5% of the data higher and 2.5% of the data lower than ±2 SD, for a total of 5% of data outside of *normal*. In this sample, 2.5% of the data are higher and 2.8% lower than ±2 SD from the mean.

D. Interpreting continuous data for clinical practice

1. From a sample study (Gagnon et al., 2005), the data can be interpreted as follows.

    a. Fact: The length of hospital stay of Canadian newborns in this study was given as a mean of 29.9 hours, with a SD of 5.4 hours. Interpretation: The typical length of hospital stay was around 29.9 hours, but 95% of the newborns stayed 29.9 hours ±2 (5.4 hours), or 19.1 to 40.7 hours (almost 1 day to almost 2 days). Clue for International Board Certified Lactation Consultants (IBCLCs): Would this generalize to your setting and clientele?

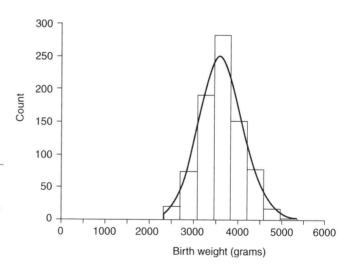

Figure 11-1
Histogram of newborn birth weights, showing frequencies of birth weight categories overlaid by a normal distribution curve.

   b. Fact: Median age at first supplementation was 8.4 hours, with a range of 1.6 to 43.9 hours. Interpretation: Fifty percent of newborns were supplemented before 8.4 hours, and 50% after 8.4 hours. Clue for IBCLCs: Although the range is interesting (i.e., the lowest and the highest values), these are the extreme values and may not represent the "typical." The median or mean is much more useful. The authors' use of a median rather than a mean implies skewed data instead of normally distributed data (most within a smaller range, but a tail of high or low values). Note: If the mean ±2 SD is an impossible value (for example, it would be impossible to have a negative length of stay), then it is skewed data and the author should report the median, not the mean or standard deviation.

E. The importance of population shift for a normal distribution
   1. According to Geoffrey Rose (1992), "A large number of people at small risk may give rise to more cases of disease than a small number who are at high risk." Epidemiologists refer to this as the Rose Theorem.
   2. For a continuous value that shows a normal distribution in the population, a small change for everyone in the population has a dramatic effect on the percentage of the population below the mean (McKinlay, 1998).
   3. A normal curve has 50% of the population below the mean. If the population mean changes upward only by a relatively small amount, such as one-quarter of an SD, the percentage of the population that is now below the original mean is only 40%, and a shift of half an SD will have only 31% below the original mean (see **Figure 11-2**).

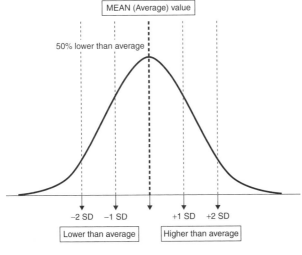

SD = Standard Deviation. Approximately 95% of the population values lie within ±2SDs of the mean value.

Figure 11-2
The normal curve distribution and the effect of population shift. Small differences in the overall mean result in large differences in the percent of the population below the mean (SD = Standard Deviation)*

* SD = Standard Deviation. Approximately 95% of the population values lie within ± 2SDs of the mean value.

a. Example: Mean IQ is 100 with a SD of 15. In Kramer et al.'s (2008) randomized hospital intervention study, breastfed babies born at Baby-Friendly Hospital Initiative (BFHI) hospitals compared to those born at non-BFHI hospitals had longer duration of exclusive breastfeeding and their mean IQ was 4.2 points higher 6.5 years later. This is $4.2 \div 15$, or approximately one-quarter of a standard deviation. So, for breastfed babies, the degree of exclusivity resulting from birth in a BFHI hospital resulted in 40% having an IQ less than 100 (compared to 50% normally). A small increase in the overall mean has a large effect at the population level for public health planners.

V. Standard Error (SE) and 95% Confidence Intervals (CI) of the Mean

A. Standard error (SE) of the mean
  1. From a sample drawn from the whole target population, SE helps you estimate a range within which you would expect *the true population mean* to be found, based on your study sample.
  2. SE is calculated from the SD and the sample size N, that is, $SE = SD \div \sqrt{N}$.
  3. Expect to find the true population mean somewhere around ±2 SE of the mean in your sample (Note: The 2 will vary by your sample size—statistical tables or statistical programs give the correct number; for general purposes with reasonable sample sizes, this is approximately 2).
  4. The larger the sample size (N), the smaller the SE, and the narrower the interval in which you can approximate the true population mean (the payoff for using large sample sizes in a study so that you have a narrower estimate of the true population mean).

B. 95% confidence interval of the mean
  1. The interval represented by the mean ±2 SE is called the 95% confidence interval (95% CI) or 95% confidence limit of the mean.
  2. We are 95% sure that the true population mean lies within this 95% CI of the mean calculated from a small sample (statistics always has uncertainty attached to its estimates).

C. Example of the normally distributed dataset of newborn birth weights for $N = 812$ newborns, where the mean = 3,624 g, SD = 464 g, and SE = 16 g.
  1. From this study, we are 95% certain that the true population mean of full-term newborns' birth weight lies somewhere between 3,592 and 3,656 g. These are the calculations.
    a. SE = SD divided by the square root of N, or $464 \div \sqrt{812} = 16$ g.
    b. 95% CI of the mean is 3,624 ±2 (SE), or 3,624 ±2 (16); that is, from 3,592 to 3,656 g.

D. Interpreting SE and 95% CI of the mean in clinical practice
  1. Use caution when reading publications showing the mean plus or minus a number. Determine whether this number is the SD, 2 SD, SE, or 95% CI. Different journals use different notations. Interpretation varies hugely. SD describes the entire dataset, with ±1 SD encompassing 68% and ±2 SD

encompassing 95% of the data points; SE describes the estimate of the population mean, with the mean ±2 SE (also called the 95% CI) giving the interval in which the researcher is 95% sure includes the true population mean.

VI. Reading Graphs

There are several ways to display data, but the most common are error bar charts, box plots, and pie charts.

  A. Error bar charts

    1. These show the mean (arithmetic average) and a line to indicate the variation.

    2. Determine what the line represents because this differs among various publications and could be specified as: ±1 SD, ±2 SD, ±1 SE, or ±2 SE (described earlier).

    3. Example: **Figure 11-3** shows mean birth weights of full-term newborns by gestational age ($N = 809$), with the lines showing ±2 SE (that is, 95% CI) indicating the estimate of the population mean for each gestational age.

      a. Wider intervals imply smaller sample size on which to base the population mean of 37 weeks gestation ($n = 32$) and 42 weeks ($n = 14$); compared to 40 weeks ($n = 300$). The larger the sample size, the narrower the SE and the narrower the estimate of the true population mean.

  B. Box plots

    1. The median is a line within the rectangle. The lower (Q1) and upper (Q3) edges of the rectangle are the 25th and 75th percentiles, respectively. Thus, Q1 and below are 25% of the data points, the median and below is 50%, and Q3 and below are 75% of the data points.

    2. The T-shaped lines extending from each end are called whiskers. Different textbooks suggest different ways to draw these, such as at the 10th and 90th percentiles, or at the most extreme low and high values, or 1.5 times the distance between Q1 and Q3 (as shown in **Figure 11-4**) where data points outside these whiskers are considered *outliers*. Outliers are considered to be very unusual values and could indicate a skewed distribution.

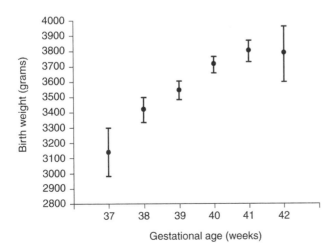

Figure 11-3
Error bar plot of birth weight by gestational age, showing 95% confidence intervals of the mean birth weight for each age.

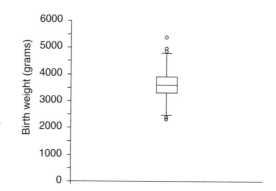

Figure 11-4
Box plot showing the
birth weights of full-term
newborns.

    3. Example: In **Figure 11-4**, the median is 3,600 g and the box is at 3,300 and
      3,900 g, so 25% of babies have birth weights below 3,300, 50% below 3,600,
      and 75% below 3,900 g. Five data points (three above, two below) lie beyond
      the whiskers, so are considered outliers.

C. Pie charts

    1. A pie chart displays the percentage of data that fits into each category, with the
      entire circle representing 100% of the data.

    2. Example: Compare **Figure 11-5** with **Figure 11-6**. **Figure 11-5** gives the
      reader the information about the relative percentage of each category. **Figure
      11-6** gives the identical information in the form of a bar chart. The reader might
      get a better idea of the relative percentages from the pie chart format.

VII. Statistical Testing and Inferential Statistics

A. Terminology

    1. *Inferential statistics*: Generalizes beyond the research sample and makes state-
      ments (inferences) about the population, with realistic uncertainty about the
      conclusions. For example, a study has a target population of interest from which
      a sample is drawn that should represent this target population. The results
      should then generalize to the target population from which you took your
      sample (you should be able to use the data to infer information about the target
      population).

    2. *Dependent and independent variables*: The dependent variable (also known as the
      outcome variable) is the measure in which you are interested as the outcome of
      your research question. The independent variable(s), also known as the *explana-*
      tory variable(s), are those measures used to help explain variation in the outcome
      measure.

      a. Example: In a study to examine factors influencing the duration of breast-
        feeding, breastfeeding duration is the outcome variable, and explanatory
        variables could include maternal age, ethnicity, parity, type of prenatal or
        postpartum counseling, and the infant's gestational age or birth weight.

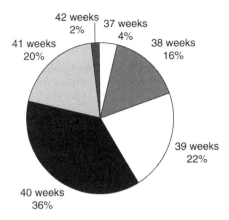

Figure 11-5
Pie chart showing the frequency of gestational age categories in a study of full-term newborns.

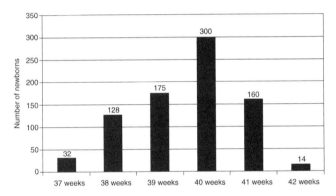

Figure 11-6
Bar chart showing frequency of gestational age categories in a study of full-term newborns.

3. *Null hypothesis and alternate hypothesis*: The "default setting" of statistics is that there is no relationship between the explanatory and outcome variables; this is called the null hypothesis. A researcher needs to find enough proof to reject the null hypothesis (that is, there is no relationship or difference) and accept the alternate hypothesis (that is, there is a relationship or difference).

4. *One-tailed versus two-tailed hypotheses*: If a hypothesis has a sense of direction, then you say it is a *one-tailed* hypothesis. If not, it is a two-tailed hypothesis. One-tailed testing is more powerful statistically, so you are less likely to make a type 2 error and more likely to find a difference if it truly exists (see definitions 6 through 8 that follow).

   a. Example: The *null hypothesis* states that there is no relationship between how long a baby is breastfed and whether the mother received postpartum support. The *alternate hypothesis* could state that "there is a relationship between breastfeeding duration and postpartum support." This is a two-tailed hypothesis because postpartum support could either increase or decrease the duration, but that isn't stated. A one-tailed hypothesis would state "Postpartum support will be associated with an increase in breastfeeding duration."

5. *P-value and the meaning of* P < .05. Statistical testing depends on the ideas of probability (italicized *P*).

   a. The *P*-value states the probability of seeing your research result based on chance alone, that is, assuming that the null hypothesis is correct and your result is simply part of a normal distribution of results when no relationship exists.

   b. $P < .05$ (read, *P* less than point zero five) states that if the null hypothesis were correct, you would see a result like this by chance only less than 5% of the time (.05 means .05 out of 1, or 5 out of 100, or 5%).

   c. If the *P*-value of a statistical test is less than 5%, you reject the null hypothesis and conclude the alternate hypothesis (that is, there is a relationship that is *statistically significant*).

   d. *P*-values less than 5%, for example, $P < .05$, $P < .01$, and $P < .001$ (less than 5%, 1% and 0.1%, respectively), conclude that there is a statistically significant finding.

   e. *P*-values greater than 5%, for example, $P < .34$, $P < .08$, and $P < .20$ (34%, 8%, and 20%, respectively), are not statistically significant (NS) and so you would conclude the null hypothesis (that is, there is no statistically significant difference or relationship).

6. *Type 1 error*: When a study concludes that there is a statistically significant difference, even though the null hypothesis was correct at the population level (could be thought of as the "overenthusiast" error; see **Table 11-1**).

   a. The *P*-value indicates the level of type 1 error, with $P < .05$, meaning that 5% of the time you could see this difference by chance alone (5% of the time, or 1 in 20 times, you could wrongly conclude a difference even though the null hypothesis was correct).

7. *Type 2 error*: When a study concludes that there is no difference (that is, concluding that the null hypothesis is correct) even though there really is a difference at the population level (could be thought of as the "skeptic" error; see **Table 11-1**) (also refer to Martens, 1995).

   a. A type 2 error may occur when the sample size (N) of a study is small.

   b. For studies that conclude no significant difference (NS), ensure that the power of the study is sufficient to find a difference if it truly exists (see *power*, described later). One possible hint is that the *P*-value is larger than 0.05; therefore, it is not statistically significant, but the value is very close (like $P=0.07$).

8. *Power of a study*: Power refers to how likely you are to find a real difference if it exists, given your sample size.

   a. Good studies are designed with a power of at least 80%.

   b. Statistical calculations prior to the study can ensure adequate power, so there is less chance of committing a type 2 error.

9. *Statistical significance versus clinical significance*: A study can show statistically significant results, but because of very large sample sizes there actually may be only a small real difference. Practitioners must decide whether the difference is *clinically significant*, that is, whether it has any clinical impact.

Table 11-1 Type I and Type II Errors

		REALITY at the population level	
		Null hypothesis is true (no difference)	Alternate hypothesis is true (real difference)
Results based on your research project	Conclude "no difference" (stick with the null hypothesis)	Correct conclusion	**Type II error**
	Conclude difference exists (reject the null hypothesis and accept the alternate hypothesis)	**Type I error**	Correct conclusion

    a. Example: In a research study involving a very large number of women, a new drug (costing twice as much as a standard drug already in use) increases milk production by a small but statistically significant amount of 1 milliliter per 24 hours (1 mL/24 h). This statistic is probably not clinically significant to justify the extra cost. Alternatively, if this drug increased a woman's milk supply by a substantial amount (50 mL/24 h, for example), then it may be clinically as well as statistically significant.

B. Statistical tests

    1. Statistical tests indicate whether there is enough proof to reject the null hypothesis and conclude the alternate hypothesis.

        a. If $P < .05$, then reject the null hypothesis and accept the alternate hypothesis (that a statistically significant relationship or difference exists).

    2. The type of statistical test chosen depends on the type of data you are analyzing. **Table 11-2** describes several commonly used statistical tests.

        a. Parametric tests assume that the data are normally distributed, whereas nonparametric tests do not assume this (for example, nonparametric tests can be used for skewed distributions of continuous data).

    3. Statistical tests can show associations between variables, but this does not necessarily mean causation (that one caused the other; see the section titled "Basic Research Designs" in Part 2 for more information on causation).

PART 2 Basic Epidemiological Concepts

I. Basic Epidemiological Terms to Determine Risk

    A. *Relative risks and odds ratios*: Statistics used to compare the risk or odds of disease for groups that are exposed or unexposed to something (see **Table 11-3** for examples).

Table 11-2 Common Statistical Tests, with Examples

Statistical Test	Type of Data	Test statistic	Example	What You Would Conclude
T-test (Student's T-test)	Compares the means of two different groups. Outcome variable: continuous data; Explanatory variable: categorical data (two "groups")	t	Is there a difference in the mean birth weight of male and female full-term newborns? Males: 3692 g (95% CI 3648–3736) ; Females: 3557 g (95% CI 3512–3602) ; t=4.18, 809 df, two-tailed, p<.001	Yes, since $p < .05$ (p is actually much less, at .001). Male newborns have a higher average birth weight compared to females.
Paired t-test	Compares two different measures of the *same* person. Outcome variable: continuous data; Explanatory variable: categorical data (one "group" measured twice)	t	Is the hospital discharge weight of a full-term newborn less than the birth weight? Mean birth weight 3629 g; Mean discharge weight 3443 g; Mean difference: −186 g (95% CI −179 to −194 g), paired t-test t = −48.5, df 771, one-tailed, $p < .00001$	Yes, since $p < .05$. There is a weight loss of full-term newborns that is probably somewhere between 179 and 194 g. Note: This is called a "one-tailed" test because it has a directional hypothesis ("less") rather than just a difference (is there any difference). A one-tailed test has more power.
Analysis of variance (anova)	Compares the means of more than two groups (are the group means different, or similar?) Outcome variable: continuous data; Explanatory variable: categorical data (several "groups") Note: If you find p < .05, a subsequent statistical test (such as a Duncan's or Tukey's multiple test) must be done to find out which of the groups differ from each other.	f	Is there a difference in birth weight for those full-term newborns who are exclusively breastfed, exclusively formula fed, or partially breastfed while in hospital? Means of groups: Formula-fed 3588 g; Partial 3648 g; Exclusively breastfed 3618 g. ANOVA test: $F = 0.71$, df 2, 810; $p = 0.49$, NS)	No, since $p > .05$ (the p-value is greater than .05 or 5%). $P = 0.49$. The notation "NS" is often used for "not statistically significant." So we would stay with the null hypothesis, i.e., conclude that there is *no* evidence to show that differences in birth weight of full-term newborns are predictors of type of feeding in hospital.

Statistical Test	Type of Data	Test Statistic	Example	What You Would Conclude
Nonparametric equivalents of the above tests are used when the outcome measure is ordinal data, or when there is a breech in the assumptions of continuous data (such as skewed data or other non-normally distributed continuous data). Nonparametric tests compare medians rather than means.				
Instead of the parametric t-test: use the nonparametric Mann Whitney U test				
Instead of the paired t-test: use the Wilcoxon test				
Instead of analysis of variance (ANOVA): use the Kruskal-Wallis test				
Chi-square test	Compares proportions (are the proportions in two or more groups different?) Explanatory and outcome variables are categorical data. Usually data are displayed in the form of a table (called a contingency table), like in Table 9-3.	χ^2	Are primiparous women more likely to experience a cesarean section birth than multiparous women? $n = 807$ (287 primips, 520 multips). 60 primips and 55 multips women had c-section births. $\chi^2 = 16.1$, df 1, p < .0001.	Yes, since $p < .05$. Primiparas were twice as likely as multiparas (20.9% versus 10.6%) to experience cesarean section birth.
Alternatives to Chi-square test:				
Fisher's Exact Test: for small counts				
McNemar Test: paired data, ie, two categorical measures of the same person				
Correlation (Pearson's correlation)	Looks at the relationship between two continuous variables (you measure two different things about the same person, over many people), and asks the question, "is it a linear relationship?" Correlation coefficients have values between −1 (strong negative relationship, with one number getting larger as the other gets smaller) and +1 (strong positive relationship, with one number getting larger as the other gets larger), with "0" meaning no relationship (the null hypothesis). The amount of variation explained by this relationship is equal to the square of the correlation coefficient r.	r	Is there a correlation between healthy, full-term newborn birth weight and the percent weight loss in hospital? $r = 0.128$, df 773; $r < .0004$	Yes. The correlation is positive (i.e., the higher the birth weight, the higher the weight loss). However, this relationship does not explain much of the variation ($r^2 = .016$, or 1.6% of the total variation).

(continues)

Table 11-2 Common Statistical Tests, with Examples (continued)

Statistical Test	Type of Data	Test statistic	Example	What You Would Conclude
Nonparametric equivalent of the Pearson's correlation: Spearman's correlation, used for continuous data that is nonnormal, or ordinal data.				
Multiple regression	Looks at the unique contribution of several explanatory variables on a continuous outcome measure. Explanatory variables can be continuous or categorical. Multiple regressions produce an equation of how each explanatory variable uniquely contributes to the outcome variable.		What are the predictors of birth weight of full-term newborns? Birth weight (grams) = −2065 + 142 (gestational age in weeks) −114 (female) + 142 (multiparous) + 129 (cesarean section birth) Model: $F = 38.5$; df 4, 798; $p < .0001$, $r^2 = 0.16$. Each explanatory variable was significant $(p < .05)$.	This model explains 16% of the variation in birth weight $(r^2 = 0.16)$, and shows the unique contribution of each explanatory variable. You can calculate the mean birth weight of a newborn from the equation. For example: for a male baby (male coded as 1, female as 0 in the equation) born at 40 weeks to a multiparous (coded as 1) mother vaginally (coded as 0): Predicted mean birth weight = −2065 + 142 (40) −114 (0) + 142 (1) + 129 (0) = 3757 g.
Logistic regression	Looks at the unique contribution of several explanatory variables on a dichotomous categorical outcome variable (yes/no; alive/dead; breastfed/not, etc.). Explanatory variables can be continuous or categorical. Odds Ratios (OR) show the unique contribution of each explanatory variable on the outcome.		What factors are associated with a breastfed baby being exclusively breastfed (this is a yes/no measure) while in hospital? Explanatory variables include: parity, sex of newborn, high birth weight (> 4000g) or not, type of delivery (cesarean section or not), and use of a spinal epidural or not during delivery n=696, model p < .001, $r^2 = 0.05$; parity (p = .71, NS); sex (p=.20, NS); type of delivery (p < .0005, OR = .42); epidural (p<.02, OR = .63); normal birth weight (p<.02, OR = 1.6)	Parity and the sex of the newborn are not statistically significant factors associated with exclusive breastfeeding. Statistically significant factors $(p < .05)$: Both cesarean section delivery and having an epidural are statistically significant factors in reducing the chance of being exclusively breastfed (the OR is less than 1); being of normal birth weight significantly increases the chance of being exclusively breastfed.

1. *Relative risk (RR)* compares the probability of getting the disease in the exposed group versus in the unexposed group. RR is an intuitive measure—an RR of 2 means that the exposed group has twice the risk of the unexposed group.
   a. Example (see **Table 11-3**): The RR of being supplemented if the baby has a high birth weight (HBW) is calculated by taking the probability of getting the "disease" (i.e., being supplemented) in the "exposed" (i.e., HBW) versus in the "unexposed" (i.e., normal weight) groups. For HBW, 67 of 142 babies were supplemented, for a probability of 0.472. For normal weight, 204 of 558 were supplemented, for a probability of 0.366. In other words, 47.2% of HBW and 36.6% of normal birth weight babies were supplemented. So, RR = (67 ÷ 142 divided by 204 ÷ 558) = (0.472 ÷ 0.366) = 1.29. This means that the risk of supplementation for HBW babies was *1.29 times the risk* for normal birth weight babies; you could also say that the risk of supplementation was 29% *higher* for HBW compared to normal birth weight babies.
2. *Odds ratio (OR)* compares the odds of getting a disease in the exposed group versus in the unexposed group. An *odds* is a calculation of the number of times an event happens divided by the number of times it did not.
   a. Example (see **Table 11-3**): The odds of being supplemented for HBW is 67 ÷ 75, or 0.893; the odds of being supplemented for normal birth weight babies is 204 ÷ 354, or 0.576. The OR = odds of getting the disease for the exposed group compared to the unexposed group = 0.893 ÷ 0.576 = 1.55. This is a much more complex idea and doesn't translate as intuitively as an RR. Sometimes people use the word *likelihood* to describe OR. For example, the likelihood of supplementation is 1.55 times greater for the HBW babies compared to normal birth weight babies. That does not translate as intuitively as RR (see the previous example).

Table 11-3 Is the Risk of Being Supplemented Associated with a Full-Term Breastfed Newborn's Birth Weight?*

	Breastfed newborns in hospital: exclusive or supplemented		
	Supplemented ("diseased")	**Exclusively breastfed ("not diseased")**	**Total**
High birth weight ("exposed")	**67 (47.2%)**	**75**	142
Normal birth weight ("not exposed")	**204 (36.6%)**	**354**	558
	429	271	700

*Chi-square = 5.38, 1 df, *p* < .025 (because the *P*-value is less than 0.05, it means there is a "statistically significant" association between high birth weight and supplementation).

3. For both RR and OR, 1 means that there is the same risk, greater than 1 (> 1) means a bigger risk, and less than 1 (< 1) means a smaller risk.
   a. RR and OR are often shown with 95% CI. If the 95% CI includes 1, then it is not statistically significant (NS), and we conclude that the exposure has no significant effect on the risk of disease.
   b. For example: RR = 1.4 (95% CI 1.3–1.5). From this example, conclude that there is a statistically significantly higher risk of disease in the exposed group because the RR is greater than 1, and the 95% CI does not include 1. When relative risk is 1.2 (95% CI 0.9–1.5, NS), because the 95% CI includes 1, it is not statistically significant (NS), so you can conclude that there is no statistically significant increase in the risk of disease. When RR = 0.5 (95% CI 0.3–0.7), conclude that there is a statistically significant lower risk of disease in the exposed group because the RR is less than 1, and the 95% CI does not include 1.
4. RR and OR are very close numerically only if the prevalence of disease is small, that is, less than 10% (< 10%; Zhang, 1998).
5. Certain types of statistical analyses (such as logistic regression) and study designs (such as case-control studies) produce OR values rather than RR. Be very careful of the interpretation of OR when the outcome is not a rare event (i.e., more than 10%) (as described earlier).
6. Various other measures are used in epidemiologic studies, such as risk difference, attributable risk (exposed), and population-attributable risk. (See **Table 11-4**.)
7. Number needed to treat (NNT)
   a. Usually used to describe a positive intervention, such as a pharmaceutical or program intervention. Calculated by 1 ÷ RD, where RD is the *risk difference* (see **Table 11-4**).
   b. How many people would you need to treat to see the effect?
   c. Example: In a longitudinal study on infant feeding and its relationship to type 2 diabetes, it was found that 10% of adults who had been exclusively breastfed and 17% of adults who had been exclusively formula-fed had adult type 2 diabetes. The RD is 17% – 10% = 7% (or 0.07 as a fraction of 1 rather than a percentage). So, the NNT = (1 ÷ .07) = 14, meaning that 14 babies must be exclusively breastfed to prevent one case of adult type 2 diabetes.

II. Basic Research Designs

A. Study designs can be described through a series of questions (see **Figure 11-7**).
   1. Is the study descriptive or analytical?
   2. If analytical, is there artificial manipulation (*experimentation*) or not?
   3. Is the artificial manipulation (in *experimental studies*), that is, intervention, under the control of the researcher?
      a. Are people or sites randomly assigned to receive or not receive the intervention (*randomized controlled trial*)? For example: Women experiencing sore nipples postpartum are randomly assigned two types of nipple cream and followed to see which produces the fastest healing.

Table 11-4 Epidemiologic Concepts, Meanings, and Examples

Measure	Other Names	What This Means	Example from Table 9-3	Interpreting the Example
Relative Risk (RR)	Risk ratio Rate ratio	Comparing two groups. What risk for disease has the exposed group compared to the unexposed group?	Of breastfed full-term newborns ($n = 700$), 47.2% of high birth weight babies were supplemented, but only 36.6% of other newborns. RR = 1.29. (OR = 1.55)	A high birth weight newborn was 1.29 times (29%) more likely to be supplemented compared to a normal birth weight newborn. Note that the OR similarly shows that there is a greater chance or "odds" of (OR = 1.55), but not as intuitive as RR. OR and RR are very close only if the outcome is rare.
Risk Difference (RD)	Rate difference Absolute risk reduction		Of breastfed full-term newborns ($n = 700$), 47.2% of high birth weight babies were supplemented, but only 36.6% of other newborns. Risk Difference (RD) = .472 − .366 = .106 (or 10.6% difference)	10.6% more babies were supplemented in the high birth weight group. This gives an idea of how LARGE the true difference is (note: you can have a large RR, but a very small risk difference. For example: if only 1% of high birth weight babies and .78% of the others were supplemented, the RR would still be 1.29, but the risk difference is a very small amount, i.e., 1% − .78% = .22%)
Attributable Risk (exposed)	Attributable fraction exposed, (or proportion exposed, or risk percent exposed)	Among those "exposed" to the risk factor, what proportion of "disease" resulted because of being exposed?	Attributable Risk (exposed) = (RR − 1) ÷ RR = (1.29-1) ÷ 1.29 = 0.225 or 22.5%	Among those having the risk factor of high birth weight, .225 or 22.5% of them were supplemented because of this risk factor. In other words, some of these babies would have been supplemented just because supplementation also occurred in the nonrisk (nonhigh birth weight) babies. So 22.5% of the high birth weight babies were supplemented due to being high birth weight.

(continues)

Table 11-4 Epidemiologic Concepts, Meanings, and Examples (continued)

Measure	Other Names	What This Means	Example from Table 9-3	Interpreting the Example
Population Attributable Risk	Etiologic Fraction, Population attributable fraction, Population attributable proportion, Population attributable risk percent	Among the WHOLE population, what proportion of the disease cases resulted because of being exposed?	Population Attributable Risk = $$P(RR-1) \div [P(RR-1) + 1] = .203(1.29 - 1) \div [.203(1.29-1) + 1] = .056 \text{ or } 5.6\%$$ Note: to calculate Population Attributable Risk, you need to know the overall proportion of high birth weight (P) in your population. In Table 9-3, P, which is 142 of the 700 babies, or 20.3%.	Of all the supplemented newborns (both high birth weight and normal birth weight), 5.6% of them were supplemented because they were "exposed" (because they were of high birth weight).

b. Are people or sites selected to be as similar as possible prior to the intervention, but not randomly assigned (*quasi-experimental comparison group*)? For example: Two very similar hospital sites are chosen, and one site begins a new rooming-in policy intervention while the other does not. In-hospital exclusive breastfeeding rates are measured at both sites over the next several months to see if the policy had an effect.

4. Is artificial manipulation used or is the research an observational study?

a. Is information collected concurrently at one point in time (that is, a *cross-sectional study*) or over time (*longitudinal study*)?

b. If cross-sectional, you cannot say that one factor "causes" the other, only that they are "associated." For example: Using national survey data collected at one point in time, you find that low income is associated with low breastfeeding rates of babies. This is an association, but one does not necessarily cause the other.

c. If longitudinal, then:

i. *Cohort study*: Do you follow people forward from "exposure" to "disease" to see the effects of exposure or nonexposure on future risk of disease? Do you start now and go forward in time (prospective), or do you have a "cohort" somewhere in the past and you follow them forward (historical prospective)? For example: Interviewing women in their third trimester about their social supports and confidence levels ("exposures") and following them through time to see if they breastfed or not ("disease").

ii. *Case-control study*: Do you go backward from "disease" to "exposure," that is, compare those people with and without the disease according to their past exposure to the risk factors being studied? For example: Selecting groups of adults with and without diabetes (disease) and taking a history

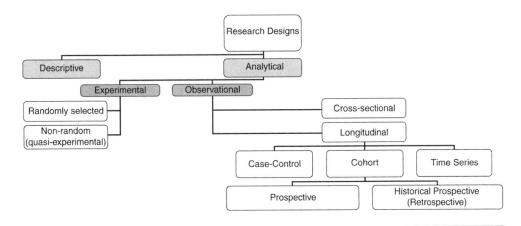

Figure 11-7 Research design schema.

of their past exposure such as breastfeeding status, eating patterns, and past exercise to see if exposure patterns differ between the two groups.

   iii. *Time series study* (with or without a comparison site): Do you measure rates of a population over time to see if any trends are occurring (and if these can be related to naturally occurring interventions in the community; called natural experiments). For example: Community breastfeeding rates are tracked year by year over 15 years, and qualitative data about occurrences in policy or programs in the community are layered on these trends to see what might have influenced the trends (time series without a comparison). The breastfeeding rates of another community that did not receive the policy or program could also be tracked over 15 years, to see the differences (*time series with a comparison*).

B. Each study design has its strengths and limitations in terms of validity. There are also various threats to validity (Campbell et al., 1963).

   1. *Internal validity*: Refers to the strength of evidence for causation. For example, does X really cause Y?

     a. Examples of threats to internal validity (see Martens 2002a, 2002b): non-blinding (the people in the experiment know which treatment group they are in); selection bias (the groups differed before the intervention even occurred); maturation (did something change naturally over time, despite the intervention?).

     b. Randomized controlled trials (RCTs) are considered to have high internal validity, but not all interventions can be randomized ethically (you can't randomize babies to be breastfed or not!).

     c. Evaluation criteria for the type of evidence: the *Clinical Guidelines for the Establishment of Exclusive Breastfeeding* (Overfield et al., 2005) considers internal validity of a research study by classifying the strength of the evidence according to a hierarchy similar to **Figure 11-8** .

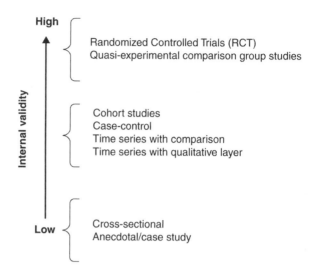

Figure 11-8
Hierarchy of internal validity
(causality) for research designs.

2. *External validity*: Refers to whether the results of the study are generalizable to settings beyond the study itself.

    a. Does the study reflect the "real world" or are the restrictions to enrollment, the setting, or the conditions of the intervention quite different than your clinical setting or the ordinary care a person would receive?

    b. Although RCTs are high in internal validity, they may be less than ideal for generalizability because of their highly restrictive enrollment and artificial setting. Thus, quasi-experimental or observational studies may better generalize into other real-world settings.

PART 3 Basic Research Tools and Instruments

I. Instruments

Measures can be derived from various sources, such as chart audits or direct measures using *instruments*. These instruments can take the form of measurement instruments such as weigh scales or tools such as surveys.

II. Instrument Reliability and Validity

A. Reliability: How reproducible are the results?

   1. Example: Weighing a baby on a scale several times should give you the same (or similar) results if the scale is *reliable*.

B. Validity: How close to the truth are the results?

   1. Example: How close is a scale to the true weight? A scale can be giving a similar weight over several weighings (reliable), but could be consistently weighing too high or too low (therefore, not valid). Only by calibrating the scale to a valid standard and then doing serial weighings would the data be valid.

C. Nonvalidity: You can "hit the mark" (that is, be close to the truth; valid) or you can get repeatable results (that is, close to each other; reliable) without being valid (**Figure 11-9**). If you have nonrepeatability (nonreliability), then you cannot have validity.

III. Survey Instruments

A. Need to be tested for reliability

1. Test–retest (that is, do people get similar results when doing the test a second time after a period when nothing has changed?); interraterreliability (if there is more than one surveyor, do they code in a similar way?); intrarater reliability (is each surveyor coding consistently over time?).

2. Statistical tests that indicate reliability include Cronbach alpha (from 0 to 1, where closer to 1 means better reliability), Cohen kappa (where two observers rate the same event to see whether there is close agreement; ≥ .7 is considered good agreement).

B. Need to be tested for validity

1. *Construct validity*: Does the tool measure all aspects of the concept it is designed to measure? You need to do a literature search to see which concepts should be included when designing a tool.

2. *Content validity, face validity*: Does the content of the survey make sense to the experts in the field and the current literature? A peer review from experts in the field is useful.

3. *Concurrent validity*: Does this tool perform similarly to another validated tool that is supposed to measure a similar construct? Example: Does a new tool to measure the effectiveness of breastfeeding in the early postpartum period give similar results to a tool already tested in the literature?

4. *Predictive validity*: Does this tool measure something that is statistically predictive of some logical variable in the future? Example: You hypothesize that a tool measuring the intent to breastfeed shows a statistically significant positive relationship with the real infant feeding choice at birth. If it does, then the tool has predictive validity.

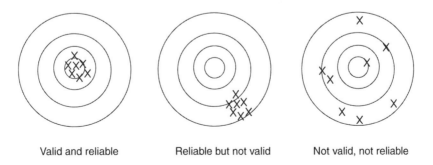

Valid and reliable   Reliable but not valid   Not valid, not reliable

Figure 11-9 A diagram illustrating validity and reliability in terms of "hitting the mark" of a target.

C. Checklist for using survey instruments
   1. Always pilot test a survey with people similar to those who will be in the study.
   2. Look for surveys that have been used before, that have been tested for validity and reliability.
   3. Avoid common problems in survey questions.
      a. Avoid double negatives. Bad example: Do you not breastfeed in situations that are not private? Better wording: Do you breastfeed in public situations?
      b. Avoid asking more than one question in an item. Bad example: Answer yes or no: Do you like cheese or pickles? Problem: If the respondent answers yes, the surveyor doesn't know whether the person likes cheese only, pickles only, or both. Better wording is to ask separate questions.
      c. Avoid overlapping categories. Bad example: Is your baby 2–4 months old or 4–6 months old? Problem: Which answer should be given if the baby is 4 months old? Better wording: Is your baby 2–4 months old or 5–6 months old?
      d. Avoid leading or biased questions.
      e. Avoid questions that are not applicable to all respondents, unless you allow people to skip questions.
      f. Avoid forcing people to answer questions for which they don't know the answer—give a "don't know" choice.
D. A survey is a tool to collect data for many different research designs (longitudinal, cross-sectional, RCTs, and so on) and not a study design itself.

IV. Importance of Definitions (Operationalizing the Construct)

A. It is important to understand the way in which a construct is operationalized, that is, how an idea or concept is actually defined for measurement.
   1. Example: In a study of health outcomes, breastfed babies are compared to babies who are not breastfed. To understand the study and critically analyze the results, it is important to understand how these constructs (breastfed and non-breastfed) were operationalized (defined).

PART 4 How to Critique the Quantitative Literature: Being a Good Consumer of Research

I. Reviewing the Literature

A. Internet search engines
   Search various web-based sources using keywords or phrases.
   1. *PubMed* (United States National Library of Medicine and the National Institutes of Health) is a free search engine of peer-reviewed health-related published articles (www.ncbi.nlm.nih.gov/pubmed). PubMed displays the abstracts and, for some articles with free access, the entire article. Most universities also provide access to the complete articles through special access to PubMed or other search engines in health and social sciences.

B. Published conference abstracts
  1. Called gray literature because they have not undergone rigorous peer review and neither are they published in a peer-reviewed journal. The abstracts might provide anecdotal evidence, preliminary or unconfirmed study results of interest, and suggestions for further research.
C. Tips for searching the literature
  1. Be careful of the single study. One study alone is probably not sufficient evidence on which to base practice. The concept of $P < .05$ implies that 5% of the time (or 1 time out of 20) you could make a type 1 error and jump to the alternate hypothesis in error. Several repeated studies that all find similar results give a much stronger case on which to base practice.
  2. Look for *systematic reviews*, which are summaries of the literature done through critical appraisals of study design and methodology for all the literature on a specific topic.
      a. The Cochrane Collaboration (www.cochrane.org) library contains systematic reviews on various medical topics compiled by worldwide experts. These reviews often rely on randomized controlled trial (RCT) evidence but also include studies with other research designs if deemed of high quality. This is an extremely valuable source both for systematic reviews and for meta-analyses (described later).
      b. Examples of systematic reviews: *Clinical Guidelines for the Establishment of Exclusive Breastfeeding* (Overfield et al., 2005), which rates the evidence for each management strategy; and Britton et al. (2007), a Cochrane review of the literature on supports for breastfeeding women
  3. Look for *meta-analyses*, which statistically combine the results from several studies as if they were all part of one big study. This increases the sample size and reduces the possibility of type 2 errors in the many smaller studies. The Agency for Healthcare Research and Quality (AHRQ; www.ahrq.gov) is an excellent source for systematic reviews and meta-analyses.
      a. For example: Arenz et al. (2009) did a meta-analysis of the relationship between breastfeeding and a decreased risk of obesity. They combined several studies to yield an adjusted odds ratio of 0.77 (0.72–0.82), showing a protective effect of breastfeeding on obesity. The AHRQ also did an extensive review of all meta-analyses examining the relationship between breastfeeding and obesity (Ip et al., 2007) and also concluded a protective effect.

II. Critiquing Quantitative Research Articles

A. Criteria for research:
  1. When critiquing research articles, or designing research yourself, you need to ensure that certain criteria are met (see also Martens, 2002b). **Table 11-5** is a summary checklist.

B. ILCA funding for research:
   1. If you are submitting a research proposal to the ILCA Research Committee, a similar checklist will be used to critique the proposal (with additional checks of the budget, the proposed timeline, and the potential for the study to further the understanding of breastfeeding issues). Information for applying is available on the ILCA website, Research section (available at www.ilca.org/i4a/pages/index .cfm?pageid=3355).

Table 11-5 Checklist for Evaluating Quantitative Studies

Section	Comments
1. Problem statement and hypothesis	Is the problem clearly stated? Are the research questions, objectives, and hypotheses clearly stated? Are the population, variables, and any relationships identified? Is the problem researchable?
2. Purpose/significance	Is there an identified and supported need for the study?
3. Abstract	Never rely solely on an abstract, since you may be missing important details. Only use abstracts as screening tools for finding which studies relate to your topic of interest. Does the abstract summarize important findings in a clear manner? Does it reflect the true findings of the actual full study?
4. Literature review and background	Is there an adequate review of the literature that outlines previous findings related to the present problem? Does it present a well-rounded review? Does the review logically guide the reader to the present study? Are there sufficient background facts? Does the literature review contain systematic reviews and meta-analyses if available?
5. Conceptual framework or theory	Is there a conceptual framework or a theory that links together the study variables and makes sense as to the problem and hypotheses being studied?
6. Methodology	
A. Design	Is the design clearly explained and appropriate for the problem? What are the strengths and limitations of this type of study design? What is the degree of internal/external validity?
B. Variables	What are the independent (explanatory) and dependent (outcome) variables, and how have these been defined and measured? Do these variables adequately operationalize the constructs?
C. Population and sampling	Are the type of sampling, the selection process, and the exclusion/inclusion criteria given? Is the representativeness of the sample (in terms of representing a certain target population) described? Does this sample generalize to your particular clinical population?
D. Sample size	Is the sample size justified? Is there adequate power to detect an expected difference (80% or more power)?

Section	Comments
6. Methodology (continued)	
E. Procedures and tools	Are data collection methods appropriate for the design and setting? If instruments and tools are used, are they described adequately, including validity and reliability of the tools?
F. Ethical considerations	Did participants have a consent process? Was this research protocol reviewed by a credible ethical review committee? Are the procedures ethical? Did the researcher ensure privacy and confidentiality of the research subjects? Are data properly stored and housed?
7. Data Analysis	
A. Statistical analysis	Are the statistical tests appropriate for the design, sample size, and type of data collected? If there are skewed data, is the median result given? Are the p-values given, so you can determine the statistical significance, and the possibility of type 2 error?
B. Loss to follow-up	Is there a careful explanation of who was "lost to follow-up" in the study, and why they did not complete the study? Would this bias the study results (i.e., were those who completed the study different from those who did not?)?
8. Results	Has the research question been answered in a clear manner? Is the result clinically significant, or only statistically significant? If the conclusion is "no difference," was there adequate sample size (i.e., did the study have sufficient power)?
9. Discussion and interpretation	Does the discussion and interpretation follow from the results given, or do they go beyond the results of the study? Are the conclusions true to the study results? Are limitations of the study discussed?
10. Generalizeability	What is the real world interpretation of the study? Does it generalize to your clientele? Is the result clinically significant, not only statistically significant? Does the additional burden justify any additional cost? Is there a calculation of the RR, RD, PAR, NNT (see Table 9-4)? If not, could you do these calculations to determine if it has real world significance?
11. Sponsorship	Who sponsored or funded the study? Could this lead to potential bias? If so, examine the definitions used, the sample sizes used (to ensure adequate power, if the conclusion is not statistically significantly different, NS), and the conclusions given.

References

Arenz, S., & von Kries, R. (2009). Protective effect of breast-feeding against obesity in childhood: Can a meta-analysis of published observational studies help to validate the hypothesis? *Advances in Experimental Medicine and Biology, 639*, 145–152.

Britton, C., McCormick, F. M., Renfrew, M. J., Wade, A., & King, S. E. (2007). Support for breastfeeding mothers. *Cochrane Database of Systematic Reviews*, 1. Art. No.: CD001141. Retrieved from http://www2.cochrane.org/reviews/en/ab001141.html. doi:10.1002/14651858. CD001141.pub3

Campbell, D. T., & Stanley, J. C. (1963). *Experimental and quasi-experimental designs for research*. Chicago, IL: Rand McNally.

Gagnon, A. J., Leduc, G., Waghorn, K., & Platt, R.W. (2005). In-hospital formula supplementation of healthy breastfeeding newborns. *Journal of Human Lactation, 21*, 397–405.

Ip, S., Chung, M., Raman, G., Chew, P., Magula, N., DeVine, D., Trikalinos, T., & Lau, J. (2007, April). *Breastfeeding and maternal and infant health outcomes in developed countries* (Evidence Report/Technology Assessment No. 153, AHRQ Publication No. 07-E007). (Prepared by Tufts-New England Medical Center Evidence-based Practice Center, under Contract No. 290-02-0022). Rockville, MD: Agency for Healthcare Research and Quality. Retrieved from http://www.ncbi.nlm.nih.gov/books/NBK38337/

Kramer, M. S., Aboud, F., Mironova, E., Vanilovich, I., Platt, R. W., Matush, L., Igumnov, S., Fombonne, E., Bogdanovich, N., Ducruet, T., Collet, J. P., Chalmers, B., Hodnett, E., Davidovsky, S., Skugarevsky, O., Trofimovich, O., Kozlova, L., & Shapiro, S. (2008). Promotion of Breastfeeding Intervention Trial (PROBIT) Study Group. Breastfeeding and child cognitive development: New evidence from a large randomized trial. *Archives of General Psychiatry, 65*(5), 578–584.

Martens, P. J. (1995). A mini-lesson in statistics: What causes treatment groups to be deemed "not statistically different"? *Journal of Human Lactation, 11*, 117–121.

Martens, P. J. (2002a). "First, do no harm": Evaluating research for clinical practice. *Current Issues in Clinical Lactation*, 37–47.

Martens, P. J. (2002b). Will your breastfeeding intervention make a difference? What the lactation consultant needs to know about program evaluation. *Journal of Human Lactation, 18*, 379–381.

McKinlay, J. B. (1998). Paradigmatic obstacles to improving the health of populations—implications for health policy. *Salud Publica de Mexico, 40*, 369–379. Retrieved from http://www.scielosp.org/scielo.php?script=sci_arttext&pid=S0036-36341998000400010

Overfield, M. L., Ryan, C. A., Spangler, A., & Tully, M. R. (Eds.). (2005). *Clinical guidelines for the establishment of exclusive breastfeeding* (2nd ed.). Raleigh, NC: International Lactation Consultant Association. Retrieved from http://www.ilca.org/files/resources/ClinicalGuidelines2005.pdf

Rose, G. (1992). *The strategy of preventive medicine*. Oxford, England: Oxford University Press.

Streiner, D. L., & Norman, G. R. (1998). *PDQ (PrettyDarnedQuick) epidemiology* (2nd ed.). Hamilton, Canada: B. C. Decker.

Zhang, J. (1998). What's the relative risk? A method of correcting the odds ratio in cohort studies of common outcomes. *Journal of the American Medical Association, 280*, 1690–1691.

Suggested Reading

Barnett, V. (2002). *Sample survey: Principles and methods* (3rd ed.). New York, NY: Oxford University Press.

Bhopal, R. (2002). *Concepts of epidemiology: An integrated introduction to the ideas, theories, principles and methods of epidemiology.* New York, NY: Oxford University Press.

Harmon-Jones, C. (2005). Reading and evaluating breastfeeding research. *Leaven, 41,* 99–103.

Last, J. M., Spasoff, R. A., Harris, S. S., & Thuriaux, M. C. (Eds.). (2001). *A dictionary of epidemiology* (4th ed.). Edited for the International Epidemiological Association. New York, NY: Oxford University Press.

Norman, G. R., & Streiner, D. L. (2003). *PDQ (PrettyDarnedQuick) statistics* (3rd ed.). Hamilton, Canada: B. C. Decker.

Shadish, W. R., Cook, T. D., & Campbell, D. T. (2002). *Experimental and quasi-experimental designs for generalized causal inference.* Boston, MA: Houghton Mifflin.

Young, T. K. (2005). *Population health: Concepts and methods* (2nd ed.). New York, NY: Oxford University Press.

CHAPTER 12
Interpretation of Research: Qualitative Methodology

Sara L. Gill, PhD, RN, IBCLC, and Lisa M. Cleveland, PhD, RN, IBCLC

OBJECTIVES

- Define qualitative research.
- Describe qualitative methodologies.
- Describe the major phases of a qualitative research project.
- Discuss issues of scientific rigor in qualitative studies.

INTRODUCTION

Qualitative research is a method of inquiry used by a variety of disciplines including sociology, anthropology, and the various health sciences. Each of these disciplines has a specific area of interest or domain. Qualitative researchers seek to develop a comprehensive understanding of human behavior and the ways in which individuals create meaning in their lives. Qualitative methodologies provide a means of exploring the depth, richness, and complexity of human phenomena. The researcher becomes the instrument used to collect data through interviews and observations from key informants known as participants or respondents. These key informants have special knowledge about the phenomena under study and often help the researcher locate information or individuals (informants) to interview.

I. Assumptions of Qualitative Research

    A. Multiple constructed realities
        1. Reality, based on perception, is different for each person.
        2. The qualitative researcher must consider multiple perspectives in an attempt to fully understand a phenomenon.
    B. Subject–object interaction
        1. Researcher and participant interact to influence each other.
    C. Participant has personal knowledge about the phenomenon of interest. This knowledge may be unwritten and unspoken and includes personal beliefs and attitudes (called tacit knowledge).

D. Simultaneous mutual shaping
   1. There is no attempt to determine causality but a belief that it is impossible to differentiate cause from effect. The researcher, when using qualitative methods, does not try to show that one thing causes another, but instead is interested in understanding a phenomenon.
E. Value-bound inquiry
   1. Influenced by the researcher in the choice of method that guides the investigation

II. Qualitative Research Traditions

Each type of qualitative method is guided by a particular philosophy. This philosophy guides research questions asked, the observations made, and the data interpretation.

A. Anthropology
   1. Domain: Culture
   2. Research tradition: Ethnography, ethnoscience
   3. Example:
      a. Everyday nursing practice values in the NICU and their reflection on breast-feeding promotion (Cricco-Lizza, 2010)
      b. In this ethnographic study, the high-control, high-tech, time-urgent nursing practice values were found to be helpful in confronting uncertainty but posed challenges to ongoing nursing efforts to promote breastfeeding.
B. Philosophy
   1. Domain: Lived experience
   2. Research tradition: Phenomenology, hermeneutics
   3. Example:
      a. Mothering an extremely low-birth-weight infant: a phenomenological study (Schenk et al., 2010)
      b. The purpose of this phenomenological study was to describe the lived experience of mothers of extremely low-birth-weight infants.
      c. The breastfeeding conversation: A philosophical exploration of support (Grassley et al. 2008)
      d. The aim of this study was to explore the language of nurse–mother conversations intended to offer breastfeeding support.
C. Sociology
   1. Domain: Social settings
   2. Research tradition: Grounded theory methods
   3. Example:
      a. Complex decisions: Theorizing women's infant feeding decisions in the first 6 weeks after birth (Sheehan et al., 2009)
      b. The purpose of this grounded theory study was to investigate the decision-making processes of both breastfeeding and formula-feeding women.

D. Sociolinguistics
    1. Domain: Human communication
    2. Research tradition: Narrative analysis, discourse analysis
    3. Example:
        a. Motherhood, ethnicity, and experience: A narrative analysis of the debates concerning culture in the provision of health services for Bangladeshi mothers in East London (Griffith, 2010)
        b. In this study, the authors explore cultural claims that mothers make about motherhood by listening to the stories (narratives) that mothers shared.

E. History
    1. Domain: Past events, behavior
    2. Research tradition: Historical
    3. Example:
        a. From social to surgical: Historical perspectives on perineal care during labor and birth (Dahlen et al., 2010)
        b. A review of key historical texts (from a.d. 98–138) was conducted to gain a historical perspective on perineal care during labor and delivery.

III. Characteristics of Qualitative Research

A. Natural setting for conducting the investigation
B. Researcher is the "instrument."
    1. The researcher gathers data through interviews and observations rather than using survey tools, measurement instruments, or observation checklists (pen and paper measures).
C. Uses tacit knowledge to understand the world of the informants
D. Often (but not exclusively) uses qualitative data and methods
    1. Deals with narrative (words)
    2. Interpretative
E. Purposive sampling
    1. Participants are selected for the study based on their knowledge about the phenomena of interest.
F. Inductive data analysis: Putting pieces together to make a whole
G. Emergent research design: The research design emerges during the course of the study.
H. Tentative application
    1. Generalizability is not a goal of qualitative research, so qualitative researchers do not make broad applications of the study findings.
I. Focus-determined boundaries
    1. The qualitative researcher sets boundaries to the inquiry based on the research question, perceptions of the participants, setting, and values.

IV. Most Commonly Used Interpretative Methodologies

Method is selected according to the nature of the problem and what is known about the phenomenon to be studied.

A. Basic qualitative description

  1. Generic form of qualitative research
  2. Offers a topical/thematic summary/survey of events
  3. Least interpreted of qualitative descriptions
  4. Example:
     a. A qualitative description of receiving a diagnosis of clefting in the prenatal or postnatal period (Nussbaum et al., 2008)
     b. The purpose of this study was to describe the experiences of parents who receive a diagnosis of clefting in the prenatal or postnatal time period.

B. Phenomenology

  1. Focus is on the discovery of meaning of people's lived experience.
  2. Goal is to describe fully the lived experience and the perceptions to which it gives rise.
  3. Source of data is in-depth conversations.
  4. Steps in the process include bracketing, intuiting, analyzing, describing.
     a. Bracketing: Researcher is aware of preconceived thoughts and opinions about the phenomena of interest.
     b. Intuiting: Researcher is open to the meaning of the phenomena from the participants' perspectives.
     c. Analyzing: Researcher identifies the structure of the phenomena under study.
     d. Describing: Researcher represents a particular perspective/interpretation of the phenomena.
  5. Example:
     a. Impact of birth trauma on breastfeeding (Beck et al., 2008)
     b. Mothers' breastfeeding experiences after a birth trauma were explored using phenomenology.

C. Ethnography

  1. Goal is to describe and interpret cultural behavior.
  2. Culture is inferred from the group's words, actions, and artifacts.
  3. Assumption is that cultures guide the way people structure their experience.
  4. Seeks an emic (insider) perspective of the culture.
  5. Sources of data: Participant observations, in-depth interviews with key informants, records, charts, and physical evidence, photographs, video recordings
  6. Steps in the process include description, analysis, and interpretation.
  7. Example:
     a. Formative infant feeding experiences and education of NICU nurses (Cricco-Lizza, 2009)
     b. Using ethnography, this researcher examined NICU nurses' perspectives about infant feeding.

D. Grounded theory
  1. Best identifies and analyzes complex processes.
  2. Generates theory from data. Theory is grounded in and connected to the data.
  3. Goal is to generate comprehensive explanations of phenomena that are grounded in reality.
  4. Data collection, data analysis, and sampling occur simultaneously.
  5. Sources of data: In-depth interviews (occasionally observations).
  6. Steps include constant comparison, categories, core category, and basic social process.
  7. Example:
     a. "I wanted to do a good job": experiences of "becoming a mother" and breastfeeding in mothers of very preterm infants after discharge from a neonatal unit (Flacking et al., 2007)
     b. The purpose of this grounded theory study was to describe the process of becoming a breastfeeding mother from the perspective of mothers with very preterm infants.

V. Phases in Qualitative Design

Qualitative methodologies use a flexible rather than linear approach.

A. Orientation and overview
  1. Identify a problem.
     a. Broad topic or focus topic
     b. No hypotheses
  2. Literature review.
  3. Address ethical issues.
     a. More of a concern than in quantitative methodologies because of the close relationship between the researcher and participants.
  4. Gaining entry (access to setting and/or participants in which the researcher is interested).
B. Focused exploration
  1. Conducting the study
  2. Data analysis after data "saturation"
     a. Data collection continues until no new information is obtained during interviews or participant observation (the point of saturation). At this point, there is redundancy in the information.
C. Confirmation and closure
  1. Exiting the setting
  2. Ensuring trustworthiness
     a. Trustworthiness is similar to reliability and validity in quantitative research. When a study is trustworthy, the reader is reassured that the findings accurately reflect the viewpoints and experiences of the participants.

3. Dissemination
   a. Dissemination of research findings is critical as a means for sharing new knowledge. This may occur through a variety of venues such as oral or poster presentations at relevant conferences or through publication in professional journals or books. Additionally, findings may be shared with the community and other populations for whom the findings may be of interest.

VI. Sampling

A. Types:
   1. *Purposive:* Seek participants who have knowledge about the phenomena and can share that information.
   2. *Convenience*: May be referred to as a volunteer sample and can be used when the researcher needs potential participants to come forward. However, this is not the preferred sampling method for qualitative research because a convenience sample may not provide the researcher with the rich data needed to understand the phenomenon.
   3. *Maximum variation sampling*: Involves intentionally selecting participants who have a wide variation of dimensions specific to the phenomenon of interest.
   4. *Snowball sampling*: Asking participants to refer other participants who have knowledge of the phenomenon being investigated.
   5. *Theoretical*: Select participants based on ongoing analysis to ensure adequacy and accuracy of the emerging categories, themes, or theory.

B. Interview/observe people who have experience.
   1. At informant's convenience because of time commitments

C. Data and/or theoretical saturation is used to decide when to stop sampling.

VII. Types of Data

A. Interviews
   1. Semistructured using open-ended questions.
   2. Examine one or two topics in detail.
   3. Follows participant's lead in asking further questions; the researcher avoids asking leading questions.
   4. Sensitive to language.
   5. Checks to make sure the researcher understands what the participant is saying.
   6. As interviews progress, researcher may add additional questions.
   7. Types of questions:
      a. Behaviors or experiences
      b. Opinions or beliefs
      c. Feelings
      d. Knowledge
      e. Sensory
      f. Background or demographics

B. Participant observation
   1. Purpose
      a. A means of describing through observations the ways in which people construct their reality.
      b. A means of describing through observations the activities and interactions of a setting.
      c. Data are recorded as field notes.
   2. Steps in participant observation
      a. Gaining entry (permission to conduct the study)
      b. Initial contact
         i. Researcher introduction
        ii. Explanation of study purpose
   3. Develop trust and a cooperative relationship with the participants
      a. Be unobtrusive.
      b. Be honest.
      c. Be unassuming.
   4. Observe
      a. Space (physical)
      b. Participants
      c. Activities
      d. Objects
      e. Events
      f. Time sequencing
      g. Feelings
C. Document review
   1. May include a review of written records such as diaries, letters, newspapers, meeting minutes, and legal documents
D. Artifacts
   1. May include an analysis of items made or used by the culture such as feeding vessels or feeding utensils

VIII. Data Analysis

A. Start data analysis when researcher begins to collect data.
B. Iterative process.
   1. Data analysis guides further data collection, sampling, and analysis.
   2. Data analysis begins with the process of comparison and the development of category schemes. Data can then be coded according to correspondence with the various categories.
C. Product is rich, thick description (a very thorough description of the setting, interactions, and features of the phenomena).
D. Computer software programs (HyperResearch, Atlas.ti, QSR NVivo, and others) are available for organization and management of qualitative data.

IX. Trustworthiness

The researcher must persuade the readers that findings accurately reflect the experiences and viewpoints of the participants. Rigor or trustworthiness in qualitative research ensures that data collection and analysis are truthful. Trustworthiness in qualitative research is similar to reliability and validity in quantitative research.

- A. Credibility
  1. Techniques are employed that make it more likely that credible findings and interpretations will be produced.
  2. Prolonged engagement in the setting that is long enough to learn the culture, develop trust, and minimize misinformation.
  3. Persistent observation to identify characteristics and elements in the situation most relevant to the problem.
  4. Triangulation involves the use of corroborating evidence to draw conclusions about the phenomena. Triangulation allows for a multidimensional perspective of the phenomena of interest. Triangulation can enhance the credibility of a study. Triangulation refers to the use of multiple and different:
     a. Data sources
     b. Data collection methods
     c. Investigators
     d. Theories
  5. Peer debriefing occurs when the researcher exposes himself or herself to a disinterested peer to keep the inquirer honest, test working hypotheses, and test the next step in the methodological design.
  6. Negative case analysis is when the researcher looks for disconfirming data (data that challenge the researcher's understanding of the phenomena) in both past and future observations/interviews. Analyzing disconfirming data provides new understanding about the emerging conceptualization.
  7. Member checks are when data and beginning interpretations are confirmed by study participants.
- B. Dependability
  1. The stability of qualitative data over time and conditions. An inquiry audit, a scrutiny of the data collection and analysis by an external reviewer, is used to ensure dependability.
- C. Confirmability
  1. Refers to the objectivity of the data. Inquiry audits are used to ensure confirmability. The researcher must develop an audit trail, materials consistently and conscientiously recorded and organized throughout the research process documenting both data collection and analysis strategies, which allows an independent auditor to come to conclusions about the data.
- D. Transferability
  1. Refers to the extent to which the researcher has provided a thorough description of the phenomenon (thick description).
  2. The researcher is responsible for providing thick description that makes transferability judgments possible on the part of the potential appliers.

X. Ethical Concerns

A. The same ethical principles for quantitative methods apply to qualitative methods. Given the nature of qualitative methods, implementation of these principles throughout the research process may be different.

B. Concern around issues of harm, consent, deception, privacy, and confidentiality of data.

C. Prior to data collection, Institutional Review Board approval must be obtained as well as permission from the data collection site.

D. Consent is ongoing in qualitative studies.

E. Anonymity must be preserved.

    1. More than changing persons' names.

    2. Remove as many identifiers as possible.

    3. Report demographic characteristics as group data.

    4. Change the name of institutions, cities, suburbs, and so forth.

F. Participants have the following rights:

    1. To be fully informed of the study's purpose

    2. To be aware of the time required and amount of involvement for participation

    3. To confidentiality and anonymity

    4. To ask questions of the investigator

    5. To refuse to participate without negative ramifications

    6. To refuse to answer any questions

    7. To withdraw from the study at any time

    8. To know what to expect during the research process

    9. To know what information is being obtained about them

    10. To know who will have access to the information

    11. To know how the information will be used

    12. To receive a copy of the findings, if desired

XI. Critiquing Qualitative Research (Beck, 2009)

A. Was the research problem clearly stated and easy to identify?

B. Were the research questions explicitly stated?

C. Did the current literature on the topic provide a solid basis for the new study?

D. Were appropriate measures taken to safeguard the rights of the participants?

E. Was the research methodology congruent with the techniques used to collect and analyze the data?

F. Was the best possible method used to ensure an adequate sample and richness of data?

G. Were the data gathering methods well described and were they appropriate?

H. Were measures taken to ensure trustworthiness of the data?

I. Were data management and analysis consistent with the methodology?

J. Was sufficient evidence presented in the written report to demonstrate a relationship between the interpretation (categories, codes, etc.) and the data (quotations)?

References

Beck, C. T. (2009). Critiquing qualitative research. *AORN Journal, 90*, 543–554

Beck, C. T., & Watson, S. (2008). Impact of birth trauma on breast-feeding. *Nursing Research, 57*, 228–236.

Cricco-Lizza, R. (2009). Formative infant feeding experiences and education of NICU nurses. *MCN, American Journal of Maternal Child Nursing, 34*(4), 236–242.

Cricco-Lizza, R. (2010). Everyday nursing practice values in the NICU and their reflection on breastfeeding promotion. *Quality Health Research, 20*, 1–12.

Dahlen, H. G., Homer, C. S., Leap, N., & Tracy, S. K. (2010). From social to surgical: Historical perspectives on perineal care during labour and birth. *Women & Birth, 164*, 1–7.

Flacking, R., Ewald, U., & Starrin, B. (2007). "I wanted to do a good job": Experiences of "becoming a mother" and breastfeeding in mothers of very preterm infants after discharge from a neonatal unit. *Social Science & Medicine, 64*(12), 2405–2416.

Grassley, J. L., & Nelms, T. P. (2008). The breast-feeding conversation: A philosophical exploration of support. *Advanced Nursing Science, 31*, E55–E66.

Griffith, L. (2010). Motherhood, ethnicity and experience: A narrative analysis of the debates concerning culture in the provision of health services for Bangladeshi mothers in East London. *Anthropology & Medicine, 17*, 289–299.

Nussbaum, R., Grubs, R., Losee, J., Weidman, C., Ford, M., & Marazita, M. (2008). A qualitative description of receiving a diagnosis of clefting in the prenatal or postnatal period. *Journal of Genetic Counseling, 17*, 336–350.

Polit, D. F., & Beck, C. T. (2012). Nursing research: Generating and assessing evidence for nursing practice (9th ed.). Philadelphia, PA: Lippincott.

Schenk, L. K., & Kelley, J. H. (2010). Mothering an extremely low birth-weight infant: A phenomenological study. *Advances in Neonatal Care, 10*, 88–97.

Sheehan, A., Schmied, V., & Barclay, L. (2009). Complex decisions: Theorizing women's infant feeding decisions in the first 6 weeks after birth. *Journal of Advanced Nursing, 66*, 371–380.

Suggested Reading

Beck, C. T. (1993). Qualitative research: The evaluation of its credibility, fittingness, and auditability. *Western Journal of Nursing Research, 15*, 263–266.

Beck, C. T. (2003). Initiation into qualitative data analysis. *Journal of Nursing Education, 42*, 231–234.

Burns, N., & Groves, S. K. (2005). *The practice of nursing research* (5th ed.). St. Louis, MO: Elsevier Saunders.

Creswell, J. W. (2007). *Qualitative inquiry and research design: Choosing among five traditions.* Thousand Oaks, CA: Sage Publications.

Denzin, N. K., & Lincoln, Y. S. (Eds.). (2005). *The Sage handbook of qualitative research.* Thousand Oaks, CA: Sage Publications.

Lincoln, Y. S., & Guba, E. G. (1985). *Naturalistic inquiry.* Newbury Park, CA: Sage Publications.

Morse, J. M. (1999). Myth #93: Reliability and validity are not relevant to qualitative inquiry. *Qualitative Health Research, 9*, 717–718.

Polit, D. F., & Beck, C. T. (2008). *Nursing research: Principles and methods* (8th ed.). Philadelphia, PA: Lippincott.

Polit, D. F., & Beck, C. T. (2010). Generalization in quantitative and qualitative research: Myths and strategies. *International Journal of Nursing Studies*, *47*, 1451–1458.

Sandelowski, M. (2000). Whatever happened to qualitative description? *Research in Nursing and Health*, *23*, 334–340.

Savage, J. (2000). Participant observation: Standing in the shoes of others? *Qualitative Health Research*, *10*, 324–339.

Spradley, J. (1979). *The ethnographic interview*. New York, NY: Holt, Rinehart and Winston.

Spradley, J. P. (1980). *Participant observation*. New York, NY: Holt, Rinehart and Winston.

Strauss, A., & Corbin, J. (1990). *Basics of qualitative research: Grounded theory procedures and techniques*. Newbury Park, CA: Sage Publications.

Van Manen, M. (1990). *Researching lived experience*. New York, NY: State University of New York Press.

CHAPTER 13
A Legal Primer for Lactation Consultants

Priscilla G. Bornmann, JD

OBJECTIVES

- List ways in which the lactation consultant–client relationship can be created.
- Describe legal actions most likely to be brought against lactation consultants.
- Define *informed consent* and discuss how it relates to the lactation consultant.
- Describe the use of technology as it relates to lactation consultant practice.
- Discuss at least three techniques a lactation consultant should use when testifying at a deposition or trial.

INTRODUCTION

This chapter is designed to provide accurate general information regarding legal matters that the lactation consultant might encounter in practice. Although the information relates specifically to the United States, the intent and general concepts in this chapter would most likely have parallels in other countries. The Jones & Bartlett Learning Core Curriculum website (www.go.jblearning.com/corecurriculum) contains forms prepared in a format that is readily convertible to personal use. Readers should feel free to reproduce or retype these forms for their personal use or for the use of their offices. However, they should not be used without reading the outline material that relates to them, and neither should they be used without the user's absolute certainty that they have not been changed to fit the user's specific circumstances (including any requirements specific to the relevant jurisdiction). These forms are not to be resold. If legal advice or other expert assistance is required, the services of a competent professional should be sought. To obtain copyright permissions, please contact the copyright holder, P. G. Bornmann and Jones & Bartlett Learning. Copyright © 2011 by Priscilla G. Bornmann, JD. All rights reserved Priscilla G. Bornmann, Esq., Cyron & Miller, LLP, 100 North Pitt Street, Suite 200, Alexandria, VA 22314. Tel: 1-703-299-0600. E-mail: pbornmann@cyronmiller.com.

I. The Lactation Consultant–Client Professional Relationship

A. Creation of the lactation consultant–client relationship

1. *There is generally no duty to render care or attention unless the lactation consultant agrees to do so.* However, if the lactation consultant "accepts" a client, duties are created that are contractual in nature.[1] The duties created exist whether or not the lactation consultant is being paid for services.[2]

    a. Duty to render the appropriate level of care (unless authorized to withdraw)

    b. Duty to refer, if unable to render appropriate care

    c. Duty not to abandon client

2. The contract creating the client relationship may be created either by an express agreement or an implied agreement:

    a. Express agreement. An express agreement is an actual agreement, the terms of which are stated either orally or in writing, as when a lactation consultant agrees to counsel participants who participate in a health plan.

    b. Implied agreement. An implied agreement is a contract inferred in law as a matter of reason and justice from the acts or conduct of the parties or the circumstances surrounding the transaction. Such a contract could result from a telephone conversation in which client asks to make an appointment for a specific condition (not merely to "see" a lactation consultant).[3]

3. *Occurrences that may create a lactation consultant–client relationship.*

    a. Periodic visits, but for different reasons: each appointment is a new contract.

    b. Ongoing visits for a chronic condition requiring client to appear for follow-up: one contract.

    c. Making an appointment. This usually constitutes an agreement to meet to determine whether to enter a client relationship. However, in some cases a client relationship is created by the act of making an appointment. For example, in a case on point, a blind woman and her 4-year-old guide dog went to a doctor's office. The doctor demanded that the guide dog be removed, refused to treat the woman, and did not assist her in finding other medical attention. The court noted that the appointment, which had been made "for the treatment of a vaginal infection" and thus created a relationship and duties . . . was more than a mere appointment to see a physician.[4] In such a case, the following questions would be relevant to a lactation consultant: (1) Did the client entrust her treatment to the lactation consultant? and (2) Did the lactation consultant accept the case?[5] Think before turning away someone who arrives pursuant to an appointment. If the person needs immediate counseling or care, give it. If not, you should make alternate arrangements or refer to another competent practitioner.

    d. Examination. Conducting a patient examination may create a limited professional relationship.[6] If you examine a client, take care not to cause harm when doing so, and if you discover a problem beyond your competency, advise the client of your concerns and about the need to obtain follow-up care, and refer to a competent practitioner.

e. Phone calls. The content of the phone call determines whether it has created a professional relationship. The following steps should help lactation consultants achieve this result:[7]

   i. The person receiving the call should identify herself or himself and obtain the name of the individual who placed the call.

   ii. The person receiving the call may listen to the caller's complaints.

   iii. If an appointment is made, it should be made clear that the appointment is being made for evaluation to determine whether the lactation consultant can accept the new client.

   iv. If no appointment is made, the person receiving the call should inform the caller of her options. For example, she may go to the local emergency room, phone an appropriate physician, or phone another lactation consultant.

   v. If the lactation consultant gives comments in the nature of advice, a lactation consultant–client relationship has been created.

4. *Occurrences that usually do not create a lactation consultant–client relationship.*

   a. A request by a physician that the lactation consultant see a client or review the client's record. However, if the physician is "relying" on the lactation consultant and the lactation consultant knows this, a relationship may be implied (see the client soon).

   b. The lactation consultant's hospital affiliation. Generally, no relationship exists as to persons who once were in the hospital, but who are no longer inpatients. However, this rule may not apply if the call is to a hospital "hotline." In an emergency, it would be best to see and/or refer.

B. Duration and termination of the lactation consultant–client relationship

1. *Duration.* Usually no duration is specified, so the law fills in by requiring the lactation consultant to continue care until one of the following conditions is met:

   a. The need for lactation consultant services no longer exists.

   b. The client withdraws from care.

   c. The lactation consultant withdraws in a manner that does not constitute "abandonment" of the client.

2. *Termination.* The relationship exists until one of the following conditions is met:

   a. The need for lactation consultant services no longer exists.

   b. The lactation consultant and client mutually agree to discontinue the relationship.

   c. The client discharges the lactation consultant either expressly or by seeking lactation consultant services from another provider.

   d. The lactation consultant unilaterally withdraws from relationship by:

     i. Giving the client appropriate notice of intent to withdraw

      (a) Talk by phone or in person

      (b) Send certified letter, return receipt requested, stating: (1) status of the client; (2) need for follow-up care; (3) intention to withdraw by definite stated date (date must give time for client to seek alternative care); (4) that the client may seek lactation consultant for emergencies until date stated; and (5) that any subsequent physician or lactation consultant can obtain a copy of all records with written permission from client. *Note*: A client's failure to pay will not justify the lactation consultant's unilateral withdrawal without giving sufficient opportunity to obtain alternative care.

    ii. Referring to a competent replacement or to a specialist when client's problem is outside the lactation consultant's competence[8]

3. *Situations that may constitute abandonment.*

  a. If lactation consultant called to consult (this is a limited contract), take three steps.

    i. Tell the client verbally and write in chart: "I have been called by Dr. ___ to evaluate ___."

    ii. Perform service needed.

    iii. Tell the client verbally and write in chart: "I am signing off this case and will no longer follow this client. However, I (or business name) will remain available if I am notified that additional consultations or assistance are required."

  b. Failure to attend the client when required under a general contract for treatment

  c. Substitution of lactation consultants. The client is not abandoned if the replacement is competent. To avoid problems:

    i. Notify replacement of case details verbally and in writing.

    ii. If possible, give notice to the client of intent to substitute.

    iii. Advise a new client of your group's rotation procedure.

  d. Client's failure to keep follow-up appointment or to follow medical advice. Under such circumstances a lactation consultant has a duty to do the following:

    i. Be sure the client understands nature of condition

    ii. Be sure the client is informed of risks of failing to seek medical attention

    iii. Provide the client with an opportunity to visit the lactation consultant for counseling or care

  e. *Practice Tip:* Call the client with the information described in the preceding section. Follow up with a letter to the client that contains the same information and send the letter by traceable means.

II. Consent, Informed Consent, and the Lactation Consultant in the United States

These comments on consent and the doctrine of informed consent, as it has been applied in the United States, are not specific to breastfeeding issues because no cases related to breastfeeding have been reported. However, it is hoped that an overview of general principles may help lactation consultants better understand this common law doctrine, which is gaining acceptance in a wide variety of medical settings.[9]

A. Consent principles. The distinction between *consent* and *informed consent* is legally significant.

    1. *Consent.* Consent occurs when the client, or one authorized on her behalf, agrees to a course of treatment or the performance of a medical procedure. It requires only that the client, or her representative, understand the nature of the proposed treatment.[10] If the lactation consultant fails to obtain consent and proceeds to touch the client, the lactation consultant may be guilty of battery (of touching the client without consent) and liable for an award of nominal damages, even though no real injury results.

    2. *Informed consent.* Even if a client's consent is given, a lactation consultant could be found liable to a client for not obtaining consent. The duty to obtain informed consent is based on the right of clients to control what will be done with their own bodies.[11] In most jurisdictions, the mere absence of a law recognizing informed consent liability at the time of a defendant's alleged breach will not preclude imposing informed consent liability if making more extensive disclosures would have been recognized as good and acceptable medical practice at the time.[12]

        a. To prevail in an action alleging failure to obtain informed consent, a plaintiff must prove not only that the medical provider breached a duty to give or obtain such consent, but also that this caused injury or damage. This usually requires that the client prove she would have elected a different treatment or course of therapy had she been properly informed.[13]

        b. What information is needed as the basis for informed consent? The courts have generally held that a client's informed consent is given only if the following areas have been discussed:
- The nature of the client's problem or illness
- The nature of the proposed therapy or treatment
- Reasonable alternative therapies or treatments
- The chance of success with the proposed therapy or treatment
- Substantial risks inherent in the therapy or treatment
- Any risks[14] related to failing to undergo therapy or treatment

        c. Although a written consent form is considered evidence that the client's informed consent was obtained, it is not usually conclusive.[15] That is because standard consent forms alone ordinarily don't provide sufficient information about the disclosures made to the client to establish that the client's consent was an adequately informed one.[16] Many states limit the application of the consent doctrine to cases involving surgical or medical procedures.[17] A few other states have held that their informed consent statutes do not apply to "routine medical procedures,"[18] and in many states only the primary treating physician has the duty to obtain the client's informed consent for treatment, and not those persons who merely consult with,[19] refer to,[20] or assist[21] the attending physician.[22] In such jurisdictions, it is doubtful that the doctrine of informed consent would be relevant to most breastfeeding situations.

However, there is case law that holds that the doctrine of informed consent applies to noninvasive, as well as invasive, medical procedures.[23]

On the other hand, a consent form will be given effect as a defense if all the evidence supports a conclusion that the client was informed about the treatment to which he or she consented.[24]

d. A suit for lack of informed consent is generally based on negligence.[25]

B. Who should consent?

1. *The duty to obtain consent is owed to the client, so it is the client who should consent.* However, if the client is a minor or under a disability, the client may not be legally competent to give consent. In such cases, the lactation consultant should obtain the consent from the patient/client's parent or guardian.

2. *In breastfeeding cases, who is the client—the mother alone or the mother and the baby?* Although there is no existing case law, because breastfeeding has physical ramifications for both mother and baby, it appears that both have "client" status.

C. Who can give consent for an infant?

1. *The general rule in the United States is that competent adults are capable of giving valid consent.* Prior to the age of majority, which usually is designated by state statute, an individual is considered incapable of consenting to medical care or treatment. Thus, it is necessary to obtain the consent of an infant's parent or guardian to consent on the infant's behalf.[26] A parent with legal custodial rights over a child has the authority to consent to medical care and treatment for that child. So, if parents are divorced or legally separated (that is, a separation agreement has been signed), the parent granted legal authority for the care, custody, and control of the child has the right to consent to treatment, to the exclusion of the other parent.

2. *If the parent herself is a minor, the legal waters are muddied and her ability to consent to treatment for her child is less clear.* Best practice would suggest that the lactation consultant receive the consent of the other parent (if that parent is not a minor) or from the minor's parents (grandparents) or guardian, unless the minor parent is considered to be "emancipated" or a "mature minor."

3. *Emancipated minors. Emancipation* has been defined as "the relinquishment by the parent of control and authority over the minor child, conferring on him (child) the right to his earnings and terminating the parents' legal duty to support the child."[27] Emancipation generally occurs when a minor lives away from her parents, supports herself, and conducts her own affairs. Some states have statutes defining particular circumstances that qualify a child as emancipated.[28] Other states, to avoid encouraging runaways, require that this relationship be consensual between the child and the parent. In the absence of such a statute, the following have been considered to confer emancipated or "mature minor"[29] status on a minor:

- Military duty[30]
- Marriage[31]
- Living apart from the child's family independently of their support and services[32]

Emancipated minors are granted the same legal status as if already at the age of full majority. They are able to provide consent for their own medical care, and so may be able to consent to such care for their children as well. However, if the emancipated minor parent has a spouse of legal age, the lactation consultant is advised to obtain the consent of the spouse for the treatment of the infant whenever possible.

D. Using information sheets to obtain informed consent. For lactation consultants in a busy practice, adequate legal protection may be obtained in relation to courses of treatment often recommended by writing up an information sheet about the treatment or procedure, *provided the information sheet is kept up to date.*

The lactation consultant should ask the mother (or both parents, if they are available) to sign and date two identical forms, below a typed statement saying that she or they acknowledge(s) receipt of the information. One copy of the form should remain in the lactation consultant's files, and the other should be given to the mother or both parents. When determining the information to include in such a form, consider the following recommendations:

- Consult with other lactation consultants to determine what risks and alternative modes they explain to their clients.
- Consult current medical literature to determine the frequency and severity of risks and the availability of reasonable alternative modes of treatment.
- Supplement the preceding with those additional risks that are serious or life threatening even though infrequently encountered.
- Add to the form additional information that you believe the average prudent client or clients would want to have explained to allow her or them to give informed consent.

III. Legal Actions Most Likely to Be Brought Against Lactation Consultants

A. Battery

1. *Description*: A technical battery occurs if a lactation consultant, in the course of treatment, exceeds the consent given by the client, even though the lactation consultant intended no wrong to aid the client (unless there is an emergency).

2. *Elements (in most states):*

   a. Duty: To respect the rights of other persons to freedom from harmful or offensive bodily contact.

   b. Intent: Lactation consultant intended to physically contact client.

   c. Breach: Unconsented to, harmful, or offensive contact with one person by another.

   d. Causation: Causation of injury presumed (no need to prove causation).

   e. Damage: Injury (to dignity) presumed (no need to prove injury only amount of damages).

3. *Example*: If a nurse gives a bottle to a baby whose parents have directed be exclusively breastfed and be given no water and no artificial nipples, she has committed battery.

4. *Exception*: In a case in which employees of the hospital mistakenly brought the wrong infant to a mother for feeding, a hospital nurse suctioned the breastmilk from the baby's stomach, because it was unclear at the time whether the infant had been exposed to the possibility of infection. Later, the mother of the child who was mistakenly fed by another claimed that the suctioning constituted a battery suffered by her child. However, the court found that consent had been given because the hospital's Newborn Care Path placed the decision to suction within the nurse's discretion, that the mother had signed a general consent for medical care when she was admitted to the hospital that authorized the hospital and its employees to perform any tests or procedures authorized by her doctor, and that the nurse had suctioned the infant's stomach pursuant to a physician's "PRN" order. *Hobbs v. Seton Corp.* (2009 WL 196040, Tenn Ct. App. 2009).

B. Professional negligence (includes failure to diagnose, initiate treatment, refer or consult, provide attention or care, or obtain informed consent).

1. *Description:* Professional negligence occurs if, when rendering professional services, a lactation consultant fails to exercise that degree of skill and learning commonly applied under all the circumstances in the community by the average prudent reputable member of the profession, with the result of injury, loss, or damage to the recipient of those services or to those entitled to rely upon them.

2. *Elements (in most states):*
   a. Duty: To use due care on rendering lactation consultant services.
   b. Breach: Act/omission causing lactation consultant to fail to provide standard of care as would be provided by the "ordinary, prudent lactation consultant" under similar circumstances.
   c. Causation: Direct or proximate causation of injury must be proved.
   d. Damage: Dollar value of resulting injury.

3. *Example: Baptist Memorial Hospital-Union County v. Johnson*, No 98-IA-00175-SCT (Supreme Court of Mississippi, 2000). Parents brought negligence action against hospital for mistakenly placing their infant with an unidentified female client, who breastfed the infant. In response to parents' request for discovery of the client's identity and medical records, the hospital affirmatively asserted the patient/client's medical privilege of confidentiality. At the hearing on the parents' motion to compel, the judge compelled discovery of the client's identity and production of her medical records and also entered an interlocutory order asking for determination of scope of statutory client–physician privilege. On appeal, the state supreme court held that: (1) the hospital must disclose identity of unidentified female client, who mistakenly breastfed the infant, as a witness to hospital's alleged conduct, and (2) the hospital must produce woman's medical records to trial court for in-camera review, subject to the issuance of protective orders to determine whether infant's health was at risk.

C. Infliction of emotional distress
    1. *Description:* A cause of action by which a person may seek redress for extreme emotional disturbance suffered as a result of the negligent or intentional conduct of another person.
    2. *Elements (these vary widely by state, but read much like the following):*
        a. Duty: To refrain from harmful conduct.
        b. Breach: The lactation consultant acts in an extreme and outrageous manner exceeding the bounds of decency observed by a civilized society.
        c. Intent: The lactation consultant knew or should have known his or her conduct was likely to cause plaintiff severe emotional distress.
        d. Causation: The lactation consultant's actions directly and proximately caused the plaintiff to suffer actual and severe emotional distress (more than embarrassment or humiliation).
        e. Damage: Dollar value of resulting severe mental distress.
    3. *Examples:*
        a. *Garcia v. Lawrence Hospital*, 5 A.D.3d 227, 773 N.Y.S.2d 59 (N.Y. 2004). The client alleged that the hospital was negligent in bringing her day-old baby to her for breastfeeding after she was medically sedated, and then leaving them alone together unsupervised after the sedative allegedly caused client to fall asleep on top of the baby, smothering him to death. The court granted the client's motion for leave to amend her complaint so as to include a cause of action for emotional injury, and hospital appealed.

            In the end, the court held that the client had cause of action for emotional injury under a zone-of-danger theory. Although the client did not observe the injury she inflicted and was never personally exposed to unreasonable risk of bodily harm, there was an especial likelihood of genuine and serious mental distress, arising from special circumstances.
        b. *Volm v. Legacy Health Systems, Inc.*, 237 F. Supp. 2d 1166 (United States District Court, D. Oregon 2002). In this case, a lactation consultant sued healthcare corporation that had banned her from all of its hospital and clinic facilities, and individual doctors and nurses. The court found that certain individual physicians' and nurses' alleged conduct was not sufficient to constitute an extraordinary transgression of bounds of socially tolerable conduct, as required to support claim for intentional infliction of emotional distress under Oregon law.
        c. *Champagne v. Mid-Maine Medical Center*, 711 A.2d 842 (Me. 1998). A mother whose newborn baby was mistakenly breastfed by another client in maternity ward at hospital sued hospital and nursing student to recover for invasion of privacy, battery, intentional infliction of emotional distress, and negligent infliction of emotional distress. The court found that: (1) the mother was not direct or indirect victim of alleged negligence, as required to recover for negligent infliction of emotional distress; (2) the mother failed to show causal relationship between the alleged failure to inform her of the risks

created by the breastfeeding incident and the emotional distress she claimed; and (3) the incident could not be characterized as so extreme and outrageous as to exceed all possible bounds of decency in a civilized community.

D. Breach of warranty

1. *Description:* A statement of fact respecting the quality or outcome or particular result to be achieved by agreeing to receive certain medical services or treatments, made by the medical service provider to induce the client to consent to those services and/or treatments, and relied upon by the client, which is not fulfilled.

2. *Elements (in most states):*

   a. Duty: Lactation consultant promises or "guarantees" a result.

   b. Intent: No proof of fraudulent intent or untruthfulness required.

   c. Breach: Promised result not achieved.

   d. Causation: Direct or proximate causation of damage must be proved.

   e. Damage: Dollar value of the difference between the value of the expected outcome and the value of the actual outcome.

3. *Example:*

   a. *Hawkins v. McGee*, 84 N.H. 114, 146 A. 641 (1929).

   b. Background: Hawkins consulted McGee, a surgeon, about scar tissue that was the result of a severe burn caused by contact with an electric wire, which Hawkins had experienced about 9 years prior. The surgeon suggested removing the scar tissue from the palm of the plaintiff's right hand and replacing it with a skin graft taken from the plaintiff's chest. Evidence was produced to the effect that before the operation was performed, Hawkins and his father went to McGee's office and that McGee, in answer to the question, "How long will the boy be in the hospital?" replied, "Three or four days, not over four; then the boy can go home and it will be just a few days when he will go back to work with a good hand." The court found these statements could only be construed as expression of opinions or predictions, even though those estimates were exceeded. However, the evidence also showed that Dr. McGee said before the operation was decided upon, "I will guarantee to make the hand a hundred per cent perfect hand or a hundred per cent good hand." Because after the operation, the boy grew hair from the palm of his hand, the result was not "perfect" or "one hundred per cent good." Thus, the court found that Dr. McGee had given a warranty as to the result of the operation, which had been breached and that damages were due Hawkins.

E. Unauthorized practice of medicine (governed by state statute)

1. *Description:* Practicing medicine (as defined in the medical practice act for the applicable state) without the authority (license) to do so. State legislatures, through licensing laws, determine what is and what is not the practice of medicine. However, legislatures often authorize several professions to practice in the same, related, or similar fields and as a result these have overlapping practice

areas. Thus, courts as well as legislatures have recognized that licensing laws don't create monopolies for professions[33] and not all practice areas are exclusive.[34]

2. *Overlapping scopes of practice:* For International Board Certified Lactation Consultants (IBCLCs) who hold no other healthcare credential, the only question is whether a lactation consultant's activity is within the scope of lactation consultant practice, defined by the International Board of Lactation Consultant Examiners (IBLCE).[35] If not, and it is reserved by statutes to one of the other professions, then it is illegal for a lactation consultant to engage in it. However, if it is the scope of lactation consultant practice, then it is not important whether other professions are also permitted to engage in it. Many lactation consultants are also registered nurses or other licensed healthcare professionals whose statutorily defined scope of practice includes some lactation care activities.

3. *The practice of medicine generally includes the right to diagnose, treat, and prescribe.* Some states' statutes specifically exempt any person licensed or certified to practice a limited field of the healing arts under their laws, if those persons strictly confine themselves to the field for which they are licensed or certified and don't assume the title of physician or surgeon, and don't hold themselves out as qualified to prescribe drugs in any form or to perform operative surgery.[36]

4. Diagnosis is generally defined as the identification of a disease based on its signs and symptoms. However, many states make a distinction between a "medical diagnosis" (the identification of a disease and its cause based on its signs and symptoms) and a "nursing diagnosis"[37] (the identification of and discrimination between physical and psychosocial signs and symptoms essential to the effective execution and management of the nursing regimen). The main difference between these two types of diagnosis is that the nursing diagnosis does not make a final conclusion about the identity and cause of the underlying disease.

F. Failure to report child neglect/abuse (governed by state statute)

1. *Reporting is required.* In most U.S. states, Canada, and Northern Ireland, healthcare workers and others who have direct contact with children and who observe something suggesting possible child abuse or neglect[38] are required by law to report suspected child abuse. Australia has mandatory reporting that varies among states and territories as to who is required to report. Many other countries have some form of voluntary reporting. This report should be made according to the laws where the lactation consultant works, as described by the procedures in place in the lactation consultant's work setting. The justification for overriding client confidentiality is the state's interest in protecting public health. Although similar in many respects, the specific requirements of each country/state's laws are different and the avenues for reporting may be different for lactation consultants in different settings, but the lactation consultant's responsibility remains the same. The protocol for notifying authorities should be taken seriously and followed to the letter. In the event no protocols are in position for the lactation consultant's workplace, the lactation consultant should first follow through by reporting to the client's physician and local authorities and,

second, follow up by taking steps to make certain a protocol is put in place (an employment lawyer can help with this).

When reporting, the lactation consultant should take care to report objective observations (and not accuse) to protect against any risk of becoming the subject of a retaliatory charge of slander.

2. *Failure to report:* If a lactation consultant fails to report as required, he or she risks being charged with a criminal offense, which most U.S. states classify as a misdemeanor.

3. *Sources of information:*

- U.S. lactation consultants can check for their state's rules by going to the Administration for Children and Families website (www.acf.hhs.gov), which maintains a database of U.S. state requirements at www.childwelfare.gov/systemwide/laws_policies/state/can/. If the appropriate state is not listed or the suspected abuse took place outside the state in which the lactation consultant practices, it is possible to use the Childhelp USA National Abuse Hotline at 1-800-4-A-CHILD (1-800-422-4453) to obtain relevant information.

- Canadian lactation consultants can refer to the website for child abuse prevention, which lists contact information for all Canadian states and territories: www.safekidsbc.ca/provincial.htm.

- Australian lactation consultants can find reporting information at www.aifs.gov.au/nch/pubs/sheets/rs3/rs3.html.

- Northern Ireland and the rest of the United Kingdom can report suspected child abuse to the National Society for the Prevention of Cruelty to Children by calling the NSPCC Helpline at 0808 800 5000.

4. *Immunity from suit if reported in good faith:* Most states' statutes confer immunity from civil and criminal suits that might otherwise be brought against those persons who report in good faith.

5. *False reports may result in a criminal conviction:* Persons who knowingly or intentionally make a false report may be convicted for a felony in the United States.

G. Violation of unfair and deceptive trade practice statutes (State "Little FTC Acts" or Consumer Protection Acts)

1. *Description*

a. Federal law: U.S. Supreme Court decisions in the 1970s established that the "learned professions" have commercial aspects and thus are not immune from antitrust law.[39] These were the forerunners of state court rulings holding that the entrepreneurial and business aspects of medical practices are not exempt from little Federal Trade Commission (FTC) act coverage.

b. States' laws: State or "little" FTC acts prohibit "unfair" or "deceptive" acts or practices in trade or commerce. Such causes of action are often included in healthcare suits because they are attractive to plaintiffs because many of these acts provide for the recovery of attorney fees and/or treble damages for willful, knowing, or bad faith violations. Brochures and websites that provide medically related information to consumers often also serve as advertisements. In addition, websites may provide hyperlinks to other sites. These raise a host of concerns, including the ethical and legal obligations governing marketing and referral practices, which could become the subject of little FTC act litigation.

2. *Examples*:

   a. *Quimby v. Fine*, 724 P.2d 403 (Wash. App. 1986). Although lack of informed consent claims are usually brought as negligence cases, some states have recognized this conduct as a violation of consumer protection law(s), particularly if the lack of informed consent "relates to the entrepreneurial aspects of the medical practice—such as setting prices, billing, collection, obtaining, retaining and dismissing clients."

   b. *Mother & Unborn Baby Care of N. Texas v. State*, 749 S.W.2d 533, 542 (Tex. App. 1988). A facility run by antiabortion activists was found to have violated the Texas act in holding itself out, in the Yellow Pages and statements to prospective clients, as an abortion clinic and then trying to dissuade clients from having abortions.

   c. *Gadsden v. Newman*, 807 F. Supp. 1412, 1420 (C.D. Ill. 1992). Plaintiff alleged that defendant psychiatrist had an undisclosed contract with a hospital that included financial incentives, self-referrals, and increased billings.

   d. *Vassolo v. Baxter Healthcare Corp.*, 696 N.E.2d 909, 915, 924 (Mass. 1998). Client brought a claim against a breast implant manufacturer based on that manufacturer's failure to disclose the risks of its product to her healthcare provider.

H. Copyright infringement

   1. *Description*: Unauthorized use of copyrighted material. See 17 U.S.C. §501.

   2. *Examples*:

      a. Making multiple copies of a journal article for numerous hospital staff members to keep at their desks for reference.

      b. Using a cartoon as a slide to illustrate a presentation for which you receive an honorarium, without first obtaining the artist's permission to use it in this way.

I. Trademark/service mark/certification mark infringement

   1. *Description:* The unauthorized use or colorable imitation of the mark already appropriated by another, on goods or services of a similar class. See U.S.C. § 1051, et seq.

      a. Trademarks apply to products. A trademark is any word, phrase, slogan, or design that is used by a person or entity to define its products and distinguish them from the products of others.[40]

      b. Service marks apply to services. A service mark is the same as a trademark except that it identifies and distinguishes services rather than products.[41] Registered service marks that are familiar to lactation consultants include the words "International Board of Lactation Consultant Examiners" and the IBLCE's logo.

c. Certification marks apply to products or services. Unlike trademarks or service marks, a certification mark[42] is not used by the owner of the mark, but instead is applied by other persons to their goods or services, with authorization from the owner of the mark. The certifier/owner of a certification mark does not produce the goods or perform the services in connection with which the mark is used, and thus does not control their nature or quality. What the certifier/owner of the certification mark does control is the use of the mark by others on their goods or in connection with their services, by taking steps to ensure that the mark is applied only to goods or services that contain the requisite characteristics or meet the specified requirements that the certifier/owner has established or adopted for the certification.

2. *Examples*: Examples of registered certification marks that are familiar to lactation consultants include the acronyms "IBCLC" and "RLC" and the phrases "International Board Certified Lactation Consultant" and "Registered Lactation Consultant."

3. *Infringement:* Identical standards govern the determination whether a trademark, service mark, or certification mark has been infringed. Thus, just as it is unlawful to market any dark-colored effervescent drink as "Coca-Cola," if a person uses the initials "IBCLC" when he or she did not successfully complete the IBLCE examination, or when he or she has failed to timely recertify as required to maintain certification as an IBCLC, that use constitutes actionable infringement of the "IBCLC" service mark, which is owned and has been registered by the IBLCE.

IV. Use of Technology in Lactation Consultant Practice

The rapid proliferation of technological advances continues to influence the way lactation consultants practice. Devices and concepts such as fax machines, video conferencing, email, the Internet, cellular phones, networked computer systems, and satellite communications shape the way lactation consultants serve their clients on a day-to-day basis. Certainly, technology provides the means for more efficient and effective methods of performing services, but these same advances that can improve a lactation consultant's ability to serve clients may also present a number of ethical pitfalls for the unwary practitioner.

A. Facsimiles (faxes) and client confidentiality. As the result of an inadvertent mistake, you or another staff member fax a medical record to the wrong number. The mistake is discovered later that afternoon after you receive a call from the pediatrician inquiring as to why he or she has not yet received the faxed records. After making a check, you discover that the fax was sent to the wrong location.
1. Has there been a breach of client confidentiality?
2. What steps should or must you take to recover the medical record from the recipient and to minimize any potential damage to your client's confidentiality?
3. Have you personally committed an ethical violation?
4. Would the issues be any different if the message had been sent to the wrong e-mail address instead?

B. Cell phones and client confidentiality. Has it occurred to you that it is possible to breach a client's confidentiality when you talk to her? This can happen if someone is eavesdropping on your conversation. In today's world, the biggest eavesdropping risk is posed not by the person lurking behind the door, but by a third party's interception of a cellular phone call. Does a lactation consultant who uses a cell phone to discuss client matters breach the ethical obligation to protect client confidentiality?[43] The answer to this question is anything but clear. In fact, the most accurate answer is, "It depends . . ."

There is no lactation consultant ethical history on which to base an answer.[44] However, parallel cases in other professional contexts indicate that whether a lactation consultant's use of a cellular phone to communicate with clients violates a duty of confidentiality "depends" on whether there is a reasonable expectation of privacy in the communication. Determining whether a lactation consultant has a "reasonable expectation of privacy" in a means of communication is a two-part inquiry: First, one must determine whether the lactation consultant has a subjective belief that the chosen mode of communication is private. Second, the belief must be objectively reasonable.[45]

There are two types of cellular phones—analog and digital—and the expected level of privacy in using each differs greatly. Conversations over analog phones are particularly susceptible to interception by third parties. On the other hand, digital cellular phones work differently and are believed to provide greater security against interception, although they are not completely secure. Moreover, even if a digital phone is used, this does not necessarily mean the call is being transmitted through a digital network.[46]

As cellular phones become more prevalent and demands on lactation consultants have become even greater, increasing numbers of lactation consultants are using cell phones to communicate with their clients. Keep in mind the following guidelines before using cell phones to discuss any confidential information.

- Tell your clients when you are using a cell phone, informing them of the risks of doing this, and providing them with the opportunity to consent.
- Consider purchasing a scrambler to prevent the interception of analog cellular calls if you frequently use a cell phone to call clients about confidential matters.
- Check to see whether the International Lactation Consultant Association (ILCA) or the IBLCE have issued ethical guidelines or whether the legislatures or courts in your jurisdiction have rules on the reasonable expectation of privacy in cellular communications.
- Check with your professional liability insurance carrier to see if it has issued any guidance on the issue.
- When possible, use a landline phone instead of a cell phone.
- If in doubt, don't use a cell phone.

C. Internet communications. Problems can arise when a lactation consultant participates on electronic bulletin boards, online services, or the Internet. Because this is a new area, the ethical rules and codes of conduct that apply to this part of a lactation consultant's practice are just beginning to evolve, so there is little precedent.[47] These tips may help lactation consultants avoid liability for false or misleading advertising, breach of confidentiality, malpractice, or the unauthorized practice of medicine as a result of their electronic communications. Because Internet sources are not equally reliable, it is imperative that you consider the purpose for which this information could possibly be used before presenting it to a client who might rely on its accuracy.

1. *False or misleading advertising*
   a. Websites: Potentially, a website is a great place to advertise to a wide audience. Just remember that all of the rules that generally govern advertising will apply to anything you say to a prospective client (by way of any medium, not just electronic communications). Generally, advertising must be truthful and incapable of misleading even an unsophisticated consumer.
   b. E-mail solicitations: No parameters for these have been established, but there seems no reason to distinguish them from other mass mailing strategies or targeted mailing tactics.
2. *Breach of confidentiality*
   a. The risks of interception, misdirection, and misforwarding.
   b. E-mail and Internet communications may be subject to interception, misdirection, and misforwarding. Therefore, be especially wary of posting any message that could be construed to be "medical advice." The safest course is to limit online communication to information, rather than advice, whether partaking in bulletin board discourse or drafting a web page.
   c. Unlike faxes or "snail mail" (i.e., regular mail services), the risk of misdirected e-mail is higher simply because one can write and send an e-mail message much faster than a letter or fax. Also, the intended recipient(s) can easily forward these communications to other unintended recipients. A partial solution to this dilemma is the "envelope within the envelope" approach. When using this approach, the entire text of the primary e-mail message is the message on unintended transmission. Then the sensitive information is added to the email message as an attachment.
   d. To minimize the possibility that your comments will be construed as medical advice, you could also decide to place a written disclaimer either at the beginning or the end of the text.[48]
   e. Consider including a message at the top or bottom of your transmissions similar to the following:
   CONFIDENTIALITY NOTE: This message does not constitute medical advice. It is intended only for the addressee(s) named herein and may contain information that is privileged and confidential. This communication may not be forwarded without the prior written permission of the original author. If the reader of this message is not the intended recipient, you are hereby notified that the disclosure, copying, distribution, or the taking of any action in reliance on the contents of this information is strictly prohibited. If you have received this communication in error, please call collect to _____ (phone number), so we may arrange to retrieve this transmission at no cost to you.

Although taking this precaution "can't hurt," it is not always a successful measure. Around the country, courts have issued varying opinions regarding the effectiveness of such a message in diminishing the sender's liability for the unintended recipient's use of information received by mistake.

3. *Professional negligence*

a. Another area of concern is the lack of professionalism that often accompanies the use of e-mail, blogs, and bulletin boards. Often people who routinely review outgoing first-class mail for spelling, grammar, style, and neatness fail to review their outgoing e-mail. It is also important to be careful with the substance of what your e-mail message says. Many courts have held that employees have no protectable privacy interest in the messages sent from their employer's computers, so it is reasonable to expect that your messages may be reviewed. In addition, e-mail results in a written record that is not completely deleted from the computer or network when you press the Delete button. The rule is simple: Unless you are comfortable having the text of your e-mail discussed on television news, don't send it over the office system. Postings by e-mail, in blogs, and on bulletin boards could inadvertently create a lactation consultant–client relationship. Whether such a relationship has been formed will be judged by the *client's* subjective belief that such a relationship exists, provided that belief is "reasonable." There are two basic issues: (1) maintaining competence and (2) avoiding negligence. Think about whether you would feel comfortable giving advice to someone who called you and gave you the same skeletal facts that you receive in an email message or in a blog. If you would want more information, be sure to ask for it or don't answer the questions. If you need to do research, do it, or don't answer the questions. If you need to observe the mother and/or baby, say so, and don't answer the question. The safest tactic is to completely avoid giving "medical advice" (refer to the information given under "confidentiality" earlier).

4. *Unauthorized practice of medicine.* Electronic communications cross state and international boundaries in seconds. Do you know where the client is located? Be aware that if your message includes a "diagnosis" or a "prescription," or any other action that falls within the state's or country's unauthorized practice statutes (as judged on the basis of 20/20 hindsight) and if the client lives in a state or country that vigorously enforces those laws, you could be risking a legal action.

D. Operating a website. The operation of a website may present certain areas of exposure for lactation consultants who own or operate one. Sources of potential liability include infringement (either in the domain name itself or in the content of the website), privacy (relating to the use of website user information or to the posting of website content containing the name or likeness of a person), defamation (in the form of web content), reliance (based on information contained on the website and the use of that information), or accessibility (for individuals with visual or hearing impairments).[49]

E. Summary: Although technology continues to change rapidly, the ethical and legal principles that govern lactation consultant practice do not. Competence, confidentiality, diligence, honesty, and service to the public are time-honored concepts that form the foundation for all lactation consultant practice.

V. ABCs of Testifying at a Deposition or a Trial

Lactation consultants occasionally become involved in litigation. If you are deposed, or called to testify at trial, try to determine whether you are being called as a "fact witness" or an "expert witness." The roles are equally important, but slightly different.

A. *Fact witness:* Fact witnesses have first-hand knowledge relevant to the issues in a case. They may testify either because they have volunteered to do so or because they have been required to testify by receiving a subpoena. If you have worked directly with the mother–infant dyad, you would be qualified to serve as a fact witness. Generally, fact witnesses must limit their testimony to facts, although courts may "let in" opinions that may be helpful to the understanding of their testimony. Although fact witnesses are not usually paid for their testimony, they are entitled to reimbursement of their expenses. (Note: A fact witness in one case may serve as an expert witness in another. Many fact witnesses have the background necessary to qualify as an expert witness.)

B. *Expert witness:* Expert witnesses testify because they have knowledge, skill, experience, training, education, or expertise that may prove helpful to the judge or jury. Expert witnesses testify voluntarily, by agreement with one of the attorneys or the court. It is best if lactation consultants testifying as expert witnesses have no prior contact with the litigants. The role of an expert witness is to review the records, know the case, suggest authorities and references that support the case, and so forth. Meetings may be held with counsel to discuss areas of contemplated interrogation and possible cross-examination, the selection of exhibits, and the documents to be introduced. Expert witnesses are entitled to payment for their services and to reimbursement of their expenses.

C. *Behavior during a deposition or trial:* The following pointers are general instructions on how to act at a deposition or at trial. You should not follow them strictly but use them as guidelines. Everyone makes mistakes; however, these suggestions should help you to avoid them.

1. *Tell the truth.*

a. Honesty. In a lawsuit, as in all other matters, honesty is the best policy. A lie may lose the case. Telling the truth, however, demands more than refraining from telling a deliberate falsehood. Telling the truth requires that witnesses testify accurately about what they know. Everything you say must be right, must be correct, and must be accurate.

b. Accuracy. To be accurate in all of your answers, you must be aware that technically you can't possibly tell what you did yesterday, what you saw yesterday, or what you heard yesterday. Technically, you can only testify to what you remember seeing yesterday, or what you remember hearing yesterday.

c. Memory. Memory is not perfect. You can talk about what you saw, what you heard, and what you did as though memory were a fact, but you are really only remembering something. That's an important distinction. Obviously, there are some things that you do remember, and you remember them clearly, and there can be no question about them. But there will probably be many things about which you may be uncertain. In those instances, you can testify only about what you remember.

2. *Do not act as the advocate for any party.* Attempt to testify objectively and only about that which you are knowledgeable. This means that you will probably answer all kinds of questions about breastfeeding. But in most cases, don't give an opinion about any other topic because it will only serve to diminish your credibility. For example: In a custody case, do you really know what is truly best for the child? Unless you are brought in as a character witness for a friend (and not as a lactation consultant), avoid taking either parent's "side."

3. *Educate "your" attorney.* Give the attorney your résumé so that he or she has the information necessary to qualify you as an expert witness. Be prepared to explain your credentials, which include formal schooling, employment history, and other relevant experience. If you are an IBCLC, give the attorney an IBLCE brochure and make sure the lawyer understands the credential. If it is foreseeable that your testimony may be countered by that of some other healthcare provider, explain in detail how little formal background in breastfeeding most professional schools include in their curricula.

4. *Ask "your" attorney about the mother and baby.* Background of the case. In many cases, you will not know the people involved, so it is important that you ask about the background of the breastfeeding dyad. For example, does the mother smoke? (If so, then be prepared to rebut any inferences to the effect that her breastmilk may be harmful to the child.) Does she drink alcohol? Take illegal drugs? Have there been any neglect or abuse issues? You know what's relevant. The attorney may not.

5. *Supply "your" attorney with copies of the references on which you will rely and other authoritative reference materials.* If you know the issues that are likely to arise during the trial, assemble copies of the most authoritative articles and other materials, and give them to the attorney to read. If possible, supply the attorney with a set of questions to ask.

6. *Be prepared to quote a fee.* The attorney will not be able to tell you precisely how long the proceeding will take. So, be prepared to quote an hourly fee and to charge 50% of that hourly fee for your travel time. This charge for testifying should be about the same as what you would charge for a private consultation of the same duration.

7. *Ask "your" attorney whether you should bring some general references when you testify.* Many times no references are necessary. But if having up-to-date respected lactation texts with you will calm your nerves, why not bring them along? Impress on the attorney that these are generally accepted as authoritative, in case they could be used in cross-examination.

8. *Be prepared for the hypothetical question, particularly hypothetical questions about practice scenarios.* An attorney may describe a scenario based on a particular set of facts and then ask you to comment on it in your "professional opinion" or to a "reasonable degree of medical certainty." Be aware that usually when this is done, they are asking about some issue very central to the case. Think about the question before answering. Then answer with clarity. If additional facts would make a difference, say so at the outset. Unless the question is very simple, avoid giving a bare "yes" or "no" answer.

9. *Educate the people in the courtroom or conference room.* Generally, you truly will be the expert on human lactation at any trial or deposition. The only time that there will be someone there who knows as much as you will is if another lactation consultant is called to testify. Try to remember how little the average person in our society knows about breastfeeding and to define basic terms and to describe simply basic processes (for example, the effect of stimulation on milk supply). When possible, give a little background about the basic anthropological/social/medical theory on which your answer is built. Judges and lawyers are usually fascinated by a lactation consultant's testimony.

10. *Admit what you do not know.* The issue here is credibility. You can't be effective if you aren't prepared to do this.

11. *Straighten out confusion.*

    a. Be clear. If you should get confused about a point, straighten the matter out while the testimony is being taken. (If you are testifying at a deposition, you will have an opportunity to read the testimony over afterward and make any necessary corrections, but it is better to make your corrections at the time of the deposition.)

    b. Example: The opposing lawyer may ask you a question that will remind you of a related question that you have already answered. The new questions may remind you that when you answered the previous one, you made a mistake. The worst tactic you can take is to try and cover up that mistake by giving an incorrect answer. The best one is to correct the mistake then and there. Say, "Excuse me, I just remembered back there you asked me X and I said Y. I was mistaken. I should have told you Z."

12. *Do not guess, give exacting answers.* If you don't remember something, admit it. If you don't know something, admit it. You may feel embarrassed. You may feel that you should be able to remember, but unless you really do remember, don't guess. There is nothing to gain by guessing. If you guess rightly, you have not won anything. If you guess wrongly, you have lost. You can't answer accurately if you don't hear or understand a question, so be sure that you hear and understand it before you try to answer it. If you don't hear it, ask to have it repeated. If you don't understand it, ask to have it explained. It is important that you understand each question the way the lawyer intends you to understand it. It is likewise important that anyone else who hears or reads your answer understand it the same way that you mean it. Language is inexact. It is much easier to be general than to be specific. Therefore, the defense attorney's questions may have

several meanings, and your answers may have several meanings. Be sure that your answers are as exact as they can be so that no one can misinterpret them.

13. *Give accurate estimates.* Beware of questions involving time and dates. If you estimate, make sure everyone understands you are estimating.

14. *Clarify multiple meanings.* You will be asked questions that have multiple meanings. You will have to answer them, so if there is any doubt in your mind as to whether a question has a multiple meaning, either make certain that you understand what the questioner means (by asking the person, "Do you mean . . .?") or make sure that what you mean is clear.

15. *Answer background questions as accurately as possible.* The lawyers will ask you for background information, which may include your address, when and where you were born, where you went to school, and what jobs you have held. You may not be able to remember all such details, but do your best. If you do not remember, tell the questioner that you don't remember or give the best possible estimate. For example, "Well I'm not sure, but it seems to me it may have been back in 1995 or 1996, about then."

16. *Beware of a question that assumes fact.*
    a. Questions. You might be asked a question that assumes a fact that isn't true or assumes that you have testified to a fact when you have not. You have heard the question, "Have you stopped beating your wife yet?" You cannot answer it "yes" or "no" without getting into trouble because it assumes a fact that is not true.
    b. Example: The questioner may ask, "When did you first see the baby?" and you may say, "Well, I'm not sure, on July 5th or 6th. I don't know, somewhere along in there." Later, the questioner will ask, "Well, after you first saw the baby on July 5th, what happened?" This assumes you had testified that you first saw the baby on July 5th when in fact you testified you weren't sure when you first saw the baby.

17. *Watch out for alternative questions.*
    a. Questions. Another type of question to watch out for is a question in the alternative, such as, "Well, now is it one or is it two? Which is it?" The danger is that you may know it isn't one, but you don't know whether it is two or not. Your mind may reason that if it is either one or two, and you know it is not one, then it must be two. So you answer, "It's two," when you really don't know.
    b. Other options. The fallacy in this type of reasoning is easy to see. "What color is this pencil? Is it red or is it blue?" You can see that it is obviously yellow. So, just because questions are put to you in the alternative doesn't mean that the given alternatives are the only options.

18. *Be alert to paraphrases.*
    a. Assert your truth and accuracy. The opposing attorney may paraphrase part of your testimony. He or she may say, "Well, now, let me see if I understand you correctly; if I am mistaken, you correct me," and then state what he or

she understands your testimony to be. If any word or phrase is used that you don't think is correct, call it to the lawyer's attention.

b. Qualify statements. Even if the paraphrase sounds perfect to you, do not give an unqualified "yes," because you may be saying "yes" to something you really did not intend. A word may have meaning that you do not understand or appreciate. The most you can say is, "Yes, that sounds about right," or "As far as I can tell, that's about right." Otherwise, you are putting your stamp of approval on every word used. You are letting the attorney tell your story in his or her words, some of which you may not have fully understood.

19. *Take your time.*

a. Consider. Give each question as much thought as is required to understand it and form your answer and then give the answer. Never give a snap answer, but bear in mind that if you take a long time to answer each question, a judge or jury may think you are making up your answers.

b. Interruptions. Don't answer while the questioner is still talking. If you are talking and the questioner is talking, you should stop. One of two things is happening:

  i. You are answering before the questioner has finished the question, in which case you should stop because you cannot listen to the question and understand it while you are answering it.

  ii. The questioner is interrupting you before you have completed your answer to the first question, in which case you should also stop.

  When you stop because you have been interrupted, pay no attention to the question being asked, but keep in mind what you were about to reply to the first question. If you don't, chances are you will forget it. When the questioner finishes talking, say, "Pardon me, I wasn't through with my last answer." Then give your answer and ask, "Now, what was your next question?"

20. *Answer concisely.*

a. Be crisp. Answer a question concisely and then wait for the next question. Say what you need to say, but don't go off on a tangent.

b. Be nonconfrontational. You should not be evasive or argumentative, nor should you nitpick about language. Don't hide anything. You are only to answer the question, but the question must be asked before you give an answer.

c. Don't invite more questions. You can do this by the inflection of your voice. For example, the questioner may ask what shoe you put on first this morning. If you answer, "Well, I don't remember which shoe I put on first this morning," with the accent on "this," you are inviting another question.

21. *Be aware of your speech and appearance.* Make a professional presentation. Talk loudly enough so that everybody can hear you. Don't chew gum, and keep your hands away from your mouth so that you can speak distinctly. Speak up so that the court reporter can hear you. You must give an audible "yes" or "no" answer. The reporter can't hear nods of the head. "Yes" or "no" sounds better than "uh-huh" or "yeah." Dress conservatively and be well groomed.

22. *Look the judge (and jurors, if any) in the eye.* Don't be afraid to make direct eye contact with the judge and jurors while you are testifying. They are naturally sympathetic to a witness and want to hear what is said. Look at them most of the time and speak frankly and openly as you would to a friend or neighbor.

23. *Do not look at "your" lawyer for approval.* Don't look for help when you are on the stand. You are on your own. If you look at your lawyer when a question is asked on cross-examination or look for approval after answering a question, the jury will notice and will get a bad impression. You must appear confident about your answers.

24. *Do not be defensive.* Don't argue with opposing lawyers. They have a right to question you, so don't become defensive or give evasive answers. You are not there to convince them how right you are or how wrong the other side is. You are not there to do anything except answer every question as accurately, courteously, and concisely as possible.

25. *Do not lose your temper.* You should appear to be completely disinterested. Don't lose your temper no matter how hard you are pressed.

26. *Be courteous.* One of the best ways to make a good impression is to be courteous. Be sure to address the judge as "Your Honor."

27. *Avoid joking.* Avoid wisecracking and joking. This is particularly true for depositions. Remarks that everyone present understands as a joke can haunt you after they are transcribed. This is because voice inflection, facial expression, and body posture made the difference. But there it is in black and white, "I could have killed her!"

28. *Do not be reluctant to admit to discussions with "your" attorney.* Be honest. If you are asked whether you have talked to "your" lawyer, admit it freely. The same thing goes for when you are asked if you are being paid. It can be particularly effective to say, "Although I am earning a fee, that will not affect the content of my answers."

29. *Beware of the "have you told me everything" question.* At the end of your testimony, the opposing attorney may decide to ask you, "Have you told me everything about how this happened?" Chances are you have not because you were not asked questions about everything. You are only required to answer what was asked, so do not "close the book" by saying, "Yes, this is all." Instead, what you can say is, "Yes, as far as I can recall, that's about all. I have tried to answer your questions. I believe I have answered them the best I know how."

30. *Relax.* If you relax and talk as you would to neighbors or friends, you will make a more credible impression.

31. *Reread these instructions the night before you testify so that you will have them firmly in your mind.*

VI. Reported Cases of Interest to Lactation Consultants

A. *Baptist Memorial Hospital v. Johnson*, 754 So. 2d 165 (Miss. 2000)

B. *Champagne v. Mid-Maine Medical Center*, 711 A.2d 842 (Me. 1998)

C. *Garcia v. Lawrence Hospital, 5 A.D.3d 227*, 773 N.Y.S.2d 59 (N.Y. 2004)

D. *Hobbs v. Seton Corp.* (2009 WL 196040, Tenn Ct. App. 2009)

E. Utah v. Draper, 128 P.3d 1220 (Utah Ct. of Appeals, 2006)

F. Volm v. Legacy Health Systems, Inc., 237 F. Supp. 2d 1166 (U.S.D.C. D. Or. 2002)

Notes

[1] *MacNamara v. Emmons*, 36 Cal. App. 2d., 199, 204-205, 97 P.2d 503, 507 (1939).

[2] Failure to pay an account may constitute grounds for a lactation consultant to terminate a client relationship, so long as the lactation consultant does not attempt to do so at a critical time, the lactation consultant provides notice to the client, and the lactation consultant gives the client an opportunity to obtain proper care elsewhere.

[3] But see *Tsoukas v. Lapid*, 191 Ill. 2d 561, 738 N.E.2d 936 (Ill. 2000), in which the court held that a health maintenance organization (HMO) patient's telephone calls to a physician listed in an HMO directory did not establish a physician–patient relationship between the parties.

[4] *Lyons v. Grether*, 218 Va. 630, 239 S.E.2d 103 (1977).

[5] *Parkell v. Fitzporter*, 301 Mo. 217, 256 S.W. 239 (1923); *Hanson v. Pock*, 57 Mont. 51, 187 P. 282 (1920); *Peterson v. Phelps*, 23 Minn. 319, 143 N.W. 793 (1913).

[6] *Green v. Walker*, 910 F.2d 291 (5th Cir. 1990); see also, *Harris v. Kreuzer*, 2006 W.L. 68765 (Va. Jan. 13, 2006) VLW#006-6-013 23 pages. (Physician's consent to examine patient formed a limited relationship for purpose of the examination imposing on the physician a duty, limited solely to the exercise of due care consistent with the applicable standard of care so as not to cause harm to the patient in the actual conduct of the examination.)

[7] *Hamil v. Bashline*, 224 Pa. Super. 407, 307 A.2d 57 (1973); but see *Fabien v. Matzko*, 235 Pa. Super 267, 344 A.2d 569 (1975) and *Childs v. Weis*, 440 S.W.2d 104 (Tex. Civ. App. 1969); but see *Tsoukas v. Lapid*, 191 Ill. 2d 561, 738 N.E.2d 936 (Ill. 2000) in which the court held that an HMO patient's telephone calls to a physician listed in an HMO directory did not establish a physician–patient relationship between the parties.

[8] *Brandt v. Grubin*, 131 N.J. Super 182, 329 A.2d 82, 89 (1974).

[9] *Ketchup v. Howard*, 247 Ga. App. 54, 00 FCDR 206, 2000 WL 1747538 (Ga. Ct. App., Nov. 29, 2000) (held that medical professionals, including dentists, must obtain informed consent from patients by advising them about procedures' known risks and available treatment alternatives); *Matthis v. Mastromonaco*, 733 A.2d 456 (1999) (held that the informed consent doctrine applies to noninvasive procedures as well as invasive ones).

[10] Note, however, the patient's consent, or even insistence on a certain treatment plan or procedure, will not relieve a healthcare provider from the obligation to treat patients within the accepted standard of care. *Metzler v. New York State Board for Professional Medical Conduct*, 610 N.Y.S.2d 334 (AD 3 Dept 1994) (homeopathic treatment).

[11] *Canterbury v. Spence*, 150 App. D.C. 263, 464 F.2d 772 (D.C. Cir. 1972) cert. denied 409 U.S. 1064 (1972); *Sard v. Hardy*, 281 Md. 432, 379 A.2d 1014 (1977); *Smith v. Shannon*, 100 Wash.2d, 666 P.2d 351 (1983). However, in many jurisdictions, this duty arises out of the fiduciary nature of the physician–patient relationship and may not apply to lactation consultants. *Nelson v. Gaunt*, 125 Cal. App. 3d 623, 178 Cal. Rptr. (1981).

[12] *Halley v. Birbiglia*, 3901 Mass. 540, 458 N.E.2d 710 (1983).

[13] *Canterbury v. Spence*, 464 F.2d 772, 780 (D.C. Cir.), cert. denied, 409 U.S. 1064 (1972); *St. Gemme v. Tomlin*, 118 Ill. App. 3d 766, 74 Ill. Dec. 264, 455 N.E.2d 294 (1983). Also see *Koegan v. Holy Family Hospital*, 95 Wash.2d 306, 622 P.2d 1246 (1980).

[14] It is well settled that only material risks need to be disclosed. There is no duty to disclose all conceivable risks (*Gouse v. Cassell*, 532 Pa. 197, 615 A.2d 33 [1992]), risks that are not reasonably foreseeable (*Hondroulis v. Schumacher*, 546, So. 2d 466 [La. 1989]), or those risks that are minimal (*Penwick v. Christensen*, 912 S.W.2d 275 [Tex. App. Houston, 14th Dist, 1995] writ denied [June 28, 1996]; rehearing of writ of error filed [July 12, 1996] rehearing of writ of error overruled [August 1, 1996]). However, establishing whether a particular risk is more than merely "conceivable," or "reasonably foreseeable," or greater than "minimal" is an imprecise exercise that has spawned much litigation.

[15] *Siegel v. Mt. Sinai Hospital*, 62 Ohio App. 2d 12, 403 N.E.2d 202 (1978).

[16] *Pegram v. Sisco*, 406 F. Supp 776 (WD Ark. 1976) aff'd 547 F.2d 1172 (8th Cir. l976); *LePelley v. Grefenson*, 101 Idaho 422, 614 P.2d 962 (1980); *Karl J. Pizzalotto MD Ltd v. Wilson*, 437 So. 2d 859 (La. 1983) remd 444 So. 2d 143 (La. App. 1983); *LaCaze v. Collier*, 434 So. 2d 1039 (1983); *Roberson v. Menorah Medical Center*, 588 S.W.2d 134 (Mo. App. 1979); *Gray v. Grunnagle*, 423 Pa. 144, 233 A.2d 633 (1966); *Cross v. Trapp*, 294 S.E.2d 446 (W.Va. 1982).

[17] *Boyer v. Smith*, 345 Pa. Super. Ct. 66, 497 A.2d 646 (1985) (holding that the defendant had no duty to obtain a patient's informed consent to the administration of a therapeutic drug).

[18] *Novak v. Texada, Miller, Masterson & Davis Clinic*, 514 So. 2d 524 (La. App. 1987) cert. denied 515 So. 2d 807 (La. (1987) (administration of a flu shot held to be a "routine" medical procedure to which Louisiana's informed consent statute did not apply); *Daniels v. State*, 532 ASo. 2d 218 (La. App. 1988) (treating a closed wrist fracture found to be a routine medical procedure to which Louisiana's informed consent statute did not apply).

[19] *Halley v. Birbiglia*, 390 Mass. 540, 458 N.E.2d 240 (1982).

[20] *Stovall v Harms*, 214 Kan. 835, 522 P.2d 353 (1974); *Llera v. Wisner*, 171 Mont. 254, 557 P.2d 805 (1976); *Johnson v. Whitehurst*, 652 S.W.2d 441 (Tex. App. 1983).

[21] *Harnish v. Children's Hospital Medical Center*, 387 Mass. 152, 439 N.E.2d 240 (1982).

[22] *Beard v. Brunswick Hospital Center*, 632 N.Y.S.2d 805 (App. Div. 2d Dept, 1995) [a physician who assisted a surgeon, but who was not the primary surgeon, found not liable]; *Foflygen v. Zemel*, 420 Pa. Super. 18, 615 A.2d 1380 (Pa. 1993) [a physician taking a patient's medical history in conjunction with the patient's admission to the hospital for medical treatment, and a nurse assisting the treating physician during the procedure held not liable]; *Barnes v. Gorman*, 605 So. 2d 805 (Miss. 1992) [consent obtained by a licensed practical nurse may not be adequate], but see *Perez v. Park Madison Professional Lab* (lst Dept., 1995) 212 App. Div. 2d 271, 630 N.Y.S.2d 37, partial summary judgment granted, cause dismd. (N.Y. App. Div. lst Dept) 1995 N.Y. App. Div. LEXIS 7844 and app. dismd. without op. 87 N.Y.S. 896, 640 N.Y.S.2d 880, 663 N.E.2d 922; *Sangiulo v. Leventhal*, 132 Misc2d 680, 505 N.Y.S.2d 507 (1986) (a "substitute physician" administering part of a course of treatment started by a physician for whom he was covering found not liable).

[23] *Matthis v. Mastromonaco*, 160 N.J. 26, 733 A.2d 456 (N.J. 1999).

[24] See *Rogers v. Brown*, 416 So. 2d 624 (La. App. 1982). In this case, the client's consent was established on the basis of a consent form where the physician and nurse testified that risks of treatment were fully explained to the client and the form was completed, signed, and given to the client.

[25] The case law of the state of Pennsylvania is an exception to this rule. In Pennsylvania, if informed consent was not given, this is treated as the legal equivalent of no consent having been given, and the action is then an action for battery (not negligence). *Gouse v. Cassel*, 532 Pa. 197, 615 A.2d 331, 334 (1992); *Sagala v. Tavares*, 533 A.2d 165(Pa. Super. 1987); *Boyer v. Smith*, 345 Pa. Super Ct. 66, 497 A.2d 646 (1985); *Salis v. United States*, 522 F. Supp 989 (MD Pa. 1981); *Gray v. Grunnagle*, 423 Pa. 144, 233 A.2d 633 (1966). Consider also *People v. Messinger*, No. 9467694FH

(Mich, Ingham County Cir. Ct. Feb. 2, 1995) (jury acquitted a father charged with involuntary manslaughter on grounds that his decision to disconnect premature infant son's respirator was the result of informed decision to withdraw life-sustaining treatment in the child's "best interests"); *Dewes v. Indian Health Service*, 504 F. Supp 203 (D S.D. 1980).

[26] In some jurisdictions, children over a certain age may consent to particular treatments for themselves, such as for infectious disease, family planning, outpatient substance abuse rehabilitation, and outpatient mental health treatment.

[27] *Wallace v. Cox*, 136 Tenn. 69, 188 S.W. 611, 612 (1916).

[28] For example, see §16.1-331, et seq., 3, Code of Virginia, which provides that a petition for emancipation may be filed for any minor who has reached his or her 16th birthday.

[29] *Belcher v. Charleston Area Medical Center*, 188 W. Va. 105, 422 S.E.2d 827 (1992).

[30] *Swenson v. Swenson*, 241 Mo. App. 21, 227 S.W.2d 103 (1950).

[31] *Bach v. Long Island Jewish Hospital*, 49 Misc.2d 207, 267 N.Y.S.2d 289 (1966).

[32] *Smith v. Seigly*, 72 Wash.2d 16, 431 P.2d 719 (1967).

[33] *In Re Carpenter's Estate*, 196 Mich. 561 (1917).

[34] *Sermchief v. Gonzales*, 600 S.W.2d 683 (Mo. 1983) ("Having found that the nurses' acts were authorized by [the Nursing Practice Act], it follows that such acts do not constitute the unlawful practice of medicine); *Professional Health Care Ina v. Bigsby*, 709 P.2d 86, 88 (Colo., 1985) (acts of a nurse practitioner who was indirectly supervised by a physician and who followed protocols and directions that he established "constituted only the practice of professional nursing and could not be construed to be the illegal practice of medicine"); *Prentice Medical Corporation v. Todd*, 145 Ill. App.3d 692, 495 N.E.2d 1044, 99 Ill. Dec. 303 (Ill. App. Ct., 1986) (nurse who practiced under standing orders and cooperated with supervising physicians was not holding herself out as practicing medicine, despite the fact that she referred to her "practice"); *Hofson v. Orenreich*, 168 A.D.2d 243, 562 N.Y.S. 2d 479 (New York 1990) (New York Supreme Court determined that a jury was justified in finding that a nurse who incised and drained three acne cysts and removed blackheads was not engaged in the unauthorized practice of medicine.).

[35] See *Scope of Practice for International Board Certified Lactation Consultants* (March 8, 2008).

[36] Examples include §71-1.103(16) of the Laws of Nebraska and Delaware Code title 24 §1702(9).

[37] See the discussion of Pennsylvania law in Kabla, Edward, J. (1998, September). Legalities of a telephone nurse triage system. *Physicians News Digest*. Retrieved from www.physiciansnews.com/law/998kabala.html. ("Registered nurses are typically authorized to make assessment of persons who are ill and to render a nursing diagnosis in their capacity as professionals. For example: a nursing diagnosis could be a situation where the nurse finds or fails to find symptoms described by a physician in standing orders or protocols. The nurse would identify symptoms for the purpose of administering courses of treatment prescribed by the physicians. The nursing regimen is always designed to function in consultation with the treating physicians or other physicians licensed in Pennsylvania. Further, the protocols used in the nursing regimen would have been developed by a facility or practice with specific knowledge as to the capability of their nursing staff and the accessibility of the physicians.").

[38] Some U.S. states, such as Iowa, recognize that what most people think of as an issue of "neglect" is covered under the child abuse category of "denial of Critical Care."

[39] *Goldfarb v. Virginia State Bar*, 421 U.S. 773 (1975); *National Society of Professional Engineers v. U.S.*, 435 U.S. 679 (1978).

[40] 15 U.S.C. § 1127.

[41] *Reddy Communications v. Environmental Action Foundation*, 477 F. Supp. 936, 943 (D.D.C. 1979) ("Service marks might just as well have been called trade marks for services, leaving conventional trade marks to be referred to as trade marks for goods, but the different term is probably more convenient....").

[42] A certification mark "certifies" the "regional or other origin, material, mode of manufacture, quality, accuracy, or other characteristics of such person's goods or services or that the work or labor on the goods or services was performed by members of a union or other organization." 15 U.S.C. § 1127.

[43] Principle #3, Code of Professional Conduct for International Board Certified Lactation Consultants (November 1, 2011).

[44] In most instances, the IBLCE's Ethics and Discipline Committee issues opinions only on matters that have come before it and this issue has not been the subject of a complaint.

[45] See generally *Katz v. United States*, 389 U.S. 347 (1967).

[46] The caller and/or recipient may be in an area in which digital service is not available or may be on an analog or cordless phone. Most digital phones have the capability of switching back and forth from digital to analog to address this very problem.

[47] Laws that expressly address advertising through "electronic media" govern advertising on the Internet.

[48] Some legal commentators claim that a disclaimer alone may not be sufficient and could even be used as evidence that you "knew" the communication was not confidential.

[49] *Nat'l Fed'n of the Blind v. Target Corp.*, 582 F. Suppl 2d 1185, 1189 (N. D. Cal. 2007). The plaintiffs in this class action on behalf of individuals with visual impairments alleged that the retailer had violated the public accommodation provision of the Americans with Disabilities Act because it had failed to make its website accessible to blind persons by including coding that would make the website compatible with screen-reading software that vocalizes text and describes graphics.

References

Bornmann, P. G., (1986). *Legal considerations and the lactation consultant—USA. Unit 3* [The Lactation Consultant Series]. Wayne, NJ: Avery Publishing Group.

Coates, M. M., & Riordan, J. (2011). *Breastfeeding and human lactation* (4th ed.) Sudbury, MA: Jones and Bartlett.

Fry, S. T., & Johnstone, M.-J. (2002). *Ethics in nursing practice: A guide to ethical decision making.* Oxford, England: Blackwell Science.

Jameton, A. (1984). *Nursing practice: The ethical issues.* Upper Saddle River, NJ: Prentice Hall.

Lawrence, R. A., & Lawrence, R. M. (2010). *Breastfeeding: A guide for the medical profession* (76th ed.). St. Louis, MO: Mosby.

Wallace, I., & Bunting, L. (2007). An examination of local, state and international arrangements for the mandatory reporting of child abuse: Implications for Northern Ireland. Belfast, Ireland: National Society for the Prevention of Cruelty to Children Northern Ireland Policy and Research Unit.. Retrieved from http://www.nspcc.org.uk/Inform/publications/downloads/mandatoryreportingNI_wdf51133.pdf

Suggested Reading

Council of Medical Specialty Societies (March 2011). *Code for Interaction with Companies.* Available from http://www.cmss.org/codeforinteractions.aspx

International Lactation Consultant Association. (2005). *Standards of practice for International Board Certified lactation consultants.* Available in English, French and German from: http://www.ilca.org/i4a/pages/index.cfm?pageid=3933

International Board of Lactation Consultant Examiners. (2008, March 8). *Scope of practice for International Board Certified lactation consultants.* Available from http://www.iblce.org/home. Under the "Professional Standards" tab at the top of the page.

International Board of Lactation Consultant Examiners. (2010, December 6). *Clinical competencies for the practice of International Board Certified lactation consultants.* Available from http/www.iblce.org/home. Under the "Professional Standards" tab at the top of the page.

International Board of Lactation Consultant Examiners. (2010, March 20). *Documentation guidelines.* Retrieved from http://www.iblce.org/upload/downloads/DocumentationGuidelines.pdf

International Board of Lactation Consultant Examiners. (2011, November). *Code of professional conduct for International Board Certified lactation consultants.* Retrieved from http://iblce.org/upload/downloads/CodeOfProfessionalConduct.pdf

National Society for Prevention of Cruelty to Children. United Kingdom. Available at nspcc.org.uk.

Pallash, B. (2002, January). Advocating effectively. *Association Management* (subscription service), *54*(1).

Smith, L. J. (1991). Expert witness: What to emphasize. *Journal of Human Lactation, 7*(3), 141.

Suhler, A., Bornmann, P., & Scott, J. (1991). The lactation consultant as expert witness. *Journal of Human Lactation, 3*, 129–140.

CHAPTER 14
Developing and Managing a Hospital Lactation Service

Rebecca Mannel, BS, IBCLC, FILCA

OBJECTIVES

- Describe best practices for hospital lactation care.
- Define lactation acuity and how it relates to patient safety and best practices.
- Identify lactation services needed and determine staffing needs.
- Identify policies needed and resources for their development.
- Describe professional competencies needed for lactation consultant staff.
- Describe breastfeeding competencies needed for other healthcare professionals.
- Describe methods to identify clinical needs of breastfeeding families.
- Explain the difference between lactation consultant documentation and nursing staff documentation.
- Identify methods for collection of essential data.
- Promote lactation support for healthcare system staff.

INTRODUCTION

In many areas of the world, the critical period for initiation of breastfeeding occurs in a hospital or birthing facility. Breastfeeding mothers and children also may experience hospital admissions because of illness or injury that can compromise or threaten the continuation of breastfeeding. The need for skilled lactation support at these sensitive periods has been identified by many healthcare organizations, including the World Health Organization (2003), the U.S. Department of Health and Human Services (Office of the U.S. Surgeon General, 2011), the European Union (2004), and the Australian Health Ministers' Conference (2009). This chapter describes the key elements of a hospital lactation program that will meet the needs of breastfeeding families during a hospital stay.

I. Proposing Lactation Service to Hospital Administrators

A. Explain best practices in the care of breastfeeding families.

  1. The Baby-Friendly Hospital Initiative (BFHI) outlines evidence-based practices for maternity services.

    a. *The Ten Steps to Successful Breastfeeding* (World Health Organization [WHO], 1998)

    b. *The International Code of Marketing of Breast-Milk Substitutes* (WHO, 1981)

  2. The *U.S. Surgeon General's Call to Action to Support Breastfeeding* (Office of the Surgeon General, 2011) lists action items for the healthcare system:

    a. Ensure that maternity care practices are fully supportive of breastfeeding.

    b. Develop systems to guarantee continuity of skilled support for lactation between hospitals and healthcare settings in the community.

    c. Provide education and training in breastfeeding for all health professionals who care for women and children.

    d. Ensure access to services provided by International Board Certified Lactation Consultants (IBCLCs).

  3. The U.S. *Surgeon General's Call to Action* also states the impact of having IBCLCs on staff:

    a. "Research shows that rates of exclusive breastfeeding and of any breastfeeding are higher among women who have had babies in hospitals with IBCLCs on staff than in those without these professionals" (Office of the Surgeon General, 2011).

  4. The U.S. Joint Commission adopted a core measure on exclusive breastmilk feeding to improve breastfeeding outcomes in maternity facilities (The Joint Commission, 2010).

    a. The Joint Commission's core measures serve as a national, standardized performance measurement system providing assessments of care delivered in given focus areas.

  5. The European Union's (2004) *Blueprint for Action on Breastfeeding* goal is "to ensure that services for the support of breastfeeding, including assistance provided by appropriately qualified lactation consultants or other suitably competent health care staff when needed, are accessible and affordable to all mothers."

  6. The *Australian National Breastfeeding Strategy* states, "The timing of breastfeeding interventions is crucial for effectiveness" and "individual level professional support" significantly increased the duration of breastfeeding (Australian Health Ministers' Conference, 2009).

B. Define the concept of lactation acuity in determining the level of clinical support needed by breastfeeding families (Mannel, 2011).

  1. Increasing maternal–infant lactation acuity leads to increased risk of poor breastfeeding outcomes, including premature weaning.

    a. See **Table 14-1**

Table 14-1 Lactation Acuity Levels[a]

Acuity level 1	Level 1 acuity patients can be cared for by nursing staff that have basic breastfeeding knowledge and competency.[31-33]
Maternal characteristics	Basic breastfeeding education, routine management
	Latch/milk transfer appear optimal
	Maternal decision to routinely supplement
	Maternal decision to pump and feed expressed breast milk
	Maternal indecision regarding breastfeeding
	Mother can latch baby with minimal assistance
	Multiparous mother with healthy-term baby and prior breastfeeding experience
Acuity level 2	Level 2 acuity patients should be cared for by Registered Lactation Consultants staff as soon as possible, or referral made to Registered Lactation Consultants in the community. Early follow-up after discharge is critical.[33-41]
Maternal characteristics	Antepartum admission with increased risk of preterm delivery[37,38,42]
	Cesarean section delivery[12,43,44]
	Delayed breastfeeding initiation (defined as after 1 hour with routine vaginal delivery and after 2 hours with routine cesarean section)[2,3,43]
	Maternal acute illnesses/conditions (eg, preeclampsia, cardiomyopathy, postpartum depression, postpartum hemorrhage)[38-40]
	Maternal age (mother < 18 years or > 35 years)[40,41]
	Maternal chronic conditions (eg, rheumatoid arthritis, systemic lupus erythematosus, hypertension, cancer, history of gastric bypass, obesity)[38,45,46]
	Maternal cognitive impairment (eg, mental retardation, Down syndrome, autism)[38,41]
	Maternal endocrine disorders (eg, polycystic ovary syndrome, infertility, thyroid disorders, diabetes)[38-40]
	Maternal medication concerns[47]
	Maternal physical disability (eg, paraplegic, cerebral palsy, visual impairment, psychiatric)[38,40]
	Maternal readmission (eg, breastfeeding well established, noncritical issues)[38,40]
	Maternal request[48]
	Multiparous mother with history of breastfeeding difficulty[37,38]
	Primiparous mother or first-time breastfeeding mother with healthy-term baby[49,50]
	Social/cultural issues (eg, communication barriers, domestic/sexual abuse)[41,51,52]

(continues)

Table 14-1 Lactation Acuity Levels[a] (continued)

Infant characteristics	Consistent LATCH score < 6 at day of discharge[53,54] Breastfeeding Assessment Score 5[27,28] Latch difficulties (eg, pain)[37-41,55] Infant readmission (breastfeeding well established, noncritical issues)[38,40] Newborn birth trauma (eg, cephalohematoma, shoulder dystocia)[12,56] Suboptimal/inadequate milk transfer leading to medical recommendation to supplement[5,37,57]
Acuity level 3	Level 3 acuity patients need to be cared for by Registered Lactation Consultant staff while in hospital. These patients will require in-depth assessment and ongoing management. Early follow-up after discharge is critical.[33-41]
Maternal characteristics	Abscess/mastitis[37,58] High maternal anxiety[38,48] Induced lactation[5,38,40] Maternal breast conditions (eg, breast/simple anomalies, glandular insufficiency, history of breast surgery)[8,38,56] Maternal illness/surgery[38,40,59] Maternal readmission (breastfeeding not well established and/or critical issues)[38,40] Pathologic engorgement[8,60]
Infant characteristics	High-risk infant on mother-baby unit (eg, late preterm, small/large for gestational age, multiples)[5,8,61-63] Hyperbilirubinemia[64-66] Hypoglycemia[67] Infant admission to neonatal intensive care[42,68] Infant congenital anomalies[38,69,70] Infant illness/surgery[8,38] Infant oral/motor dysfunction (eg, tight frenulumn, hypotonia/hypertonia)[70-72] Infant readmission (breastfeeding not well established and/or critical issues)[38,40,41] Infant weight loss > 7% of birth weight before discharge[8,73]

[a]Acuity levels can change on the basis of assessment by the Registered Lactation Consultant or other health care team members.

2. Patient safety is compromised when hospitals fail to provide adequate support for high-acuity lactation situations.

    a. Inappropriate care can increase risk of maternal infection, newborn dehydration and jaundice, and delayed discharge resulting from poor feeding (Martin et al., 2002; Moritz et al., 2005).

3. Risk management issues increase when staff do not have appropriate training and skills to care for higher lactation acuity.

    a. Compromised breastfeeding or lactation increases risk of hospital readmissions and increased length of stay for infants in neonatal intensive care units (NICUs) (Martens et al., 2004; Paul et al., 2006).

    b. Many registered nurses (RNs) in the United States have not had adequate training or education to care for breastfeeding patients (Centers for Disease Control and Prevention [CDC], 2009).

    c. Nursing staff should have training to manage the care of low-acuity breastfeeding patients while higher lactation acuity situations should be referred to IBCLCs.

    d. There have been legal cases involving poor lactation care in the United States.

        i. *Clements v. Lima Memorial Hospital*, 2010 WL 597368

        ii. *Hall-ex rel Wade v. Henry Ford Health System*, 2005 WL473683

        iii. *Garcia v. Lawrence Hospital*, 773 N.Y.S.2d 59 (2004)

        iv. *Baptist Memorial Hospital-Union County v. Johnson*, No. 98-IA-00175-SCT. 2000

II. Determine Resources Needed

A. The lactation service varies depending on the level of service provided by the hospital in other areas (Mannel & Mannel, 2006). For example, does the hospital have a Level III NICU or are all high-acuity newborns transferred to a regional center?

1. Inpatient lactation service is most commonly provided and should provide clinical care and support to breastfeeding patients admitted to any area of the facility.

    a. Lower-level community hospitals may focus most of their support in the maternity area of the hospital.

    b. Higher-level regional centers require lactation support in maternity areas, neonatal intensive care areas, pediatric units, and general medical/surgical areas where maternal admissions might occur.

        i. Average mother/baby consult times (includes documentation time) (Mannel et al., 2006):

            (a) Initial visits: 35 minutes

            (b) Follow-up visits: 32 minutes

     ii. Average NICU consult times (includes documentation time) (Mannel, unpublished):

        (a) Initial visits: 67 minutes

        (b) Transition to direct breastfeeding: 68 minutes

        (c) Discharge teaching: 73 minutes

   c. Pediatric hospitals with no maternity services also require professional lactation support (Lessen, 2009).

2. Outpatient lactation service may be provided by the hospital or referral made to professional lactation services in the community.

   a. Outpatient lactation services may be available in community clinics, in public health agencies, and in the home via private practice lactation consultants or public health programs.

     i. Average outpatient lactation consult time (includes documentation time) (Mannel et al., 2006):

        (a) Initial visit: 95 minutes

3. Telephone lactation support is an important postdischarge element of patient care (Mannel et al., 2006; Murray et al., 2007).

   a. Hospital lactation services may provide on-demand telephone support or may proactively contact all breastfeeding mothers after discharge for early follow-up.

     i. Data from Mannel et al. (2006) indicate average length of telephone consults is 20 minutes. This length is consistent with data from the U.S. Oklahoma Breastfeeding Hotline, where average phone consults are 25 minutes (Oklahoma State Department of Health, 2011).

     ii. If all breastfeeding patients received at least one follow-up call from an IBCLC after discharge, 1.0 full-time equivalent (FTE) per 3,915 deliveries would be required (Mannel et al., 2006).

   b. If not provided by the hospital, referral to community telephone support is essential.

   c. Some countries have national breastfeeding support lines. In the United States, some states have separately funded breastfeeding helplines.

B. Calculate staffing needs for a hospital lactation service.

1. Data from a U.S. survey of hospital lactation programs demonstrate a significant relationship among breastfeeding rates (initiation and exclusive breastfeeding [EBF]), number of deliveries, and number of days per week that lactation consultants were available (Mannel et al., submitted for publication).

   a. More full-time equivalent (FTE) positions for lactation consultants were significantly related to increased breastfeeding initiation.

   b. Increased FTEs were significantly related to increased lactation education hours for hospital nursing staff.

2. Recommendations for staffing a tertiary-level hospital lactation service are provided in **Table 14-2**.

   a. The variety and level of services determine the staffing recommendations.

Table 14-2 Staffing Ratios

Service	FTE Ratio
Mother/baby coverage (inpatient)	1:783 breastfeeding couplets
NICU coverage (inpatient)	1:235 infant admits
Postdischarge coverage	
Mother/baby outpatients	1:1292 breastfeeding couplets
Mother/baby telephone follow-up	1:3915 breastfeeding couplets
NICU outpatients	1:8181 breastfeeding infants
Education	0.1:1000 deliveries
Program development/administration	0.1:1000 deliveries
Research	0.1–0.2 FTE total

FTE = full-time equivalent; NICU = neonatal intensive care unit.

      3. The U.S. Lactation Consultant Association (USLCA) and the Association for Women's Health, Obstetric and Neonatal Nurses (AWHONN) provide the following staffing guidelines (AWHONN, 2010; USLCA, 2010):

        a. 1.9 FTE: 1,000 deliveries (tertiary care center)

        b. 1.3 FTE: 1,000 deliveries (no neonatal service)

        c. 1.0 FTE: 235 infant transfers/admissions to neonatal service

III. Policy Development

    A. Every maternity and pediatric facility needs a policy that addresses evidence-based care and practice for breastfeeding patients (CDC, 2009; WHO, 1998).

    B. Numerous resources exist for hospital breastfeeding policies:

      1. International Lactation Consultant Association's (ILCA) *Clinical Guidelines for the Establishment of Exclusive Breastfeeding* (ILCA, 2005)

      2. Academy of Breastfeeding Medicine's (ABM) "Protocol #7, Model Hospital Breastfeeding Policy" (ABM, 2010)

        a. ABM has numerous protocols that can be used to develop more situation-specific policies.

      3. American Academy of Pediatrics "Sample Hospital Breastfeeding Policy" (American Academy of Pediatrics Section on Breastfeeding, 2009)

      4. The Human Milk Banking Association of North America has information for policy development on use of donor milk, milk collection and storage, and human milk feeding errors available at www.hmbana.org.

      5. The U.S. Breastfeeding Committee (USBC) provides guidance on implementing the new core measure on EBF at discharge (USBC, 2010).

6. Hospitals and healthcare facilities also should address the needs of breastfeeding employees and clinicians. A human resources policy outlines the expectations for both employer and employees. A sample HR policy on breastfeeding is available at www.go.jblearning.com/corecurriculum.

C. Lactation service–specific policies may also be indicated.

1. See sample policies at www.go.jblearning.com/corecurriculum.

IV. Lactation Program Management

A. A well-functioning lactation program must have dedicated FTEs for lactation consultants to ensure access to care in a timely fashion by breastfeeding families.

1. The International Board Certified Lactation Consultant (IBCLC) credential for lactation consultants is the only credential that is awarded by a certification program that is accredited by the National Commission for Certifying Agencies. The U.S. Surgeon General's *Call to Action* states that IBCLCs are "the only health care professionals certified in lactation management" (p. 27).

   a. IBCLCs must adhere to the International Board of Lactation Consultant Examiners (IBLCE) Scope of Practice and Code of Professional Conduct for IBCLCs (IBLCE, 2008, 2011).

   b. IBCLCs must adhere to the ILCA Standards of Practice for IBCLCs (ILCA, 2006).

   c. IBCLCs are also known as Registered Lactation Consultants (RLCs) in the United States.

2. Newly hired IBCLCs need adequate orientation and training.

   a. IBLCE (2010) has published the Clinical Competencies for IBCLC Practice, which can be used during orientation to verify competency of an IBCLC.

3. IBCLCs, along with other healthcare staff caring for breastfeeding families, need lactation-specific annual competencies and education.

4. Some hospital lactation programs have implemented annual peer review of IBCLCs during lactation consults. Peer reviews are typically done by an IBCLC in a supervisory position.

B. Identifying patients needing to be seen by the IBCLC staff can be done in the following ways:

1. *Referral system*: Referrals may be generated by clinicians, nursing staff, other healthcare team members, and patients/families.

2. *Lactation rounds system:* IBCLC staff round on newly delivered mothers to identify high-acuity breastfeeding couplets (Mannel, 2010).

C. Documentation:

1. IBCLCs typically document separately from nursing staff.

   a. IBCLCs function as interdisciplinary care team members rather than an extension of the nursing team.

   b. IBLCE has *Documentation Guidelines* (IBLCE, 2010).

    c. IBCLCs should follow documentation guidelines for abbreviations. Most hospitals have designated references for approved abbreviations (e.g., *Stedman's Medical Dictionary*).

       i. Breastfeeding should be accurately defined (Labbok et al., 1990).

         (a) *Exclusive breastfeeding* is no other foods or liquids; breastfeeding or breastmilk only.

         (b) *Partial breastfeeding* includes other liquids or foods, including breastmilk substitutes.

           (i) High = more than 80% of feeds are breastmilk.

           (ii) Medium = 20–80% of feeds are breastmilk.

           (iii) Low = less than 20% of feeds are breastmilk.

         (c) *Token breastfeeding* is irregular, minimal breastfeeding, not for major nutritive purposes.

         (d) *Exclusive formula feeding* is all feeds consisting of breastmilk substitutes.

  2. IBCLCs and nursing staff should document latch through a standardized latch assessment process (CDC, 2009). See Chapter 28, Guidelines for Facilitating and Assessing Breastfeeding, for latch assessment tools.

    a. Nurses are responsible for documenting each infant feeding while IBCLCs document an assessment and plan of care for the mother–infant dyad.

    b. IBCLCs typically document on both mother and child if both are hospital patients.

  3. Breastfeeding mothers are often referred to IBCLCs for information on safety of medications during lactation. IBCLCs can provide evidence-based information about medications to healthcare providers and families. See sample medication note at www.go.jblearning.com/corecurriculum.

D. Data collection/reporting:

  1. Breastfeeding data are health outcomes that are reportable and tracked annually in a few countries.

    a. The U.S. CDC monitors state and national breastfeeding rates, including any and exclusive breastfeeding rates. This information is available at www.cdc.gov/breastfeeding/data.

       i. Many hospitals do not have a system for routinely tracking breastfeeding outcomes (CDC, 2009).

    b. California monitors any breastfeeding and EBF rates at hospital discharge and publicly reports by hospital. Data are collected from newborn screening information (California WIC Association and University of California, Davis, 2008).

    c. The U.S. Joint Commission defines exclusive breastmilk feeding at discharge as the percentage of newborns receiving only breastmilk or breastfeeding out of the total number of newborns during their entire hospital stay.

    d. The United Kingdom monitors national breastfeeding rates, including initiation and prevalence at 6–8 weeks. This information is available at www.dh.gov.uk.

        e. Canada and Australia periodically report national breastfeeding rates.

           i. Canadian data are available at http://www.hc-sc.gc.ca/fn-an/surveill/ nutrition/commun/prenatal/duration-duree-eng.php.

          ii. Australian data are on page 9 of the Australian National Breastfeeding Strategy 2010-2015 available at www.health.gov.au/internet/main/ publishing.nsf/Content/49F80E887F1E2257CA2576A10077F73F/ $File/Breastfeeding_strat1015.pdf.

        f. The United Nations Children's Fund (UNICEF) tracks national breastfeeding data by country. This information is available at http://www.childinfo. org/breastfeeding_infantfeeding.html.

    2. The World Health Organization maintains a breastfeeding data bank with data available from 93 countries at http://www.who.int/nutrition/databases/ infantfeeding/countries/en/index.html.

    3. Other data points depend on level of service of the facility.

        a. Percentage of NICU infants receiving own mother's milk feedings

        b. Percentage of NICU infant feeds that are expressed breastmilk or pasteurized donor milk

        c. Percentage of NICU infants transitioning to direct breastfeeding before discharge

        d. Percentage of high-acuity lactation consults

        e. Readmission rates of breastfeeding patients

V. Staff Education

A. Hospital lactation services often provide basic lactation education and training to other healthcare team members.

    1. IBCLCs are recognized experts in the management of breastfeeding and lactation.

B. Nursing staff working in maternal–child health areas need basic breastfeeding education and training to equal 20 hours in their first year with annual updates (WHO, 1998).

    1. WHO Baby-Friendly Hospital Initiative (BFHI) curriculum (WHO, 2009b)

    2. U.S. Breastfeeding Committee *Core Competencies in Breastfeeding Care and Service for all Health Care Professionals* (USBC, 2009)

    3. Association of Women's Health, Obstetric and Neonatal Nurses' *Position Statement: Breastfeeding* (AWHONN, 2008)

C. Physicians/clinicians need education in basic breastfeeding care and management (WHO, 1998).

    1. Resources available include the following:

        a. Wellstart lactation management self-study module for physicians (Wellstart International, 2009)

        b. WHO infant and young child feeding model chapter for medical and other student textbooks (WHO, 2009a). Available in English and Spanish.

c. American Academy of Pediatrics (AAP) breastfeeding residency curriculum for medical residents (AAP, 2009)

d. Video clips available from Stanford University, California, USA. Available at http://newborns.stanford.edu/Breastfeeding/

e. See list of additional resources at www.go.jblearning.com/corecurriculum

VI. Hospital Lactation Support for Employees

A. Hospitals should develop policies and practices to support their own breastfeeding employees and clinicians (Wiseman et al., 2012).

1. Hospitals are often leaders of health and wellness promotion efforts.

2. Hospitals are often major employers in their communities.

3. The U.S. Department of Labor (2010) passed new regulations requiring workplace support of breastfeeding employees.

4. Hospital policies and environments affect the health and wellness of patients, visitors, and healthcare professionals and staff.

   a. Many hospitals around the world are now tobacco-free environments.

   b. Some hospitals are now recognized as breastfeeding-friendly worksites or employers.

B. Lactation consultants are skilled in management of breastfeeding and lactation, including support of breastfeeding mothers who are employed. (See Chapter 7, Breastfeeding and Working Women.)

1. Hospital staff and physicians logically refer to the hospital lactation service when experiencing challenges with breastfeeding after return to work.

2. Lactation consultants have the knowledge and skill to promote development of hospital policies supportive of working breastfeeding women.

3. Lactation consultants can be instrumental in designing staff lactation rooms with appropriate space and equipment.

References

Academy of Breastfeeding Medicine. (2010). Clinical protocol #7: Model breastfeeding policy. *Breastfeeding Medicine*, *4*(5).

American Academy of Pediatrics. (2009). *Breastfeeding promotion in physicians' office practices, phase III, breastfeeding residency curriculum*. Retrieved from http://www2.aap.org/breastfeeding/curriculum/

American Academy of Pediatrics Section on Breastfeeding. (2009). Sample hospital policy on breastfeeding for newborns. AAP 2009. Available at https://www2.aap.org/breastfeeding/curriculum/documents/pdf/Hospital%20Breastfeeding%20Policy_FINAL.pdf

Association of Women's Health, Obstetric and Neonatal Nurses. (2008). *Position statement: Breastfeeding*. Retrieved from http://www.awhonn.org/awhonn/content.do?name=02_PracticeResources%2F2C1_Breastfeeding.htm

Association of Women's Health, Obstetric and Neonatal Nurses. (2010). *Guidelines for professional registered nurse staffing for perinatal units*. Washington, DC: Author.

Australian Health Ministers' Conference. (2009). *The Australian National Breastfeeding strategy 2010–2015*. Canberra, Australia: Australian Government Department of Health and Ageing.

California WIC Association and University of California, Davis. (2008). Depends on where you are born: California hospitals must close the gap in exclusive breastfeeding rates. Retrieved from http://www.calwic.org/storage/documents/wellness/bfhospital2008.pdf

Centers for Disease Control and Prevention. (2008). Breastfeeding-related maternity practices at hospitals and birth centers, United States, 2007. *Morbidity and Mortality Weekly Report, 57*, 621–625. Retrieved from http://www.cdc.gov/mmwr/preview/mmwrhtml/mm5723a1.htm

Centers for Disease Control and Prevention. (2009). Maternity practices in infant nutrition and care survey results. Retrieved from http://www.cdc.gov/breastfeeding/data/mpinc/results.htm

European Union, EU Project on Promotion of Breastfeeding in Europe. (2004). *Protection, promotion and support of breastfeeding in Europe: A blueprint for action*. Luxembourg, Belgium: European Commission, Directorate Public Health and Risk Assessment. Retrieved from http://ec.europa.eu/health/ph_projects/2002/promotion/fp_promotion_2002_frep_18_en.pdf

International Board of Lactation Consultant Examiners. (2008). *Scope of practice for International Board Certified Lactation Consultants (IBCLCs)*. Retrieved from http://iblce.org/upload/downloads/ScopeOfPractice.pdf

International Board of Lactation Consultant Examiners. (2010). *Documentation guidelines*. Retrieved from http://iblce.org/upload/downloads/DocumentationGuidelines.pdf

International Board of Lactation Consultant Examiners. (2011). *Code of Professional Conduct for International Board Certified lactation consultants*. Retrieved from http://iblce.org/upload/downloads/CodeOfProfessionalConduct.pdf

International Board of Lactation Consultant Examiners. (2010). *Clinical competencies for IBCLC practice*. Retrieved from http://iblce.org/upload/downloads/ClinicalCompetencies.pdf

International Lactation Consultant Association. (2005). *Clinical guidelines for the establishment of exclusive breastfeeding*. Rockville, MD: Maternal and Child Health Bureau. Retrieved from http://www.ilca.org/files/resources/ClinicalGuidelines2005.pdf

International Lactation Consultant Association. (2006). *Standards of practice for International Board Certified lactation consultants*. Retrieved from http://www.ilca.org/files/resources/Standards-of-Practice-web.pdf

The Joint Commission. (2010, September). *Specifications manual for Joint Commission national quality measures*. Retrieved from http://manual.jointcommission.org/releases/TJC2010B/MIF0170.html

Labbok, M., & Krasovec, K. (1990). Towards consistency in breastfeeding definitions. *Studies in Natural Family Planning, 21*(4).

Lessen, R. (2009, December). Use of skim breast milk for an infant with chylothorax. *Infant, Child, and Adolescent Nutrition, 1*(6),303-310.

Mannel, R. (2010). Lactation rounds: A system to improve hospital productivity. *Journal of Human Lactation, 26*, 393–398.

Mannel, R. (2011). Defining lactation acuity to improve patient safety and outcomes. *Journal of Human Lactation, 27*, 163–170.

Mannel, R., & Mannel, R. (2006). Staffing for hospital lactation programs: Recommendations from a tertiary care teaching hospital. *Journal of Human Lactation, 22*, 409–417.

Mannel, R., Godman, B. and Stehel, E. (2012). National survey of hospital lactation services. Manuscript in preparation in 2011 and submitted for publication 2012.

Martens, P. J., Derksen, S., & Gupta, S. (2004, September). Predictors of hospital readmission of Manitoba newborns within six weeks postbirth discharge: A population-based study. *Pediatrics, 114*(3), 708–713.

Martin, T. C., Shea, M., Alexander, D., Bradbury, L., Lovell-Roberts, L., & Francis, V. (2002, June). Did exclusive breast-feeding and early discharge lead to excessive bilirubin levels in newborns in Antigua and Barbuda? *West Indian Medical Journal, 51*(2), 84–88.

Moritz, M. L., Manole, M. D., Bogen, D. L., & Ayus, J. C. (2005). Breastfeeding-associated hypernatremia: Are we missing the diagnosis? *Pediatrics, 116*, e343. doi:10.1542/peds.2004-2647

Murray, E., Ricketts, S., & Dellaport, J. (2007). Hospital practices that increase breastfeeding duration: Results from a population-based study. *Birth, 34*, 3.

Office of the U.S. Surgeon General. (2011). *The Surgeon General's call to action to support breastfeeding.* Washington, DC: U.S. Department of Health and Human Services. Retrieved from http://www.surgeongeneral.gov/topics/breastfeeding/.

Oklahoma State Department of Health. (2011). *Oklahoma breastfeeding hotline annual report.* Contact Rebecca-mannel@ouhsc.edu.

Paul, I. M., Lehman, E. B., Hollenbeak, C. S., & Maisels, M. J. (2006, December). Preventable newborn readmissions since passage of the Newborns' and Mothers' Health Protection Act. *Pediatrics, 118*(6), 2349–2358.

United States Breastfeeding Committee. (2009). *Core competencies in breastfeeding care and services for all health professionals.* Washington, DC: Author. Retrieved from http://www.usbreastfeeding.org/LinkClick.aspx?link=Publications%2fCore-Competencies -2010-rev.pdf&tabid=70&mid=388

United States Breastfeeding Committee. (2010). *Implementing the Joint Commission perinatal core measure on exclusive breast milk feeding.* Washington, DC: Author. Retrieved from http://www. usbreastfeeding.org/Portals/0/Publications/Implementing-TJC-Measure-EBMF-2010-USBC.pdf

U.S. Department of Labor, Wage and Hour Division. (2010). Fact sheet #73: Break time for nursing mothers under the FLSA. Retrieved from http://www.dol.gov/whd/regs/compliance/whdfs73.htm

U.S. Lactation Consultant Association. (2010). International Board Certified lactation consultant staffing recommendations for the inpatient setting. Retrieved fromhttp://www.ilca.org/files/ USLCA/Resources/Publications/IBCLC_Staffing_Recommendations_July_2010.pdf

Wellstart International. (2009). *Lactation management self-study modules*, Level I (3rd Ed., Rev.), Shelburne, VT: Wellstart International. Retrieved from http://www.wellstart.org/Self-Study-Module.pdf

Wiseman, A., Boothe, A., Belay, B., & Reynolds, M. (2012). A policy and environmental approach to hospital food, physical activity, breastfeeding and tobacco environments: Recommendations from an expert panel. Atlanta, GA: Division of Nutrition and Physical Activity, Centers for Disease Control and Prevention. Retrieved from www.cdc.gov/nccdphp/dnpao/hwi/resources/ hospital_p2p.htm

World Health Organization. (1981). *International code of marketing of breast-milk substitutes.* Geneva, Switzerland: Author. Retrieved from http://www.who.int/nutrition/publications/code_english.pdf

World Health Organization. (1998). *Evidence for the ten steps to successful breastfeeding.* Geneva, Switzerland: Author.

World Health Organization. (2003). *The global strategy for infant and young child feeding.* Geneva, Switzerland: Author.

World Health Organization. (2009a). Infant and young child feeding: Model Chapter for textbooks for medical student and allied health professionals. Retrieved from http://www.who.int/ maternal_child_adolescent/documents/9789241597494/en/index.html

World Health Organization. (2009b). Section 3: Breastfeeding promotion and support in a baby-friendly hospital. A 20-hour course for maternity staff. Retrieved from http://whqlibdoc.who.int/ publications/2009/9789241594981_eng.pdf

Section II

Science of Lactation

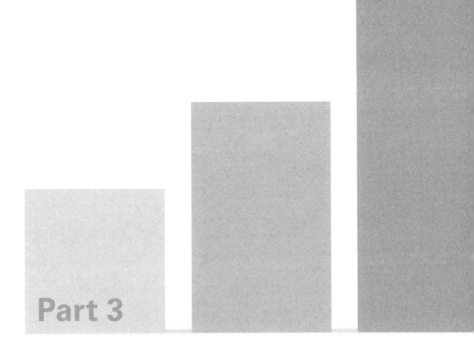

Part 3

Breastfeeding Anatomy and Physiology

CHAPTER 15
Maternal Breastfeeding Anatomy

Judith Lauwers, BA, IBCLC, FILCA

> *Such a spectacular survival strategy that we call ourselves after the mammary gland, mammals... animals that suckle their young.*
>
> —GABRIELLE PALMER, AUTHOR AND ACTIVIST

OBJECTIVES

- Describe the process of breast development.
- Locate the major structures of the breast.
- Describe the function of the major structures of the breast.
- Discuss variations of breast anatomic structures.

INTRODUCTION

The medical term for the breast is *mammary gland*, which comes from the Latin word *mamma*, meaning "the breast." The mammary gland is the only organ that is not fully developed at birth. It undergoes four major phases of growth and development: in utero, during the first 2 years of life, at puberty, and finally during pregnancy and lactation. The breast provides both nutrition and nurturing. The lactation consultant requires a basic understanding of the structures and functions of the breast to provide proper breastfeeding management guidelines and to troubleshoot problems.

I. Breast Development

A. Embryo and neonate
1. Weeks 3 to 4: Breast development begins with a primitive milk streak running bilaterally from the axilla to the groin.
2. Weeks 4 to 5: Milk streak becomes mammary milk ridge, or milk line. Paired breasts develop from this line of glandular tissue.
3. Weeks 7 to 8: Thickening and inward growth into the chest wall continue.
4. Weeks 12 to 16: Specialized cells differentiate into smooth muscle of nipple and areola.
   a. Epithelial cells develop into mammary buds.
   b. Epithelial branches form to eventually become alveoli (Vorherr, 1974).

5. Weeks 15 to 25: Epithelial strips are formed, which represent future secretory alveoli.
   a. Lactiferous ducts and their branches form and open into a shallow epithelial depression known as the mammary pit.
   b. The mammary pit becomes elevated, forming the nipple and areola.
   c. An inverted nipple results when the pit fails to elevate.
6. After 32 weeks: A lumen (canal) forms in each part of the branching system.
7. Near term: 15 to 25 mammary ducts form the fetal mammary gland.
8. Neonate:
   a. Galactorrhea (also called witch's milk): Secretion of colostral-like fluid from neonate mammary tissue resulting from influence of maternal hormones (Collaborative Group, 2002; Lee et al., 2003; Madlon-Kay, 1986).
   b. Recommend not to express neonatal colostrum because this might lead to mastitis in the newborn (Collaborative Group on Hormonal Factors in Breast Cancer, 2002; Lee et al., 2003).

B. Puberty
1. Breasts keep pace with general physical growth.
2. Growth of the breast parenchyma produces ducts, lobes, alveoli, and surrounding fat pad.
3. Onset of menses at 10 to 12 years of age continues development of the breast.
   a. Primary and secondary ducts grow and divide.
   b. Terminal end buds form, which later become alveoli (small sacs where milk is secreted) in the mature female breast.
   c. Proliferation and active growth of ductal tissue takes place during each menstrual cycle and continues to about age 35 years.

C. Pregnancy
1. Complete development of mammary function occurs only in pregnancy.
2. Breast size increases, skin appears thinner, and veins become more prominent.
3. Areola diameter increases (Hytten, 1954), Montgomery glands enlarge, and nipple pigment darkens.

D. Anomalies in breast development
1. Some illnesses, chemotherapy, therapeutic radiation to the chest, chest surgery, or injuries to the chest might affect development.
2. Programmed apoptosis (cell death) has been suggested as one theory for lower breast cancer rates in women who have breastfed (Collaborative Group, 2002; Lee et al., 2003; Tryggvadottir et al., 2001).

II. General Anatomy of a Mature Breast

A. Exterior breast (**Figure 15-1**)
1. Located in the superficial fascia (fibrous tissue beneath the skin) between the second rib and the sixth intercostal space.

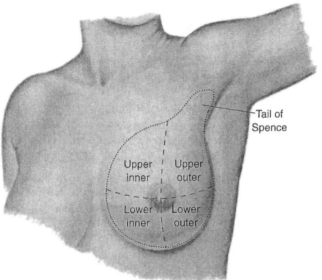

Figure 15-1
Breast quadrants and axillary
Tail of Spence.

2. Tail of Spence: Mammary glandular tissue that projects into the axillary region.
   a. Distinguished from supernumerary tissue because it connects to the duct system
   b. Potential area of milk pooling and mastitis (Lee et al., 2003)
3. Skin surface contains the nipple, areola, and Montgomery glands.
4. Size is not related to functional capacity.
   a. Fat composition of the breast gives it its size and shape.
   b. Size may indicate milk storage potential (Daly et al., 1995; Hartmann et al., 1996).
B. Nipple areola complex (**Figure 15-2**)
   1. Nipple
      a. Conical elevation located slightly below the center of the areola
      b. Nipple features
         i. Average diameter of a nipple is 1.6 cm; average length is 0.7 cm (Ziemer, 1993).
         ii. There are 5 to 10 milk duct openings (Ramsay, Kent et al., 2005; Walker, 2011).
         iii. Smooth muscle fibers function as a closure mechanism to keep milk from continuously leaking from the nipple.
         iv. The nipple is densely innervated with sensory nerve endings.
      c. Nipple erection
         i. Longitudinal inner muscles and outer circular and radial muscles make the nipple erect when contracted.

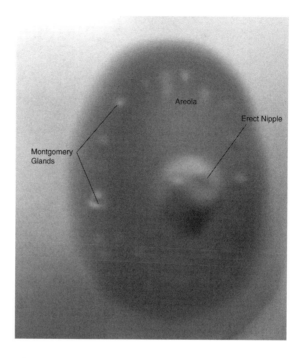

Figure 15-2
Nipple areolar complex.

      ii. Venostasis slows blood flow and decreases surface area.

      iii. The nipple becomes smaller, firmer, and more prominent to aid the infant in latching.

  2. Areola

    a. Circular, dark pigmented area that surrounds the nipple.

      i. Elastic like the nipple.

      ii. Average diameter is 6.4 cm (Ziemer, 1993).

      iii. Constructed of smooth muscle and collagenous, elastic, connective tissue fibers in radial and circular arrangement.

      iv. Usually darkens and enlarges during pregnancy.

    b. Montgomery's tubercles are located around the areola.

      i. Contain ductal openings of sebaceous and lactiferous glands and sweat glands.

      ii. Enlarge during pregnancy and resemble small, raised pimples.

      iii. Secrete a substance that lubricates and protects the nipples.

      iv. Some secrete a small amount of milk.

      v. Secretions may produce a scent to help the infant locate the nipple (Doucet et al., 2009; Schall et al., 2006).

 C. Parenchyma: Functional parts of the breast (**Figure 15-3**)

  1. Alveoli (also called acini) are the basic components of the mature mammary gland.

    a. Alveoli are secretory cells in which the milk is produced (**Figure 15-4**).

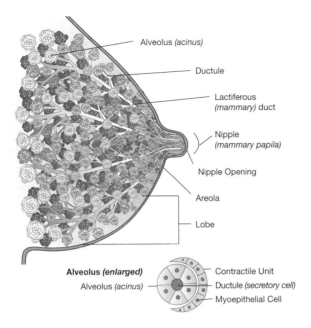

Figure 15-3
Structure of a lactating breast.

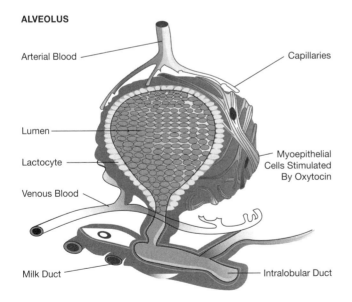

Figure 15-4
Cross section of an alveolus.

Source: Riordan, J., & Wambach, K. (2010). *Breastfeeding and human lactation* (4th ed.). Sudbury, MA: Jones and Bartlett.

         i. Lactocytes, specialized epithelial cells that line the interior of the alveolus, absorb nutrients, immunoglobulin, and hormones from the mother's blood stream to compose milk.

        ii. Prolactin receptor sites in the lactocytes allow prolactin to be absorbed from the blood and enter into the alveoli to stimulate milk production.

    b. Myoepithelial cells encase the alveoli and contract in response to oxytocin to eject milk into ductules.

2. The breast contains from 15 to 25 lobes that carry milk through the ductules from the alveoli to the nipple.

    a. Each lobe contains from 10 to 100 alveoli in an intricate system of ductules that branch out from the lobes to converge into lactiferous ducts behind the nipple.

    b. Ultrasound imaging shows connections between lobes (Geddes, 2007).

    c. Ducts widen temporarily in response to milk ejection and narrow when the duct is drained (Ramsay et al., 2004; Ramsay, Mitoulas, et al., 2005).

    d. Milk that is not removed flows backward up the collecting ducts.

3. Lactiferous ducts lead to 5 to 10 openings in the nipple.

D. Stroma: Supporting tissues of the breast

    1. Connective tissue, fat tissue, blood vessels, nerves, and lymphatics

    2. Cooper's ligaments

        a. Suspensory ligaments running vertically through the breast

        b. Attach the deep layer of subcutaneous tissue to the dermis layer of the skin

E. Vascular anatomy (**Figure 15-5**)

    1. The breast is highly vascular.

    2. Internal mammary artery supplies 60% of blood to the breast.

    3. Lateral thoracic artery supplies 30% of blood to the breast.

    4. Blood vessels within the breast enlarge.

    5. Surges of estrogen stimulate growth of the ducts.

    6. Surges of progesterone cause glandular tissue to expand.

F. Lymphatic system (**Figure 15-6**)

    1. Collects excess fluids from tissue spaces, bacteria, and cast-off cell parts

    2. Drains mainly to the axillary lymph nodes

G. Innervation (**Figure 15-7**)

    1. Breast innervation derives mainly from branches of the fourth, fifth, and sixth intercostal nerves.

    2. Nerve supply to the innermost areas of the breast is sparse.

    3. The fourth intercostal nerve penetrates the posterior aspect of the breast.

        a. It supplies the greatest amount of sensation to the areola, at the four o'clock position on the left breast and at the eight o'clock position on the right breast.

        b. It becomes more superficial as it reaches the areola, where it divides into five branches.

Key
1. Subclavian artery
2. Superior thoracic artery
3. Internal thoracic artery
4. Major pectoralis muscle
5. Perforating branches of the
    internal mammary artery
6. Arterial plexus around areola
7. Intercoastal arteries
8. Pectoral branches of the lateral
    thoracic artery
9. Circumflex scapular artery
10. Minor pectoralis muscle
11. Subscapular artery
12. Lateral thoracic artery
13. Pectoral branch of the
    thoracoacromial artery
14. Axillary artery
15. Deltoid branch of the
    thoracoacromial artery

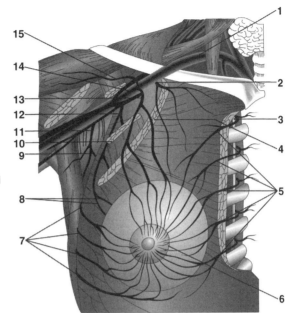

Figure 15-5 Arterial blood supply to the breast.

    c. The lowermost branch penetrates the areola at the five o'clock position on the left breast and at the seven o'clock position on the right breast.

    d. Trauma to this nerve might result in some loss of sensation in the breast.

    e. If the lowermost branch is severed, loss of sensation to the nipple and areola might result.

    f. Aberrant sensory or autonomic nerve distributions in the nipple/areola complex.

        i. Could affect the milk ejection reflex and secretion of prolactin and oxytocin.

        ii. Trauma or severing of this nerve could result from breast augmentation or reduction surgery.

III. Variations

    A. Breasts vary in size, shape, color, and placement on the chest wall (**Table 15-1**; **Figure 15-8**).

      1. Weight increases through pregnancy and lactation

        a. Nonpregnant woman: Mature breast weighs about 200 g.

        b. Pregnancy near term: Breast weighs between 400 and 600 g.

        c. Lactation: Breast can weigh 600 to 800 g.

      2. Asymmetry is common, with the left breast often larger than the right breast.

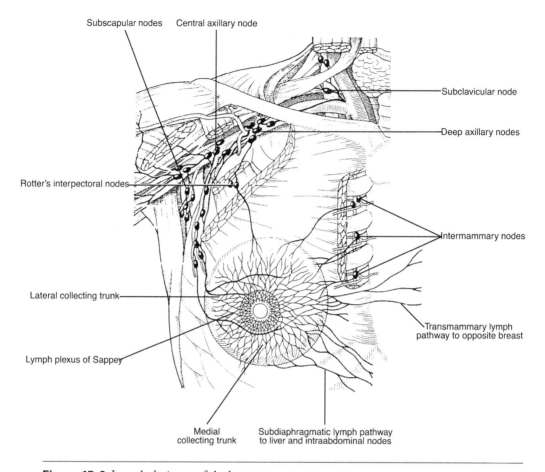

Figure 15-6 Lymph drainage of the breast.

B. Breast malformations:
  1. Hypermastia: Presence of an accessory mammary gland
     a. Accessory or supernumerary nipple develops along the milk line between the axilla and the groin (Schmidt, 1998; Velanovich, 1995).
     b. Often prominent during pregnancy and lactation.
     c. May be associated with renal or other organ-system anomalies (Berman et al., 1994).
     d. Accessory glandular tissue can lactate and undergo malignant changes (Collaborative Group, 2002; Lee et al., 2003).
  2. Hyperthelia: Nipple without accompanying mammary tissue
  3. Hypertrophy: Abnormally large breast
  4. Hypomastia: Abnormally small breast
  5. Hyperplasia: Overdevelopment of the breast—hyperplastic breast

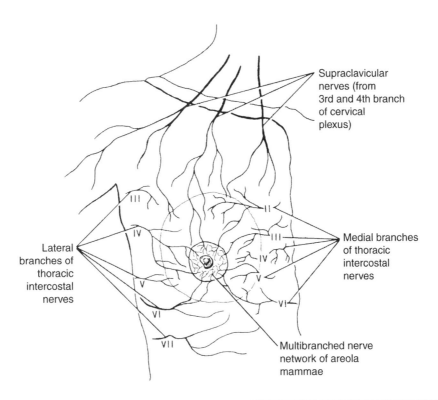

Figure 15-7 Innervation of the breast.

6. Hypoplasia: Underdevelopment of the breast—hypoplastic breast
   a. Tubular or tuberous shape because of lack of glandular tissue.
   b. Breasts may have large areolas.
   c. Breasts are frequently asymmetric and widely spaced.
   d. May present increased risk for insufficient milk (Huggins et al., 2000).
   e. Unilateral hypoplasia of the breast combined with hypoplasia of the thorax and pectoral muscles—Poland's syndrome.

Table 12-1 Breast Types Classified by Physical Characteristics

Type 1	Round breasts, normal lower, medial, and lateral quadrants
Type 2	Hypoplasia of the lower medial quadrant
Type 3	Hypoplasia of the lower medial and lateral quadrants
Type 4	Severe constrictions, minimal breast base

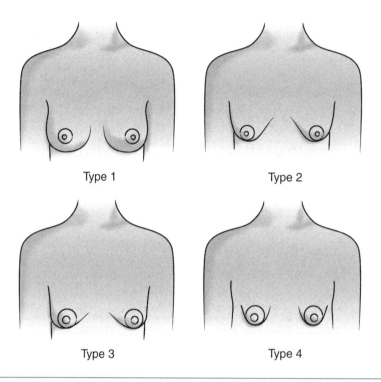

Type 1   Type 2

Type 3   Type 4

Figure 15-8 Breast classifications.

C. Nipple variations (**Figure 15-9**):
1. Restricted protractility
   a. The nipple should evert and become protractile when compressed or stimulated.
   b. The incidence of poor protractility in primigravid women ranges from 10% to 35% (Alexander et al., 1992; Blaikeley et al., 1953; Hytten et al., 1958; Waller, 1946).
   c. Protractility improves during pregnancy. The effect on latch is minimal when the baby has a large mouthful of breast tissue.
   d. Nipple inversion occurs in about 3% of women and is usually bilateral (Park et al., 1999).
      i. A truly inverted nipple remains inverted when compressed or stimulated.
      ii. A pseudo-inverted nipple appears inverted but everts when compressed or stimulated.
      iii. A short-shanked nipple appears everted but retracts when compressed or stimulated.

Type of Nipple	Before Stimulation	After Stimulation
Common nipple The majority of mothers have what is referred to as a *common nipple*. It protrudes slightly when at rest and becomes erect and more graspable when stimulated. A baby has no trouble finding and grasping this nipple in order to pull in a large amount of breast tissue and stretch it to the roof of his mouth.	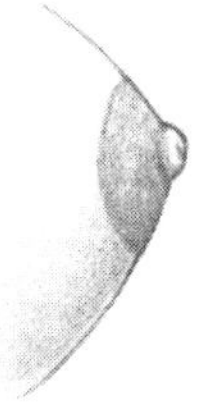	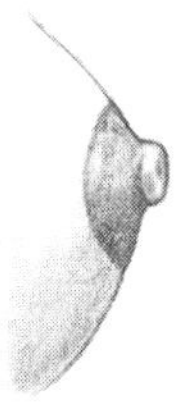
Flat and/or Short Shanked nipple The *flat nipple* may be soft and pliable and have the ability to ridge, therefore it molds to the infants mouth without problem. The *flat nipple may have a short shank* that makes it less easy to ridge and for the baby to find and grasp. In response to stimulation, this nipple may remain unchanged or may retract with compression. Slight movement inward or outward may be present, but not enough to aid the baby in finding and initially grasping the breast on center. This nipple may benefit from the use of a syringe to increase protractility.	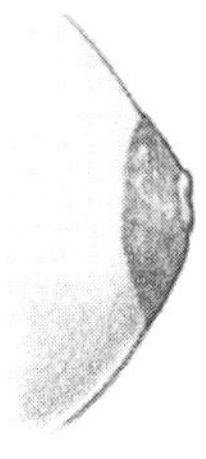	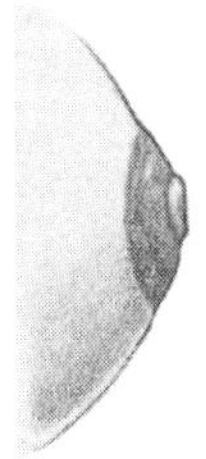
Pseudo-inverted nipple An *pseudo-inverted* nipple may appear inverted but becomes erect after compression and/or stimulation. This nipple needs no correction and presents no problems with grasp ability.	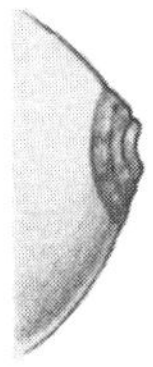	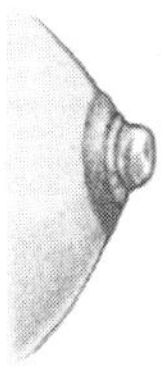
Retracted nipple The *retracted nipple* is the most common type of inverted nipple. Initially, this nipple appears to be graspable. However, on stimulation, it retracts, making attachment difficult. This nipple responds well to techniques that increase nipple protrusion.	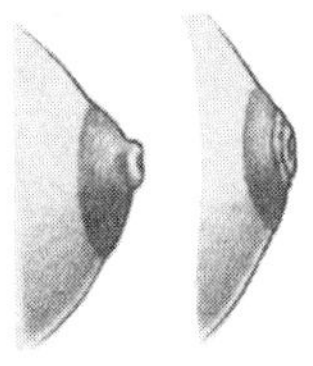	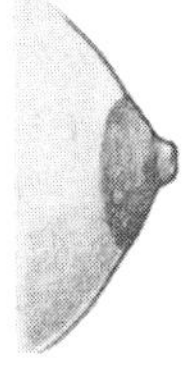
Inverted nipple The truly *inverted nipple* is retracted both at rest and when stimulated. Such a nipple is very uncommon and more difficult for the baby to grasp. All techniques used to enhance protractility of breast tissue can be used to improve attachment. Even if the nipple remains retracted, the baby should be able to latch on if the mother helps form her breast into the mouth	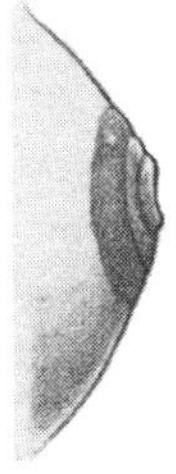	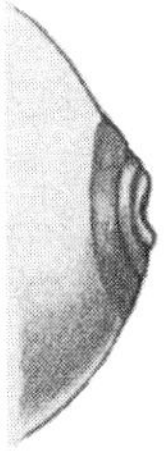

Figure 15-9 Five basic types of nipples.

2. Other nipple variations
   a. Bulbous: Large nipple that may be difficult for a baby to grasp
   b. Dimpled: Increases the risk for maceration as the nipple lies enveloped by the areola
   c. Bifurcated
   d. Double and/or multiple nipples close together
   e. Skin tag: More prevalent during pregnancy

References

Alexander, J. M., Grant, A. M., & Campbell, M. J. (1992). Randomized controlled trial of breast shells and Hoffman's exercises for inverted and non-proctractile nipples. *British Medical Journal, 304*, 1030–1032.

Berman, M. A., & Davis, G. D. (1994). Lactation from axillary breast tissue in the absence of a supernumerary nipple: A case report. *Journal of Reproductive Medicine, 39*, 657–659.

Blaikeley, J., Silas, C., MacKeith, D., et al. (1953). Breastfeeding: Factors affecting success. *Journal of Obstetrics and Gynaecology of the British Empire, 60*, 657–669.

Collaborative Group on Hormonal Factors in Breast Cancer. (2002). Breast cancer and breastfeeding: Collaborative reanalysis of individual data from 47 epidemiological studies in 30 countries. *Lancet, 360*, 187–195.

Cregan, M. D., & Hartmann, P. E. (1999). Computerized breast measurement from conception to weaning: Clinical implications. *Journal of Human Lactation, 15*(2), 89–96.

Daly, S., & Hartmann, P. (1995). Infant demand and milk supply. Part 1: Infant demand and milk production in lactating women. *Journal of Human Lactation, 11*, 21–26.

Doucet, S., Soussignan, R., Sagot, P., & Schaal, B. (2009). The secretion of areolar (Montgomery's) glands from lactating women elicits selective, unconditional responses in neonates. *PLoS One, 4*(10), e7579.

Geddes, D. T. (2007). Inside the lactating breast: The latest anatomy research. *Journal of Midwifery and Women's Health, 52*, 556–563.

Hartmann, P. E., Owens, R. A., Cox, D. B., & Kent, J. C. (1996). Breast development and control of milk synthesis. *Food and Nutrition Bulletin, 17*, 292–304.

Huggins, K. E., Petok, E. S., & Mireles, O. (2000). Markers of lactation insufficiency: A study of 34 mothers. In *Current issues in clinical lactation–2000* (pp. 25–35). Sudbury, MA: Jones and Bartlett.

Hytten, F. E. (1954). Clinical and chemical studies in lactation: IX. Breastfeeding in hospital. *British Medical Journal, 18*, 1447–1452.

Hytten, F. E., & Baird, D. (1958). The development of the nipple in pregnancy. *Lancet, 1*, 1201–1204.

Lee, S. Y., Kim, M. T., Kim, S. W., et al. (2003). Effect of lifetime lactation on breast cancer risk: A Korean women's cohort study. *International Journal of Cancer, 105*, 390–393.

Madlon-Kay, D. J. (1986). "Witch's milk." Galactorrhea in the newborn. *American Journal of Diseases of Children, 140*, 250–253.

Park, H. S., Yoon, C. H., & Kim, H. J. (1999). The prevalence of congenital inverted nipple. *Aesthetic Plastic Surgery, 23*, 1446.

Ramsay, D. T., Kent, J. C., Owens, R. A., & Hartmann, P. E. (2004). Ultrasound imaging of milk ejection in the breast of lactating women. *Pediatrics, 113*, 361–367.

Ramsay, D. T., Mitoulas, L. R., Kent, J. C., et al. (2005). The use of ultrasound to characterize milk ejection in women using an electric breast pump. *Journal of Human Lactation, 21,* 421–428.

Ramsay, J. C., Kent, C., Hartmann, R. A., & Hartmann, P. E. (2005). Anatomy of the lactating human breast redefined with ultrasound imaging. *Journal of Anatomy, 206,* 525.

Rusby, J., Brachtel, E., Michaelson, J., et al. (2007). Breast duct anatomy in the human nipple: Three-dimensional patterns and clinical implications. *Breast Cancer Research and Treatment, 106*(2), 171–179.

Schaal, B., Doucet, S., Sagot, P., et al. (2006). Human breast areolae as scent organs: Morphological data and possible involvement in maternal-neonatal coadaptation. *Developmental Psychobiology, 18*(2), 100–110.

Schmidt, H. (1998). Supernumerary nipples: Prevalence, size, sex and side predilection—a prospective clinical study. *European Journal of Pediatrics, 157,* 821–823.

Tryggvadottir, L., Tulinius, H., Eyfjord, J. E., & Sigurvinsson, T. (2001). Breastfeeding and reduced risk of breast cancer in an Icelandic cohort study. *American Journal of Epidemiology, 154,* 37–42.

Velanovich, V. (1995). Ectopic breast tissue, supernumerary breasts, and supernumerary nipples. *Southern Medical Journal, 88,* 903–906.

Vorherr, H. (1974). Development of the female breast. In H. Vorherr (Ed.), *The breast* (pp. 1–18). New York, NY: Academic.

Walker, M. (2011). *Breastfeeding management for the clinician: Using the evidence.* Sudbury, MA: Jones and Bartlett.

Waller, H. (1946). The early failure of breastfeeding. *Archives of Disease in Childhood, 21,* 1–12.

Ziemer, M. (1993). Nipple skin changes and pain during the first week of lactation. *JOGN Nursing, 22,* 247–256.

Suggested Reading

Auerbach, K. G., & Riordan, J. (2000). *Clinical lactation: A visual guide.* Sudbury, MA: Jones and Bartlett.

Harris, J. R., Lippman, M. E., Morrow, M., & Osborne, C. K. (2004). *Diseases of the breast.* Baltimore, MD: Lippincott Williams & Wilkins.

Imaginis. (2012). Breast anatomy and physiology. Retrieved from http://imaginis.com/breasthealth/breast_anatomy.asp

Lauwers, J., & Swisher, A. (2010). *Counseling the nursing mother: A lactation consultant's guide* (5th ed.). Sudbury, MA: Jones and Bartlett.

Lawrence, R. A., & Lawrence, R. M. (2011). *Breastfeeding: A guide for the medical profession* (7th ed.). St. Louis, MO: Mosby.

Love, S., & Lindsey, K. (2000). *Dr. Susan Love's breast book* (3rd ed.). Cambridge, MA: Da Capo Press.

Osborne, M. P. (2000). Breast development and anatomy. In J. R. Harris, I. C. Henderson, S. Hellman, & D. W. Kinney (Eds.), *Diseases of the breast* (pp. 1–14). Philadelphia, PA: Lippincott.

Riordan, J., & Wambach, K. (2010). *Breastfeeding and human lactation* (4th ed.). Sudbury, MA: Jones and Bartlett.

Wilson-Clay, B., & Hoover, K. (2008). *The breastfeeding atlas* (4thd ed.). Manchaca, TX: LactNews Press.

CHAPTER 16
Infant Anatomy for Feeding

Catherine Watson Genna, BS, IBCLC

OBJECTIVES

- Locate and name the cranial and facial bones, sutures, fontanelles, joints, and processes on the infant skull.
- Name and describe the function of the 12 pairs of cranial nerves.
- Locate, name, and describe the function and innervation of the muscles of sucking and mastication.
- Locate, name, and describe the anatomic features of an infant's oral cavity.
- Identify the reference, atypical, and abnormal infant head and oral cavity.
- Describe the oral reflexes related to breastfeeding.

INTRODUCTION

Familiarity with the anatomy of the infant's head is important as a basis for understanding the normal structure and function in infant feeding and as a reference for analyzing and correcting breastfeeding problems. The term *reference* is a nonjudgmental word used to describe the most common example or the greatest representation of a population, rather than the term *norm*. It is necessary to distinguish between normal variations and abnormalities, both of which might cause breastfeeding problems. The lactation consultant requires an understanding of how infant anatomic structures and motions combine to enable the infant to take in nutrients and to determine his or her requisite milk supply. The newborn's oral anatomy is his or her primary way of relating to the world (Bosma, 1972; Brazelton, 1995). Appropriate and accurate anatomic assessment aids the lactation consultant in assessing the normal and recognizing deviations that are amenable to intervention.

I. Basic Concepts of Anatomic Terminology

    A. *Reference*: Used to describe the most common example

    B. *Body planes*: Used to facilitate uniformity in descriptions of the body (Kapit et al., 1993)

        1. *Midsagittal*: The plane vertically dividing the body through the midline into right and left halves

2. *Sagittal*: Any plane that is parallel to the midsagittal line, vertically dividing the body into right and left portions

3. *Coronal* (*frontal*): Any plane dividing the body into anterior (ventral) and posterior (dorsal) portions at right angles to the sagittal plane

4. *Transverse* (*cross, horizontal*): Plane dividing the body into superior (upper) and inferior (lower) portions

C. *Directions and positions*:

1. *Cranial, superior, rostral*: Uppermost or above

2. *Caudal, inferior*: Lowermost or below

3. *Anterior, ventral*: Toward the front

4. *Posterior, dorsal*: Toward the back

5. *Medial*: Nearest the midline of the body

6. *Lateral*: Toward the side

7. *Proximal*: Nearest the point of attachment or origin

8. *Distal*: Away from the point of attachment or origin

9. *Superficial*: On the surface

10. *Deep*: Below the surface

11. *Ipsilateral*: Pertaining to the same side

12. *Contralateral*: Pertaining to the opposite side

D. *Terms*:

1. *Alveolus*: A small cavity—in breast, a spherical arrangement of lactocytes (milk-producing cells) around a central lumen, drained by a ductule

2. *Process*: Projections on a bone

3. *Meatus*: A passage or channel, especially the external opening of a canal

4. *Foramen*: A natural hole or passage, especially one into or through a bone

5. *Lumen*: The cavity or channel within a tube or tubular organ

6. *Sinus*: A recess, cavity, or hollow space

7. *Protuberance*: A projecting part, process, or swelling (on bone, for the connection of a muscle, tendon, or ligament)

8. *Fontanel*: Junctions of cranial bones covered by a tough membrane

E. *Body positions*:

1. *Prone*: Lying face down

2. *Supine*: Lying on the back

F. *Joints*:

1. *Temporomandibular*: Opens and closes the jaw; lateral displacement of the mandible

2. *Suture*: A joint that does not move; the bones are united by a thin layer of fibrous tissue

G. *Muscles*:

1. *Involuntary*: Contraction controlled by autonomic nervous system, no willful control

2. *Voluntary*: Movement using willful control, central nervous system

3. *Visceral/smooth*: Found in digestive and respiratory tracts

4. *Cardiac/striated*: Involuntary muscle possessing a striated appearance of voluntary muscles but with incomplete separation between the cells, allowing coordination of contraction

5. *Skeletal/striated*: Voluntary, striated; gross and fine motor movements

6. *Origin*: The more fixed attachment of a muscle that serves as a basis of action

7. *Insertion*: The movable attachment where the effects of movement are produced

H. *Systems*: Groups of organs that form the general structural plan of the body

1. *Skeletal*: Bones, cartilage, and membranous structures that protect and support the soft parts of the body and that supply levers for movement

2. *Muscular*: Facilitates movement

3. *Cardiovascular*: Pumps and distributes blood

4. *Lymphatic*: Drains tissue spaces, provides for intercellular waste disposal, and carries absorbed fat in the blood

5. *Nervous*: Controlling system for cognition, movement, and autonomic functions

6. *Endocrine*: Chemical regulator of body functions

7. *Integument*: Skin (hair, nails, sebaceous, and sweat glands); insulation, temperature, and water regulation

8. *Respiratory*: Brings oxygen to and eliminates carbon dioxide from the blood

9. *Digestive*: Converts food into substances that the body can absorb and utilize

10. *Urinary*: Forms and eliminates urine and maintains homeostasis

11. *Immune*: Protection from and reaction to disease and infection

12. *Reproductive*: Perpetuation of the species

II. Skeletal System of the Infant's Head, Face, and Neck

A. Bones (Diamond et al., 1991; Grant, 1956)

1. *Occipital*: Forms the back and base of the cranium; contains the foramen magnum through which the spinal cord passes

2. *Frontal*: Forms the forehead, roof of the nasal cavity, and orbits (bony sockets containing the eyes)

3. *Parietal*: Sides and roof of the cranium

4. *Temporal*: Sides and base of the cranium; houses the middle and inner ear structures

5. *Sphenoid:* Butterfly-shaped bone bridging other cranial bones internally, forming part of temple, floor of skull (sella turcica—seat of pituitary), nasal septum, posterior walls of orbits

6. *Ethmoid*: Between the nasal bones and sphenoid; forms part of the anterior cranial floor, medial walls of the orbits, and part of the nasal septum

7. *Nasal*: Upper bridge of the nose

8. *Vomer*: Posterior nasal cavity; forms a portion of the nasal septum

9. *Lacrimal*: Anterior, medial wall of the orbit

10. *Zygomatic arch*: Prominence of the cheeks and part of the lateral wall and floor of the orbits
11. *Palatine*: Posterior nasal cavity between the maxillae and sphenoid
12. *Maxilla*: Upper jaw
13. *Mandible*: Lower jaw
14. *Inferior nasal concha*: Lateral wall of the nasal cavity
15. *Hyoid bone*: Horseshoe-shaped bone suspended from the styloid process of the temporal bone

B. Passages
1. *Choanae*: Posterior nasal apertures, paired passages from the nasal cavity to the nasopharynx. Breastfeeding widens the choanae, unless tongue tie is present (Palmer, 1998).

C. *Sutures*: Found only in the skull
1. *Coronal*: Line of articulation between the frontal bone and the two parietal bones
2. *Sagittal*: Line of articulation between the two parietal bones in the midline
3. *Lambdoidal*: Anterior articulation between the occipital and parietal bones

D. Fontanels: The membranous intervals between the angles of the cranial bones in infants
1. *Anterior fontanel*: A diamond-shaped interval where the frontal angles of the parietal bones meet the two separate halves of the frontal bones
2. *Posterior fontanel*: A triangular interval at the union of the lambdoid and sagittal sutures
3. *Sphenoidal fontanel*: Irregularly shaped interval on either side of the skull
4. *Mastoid fontanel*: Interval on either side of the posterior skull

III. Innervation of the Mouth and Suckling Motion (Netter, 2006)

A. Cranial nerves
1. CN I olfactory: Smell
2. CN II optic: Sight
3. CN III oculomotor: Innervates external muscles for several movements of the eye
4. CN IV trochlear: Innervates muscles that move the eye up and down
5. CN V trigeminal: Three branches; muscles of mastication
6. CN VI abducens: Moves the eye away from the center of the body
7. CN VII facial: Muscles of facial expression
8. CN VIII vestibulocochlear: Hearing and equilibrium
9. CN IX glossopharyngeal: Taste, sensation in pharynx (important for swallowing)
10. CN X vagus: Larynx, pharynx
11. CN XI spinal accessory: Muscles of the neck and shoulder.
12. CN XII hypoglossal: Muscles of the tongue

B. Cranial nerves related to suckling (**Table 16-1**)
1. Cranial nerves related to swallowing; 26 muscles and six cranial nerves must coordinate for swallowing (**Table 16-2**).

Table 16-1 Cranial Nerves Related to Suckling

Structure	Cranial Nerve/Sensory	Cranial Nerve/Motor
Mouth	CN V (shape/texture)	CN VII
Tongue	CNVII, IX (taste)	CN XII
Jaw	CN V (position of TMJ)	CN V

Source: Adapted from Wolf, L. S., & Glass, R. P. (1992). *Feeding and swallowing disorders in infancy: Assessment and management*. Tucson, AZ: Therapy Skill Builders.

Table 16-2 Cranial Nerves Related to Swallowing

Structure	Cranial Nerve/Sensory	Cranial Nerve/Motor
Palate	CN V, IX	CN V, VII, IX, X
Tongue	CN IX	CN V, VII, XII
Pharynx	CN V, X	CN IX, X
Larynx	CN X	CN IX, X

Source: Adapted from Wolf, L. S., & Glass, R. P. (1992). *Feeding and swallowing disorders in infancy: Assessment and management*. Tucson, AZ: Therapy Skill Builders.

IV. Muscles Related to Suckling

A. Muscles used in mastication and suckling (**Figure 16-1**; **Figure 16-2**)
   1. *Temporalis*: Raises the mandible; closes the mouth; draws the mandible backward
   2. *Masseter*: Closes the jaw (Gomes et al., 2006)
   3. *Medial pterygoid*: Raises the mandible; closes the mouth
   4. *Lateral pterygoid*: Brings the jaw forward
   5. *Buccinator*: Compresses the cheek and retracts the angle (Gomes et al., 2006)
   6. *Orbicularis oris*: Closes the lips
   7. *Mentalis*: Elevates center of lower lip (Rodriguez Jacinto-Goncalves et al., 2004)
B. Muscles that move the tongue (Takemoto, 2001)
   1. *Genioglossus*: Depresses and extends/protrudes tongue forward
   2. *Styloglossus*: Draws the tongue upward and backward
   3. *Stylohyoid*: Draws the hyoid and tongue upward
   4. *Digastric*: Raises the hyoid or opens the mouth
   5. *Mylohyoid*: Elevates the hyoid; supports the mouth floor
   6. *Hyoglossus*: Depresses the tongue
   7. *Geniohyoid*: Elevates and draws the hyoid forward

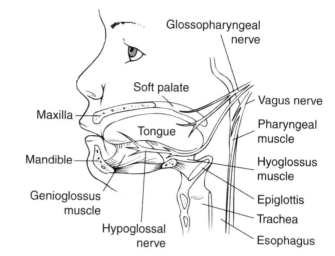

Figure 16-1
Muscles and nerves used in suckling and swallowing, sagittal section.

Source: Adapted from Biancuzzo, M. (2010). *Breastfeeding the newborn: Clinical strategies for nurses*. St. Louis: Mosby, Inc.

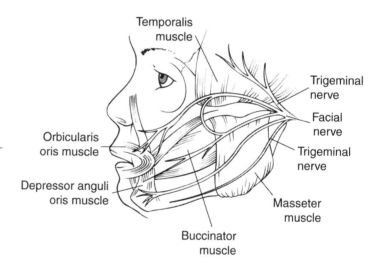

Figure 16-2
Lateral view.

Source: Adapted from Biancuzzo, M. (2010). *Breastfeeding the newborn: Clinical strategies for nurses*. St. Louis: Mosby, Inc.

    8. *Intrinsic musculature of tongue*: Shapes the tongue
        a. *Superior longitudinal*: Elevates tip and sides of tongue, makes tongue concave
        b. *Inferior longitudinal*: Curls tongue tip downward, makes tongue convex
        c. *Transverse lingual*: Narrows and increases thickness of tongue
        d. *Vertical lingual*: Broadens and lengthens tongue
  C. Muscles that move in the throat (important for swallowing)
    1. *Sternohyoid*: Depresses the hyoid and larynx
    2. *Omohyoid*: Depresses the hyoid
    3. *Sternothyroid*: Depresses the thyroid cartilage
    4. *Thyrohyoid*: Raises and changes the form of the larynx

V. Anatomy of the Head, Mouth, and Pharynx of the Newborn as It Relates to Feeding (Morris et al., 2000)

A. Oral cavity (mouth)

1. Bounded by the roof, floor, lips, and cheeks.
2. Roof consists of the palatine process of the maxilla and the palatine bone (hard palate).
3. Transitions posteriorly into the soft palate and uvula.
4. Floor consists of the mandible spanned by the mylohyoid, geniohyoid, and front of the digastric muscle.
5. The orbicularis oris surrounds the lips.
6. Cheeks are defined by the buccinator and masseter muscles; sucking pads that consist of fatty tissue are encased in the cheek to provide stability for the cheek during sucking, lateral borders for the tongue.
7. Mandible is small and retracted.
8. The tongue fills the entire oral cavity and touches the roof and floor of the mouth as well as the lateral gum lines and cheeks.
9. Lingual frenulum: A fold of mucous membrane extending from the floor of the mouth to the midline of the under surface of the tongue, should regress during midgestation (Dollberg et al., 2006, Geddes et al., 2008, 2009; Hogan et al., 2005).
10. Labial frenae: The membranes that attach the lips to the gum ridges, inferiorly and superiorly (Oldfield, 1955).

B. Pharynx: A soft muscular tube at the back of the throat

1. *Oropharynx*: Composed of the area between the elevated soft palate and the epiglottis
2. *Nasopharynx*: Section of the pharynx between the nasal choanae and the elevated soft palate; the eustachian tubes originate in the nasopharynx
3. *Hypopharynx*: Extends from the base of the epiglottis to the cricopharyngeal sphincter

C. Larynx: Gateway to the trachea composed of cartilage suspended by muscles and ligaments to the hyoid bone and cervical vertebrae

1. Contains the epiglottis, which folds down to cover the airway during swallowing
2. Contains the vocal folds or cords, which also close during swallowing to protect the airway

D. Trachea: A semirigid tube that branches into the primary bronchi leading to each lung; the posterior aspect is a membranous wall that abuts the soft tissue of the esophagus

E. Esophagus: A thin, muscular tube that extends to the stomach and distends as food is propelled through it by peristaltic motion

VI. Palate

A. Function

1. The hard palate assists with positioning and stability of the nipple within the mouth.
2. The soft palate works with the tongue to create the posterior seal of the oral cavity.
3. The soft palate elevates during the swallow, contacting the pharyngeal walls and closing off the nasal cavity, directing the bolus toward the hypopharynx.

B. Reference palate

1. The hard palate should be intact and smoothly contoured.
   a. In utero and after birth, the shape of the hard palate is contoured by the continual pressure of the tongue as it rests and moves against the palate.
2. Submucous clefts of the soft palate cannot be directly visualized.
   a. Might see a translucent zone in the middle of the soft palate
   b. Bifid uvula
   c. Absent or notched posterior nasal spine
   d. Paranasal bulge (transverse bony ridge alongside the nose) (Stahl, 1998)

C. Variations and abnormalities of the palate. Note that tongue movements shape the palate (Palmer, 1998).

1. *High palate*: The palate or a portion of the palate is very high, altering the shallow saucer shape. See **Figure 16-3**.
2. *Wide palate or flat palate*: Reduced arch.
3. *Narrow palate*: Reduced horizontal spread of palate.
4. *Short and long palates*: Shorter or longer than the typical 1 inch from the alveolar ridge (gum ridge) to the point where the soft palate folds.
5. *Channel palate*: Midline groove usually from the prolonged presence of orotracheal tubes.
6. *V-shaped arch*: A high, narrow palate that is narrower anteriorly.
7. *Bony prominences*: Uncommon; more common is an Epstein pearl (accumulation of epithelial cells; also called a retention cyst) located at the juncture of the hard and soft palates.
8. *Sloped palate*: Sudden declines in the normal curve.
9. *Bubble palate*: Concavities of the hard palate confined with a rim.
10. *Cleft*: A complete opening in the hard or soft palate resulting from the failure of the primary palate and/or palatal shelves to meet and fuse during the seventh to eighth week of gestation (Danner et al., 1986; Miller et al., 1996; Mohrbacher, 1994).

VII. Mandible Placement

A. Reference

1. Upper and lower jaw loosely opposed
2. Both gum ridges in direct opposition

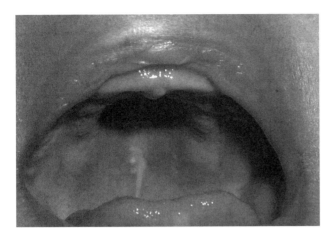

Figure 16-3 A high, narrow palate associated with ankyloglossia (tongue-tie).

B. Deviations
   1. *Recessed jaw*: The lower gum ridge is posterior to the upper gum ridge.
   2. *Micrognathia*: An excessively small or posteriorly positioned mandible; internally, the tongue is also posteriorly positioned in relation to the oral cavity.

VIII. Tongue
   A. Reference
      1. Brings the nipple into the mouth, shaping it and stabilizing its position.
      2. When the posterior tongue and mandible drop, negative pressure in the mouth causes milk to flow from the nipple (Ramsay et al., 2005). Wave of compression from front to back exerts positive pressure to initiate swallow, moving bolus back into pharynx (Kennedy et al., 2010).
      3. Forms a central groove to stabilize the teat and channel fluid toward the pharynx.
      4. Assists in forming a bolus in preparation for the swallow.
      5. The tongue is soft with a rounded tip.
      6. Lies on the bottom of the mouth with a slight central groove and the tip over the lower gum.
   B. Variations and anomalies
      1. *Tongue tip elevation*: The tip of the tongue is in opposition to the upper gum ridge or the palate behind the alveolar ridge. See **Figure 16-4**.
      2. *Humped*: In an anterior-posterior direction.
      3. *Bunched*: Compressed in a lateral direction.
      4. *Retracted*: Held posteriorly in the mouth behind the inferior alveolar ridge.
      5. *Protruded*: The tip rests forward, well past the lips.
      6. *Tongue-tie or ankyloglossia*: A short or tight lingual frenulum (Amir et al., 2005; Coryllos et al., 2004; Griffiths, 2004; Jain, 1996; Messner et al., 2000; Riche et al., 2005).
      7. See **Figure 16-5**.

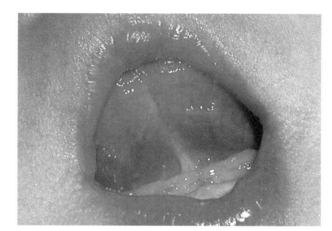

Figure 16-4
Tongue tip elevation. This posture is common in infants with retrognathia (short lower jaw) or respiratory difficulties.

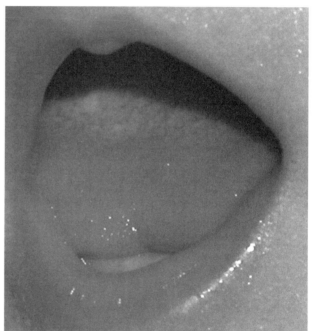

Figure 16-5
Restriction of tongue protrusion due to ankyloglossia.

IX. Oral Reflexes

A. Adaptive

1. *Rooting response*: Touching or stroking the baby's lips or cheek causes turning of the head toward the stimulus and opens the mouth (gape response).

2. *Sucking reflex*: A light touch of the nipple or a finger to the lips or tongue initiates the complex movements of the suckle.

3. *Swallowing*: Elicited by a bolus of fluid impacting the sensory receptors of the soft palate and back of the mouth; has both reflexive and voluntary properties triggered at the valeculae in newborns.

4. *Protrusion reflex*: Baby's tongue moves down and forward in anticipation of grasping and drawing the breast into the mouth.

B. Protective

1. *Gag reflex*: Protects the baby from ingesting items that are too large for the esophagus; is elicited in the newborn at the midtongue area.

2. *Cough reflex*: Mechanism that protects the airway from the aspiration of liquids.

C. Other feeding-related behaviors

1. *Scanning*: Searching for the breast with the cheeks by moving the head from side to side

2. *Stepping reflex*: Using the stepping reflex to crawl to the breast (Colson et al., 2008)

3. *Hand movements*: Predictable hand movements to stimulate (Matthiesen, 2001), move, and shape the breast (Genna et al., 2010)

References

Amir, L. H., James, J. P., & Beatty, J. (2005). Review of tongue tie release at a tertiary maternity hospital. *Journal of Paediatrics and Child Health*, *41*, 243–245.

Bosma, J. F. (Ed.). (1972). *Oral sensation and perception: The mouth of the infant*. Springfield, IL: Charles C. Thomas.

Brazelton, T. B. (1995). Neonatal behavioral assessment scale. In *Clinics in developmental medicine* (No. 88). Philadelphia, PA: Lippincott.

Colson, S. D., Meek, J. H., & Hawdon, J. M. (2008). Optimal positions for the release of primitive neonatal reflexes stimulating breastfeeding. *Early Human Development*, *84*, 441–449.

Coryllos, E., Genna, C. W., & Salloum, A. C. (2004). Congenital tongue-tie and its impact on breastfeeding. AAP Breastfeeding Section: Breastfeeding, Best for Baby and Mother. Retrieved from http://www.tongue-tie.org/Congenital-Tongue-Tie-and-its-Impact-on-Breastfeeding.html

Danner, S., & Wilson-Clay, B. (1986). Breastfeeding the infant with cleft lip/palate. In K. G. Auerbach (Ed.), *Lactation consultant series* (Unit 10). Schaumburg, IL: La Leche League International.

Diamond, M. D., Scheibel, A. B., & Elson, L. M. (1991). *The human brain coloring book*. New York, NY: Harper Collins.

Dollberg, S., Botzer E., & Grunis, E. (2006). Immediate nipple pain relief after frenotomy in breast-fed infants with ankyloglossia: A randomized, prospective study. *Journal of Pediatric Surgery*, *41*(9), 1598–1600.

Geddes, D. T., Langton, D. B., Gollow, I., et al. (2008). Frenulotomy for breastfeeding infants with ankyloglossia: Effect on milk removal and sucking mechanism as imaged by ultrasound. *Pediatrics*, *122*(1), e188–e194.

Geddes, D. T., Kent, J. C., McClellan, H. L., et al. (2009). Sucking characteristics of successfully breastfeeding infants with ankyloglossia: A case series. *Acta Paediatrica*, *99*(2), 301–303.

Genna, C. W., and Barak, D. (2010). Facilitating autonomous infant hand use during breastfeeding. *Clinical Lactation*, *1*(1), 15–20.

Gomes, C. F., Trezza, E., Murade, E., et al. (2006). Surface electromyography of facial muscles during natural and artificial feeding of infants. *Journal of Pediatrics (Rio J)*, *82*(2), 103–109.

Grant, J. C. B. (1956). *An atlas of anatomy.* Baltimore, MD: Williams & Wilkins.

Griffiths, D. M. (2004). Do tongue ties affect breastfeeding? *Journal of Human Lactation, 20,* 409–414.

Hogan, M., Westcott, C., & Griffiths, M. (2005). Randomized, controlled trial of division of tongue-tie in infants with feeding problems. *Journal of Paediatrics and Child Health, 41,* 246–250.

Jain, E. (1996). *Tongue-tie: Impact on breastfeeding. Complete management including frenotomy* [Video]. Calgary, Alberta, Canada: Lakeview Breastfeeding Clinic.

Kapit, W., & Elson, L. (1993). *The anatomy coloring book.* New York, NY: Addison Wesley.

Kennedy, D., Kieser, J., Bolter, C., Swain, M., Singh, B., & Waddell, J. N. (2010). Tongue pressure patterns during water swallowing. *Dysphagia, 25,* 11–19.

Matthiesen, A. S., Ransjo-Arvidson, A. B., Nissen, E., & Uvnas-Moberg, K. (2001). Postpartum maternal oxytocin release by newborns: Effects of infant hand massage and sucking. *Birth, 28,* 13–19.

Messner, A. H., Lalakea, M. L., Aby, J., et al. (2000). Ankyloglossia: Incidence and associated feeding difficulties. *Archives of Otolaryngology—Head & Neck Surgery, 126,* 36–39.

Miller, J. G., & Miller, J. H. (1996). *The controversial issue of breastfeeding for infants with cleft palate.* St. Innisfail, Alberta, Canada: Med Medical Research and Publishing.

Mohrbacher, N. (1994, March–April). Nursing a baby with a cleft lip or palate. *Leaven,* 19–23.

Morris, S., & Klein, M. (2000). *Pre-feeding skills* (2nd ed.). Tucson, AZ: Therapy Skill Builders.

Netter, F. (2006). *Atlas of human anatomy.* Philadelphia, Elsevier Health Sciences.

Oldfield, M. C. (1955). Congenitally short frenula of the upper lip and tongue. *Lancet, 1,* 528–530.

Palmer, B. (1998). The influence of breastfeeding on development of the oral cavity: A commentary. *Journal of Human Lactation, 14,* 93–98.

Ramsay, D. T., & Hartmann, P. (2005, March). Milk removal from the breast. *Breastfeeding Review, 13*(1), 5–7.

Riche, L. A., Baker, N. J., Madlon-Kay, D. J., & DeFor, T. A. (2005). Newborn tongue-tie: Prevalence and effect on breast-feeding. *Journal of the American Board of Family Practitioners, 18,* 1–7.

Rodriguez Jacinto-Goncalves, S., Duarte Gavião, M. B., Fausto, B., Siriani de Oliveira, A., & Adamov Semeguini, T. (2004). Electromyographic activity of perioral muscle in breastfed and non-breastfed children. *Journal of Clinical Pediatric Dentistry, 29,* 57–62.

Stahl, S. (1998). Classic and occult submucous cleft palates: A histopathologic analysis. *Cleft Palate–Craniofacial Journal, 35,* 351–358.

Takemoto, H. (2001). Morphological analyses of the human tongue musculature for three-dimensional modeling. *Journal of Speech, Language, and Hearing Research, 44*(1), 95–107.

Suggested Reading

Bly, L. (1983). *The components of normal movement during the first year of life and abnormal motor development* [Monograph]. Oak Park, IL: Neuro-Developmental Treatment Association.

Genna, C. W. (2013). *Supporting sucking skills in breastfeeding infants (2nd ed.).* Sudbury, MA: Jones and Bartlett.

Gray, H. (2005). *Gray's anatomy.* New York, NY: Barnes and Noble Books.

Ingram, T. T. S. (1962). Clinical significance of the infantile feeding reflexes. *Physiology & Behavior, 26,* 327–329.

Marmet, C., & Shell, E. (1984). Training neonates to suck correctly. *MCN: The American Journal of Maternal/Child Nursing, 9,* 401–407.

Milani-Comparetti, A. (1981). The neurophysiologic and clinical implications of studies on fetal motor behavior. *Seminars in Perinatology, 5,* 183–189.

CHAPTER 17
Physiology of the Breast During Pregnancy and Lactation

Second edition revision by Gini Baker, RN, MPH, IBCLC
Third edition revision by Marion ("Lou") Lamb, RN, MS, IBCLC

> *A pair of substantial mammary glands has the advantage over
> the two hemispheres of the most learned professor's brain, in the
> art of compounding a nutritious fluid for infants.*
>
> —DR. OLIVER WENDELL HOLMES, SR.

OBJECTIVES

- Discuss the hormonal control of mammary growth during pregnancy.
- Describe the processes of lactogenesis I, II, and III.
- List the hormones of lactation and their function.
- Describe the neuroendocrine control of milk ejection.
- Discuss the feedback inhibitor of lactation.
- Define autocrine (local) control of milk synthesis.
- Explain the process of milk synthesis.

INTRODUCTION

The breast is a remarkable endocrine organ that experiences growth, differentiation, and lactation in response to a complex interplay of hormones and stimulation. Mammogenesis, which is the development of the mammary gland and related structures within the breast, occurs throughout fetal, adolescent, and adult life. It is a time of growth, functional differentiation, and regression. Lactation is the physiologic completion of the maternal reproductive cycle (Creasy et al., 2004). The stages of breast changes during pregnancy and breastfeeding are: (1) *mammogenesis*; (2) *lactogenesis I* (also known as *secretory differentiation*); (3) *lactogenesis II* (or *secretory activation*); (4) *lactogenesis III* (previously called galactopoesis); and (5) *involution* (or weaning).

The hormonal environment of pregnancy finishes preparing the breasts to assume the role of nourishing the infant following birth. After delivery, a profound change occurs in the hormonal milieu, enabling an elaborate system of neuroendocrine

(continues)

287

feedback to produce and deliver milk of a changing volume and composition to meet the needs and stores of the infant as he or she grows and develops. The breasts are capable of full lactation from about 16 weeks of pregnancy onward. Milk does not "come in" because it is already present before delivery during lactogenesis I in the form of colostrum.

Milk production is under endocrine or hormonal control before delivery of the placenta and changes to autocrine (or local) control during lactogenesis II. Abundant production is suppressed during pregnancy by inhibiting hormones until placental delivery, when the change in hormonal checks and balances followed by the stimulus of infant suckling signal the breasts to produce copious amounts of milk. The lactation consultant benefits from a familiarity with this cascade of events and its influence on lactation. In addition, awareness of select primary factors (i.e., maternal health) and secondary factors (i.e., mismanagement of early breastfeeding) that can affect this robust but critical and carefully programmed physiologic process is crucial for the practicing lactation consultant.

I. Mammogenesis: Prenatal Breast Development

A. The breasts during pregnancy
   1. Final preparation for lactation
      a. Early in the first trimester, mammary epithelial cells proliferate, ductal sprouting and branching are initiated, and lobular formation occurs.
      b. Ducts proliferate into the fatty pad, and the ductal end buds differentiate into alveoli.
      c. Increases occur in mammary blood flow, interstitial water, and electrolyte concentrations.
      d. Mammary blood vessels increase their luminal diameters and form new capillaries around the lobules.
      e. During the last trimester, secretory cells fill with fat droplets and the alveoli are distended with colostrum.
      f. Mammary cells become competent to secrete milk proteins at midpregnancy but are kept in check by high circulating levels of steroids, particularly progesterone.
      g. Most milk products secreted during pregnancy find their way back into the plasma via the leaky junctions (spaces between the mammary alveolar cells).
   2. Hormonal control of prenatal breast changes
      a. Lactogenesis is hormonally driven: endocrine control system.
      b. Human placental lactogen, prolactin, and human chorionic gonadotropin: accelerate growth.
      c. A form of estrogen, 17 beta-estradiol, is required for mammary growth and epithelial proliferation during pregnancy.

    d. Glucocorticoids enhance formation of the lobules during pregnancy.

    e. Estrogen:

        i. Increases during pregnancy

        ii. Stimulates ductal sprouting

    f. Prolactin:

        i. Necessary for complete growth of the gland (Uvnas-Moberg et al., 1990).

        ii. Secreted by the anterior pituitary gland.

        iii. Stimulates prolactin receptor sites for the initiation of milk secretion located on the alveolar cell surfaces.

        iv. Levels rise throughout pregnancy and during sleep (Cregan et al., 2002).

        v. Prolactin is prevented from exerting its positive influence on milk secretion during pregnancy by the elevated levels of circulating progesterone.

        vi. Prolactin-inhibiting factor is secreted by the hypothalamus to negatively control prolactin's effects.

    g. Progesterone:

        i. Increases during pregnancy.

        ii. Progesterone stimulates lobuloalveolar growth while suppressing secretory activity.

        iii. Sensitizes mammary cells to the effects of insulin and growth factors.

        iv. May be involved in the final preparation of the gland for copious milk production (lactogenesis II).

II. Lactogenesis I or Secretory Differentiation

    A. Beginning of secretory cellular activity and milk production.

    B. Occurs around 16 weeks prenatally (Lawrence et al., 2011).

    C. Breast is first capable of synthesizing unique milk components; human placental lactogen and growth factors are thought to be responsible (Buhimschi, 2004).

    D. Thyroid hormones increase the responsiveness of mammary cells to prolactin and can improve lactation performance.

    E. Main reproductive hormones necessary for secretory differentiation include estrogen, progesterone, placental lactogen, and prolactin.

    F. Supportive metabolic hormones include glucocorticoids such as cortisol, insulin, thyroid-parathyroid hormone, and growth hormone (Hurst, 2007).

    G. The antepartum secretion, or colostrum, shows a gradually increasing presence of lactose, casein, and alpha-lactalbumin.

    H. Colostrum (milk) is available to the infant at delivery (milk does not have to "come in"). In addition, an increase in the concentrations of two immunoprotective proteins in colostrum, sIgA and lactoferrin, occurs after delivery.

III. Lactogenesis II or Secretory Activation

A. Lactogenesis II is the onset of copious milk secretion.
1. Between 30 and 72 hours following delivery of the placenta.
2. Women do not typically begin feeling breast fullness until 50 to 72 hours (2–3 days) after birth (Riordan, 2005).
3. Initially under endocrine control and now under autocrine, or local, control (De Coopman, 1993; Wilde, Addey et al., 1995; Wilde, Prentice et al., 1995).

B. Placental expulsion following delivery precipitates an abrupt decline in levels of human placental lactogen, estrogen, and progesterone.
1. Decline in progesterone levels is thought to be the initiating event for lactogenesis II because progesterone is a prolactin inhibitor.
2. This decline in progesterone acts in the presence of a lactogenic complex of hormones, including prolactin, insulin, and cortisol, for full secretory activation (Pang et al., 2007).
3. Changes in milk composition occur including a sharp rise in citrate and alpha-lactalbumin.

C. Risk factors for delayed onset of lactation include
1. Maternal fluid loads in labor (Chantry et al., 2011; Cotterman, 2004; Lauwers et al., 2005).
2. Method of delivery: cesarean section (Dewey et al., 2007), stressful vaginal birth with long stage II labor (Neville et al., 2001).
3. Maternal health status: Type 1 diabetes mellitus may cause a temporary imbalance in the amount of insulin required for glucose homeostasis, a requirement for the initiation of lactation (Oliveira et al., 2008). Other health conditions of concern include obesity (Nommsen-Rivers et al., 2010; Rasmussen et al., 2004), history of reduction mammoplasty, hypoplasia (insufficient mammary tissue), polycystic ovarian syndrome, infertility (Riordan, 2005), and thyroid dysfunction.
4. Any maternal illness or situation interfering with early milk removal (Neville et al., 2001).
5. Sheehan's syndrome: A pituitary infarct caused by severe postpartum hemorrhage.
6. Parity: Primiparas are at increased risk of delayed lactogenesis (Scott et al., 2007).
7. Retained placental fragments.

D. Prolactin:
1. Plasma prolactin levels increase sharply after placenta delivery and rise and fall with the frequency, intensity, and duration of nipple stimulation. Prolactin levels fall about 50% in the first week postpartum. Prolactin has been detected in mature milk up to 40 weeks postpartum (Riordan, 2005). In addition, there is a prolactin circadian rhythm with prolactin release being higher at night, surging in response to baby's suckling or the breast pump.
2. Frequent feeding in early lactation stimulates development of prolactin receptor sites in the mammary gland. The theory is that the controlling factor in

breastmilk production is the number of prolactin receptor sites and not the amount of prolactin in circulating blood (Riordan, 2005). However, a recent small study did show an increase in milk volume with administration of recombinant prolactin (Powe et al., 2011).

3. Lactogenesis II occurs earlier if the woman has breastfed before, possibly because of the increased number of prolactin receptor sites (Zuppa et al., 1988).

4. In nonnursing mothers, prolactin drops to prepregnant levels at 2 weeks postpartum.

5. Although prolactin is necessary for milk secretion, its levels are not directly related to the volume of milk produced; that is, prolactin becomes "permissive" in its function.

6. Prolactin release occurs only in response to direct stimulation of the nipple/areola in a neurohormonal feedback pathway. (See **Figure 17-1**.) This autocrine control is responsible for the next stage of milk production: lactogenesis III.

IV. Lactogenesis III

A. The stage of mature milk production and supply (also known as galactopoesis), which is defined as later than 9 days after birth to the beginning of involution; Uvnas-Moberg et al., 1996); is the maintenance phase of lactation, dependent on autocrine, or local, control.

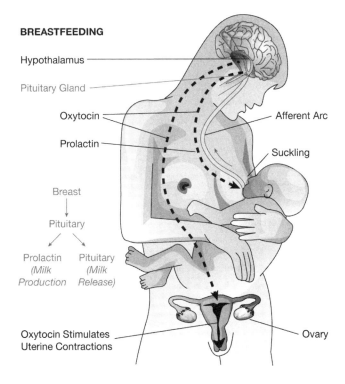

Figure 17-1
Neuroendocrine Reflex Arc.

Courtesy of Lactation Education Resources

B. Milk synthesis is controlled by two mechanisms. (See **Figure 17-2**.)

　1. Feedback inhibitor of lactation (FIL): A small active whey protein synthesized by the lactocytes, which accumulates in the alveolar lumen.

　　a. Role of FIL appears to be to moderate milk synthesis locally, based on the fullness of the breast.

　　b. Rate of milk synthesis slows when milk accumulates in the breast because more FIL is present in the milk, which initiates this chemical feedback loop.

　　c. Rate of milk synthesis speeds up when milk is removed from the breast and less FIL is present.

　　d. More frequent and complete milk removal, theoretically, will produce more milk.

　2. Prolactin receptor theory: Another, less understood, local mechanism regulating the rate of milk synthesis involves prolactin receptors in the basement membrane of the alveoli to which the lactocytes are attached.

　　a. As milk accumulates in the breast, the shape of the lactocyte is distorted and prolactin cannot bind to its receptor, creating an inhibitory effect on level of milk production (van Veldhuizen-Staas, 2007; Zoubiane et al., 2003).

　　b. Prolactin uptake is inhibited by alveolar distension, downregulating milk synthesis (Hale et al., 2007).

C. Foremilk and hindmilk:

　1. All milk starts out as concentrated milk, sometimes referred to as hindmilk (Hale et al., 2007).

　2. When milk remains in the breast, it draws in water and lactose and becomes more dilute foremilk.

　3. Hindmilk has a higher fat content than does foremilk.

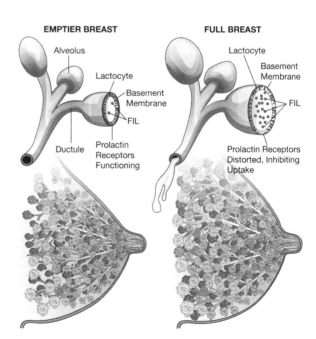

Figure 17-2

Milk Synthesis Control: Feedback Inhibitor of Lactation (FIL) and Prolactin Receptor Theory.

Courtesy of Lactation Education Resources

D. Calorie and fat content of mature milk (Cregan et al., 1999; Cregan et al., 2002; Daly et al., 1995a, 1995b; Daly et al., 1992; Kent et al., 2006; Mitoulas et al., 2002; Ramsay et al., 2005; Ramsay & Mitoulas, et al., 2005; Walker, 2011):
  1. Colostrum mean energy value is 67 kcal/dL, or 18.76 kcal/oz.
  2. Mature milk mean energy value is 75 kcal/dL, or 21 kcal/oz.
  3. Caloric content varies widely throughout each feeding and the time of day because of changing fat content.
  4. The amount of fat in human milk changes during each feeding depending on the time since the last feeding.
  5. Fat type and content in human milk are also influenced by several factors including maternal metabolism, maternal weight (Anderson et al., 2005), maternal diet (Kent, 2007), gestational age of infant (Moltó-Puigmartí et al., 2011), and duration of breastfeeding (Mandel et al., 2005).

V. Involution

A. Occurs when the milk-producing system in the breast is no longer being used, which results in secretory epithelial apoptosis, or cell death.
B. Complete involution varies among women and is typically defined as occurring approximately 40 days after complete cessation of breastfeeding.
C. Depends on type of weaning process, whether abrupt or gradual.
D. Anecdotally, women report that the longer they are actively producing milk, the longer it takes for the production to completely cease.

VI. General Information

A. Milk production
  1. Volume of milk removed from the breast at a feeding or expression is correlated to the needs of the baby, an elegant example of the concept of supply and demand.
  2. Studies show an increased sensitivity of prolactin receptors in multiparous women that can affect overall milk production (Zuppa et al., 1988).
  3. Affected by influences such as breast hypoplasia, obesity, maternal disease, rate of metabolism, and maternal medications (specifically, prolactin-inhibiting factors also known as dopamine agonists, such as bromocriptine and ergotamine, which inhibit prolactin secretion; Riordan, 2005).
B. Milk synthesis (accumulation of milk within the breast)
  1. Rate of milk synthesis: Rate at which newly manufactured milk is accumulating within the breast.
  2. Local, or autocrine, control regulates short-term milk synthesis.
  3. Milk synthesis responds to the varying amount of residual milk remaining in the breast after a feeding (FIL factor). (See **Figure 17-2**.)
  4. Degree to which milk is removed signals the amount of milk to be made for the next feeding.
  5. Milk synthesis is controlled independently in each breast.

6. Storage capacity of breasts varies greatly among women.

7. Measured storage capacity of a breast increases with breast size.

8. Small breasts are capable of secreting as much milk over a 24-hour period as large breasts (Ramsay, Kent, et al., 2005).

C. Milk synthesis process

1. Cells lining both the alveoli and the smaller ductules appear capable of secreting milk.

2. Degree of fullness in breast and rate of short-term synthesis are inversely related (Daly, Owens et al., 1993; Daly et al., 1996; Daly et al., 1992; Walker, 2011).

3. Wide variability in rate of milk synthesis, ranging from 17 to 33 mL/h (Arthur, Smith et al., 1989; Arthur, Jones et al., 1989).

4. The milk is stored in the alveoli and in small ducts adjacent to the cells that secrete it, compressing and flattening the cells.

5. Milk synthesis occurs in the lactocyte (or secretory epithelial cell) after the uptake of substrates from maternal blood necessary for milk production (Hale et al., 2007). Five pathways are involved in milk synthesis (Arthur, Smith, et al., 1989; Arthur, Jones, et al., 1989; Daly et al., 1996):

   a. Pathway I: Protein secretion

      i. Most important proteins synthesized by the mammary cell are casein, lactoferrin, alpha-lactalbumin, and lysozyme.

   b. Pathway II: Lactose secretion

   c. Pathway III: Milk fat synthesis

   d. Pathway IV: Monovalent ion secretion into milk

      i. Sodium, potassium, and chloride

   e. Pathway V: Plasma protein secretion

      i. Plasma immunoglobulin A (IgA) binds to the mammary alveolar cell and is released into the milk and is involved in disease protection.

D. Milk release (also referred to as milk ejection reflex or letdown reflex)

1. Neuroendocrine involvement in milk ejection

   a. Occurs with:

      i. Direct stimulation by the infant to sensory neurons in the areola, which initiate a neuroendocrine arc to the posterior pituitary to release oxytocin into the bloodstream. (See **Figure 17-1**.)

      ii. Impulses from the cerebral cortex, ears, and eyes can also elicit the release of oxytocin through exteroceptive stimuli (such as hearing a baby cry) (Uvnas-Moberg et al., 1990).

   b. Some women feel the milk ejection reflex as increased pressure or tingling within the breast or as shooting pains, whereas some women never feel the milk ejection reflex.

    c. Response to oxytocin release from the posterior pituitary:

        i. Mothers, especially multiparous women, with each breastfeeding will also feel uterine cramping for the first few days after birth (also known as *afterbirth pains*). (See **Figure 17-1**.)

        ii. Mothers might also report increased thirst, a warm or flushed feeling, increased heat from the breasts, or a feeling of sleepiness or calmness.

    d. Milk ejection signs can be seen with dripping of milk from the breast or when the baby begins gulping milk (when the rapid pattern of two sucks per second decreases to one suck or so per second with swallowing).

    e. Milk ejection reflex serves to increase the intraductal mammary pressure and to maintain it at levels that are sufficient to overcome the resistance to the outflow of milk from the breast.

    f. The amount of milk transferred by the infant is correlated to the number of milk ejections per feeding and is independent of the amount of time spent at the breast (Ramsay et al., 2004).

2. Oxytocin

    a. A simultaneous and closed secretion of oxytocin occurs into brain regions of the lactating mother (Febo et al., 2005; Jonas et al., 2007; Mezzacappa et al., 2001; Uvnas-Moberg et al., 2004; Winberg, 2005).

        i. Has a calming, analgesic affect

        ii. Lowers maternal blood pressure

        iii. Decreases cortisol levels, decreases anxiety and aggressive behavior

        iv. Permeates the areas of the brain associated with mothering and bonding behaviors

    b. Causes a contraction of the myoepithelial cells surrounding the alveoli, forcing milk into the collecting ducts of the breast.

    c. Nipple stimulation causes oxytocin release of brief 3- to 4-second pulsatile bursts into the bloodstream every 5 to 15 minutes (Neville, 2001).

    d. Variable and intermittent bursts of oxytocin are also seen from prenursing stimuli and mechanical stimulation from a breast pump (Fewtrell et al., 2001).

    e. Oxytocin causes shortening of the ducts without constricting them, thus increasing milk pressure (Neville, 2001).

    f. Oxytocin secretion can be inhibited by pain or stress (Lawrence, 2005; Newton et al., 1948); alcohol (Cobo, 1973; Menella et al., 2005); and certain labor practices because induction or augmentation of labor with synthetic oxytocin has been found to interfere with the release of endogenous oxytocin (Jonas et al., 2009; Jordan et al., 2009).

References

Anderson, N., Beerman, K., & McGuire, M.A., et al. (2005). Dietary fat type influences total milk fat content in lean women. *Journal of Nutrition*, *135*(3), 416–421.

Arthur, P. G., Smith, M., & Hartmann, P. E. (1989). Milk lactose, citrate, and glucose as markers of lactogenesis in normal and diabetic women. *Journal of Pediatric Gastroenterology and Nutrition*, *9*, 488–496.

Arthur, P. G., Jones, T. J., Spruce, J., & Hartmann, P. E. (1989). Measuring short-term rates of milk synthesis in breast-feeding mothers. *Quarterly Journal of Experimental Physiology*, *74*, 419–428.

Buhimschi, C. S. (2004). Endocrinology of lactation. *Obstetrics and Gynecology Clinics of North America*, *31*(4), xii, 963–979.

Chantry, C. J., Nommsen-Rivers, L. A., Peerson, J. M., et al. (2011). Excess weight loss in first-born breastfed newborns relates to maternal intrapartum fluid balance. *Pediatrics*, *127*(1), 171–179.

Cobo, E. (1973). Effect of different doses of ethanol on the milk ejection reflex in lactating women. *American Journal of Obstetrics and Gynecology*, *115*, 817–821.

Cotterman, K. (2004). Reverse pressure softening: A simple tool to prepare areola for easier latching during engorgement. *Journal of Human Lactation*, *20*, 227–237.

Cox, D. B., Owens, R. A., & Hartmann, P. E. (1996). Blood and milk prolactin and the rate of milk synthesis in women. *Experimental Physiology*, *81*, 1007–1020.

Cox, D. B., Owens, R. A., & Hartmann, P. E. (1998). Studies on human lactation: The development of the computerized breast measurement system. Retrieved from http://mammary.nih.gov/reviews/lactation/Hartmann001/

Creasy, R., & Resnik, R. (Ed.). (2004). *Maternal and fetal medicine: Principles and practice* (5th ed.). Philadelphia, PA: W. B. Saunders.

Cregan, M. D., & Hartmann, P. E. (1999). Computerized breast measurement from conception to weaning: Clinical implications. *Journal of Human Lactation*, *15*, 89–96.

Cregan, M. D., Mitoulas, L. R., & Hartmann, P. E. (2002). Milk prolactin, feed volume and duration between feeds in women breastfeeding their full-term infants over a 24 h period. *Experimental Physiology*, *87*, 207–214.

Daly, S. E. J., Di Rosso, A., Owens, R. A., & Hartmann, P. E. (1993). Degree of breast emptying explains changes in the fat content, but not fatty acid composition, of human milk. *Experimental Physiology*, *78*, 741–755.

Daly, S. E. J., & Hartmann, P. E. (1995a). Infant demand and milk supply. Part 1: Infant demand and milk supply in lactating women. *Journal of Human Lactation*, *11*, 21–31.

Daly, S. E. J., & Hartmann, P. E. (1995b). Infant demand and milk supply. Part 2: The short-term control of milk synthesis in lactating women. *Journal of Human Lactation*, *11*, 27–37.

Daly, S. E. J., Kent, J. C., Owens, R. A., & Hartmann, P. E. (1996). Frequency and degree of milk removal and the short-term control of human milk synthesis. *Experimental Physiology*, *81*, 861–875.

Daly, S. E. J., Kent, J. C., Owens, R. A., et al. (1992). The determination of short-term volume changes and the rate of synthesis of human milk using computerized breast measurement. *Experimental Physiology*, *77*, 79–87.

Daly, S. E. J., Owens, R. A., & Hartmann, P. E. (1993). The short-term synthesis and infant-regulated removal of milk in lactating women. *Experimental Physiology*, *78*, 209–220.

De Coopman, J. (1993). Breastfeeding after pituitary resection: Support for a theory of autocrine control of milk supply? *Journal of Human Lactation*, *9*, 35–40.

DeCarvalho, M. D., Robertson, S., Friedman, A., & Klaus, M. (1983). Effect of frequent breast-feeding on early milk production and infant weight gain. *Pediatrics, 72*, 307–311.

Dewey, K. G., Nommsen-Rivers, L. A., Heinig, M. J., & Cohen, R. J. (2003). Risk factors for suboptimal infant breastfeeding behavior, delayed onset of lactation, and excess neonatal weight loss. *Pediatrics, 112*, 607–619.

Dökmetaş, H. S., Kilicli, F., Korkmaz, S., & Yonem, O. (2006). Characteristic features of 20 patients with Sheehan's syndrome. *Gynecological Endocrinology, 22*(5), 279–283.

Febo, M., Numan, M., & Ferris, C. F. (2005). Functional magnetic resonance imaging shows oxytocin activates brain regions associated with mother–pup bonding during suckling. *Journal of Neuroscience, 25*, 11637–11644.

Fewtrell, M., Lucas, P., Collier, S., & Lucas, A. (2001). Randomized study comparing the efficacy of a novel manual breast pump with a mini-electric breast pump in mothers of term infants. *Journal of Human Lactation, 17*, 126–131.

Geddes, D. T. (2007). Inside the lactating breast: The latest anatomy research. *Journal of Midwifery & Women's Health, 52*(6), 556–563.

Hale, T., & Hartmann, P. (2007). *Textbook of human lactation*. Amarillo, TX: Hale.

Hurst, M. (2007). Recognizing and treating delayed or failed lactogenesis II. *Journal of Midwifery and Women's Health, 52*(6), 588–594.

Jonas, K., Johansson, L. M., Nissen, E., Eideback, M., Ransio-Arvidson, A. B., & Uvnas-Moberg, K. (2009). Effects of intrapartum oxytocin administration and epidural analgesis on the concentration of plasma oxytocin and prolactin, in response to suckling during the second day postpartum. *Breastfeeding Medicine, 4*(2), 71–82.

Jonas, W., Wiklund, I., & Nissen, E., et al. (2007). Newborn skin temperature two days postpartum during breastfeeding related to different labour ward practices. *Early Human Development, 83*(1), 55–61.

Jordan, S., Emery, S., Watkins, A., Evans, J. D., Storey, M., & Morgan, G. (2009). Associations of drugs routinely given during labor with breastfeeding at 48 hours: Analysis of the Cardiff Birth Survey. *BJOG: An International Journal of Obstetrics and Gynaecology, 116*(12), 1622–1632.

Kent, J. C. (2007). How breastfeeding works. *Journal of Midwifery and Women's Health, 52*(6), 564–570.

Kent, J. C., Mitoulas, L. R., Cregan, M. D., Ramsay, D. T., Doherty, D. A., & Hartmann, P. E. (2006). Volume and frequency of breastfeedings and fat content of breast milk throughout the day. *Pediatrics, 117*, e387–e395.

Lauwers, J., & Swisher, A. (2005). *Counseling the nursing mother: A lactation consultant's guide*. Sudbury, MA: Jones and Bartlett.

Lawrence, R. A., & Lawrence, R. M. (2005). *Breastfeeding: A guide for the medical profession*. 6th ed. Philadelphia, PA: Elsevier Mosby.

Mandel, D., Lubetzky, R., Dollberg, S., Barak, S., & Mimouni, F. B. (2005). Fat and energy contents of expressed human breast milk in prolonged lactation. *Pediatrics, 116*, e432–e435.

Mennella, J., Yanino, M., & Teff, K. (2005). Acute alcohol consumption disrupts the hormonal milieu of lactating women. *Clinical Endocrinology and Metabolism, 90*(4), 1979–1985.

Mezzacappa, E. S., Kelsey, R. M., Myers, M. M., & Katkin, E. S. (2001). Breast-feeding and maternal cardiovascular function. *Psychophysiology, 38*, 988–997.

Mitoulas, L. R., Kent, J. C., Cox, D. B., et al. (2002). Variation in fat, lactose and protein in human milk over 24 h and throughout the first year of lactation. *British Journal of Nutrition, 88*, 29–37.

Moltó-Puigmartí, C., Castellote, A. I., Carbonell-Estrany, X., & López-Sabater, M. C. (2011). Differences in fat content and fatty acid proportions among colostrum, transitional, and mature milk from women delivering very preterm, preterm, and term infants. *Clinical Nutrition*, *30*(1), 116–123.

Neville, M. C. (2001). Anatomy and physiology of lactation. *Pediatric Clinics of North America*, *48*(1), 13–34.

Neville, M. C., & Morton, J. (2001). Physiology and endocrine changes underlying human lactogenesis II. *Journal of Nutrition*, *131*(11), 30055–30085.

Newton, M., & Newton, N. (1948). The let-down reflex in human lactation. *Journal of Pediatrics*, *33*(6), 698–704.

Nommsen-Rivers, L. A., Chantry, C. J., Peerson, J. M., Cohen, R. J., & Dewey, K. G. (2010). Delayed onset of lactogenesis among first-time mothers is related to maternal obesity and factors associated with ineffective breastfeeding. *American Journal of Clinical Nutrition*, *92*(3), 574–584.

Oliveira, A. M., Cunha, C. C., Penha-Silva, N., Abdallah, V. O., & Jorge, P. T. (2008). Interference of the blood glucose control in the transition between phases I and II of lactogenesis in patients with type 1 diabetes mellitus. *Brazilian Archives of Endocrinology & Metabolism*, *52*(3), 473–481. (in Portugese).

Pang, W., & Hartmann, P. (2007). Initiation of human lactation: Secretory differentiation and secretory activation. *Journal of Mammary Gland Biology and Neoplasia*, *12*, 211–221.

Powe, C. E., Puopolo, K. M., Newburg, D. S., et al. (2011). Effects of recombinant human prolactin on breast milk composition. *Pediatrics*, *127*(2), 359–366.

Ramsay, D. T., & Hartmann, P. E. (2005). Milk removal from the breast. *Breastfeeding Review*, *13*, 5–7.

Ramsay, D. T., Kent, J. C., Hartmann, R. A., Hartmann, P. E. (2005). Anatomy of the lactating breast redefined with ultrasound imaging. *Journal of Anatomy*, *206*(6), 525–534.

Ramsay, D. T., Kent, J. C., Owens, R. A., et al. (2004). Ultrasound imaging of milk ejection in the breast of lactating women. *Pediatrics*, *113*, 361–367.

Ramsay, D. T., Mitoulas, L. R., Kent, J. C., et al. (2005). The use of ultrasound to characterize milk ejection in women using an electric breast pump. *Journal of Human Lactation*, *21*, 421–428.

Rasmussen, K. M., & Kjolhede, C. L. (2004). Prepregnant overweight and obesity diminish the prolactin response to suckling in the first week postpartum. *Pediatrics*, *113*, 465–471.

Riordan, J. (2005). *Breastfeeding and human lactation* (2nd ed.). Sudbury, MA: Jones and Bartlett.

Scott, J., Binns, C., & Oddy, W. (2007, July). Predictors of delayed onset of lactation. *Maternal and Child Nutrition*, *3*(3), 186–193.

Uvnas-Moberg, K., & Eriksson, M. (1996). Breastfeeding: Physiological, endocrine and behavioral adaptations caused by oxytocin and local neurogenic activity in the nipple and mammary gland. *Acta Paediatrica*, *85*, 525–530.

Uvnas-Moberg, K., & Petersson, M. (2004). Oxytocin—biochemical link for human relations. Mediator of antistress, well-being, social interaction, growth, healing. *Lakartidningen*, *101*, 2634–2639. (in Swedish).

Uvnas-Moberg, K., Widstrom, A.-M., Werner, S., et al. (1990). Oxytocin and prolactin levels in breast-feeding women. *Acta Obstetricia et Gynecologica Scandinavica*, *69*, 301–306.

van Veldhuizen-Staas, C . (2007, August). Overabundant milk supply: An alternative way to intervene by full drainage and block feeding. *International Breastfeeding Journal*, *2*, 11.

Walker, M. (2011). *Breastfeeding management for the clinician* (2nd ed.). Sudbury, MA: Jones and Bartlett.

Wilde, C. J., Addey, C. V. P., Boddy, L. M., & Peaker, M. (1995). Autocrine regulation of milk secretion by a protein in milk. *Biochemical Journal*, *305*, 51–58.

Wilde, C. J., Prentice, A., & Peaker, M. (1995). Breastfeeding: Matching supply with demand in human lactation. *Proceedings of the Nutrition Society*, *54*, 401–406.

Winberg, J. (2005). Mother and newborn baby: Mutual regulation of physiology and behavior—a selective review. *Developmental Psychobiology*, *47*, 217–229.

Zoubiane, G. S., Valentijn, A., Lowe, E. T. et al. (2003). A role for the cytoskeleton in prolactin-dependent mammary epithelial cell differentiation. *Journal of Cell Science*, *117*(2), 271–280.

Zuppa, A. A., Tornesello, A., Papacci, P., et al. (1988). Relationship between maternal parity, basal prolactin levels and neonatal breast milk intake. *Biology of the Neonate*, *53*, 144–147.

CHAPTER 18
Anatomy and Physiology of Infant Suckling

Amy Spangler, MN, RN, IBCLC, and Maeve Howett, PhD, APRN, IBCLC

OBJECTIVES

- Define sucking and suckling.
- Define nutritive and nonnutritive modes of suckling.
- Describe oral motor and feeding development.
- Describe the suckling cycle.
- List factors that can influence or contribute to suckling abnormalities.
- Understand the unique vulnerabilities of the preterm infant in regard to feeding.

INTRODUCTION

Knowing that respiration and nutrition are essential to newborn survival, the transition to extrauterine life requires that newborn infants can breathe, locate and attach to the breast, and effectively suckle and swallow. The dynamic and intricate coordination of sucking, swallowing, and breathing superimposed on a background of the infant's behavioral state arguably make infant feeding the most complex skill a newborn infant must master in establishing life outside the mother's womb (Reynolds et al., 2010; Wolf et al., 1992). During pregnancy, the developing fetus receives nutrients through the placental circulation, and waste products are excreted through the maternal circulation. After birth, the newborn must independently ingest food by mouth, digest and absorb nutrients, and excrete metabolic wastes. All of these activities occur during a period of rapid growth, high nutritional needs, and body systems that are operationally immature. The lactation consultant benefits from an understanding of oral motor development, the mechanism of suckling, and the processes that control effective suckling behavior. Poor feeding can be a sign of neurological damage and a sensitive indicator of central nervous system disease (Reynolds et al., 2010). Knowledge of normal fetal and infant anatomy and development provides a standard against which variations can be assessed, allowing for earlier identification of infants at risk for neurodevelopmental delay and feeding problems.

I. Oral Anatomy

The oral anatomy consists of the nose, mouth, pharynx, airways, and esophagus. Muscular activity and changing pressure gradients combine to move air and food from the nasal and oral cavities to the stomach (Kennedy et al., 1988; Ramsay et al., 2004). To facilitate the safe transport of air and food through the same and adjacent structures, a system of valves that includes the lips, soft palate, tongue, epiglottis, and cricopharyngeal sphincter channels food and air in the proper direction at the proper time (Morris, 1982). The default position of the valves favors respiration, with most of the valves changing position to allow swallowing. As the fetus develops, soft pliable tissues gradually can provide the mechanical stability needed for breathing and feeding. As the newborn grows, the method of stabilization shifts from positional to postural. The closeness of the anatomic structures and a large amount of subcutaneous fat provide positional stability in the newborn. As the infant matures, larger amounts of connective tissue, cartilage, and highly specialized muscle control provide postural stability. There is also a maturational progression in the suck-swallow-breathe interaction clearly seen in preterm infants but less pronounced in infants born full term (Reynolds et al., 2010).

A. Birth (at 37–42 weeks gestation) to 6 months of age
   1. Oral cavity is short from top to bottom and bounded by the roof, floor, lips, and cheeks.
   2. Hard palate is short, wide, and slightly arched with a corrugated surface (rugae).
   3. Soft palate and epiglottis are closely approximated.
   4. Sucking fat pads are present in the cheeks.
   5. Tongue fills the oral cavity; tongue tip protrudes past the alveolar ridge, maintaining contact with the lower lip.
   6. Frenulum anchors the tongue to the floor of the mouth.
   7. Jaw is recessed with the lower gum line slightly behind the upper gum line.
B. Six months to 1 year of age
   1. Oral cavity elongates vertically and becomes more spacious.
   2. Soft palate and epiglottis are no longer in close proximity. Larynx must elevate farther to allow epiglottis to seal completely during swallowing.
   3. Tongue positioned more toward the back of the mouth; tongue tip is behind the alveolar ridge. Lateral tongue movements facilitate manipulation of food.
   4. Sucking fat pads and other adipose tissue in the cheeks diminish. This allows for greater movement of the lips and cheeks.
   5. Teeth erupt.

II. Oral Reflex Development (Delaney et al., 2008; Wolf et al., 1992)

A. Sucking and swallowing: Sucking and swallowing play a crucial role in infant survival and are facilitated by infantile reflexes that develop at an early age (Bosma, 1985; Pritchard, 1966). The fetus exhibits:
   1. Swallowing at 12 to 14 weeks gestation (Bosma, 1985; Ianniruberto et al., 1981).
   2. Sucking as early as 15 to 18 weeks gestation (Ianniruberto et al., 1981).

3. In the extrauterine environment, sucking activity has been observed in infants.

    a. At 27 to 28 weeks gestation, sucking activity is present but the pattern is disorganized and random.

    b. At 32 weeks gestation, a burst–pause pattern is emerging but still lacks coordination.

    c. At 34 to 35 weeks gestation, sucking and related components for effective feeding are present (Delaney et al., 2008).

B. Oral reflexes: Two categories of oral reflexes serve to assist the infant in feeding while protecting the airway:

    1. Adaptive (rooting and sucking)

    2. Protective (gag and cough)

C. When a reflex loses its functional significance, it diminishes or disappears. Reflexes that are essential to survival persist, such as the gag and cough reflexes.

D. Swallowing plays a role in the regulation of amniotic fluid volume and composition, recirculation of solutes from the fetal environment, and maturation of the fetal gastrointestinal tract (Ross et al., 1998).

    1. Near term, the normal fetus swallows approximately one-half of the total volume of amniotic fluid each day (Diamant, 1985).

    2. Amniotic fluid volume is directly correlated with perinatal mortality and morbidities including trachea-esophageal fistula, duodenal atresia, renal anomalies, and intrauterine growth restriction (IUGR). Inability to swallow because of obstruction or neurological defect results in polyhydramnios, while urinary tract anomalies are often related to oligohydramnios (Harman, 2008).

E. Gag reflex:

    1. Stimulus: Posterior tongue/pharynx

    2. Appears: 18 weeks gestation and peaks at 40 weeks gestation (Ianniruberto et al., 1981; Tucker, 1985)

    3. Diminishes: 6 months but persists into adulthood

F. Phasic bite reflex:

    1. Stimulus: Gums

    2. Appears: 28 weeks gestation

    3. Disappears: 9 and 12 months

G. Rooting reflex:

    1. Stimulus: Mouth corner/lips/cheek

    2. Appears: 32 weeks gestation and peaks at 40 weeks gestation

    3. Disappears: 3 to 6 months

H. Sucking reflex:

    1. Stimulus: Mouth/tongue

    2. Appears: 15 to 18 weeks gestation

    3. Disappears: 6 to 12 months

I. Swallowing reflex:
   1. Stimulus: Pharynx
   2. Appears: 12 to 14 weeks gestation
   3. Persists: Into adulthood
J. Tongue protrusion reflex:
   1. Stimulus: Tongue/lips
   2. Appears: 28 weeks gestation
   3. Disappears: 6 months

III. Science of Suckling

Suckling and *sucking* are often used interchangeably to describe infant mouth movements that occur with or without the ingestion of food (Lawrence, 2011).

- Some authors make a clear distinction between *suckling* and the more mature *sucking* (Arvedson et al., 1993; Lawrence, 2011; Wolf et al., 1992).
- During the first weeks after birth, the physiologic flexion into a fetal position (acquired as a result of the limited space inside the uterus) contributes to successful oral feeding (Arvedson et al., 1993). Arvedson et al. (1993) describe two distinct suck phases, suckling and sucking.

   A. Suckling:
      1. The first pattern to develop.
      2. Involves a backward and forward movement of the tongue.
      3. The tongue moves forward for half of the suckle pattern, with the backward phase being the most pronounced.
      4. Tongue protrusion does not extend beyond the border of the lips (Arvedson & Brodsky, 1993).
      5. The sides of the tongue move upward to form a central groove, helping to form the liquid bolus and move the bolus posteriorly.
   B. Sucking:
      1. Second phase develops between 6 and 9 months of age when the tongue has more room for movement because of the downward and forward growth of the oral cavity.
      2. During sucking, the tongue raises and lowers, and the jaw makes smaller vertical excursions.
   C. Lawrence (2011) differentiates between suckling and sucking as follows:
      1. Suckling is the means by which the infant takes nourishment at the breast, that is, breastfeeding.
      2. Sucking is the drawing of food into the mouth by means of a partial vacuum, that is, what the infant does to bottle-feed.
   D. Wolf et al. (1992) use sucking to describe the rhythmic movements of the infant's mouth and tongue in either of the following situations:
      1. On a bottle or breast to obtain nourishment
      2. On a pacifier, finger, or other object to modulate state or explore the environment (Arvedson et al., 1993; Lawrence, 2011)

E. Mammalian suckling: All mammals are characterized by their ability to lactate.

1. Suckling patterns are unique to each mammal species.

2. When healthy, unmedicated, full-term infants are placed on their mother's abdomen immediately after birth, they can seek and find the breast, latch on, and suckle within the first hour (Righard et al., 1990). This raises the question of the impact of separation of a mother and infant on breastfeeding initiation and duration and the extent to which the interruption produces lasting harm (Faturi et al., 2009; Illingworth et al., 1964; Righard et al., 1990). The principal mechanism of milk removal common to all mammals is the contractile response of the mammary myoepithelium under the hormonal influence of oxytocin from the posterior pituitary, a phenomenon known as the milk ejection reflex (MER; Lawrence, 2011).

   a. Infant suckling is the stimulus for the MER.

   b. Milk ejection causes the suckling pattern to change from nonnutritive to nutritive (Mizuno et al., 2005).

3. Central nervous system (CNS) control of milk ejection contributes to the MER occurring under circumstances that are conducive to effective milk removal (Lawrence, 2011).

4. Effective provision of milk requires:

   a. A storage system (alveoli)

   b. Exit channels (ducts)

   c. A prehensile appendage (areola)

   d. An expulsion mechanism (the MER)

   e. A retention mechanism (Lawrence, 2011)

IV. Nonnutritive and Nutritive Sucking

A. Nutritive sucking is the process of obtaining nutrients.

B. Nonnutritive sucking occurs in the absence of nutrient flow and may be used to satisfy an infant's basic sucking urge or as a mechanism for regulating state (Wolf et al., 1992).

C. Nonnutritive sucking such as the spontaneous sucking that occurs when a finger, pacifier, or dummy is placed in an infant's mouth can function in the following ways:

1. Increase peristalsis of the gastrointestinal tract (Widstrom et al., 1988)

2. Enhance secretion of digestive fluids (Widstrom et al., 1988)

3. Decrease infant crying and help an infant reorganize to a calm state

4. Reduce the risk for sudden infant death syndrome (SIDS; Hauck et al., 2003; Kahn et al., 2003)

D. Pacifier use:

1. The American Academy of Pediatrics (AAP) recommends the use of pacifiers when infants are put to sleep as a means of reducing the risk for SIDS (AAP Task Force on Sudden Infant Death Syndrome, 2005). Why this strategy is protective is unclear. More data are needed before definitive statements can be made about the impact of pacifier use on breastfeeding, fertility, and dentition (Ingram et al., 2004; Ullah et al., 2003; Viggiano et al., 2004).

2. The AAP currently recommends delaying the use of pacifiers until infants are 1 month of age to ensure that breastfeeding is well established (AAP Task Force on Sudden Infant Death Syndrome, 2005; Howard et al., 2003).

V. The Mechanisms of Suckling

Before the advent of ultrasound imaging, infant feeding data were collected on bottle-feeding infants. Using advanced ultrasound technology, researchers can now visualize the lactating breast and the breastfeeding infant and make clear distinctions between breastfeeding and bottle-feeding infants (Ramsay et al., 2004; Taki et al., 2010).

A. Historically, the baby sucked and the mother suckled. Definitions have changed in modern times as noted previously.

B. *Suckling* describes the removal of milk from the breast by the infant, that is, breastfeeding.

C. The volume of milk removed is determined by milk flow. The milk ejection reflex (MER) controls milk flow. If the MER does not occur, the infant is unable to get enough milk (Taki et al., 2010).

   Additional mechanisms that facilitate milk removal include:

   1. Negative pressure within the oral cavity
   2. Positive pressure of the tongue against the teat (nipple and areola)
   3. Increased intraductal pressure (Ramsay et al., 2004)

D. Milk ejection is under neuroendocrine control.

   1. Infant suckling stimulates the release of oxytocin by the posterior pituitary gland. Oxytocin causes the myoepithelial cells surrounding the alveoli to contract, forcing milk from the alveoli into the milk ducts (Ramsay et al., 2004; Taki et al., 2010).
   2. Neither the negative or positive pressure exerted by suckling stimulate milk ejection.

E. Effective suckling:

   1. Effective suckling requires that the infant be able to coordinate three complex tasks: sucking, swallowing, and breathing. Bu'Lock and colleagues (1990) conclude that this neuromuscular coordination is more a function of gestational maturity than postnatal sucking experience after observing that a group of term infants (37+ weeks) did not exhibit the apneic pause in breathing seen in near-term and preterm infants. Taki and colleagues (2010) found that feeding efficiency (total feeding time and volume of milk ingested) increased over time, supporting a theory of maturation.
   2. Data show that although nasal breathing is preferred, it is not obligatory (Rodenstein et al., 1985).
      a. Infants were once categorized as obligate nose breathers—unable to breathe through their mouths.
      b. Infants have the ability to breathe through their mouth, albeit at the expense of respiratory efficiency (Miller et al., 1985).

3. For many years it was believed that sucking and swallowing occurred in isolation from breathing.

   a. Wilson and colleagues (1980) were the first to report that swallowing coincided with cessation of nasal airflow, that is, breathing stops when swallowing occurs.

   b. Weber and colleagues (1986) reported similar findings, that is, the rhythmic swallowing accompanying sucking interrupts breathing.

   c. These findings support the current view that sucking, swallowing, and breathing must be coordinated in infant feeding. In a perfectly coordinated cycle, suck, swallow, breathe movements are related in a 1:1:1 sequence and breathing is continuous and uninterrupted (Bu'Lock et al., 1990). During feeding that is less well coordinated, breathing is always interrupted by swallowing and may actually be subordinate to it (Bu'Lock et al., 1990; Reynolds et al., 2010). Taki and colleagues (2010) found that the sucking pattern (number of sucks per burst and burst duration) in bottle-fed infants was outside the physiologically appropriate range as defined by the sucking pattern of breastfed infants. Furthermore, they found that even though some bottle-feeding infants may tolerate long periods of continuous sucking, once they suffer upper respiratory problems they tend to exhibit difficulty bottle-feeding (Taki et al., 2010).

F. Rate of suckling:

   1. Term infants often exhibit a transient, immature suck pattern during their first feeding attempts (Gryboski, 1975). This pattern is characterized by short bursts of 3–5 sucks followed by swallows. Over the next 24–48 hours, the number of sucks per burst increases to 10–30, and swallows occur during the sucking burst (Gryboski, 1975). Taki and colleagues (2010) found that breastfed infants averaged 17.8 sucks per sucking burst at 1 month of age, increasing to 32.4 sucks per sucking burst at 6 months. The sucking rate varies from 55 per minute (slightly less than 1 suck per second) in the immediate postnatal period to just more than 1 suck per second (70 per minute) by the end of the first month (Qureshi et al., 2002).

   2. The infant may exhibit interruptions (pauses) of various lengths.

      a. These interruptions might be part of the total suckling sequence (e.g., a few seconds of interruption after every 8 to 12 suck/swallow sequences) or they may be less predictable (Arvedson et al., 1993).

   3. The sucking rate is faster in nonnutritive sucking, averaging about 2 sucks per second (Wolf et al., 1992).

G. There is an inverse relationship between rate and flow. The higher the milk flow, the lower the rate of suckling (Bowen-Jones et al., 1982; Ramsay et al., 2004).

H. The rate of suckling may also be related to the size of the oral cavity. As the infant ages, the oral cavity enlarges, which might allow the infant to hold a greater amount of fluid before a swallow is needed (Wolf et al., 1992).

I. Qureshi and colleagues (2002) in a study of 16 bottle-fed infants found that the average volume of milk per suck and per swallow nearly doubled during the first month—average suck volume increased from 0.17 mL to 0.30 mL; average swallow volume increased from 0.23 mL to 0.44 mL. Qureshi and colleagues (2002) also found that over time infants gain the ability to adjust their feeding patterns to improve efficiency by adding suck:swallow ratios of 2:1, 3:1, and so on. Similar results were reported by Taki and colleagues (2010) in a study of 16 breastfed infants and 8 bottle-fed infants. They found that the average milk volume per suckle nearly doubled between 1 and 6 months of age in the breastfed infants, increasing from 0.15 mL per suck at 1 month to 0.25 mL at 3 months. Taki and colleagues (2010) also found that feeding efficiency (milliliters per minute) increased from an average of 6.6 mL/min at 1 month to 21.2 mL/min at 6 months.

J. Milk intake is positively correlated with the number of milk ejections (Ramsay et al., 2004).

K. Bowen-Jones and colleagues (1982) found that milk ejection occurs on average 2.2 minutes after the infant begins to suckle. However, Ramsay and colleagues (2004) reported milk ejection on average 56 seconds after the start of suckling, with each ejection lasting on average 1.5 minutes as defined by duct dilation. Milk ejection as demonstrated by an increase in duct diameter coincided with a change in the sucking pattern of the infant (Ramsay et al., 2004).

L. Control of milk intake comes under intrinsic control of the infant during the first month (Woolridge et al., 1982). Consistent with the theory that the infant's appetite regulates milk intake, Ramsay and colleagues (2004) found that in 39% of women with multiple milk ejections, the infant terminated a breastfeed during a milk ejection.

M. The wide range in breastmilk volume in well-nourished populations is the result more of variation in infant demand than it is to insufficient milk production (Dewey et al., 1986).

N. Sucking pressure plays an important role in modulating milk flow. It appears that infants generate more pressure through negative intraoral pressure (suction) than by positive pressure (compression) on the nipple (Ramsay et al., 2004).

O. Sucking pressures also vary with state and behavioral factors (Delaney et al., 2008). A sleepy infant generates less pressure than an alert infant does, and a hungry infant generates more pressure than an infant who is full. Gestational age also is important, with preterm infants, including late preterm infants, generating less vacuum than full-term infants, suggesting that feeding behavior matures over time (Lang et al., 2010).

VI. Suckling Cycle (Figure 18-1)

Ardran et al. (1958a, 1958b), using x-ray cineradiography, proposed a stripping theory of infant suckling and milk removal. This theory proposes that compression of the lactiferous sinuses and peristaltic tongue movements facilitate milk removal. Later descriptions based on ultrasound imaging revised our understanding of the anatomy of the breast and the mechanisms of milk removal, giving rise to a second theory described as the intraoral vacuum theory

(Geddes et al., 2008; Smith et al., 1988; Taki et al., 2010). Because the milk ducts were smaller in diameter than originally described (approximately 2 mm) and branch close to the nipple, the ductal system serves to transport rather than store milk (McClellan et al., 2010; Ramsay et al., 2008). Unlike the stripping theory, the intraoral vacuum theory does not rely on the presence of lactiferous sinuses within the breast.

A. The nipple, surrounding areola, and underlying tissue elongate to form a highly elastic teat.

B. The infant draws the teat into the mouth by means of a vacuum (baseline vacuum).

C. Application of a baseline vacuum places the nipple in the optimal position for removing milk from the breast and clearing it from the oral cavity (nipple approximately 6–8 mm from the junction of the hard and soft palates [HSPJ]). (See **Figure 18-1**.)

D. The lips and cheeks facilitate the formation of a seal and the creation of negative pressure in the oral cavity.

E. Negative pressure in the oral cavity functions to hold the teat in place. The jaw provides a stable base for the movements of other structures including the tongue, lips, and cheeks.

F. The tongue is then drawn down in a piston-like fashion, evenly expanding the nipple, increasing nipple duct diameter, moving the nipple closer to the HSPJ (4–5 mm), and increasing vacuum. As a result, milk flows into the infant's oral cavity (first half of the suck cycle).

G. As the tongue is drawn downward, the soft palate is also drawn down in apposition with the tongue creating a space for the milk bolus.

H. The tongue is then raised (tip first) and the milk bolus is cleared from the oral cavity under the soft palate. During this phase (second half of the suck cycle), vacuum reduces and the nipple is compressed.

I. The tongue then remains in apposition with the palate (no milk is evident) until the beginning of the next suck cycle.

VII. Factors That Affect Suckling and/or Contribute to Ineffective Suckling

Although it is difficult to list all the possible causes of dysfunction, several categories can be described along with examples.

A. Anomalies of the face, mouth, or pharynx
   1. Cleft lip/palate
   2. Macroglossia: Excessively large tongue
   3. Micrognathia: Recessed jaw and posteriorly placed tongue
   4. Ankyloglossia: Short/tight frenulum, commonly known as tongue-tie
   5. High palatal arch: Bubble palate

B. Dysfunction of the central or peripheral nervous system or musculature
   1. Prematurity
   2. Down syndrome or other genetic syndromes
   3. Asphyxia

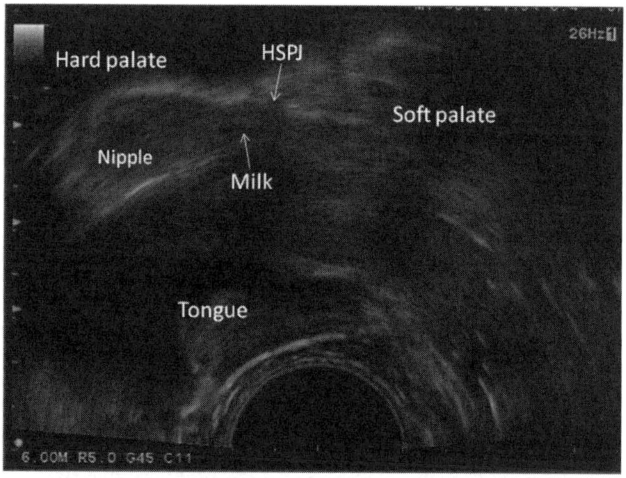

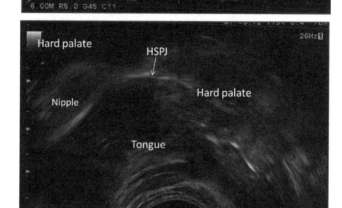

Figure 18-1a
Tongue up: A baseline vacuum is applied and the nipple is positioned about 7–8mm from the HSPJ. The nipple is compressed and elongated. No milk is evident as the tongue is in apposition with the palate. (Ramsay et al., 2004)

Figure 18-1b
Tongue down: in the first half of the suck cycle the nipple expands and moves closer to the HSPJ and milk flows into the oral cavity as vacuum strength increases. (Ramsay et al., 2004)

    4. Intracranial hemorrhage
    5. CNS infection (toxoplasmosis, cytomegalovirus, bacterial meningitis, and so forth)
  C. Miscellaneous factors
    1. Early use of artificial nipples
    2. Hyperbilirubinemia/kernicterus (Bertini et al., 2001; Hall et al., 2000; Nylander et al., 1991)
    3. Pain
      a. Oral herpes simplex lesions
      b. Oral candidiasis (thrush)
      c. Birth trauma secondary to forceps, vacuum extraction, suctioning, intubation, or other procedures
      d. Maternal anesthesia (with concomitant secondary depression of neonatal reflexes)

VIII. Conclusion

Through the use of advanced ultrasound technology, researchers can now visualize the breastfeeding infant and the lactating breast. Clear distinctions between breastfeeding and bottle-feeding are emerging. The importance of a neurologically mature infant is now well established, and understanding fetal development assists the lactation consultant in supporting preterm and near-term infants. Foremost among the findings is the remarkable adaptability of the human infant to effectively coordinate breathing, suckling, and swallowing.

References

American Academy of Pediatrics Task Force on Sudden Infant Death Syndrome. (2005). The changing concept of sudden infant death syndrome: Diagnostic coding shifts, controversies regarding the sleeping environment, and new variables to consider in reducing risk. *Pediatrics*, *116*(5), 1245–1255.

Ardran, G., Kemp, F., & Lind, J. (1958a). A cineradiographic study of bottle-feeding. *British Journal of Radiology*, *31*, 11–22.

Ardran, G., Kemp, F., & Lind, J. (1958b). A cineradiographic study of breast-feeding. *British Journal of Radiology*, *31*, 156–162.

Arvedson, J., & Brodsky, L. (1993). *Pediatric swallowing and feeding*. San Diego, CA: Singular.

Bertini, G., Dani, C., Tronchin, M., & Rubaltelli, F. F. (2001). Is breastfeeding really favoring early neonatal jaundice? *Pediatrics*, *107*, E41.

Bosma, K. (1985). Postnatal otogeny of performances of the pharynx, larynx and mouth. *American Review of Respiratory Diseases*, *131*, S10–S15.

Bowen-Jones, A., Thompson, C., & Drewett, R. F. (1982). Milk flow and sucking rates during breast-feeding. *Developmental Medicine and Child Neurology*, *24*, 626–633.

Bu'Lock, F., Woolridge, M. W., & Baum, J. D. (1990). Development of coordination of sucking, swallowing and breathing: Ultrasound study of term and preterm infants. *Developmental Medicine and Child Neurology*, *32*, 669–678.

Delaney, A., & Arvedson, J. (2008). Development of swallowing and feeding: Prenatal through first year of life. *Developmental Disabilities Research Reviews*, *14*, 105–117.

Dewey, K. G., & Lonnerdal, B. (1986). Infant self-regulation of breast milk intake. *Acta Paediatrica Scandinavica*, *75*, 893–898.

Diamant, N. (1985). Development of esophageal function. *American Review of Respiratory Disease*, *131*, S29–S32.

Faturi, C. B., Tiba, P. A., Kawakami, S. E., Catallani, B., Kerstens, M., Suchecki, D., et al. (2010). Disruptions of the mother–infant relationship and stress-related behaviours: Altered corticosterone secretion does not explain everything. *Neuroscience and Biobehavioral Reviews*, *34*, 6, 821–834.

Geddes, D., et al. (2008). Tongue movement and intra-oral vacuum in breastfeeding infants. *Early Human Development*, 84, 7, 471-477.

Gryboski, J. (1975). Gastrointestinal problems in the infant. Major problems in clinical pediatrics. *XIII*, 17–47.

Hack, M., Estabrook, M., & Robertson, S. (1985). Development of sucking rhythms in preterm infants. *Early Human Development*, *11*, 133–140.

Hall, R. T., Simon, S., & Smith, M. T. (2000). Readmission of breastfed infants in the first 2 weeks of life. *Journal of Perinatology*, *20*, 432–437.

Harman, C. (2008). Amniotic fluid abnormalities. *Seminars in Perinatology*, *32*(4), 288–294.

Hauck, F. R., Herman, S. M., Donovan, M., et al. (2003). Sleep environment and the risk of sudden infant death syndrome in an urban population: The Chicago Infant Mortality Study. *Pediatrics*, *111*, 1207–1214.

Howard, C. R., Howard, F. M., Lanphear, B., et al. (2003). Randomized clinical trial of pacifier use and bottle-feeding or cupfeeding and their effect on breastfeeding. *Pediatrics*, *111*, 511–518.

Ianniruberto, A., & Tajani, E. (1981). Ultrasonographic study of fetal movements. *Seminars in Perinatology*, *5*, 175–181.

Illingworth, R. S., & Lister, J. (1964). The critical or sensitive period, with special reference to certain feeding problems in infants and children. *Journal of Pediatrics*, *65*, 839–848.

Ingram, J., Hunt, L., Woolridge, M., & Greenwood, R. (2004). The association of progesterone, infant formula use and pacifier use with the return of menstruation in breast-feeding women: A prospective cohort study. *European Journal of Obstetrics and Gynecology and Reproductive Biology*, *114*, 197–202.

Kahn, A., Groswasser, J., Franco, P., et al. (2003). Sudden infant deaths: Stress, arousal and SIDS. *Early Human Development*, *75*(Suppl.), S147–S166.

Kennedy, J., & Kent, R. (1988). Physiologic substrates of normal deglutition. *Dysphagia*, *3*, 24–27.

Lang, C. L., Buist, N. R. M., Geary, A., Buckley, S., Adams, E., Jones, A. C., et al. (2010). Quantification of intraoral pressures during nutritive sucking: Methods with normal infants. *Dysphagia*, 26.

Lawrence, R. A. (2011). *Breastfeeding: A guide for the medical profession* (7th ed.). St. Louis, MO: Mosby.

McClellan, H. L., Sakalidis, V. S., Hepworth, A. R., Hartman, P. E., & Geddes, D. T. (2010). Validation of nipple diameter and tongue movement measurements with b-mode ultrasound during breastfeeding. *Ultrasound in Medicine and Biology*, *36*, 1797–1807.

Miller, M., Martin, R., & Carlo, W. (1985). Oral breathing in newborn infants. *Journal of Pediatrics*, *107*, 465–469.

Mizuno, K., & Ueda, A. (2005). Changes in sucking performance from nonnutritive sucking to nutritive sucking during breast- and bottle-feeding. *Pediatric Research*, *59*, 728–731.

Morris, S. (1982). *The normal acquisition of oral feeding skills: Implications for assessment and treatment.* Central Islip, NY: Therapeutic Media.

Nylander, G., Lindemann, R., Helsing, E., & Bendvold, E. (1991). Unsupplemented breastfeeding in the maternity ward. Positive long-term effects. *Acta Obstetricia et Gynecologica Scandinavica*, *70*, 205–209.

Pritchard, J. (1966). Fetal swallowing and amniotic fluid volume. *Obstetrics and Gynecology*, *28*, 606–610.

Qureshi, M. A., Vice, F. L., Taciak, V. L., Bosma, J. F., & Gewolb, I. H. (2002). Changes in rhythmic suckle feeding patterns in term infants in the first month of life. *Developmental Medicine and Child Neurology*, *44*, 34–39.

Ramsay, D. T., Kent, J. C., Owens, R. A., & Hartmann, P. E. (2004). Ultrasound imaging of milk ejection in the breast of lactating women. *Pediatrics*, *113*, 361–367.

Reynolds, E. W., Grider, D., Caldwell, R., Capilouto, G., Vijaygopal, P., Patwardhan, A., & Charnigo, R. (2010). Swallow–breath interaction and phase of respiration with swallow during nonnutritive suck among low-risk preterm infants. *American Journal of Perinatology*, *27*(10), 831–840.

Righard, L., & Alade, M. O. (1990). Effect of delivery room routines on success of first breast-feed. *Lancet*, *336*, 1105–1107.

Rodenstein, D., Perlmutter, N., & Stanescu, D. (1985). Infants are not obligatory nose breathers. *American Review of Respiratory Disease*, *131*, 343–347.

Ross, M. G., & Nyland, M. J. M. (1998). Development of ingestive behavior. *American Journal of Physiology*, *43*, R879–R893.

Smith, W. L., Erenberg, A., & Nowak, A. (1988). Imaging evaluation of the human nipple during breast-feeding. *American Journal of the Disease of Children*, *142*, 76–78.

Taki, M., Minuzo, K., Murase, M., Nishida, Y., Itabashi, K., & Mukai, Y. (2010). Maturational changes in the feeding behavior of infants—a comparison between breast-feeding and bottle-feeding. *Acta Paediatrica*, *99*, 61–67.

Tucker, J. (1985). Perspective of the development of the air and food passages. American Review of Respiratory Disease, *131*, S7–S9.

Ullah, S., & Griffiths, P. (2003). Does the use of pacifiers shorten breastfeeding duration in infants? *British Journal of Community Nursing*, *8*, 458–463.

Viggiano, D., Fasano, D., Monaco, G., & Strohmenger, L. (2004). Breast feeding, bottle feeding, and non-nutritive sucking; effects on occlusion in deciduous dentition. *Archives of Disease in Childhood*, *89*, 1121–1123.

Weber, F., Woolridge, M., & Baum, J. (1986). An ultrasonographic study of the organization of sucking and swallowing by newborn infants. *Developmental Medicine and Child Neurology*, *28*, 19–24.

Widstrom, A. M., Wahlberg, V., Matthiesen, A. S., et al. (1990). Short-term effects of early suckling and touch of the nipple on maternal behaviour. *Early Human Development*, *21*, 153–163.

Wilson, S., Thach, B., & Brouillet, R. (1980). Upper airway patency in the human infant: Influence of airway pressure and posture. *Journal of Applied Physiology*, *48*, 500–504.

Wolf, L., & Glass, R. (1992). *Feeding and swallowing disorders in infancy: Assessment and management.* San Antonio, TX: Therapy Skill Builders.

Woolridge, M. W., How, T. V., Drewett, R. F., et al. (1982). The continuous measurement of milk intake at a feed in breast-fed babies. *Early Human Development*, *6*, 365–373.

Suggested Reading

Anderson, G. (1982). Development of sucking in term infants from birth to four hours post birth. *Research in Nursing and Health*, *5*, 21–27.

Awi, D. D., & Alikor, E. A. (2004). The influence of pre- and post-partum factors on the time of contact between mother and her new-born after vaginal delivery. *Nigerian Journal of Medicine*, *13*, 272–275.

Bader, A. M., Fragneto, R., Terui, K., et al. (1995). Maternal and neonatal fentanyl and bupivacaine concentrations after epidural infusion during labor. *Anesthesia and Analgesia*, *81*, 829–832.

Bader, A. M., Ray, N., & Datta, S. (1992). Continuous epidural infusion of alfentanil and bupivacaine for labor and delivery. *International Journal of Obstetric Anesthesia*, *1*, 187–190.

Baumgarder, D., Muehl, P., Fischer, M., & Pribbenow, B. (2003). Effect of labor epidural anesthesia on breastfeeding of healthy full-term newborns delivered vaginally. *Journal of the American Board of Family Practitioners*, *16*, 7–13.

Blomquist, H. K., Jonsbo, F., Serenius, F., & Persson, L. A. (1994). Supplementary feeding in the maternity ward shortens the duration of breast feeding. *Acta Paediatrica*, *83*, 1122–1126.

Brake, S., Fifer, W., Alfasi, G., & Fleischman, A. (1988). The first nutritive sucking responses of premature newborns. *Infant Behavior and Development, 11*, 1–9.

Braun, M. L., Giugliani, E. R., Soares, M. E., et al. (2003). Evaluation of the impact of the Baby-friendly Hospital Initiative on rates of breastfeeding. *American Journal of Public Health, 93*, 1277–1279.

Bunik, M., et al. (2011). ABM clinical protocol #10: Breastfeeding the late preterm infant (34(0/7) to 36(6/7) weeks gestation) (first revision June 2011). *Breastfeeding Medicine, 6*(3), 151–156.

Buranasin, B. (1991). The effects of rooming-in on the success of breastfeeding and the decline in abandonment of children. *Asia Pacific Journal of Public Health, 5*, 217–220.

Casaer, P., Daniels, H., Devlieger, H., et al. (1982). Feeding behavior in preterm neonates. *Early Human Development, 7*, 331–346.

Casiday, R. E., Wright, C. M., Panter-Brick, C., & Parkinson, K. N. (2004). Do early infant feeding patterns relate to breast-feeding continuation and weight gain? Data from a longitudinal cohort study. *European Journal of Clinical Nutrition, 58*, 1290–1296.

Centuori, S., Burmaz, T., Ronfani, L., et al. (1999). Nipple care, sore nipples, and breastfeeding: A randomized trial. *Journal of Human Lactation, 15*, 125–130.

Ellison, S., Vidyasagar, V., & Anderson, G. (1979). Sucking in the newborn infant during the first hour of life. *Journal of Nurse Midwifery, 24*, 18–25.

Fisher, S., Painter, M., & Milmoe, G. (1981). Swallowing disorders in infancy. *Pediatric Clinics of North America, 28*, 845–853.

Hall, R. T., Mercer, A. M., Teasley, S. L., et al. (2002). A breastfeeding assessment score to evaluate the risk for cessation of breastfeeding by 7 to 10 days of age. *Journal of Pediatrics, 141*, 659–664.

Hill, P. D., Humenick, S. S., Brennan, M. L., & Woolley, D. (1997). Does early supplementation affect long-term breastfeeding? *Clinical Pediatrics (Philadelphia), 36*, 345–350.

Hodgkinson, R., Bhatt, M., & Wang, C. (1978). Double-blind comparison of the neurobehavior of neonates following the administration of different doses of meperidine to the mother. *Canadian Anaesthetists Society Journal, 25*, 405–411.

Kramer, M. S., Barr, R. G., Dagenais, S., et al. (2001). Pacifier use, early weaning, and cry/fuss behavior: A randomized controlled trial. *Journal of the American Medical Association, 286*, 322–326.

Kurinij, N., & Shiono, P. H. (1991). Early formula supplementation of breast-feeding. *Pediatrics, 88*, 745–750.

Lindenberg, C. S., Cabrera Artola, R., & Jimenez, V. (1990). The effect of early post-partum mother–infant contact and breast-feeding promotion on the incidence and continuation of breast-feeding. *International Journal of Nursing Studies, 27*, 179–186.

Medoff-Cooper, B., Bilker, W., & Kaplan, J. (2010). Sucking patterns and behavioral state in 1- and 2-day-old full-term infants. *Journal of Obstetric, Gynecologic, and Neonatal Nursing, 39*, 519–524.

Meites, J. (1974). Neuroendocrinology of lactation. *Journal of Investigative Dermatology, 63*, 119–124.

Murray, A., Dolby, R., Nation, R., & Thomas, D. B. (1981). Effects of epidural anesthesia on newborns and their mothers. *Child Development, 52*, 71–82.

Nordeng, H., & Havnen, G. C. (2004). Use of herbal drugs in pregnancy: A survey among 400 Norwegian women. *Pharmacoepidemiology and Drug Safety, 13*, 371–380.

Nordeng, H., Lindemann, R., Perminov, K. V., & Reikvam, A. (2001). Neonatal withdrawal syndrome after in utero exposure to selective serotonin reuptake inhibitors. *Acta Paediatrica, 90*, 288–291.

Nysenbaum, A., & Smart, J. (1982). Sucking behavior and milk intake of neonates in relation to milk fat content. *Early Human Development, 6*, 205–213.

Palmer, M. M., Crawley, K., & Blanco, I. A. (1993). Neonatal oral-motor assessment scale: A reliability study. *Journal of Perinatology, XIII*(1), 28–35.

Perez-Escamilla, R., Pollitt, E., Lonnerdal, B., & Dewey, K. G. (1994). Infant feeding policies in maternity wards and their effect on breast-feeding success: An analytical overview. *American Journal of Public Health, 84*, 89–97.

Philipp, B. L., Malone, K. L., Cimo, S., & Merewood, A. (2003). Sustained breastfeeding rates at a US baby-friendly hospital. *Pediatrics, 112*, 234–236.

Philipp, B. L., & Merewood, A. (2004). The baby-friendly way: The best breastfeeding start. *Pediatric Clinics of North AmErica, 51*, xi, 761–783.

Ramsay, D. T., Kent, J. C., Hartmann, R. A., & Hartmann, P. E. (2005). Anatomy of the lactating human breast redefined with ultrasound imaging. *Journal of Anatomy, 206*, 525–534.

Riordan, J., Gross, A., Angeron, J., et al. (2000). The effect of labor pain relief medication on neonatal suckling and breastfeeding duration. *Journal of Human Lactation, 16*, 7–10.

Rosen, A., & Lawrence, R. (1994). The effect of epidural anesthesia on infant feeding. *Journal of the University of Rochester Medical Center, 6*, 3.

Sievers, E., Haase, S., Oldigs, H. D., & Schaub, J. (2003). The impact of peripartum factors on the onset and duration of lactation. *Biology of the Neonate, 83*, 246–252.

Strembel. S., Sass, S., Cole, G., Hartner, J., & Fischer, C. (1991). Breast-feeding policies and routines among Arizona hospitals and nursery staff: Results and implications of a descriptive study. *Journal of the American Dietetic Association, 91*, 923–925.

Torvaldsen, S., Roberts, C. L., Simpson, J. M., Thompson, J. F., & Ellwood, D. A. (2006). Intrapartum epidural analgesia and breastfeeding: A prospective cohort study. *International Breastfeeding Journal, 1*, 24.

Vestermark, V., Hogdall, C., & Birch, M. (1990). Influence of the mode of delivery on initiation of breastfeeding. *European Journal of Obstetrics and Gynecology and Reproductive Biology, 38*, 33.

Voloschin, L. M., Althabe, O., Olive, H., et al. (1998). A new tool for measuring the suckling stimulus during breastfeeding in humans: The orokinetogram and the Fourier series. *Journal of Reproduction and Fertility, 114*, 219–224.

Widstrom, A. M., Marchini, G., Matthiesen, A. S., et al. (1988). Nonnutritive sucking in tube-fed preterm infants: Effects on gastric motility and gastric contents of somatostatin. *Journal of Pediatric Gastroenterology and Nutrition, 7*, 517–523.

Wolff, P. (1968). The serial organization of sucking in the young infant. *Pediatrics, 42*, 943–956.

Wolff, P. (1972). The interaction of state and non-nutritive sucking. In J. Bosma (Ed.), *Oral sensation and perception* (pp. 293–312). Springfield, MO: Charles C. Thomas.

Woolridge, M. W. (1986). The anatomy of infant suckling. *Midwifery, 2*, 164–171.

Woolridge, M. W., Baum, J. D., & Drewett, R. F. (1980). Does a change in the composition of human milk affect sucking patterns and milk intake? *Lancet, 2*, 1292–1293.

World Health Organization. (1998). *Evidence for the Ten Steps to Successful Breastfeeding* (Rev. ed.). Unpublished manuscript.

World Health Organization/United Nations International Children's Emergency Fund. (1990). Protecting, promoting and supporting breastfeeding: The special role of maternity services. A joint WHO/UNICEF statement. *International Journal of Gynaecology and Obstetrics, 31*(Suppl. 1), 171–183.

Yamauchi, Y., & Yamanouchi, I. (1990). The relationship between rooming-in/not rooming-in and breast-feeding variables. *Acta Paediatrica Scandinavica, 79*, 1017–1022.

Part 4

Nutrition and Biochemistry

CHAPTER 19
Nutrition for Lactating Women

Michelle Scott, MA, RD/LD, IBCLC

OBJECTIVES

- Discuss how lactating women's diet is different from a healthy diet for women of the same age, including special considerations for lactating teenage mothers.
- Understand how certain disease states may affect the nutritional status of lactating women.
- Describe how overweight or underweight might affect ability to nurse and quality of milk.
- Distinguish levels of individual nutrients in lactating women's diet that affect the quantity of those nutrients in the breastmilk.
- Help mothers determine whether particular foods might affect breastmilk and perhaps should be eliminated or added and the use of nutritional supplements.
- Help mothers evaluate a healthy diet and understand what they need to improve through making healthier choices and perhaps accessing food through community resources.
- Evaluate the need for referral to a dietitian or nutritionist who has expertise with lactating women or other health professionals, such as social workers or therapists, for help with eating disorders.

INTRODUCTION

The prenatal period is frequently a prime time when women become more interested in their nutritional status (Olson, 2005). Similarly, the lactating woman often has a continuing interest in nutrition for providing high-quality breastmilk. During lactation, cultural and social influences might need to be honored and the lactation consultant might need to discuss myths, with or without scientific foundation, with mothers so that they can make their own decisions. Breastmilk quality is influenced by nutrient intake, and a healthy diet contributes to the energy level and well-being of women. Mothers frequently ask what they can and cannot eat. During lactation, there are no general food restrictions as long as the mother is not allergic to certain foods and tolerates the food or beverage. There is no need to make breastfeeding seem difficult by

(continues)

providing lists of foods to avoid. Women should not hesitate to nurse their babies if their diet is not good or ideal because most key nutrients are available in breastmilk. The goal in this chapter is to help the lactation consultant evaluate the risks of poor nutrition in patients/clients through an understanding of basic requirements, address common questions regarding nutrition and lactation, and make referrals as needed.

I. Assessment and Referral

A. The interview: How to assess. Consider prenatal and pregnancy nutrition issues or concerns, infant issues about weight gain and irritability, and mother's concerns about nutrition and food.

   1. Use open-ended questions to give the mother a chance to describe her diet and food-related concerns (Miller et al., 2002).
   2. Ask for information such as, "Tell me what you usually eat for breakfast. Tell me what you ate and drank yesterday over the whole day, meals and snacks."
   3. Avoid questions with yes or no or one-word answers, for example, "How is your diet?"
   4. As a health professional, go through the mother's day with her, asking how many times the baby fed, how she thinks the feedings are going, when and what the mother ate and drank.
   5. Generally, there should be at least four servings of protein foods such as milk, cheese, meat, eggs, nuts, and beans (legumes) and at least four to five servings of fruit or vegetables. Carbohydrates are seldom an issue, but four to six servings should include some whole grains.
   6. By finding out what the mother eats, the lactation consultant can determine whether there is an eating disorder, neglect of self, or other concern.
   7. The lactation consultant should be sure to ask about supplements and any medications (both prescribed and over-the-counter medications and any herbal supplements) the mother may be taking.

B. Risk factors

   1. Body mass index (BMI) is a measure of percentage of body fat. It gives a good indication of risk at the upper and lower ends, and normal has a wide range. For example: For someone 5 ft 5 in., or 162 cm—the normal ranges from 120 to 155 lb, or 54.5 to 70.4 kg. See **Table 19-1**.
      a. Normal between 18.5 and 25
      b. Underweight: BMI <18.5
      c. Overweight: BMI ≥ 25 to < 30
      d. Obese: BMI ≥ 30

Table 19-1 The International Classification of adult underweight, overweight, and obesity according to BMI

Classification	BMI (kg/m)	
	Principal cut-off points	**Additional cut-off points**
Underweight	**< 18.50**	**< 18.50**
Severe thinness	< 16.00	< 16.00
Moderate thinness	16.00–16.99	16.00–16.99
Mild thinness	17.00–18.49	17.00–18.49
Normal range	**18.50–24.99**	**18.50–22.99**
		23.00–24.99
Overweight	**> 25.00**	**> 25.00**
Pre-obese	25.00–29.99	25.00–27.49
		27.50–29.99
Obese	**> 30.00**	**> 30.00**
Obese class I	30.00–34.99	30.00–32.49
		32.50–34.99
Obese class II	35.00–39.99	35.00–37.49
		37.50–39.99
Obese class III	> 40.00	> 40.00

Source: Adapted from WHO, 1995, WHO, 2000 and WHO 2004.

2. Weight issues: Underweight:
   a. May have insufficient micronutrients because of low maternal storage resulting from poor diet.
   b. Ask about surgical history for bariatric patients, malabsorption diseases such as Crohn's disease, and other gastrointestinal (GI)-related history.
   c. Underweight might be indicative of disordered eating with consequences affecting lactation such as very low fat in milk and low levels of some nutrients.
3. Weight issues: Overweight:
   a. Women might have a healthy diet (Durham et al., 2011).
   b. Delayed lactogenesis II has been reported in obese mothers, making it necessary to provide breastfeeding guidelines for use during a prolonged colostral phase (Jewitt et al., 2007).
   c. Lactogenesis II can be delayed by cesarean births with postnatal complications and/or prolonged labor.

    d. Although lactation might reduce obesity of both mother and infant, obese women are statistically less likely to initiate and maintain lactation because of birth complications and/or short or flat nipples resulting from oversized breasts (Jewitt et al., 2007).

    e. Obese mothers have a greater risk of a macrosomic baby and tend to breast-feed (and exclusively breastfeed) for shorter periods of time than do normal-weight mothers (Leonard et al., 2011).

    f. Obese mothers may be at risk for nutrient deficiencies of vitamins A, E, C, and folate if they consume a diet typical of American women. Women from other countries can have different concerns (Durham et al., 2011; (Kimmons et al., 2006).

4. Teenagers who are less than 4 years from menarche:

    a. Diets of teens are frequently low in iron, calcium, and other nutrients as a result of eating habits or their own growth issues as well as the fetal demands, but teens can and should be encouraged to breastfeed (Institute of Medicine [IOM] Food and Nutrition Board, 2010).

5. Medical conditions—type 1 or type 2 diabetes, gestational diabetes, bariatric surgery, gastrointestinal malabsorption (Crohn's disease, irritable bowel syndrome [IBS], metabolic conditions such as phenylketonuria [PKU]), or eating disorders:

    a. Birth has some effects on insulin: Imbalances change after pregnancy and need lowering under most circumstances because there is no fetus making demands internally. Monitor blood glucose postpartum. Lactogenesis may be delayed in type 1 diabetes (Hartmann et al., 2001). See Chapter 39, Insufficient Milk Supply, for more information.

    b. Women who have had bariatric surgery are at increased risk of nutritional deficiencies, especially vitamin B_{12}, because of insufficient calories or absorptive issues.

    c. Allergies might restrict food intake, and self-imposed dietary restrictions might limit certain nutrients.

    d. Twin and triplet births may increase protein and nutrient demands—refer mothers to a dietitian to evaluate their diet.

    e. Present weight may be within normal limits, but recent weight loss or gain might present a risk resulting from nutrient stores or restricted or unusual eating patterns.

    f. Pregnancies less than 18 months apart (including miscarriages) create high nutrient demand (King, 2003).

    g. Poor diet may be an indicator or marker of other health issues.

    h. Poverty, physical disability, single mothers, mental illness, or limited intellectual ability can all affect diet intake.

i. Not enough food or available food: Refer to a dietitian or nutritionist for specific dietary guidance. Refer to social services for help with other issues that affect food intake and choices. The U.S. Department of Agriculture Special Supplemental Nutrition Program for Women, Infants and Children (WIC) can help provide nutritious foods for mothers. Other sources of supplemental foods include food banks and pantries, soup kitchens, and regional or local family support programs.

II. General Nutrition Recommendations for Lactation

A. Preconception nutrition and weight status can affect pregnancy and lactation by such factors as low vitamin/mineral stores and continuing poor diet. Reduce weight before pregnancy to near normal BMI range, assess iron and folic acid status, and discuss steps to reduce foodborne illness (see U.S. Food and Drug Administration [FDA] website on food safety or Food Standards Agency in the United Kingdom; most other countries have similar agencies).

B. Nutrition support and assessment need to be included in postpartum support.

   1. Lactation—general recommendations for women: Lactation is a normal physiologic process for a woman who is generally healthy. Mothering is hard work, but women seem designed to make the adaptation without needing major adjustments in diet or special diets (Butte et al., 2001). All mothers who are caring for young children need to eat well, although not perfectly, every day.

   2. Lactation and pregnancy increase the body's efficiency in use of energy and the uptake of some nutrients (e.g., calcium).

   3. Women should eat a variety of foods. See the USDA My Plate at www.choosemyplate.gov/mypyramidmoms for typical recommendations, including those for vegetarian and other special diets.

   4. Mothers should drink to satisfy thirst, using water first, as well as other healthy beverages such as milk and juice. Small quantities of coffee, tea, and soda can be included. Pale urine is an indicator of adequate fluids. More fluids do not increase breastmilk quantity, and excessive fluids can actually cause a decrease in milk production (Morse et al., 1992).

   5. Weight loss postpartum is more likely to occur for women who breastfeed (Onyango et al., 2011) but depends on activity level, food choices, calories consumed, and individual metabolism.

   6. Lactating women's diets should be in the range of 50–55% carbohydrates (mostly unrefined carbohydrates are recommended), 12–15% protein (about 1 g per kilogram of normal weight), and 20–30% fats (most fats should be unsaturated, non trans fatty acids) (Mozaffarian et al., 2006).

C. Energy and weight patterns:
1. Pregnancy calorie recommendations are based on an average calorie per kilogram of normal and overweight (BMI 20–29), with none or few extra calories in the first trimester, 300/day for the second and third trimesters.
2. In lactation, about 500 extra calories per day (approximately the calories contained in one peanut butter and jelly sandwich or meat sandwich) are required during the first 6 months, with some calories supplied by the body fat stored during pregnancy. No prescription for a set calorie level is usually made (IOM Food and Nutrition Board, 2005).
3. Calorie cost of 1 L of breastmilk is about 940 calories, with most women producing about 750 mL/day.
4. Each milliliter is about 0.67 calories plus some energy for the metabolic cost of synthesis.
5. The 500-calorie-per-day "cost" of breastmilk is an average that depends on the woman's fat stores and foods consumed (Butte et al., 2001).
D. Protein needs: Average requirement is 65 g/day in first 6 months of lactation, 62 g for the next 6 months. Example: 4 oz meat is 28 g of protein; 24 oz milk is 24 g of protein; four servings of carbohydrates is 15 g of protein: 28 g + 24 g +15 g = total of 67 g of protein.
E. Vegetarians, vegans, and lacto-ovo diets: Vegetarians get most protein from dairy, legumes, nuts, and carbohydrates. Vegans eat no animal products and are at risk for vitamin B_{12} deficiency. Some vegetarians eat seafood, eggs, and some occasionally include meats such as chicken (Butte et al., 2005). Evaluate diets for protein and B_{12} (IOM Food and Nutrition Board, 2005).
F. Fats: Adequate intake of fats is about 20–35% of total calories. Recommended types of fats are small amounts of saturated fats (animal fats), no recommendation for trans fats, and small amounts of omega-3 fatty acids (α-linolenic), which include DHA, in the form of seafood (from nonmercury sources), eggs, or a supplement. Consumption of 1.3 g of DHA is recommended (IOM Food and Nutrition Board, 2005) for lactating women.
G. Vitamins and minerals—see **Table 19-2**.
1. During lactation, the need for some vitamins and minerals is increased, but so is food intake.
2. Taking a vitamin supplement is often recommended. Supplements should not exceed the Recommended Daily Intake (RDI) by more than 20% because some vitamins can accumulate in tissue and cause toxicity (IOM Food and Nutrition Board, 2005).
3. Refer mothers to a dietitian if there is any concern for micronutrient intake, either deficiency or excess. Use discretion because women need not become overly concerned to the point of giving up breastfeeding.
4. In general, the following micronutrients in breastmilk are affected by low maternal status: thiamin, riboflavin, vitamin B_6, vitamin B_{12}, vitamins D and A, and selenium. Unless a known deficiency is found, most are rapidly restored by increasing the mother's intake.

5. Nutrients not generally affected by the mother's status are zinc, iron, folate, calcium, and copper.
6. A more recent concern among well-nourished women is the use of megadoses of micronutrients through the use of supplements or fortified energy bars and drinks. See **Table 19-2** for information.
7. Vitamin D deficiencies may be corrected by the use of megadoses, and these should be taken under a physician's guidance and reduced when the blood levels are normalized (Basile et al., 2006; Hollis, 2007).
8. Iron:
   a. Ideally, anemia should be corrected preconception.
   b. Testing ferritin level is more accurate than is measuring hemoglobin because of hemodilution during pregnancy. Supplements should be used cautiously because there are side effects of constipation or diarrhea and teratogenicity (Tran et al., 2000).
   c. During lactation, little extra iron is needed because small amounts are secreted into milk, and the woman is no longer growing a fetus or menstruating. A multivitamin is recommended for all women of childbearing age because this helps to ensure adequate levels of micronutrients for breastmilk and the woman herself, as well as the possibility of an unplanned pregnancy.
9. Calcium:
   a. Because of phytates in whole grains that bind calcium, a diet that is mostly whole grains can be deficient in calcium. This is mainly a concern in countries where people's diets depend mostly on whole grains or in certain disordered eating patterns.
   b. If a woman is allergic or intolerant to dairy products, she may want to take a calcium supplement of 600 mg. Calcium citrate is preferred over calcium carbonate for better absorption. Calcium should be taken separately from iron supplements.
   c. Bone loss occurs during lactation even when dietary calcium is thought to be adequate. To some extent, remineralization takes place in breastfeeding women following the return of the menses, which ultimately results in more dense bones. Studies have shown that multipara women who breastfeed are not at higher risk for osteoporosis and might even have less risk (Henderson et al., 2000; Lenora et al., 2009).

H. Exercise: The mother who exercises strenuously for more than 1 hour per day might have increased calorie needs. Breast refusal by the infant following a mother's extremely heavy exercise has been suggested to be caused by elevated levels of lactic acid, but this has been refuted by two recent studies (Lovelady, 2011; Wright et al., 2002).

I. Special needs during lactation:
   1. Young women younger than 20 years of age, especially those who are fewer than 4 years past menarche: Diet evaluation by dietitian is recommended because of risk of low iron, folic acid, and calcium. Lack of knowledge of nutrition may coincide with a desire to do the best for the baby, making this an opportunity for nutrition education.

Table 19-2 Vitamins and Minerals For Lactating Women

Vitamin or Mineral	RDA	RDA during lactation	Upper Tolerable Limits (UL)	Comments on levels in breast-milk, and woman's status	Food Sources
Vitamins					
Vitamin A	700 RE	1300 RE first 6 mo 1200 RE 6–12 mo of lactation	50,000 IU in women	Vitamin A will be present in brmilk at expense of mother's stores, unless mother is deficient as in some developing countries, then should be supplemented. Carotenes are converted to Vit A.	Any leafy greens or green herb, pumpkin, other dark orange vegetables, fortified cereals and dairy products. Beta carotenes (and other carotenes) have no known upper limit, but supplements of vitamin A >UL can be teratrogenic, and for the mother and/or infant may cause liver damage or neurological problems.
Vitamin D	600 IU	400–600 IU for lactation 400 IU for infants	4000 IU for women 1,000 for infants	Mother's milk is increased in vit D only when 1,000 to 4,000 IU are given. Infants can be given 400 IU, and mother's will get 600 400++ in a vitamin supplement + sunshine, with no risk of vit D toxicity	Eggs, fatty fish such as salmon or sardines, and vitamin D fortified milk. Some 'energy' bars are also fortified. Caution with consumption of fish due to mercury and PCB contamination. See www.montereybayaquarium.org for healthy seafood choices.
Vitamin E	15mg	19mg	100–800 mg	Deficiency rare, no known benefit for high doses.	Nuts, green leafy vegetables, wheat germ and oils such as soy, corn and safflower.
Vitamin K	90mcg	90mcg	None stated	Deficiency in newborns prevented by vit K admin at birth. Breastmilk contains small amt not changed by average supplement	Leafy greens provide from 50 to 800 mcg per 100 g serving. Very small amt in other foods. Present in multivitamins.
Folate	400mcg	500mcg	800mcg,	Under most circumstances, breastmilk will be sufficient at expense of mother's stores. Caution with continuing very high dose given to prevent neural tube defects in pregnancy.	Legumes such as kidney beans, soybeans, chick peas, spinach and other dark leafy greens, orange juice, cantaloupe, sweet potato. Caution with highly fortified foods, while taking supplements.
Thiamin	1.1mg	1.4mg	None Known	Deficiencies are rare, thiamin in breastmilk is usually 0.2mg in 750ml of breastmilk.	Unrefined whole grains like whole wheat, or oats, lean pork, legumes, seeds, and nuts. Enriched flour and cereal have thiamin added.
Riboflavin	1.1mg	1.4mg	None known excess poorly absorbed	Deficiencies rare, small amounts in breastmilk available for infant.	Animal protein, enriched grain products, most green vegetables, like broccoli, turnip greens, asparagus, spinach.
Niacin	14mg	18mg	35mg	Very high doses given for cholesterol reduction may not be appropriate during lactation.	In a diet with meats/eggs/dairy products there will be sufficient niacin. A diet lacking these, would need a higher level of niacin by ingestion of fortified grains, or a supplement.

Pantothenic acid	5mg	7mg	None known	Much of the pantothenic acid is secreted into breastmilk, deficiencies very rare except for very malnourished women.	Available in grains, animal tissues, and legumes, with smaller amounts in milk, vegetables and fruits.
Vitamin B$_6$	1.2mg	2.0mg	80mg high levels cause neurological, GI, and skin problems	B$_6$ levels in milk depend on maternal intake and increases readily with foods/supplements.	Richest sources: chicken, fish, kidney, liver, pork, and eggs. Brown rice, soy beans, oats, and whole wheat products, peanuts, and walnuts.
Vitamin B$_{12}$	2.6mcg	2.8mcg	None determined	Deficiencies mostly in women not eating animal products, or in disturbances of intrinsic factor in the case of GI issues. Urinary excretion of methylmalanoic acid is indicative of deficiency.	Animal products where it has accumulated from bacterial synthesis. Plant foods are essentially devoid of B$_{12}$ except for microbially formed B$_{12}$ as seen in the case of some fermented foods.

Minerals

Iron	15mg	15mg	45 mg	Even women low in iron will provide the same amount for their infants as women with adequate iron.	Two kinds of iron exist: heme iron from meats which is absorbed more efficiently, and nonheme iron from plant foods which is also absorbed but not as efficiently. Meats, breads, watermelon, nuts/seeds, legumes are all sources of iron.
Zinc	8mg	12mg	40mg	Chronic high dose can interfere with copper absorption, interfere with immune suppression, and lower HDL.	Oysters, meats/chicken, fortified cereals, oatmeal, some legumes and nuts.
Calcium	1300 for <19yr 1000 for >19 yr	same as RDI for non-lact	2500mg	Calcium content of breastmilk not affected by maternal diet	Dairy, leafy dark greens, sesame seeds, broccoli, and small amounts in many foods including the use of some preservatives
Copper	900 μgm	1300 μgm	10000 μgm	Rarely a concern, except for dx of Wilson's disease which results in low serum copper	Copper is present in organ meats, seafoods, nuts, and seeds. May be available if copper pipes used for conduit of drinking water
Magnesium	310mg	310mg	350mg as a supplement	Magnesium in foods is not a concern for overdose	Whole grains, nuts, beans, and greens are best sources
Selenium	55mg	70mg	400mg	If mother is supplemented, the increase is available to infant	Present in seafoods, kidney, and liver, and in some meats, as well as grains, but varies according to soil types.
Manganese	2.6mg	2.6mg	11mg	Not usually a concern	Black tea, wheat germ and oat bran, nuts, shellfish, dark chocolate, pumpkin seeds, sesame, flax, sunflower seeds

RDA: The average daily dietary nutrient intake level sufficient to meet the nutrient requirement of nearly all (97 to 98 percent) healthy individuals in a particular life stage and gender group.

UL: The highest average daily nutrient intake level that is likely to pose no risk of adverse health effects to almost all individuals in the general population. As intake increases above the UL, the potential risk of adverse effects may increase.

Retrieved from http://fnic.nal.usda.gov/dietary-guidance/dietary-reference-intakes

2. Effects of various disease states:

   a. Diabetes: Type 1 is caused by pancreas not producing insulin; need to count carbohydrates and take insulin. Type 2 diabetes is an inability of cell receptors for glucose to function properly; patients need to use medication and diet. Gestational diabetes can be a combination of the two and responds to dietary modifications and/or insulin. Lack of control of glucose in pregnancy results in macrosomic infants.

   b. Gastrointestinal diseases such as Crohn's disease, IBS, bypass/bariatric surgery patients: These patients need to have careful evaluation because of various absorptive issues, avoidance of certain foods, and in the case of bypass/bariatric surgery, insufficient intake.

   c. PKU or other metabolic disease and cystic fibrosis: These diseases should trigger the lactation consultant to inquire into the management of the condition and make referrals to a dietitian who specializes in these conditions.

3. Malnourished women:

   a. Because micronutrient levels are quickly reflected in breastmilk, renourishment of the woman is effective for mother and infant. It is less expensive and safer to nourish the mother than it is to give the infant artificial baby milk.

   b. It is necessary to address the reason(s) for the malnourished condition of the mother to continue to sustain the breastfeeding dyad. Referrals should be made as appropriate to social supports providing assistance.

   c. Babies who have undernourished mothers *usually* do not reflect the same state of malnourishment because they can draw much of what they need from breastmilk at the expense of the mother. See **Table 19-2** for information on nutrients that are affected by dietary level.

4. Eating disorders:

   a. A woman who has anorexia or bulimia or a history of either needs to be under the care of suitable healthcare and counseling professionals. Concern for the infant can be a motivating factor for change (Micali, Simonoff, & Treasure, 2009). If the lactation consultant suspects either of these conditions, a referral should be made as diplomatically as possible and a follow-up call or visit should be made.

   b. In anorexia, breastmilk may be affected by low amounts of some water-soluble vitamins, lactose, and fat concentration.

   c. Bulimia patients have a wide variation in diet, and few data exist describing lactation effects.

5. Multiples:

   a. During pregnancy, especially in the last trimester, the mother may need to eat small, frequent meals because of limited stomach capacity.

   b. During breastfeeding, nutrient needs are increased above the needs of a mother who is breastfeeding a singleton, but doubling the micronutrient supplement can be unsafe (vitamin A is too high), and there is no research to support such recommendations. Most nutrients can be increased by increasing foods to meet caloric needs. If the mother's diet is suspected to be inadequate, refer to a nutritionist. Monitor to help avoid excessive weight loss or gain.

6. Breastfeeding and pregnancy:
    a. Nutrient needs are generally increased, though very little for the first trimester, depending on the age of the nursing infant. Doubling the vitamin/mineral supplement is not recommended because of possible teratogenic results from excess vitamin A.
    b. It is common for women to continue nursing when they are pregnant with another child. The decision whether to continue to breastfeed depends on the health condition of the mother, the physician's recommendation, and the mother's desire to continue. Some infants spontaneously wean. This as well as factors such as frequency of breastfeeding, age and medical condition of the baby, and the mother's risks for miscarriage should be discussed by the woman and her care providers, with support from lactation consultants (Lawrence et al., 2005; Merchant et al., 1990).

7. Vegetarian women:
    a. Vegetarians can have healthy diets, or they might not. A healthy vegetarian diet does not rely heavily on dairy products, but includes a variety of legumes, nuts, and seeds, as well as soy protein if desired.
    b. The following are types of vegetarian diets seen in a practice:
        i. *Vegan*: No animal proteins or products (no eggs or milk).
        ii. *Semivegetarian*: Eats vegetables, legumes, milk products, seafood, and poultry.
        iii. *Lactovegetarian:* Consumes milk and milk products in addition to plant proteins.
        iv. *Lacto-ovo vegetarian:* Consumes eggs in addition to dairy products and plant proteins.
        v. *Fruitarian:* Consumes fruits, nuts, olive oil, and honey.
        vi. *Macrobiotic:* Eats foods that are organic, fresh, and seasonal. Does not eat dairy or animal products. The advanced diet form is not usually nutritionally adequate for vitamin B_{12} for lactating women but can be adapted if the mother is willing.
    c. Vegetarians who are not consuming vitamin D–fortified milk and who have little sun exposure are at risk for vitamin D deficiency. Most vitamin supplements have 400–600 IU added (IOM Food and Nutrition Board, 2010).
    d. Vitamin B_{12} can be low in women who do not consume animal products and should be supplemented. They can also use nutritional yeast, fortified cereals, and soy milk.

8. Socioeconomic effects on food choices:
    a. Higher levels of education often correlate with better diets.
    b. A lack of money might limit the food that is available as well as the facilities to store and prepare the food. Ask questions like: "Do you have a working stove, oven, microwave, or refrigerator?"

    c. Provide phone numbers and information to the mother for food assistance programs (such as WIC in the United States or equivalent programs throughout the world), food stamps, local food banks, or other agencies that might include this kind of assistance. Provide follow-up contact to see whether the family gained access to services.

    d. Many, if not most, people's nutrition information might come from advertisements.

    e. An opinion of what a healthy diet consists of might vary considerably, such as what is eaten and when/where meals are eaten.

    f. Rigid rules regarding foods can make breastfeeding seem too difficult. A more supportive approach is to present options and suggestions and to find out what the woman is willing to do.

    g. Ask about cooking skills. If the woman or the family is willing to learn, refer to classes or appropriate recipes and resources.

9. Time:

    a. Time is needed to shop for food, prepare, and eat food. A mother has many demands on her time, and snacking on convenience foods might be the only way she feels she can manage.

    b. Help guide her to healthy ways to save time by eating more fresh, uncooked foods because cooked, highly processed foods are higher in cost and lower in nutrients.

III. Effects of Maternal Food Intake on the Breastfeeding Infant

(*See also* Chapter 20, Nutrition for the Breastfeeding Child.)

A. Increasing maternal energy intake and fluid does not influence milk volume unless the mother was significantly malnourished (Morse et al., 1992).

B. The type of fat, but not the amount of fat, is influenced by the mother's diet, so a mother on a low-fat diet should still provide adequate fats for the infant. Avoiding trans fatty acids is recommended. (See Chapter 21, Biochemistry of Human Milk.)

C. Breastmilk carbohydrate levels are not affected by dietary levels, including for diabetics.

D. Factors other than nutrition, particularly nursing behavior and stress, have a greater effect on milk supply. Emphasize healthy food choices as being good for the mother's energy level and sense of well-being.

E. Immunological effects:

    1. Iron in breastmilk has immunological benefits and is preferentially deposited in breastmilk at the expense of the mother's iron stores.

    2. Colic and allergy to breastmilk or substances in breastmilk: There is little evidence to support the avoidance of particular foods during breastfeeding, except for possibly cow's milk. However, some mothers do report that a particular food seems to cause distress in the infant, and it is wise to acknowledge this information.

3. Some cultural traditions limit the mother's foods or recommend particular foods for the first few weeks postpartum. In most cultures, however, women return to their usual foods within hours after birth.

4. If a food is suspected of causing a problem, it can be eliminated for 2 weeks. If symptoms reappear when the food is reintroduced, the mother can avoid the food for a few months. Mothers who avoid a major food group such as dairy must eliminate all dairy proteins, whey and casein, in all products by reading labels carefully. Although breastmilk contains some of these same proteins, they are not likely to be the cause of blood in the stool because they are not bovine whey or casein.

5. If dairy is to be removed from the mother's diet, inquire as to how much difficulty this will cause. If she has been eating cereal with milk, cheese pizza, cheese and crackers, creamy salad dressing, macaroni and cheese, and smoothies, she may need the help of a dietitian to find alternatives because casein and whey appear in many processed foods. One study showed that infants testing positive to a milk allergy skin test benefited when their mothers eliminated dairy (Moravei et al., 2010).

6. Eczema: This condition is usually not caused by diet. Some providers may mistakenly think that breastmilk is the issue and the mother may be advised to temporarily stop breastfeeding. She should consider seeking a second opinion (The Joint Commission, 2011). If the mother chooses to wean temporarily, she should express milk regularly to maintain her supply, while the baby will probably be put on an amino acid formula for a 5- to 7-day trial; then breastfeeding should be reinstated immediately.

7. Allergies and breastfeeding: Recent recommendations from the American Academy of Pediatrics suggest that it is not necessary to avoid highly allergic foods while pregnant or breastfeeding, but the studies are mixed in terms of recommendations (Greer et al., 2008). It can be helpful to support the mother with a history of allergies in avoiding milk, eggs, and peanuts during pregnancy and breastfeeding by helping her choose nutritious foods in their place. Introduce those foods in the infant diet after 18 months. There is no harm in doing this until the research is more conclusive (West et al., 2010).

8. Caffeine:
   a. Caffeine ingested by the mother at less than 300 mg/day does not likely cause a problem for most infants because the dose of caffeine available to the infant is approximately 0.96% to 1.5% of the maternal dose (Hale, 2010).
   b. Preterm or ill infants might not metabolize caffeine well, leading to accumulation and wakefulness or irritability.
   c. Coffee has 80 to 100 mg of caffeine per 8 oz cup. Black and green teas contain 30 to 60 mg of caffeine per 8 oz cup. The theobromines in chocolate cause a similar effect on the nervous system. Most infants are not bothered, but fussiness may be a symptom of sensitivity.

9. Herbs and herbal teas:
   a. Normal amounts of herbs used in cooking do not usually affect the infant.
   b. Herbal teas are used in many cultures for lactating women. Caution should be exercised because some herbs such as chaparral, comfrey, germander, pennyroyal, and blue cohosh have been documented to cause problems in the infant such as hepatotoxicity, anticholinergic symptoms, and caridotoxicity. The resource *Medications and Mothers' Milk* by Thomas Hale is a good resource for lactation consultants because it includes information on herbs. Lactation textbooks also contain discussions and tables on herbs (Lawrence et al., 2005; Riordan, 2010).
   c. Healthcare professionals and parents should exercise caution because sometimes the origin of the herbs and the conditions under which they were grown, mixed, or packaged are unknown. The U.S. Food and Drug Administration does not regulate herbs.

10. Alcohol:
   a. High intakes can impair the milk ejection reflex. Doses of more than 2 g/kg (for a 132-lb woman, this is about 4 oz of liquor) can completely block the milk ejection reflex (Breslow et al., 2007; Chien et al., 2009).
   b. A number of factors influence maternal blood alcohol concentrations, including body weight, amount of adipose tissue, stomach contents, how fast the alcohol is consumed, and the amount of alcohol consumed.
   c. Peak alcohol levels in milk occur in 30 to 60 minutes on an empty stomach, and in 60 to 90 minutes when consumed with food. It takes about 1.5 to 2 hours per ounce to metabolize alcohol in the adult. The alcohol content of milk falls as the blood levels fall as a result of back diffusion of alcohol from the milk to the maternal blood stream.
   d. Alcohol passes freely into the milk, and in large amounts it can cause drowsiness, slow growth, and neurodevelopmental delays in the infant.
   e. Infants detoxify alcohol in the first 4 weeks of life at approximately half the rate of an adult. Near-term and preterm infants are at higher risk for toxicity.
   f. A high alcohol intake impairs the mother's ability to care for her child safely.

11. Taste:
   a. Breastmilk flavor changes depending on the foods and spices that the mother consumes, and this has a positive effect when the infant begins to eat solid foods because they tend to be more accepting of greater variety (Mennella et al., 2011); Sullivan & Birch, 1994).
   b. Infants sucked for 50% longer when milk was garlic flavored, and even longer when exposed to vanilla-flavored milk (Mennella, 1995).

12. Artificial sweeteners and food additives:
   a. Aspartame metabolizes to the amino acids phenylalanine and aspartic acid. It is dangerous for persons with PKU, and most products containing aspartame carry a warning label.

   b. The consumption of artificial sweeteners has not reduced the incidence of obesity since their introduction. In fact, review articles show that the increase in obesity and the use of a variety of artificial sweeteners have risen together even as more types of sweeteners are introduced (Yang, 2010).

   c. Moderate amounts of beverages or foods sweetened with aspartame might not be harmful, although research is lacking. Hale (2010) cites a level of 50 mg/kg for a woman as producing three to four times the normal dose used, which would still be a small dose in breastmilk.

   d. Caution should be taken with all artificial additives and sweeteners because many are on the market without research regarding their effects on rapidly growing infants (Soffritti et al., 2007).

IV. Consultation

For a lactation consultant who is carrying out a consultation with a nutritional focus, it is helpful to have the following:

   A. Basic knowledge of nutrition to assess the mother's intake. Ask the mother about a day's food and beverage intake.

   B. Awareness of the diversity of cultural practices. If you are not familiar with the culture, ask lots of questions.

   C. Counseling skills to gather information and discuss choices, using motivational interviewing skills.

   D. Simple charting capabilities to record information that is gathered.

   E. Education strategies to provide information to the mother.

   F. Knowledge of other food-related and education services and how to refer to them.

   G. Lactation consultants can get to know dietitians and nutritionists in their area to refer patients to so that they can be a part of a team of healthcare providers.

References

Basile, L. A., Taylor, S. N., Wagner, C. L., Horst, R. L., & Hollis, B. W. (2006). The effect of high-dose vitamin D supplementation on serum vitamin D levels and milk calcium concentration in lactating women and their infants. *Breastfeeding Medicine, 1*(1), 27–35.

Breslow, R. A., Falk, D. E., Fein, S. B., & Brummer-Strawn, L. M. (2007). Alcohol consumption among breastfeeding women. *Breastfeeding Medicine, 2*(3), 152–157.

Butte, N. F., & King, J. C. (2005). Energy requirements during pregnancy and lactation. *Public Health Nutrition, 8*(7A), 1010–1027.

Butte, N. F., Wong, W. W., & Hopkinton, J. M. (2001). Energy requirements of lactating women derived from doubly labeled water and milk energy output. *Journal of Nutrition, 131*, 53–58.

Chien, Y. C., Huang, Y. J., Hsu, C. S., Chao, J. C., & Liu, J. F. (2009). Maternal lactation characteristics after consumption of an alcoholic soup during postpartum "doing-the-month" ritual. *Public Health Nutrition, 12*(3), 382–388.

Durham, H. A., Lovelady, C. A., Brouwer, R. J., Krause, K. M., & Ostbye, T. (2011). Comparison of dietary intake of overweight postpartum mothers practicing breastfeeding or formula feeding. *Journal of the American Dietetic Association, 111*(1), 67–74.

Grandjean, P., Poulsen, L. K., Heilmann, C., Steuerwald, U., & Weihe, P. (2010). Allergy and sensitization during childhood associated with prenatal and lactational exposure to marine pollutants. *Environmental Health Perspectives, 118*(10), 1429–1433.

Greer, F. R., Sicherer, S. H., & Burks, A. W. (2008). Effects of early nutritional interventions on the development of atopic disease in infants and children: The role of maternal dietary restriction, breastfeeding, timing of introduction of complementary foods, and hydrolyzed formulas. *Pediatrics, 121*(1), 183–191.

Hale, T. W. (2010). *Medications and mothers' milk* (13th ed.). Amarillo, TX: Hale Publishing.

Hartmann, P., & Cregan, M. (2001). Lactogenesis and the effects of insulin-dependent diabetes mellitus and prematurity. *Journal of Nutrition, 131*(11), 3016S–3020S.

Henderson, P. H., III, Sowers, M., Kutzko, K. E., & Jannausch, M. L. (2000). Bone mineral density in grand multiparous women with extended lactation. *American Journal of Obstetrics and Gynecology, 182*(6), 1371–1377.

Hollis, B. W. (2007). Vitamin D requirement during pregnancy and lactation. *Journal of Bone Mineral Research, 22*(Suppl. 2), V39–V44.

Institute of Medicine, Food and Nutrition Board. (2005). *Dietary reference intakes for energy, carbohydrate, fiber, fat, fatty acids, cholesterol, protein, and amino acids.* Washington, DC: National Academy Press.

Institute of Medicine, Food and Nutrition Board. (2010). *Dietary reference intakes for calcium and vitamin D.* Washington, DC: National Academy Press.

Jewitt, C., Hernandez, I., & Groer, M. (2007). Lactation complicated by overweight and obesity: Supporting the mother and newborn. *Journal of Midwifery and Women's Health, 52*(6), 606–613.

The Joint Commission. (2011). Speak up: What you need to know about breastfeeding. Retrieved from http://www.jointcommission.org/speakup_breastfeeding.

Kimmons, J. E., Blanck, H. M., Tohill, B. C., Zhang, J., & Khan, K. L. (2006). Associations between body mass index and the prevalence of low micronutrient levels among US adults. *Medscape General Medicine, 8*(4), 59.

Lawrence, R. A., & Lawrence, R. M. (2011). *Breastfeeding: A guide for the medical profession.* Philadelphia, PA: Elsevier Mosby.

Lenora, J., Lekamwasam, S., & Karlsson, M. K. (2009). Effects of multiparity and prolonged breastfeeding on maternal bone mineral density: A community-based cross-sectional study. *BMC Women's Health, 1*(9), 19.

Leonard, S. A., & Rasmussen, K. M. (2011). Larger infant size at birth reduces the negative association between maternal prepregnancy body mass index and breastfeeding duration. *Journal of Nutrition, 141*(4), 645–653.

Lovelady, C. (2011). Balancing exercise and food intake with lactation to promote post-partum weight loss. *Proceedings of the Nutrition Society, 24*, 1–4.

Merchant, K., Martorell, R., & Haas, J. (1990). Maternal and fetal responses to the stresses of lactation concurrent with pregnancy and of short recuperative intervals. *American Journal of Clinical Nutrition, 52*(2), 280–288.

Micali, N., Simonoff, E., & Treasure, J. (2009). Infant feeding and weight in the first year of life in babies of women with eating disorders. *Journal of Pediatrics, 154*(1), 55–60.e1.

Miller, W. R., & Rollnick, S. (2002). *Motivational interviewing.* New York, NY: Gilford Press.

Moravej, H., Imanieh, M. G., Kashef, S., Handjani, F., & Eghterdari, F. (2010). Predictive value of the cow's milk skin prick test in infantile colic. *Annals of Saudi Medicine, 30*(6), 468–470.

Morse, J. M., Ewing, G., Gamble, D., & Donahue, P. (1992). The effect of maternal fluid intake on breast milk supply: A pilot study. *Canadian Journal of Public Health, 83*(3), 213–216.

Mozaffarian, D., Katan, M. B., Ascherio, A., et al. (2006). Trans fatty acids and cardiovascular disease. *New England Journal of Medicine, 354*(13), 1601–1613.

Olson, C. M. (2005). Tracking food choices across the transition to motherhood. *Journal of Nutrition Education and Behavior, 37*, 129–136.

Onyango, AW, Nommsen-Rivers, L, Siyam A, Borghi, E, deOnis, M, Lartey, A, Baeru, A, Bhandan, N, Dewey, KG, Araujo, CL, Mohamed, AJ, VandenBroeck, J, WHO Multicentre Growth Reference. (2011). Postpartum weight change patterns in the WHO Multicentre Growth Reference Study. *Maternal Child Nutrition, 7*(3):228-40.

Riordan, J. (2010). *Breastfeeding and human lactation* (4th ed.). Sudbury, MA: Jones and Bartlett.

Soffritti, M., Belpoggi, F., Tibaldi, E., Esposti, D. D., & Lauriola, M. (2007). Life-span exposure to low doses of aspartame beginning during prenatal life increases cancer effects in rats. *Environmental Health Perspec*tives, *115*(9), 1293–1297.

Sullivan, S. A., & Birch, L. L. (1994). Infant dietary experience and acceptance of solid foods. *Pediatrics, 93*, 271–277.

Tran, T., Wax, J. R., Philput, C., Steinfeld, J. D., & Ingardia, C. J. (2000). Intentional iron overdose in pregnancy—management and outcome. *Journal of Emergency Medicine, 18*(2), 225–228.

West, C. E., Videky, D. J., & Prescott, S. L. (2010). Role of diet in the development of immune tolerance in the contest of allergic disease. *Current Opinions in Pediatrics, 22*(5), 635–641.

Wright, K. S., Quinn, T. J., & Carey, G. B. (2002). Infant acceptance of breast milk after maternal exercise. *Pediatrics, 109*(4), 585–589.

Yang, Q. (2010). Gain weight by "going diet?" Artificial sweeteners and the neurobiology of sugar. *Yale Journal of Biology and Medicine, 83*(2), 101–108.

CHAPTER 20
Nutrition for the Breastfeeding Child

Rachelle Lessen, MS, RD, IBCLC

OBJECTIVES

- Discuss the nutrition recommendations for normal infant feeding.
- Discuss adequate intake of key nutrients for the breastfed child, including energy, protein, fatty acids, iron, zinc, and vitamin D.
- Describe caregiver behaviors that can affect normal transitioning from an all-milk infant diet to a diet of family foods.
- Evaluate the need for referral to a nutrition specialist or other healthcare provider.

INTRODUCTION

Human milk provides sufficient nutrition for optimal growth, development, and health for the first 6 months of life. The exclusively breastfed infant is the standard for growth because human milk provides the ideal amount of calories and protein required for the healthy term infant. In the first 6 months of life, breastfed infants do not need any additional foods or fluids, and healthy term infants from well-nourished mothers do not require vitamin or mineral supplements, with the exception of supplemental vitamin D. Complementary foods are introduced to the breastfed child around 6 months when additional nutrients are needed to supplement human milk intake and to accustom the child to eating a variety of family foods. In particular, foods high in iron and zinc should be included in the child's diet because iron and zinc requirements increase as the amount of these minerals in human milk decreases. Human milk continues to provide key amounts of important nutrients beyond the 6-month period of exclusive breastfeeding. Intake of human milk will gradually decrease as larger quantities of complementary food are introduced into the child's diet. To meet the nutritional needs of the growing breastfed child, complementary foods should be timely, adequate, safe, and properly fed, and caregivers should practice responsive feeding techniques.

I. World Health Organization Nutrition Recommendations for Normal Infant Feeding (Pan American Health Organization & World Health Organization [PAHO & WHO], 2003)

A. Guidelines for infant and young child feeding
   1. Exclusive breastfeeding for the first 6 months of life
   2. Complementary foods introduced at 6 months
   3. Continue frequent cue-based breastfeeding until 2 years or beyond
B. Nutritional concerns
   1. Infants are at nutritional risk during the transition period when complementary feeding begins.
   2. Children in poor, developing countries and those in the resource-rich, developed world can be inappropriately fed (Palmer, 2011).
   3. Reliance on starchy local foods such as cereals and gruels or commercially prepared baby food fruits, vegetables, and cereals may replace rather than complement breastmilk intake without supplying needed nutrients such as iron and zinc (Palmer, 2011).
   4. To meet nutritional needs, complementary foods should be:
      a. Timely: Introduced after 6 months when it can become increasingly difficult to meet all nutritional needs with breastmilk alone and when most infants are developmentally ready for other foods
      b. Adequate: Provide sufficient energy, protein, and micronutrients to meet a growing child's nutritional needs
      c. Safe: Hygienically stored and prepared and fed with clean hands using clean utensils, and not bottles and teats
      d. Properly fed: Given consistent with a child's signals of appetite and satiety, and with a meal frequency and feeding method suitable for age
   5. Healthy dietary behaviors and obesity prevention
      a. Healthy dietary behaviors must begin early (Horodynski et al., 2011).
      b. Early eating experiences can influence the development of lifelong harmful eating practices leading to overweight, obesity, and eating disorders (Palmer, 2011).
      c. Taste preferences develop early in life, and overly sweet or salty foods or energy-dense/nutrient-poor foods should be avoided.
      d. Healthy diets include increased fruit and vegetable consumption and avoidance of sweetened beverages.
      e. Nonresponsive feeding such as excessive control by caregiver (forcing/pressuring food intake), allowing the child complete control of feeding situation (indulgent feeding), or uninvolved caregiver during meals may be associated with overweight or obesity (Hurley et al., 2011).

C. Responsive feeding techniques (according to the "Guiding Principles of Complementary Feeding for the Breastfed Child" [PAHO & WHO, 2003])

1. Human milk alone typically meets all the nutrient needs during the first 6 months. After this time, complementary foods are needed to ensure adequate intake of nutrient requirements.
2. Infants should be fed directly and older children assisted to feed themselves.
3. Caregivers need to be sensitive to hunger and satiety cues.
4. Children should be fed slowly and patiently with encouragement but not force.
5. If children refuse many foods, experimenting with different food combinations, tastes, textures, and methods of encouragement can be helpful.
6. Distractions should be minimized if child loses interest easily. There should be a positive mealtime environment (no TV and family sitting down together).
7. Feeding times should be periods of learning and love. Children should be talked to during feeding with eye-to-eye contact.
8. The number of times that the child is fed complementary foods should be increased as he or she gets older. Recommendations include:
   a. Two to three meals of complementary foods at 6 to 8 months
   b. Three to four meals of complementary foods from 9 to 24 months with nutritious snacks one to two times per day
9. A variety of foods should be offered to ensure that nutrient needs are met.
   a. Meat, poultry, fish, or eggs should be eaten daily or as often as possible (Greer et al. & the Committee on Nutrition and Section on Allergy and Immunology of the American Academy of Pediatrics, 2008).
   b. Vitamin A–rich fruits and vegetables should be eaten daily.
   c. Adequate fat is needed to provide essential fatty acids, facilitate absorption of fat-soluble vitamins, and provide energy.
10. Fortified complementary foods or vitamin–mineral supplements for the infant can be used as needed.

II. Nutrition for Breastfed Children

A. Average intake of most nutrients (exception: vitamin D) of full-term infants born to healthy, well-nourished mothers is based on exclusive breastfeeding in the first 6 months and continued breastfeeding with complementary foods from 6 to 12 months.

B. From 0 to 6 months: Nutrient requirements are based on average concentration of nutrients in human milk from 2 to 6 months and average intake of 780 mL/day (Otten et al., 2006).

C. During the period of exclusive breastfeeding, intake of human milk increases rapidly from birth through the first month and then continues to increase more slowly through 6 months (Neville et al., 1988).

D. Vitamin deficiencies are rare in exclusively breastfed infants, but when maternal diet is deficient, infants may have low intakes of vitamin A, riboflavin, vitamin B_6, and vitamin B_{12}. Improving maternal diet or giving mothers supplements is preferable to providing complementary foods to younger infants (PAHO & WHO, 2003).

E. There is no evidence for increased nutrient needs in the second 6 months except for high requirements of iron and zinc.

F. From 7 to 12 months: Adequate intake of nutrients is based on average amount of nutrients provided in 600 mL/day of human milk and the usual intake of complementary foods.

III. Key Nutrient Requirements

A. Energy

1. Energy needs are based on the requirement to sustain the body's functions, respiration, circulation, activity, metabolism and protein synthesis, growth and deposition of tissues.

2. Estimated energy (calorie) requirements are based on energy expenditure plus energy deposition (that is, growth) and are calculated based on infant age and current weight.

   a. 0 to 3 mo = (89 × wt [kg] − 100) + 175
   b. 4 to 6 mo = (89 × wt [kg] − 100) + 56
   c. 7 to 12 mo = (89 × wt [kg] − 100) + 22
   d. 13 to 35 mo = (89 × wt [kg] − 100) + 20

3. Recommended energy (calorie) intakes for the breastfed child are shown in the following table (Dewey, 2001).

Age	Estimated Daily Calorie Needs	Calories from Human Milk	Calories from Complementary Foods
6–8 months	682	486	196
9–11 months	830	375	455
12–24 months	1,092	313	779

B. Protein (Otten et al., 2006)

1. Protein requirements from 0–6 months are based on the average consumption of protein from human milk. After 6 months, protein requirements are based on nitrogen balance and protein deposition for growth of new tissue. From 1–3 years, 5–20% of total calories are derived from protein.

2. Estimated daily protein requirements are calculated based on infant age and current weight. Protein requirements per kilogram decrease with age.

   a. 7 to 12 months: 1.0 g/kg/day
   b. 1 to 3 years: 0.87 g/kg/day
   c. 4 to 8 years: 0.76 g/kg/day

3. Sources of protein
   a. Human milk provides approximately 0.9 g protein per 100 mL.
   b. Complete proteins provided from animal sources containing all nine indispensable amino acids: meat, poultry, eggs, fish, milk, cheese, and yogurt.
   c. Incomplete proteins provided from vegetable sources that are deficient in one or more indispensable amino acids: legumes, grains, nuts, seeds, and vegetables.
4. Deficiency
   a. Both protein and nonprotein energy (carbohydrates and fat) must be available to prevent protein-energy malnutrition (PEM) (Otten et al., 2006).
   b. Amino acids must be present in the right balance to utilize proteins.
   c. Worldwide, PEM is common and is associated with the death of 6 million children each year.
   d. Protein deficiency affects brain and brain function, immunity, gut function, and gut permeability.
   e. Physical signs of protein deficiency are edema, failure to thrive, poor musculature, dull skin, thin and fragile hair.

C. Fluid
   1. Adequate intake for 0 to 6 months is 700 mL/day and is based on average intake of 780 mL/day of human milk. Human milk is approximately 87% water.
   2. Adequate intake for 7 to 12 months is based on average intake of human milk plus complementary foods and other beverages (800 mL/day).
   3. Adequate intake for 1 to 3 years is 1,300 mL/day, and for 4 to 8 years is 1,700 mL/day and includes all water contained in food, beverages, and drinking water.
   4. Water is vital for life and is the single largest constituent of the human body. Human milk provides infants with adequate water for growth and replacement of water lost through the skin, lungs, feces, and urine (Centers for Disease Control and Prevention [CDC], 1994).
   5. Inadequate fluid intake leads to dehydration.
   6. Fever, diarrhea, and heat exposure increase fluid losses.
   7. Excessive fluid intake leads to hyponatremia (low levels of sodium in the blood). Oral water intoxication in infants is the most common cause of seizures that have no apparent cause in infants younger than 6 months (Moritz & Ayus, 2002). Infants younger than 6 months should not receive any supplemental water (tap or bottled) (CDC, 1994).

IV. Vitamins

A. Vitamin A
   1. Vitamin A is important for normal vision, growth, and immune function.
   2. Available as preformed (retinol) in animal-based foods or as carotenoids that are converted to vitamin A in the body. Vitamin A is stored in the liver, and toxicity can occur with excess intake of preformed vitamin A from supplements or fortified foods. High intake of carotenoids has not been shown to result in toxicity.

3. Good sources of vitamin A include dairy, meat, carrots, broccoli, squash, peas, spinach, and cantaloupe. Cooking vegetables enhances absorption.

4. Deficiency results in xerophthalmia, an irreversible drying of the conjunctiva and cornea leading to blindness that affects 3 million to 10 million children annually. Decreased immune function and increased infection risk also result from vitamin A deficiency.

B. B vitamins

   1. Folate
      a. Coenzyme in metabolism of nucleic and amino acids
      b. Food sources: fortified grain products, dark green vegetables, beans and legumes

   2. B_{12} (cobalamin)
      a. Coenzyme for critical reaction that converts homocysteine to methionine and for metabolism of fatty acids and amino acids.
      b. Essential for normal blood formation and neurological function.
      c. B_{12} deficiency in breastfed children of vegan mothers can manifest at ages 4 to 8 months as failure to thrive, developmental delay, severe macrocytic anemia, weakness, muscle atrophy, psychomotor regression, hypotonia, and loss of developmental milestones (CDC, 2003).
      d. Infants of vegan mothers should be supplemented with 400 µg/day B_{12} from birth to 6 months and 500 µg/day from 7 to 12 months because their stores are low and their mother's milk may supply only small amounts. Children 1 to 3 years need 900 µg/day.
      e. B_{12} is naturally found in foods of animal origin. Particularly rich sources are organ meats, game meats, herring, sardines, and trout. Milk and beef contain B_{12}. Vegetarian sources include fortified cereals, fortified rice or soy milk, nutritional yeast, and fortified meat substitutes.

C. Vitamin C

   1. Water-soluble nutrient that acts as an antioxidant and cofactor in enzymatic and hormonal processes.
   2. Enhances iron absorption.
   3. Severe vitamin C deficiency (scurvy) is rare in industrialized nations.
   4. Vitamin C deficiency in infants (infantile scurvy) can result in bone abnormalities, hemorrhagic symptoms, and anemia. Human milk provides adequate vitamin C (PAHO & WHO, 2003).
   5. Fruits and vegetables are a rich source of vitamin C, particularly citrus fruits and juices, tomatoes and tomato juice, potatoes, Brussels sprouts, cauliflower, broccoli, strawberries, cabbage, and spinach.

D. Vitamin D
1. Involved in bone health. Aids in intestinal absorption of calcium and phosphorus, thus helping maintain normal serum levels of these minerals.
2. Vitamin D receptors are in most cells and tissues in the body. Vitamin D deficiency can be associated with many chronic diseases, including cancers, autoimmune diseases, and cardiovascular disease (Holick, 2007).
3. Naturally found in very few foods: flesh of fatty fish and some fish liver oils. Fortified milk products and breakfast cereals are good sources.
4. Fat soluble. Synthesized in the skin through exposure to ultraviolet B rays in sunlight. Synthesis is limited by sunscreen use, darker skin, greater distance from the equator, time of day, and season of the year (Otten et al., 2006).
5. Vitamin D deficiency results in rickets. Most infants are not exposed to sufficient sunlight to produce adequate vitamin D in their skin. Human milk usually does not contain sufficient vitamin D to meet an infant's needs, although high-dose maternal supplementation has been shown to increase vitamin D levels in human milk (Hollis et al., 2004; Saadi et al., 2009; Taylor et al., 2008).
6. To prevent rickets and vitamin D deficiency in healthy infants, children, and adolescents a vitamin D intake of at least 400 IU/day is recommended (Chehade et al., 2011; Hatun et al., 2011; Lowdon, 2011; Misra et al., 2008; Narchi et al., 2011; Pludowski et al., 2011; Rajakumar et al., 2005; Wagner et al. & Section on Breastfeeding & Committee on Nutrition of the American Academy of Pediatrics, 2008; Ward et al., 2007). Breastfed or partially breastfed infants should begin supplementation in the first few days of life. Supplementation should continue until the child is weaned to at least 1 L/day of vitamin D–fortified whole milk or infant formula.
7. Vitamin D deficiency is associated with increased risk of asthma and allergic disease (Ehlayel et al., 2011; Kozyrskyj et al., 2011).
8. Excess vitamin D from supplements can cause hypercalcemia and hypercalciuria.

V. Minerals

A. Iron
1. Because of rapid growth in the first year of life, the need for iron is relatively high (0.7 mg iron absorbed per day).
2. Infants use birth stores during their first 4 to 6 months.
3. Eighty percent of iron present in a term newborn is received during the third trimester.
4. Maternal conditions such as anemia, smoking, hypertension with intrauterine growth restriction, or diabetes can result in reduced fetal stores (Baker et al. & Committee on Nutrition of the American Academy of Pediatrics, 2010; Rao et al., 2007). Maternal intervention is the best way to prevent iron deficiency in newborns (Rao et al., 2007).

5. Infants born with diminished stores can exhaust their iron stores earlier. Delayed cord clamping for 30–120 seconds at birth improves iron status at 2–3 months (Hutton et al., 2007; Van Rheenan et al., 2004).

6. Bioavailability of iron in human milk is high. Iron content of human milk varies from 0.2–0.8 mg/L with an absorption rate of 20–50%, compared to absorption of 4–20% from formula (Rao et al., 2007). Exclusive breastfeeding and avoidance of cow's milk and low-iron formula are the most effective strategies for preventing iron deficiency in healthy term infants (Rao & Georgieff, 2007).

7. The prevalence of iron-deficiency anemia is low (3%) among unsupplemented breastfed infants in the first 6 months of life (Ziegler et al., 2009).

8. Iron in human milk decreases progressively and significantly over the first 6 months (Raj et al., 2008).

9. Iron deficiency and iron-deficiency anemia are worldwide concerns. Screening at-risk breastfed infants can determine need for supplementation.

10. Iron-deficiency anemia and iron deficiency without anemia are serious conditions that can result in delayed psychomotor development and impaired cognitive function that might not be reversible with iron treatment (Baker et al., 2010; Otten et al., 2006).

11. Iron deficiency can increase lead absorption, further increasing the risk of neurological and developmental deficits.

12. Recommended Dietary Allowance for iron for infants 7 to 12 months is 11 mg/day and for 1 to 3 years is 7 mg/day.

13. Preterm infants are at increased risk for iron deficiency because of reduced iron stores at birth and accelerated growth in infancy. Preterm breastfed infants should be given 2 mg/kg/day supplemental oral iron starting at 1 month and continuing through 12 months of age (Dee et al., 2008).

14. Introduction of meat as an early complementary food is recommended for exclusively breastfed infants as an excellent source of iron and zinc (Krebs et al., 2006; Palmer, 2011). When iron-rich foods are not included in the diet breastfed infants can be at risk for iron deficiency and iron-deficiency anemia after 6 months of age that persists into the second year of life (Chantry et al., 2007; Domellöf et al., 2002; Dube et al., 2010; Yang et al., 2009).

15. Heme iron from meat, poultry, and fish is well absorbed. Organ meats, clams, and oysters are especially high in iron (Baker et al., 2010; Krebs et al., 2006; Palmer, 2011).

16. Nonheme iron is present in all foods, including meat. Absorption is influenced by interactions with other dietary substances (Otten et al., 2006).
    a. Ascorbic acid enhances iron absorption.
    b. Animal muscle tissue (meat, fish, poultry) improve nonheme iron absorption.
    c. Phytates in legumes, unrefined rice, and grains inhibit iron absorption.

17. Bioavailability of iron from complementary foods for children younger than 1 year is estimated at 10% because of limited meat and high consumption of cereal and vegetables, and 18% for children older than 1 year who consume more meat.

18. Iron supplementation of iron-sufficient infants can be deleterious and should be avoided (Rao et al., 2007; Schanler et al., 2011). Poor growth is associated with iron supplementation in breastfed infants with normal hemoglobin (Dewey et al., 2002).

B. Zinc

1. Globally there is a widespread prevalence of zinc deficiency, often along with iron deficiency, in infants and young children (Krebs et al., 2006).
2. Zinc is crucial for growth and development (Otten et al., 2006).
3. Zinc in human milk is sufficient to meet requirements in the first 6 months of life (Brown et al., 2009).
4. Zinc in human milk declines over time and although not sufficient to meet requirements after 6 months, it is still an important source of dietary zinc (Otten et al., 2006).
5. Meat is an excellent source of zinc (Krebs et al., 2006) and provides adequate amounts to meet requirements of breastfed infants 7 to 12 months of age.
6. Recommended Dietary Allowance for zinc for 7 months to 3 years is 3 mg/day.
7. Other dietary sources of zinc include whole grains, some shellfish, and some fortified cereals.
8. There is greater bioavailability of zinc in human milk than cow's milk (Otten et al., 2006).

C. Calcium

1. Primary role in the body is to form structure of bones and teeth. More than 99% of body calcium is stored in bones and teeth. Calcium is also important in vascular contraction and vasodilation, muscle contractions, neural transmission, and glandular secretions.
2. Inadequate calcium intake can result in osteopenia (lower than normal bone mineral density) and increased risk of fractures.
3. Preterm infants have higher calcium requirements and might require fortification of human milk (Kleinman, 2009).
4. Foods rich in calcium include milk, yogurt, cheese, cabbage, kale, and broccoli. Calcium is poorly absorbed in foods rich in oxalic acid (spinach, sweet potatoes, rhubarb, and beans) and rich in phytates (seeds, nuts, and grains).
5. Meeting calcium requirements during transition to complementary foods can be difficult if dairy products are not part of the diet (Kleinman, 2009).

D. Fluoride

1. Vital for health of teeth and bones.
2. Inadequate intake results in increased risk of dental caries.
3. Primary source is fluoridated water.
4. Chronic excess intake in the preeruptive development of teeth can lead to enamel fluorosis in the form of discolored or pitted teeth (CDC, 2001; Institute of Medicine of the National Academies, 2006; Ismail et al., 1999). Exposure to high levels of fluoride in drinking water can adversely affect children's IQ (Tang et al., 2008).

5. Human milk contains adequate fluoride when the mother drinks fluoridated water or consumes adequate supplements. Use of fluoride supplements by pregnant women does not reduce dental caries in children (Leverett et al., 1997).

6. Infants older than 6 months may need fluoride supplements if water is not fluoridated. Supplementation for children at high risk of dental caries with 0.25 mg/day in areas where fluoride concentration in community water is less than 0.3 ppm is recommended (CDC, 2001; Kleinman, 2009; Otten et al., 2006), although accurate assessment of all sources of fluoride is crucial to prevent fluorosis.

VI. Beverages

A. Cow's milk
   1. Cow's milk should not be given before 1 year (Kleinman, 2009).
   2. Cow's milk does not have adequate nutrients to support the rapidly growing infant.
   3. When introduced at 1 year, only whole cow's milk, not reduced-fat, should be offered.

B. Juice and other drinks
   1. Juice should not be given before 6 months.
   2. Only 100% juice should be offered in a cup.
   3. Juice should be limited to 4 to 6 oz daily for children 6 months to 6 years of age.
   4. Drinks with low nutritive value such as tea, coffee, and sugary drinks should be avoided.

VII. Special Considerations

A. Vitamin and mineral supplements
   1. Many children are supplemented with vitamins and minerals in the first 2 years of life. Most young children receive adequate nutrients from diet alone, with the exception of vitamin D (Gilmore et al., 2005).
   2. Vitamin D drops for infants and toddlers can be given separately to meet recommendations. There is no evidence that older infants and young children require multiple vitamin supplements.
   3. If infants and toddlers do not consume adequate iron from food, iron drops or chewable iron tablets can be offered (Baker et al., 2010).

B. Vegetarian children (American Dietetic Association, 2003)
   1. At risk for B_{12} deficiency if mother does not consume dairy products or foods fortified with B_{12} or take B_{12} supplements.
   2. Guidelines for iron and vitamin D do not differ from nonvegetarian children.
   3. Poor growth may be seen on very restricted diets. Provision of supplemental zinc may be required.
   4. Average protein intake is usually adequate. Protein needs may be slightly higher for vegan children because of protein differences in plant food proteins.

5. Nutrient-rich complementary foods for vegetarian children include mashed or pureed tofu, legumes, soy or dairy yogurt, eggs, cottage cheese, cheese, mashed avocado, and legume spreads.
6. Commercial, full-fat fortified soymilk or cow's milk can be introduced as a primary beverage after 1 year of age.

C. Docosahexaenoic acid (DHA)
1. DHA is a polyunsaturated long-chain omega-3 fatty acid that is essential for brain development and visual acuity through 2 years of age. Nonhuman primate studies have demonstrated poor cognitive function and visual acuity with DHA deficiency (Neuringer et al., 1986).
2. DHA influences growth, metabolic, and immune outcomes in childhood (Gibson et al., 2011).
3. Levels in human milk vary based on maternal diet. The types of fatty acids consumed by the mother along with those stored in adipose tissue influence the fatty acid content of human milk. Women who eat greater amounts of fish or supplement their diet with fish oil have higher levels of DHA in their milk (Bergmann et al., 2008; Francois et al., 1998; Ruan et al., 1995). Human milk fatty acid composition has changed dramatically in the past 30 to 40 years as consumption of omega-6 fatty acids has increased (Gibson et al., 2011). (See Chapter 19, Nutrition for Lactating Women.)
4. There is limited evidence that maternal supplementation of lactating mothers will improve neurodevelopment or growth (Delgado-Noguera et al., 2010; Helland et al., 2003; Innis, 2007; Innis et al., 2001). Benefits may be more pronounced in preterm infants.
5. Complementary foods containing DHA include egg yolk, chicken, and oily fish (Hoffman et al., 2004).

VIII. Safety

A. Nitrate poisoning (methemoglobinemia) (Greer et al., 2005).
1. Greatest risk of nitrate poisoning resulting in cyanosis in infants occurs when contaminated well water is used to prepare infant formula.
2. Naturally occurring nitrates are present in foods such as green beans, carrots, squash, spinach, and beets and should not be given to children under 3 months of age. There is no nutritional indication for complementary foods to be given to healthy term infants before 6 months; therefore, there is no risk when these foods are offered at the appropriate time.
3. Breastfed infants are not at risk of nitrate poisoning from mothers who ingest water with high nitrate content because nitrate content does not concentrate in human milk.

B. Appropriate textures
1. Foods should be soft, semisolid, mashed, or pureed for infants 12 months or younger so that infants can swallow the foods without risk of aspiration (AAP, 2009). The use of commercial baby food is not necessary. Children can be offered soft family foods when they have developed appropriate chewing skills (Palmer, 2011).
2. By 8 months of age, most infants can eat "finger foods" that they feed themselves.
3. By 12 months of age, most children can eat the same types of foods as consumed by the rest of the family.
4. Food consistency should be gradually increased by age. There may be a "critical window" for introduction of lumpy foods. Delay beyond 10 months can risk later feeding difficulties.
5. Choking risks for children younger than 4 years include hot dogs, nuts, grapes, raisins, raw carrots, popcorn, and rounded or hard candies.
C. Hygiene and food handling
1. Caregiver's and children's hands should be washed before food preparation and eating.
2. Foods should be stored safely and served immediately after preparation.
3. Clean cups and bowls should be used.
4. Clean utensils should be used to prepare and serve food.

IX. Recommended Feeding Practices

A. One food at a time should be offered when first introducing complementary foods and caregivers should wait 3 to 5 days between new foods to observe for possible allergies (AAP, 2009).
B. Complementary feeding and allergies:
1. There is no current convincing evidence that delaying introduction of solid foods beyond 6 months has a significant protective effect on development of atopic disease, including the introduction of foods considered highly allergenic, such as fish, eggs, and peanuts (Greer et al., 2008). Exposure to traces of foods can induce tolerance. Some research shows delayed introduction of cow's milk products and other foods beyond 7 months is associated with increased risk of for eczema and atopic development (Kneepkens et al., 2010; Snijders et al., 2008; Zutavern et al., 2004).
2. Introduction of small amounts of gluten-containing foods (wheat, barley, rye) before 7 months while the infant is breastfeeding and continues to breastfeed may reduce the risk for celiac disease (Agostoni et al., 2008; Radiovic et al., 2010).
C. A variety of foods should be offered by the end of the first year.
D. Sugar and salt should not be added to complementary foods and are not necessary for acceptance. Addition of flavor enhancers such as garlic, vanilla, cinnamon, lemon, and other herbs and spices may improve acceptance.

E. Illness:

    1. During illness, fluid intake should be increased, including more frequent breastfeeding, and the child should be encouraged to eat soft, varied, appetizing, favorite foods.

    2. Fluid needs often increase during illness.

    3. Sick children seem to prefer breastfeeding, and frequent breastfeeding is advised.

    4. After illness, greater intake of food is needed to regain weight lost and replenish nutrient losses.

X. When to Refer

A. If a child is not achieving normal growth patterns (see Chapter 31, Breastfeeding and Growth: Birth Through Weaning), a referral can be made to the primary care provider or a specialist in pediatric nutrition.

B. If the child is refusing to eat age-appropriate complementary foods, is eating very few foods, or is consuming insufficient quantities, a referral can be made for an evaluation by a feeding team or a pediatric feeding specialist.

C. If the child is exhibiting signs of food intolerances, including but not limited to vomiting, blood in stools, diarrhea, hives, or eczema, a referral can be made to the primary care provider, an allergist, or a gastroenterologist.

D. Parents who have limited financial resources to purchase appropriate foods for their family may need a referral to social services for assistance.

References

Agostoni, C., Decsi, T., Fewtrell, M., Kolacek, S., Koletzko, B., Michaelson, K. F., Moreno, L., Puntis, J., Rigo, J., Shamir, R., Szajewska, H., Turck, D., van Goudoever, J., & ESPGHAN Committee on Nutrition. (2008). Complementary feeding: A commentary by the ESPGHAN Committee on Nutrition. *Journal of Pediatric Gastroenterology and Nutrition, 46*, 99–110.

American Dietetic Association. (2003). Position of the American Dietetic Association and Dietitians of Canada: Vegetarian diets. *Journal of the American Dietetic Association, 103*, 748–765.

Baker, R. D., Greer, F. R., & Committee on Nutrition of the American Academy of Pediatrics. (2010). Clinical report—diagnosis and prevention of iron deficiency and iron-deficiency anemia in infants and young children (0–3 years of age). *Pediatrics, 126*(5), 1–11.

Bergmann, R. L., Haschke-Becher, E., Klassen-Wigger, P., Bergmann, K., Richter, R., Dudenhausen, J. W., Grathwohl, D., & Haschke, F. (2008). Supplementation with 200 mg/day docosahexaenoic acid from mid-pregnancy through lactation improves the docosahexaenoic acid status of mothers with a habitually low fish intake and of their infants. *Annals of Nutrition & Metabolism, 52*, 157–166.

Brown, K. H., Engle-Stone, R., Krebs, N., & Peerson, J. M. (2009). Recent advances in knowledge of zinc nutrition and human health. *Food and Nutrition Bulletin, 30*(1 Suppl.), S144–S169.

Centers for Disease Control and Prevention. (1994, September 9). Hyponatremic seizures among infants fed with commercial bottled drinking water—Wisconsin, 1993. *Morbidity and Mortality Weekly Report, 43*(35), 641–644.

Centers for Disease Control and Prevention. (2001, August 17). Recommendations for using fluoride to prevent and control dental caries in the United States. *Morbidity and Mortality Weekly Report, 50*(RR-14), 1–42.

Centers for Disease Control and Prevention. (2003, January 31). Neurologic impairment in children associated with maternal dietary deficiency of cobalamin—Georgia, 2001. *Morbidity and Mortality Weekly Report, 52*(4), 61–64.

Chantry, C. J., Howard, C. R., & Auinger, P. (2007). Full breastfeeding duration and risk of iron deficiency in U.S. infants. *Breastfeeding Medicine, 2*, 63–73.

Chehade, H., Girardin, E., Rosato, L., Cachat, F., Cotting, J., & Perez, M. H. (2011). Acute life-threatening presentation of vitamin D deficiency rickets. *Journal of Clinical Endocrinology and Metabolism, 96*(9), 2681–2683.

Dee, D. L., Sharma, A. J., Cogswell, M. E., Grummer-Strawn, L. M., Fein, S. B., & Scanlon, K. S. (2008). Sources of supplemental iron among breastfed infants during the first year of life. *Pediatrics, 122*, S98–S104.

Delgado-Noguera, M. F., Calvache, J. A., & Bonfil Cosp, X. (2010, December 8). Supplementation with long chain polyunsaturated fatty acids (LCPUFA) to breastfeeding mothers for improving child growth and development. *Cochrane Database Systematic Reviews, 12*, CD007901.

Dewey, K. G. (2001). Nutrition, growth, and complementary feeding of the breastfed infant. *Pediatric Clinics of North America, 48*(1), 87–104.

Dewey, K. G., Domellöf, M., Cohen, R. J., Rivera, L. L., Hernell, O., & Lönnerdal, B. (2002). Iron supplementation affects growth and morbidity of breast-fed infants: Results of a randomized trial in Sweden and Honduras. *Journal of Nutrition, 132*, 3249–3255.

Domellöf, M., Lönnerdal, B., Abrams, S. A., & Hernell, O. (2002). Iron absorption in breast-fed infants: Effects of age, iron status, iron supplements, and complementary foods. *American Journal of Clinical Nutrition, 76*, 198–204.

Dube, K., Schwartz, J., Mueller, M. J., Kalhoff, H., & Kersting, M. (2010). Iron intake and iron status in breastfed infants during the first year of life. *Clinical Nutrition, 29*(6), 773–778.

Ehlayel, M. S., Bener, A., & Sabbah, A. (2011). Is high prevalence of vitamin D deficiency evidence for asthma and allergy risks? *European Annals of Allergy & Clinical Immunology, 43*(3), 81–88.

Francois, C. A., Connor, S. L., Wander, R. C., & Connor, W. E. (1998). Acute effects of dietary fatty acids on the fatty acids of human milk. *American Journal of Clinical Nutrition, 67*, 301–308.

Gibson, R. A., Muhlhausler, B., & Makrides, M. (2011). Conversion of linoleic acid and alpha-linolenic acid to long-chain polyunsaturated fatty acids (LCPUFAs), with a focus on pregnancy, lactation and the first 2 years of life. *Maternal and Child Nutrition, 7*(Suppl. 2), 17–26.

Gilmore, J. M. E., Hong, L., Broffitt, B., & Levy, S. M. (2005). Longitudinal patterns of vitamin and mineral supplement use in young white children. *Journal of the American Dietetic Association, 105*,763–772.

Greer, F., Shannon, M., the Committee on Nutrition, & the Committee on Environmental Health of the American Academy of Pediatrics. (2005). Infant methemoglobinemia: The role of dietary nitrate in food and water. *Pediatrics, 116*, 784–786.

Greer, F. R., Sicherer, S. H., Burks, A. W., & the Committee on Nutrition and Section on Allergy and Immunology of the American Academy of Pediatrics. (2008). Effects of early nutritional interventions on the development of atopic disease in infants and children: The role of maternal dietary restriction, breastfeeding, timing of introduction of complementary foods, and hydrolyzed formulas. *Pediatrics, 121*(1), 183–191.

Hatun, S., Ozkan, B., & Bereket, A. (2011). Vitamin D deficiency and prevention: Turkish experience. *Acta Paediatrica, 100*(9), 1195–1199.

Helland, I. B., Smith, L., Saarem, K., Saugsad, O. D., & Drevon, C. A. (2003). Maternal supplementation with very-long-chain-n-3 fatty acids during pregnancy and lactation augments children's IQ at 4 years of age. *Pediatrics, 111*, E39 E44.

Hoffman, D. R., Theuer, R. C., Casteñeda, Y. S., Wheaton, D. H., Bosworth, R. G., O'Connor, A. R., Morale, S. E., Wiedemann, L. E., & Birch, E. E. (2004). Maturation of visual acuity is accelerated in breast-fed term infants fed baby food containing DHA-enriched egg yolk. *Journal of Nutrition, 134*, 2307–2313.

Holick, M. F. (2007). Vitamin D deficiency. *New England Journal of Medicine, 357*, 266–281.

Hollis, B., & Wagner, C. L. (2004). Vitamin D requirements during lactation: High-dose maternal supplementation as therapy to prevent hypovitaminosis D for both the mother and the nursing infant. *American Journal of Clinical Nutrition, 80*(Suppl.), 1752S–1758S.

Horodynski, M. A., Baker, S., Coleman, G., Auld, G., & Lindau, J. (2011). The healthy toddlers trial protocol: An intervention to reduce risk factors for childhood obesity in economically and educationally disadvantaged populations. *BMC Public Health, 11*, 581.

Hurley, K. M., Cross, M. B., & Hughes, S. O. (2011). A systematic review of responsive feeding and child obesity in high-income countries. *Journal of Nutrition, 141*, 495–501.

Hutton, E. K., & Hassan, E. S. (2007). Late vs. early clamping of the umbilical cord in full term neonates: Systemic review and meta-analysis. *Journal of the American Medical Association, 297*, 1241–1252.

Innis, S. M. (2007). Dietary (n-3) fatty acids and brain development. *Journal of Nutrition, 137*, 855–859.

Innis, S. M., Gilley, J., & Werker, J. (2001). Are human milk long-chain polyunsaturated fatty acids related to visual and neural development in breast-fed term infants? *Journal of Pediatrics, 139*, 532–538.

Ismail, A. I., & Bandekar, R. R. (1999). Fluoride supplements and fluorosis: A meta-analysis. *Community Dentistry and Oral Epidemiology, 27*(1), 48–56.

Kleinman, R. E. (Ed.). (2009). *Pediatric nutrition handbook* (6th ed.). Elk Grove, IL: American Academy of Pediatrics.

Kneepkens, C. M. F., & Brand, P. L. P. (2010). Breastfeeding and the prevention of allergy. *European Journal of Pediatrics, 169*(8), 911–917. doi:10.1007/s00431-010-1141-7

Kozyrskyj, A. L., Bahreinian, S., & Azad, M. B. (2011). Early life exposures: Impact on asthma and allergic disease. *Current Opinion in Allergy and Clinical Immunology*, 11(5), 400–406.

Krebs, N. F., Westcott, J. E., Butler, N., Robinson, C., Bell, M., & Hambidge, K. M. (2006). Meat as a first complementary food for breastfed infants: Feasibility and impact on zinc intake and status. *Journal of Pediatric Gastroenterology and Nutrition, 42*(2), 207–214.

Leverett, D. H., Adair, S. M., Vaughan, B. W., Proskin, H. M., & Moss, M. E. (1997). Randomized clinical trial of the effect of prenatal fluoride supplements in preventing dental caries. *Caries Research, 31*, 174–179.

Lowdon, J. (2011). Rickets: Concerns over the worldwide increase. *Journal of Family Health Care, 21*(2), 25–29.

Misra, M., Pacaud, D., Petryk, A., Collett-Solberg, P. F., & Kappy, M. (2008). Vitamin D deficiency in children and its management: Review of current knowledge and recommendations. *Pediatrics, 122*, 398–417.

Moritz, M. L. & Ayus, J. C. (2002). Disorders of water metabolism in children: Hyponatremia and hypernatremia. *Pediatrics in Review, 23*, 371–379.

Narchi, H., Kochiyil, J., Zayed, R., Abdulrazzak, W., & Agarwal, M. (2011). Longitudinal study of vitamin D status in the 1st 6 months of life. *Annals of Tropical Paediatrics, 31*(3), 225–230.

Neuringer, M., Connor, W. E., Lin, D. S., Barstad, L., & Luck, S. (1986). Biochemical and functional effects of prenatal and postnatal omega 3 fatty acid deficiency on retina and brain in rhesus monkeys. *Proceedings of the National Academy of Sciences of the United States of America*, *83*, 4021–4025.

Neville, M. C., Keller, R., Seacat, J., Lutes, V., Neifert, M., Casey, C., Allen, J., & Archer, P. (1988). Studies in human lactation: Milk volumes in lactating women during the onset of lactation and full lactation. *American Journal of Clinical Nutrition*, *48*, 1375–1386.

Otten, J. J., Hellwig, J. P., & Meyers, L. D. (Eds.). (2006). *Dietary reference intakes: The essential guide to nutrient requirements*. Washington, DC: National Academies Press.

Palmer, G. (2011). *Complementary feeding: Nutrition, culture and politics*. London, England: Pinter and Martin.

Pan American Health Organization & World Health Organization. (2003). Guiding principles of complementary feeding of the breastfed child. Retrieved from http://www.who.int/child_adolescent_health/documents/a85622/en/index.html

Pludowski, P., Socha, P., Karczmarewicz, E., Zagorecka, E., Lukaszkiewicz, J., Stolarczyk, A., Piotrowska-Jastrzebska, J., Kryskiewicz, E., Lorenc, R. S., & Socha. J. (2011). Vitamin D supplementation and status in infants: A prospective cohort observational study. *Journal of Pediatric Gastroenterology and Nutrition*, *53*(1), 93–99.

Radiovic, N. P., Mladenovic, M. M., Lekovic, Z. M., Stojsic, Z. M., & Radiovic, V. N. (2010). Influence of early feeding practices on celiac disease in infants. *Croatian Medical Journal*, *51*, 417–422.

Raj, S., Faridi, M., Rusia, U., & Singh, O. (2008). A prospective study of iron status in exclusively breastfed term infants up to 6 months of age. *International Breastfeeding Journal*, *3*, 3.

Rajakumar, K., & Thomas, S. B. (2005). Reemerging nutritional rickets. *Archives of Pediatric and Adolescent Medicine*, *159*, 335–341.

Rao, R., & Georgieff, M. K. (2007). Iron in fetal and neonatal nutrition. *Seminars in Fetal and Neonatal Medicine*, *12*(1), 54–63.

Ruan, C., Liu, X., Man, H., Ma, X., Lu, G., Duan, G., DeFrancesco, C. A., & Connor, W. E. (1995). Milk composition in women from five different regions of China: The great diversity of milk fatty acids. *Journal of Nutrition*, *125*, I2993–I2998.

Saadi, H. F., Dawodu, A., Afandi, B., Zayed, R., Benedict, S., Nagelkerke, N., & Hollis, B. (2009). Effect of combined maternal and infant vitamin D supplementation on vitamin D status of exclusively breastfed infants. *Maternal and Child Nutrition*, *5*, 25–32.

Schanler, R. J., on behalf of the AAP Section on Breastfeeding, Executive Committee, Feldman-Winter, L., Landers, S., Noble, L., Szucs, K. A., & Viehmann, L. (2011). Concerns with early universal iron supplementation of breastfeeding infants. *Pediatrics*, *127*, e1097.

Snijders, B. E., Thijs, C., van Ree, R., & van den Brandt, P. A. (2008). Age at first introduction of cow milk products and other food products in relation to infant atopic manifestations in the first 2 years of life: The KOALA birth cohort study. *Pediatrics*, *122*(1), e115–e122.

Tang, Q. Q., Du, J., Ma, H. H., Jiang, S. J., & Zhou, X. J. (2008). Fluoride and children's intelligence: A meta-analysis. *Biological Trace Element Research*, *126*(1–3), 115–120.

Taylor, S. N., Wagner, C. L., & Hollis, B. W. (2008). Vitamin D supplementation during lactation to support infant and mother. *Journal of the American College of Nutrition*, *27*, 690–701.

Van Rheenen, P., & Brabin, B. J. (2004). Late umbilical cord-clamping as an intervention for reducing iron deficiency anaemia in term infants in developing and industrialized countries: A systematic review. *Annals of Tropical Paediatrics*, *24*, 3–16.

Wagner, C. L., Greer, F., Section on Breastfeeding & Committee on Nutrition of the American Academy of Pediatrics. (2008). Prevention of rickets and vitamin D deficiency in infants, children, and adolescents. *Pediatrics*, *122*(5), 1142–1152.

Ward, L. M., Gaboury, I., Ladhani, M., & Zlotkin, S. (2007). Vitamin D–deficiency rickets among children in Canada. *Canadian Medical Association Journal*, *177*(2), 161–166.

World Health Organization. (2003). *Global strategy for infant and young child feeding.* Geneva, Switzerland: Author.

Yang, Z., Lönnerdal, B., Adu-Afarwuah, S., Brown, K. H., Chaparro, C. M., Cohen, R. J., Domellöf, M., Hernell, O., Lartey, A., & Dewey, K. (2009). Prevalence and predictors of iron deficiency in fully breastfed infants at 6 mo of age: Comparison of data from 6 studies. *American Journal of Clinical Nutrition*, *89*, 1433–1440.

Ziegler, E. E., Nelson, S. E., & Jeter, J. M. (2009). Iron status of breastfed infants is improved equally by medicinal iron and iron-fortified cereal. *American Journal of Clinical Nutrition*, *90*, 76–87.

Zutavern, A., von Mutius, E., Harris, J., Mill, P., Moffatt, S., White, C., & Cullinan, P. (2004). The introduction of solids in relation to asthma and eczema. *Archives of Disease in Childhood*, *89*, 303–308.

CHAPTER 21

Biochemistry of Human Milk

Linda J. Smith, MPH, IBCLC, FILCA

OBJECTIVES

- Describe human milk synthesis and composition over the continuum of lactation.
- Discuss components of human milk and their functions.
- Discuss maternal nutrition in relation to milk volume and composition.
- Compare human milk with other products and manufactured milks.

INTRODUCTION

Human milk is a unique food designed specifically for the needs of a human infant. Nutritional and anti-infective components are woven into a tapestry of growth-promoting elements, enzymes to aid in the digestion and absorption of nutrients, and a fatty acid profile that optimizes brain growth and development. The ingredients of breastmilk are not interchangeable with, nor equivalent to, manufactured milks or nutrients from other animal species or nutritional products made from plant sources, including soy. The protein and fat content of human milk reflect the identity of a species that requires close contact and frequent feedings. Human milk is far more than a means of supplying added benefits to an infant's diet. It is the reference food and the plan in nature for nourishing young humans while simultaneously providing immune protection, regulatory hormones, living cells, bioactive enzymes, and other components. The lactation consultant benefits from knowledge of human milk composition to inform parents and professionals of the importance of supplying human milk for their baby directly from the breast or indirectly using feeding equipment.

I. Milk Synthesis and Milk Composition over the Continuum of Lactation

A. Mammogenesis is the development of duct structure from the woman's birth through her first pregnancy. (See Chapter 17, Physiology of the Breast During Pregnancy and Lactation.)

B. Lactogenesis I is driven by the endocrine system during pregnancy and beyond.

    1. Lactocytes develop on the duct structure (basement membranes) in a single layer, forming a hollow sphere (alveoli) of one layer of cells with a central lumen, surrounded by capillary vessels and myoepithelial cells.

    2. Milk secretion begins in the first trimester at approximately 16 weeks of gestation (Lawrence et al.,2011).

    3. There are five pathways for synthesis of milk components.

        a. Exocytosis: Proteins, lactose, citrate; part of feedback system.

        b. Lipid (fat) released in droplets; lipases are released at the same time, aiding digestion.

        c. Osmosis through membrane contributes ions and water.

        d. Transport of immunoglobulins across cell membranes.

        e. Paracellular (junctures between cells) pathways for white cells and water-soluble compounds.

C. Lactogenesis II is the onset of copious milk secretion (milk coming in).

    1. Trigger is delivery of placenta, which withdraws progesterone; prolactin is then unopposed; insulin, cortisol, and citrate are permissive.

    2. Changes begin 30 to 40 hours postpartum; the timing is not related to sucking stimulus and occurs regardless of the baby's status.

    3. Unopposed prolactin turns on alpha-lactalbumin, which triggers lactose synthesis in lactocytes; the increased lactose draws water into secretion via osmosis; milk volume often exceeds baby's needs.

D. Lactogenesis III (galactopoiesis) is ongoing maintenance of milk secretion.

    1. Upper limit appears to be established in first several weeks. Oxytocin pushes out already-made milk. Prolactin surges finish cell growth and continue to influence and maintain milk production.

    2. Autocrine feedback takes on dominant role in short-term regulation of milk secretion. Three components have been identified to date, collectively referred to as feedback inhibitors of lactation (FIL): Retained peptides (proteins) suppress the protein-producing exocytosis process, fatty acid accumulation slows fat synthesis, and prolactin in milk downregulates prolactin receptors on lactocyctes.

    3. Milk synthesis is controlled by the milk (autocrine control). As milk accumulates in the alveolar lumen, the rate of synthesis slows down as a result of chemical feedback from FIL components and physical pressure of retained milk, which changes the shape of the lactocyte.

    4. The degree of fullness/emptiness of the breast determines rate of milk synthesis. "Empty" breasts try to refill quickly: up to 58 mL (2 oz) per hour; "full" breasts secrete milk slowly at about 11 mL (0.33 ounce) per hour. Babies consume an average of 67.3–67.8% of available milk per feed (Kent et al., 2006).

E. Changes over time:
    1. Milk expressed in the second year of lactation has significantly increased fat and energy (Mandel et al., 2005).
    2. Serotonin and lysozyme increase over time; zinc decreases over time.
    3. As volume drops during weaning, the protective factors increase in importance and proportion to total fluid volume, providing protection to the child and the breast throughout the entire duration of lactation. Human milk is important to the infant at all stages of lactation and in any amount.

II. Components of Milk and Their Functions

A. Colostrum: Secretion begins at approximately 16 weeks of gestation (Lawrence et al., 2011).
    1. High density; thick, almost gel-like; generally yellow-colored (beta-carotene).
    2. Rapid increase in milk volume parallels newborn's increasing stomach capacity (Scammon et al., 1920; Zangen et al., 2001).
        a. Day 1 volume: Mean 37.1 mL (range 7–122.5 mL); stomach capacity 7 mL (2 mL/kg) (colostrum).
        b. Day 3 volume: Mean 408 mL (range 98.3–775 mL); stomach capacity 27 mL (8 mL/kg).
        c. Day 5 volume: Mean 705 mL (range 425.5–876 mL); stomach capacity 57 mL (17 mL/kg) (transitional milk).
        d. Calories, mean: 67 kcal/dL (18.76 kcal/oz; 2% fat).
    3. Primary function is protective: Coats the gut to prevent adherence of pathogens; promotes gut closure.
    4. Secretory immunoglobulin A (SIgA) is especially high in the first 72 hours post delivery.
    5. White cells, especially polymorphonucleocytes (90% of cells in colostrum).
    6. Lactoferrin, lysozyme epidermal growth factor, interleukin 10.
    7. Laxative effect; clears meconium with its reservoir of bilirubin.
    8. Growth factors stimulate infant's system; 21 antioxidants.
    9. Helps establish bifidus flora (nonpathogenic) in gastrointestinal (GI) tract.
    10. Compared with mature milk: lower in lactose, fat, and water-soluble vitamins; higher in vitamins A and E, carotenoids, protein, sodium, zinc, chloride, and potassium.

B. Water
    1. Water makes up the majority (87.5%) of human milk.
    2. All other components are dissolved, dispersed, or suspended in water.
    3. Human milk provides all the water a baby needs, even in hot and arid climates.

C. Proteins and nonprotein nitrogen compounds in mature milk
    1. Whey to casein ratio:
        a. Varies with stage of lactation from 90:10 in early lactation, 60:40 in mature milk, and 50:50 in late lactation (Kunz et al., 1992).
        b. Whey predominates in human milk and casein predominates in bovine (cow) milk.

2. Total protein in mature milk is 0.8% to 1.0%; lowest of all mammals.
3. Nineteen amino acids are essential to human development.
   a. Taurine: Develops brain and retina, membrane stabilization, inhibitory neurotransmitter; not found in bovine milk
   b. Tyrosine: Low in human breastmilk
   c. Phenylalanine: Much higher in bovine milk
4. Casein proteins:
   a. Phosphoproteins bind calcium, resulting in cloudy/opaque/white color.
   b. Forms soft, flocculent curds that are easily digested.
5. Whey proteins are available for digestion and perform specific functions.
   a. Alpha-lactalbumin
      i. Bovine milk is high in beta-lactoglobulin, which is not found in human milk.
      ii. Regulates milk synthesis.
      iii. Mucins bind pathogens; kill cancer cells (Aits et al., 2009).
   b. Lactoferrin
      i. Iron transport and absorption
      ii. Competes with bacteria to bind iron
      iii. Antibacterial
      iv. Essential growth factor for B- and T-cell lymphocytes
      v. Promotes growth of lactobacilli
      vi. Produced in mammary epithelial cells, milk ducts, and other regions of the body; speculated to have local as well as systemic protective properties
   c. Secretory immunoglobulin A (SIgA)
      i. Other immunoglobulins are IgG, IgM, and IgE.
      ii. SIgA is most important immunoglobulin because it coats mucosal surfaces to prevent adherence and penetration by pathogens.
   d. Enzymes (> 401 identified to date)
      i. Aid in digestion of the nutrients in milk.
      ii. Compensatory digestive enzymes.
      iii. Stimulate neonatal development.
      iv. Lipase digests fats, breaks down fatty acid chains.
      v. Bile salt–stimulated lipase is antiprotozoan; acts on Giardia and other organisms that cause diarrhea.
      vi. Lysozyme attacks cell walls of pathogens (apoptosis) without triggering inflammation; increases over time.
      vii. Amylase digests polysaccharides/starch.
      viii. Alkaline phosphatase.
      ix. Peroxidases act like hydrogen peroxide and oxidize bacteria.
         (a) Xanthine oxidase, sulfhydryl oxidase, and glutathione peroxidase

   e. Hormones and hormone-like substances
      i. Prolactin in milk (not the same as prolactin derived from mother's serum prolactin)
      ii. Prostaglandins, with anti-inflammatory properties
      iii. Oxytocin, adrenal and ovarian steroids, relaxin, and insulin
      iv. Thyroid hormones: TRH, TSH, thyroxine (T4)
   f. Growth factors
      i. Epidermal growth factors aid gut and other tissue maturity.
      ii. Nerve growth factor may help heal central nervous system (CNS) from birth-related injury.
      iii. Insulin-like growth factor.
6. Nonprotein nitrogen compounds
   a. Urea, creatine, creatinine, uric acid, glucosamine, and alpha-amino nitrogen
   b. Nucleic acids, nucleotides and polyamines
7. Carbohydrates
   a. Principal carbohydrate in human milk is lactose: disaccharide (galactose + glucose) found only in milk.
      i. Supplies 40% of baby's energy needs.
      ii. Synthesis begins at lactogenesis II, approximately 30 to 40 hours postpartum.
         (a) Rise in lactose secreted in cell draws water by osmosis and directly influences milk volume.
         (b) Colostrum is 4% lactose on day 1; rapidly increases.
      iii. Human milk is highest in lactose of all mammals.
         (a) Largest brain of all animals at birth. Larger brains need higher amounts of milk lactose (Hale et al., 2007).
         (b) There are 7.2 g/100 mL, and human milk is the sweetest of all milks.
         (c) Component of galactolipids needed for CNS structural development.
      iv. Lactose is the primary carbohydrate in milk and least variable (most consistent).
         (a) Humans produce an abundance of lactase (the enzyme that digests lactose) until age 2.5 to 7 years or more.
         (b) Lactase is a brush border intestinal enzyme present by 24 weeks of fetal life.
         (c) Concentration at delivery is two to four times higher than at 2 to 11 months postpartum. Persistence of lactase production is genetically determined and decreases with age.
         (d) Lactose assists in the absorption of calcium and iron.
         (e) Primary lactose intolerance is extremely rare; infants of all races typically display a high degree of lactose tolerance.

b. Oligosaccharides: Over 130 specific compounds active against pathogens.
   i. Stimulate Lactobacillus bifidus
   ii. Block pathogens from attaching to gut
   iii. Protect against enterotoxins in the gut, bind to bacteria
c. Bifidus factor: A combination of several different oligosaccharides.
   i. With lactose, growth in infant gut of L. bifidus, which occupies the intestine, crowds out pathogens, and produces an acid detrimental to pathogen growth, is promoted.
   ii. Suppresses pathogens and is thought to contribute to unique aroma of exclusively breastmilk stools.
d. Other carbohydrates:
   i. Glycopeptides, fructose, and galactose
8. Fats (lipids): Most variable compound in human milk and provide up to 50% of calories.
   a. Fat content of mature milk is 41.1 g/L (range 22.3–61.6 g/L), which is independent of breastfeeding frequency (Kent et al., 2006) and is directly related to the relative fullness or emptiness of the breast. As a breast empties during an individual feed and/or over a day, the proportion of fat increases.
   b. Ratio of saturated to unsaturated is relatively stable at 42% saturated; 57% unsaturated; smoking decreases the levels of some essential fatty acids in milk (Agostoni et al., 2003).
   c. Lipases (enzymes) are released simultaneously.
      i. Break down long-chain fatty acids; aid digestion.
      ii. Free fatty acids kill bacteria and parasites, including Giardia, and inactivate viruses.
   d. Ninety-eight percent of lipids are encased in globules; membrane coating prevents clumping.
   e. Variation in fat levels:
      i. Total fat is only somewhat related to mother's diet; profile of fatty acid chain length varies with maternal diet (discussed later).
      ii. Fat levels increase within each feed (foremilk to hindmilk) and increase as breast empties.
      iii. Approximately 70% of fat variation is related to relative fullness or emptiness of the breast.
      iv. Fat levels significantly increase in second year of lactation.
   f. Triglycerides predominate.
      i. Lipases break down triglycerides into free fatty acids.
   g. Cholesterol in human milk:
      i. Unique metabolic effects.
      ii. Essential part of all membranes.

        iii. Cholesterol is an important constituent of brain tissue, being necessary for the laying down of the myelin sheath, which is involved in nerve conduction in the brain, along with docosahexaenoic acid (DHA) and arachidonic acid (AA).

        iv. Breastfed babies have higher cholesterol levels than formula-fed infants.

   h. Fatty acids:

        i. Long-chain polyunsaturated fatty acids specific to infant needs:

           (a) Central role in cognitive development, vision, nerve myelinization.

           (b) May be conditionally essential to newborns (Koletzko et al., 2000).

           (c) DHA and AA are especially important to brain maturation.

        ii. Poorly synthesized from precursors (linolenic and linoleic acids).

        iii. Preformed dietary DHA is better synthesized into nervous tissue than that synthesized from linolenic acid.

   i. Phospholipids.

   j. Sterols, a component of lipid membranes.

9. Fat-soluble vitamins:

   a. Vitamin A and carotene.

   b. Vitamin D is a group of related fat-soluble compounds with antirachitic (rickets) activity and is also found in milk in an aqueous form.

   c. Exclusive breastfeeding results in normal infant bone mineral content when the maternal vitamin D status is adequate and the infant is regularly exposed to sunlight; breastfed infants require about 30 minutes of sunlight exposure per week if wearing only a diaper, or 2 hours per week if fully clothed without a hat; darkly pigmented infants require a greater exposure to sunlight (Specker et al., 1985). Only if the infant or mother (especially those with darker skin pigment or those who live in a geographic area with little sunlight) is not regularly exposed to sunlight, or if the mother's intake of vitamin D is low and cannot be raised, would supplements to the mother or infant be indicated (Lawrence et al., 2011, pp. 299–300). Supplementing the mother with high doses of vitamin D (6,400 IU daily) is effective in raising vitamin D levels in her milk (Basile et al., 2006; Hollis et al., 2004; Wagner et al., 2006; Wagner et al., 2008).

   d. Vitamin E: Functions as an antioxidant.

   e. Vitamin K: Highest in colostrum; later manufactured in infant gut.

        i. Localized in the milk fat globule with hindmilk containing a twofold higher vitamin K concentration than milk from a full pumping

10. Water-soluble vitamins: These vary with the stage of lactation, maternal intake, and if delivery takes place before term; the breast does not synthesize these water-soluble vitamins, so their origin is maternal plasma derived from the maternal diet.

   a. Thiamin, riboflavin, niacin, pantothenic acid, biotin, folate, and vitamin B_6.

    b. Vitamin B_{12}; needed by the baby's developing nervous system. Vitamin B_{12} occurs exclusively in animal tissue, is bound to protein, and is minimal to absent in plant protein. A vegetarian mother who consumes no animal products could have milk deficient in vitamin B_{12} and might need an acceptable source of intake.

    c. Vitamin C (higher in milk than maternal plasma).

    d. Inositol.

    e. Choline.

11. Cells:

    a. Macrophages:

       i. Contain IgA

       ii. Ninety percent of cells in mature milk

       iii. Phagocytosis (actively destroy microbial pathogens)

       iv. Make/facilitate lactoferrin, complement

    b. Leukocytes.

    c. Lymphocytes: 10% of cells; T cells and B cells; humoral immunity.

    d. Epithelial cells.

    e. Neutrophil granulocytes.

    f. Chemical mediators released by cells in the milk and injured/inflamed tissue cause more white cells to move into the area to facilitate healing and prevent infection.

    g. Multipotent stem cells (Patki et al., 2010).

12. Minerals:

    a. Macronutrient elements

       i. Numerous factors affect the levels of minerals in human milk; during pregnancy, involution, and mastitis, the junctions between the alveolar cells are open, allowing sodium and chloride to enter the milk space, drawing water with them; under these conditions, milk has much higher concentrations of sodium and chloride and decreased concentrations of lactose and potassium.

       ii. The presence of elevated sodium concentrations in human milk can be diagnostic of mastitis, other pathology, or low milk volume secretion.

       iii. Calcium, phosphate, magnesium, potassium, sodium, chloride, sulfate, and citrate.

    b. Trace elements

       i. Copper, chromium, and cobalt

       ii. Iron

          (a) Full-term infants are born with sufficient physiologic stores of iron in the liver and hemoglobin, which along with the iron in breastmilk is sufficient to meet the requirements for iron for at least the first 6 to 9 months if babies are exclusively breastfed.

(b) Approximately 50% of iron is absorbed from breastmilk compared with less than 7% from fortified infant formulas, and less than 4% from fortified infant cereals.

(c) Iron concentrations in breastmilk are not influenced by the maternal iron status or intake. Lactose, which promotes iron absorption, is higher in breastmilk, especially compared to some commercial formulas, some of which contain no lactose at all.

iii. Iodine, fluoride, zinc, manganese, and selenium

13. Constituents have multiple functions in addition to nutrition.

a. "The unique feature of human milk is that virtually every component examined plays some extra-nutritional role. The elegance of the system is remarkable—the more so the more we learn about it" (J. Hopkinson).

b. Alpha-lactalbumin:
   i. Nutrient synthesis
   ii. Carries metals
   iii. Prevents infection

c. Lactoferrin:
   i. Transports iron
   ii. Prevents infection
   iii. Prevents inflammation including necrotizing enterocolitis (NEC)
   iv. Promotes tissue growth and growth of lactobacilli in gut

d. SIgA, the most important immunoglobulin:
   i. Infant receives 0.5–2.5 g/dL in first month, which gradually decreases over time as the infant's own SIgA develops. SIgA concentration in colostrum is even higher in the first 24 hours (Goldman et al., 1982; Hennart et al., 1991).
   ii. Prevents inflammation.
   iii. Active against enveloped viruses, rotaviruses, polioviruses, respiratory syncytial virus, enteric and respiratory bacteria, and intestinal parasites.
   iv. Stimulates infant production of SIgA.
   v. General and specific protection against pathogens.

e. Epidermal growth factor:
   i. Prevents inflammation
   ii. Promotes growth
   iii. Catalyzing reactions

f. Lipids: Break down products (free fatty acids) active against enveloped viruses and intestinal parasites.

g. Oligosaccharides: Active against enteric and respiratory bacteria.

h. Beta-carotene: Antioxidant and nutrient.

i. Anti-inflammatory and pharmacologically active components:
   i. Prostaglandins, ovarian steroids, gonadotropins, somatostatin, prolactin, insulin

j. Differentially regulates gene expression (Chapkin et al., 2010)

k. Free oligosaccharides protect infant gut (Zivkovic et al., 2010).

l. Colostrum and human milk effectively relieves procedural pain in neonates (Shah et al., 2006, 2007; Zanardo et al., 2001).

14. Anti-infectious agents are found in many components of milk.
    a. Lipids
    b. Proteins
       i. Lactoferrin, secretory IgA, lysozyme.
       ii. Enzymes. Bile salt–stimulated lipase is active against protozoa.
    c. Nonspecific factors
       i. Complement, interferon, bifidus factor, antiviral factors
    d. White blood cells
       i. T and B lymphocytes
       ii. Macrophages
       iii. Neutrophils
15. Variations in human milk composition:
    a. Changes within a feed (e.g., fat increases during each feed)
    b. Differences between breasts; changes over the 24-hour day
       i. Fat levels increase as breast empties.
    c. Changes over short and long term of a lactation cycle (days to months to years)
       i. Zinc decreases slightly.
       ii. Whey-to-casein ratio changes, that is, casein increases proportionally to whey.
       iii. Calcium decreases.
       iv. DHA levels change somewhat in relationship to maternal intake.
    d. Preterm milk
       i. Higher protein, sodium, chloride than mature milk.
       ii. Lower lactose than mature milk.
       iii. Fatty acids parallel intrauterine levels and profiles.
    e. Colored milk
       i. May be caused by something in maternal diet or medication.
       ii. No known harmful effect on infant.
       iii. If bright red or rusty colored, investigate the cause while continuing to breastfeed/provide milk to baby. Frank blood may need follow-up by the mother's physician.
    f. Odor and flavor influenced by mother's diet, which is important to the infant in adapting to the family nutrition styles and preferences (Mizuno & Ueda, 2004).

III. Influence of Mother's Diet on Milk Volume and Composition

    A. **Table 21-1** summarizes the influence of maternal diet on milk composition and volume.

IV. Comparison of Human Milk to Manufactured Milks (Human Milk Is Species Specific)

    A. "Formula is adequate, not optimal, and is not perfectly acceptable. It does not resemble breast milk except that it contains protein, fat, and carbohydrates from bovine sources. It has none of the enzymes, ligands, immune properties or infection protection properties. It will stave off starvation and predispose to obesity" (R. A. Lawrence, 2006).

    B. Mother's milk matches much more than 50% of baby's genetic material. Milk from other species and plant-based fluids are genetically different from the infant. Breastmilk has a unique balance of nutrients and other components; it most closely matches milks of species with high maternal investment and frequent feedings.

    C. Human milk composition is not static or uniform like artificial baby milks are. Colostrum (1–5 days post birth) evolves to transitional milk (6–13 days post birth) and then into mature milk (14 days and beyond). The component called colostrum in the early weeks is more accurately described as an "immune layer" that persists throughout the duration of lactation.

    D. Bioavailability is low for all other milks.

        1. Human milk has little residue, and low solute load; nutrients are utilized efficiently.

        2. Iron absorption is greater in human milk. (See discussion earlier in this chapter in the "Minerals" section.)

Table 21-1 Influence of Mother's Diet on Milk Volume and Composition

Milk Component	Affected by Mother's Diet?
Total milk volume	No, except possibly in maternal starvation conditions
Carbohydrates	No
Proteins	No
Lipids	Fatty acid profile only (total fats unaffected)
Cellular components	No
Immune factors	No
Fat-soluble vitamins	Slight variance related to fat levels in milk
Water-soluble vitamins	Yes, deficiencies can occur if maternal diet is inadequate (esp. Vitamin B_{12})
Minerals	No: Macronutrient elements; iron, chromium, cobalt
Lead	Slight/possible: iodine, fluoride; zinc, manganese, selenium

E. Milk from other animals contains deficiencies and excesses of one or more components, only some of which can be modified for infant consumption.

    1. One hundred percent foreign proteins, derived from ruminant animals (cows, goats) or plants.

        a. Increased incidence of allergy; cow's milk protein and soy are known triggers for diabetes in genetically susceptible infants (American Academy of Pediatrics Committee on Nutrition, 1998; American Academy of Pediatrics Work Group on Cow's Milk Protein and Diabetes Mellitus, 1994; Vaarala et al., 1999).

        b. Decreased arousability, which has been implicated in sudden infant death syndrome (Horne et al., 2004); compromised heart rhythms (Zeskind et al., 1991).

        c. Bovine milk is high in phenylalanine, which increases risks of complications of phenylketonuria, such as neurodevelopmental problems (Riva et al., 1996).

    2. Soy "milk" has bioactive components including phytoestrogens (13,000–20,000 higher), aluminum, and magnesium.

    3. Nonhuman fats with no capacity to protect myelin sheath, heal from injury, or develop CNS. Increased risk of multiple sclerosis (Pisacane et al., 1994), altered cholesterol metabolism, vision, and cognitive development.

    4. Absence or deficiency of lactose, which is needed for CNS and cognitive development.

    5. Some components and special formulas are unregulated; recalls for mistakes and contamination.

        a. Powdered formulas are not sterile; approximately 14% are contaminated with Cronobacter sakazakii (formerly Enterobacter), which has caused fatal infections.

        b. Manufacturing errors.

        c. Experimental nature of product, including additions of DHA and AA from manufactured sources, with no evidence to support efficacy or safety.

        d. The U.S. Food and Drug Administration (FDA) categorizes infant formulas as GRAS (Generally Recognized As Safe).

    6. Suboptimal growth patterns (World Health Organization, 2006):

        a. Formula-fed children are fatter per length, with smaller head circumference, and meet developmental milestones later. (See Chapter 22, Infant Formulas: Artificial Baby Milk.)

        b. Increased incidence of short-term illness. (See Chapter 23, Immunology, Infectious Disease, and Allergy Prophylaxis.)

        c. Increased incidence of long-term and chronic illness. (See Chapter 24, Protection Against Chronic Disease for the Breasted Infant and Lactating Mother.)

        d. Altered metabolism for women who do not sustain lactation. (See Chapter 24.)

F. There are no benefits of human milk, rather deficiencies of infants not being breast-fed. Every other substance that can be used to feed human infants has deficiencies and documented problems.

References

Agostoni, C., Marangoni, F., Grandi, F., et al. (2003). Earlier smoking habits are associated with higher serum lipids and lower milk fat and polyunsaturated fatty acid content in the first 6 months of lactation. *European Journal of Clinical Nutrition, 57*, 1466–1472.

Aits, S., Gustafsson, L., Hallgren, O., et al. (2009). HAMLET (human alpha-lactalbumin made lethal to tumor cells) triggers autophagic tumor cell death. *International Journal of Cancer, 124*(5), 1008–1019.

American Academy of Pediatrics Committee on Nutrition. (1998). Soy protein–based formulas: Recommendations for use in infant feeding. *Pediatrics, 101*(1), 148–153.

American Academy of Pediatrics Work Group on Cow's Milk Protein and Diabetes Mellitus. (1994). Infant feeding practices and their possible relationship to the etiology of diabetes mellitus. *Pediatrics, 94*(5), 572–574.

Basile, L. A., Taylor, S. N., Wagner, C. L., Horst, R. L., & Hollis, B. W. (2006). The effect of high-dose vitamin D supplementation on serum vitamin D levels and milk calcium concentration in lactating women and their infants. *Breastfeeding Medicine, 1*(1), 27–35.

Chapkin, R. S., Zhao, C., Ivanov, I., et al. (2010). Noninvasive stool-based detection of infant gastrointestinal development using gene expression profiles from exfoliated epithelial cells. *American Journal of Physiology—Gastrointestinal and Liver Physiology, 298*(5), G582–589.

Goldman, A. S., Garza, C., Nichols, B. L., & Goldblum, R. M. (1982). Immunologic factors in human milk during the first year of lactation. *Journal of Pediatrics, 100*(4), 563–567.

Hale, T. W., & Hartmann, P. E. (2007). *Textbook of human lactation*. Amarillo, TX: Hale Publishing.

Hartmann, P., & Cregan, M. (2001). Lactogenesis and the effects of insulin-dependent diabetes mellitus and prematurity. *Journal of Nutrition, 131*(11), 3016S–3020S.

Hennart, P. F., Brasseur, D. J., Delogne-Desnoeck, J. B., Dramaix, M. M., & Robyn, C. E. (1991). Lysozyme, lactoferrin, and secretory immunoglobulin A content in breast milk: Influence of duration of lactation, nutrition status, prolactin status, and parity of mother. *American Journal of Clinical Nutrition, 53*(1), 32–39.

Hollis, B. W., & Wagner, C. L. (2004). Vitamin D requirements during lactation: High-dose maternal supplementation as therapy to prevent hypovitaminosis D for both the mother and the nursing infant. *American Journal of Clinical Nutrition, 80*(6), 1752–1758.

Horne, R. S., Parslow, P. M., Ferens, D., et al. (2004). Comparison of evoked arousability in breast and formula fed infants. *Archives of Disease in Childhood, 89*, 22–25.

Kent, J. C., Mitoulas, L. R., Cregan, M. D., et al. (2006). Volume and frequency of breastfeedings and fat content of breast milk throughout the day. *Pediatrics, 117*, e387–e395.

Koletzko, B., Michaelson, K. F., & Hernell, O. (2000). *Short and long term effects of breastfeeding on child health*. New York, NY: Kluwer Academic/Plenum Publishers.

Kunz, C., & Lonnerdal, B. (1992). Re-evaluation of the whey protein/casein ratio of human milk. *Acta Paediatrica, 81*, 107–112.

Lawrence, R. A., & Lawrence, R. M. (2011). Breastfeeding: A guide for the medical profession (7th ed.). Philadelphia, PA: Elsevier Mosby.

Mandel, D., Lubetzky, R., Dollberg, S., et al. (2005). Fat and energy contents of expressed human breast milk in prolonged lactation. *Pediatrics, 116*, e432–435.

Mizuno, K., & Ueda, A. (2004). Antenatal olfactory learning influences infant feeding. *Early Human Development, 76*, 83–90.

Patki, S., Kadam, S., Chandra, V., & Bhonde, R. (2010). Human breast milk is a rich source of multipotent mesenchymal stem cells. *Human Cell, 23*(2), 35–40.

Pisacane, A., Impagliazzo, N., Russo, M., Valiani, R., Mandarina, A., Florio, C., & Vivo, P. (1994). Breastfeeding and multiple sclerosis. *British Medical Journal, 308,* 1411–1412.

Riva, E., Agostoni, C., Biasucci, G., et al. (1996). Early breastfeeding is linked to higher intelligence quotient scores in dietary-treated phenylketonuric children. *Acta Paediatrica, 85,* 56–58.

Scammon, R., & Doyle, L. (1920). Observations on the capacity of the stomach in the first ten days of postnatal life. *American Journal of Diseases of Children, 20,* 516–538.

Shah, P. S., Aliwalas, L. I., & Shah, V. (2006). Breastfeeding or breast milk for procedural pain in neonates. *Cochrane Database of Systematic Reviews, 3,* CD004950.

Shah, P. S., Aliwalas, L., & Shah, V. (2007). Breastfeeding or breastmilk to alleviate procedural pain in neonates: A systematic review. *Breastfeeding Medicine, 2*(2), 74–82.

Specker, B. L., Valanis, B., Hertzberg, V., Edwards, N., & Tsang, R. C. (1985). Sunshine exposure and serum 25-hydroxyvitamin D concentrations in exclusively breast-fed infants. *Journal of Pediatrics, 107*(3), 372–376.

Vaarala, O., Knip, M., Paronen, J., et al. (1999). Cow's milk formula feeding induces primary immunization to insulin in infants at genetic risk for type 1 diabetes. *Diabetes, 48*(7), 1389–1394.

Wagner, C. L., Hulsey, T. C., Fanning, D., Ebeling, M., & Hollis, B. W. (2006). High-dose vitamin D_3 supplementation in a cohort of breastfeeding mothers and their infants: A 6-month follow-up pilot study. *Breastfeeding Medicine, 1*(2), 59–70.

Wagner, C. L., Taylor, S. N., & Hollis, B. W. (2008). Does vitamin D make the "world go 'round"? *Breastfeeding Medicine, 3*(4), 239–250.

World Health Organization. (2006). The WHO child growth standards. Geneva, Switzerland: Author. Retrieved from http://www.who.int/childgrowth/en/.

Zanardo, V., Nicolussi, S., Giacomin, C., Faggian, D., Favaro, F., & Plebani, M. (2001). Labor pain effects on colostral milk beta-endorphin concentrations of lactating mothers. *Biology of the Neonate, 79*(2), 87–90.

Zangen, S., Di Lorenzo, C., Zangen, T., et al. (2001). Rapid maturation of gastric relaxation in newborn infants. *Pediatric Research, 50,* 629–632.

Zeskind, P. S., Goff, D. M., & Marshall, T. R. (1991). Rhythmic organization of neonatal heart rate and its relation to atypical fetal growth. *Developmental Psychobiology, 24,* 413–429.

Zivkovic, A. M., German, J. B., Lebrilla, C. B., & Mills, D. A. (2010). Human milk glycobiome and its impact on the infant gastrointestinal microbiota. *Proceedings of the National Academy of Sciences, 2011, 108*(Suppl. 1), 4653–4658.

Suggested Reading

Cregan, M. D., De Mello, T. R., Kershaw, D., et al. (2002). Initiation of lactation in women after preterm delivery. *Acta Obstetricia et Gynecologica Scandinavica, 81,* 870–877.

Cregan, M. D., & Hartmann, P. E. (1999). Computerized breast measurement from conception to weaning: Clinical implications. *Journal of Human Lactation, 15,* 89–96.

Daly, S. E., Kent, J. C., Huynh, D. Q., et al. (1992). The determination of short-term breast volume changes and the rate of synthesis of human milk using computerized breast measurement. *Experimental Physiology, 77,* 79–87.

Daly, S. E., Kent, J. C., Owens, R. A., & Hartmann, P. E. (1996). Frequency and degree of milk removal and the short-term control of human milk synthesis. *Experimental Physiology, 81*, 861–875.

Goldman, A. S., & Garza, C. (1983). Immunologic components in human milk during the second year of lactation. *Acta Paediatrica Scandinactiva, 72*, 461–462.

Hanson, L. A. (2004). *Immunobiology of human milk: How breastfeeding protects babies*. Amarillo, TX: Pharmasoft Publishing.

Hartmann, P. E., Cregan, M. D., Ramsay, D. T, et al. (2003). Physiology of lactation in preterm mothers: Initiation and maintenance. *Pediatric Annals, 32*, 351–355.

Hartmann, P. E., Rattigan, S., Saint, L., & Supriyana, O. (1985). Variation in the yield and composition of human milk. *Oxford Review of Reproductive Biology, 7*, 118–167.

Jensen, R. G. (1995). *Handbook of milk composition*. San Diego, CA: Academic Press.

Kent, J. C., Arthur, P. G., Retallack, R. W., & Hartmann, P. E. (1992). Calcium, phosphate and citrate in human milk at initiation of lactation. *Journal of Dairy Research, 59*, 161–167.

Kent, J. C., Mitoulas, L., Cox, D. B., et al. (1999). Breast volume and milk production during extended lactation in women. *Experimental Physiology, 84*, 435–447.

Kramer, M. S., & Kakuma, R. (2002). Optimal duration of exclusive breastfeeding. *Cochrane Database Systematic Reviews, 1*, CD003517.

Labbok, M. H. (2001). Effects of breastfeeding on the mother. *Pediatric Clinics of North America, 48*, 143–158.

Mitoulas, L. R., Kent, J. C., Cox, D. B., et al. (2002). Variation in fat, lactose and protein in human milk over 24 h and throughout the first year of lactation. *British Journal of Nutrition, 88*, 29–37.

Neville, M. C., Allen, J. C., Archer, P. C., et al. (1991). Studies in human lactation: Milk volume and nutrient composition during weaning and lactogenesis. *American Journal of Clinical Nutrition, 54*, 81–92.

Picciano, M. F. (2001). Nutrient composition of human milk. *Pediatric Clinics of North America, 48*, 53–67.

Saint, L., Smith, M., & Hartmann, P. E. (1984). The yield and nutrient content of colostrum and milk of women from giving birth to 1 month post-partum. *British Journal of Nutrition, 52*, 87–95.

World Health Organization. (2003). *Global strategy for infant and young child feeding*. Geneva, Switzerland: Author.

CHAPTER 22
Infant Formulas: Artificial Baby Milk

Marsha Walker, RN, IBCLC

OBJECTIVES

- Compare the components of breastmilk and infant formula (also known as artificial baby milk).
- Identify the effect of formula-feeding on the brain, immune system, and acute and chronic diseases in breastfed and formula-fed infants.
- Explain some of the hazards of infant formula.
- Evaluate the criteria for the complementary feeding of infants.

INTRODUCTION

Infant formula differs from human milk because human milk is species specific and has evolved through the millennia to facilitate the normal growth and development of human infants. Human milk is extremely complex, and its composition is most likely programmed by chemical communication between the mother and the infant, both prenatally and postnatally. Infant formula does not duplicate the complexity, cannot provide the multiple tiers of disease protection, and cannot operate in the dynamic manner of human milk. Infant formula simply fulfills the role of maintaining growth and development within normal limits.

I. Components of Infant Formula

A. General concepts
  1. Human milk is used as a general guide for the nutrient content in infant formula.
  2. Although infant formula contains similar categories of nutrients that are in breastmilk, such as proteins, fats, carbohydrates, vitamins, and minerals, it does not duplicate them.
  3. Infant formula is an inert medium, with most types containing no bioactive components.
    a. Infant formula does not alter its composition to meet the changing needs of a growing infant.
    b. Unlike breastmilk, infant formula does not contain growth factors, hormones, live cells, immunologic agents, or enzymes.

4. The fatty acid profile of infant formula differs from that of breastmilk.

5. In general, the concentrations of nutrients in infant formula are higher than those in human milk to compensate for their reduced bioavailability and to ensure their presence throughout the entire shelf life of the product.

6. Commercial infant formula brands have many similarities to each other but can differ significantly from each other in the quality and quantity of nutrients and in other additives.

7. A number of bodies worldwide either oversee or make recommendations for the nutrient content of infant formula.

    a. The American Academy of Pediatrics, Committee on Nutrition.

    b. The European Society of Paediatric Gastroenterology and Nutrition (ESPGHAN).

    c. The Food and Agriculture Organization, a part of the United Nations.

    d. Codex Alimentarius.

    e. European Communities.

    f. The United States Food and Drug Administration (FDA).

    g. Safety evaluations of new ingredients added to infant formulas in the United States have been found to be inadequate and lacking in rigor. The Institute of Medicine (IOM, Committee on the Evaluation of the Addition of Ingredients New to Infant Formula, Food and Nutrition Board, 2004) recommends more thorough guidelines.

8. There are numerous types of infant formulas.

    a. Standard cow's milk based.

    b. Cow's milk based with reduced or no lactose.

    c. Soy.

    d. Follow-on. These are formulas marketed for infants older than age 6 months.

    e. Extensively hydrolyzed (hypoallergenic).

    f. Partially hydrolyzed.

    g. Preterm.

    h. Special formulations for metabolic problems.

    i. Amino acid based.

    j. With added soy fiber (for diarrhea).

    k. With added rice solids (for reflux).

    l. Follow-on preterm.

9. Infant formula is available in three forms: ready-to-feed, concentrated liquid, and powder.

    a. The composition of infant formula within each of these forms can differ, even among those from the same manufacturer.

    b. The composition of infant formula differs between manufacturers and varies from country to country, depending on the legal requirements for content.

10. Infant formula products frequently change composition, receive new labels, change scoop sizes in the powdered variety, are discontinued, or experience changes in their recommended usage (Walker, 2001).

11. Infant formula has an expiration date after which it should be discarded.

12. Infant formula labels state the minimum amount of ingredients that are supposed to be present at any one time.

13. Overages (additional amounts) of some components are added to compensate for their degradation over the shelf life of the product.

14. Infant formula is frequently recalled or withdrawn from the market because of health and safety issues.

    a. A list of recalled formulas in the United States can be found at www.naba-breastfeeding.org.

II. Selected Differences in Macronutrients

A. Protein

1. Infant formula can have up to 50% more protein than human milk contains.

2. Protein intake per kilogram of body weight is 55–80% higher in formula-fed infants than in breastfed infants. High early protein intake enhances weight gain in infancy and can increase later obesity risk (Koletzko et al., 2005).

3. The whey-to-casein ratio of human milk changes over time from 90:10 in the early milk to 60:40 in mature milk, and to 50:50 in late lactation.

4. In infant formula, cow's milk protein remains static, and, depending on the brand, the levels could be 18:82, 60:40, or 100% whey.

5. Bovine casein is less easily digested and forms a tough, rubbery curd in the infant's stomach, partially accounting for the slower gastric emptying time in formula-fed babies.

6. There are compositional and functional differences between the casein and whey proteins in human milk and infant formula. In infant formula:

    a. Bovine alpha-lactalbumin is not well digested.

    b. There is no lactoferrin, a protein that aids in bacterial cell destruction (Hanson, 2004).

    c. There are no immunoglobulins, such as secretory IgA.

    d. There are no enzymes (digestive or defensive).

    e. There are few of the nonprotein nitrogen components found in human milk.

7. Cow's milk–based infant formula uses processing procedures that exclude from the final product colostrum, milk fat globule membranes, and fractions that contain DNA—components that provide disease protection that is species specific to the calf.

B. Lipids (fat)

1. Lipids provide 40–50% of the energy in cow's milk infant formula.

2. During processing, cow's milk fat (butterfat) is removed and replaced with vegetable oils or a mixture of vegetable and animal fats for better digestibility and absorption.

3. These fats include coconut oil, palm oil, soy oil, corn oil, safflower oil, palm olein, high-oleic safflower oil, high-oleic sunflower oil, oleo (destearinated beef fat), and medium-chain triglycerides oil.

4. The fatty acid profile and stereospecific structures differ significantly among various brands of infant formula as well as between infant formula and human milk (Straarup et al., 2006).

   a. Positional distributions of plant-based long-chain polyunsaturated fatty acids (LCPUFAs) on triacylglycerols are different from those of human milk triglycerides. Triacylglycerols or triglycerides are the form in which the body stores fat. They consist of a glycerol spine with three attached fatty acids.

   b. The location of the fatty acid on the glycerol spine is identified by stereospecific numbering (sn). Certain fatty acids have preferences for binding at certain positions.

   c. Infant formula attempts to duplicate the overall fatty acid composition of human milk, but it cannot duplicate the triacylglycerol structure that alters lipid metabolism in infants not fed human milk (Nelson et al., 1999). Even though the formula is supplemented with docosahexaenoic acid (DHA) and arachidonic acid (AA), the shape of the molecule is different from that of the DHA and AA found in human milk.

   d. AA and DHA in human milk are present in the sn-1 or sn-2 positions but can be present in all three positions in the single cell oils (Myher et al., 1996). In human milk, 55% of DHA is found in the sn-2 position.

   e. Human milk triglycerides usually contain no more than one molecule of DHA or AA, whereas some single-cell triglycerides contain two or even three such molecules. Most of the LCPUFAs in formula are located in the outer positions of the triacylglycerol molecule, placing them at potential risk for slow and low absorption (Straarup et al., 2006).

   f. DHA and AA added to infant formula can act differently in the body from human DHA and AA, depending on where and in what proportion they are found on the triglyceride molecule. It is unknown how these differences in molecular shape and triglyceride positioning could affect their metabolism and functioning.

5. Infant formula fats do not contain DHA and AA, the long-chain polyunsaturated fatty acids (LCPUFAs) found in human milk that are thought to be necessary for normal brain growth and development.

   a. Addition of these LCPUFAs to infant formula does not replicate the complex human milk fatty acid pattern.

   b. Sources of these additives include fish oils, egg yolks, evening primrose oil, micro algae, and fungal sources and must be provided in the correct ratio to avoid growth problems.

   c. Clinical trials have failed to show efficacy in terms of improved mental and motor development, with little evidence to support any beneficial effects of adding DHA/AA to infant formulas relative to visual or general development (Simmer, 2003; Wright et al., 2006).

      d. The FDA does not approve infant formulas before they can be marketed. However, all formulas marketed in the United States must meet federal nutrient requirements, and infant formula manufacturers must notify the FDA prior to marketing a new formula (U.S. Department of Health and Human Services, Food and Drug Administration, Center for Food Safety and Applied Nutrition, 2006).

  6. The brain composition of formula-fed babies is measurably and chemically different from the brain compositions of breastfed babies, with DHA levels in formula-fed term babies remaining static, decreasing in preterm infants, and increasing in breastfed babies (Cunnane et al., 2000).

  7. Infant formula contains little to no cholesterol. Cholesterol is present in human milk and increases during the course of lactation. Cholesterol is an essential part of all membranes and is involved with the laying down of the myelin sheath, which facilitates nerve conduction in the brain.

C. Carbohydrates

  1. Lactose is the principal sugar in human milk and in most other mammals' milk.

  2. Human milk lactose:

      a. Favors the colonization of the infant's intestine with microflora that compete with and exclude pathogens

      b. Ensures a supply of galactocerebrosides that are major components of brain growth

      c. Enhances calcium absorption

  3. The use of cow's milk–based infant formula with the lactose removed, all soy preparations, and some of the hydrolyzed formula brands that have no lactose has an unknown effect on both brain development and disease outcomes in formula-fed babies.

  4. There are approximately 130 oligosaccharides (nonlactose carbohydrates) in human milk. Cow's milk contains about 10% of this amount.

  5. Human oligosaccharides inhibit pathogens from binding to their receptor sites in the gut and on mucous membranes.

  6. Human oligosaccharides contain human blood group antigens, with women from different blood groups having distinct patterns contributing to the tailor-made disease protection within each mother–baby unit.

  7. Oligosaccharides in the milk of other species confer protection to the young of that species. Oligosaccharides in breastmilk are unique to human milk and have not been replicated synthetically.

D. Vitamins and minerals

  1. Infant formula is fortified with water- and fat-soluble vitamins.

  2. There are upper and lower limits for most of these vitamins.

  3. Most brands of infant formula contain significantly higher amounts of vitamins than does human milk to offset their reduced absorption.

  4. Excesses, deficiencies, and omissions of ingredients can and do occur in the manufacturing process.

5. Approximately 50% of the iron in human milk is absorbed compared to 7% from iron-fortified formula and 4% from iron-fortified cereals (American Academy of Pediatrics [AAP] Committee on Nutrition, 1999).

E. Defense agents

1. Infant formula contains no defense agents to protect human babies from acute and chronic disease.

2. Some brands of formula contain added nonhuman nucleotides or oligosaccharides, enabling the claim of enhanced immune response. The clinical significance of this addition has not been demonstrated.

III. Effects of Formula Feeding on the Brain and Immune System

A. Formula-fed infants and children demonstrate less-advanced cognitive development compared with breastfed children (Anderson et al., 1999).

1. The development of brain electrical activity during infancy differs between those who are breastfed compared with those fed either milk or soy formula but is generally similar for formula-fed groups. These variations in electroencephalographic (EEG) activity reflect diet-related influences on the development of brain structure and function that could put infants on different neurodevelopmental trajectories along which cognitive and brain function development proceed (Jing et al., 2010).

B. Lower mental development and IQ scores are seen at all ages through adolescence in formula-fed children.

C. Infants who are fed formula have significantly lower DHA in the gray and white matter of the cerebellum, the area of the brain that coordinates movement and balance (Jamieson et al., 1999).

D. A deficiency of IQ points in formula-fed subjects is reported in most studies (Angelsen, Vik, Jacobsen, & Bakketeig, 2001; (Angelsen et al., 2001; Kramer et al., 2008).

E. Central to this discrepancy are particular fatty acids (DHA and AA) that are found in human milk absent in formula.

F. DHA and AA are found in abundance as structural lipids in the brain, retina, and central nervous system of infants.

G. Unsupplemented formula contains precursors of DHA and AA, linolenic and linoleic acid, from which an infant's immature liver is supposed to synthesize enough of these LCPUFAs to meet the needs of the rapidly developing brain.

H. IQ studies are remarkably consistent in their demonstration of higher IQs that are dose dependent relative to the number of months that a child has been exclusively breastfed (Lucas et al., 1992).

I. Formula-fed 1-week-old infants demonstrate suboptimal neurobehavioral organization (Hart et al., 2003).

J. Neural maturation of formula-fed preterm infants shows a deficit compared with neural maturation of those who are fed human milk (Rao et al., 2002). Lack of breastfeeding in preterm infants is a significant predictor of cognitive deficiencies at 5 years of age (Beaino et al., 2011).

K. Delayed maturation in visual acuity can occur in both term and preterm formula-fed infants (Birch et al., 1993; Williams et al., 2001).

L. Delayed maturation in visual acuity might affect other mental and physical functions later in development that are linked to the quality of early visual processing.

M. An IQ increase of as little as three points (one-fifth of a standard deviation) from 100 to 103 would move a person from the 50th to the 58th percentile of the population and would potentially be associated with higher educational achievement, occupational achievement, and social adjustment.

    1. One IQ point has been estimated to be worth $14,500 in lifetime earning power and economic productivity (Grosse et al., 2002).

N. Defense agents are poorly represented in cow's milk (Jensen, 1995).

O. Bovine colostrum and its antimicrobial agents are specific for the cow and are removed from milk during processing.

P. Human milk not only provides passive protection, but also directly modulates the immunologic development of the recipient infant (Goldman et al., 1998).

Q. Formula-fed infants and children have increased risks and rates of the following conditions:

    1. Allergic disease (van Odijk et al., 2003). Prolonged breastfeeding in African American infants reduced the risk of allergic rhinitis at age 3 years (Codispoti et al., 2010).

    2. Necrotizing enterocolitis (NEC; Christensen et al., 2010; Updegrove, 2004).

    3. Diarrheal disease (Duijts et al., 2010; Scariati et al., 1997).

    4. Otitis media (Scariati et al., 1997). Formula-fed infants have higher rates of otitis media and lower antibody titres to Haemophilus influenza (Sabirov et al., 2009).

    5. Lower respiratory tract illness (bronchiolitis, croup, bronchitis, and pneumonia) (Duijts et al., 2010).

    6. Sudden infant death syndrome (Vennemann et al., 2005). Breastfeeding reduced the risk of sudden infant death syndrome by approximately 50% at all ages throughout infancy (Vennemann et al., 2009).

    7. Sepsis (Hanson et al., 2002). There is a strong positive association between the intake of formula and/or nonbreastmilk supplements and the risk of hospitalization for infectious causes (Hengstermann et al., 2010).

    8. Urinary tract infections (Levy et al., 2009; Pisacane et al., 1992).

    9. *Salmonella* infection (Rowe et al., 2004).

R. Humoral and cellular immune responses to specific antigens (such as vaccines) given during the first year of life appear to develop differently in breastfed and formula-fed babies (Dòrea, 2009).

S. Formula-fed babies can show lower or absent antibody levels to their immunizations (Hahn-Zoric et al., 1990; Zoppi et al., 1983).

T. Infants who are fed soy formula can have even lower antibody titres, with some showing no response at all to some of their vaccines.

U. Infants who have never been breastfed are 50% more likely to have gross motor coordination delays than are infants who have been breastfed exclusively for at least 4 months (Sacker et al., 2006).

V. Exclusively formula-fed infants are more often colonized with pathogenic bacteria such as *Escherichia coli*, *Clostridium difficile*, *Bacteroides*, and lactobacilli compared with breastfed infants (Penders et al., 2006).

W. In susceptible families, breastfed infants can be sensitized to cow's milk protein by the giving of just one bottle in the newborn nursery during the first 3 days of life (Cantani et al., 2005; Host, 1991; Host et al., 1988). Small doses of allergens can serve to sensitize an infant to subsequent challenges compared with large doses, which induce tolerance.

X. If breastmilk is not available and if supplemental feeding is medically necessary, breastfed infants from atopic families should be supplemented with a hydrolyzed infant formula for the first 6 months of life (Miniello et al., 2008).

Y. A bacterial group found in breastfed infants that is almost as extensive as bifidobacteria is the genus Ruminococcus (Morelli, 2008). Ruminococcus delivers a protective function, producing ruminococcin, a substance that inhibits the development of many of the pathologic species of Clostridium (Dabard et al., 2001). One of the many differences between the microflora of breastfed and formula-fed infants is the low presence of clostridia in breastfed infants as compared with formula-fed infants. New molecular biology techniques have detected the presence of the genus Desulfovibrio mainly in formula-fed infants (Hopkins et al., 2005; Stewart et al., 2006). These organisms have been linked with the development of inflammatory bowel disease.

IV. Hazards of Infant Formula

A. Genetically modified ingredients
  1. Genetically engineered corn and soy have been found in numerous brands of infant formula.
  2. Transgenic ingredients pose the risk of introducing novel toxins, new allergens, and increased antibiotic resistance in infants.
  3. Labeling of genetically modified ingredients in the United States is not required, so parents are unaware of whether they are feeding their baby transgenic foods.
  4. The long-term effects of these ingredients on formula-fed infants are unknown.
B. Soy-based infant formula
  1. Twenty-five percent of all infant formula sold in the United States is soy.
  2. Soy infant formula is used much less extensively outside the United States.
  3. Soy formula might be allergenic in infants who are allergic to cow's milk protein (ESPGHAN Committee on Nutrition et al., 2006).
  4. Many soy preparations contain sucrose, which is a contributor to dental caries in babies who are fed soy formula by bottle.

5. Soy is not recommended for preterm infants who have birth weights lower than 1,800 g, for the prevention of colic or allergy, or with infants who have cow's milk protein-induced enterocolitis or enteropathy (ESPGHAN Committee on Nutrition et al., 2006).

   a. Infants who are fed soy formula can have circulating phytoestrogen concentrations that are 13,000 to 22,000 times higher than normal levels in early life (Setchell et al., 1997).

   b. This dose represents a 6- to 11-fold higher level of intake of isoflavones than that found to cause significant modifications to the hormonal regulation of the menstrual cycle in Western women.

   c. High circulating levels of genistein in the neonate might predict future adverse female reproductive outcomes (Jefferson et al., 2010).

6. The consumption of soy formula was associated with an increased occurrence of premature thelarche (breast development in girls younger than 8 years of age) in Puerto Rico and specifically in many girls before they were 18 months of age (Fremi-Titulaer et al., 1986).

7. It is unknown what other effects these bioactive compounds might produce by creating steroid hormone imbalances through competition with enzymes that metabolize steroids and drugs or by influencing gonadal function.

8. Infant formula, especially soy and some hydrolyzed formula, contains 35 to 1,500 times the amount of aluminum as in breastmilk.

9. Aluminum can accumulate in bones and in the brain, and the effect of large amounts in infancy is unknown.

10. A positive association has been found between feeding infants soy formula and the development of autoimmune thyroid disease (Fort et al., 1990).

11. Soy formula components can act against the thyroid by inhibition of thyroid peroxidase and can have the potential to disrupt thyroid function even in the presence of added iodine (Divi et al., 1997).

C. Follow-on formula

   1. Follow-on formula is marketed for infants who are 4 months of age and older who are also receiving cereal and other solid foods.

   2. The most significant difference in this category of products is that they are lower in fat than both breastmilk and standard starter formula.

   3. Regular formula and breastmilk contribute 45–50% of the energy from fat.

   4. Follow-on formula can contribute as little as 37% energy from fat.

   5. Current pediatric nutrition recommendations advise against lowering the fat intake of infants and children younger than age 2 years (Kleinman, 2004).

   6. There are few additional sources of fat in the first year of life, and this period includes rapid growth and development with high energy requirements.

D. Neurotoxins and altered behavior patterns
   1. Toxic pollutants can affect the brain in different ways.
   2. The manganese (Mn) concentration in breastmilk is very low (4–8 mg/L). Cow's milk formula is 10 times higher in manganese concentration (30–60 mg/L) than is breastmilk, whereas soy formula has about a 50–75 times higher concentration than breastmilk does.
   3. Manganese lowers the levels of serotonin and dopamine–brain neurotransmitters that are associated with planning and impulse control.
   4. Low levels of brain serotonin are known to cause mood disturbances, poor impulse control, and increased aggressive behavior.
   5. There is little regulation of manganese uptake at young ages, and formula-fed infants—especially those who are fed soy formula—will have a much larger body burden of manganese. Breastmilk contains 4–6 mcg/L of manganese, whereas milk-based infant formula contains about 30–50 mcg/L and soy formula contains 200–300 mcg/L. Manganese is a mineral that helps the cells obtain energy and it is essential for life but can be toxic at very high levels. Soy formula contains approximately 80 times the manganese level of human breastmilk. Excess manganese that the baby cannot metabolize is stored in body organs and about 8% is stored in the brain in proximity to dopamine-bearing neurons responsible, in part, for adolescent neurological development.
   6. Ingredients that contain processed free glutamic acid (monosodium glutamate) and free aspartic acid (known neurotoxins) are used in formula.
      a. These are found in high levels in some brands of hypoallergenic formula and are cause for concern because the underdeveloped blood–brain barrier renders the brain more accessible to neurotoxins.
   7. Schizophrenic patients are less likely to have been breastfed (McCreadie, 1997). Early weaning (breastfeeding less than 2 weeks) was associated with an elevated risk of schizophrenia (Sørensen et al., 2005).
   8. Some infants who were fed a chloride-deficient brand of formula in 1978–1979 showed cognitive delays, language disorders, visual motor and fine motor difficulties, and attention deficit disorders at ages 8 and 9 years (Kaleita et al., 1991).
E. Contaminants in formula and water used for reconstitution
   1. Silicon contamination can be seen in formula with levels ranging from 746 to 13,811 ng/mL. Breastmilk of women who do not have silicone implants contains approximately 51.05 ng/mL of silicon, whereas those who have implants show 55.45 ng/mL (Semple et al., 1998).
   2. Lead intoxication can occur when hot tap water or lead-containing water is boiled and is used to reconstitute concentrated or powdered formula (Shannon et al., 1992).

3. Boiling concentrates lead, arsenic, cadmium, and other contaminants in water.
4. Infants who are fed formula that has been reconstituted with nitrate-contaminated water or untested well water are at risk for potentially fatal methemoglobinemia. The baby's system converts nitrates to nitrites, resulting in hemoglobin being converted to methemoglobin that cannot bind molecular oxygen (Dusdieker et al., 1994).
    a. Breastfed infants are not at risk of nitrate poisoning from mothers who ingest water with high nitrate content because nitrate does not concentrate in the milk (Greer et al., 2005).
    b. This risk increases if babies are younger than 6 months of age and are also fed baby food that has high concentrations of nitrates, such as green beans and bananas.
5. Atrazine is a weed killer found in the water supplies in agricultural areas; it is a carcinogen at high levels. Formula-fed infants can obtain a lifetime dose by age 5 years. Most ready-to-feed formula contains water that has atrazine filtered out of it before it is used for processing (Houlihan et al., 1999).
6. Powdered infant formula is not sterile and has been implicated in a number of cases of meningitis, NEC, and sepsis in term and preterm infants (Centers for Disease Control and Prevention [CDC], 2002, 2009). The formula can be contaminated with Cronobacter (formerly called Enterobacter sakazakii), a pathogen that is not seen in ready-to-feed or liquid concentrated formula.
    a. It has been recommended that no infant under the age of 4 weeks receive the powdered version of infant formula (Bowen et al., 2006; European Food Safety Authority, 2004).
    b. To reconstitute powdered infant formula, water should be brought to a rolling boil, cooled to a temperature of 70°C (158°F), and then added to the formula; this reconstituted formula should be further cooled to body temperature before feeding (Drudy et al., 2006).
7. Bovine milk–based powdered infant formulas with lactose have a significantly higher concentration of perchlorate compared with other forms and types of formula.
    a. Perchlorate was a contaminant of all commercially available powdered infant formulas tested by Schier and colleagues (2010).
    b. Cow's milk–based powdered formula with lactose had a significantly higher perchlorate concentration than did soy, lactose-free, and elemental powdered formulas.
    c. The perchlorate reference dose may be exceeded when certain cow's milk–based powdered formulas are consumed and/or when powdered formulas are reconstituted with perchlorate-contaminated water.

F. Container hazards
   1. Phthalates are used as plasticizers and are testicular toxins and estradiol imitators; many tested brands of formula have been shown to contain phthalates (Nollet et al., 2011).
   2. Bisphenol-A is used in the production of polycarbonate plastics and has been found in plastic baby bottles; this chemical can leach from the container and has been known since 1938 to be estrogenic (Larkin, 1995).
      a. Bisphenol-A resins are used as lacquers to coat metal products such as food cans. This chemical can leach into the contents of cans during autoclaving. Some of the tested cans were concentrated milk-based formula.
   3. Bottle-fed babies are at risk for scald and burn injuries from bottles heated on the stove or in a microwave oven.
   4. Babies who are fed by bottle have increased rates of malocclusion (Labbok et al., 1990). Muscles involved with breastfeeding are either immobilized (masseter and obicularis oris), overactive (chin muscle), or malpositioned (the tongue is pushed backward) during artificial feeding (Inoue et al., 1995), contributing to abnormal dentofacial development in the child (Palmer, 1998).
   5. Bottle-feeding is positively correlated with finger sucking, which can deform the maxillary arch and palate (Viggiano et al., 2004).
   6. Formula is acidogenic and might play a significant role in the development of early dental caries in infants (Sheikh et al., 1996).
G. Errors in formula preparation and inappropriate foods
   1. Babies who are fed powdered formula are at risk for hyperosmolar (overconcentrated) feedings. Reports have been noted of mothers losing the measuring scoop, using graduated markings on a bottle that was brought home from the hospital, adding extra formula to help a small baby grow faster, diluting formula to make it last longer, using warm tap water to reconstitute powdered formula, heating bottles in a microwave, leaving bottles out at room temperature, and so on (Fein et al., 1999).
   2. Babies are also at risk for underconcentrated feedings if mothers use less powdered formula per bottle to make the supply last longer.
   3. Oral water intoxication can result not only from overly dilute formula, but also from supplemental feedings of solute-free tap water, juice, tea, soda, and bottled drinking water marketed for infants (Keating et al., 1991).
   4. Rapid ingestion of water over a short period of time can cause hyponatremic seizures and brain swelling.
   5. Infants who ingest 260–540 mL (9–19 oz) of solute-free water can become symptomatic over a relatively short period of time (90 minutes to 48 hours).
   6. The Infant Feeding Practices Study II (Labiner-Wolfe et al., 2008) showed the following results:
      a. Seventy-seven percent of mothers did not receive instructions on formula preparation or storage from a health professional.
      b. Fifty-five percent did not always wash their hands with soap before preparing formula.

  c. Thirty percent did not read preparation instructions on the label.

  d. Thirty-two percent did not always adequately wash bottle nipples between uses.

  e. Thirty-five percent heated formula bottles in a microwave.

  f. Six percent did not always discard formula left standing for longer than 2 hours.

H. Costs

 1. The direct cost of formula to families for 1 year in the United States ranges from $1,000 to $3,000 or more. In some developing countries, the cost of formula can exceed 100% of the yearly family income (UNICEF, 1999).

 2. The U.S. government is the single largest purchaser of formula in the world for the Women, Infants, and Children supplemental food program.

V. Feeding: Breastmilk and Foods

A. Exclusive versus partial breastfeeding

 1. The absence of standard definitions for breastfeeding can prevent precision and comparability in research, causing inaccuracies and confusion at both policy-making and clinical levels.

 2. A schema for defining breastfeeding has been devised. By using and describing the terms full, partial, and token, Labbok et al., (1990) further subdivide these terms based on patterns of feedings.

 3. These breastfeeding patterns might occur at any stage of the child's life and are not associated with age.

 4. Precise definitions of breastfeeding in well-controlled research show that the protective effects of breastmilk are afforded in a dose-response manner.

 5. The less breastmilk a baby receives, the higher the risk for disease and adverse cognitive development.

 6. Even partial breastfeeding confers some measure of disease protection.

 7. Exclusive breastfeeding rates for infants who are younger than 4 months old range from 19% in Africa to 49% in Southeast Asia.

 8. Although U.S. breastfeeding rates have risen, exclusive breastfeeding rates have remained unchanged. (See **Table 22-1**.) There has been a steady rise in the number of infants who are being supplemented with formula in the hospital. (See **Table 22-2**.)

 9. Healthy, full-term breastfeeding infants should not be given supplements of water, glucose water, formula, or other fluids unless ordered by a physician when a medical indication exists (AAP Section on Breastfeeding, 2005).

 10. Supplements displace breastmilk intake and can lead to increased morbidity, early cessation of breastfeeding, and interference with the bioavailability of certain key nutrients and disease-protective factors in breastmilk.

 11. Some babies will receive culturally valued supplements or ritual foods in very small amounts, such as tea, vitamin drops, honey, and butter. Whereas these supplements and foods are not necessary, most pose no problem to breastfeeding. Honey can carry the possibility of infecting the infant with botulism, however, and should not be given to infants who are younger than 1 year of age (Brook, 2007).

Table 22-1 Percentage of U.S. children who were breastfed, by birth year, National Immunization Survey, United States (percent ±half 95% Confidence Interval).

	1999	2000	2001	2002	2003	2004	2005	2006	2007 (provisional[1])
Early post-partum	68.3 ±2.9	70.9 ±1.9	71.6 ±1.0	71.4 ±0.9	72.6 ±0.9	73.1 ±0.8	74.1 ±1.0	74.0 ±0.9	75.0 ±1.2
6 months	32.6 ±2.9	34.2 ±2.0	36.9 ±1.2	37.6 ±1.0	39.1 ±0.9	42.1 ±0.9	42.9 ±1.1	43.5 ±1.1	43.0 ±1.3
12 months	15.0 ±2.1	15.7 ±1.5	18.2 ±0.9	19.0 ±0.8	19.6 ±0.8	21.4 ±0.8	21.5 ±0.9	22.7 ±0.9	22.4 ±1.1
Exclusively through 3 months	—	—	—	—	29.6 ±1.5	31.5 ±0.9	32.1 ±1.0	33.6 ±1.0	33.0 ±1.2
Exclusively through 6 months	—	—	—	—	10.3 ±1.0	12.1 ±0.7	12.3 ±0.7	14.1 ±0.8	13.3 ±0.9

[1] Interviews with caregivers of children born in 2007 will continue through November 2010; final estimates for children born in 2007 will be available in August 2011. See survey methods for details on study design.

Table 22-2 Percentage of U.S. Breastfed infants who are supplemented with infant formula, by birth year, National Immunization Survey, United States (percent ± half 95% Confidence Interval).

	2003	2004	2005	2006	2007 (provisional[1])
Before 2 days	22.3±1.6	23.5±1.0	24.9±1.1	24.2±1.1	25.4±1.4
Before 3 months	38.1±2.2	37.4±1.3	38.1±1.4	36.7±1.4	37.2±1.8
Before 6 months	47.4±2.6	44.5±1.5	45.9±1.7	43.6±1.6	43.8±2.0

[1] Interviews with caregivers of children born in 2007 will continue through November 2010; final estimates for children born in 2007 will be available in August 2011. See survey methods for details on study design.

    B. Complementary feeding: Starting solids

        1. For several decades, the World Health Organization (WHO) has issued recommendations regarding the appropriate age to begin complementary feeding (WHO, 1998).

        2. These recommendations have varied and have sparked debate about whether recommendations should be the age range of 4 to 6 months or if the phrase "at about 6 months" expresses the desired flexibility and protection of infant health.

        3. Studies show that in affluent populations, introducing solid foods before 6 months of age has little impact on the total energy intake or growth.

4. Studies show that there is no growth advantage in the complementary feeding of breastfed infants in developing countries prior to 6 months of age. The results of a systematic review support the recommendation of exclusive breastfeeding for about 6 months (Kramer et al., 2009).

5. The American Academy of Pediatrics states that exclusive breastfeeding is ideal nutrition and is sufficient to support optimal growth and development for approximately the first 6 months after birth (AAP Section on Breastfeeding, 2012).

6. At about 6 months of age, the normal infant begins using his or her iron stores.

7. Exclusively breastmilk-fed infants may need additional sources of iron, energy, zinc, vitamin A, and calcium after 6 months of age.

8. The neuromuscular and gastrointestinal systems are beginning to mature around 6 months of age.
   a. Although infants at this age can physically manage food, the efficiency of consumption of different types of foods varies considerably with age.

9. It is practically impossible to supply enough iron from unmodified complementary foods to meet the calculated needs of an infant who is between 6 and 11 months of age without unrealistically high intakes of animal products.

10. Iron-fortified cereals or other iron-containing foods (such as meat) are usually introduced as the first solids where available.

11. Iron deficiency can result when using iron-fortified cereal and whole cow's milk during the second 6 months of life. This condition results from a combination of poor bioavailability of electrolytic iron in some cereals and the composition of cow's milk, which makes iron less available to the infant.

12. Giving infants coffee or tea can have a strong inhibitory effect on iron absorption from foods that are consumed in the same meal or from iron supplements.

13. Once complementary foods are introduced at about 6 months of age, special transitional foods (for example, with semisolid consistency and adequate energy and nutrient densities) are recommended.

14. Breastfed infants from 6 to 8 months of age can receive (in addition to breastmilk) two to three meals per day depending on the population's nutritional status and the energy density of the complementary foods.

15. Children who are older than 8 months can receive at least three meals per day.

C. Inappropriate foods (WHO/UNICEF, 2003)

1. The definition of inappropriate foods varies with the population that is being discussed.

2. Generally, cow's milk or the fluid milk of other species is not recommended during infancy because of its displacement of breastmilk, possible microbial contamination, inappropriate blends of nutrients, and gastrointestinal blood loss when fresh milk is consumed.

3. Local foods that have a low nutrient density might need to be fortified.

4. Solid foods, such as cereals, should not be given to young babies to make them sleep through the night (Hall et al., 2000).

5. Solid foods should not be diluted and put in bottles for young babies to consume.

6. Acceptance of semisolid food is not an indication of maturity.

7. Parents might need help in resisting the pressure from healthcare providers, baby food manufacturers, and grandparents to introduce solids before 6 months.

8. Water and fruit juices are unnecessary for exclusively breastfed babies during their first 6 months, even in hot weather climates (American Academy of Pediatrics, 2012).

9. If commercial baby foods are used, parents should be counseled to avoid those that contain modified food starch or added sugar or salt, or those that have multiple ingredients.

10. Soy milk that is used in addition to or in place of formula is inappropriate.

11. Coffee creamers, flour and water mixtures, adult beverages, and carbonated or alcoholic drinks are inappropriate and could severely jeopardize the health of the infant.

References

American Academy of Pediatrics Committee on Nutrition. (1999). Iron fortification of infant formula. *Pediatrics*, *104*, 119–123.

American Academy of Pediatrics Section on Breastfeeding. (2012). Breastfeeding and the use of human milk. *Pediatrics*, *129*, e827–e841.

Anderson, J. W., Johnstone, B. M., & Remley, D. T. (1999). Breastfeeding and cognitive development: A meta-analysis. *American Journal of Clinical Nutrition*, *70*, 525–535.

Angelsen, N. K., Vik, T., Jacobsen, G., & Bakketeig, L. S. (2001). Breast feeding and cognitive development at age 1 and 5 years. *Archives of Disease in Childhood*, *85*, 183–188.

Beaino, G., Khoshnood, B., Kaminski, M., Marret, S., Pierrat, V., Vieux, R., Thiriez, G., Matis, J., Picaud, J. C., Rozé, J. C., Alberge, C., Larroque, B., Bréart, G., Ancel, P. Y., & EPIPAGE Study Group. (2011). Predictors of the risk of cognitive deficiency in very preterm infants: The EPIPAGE prospective cohort. *Acta Paediatrica*, *100*, 370–378.

Bener, A., Hoffmann, G. F., Afify, Z., Rasul, K., & Tewfik, I. (2008). Does prolonged breastfeeding reduce the risk for childhood leukemia and lymphomas? *Minerva Pediatrica*, *60*, 155–161.

Birch, E., Birch, D., Hoffman, D., et al. (1993). Breastfeeding and optimal visual development. *Journal of Pediatric Ophthalmology and Strabismus*, *30*, 30–38.

Bowen, A. B., & Braden, C. R. (2006). Invasive *Enterobacter sakazakii* disease in infants. *Emerging Infectious Diseases*, *12*, 1185–1189.

Brook, I. (2007). Infant botulism. *Journal of Perinatology, 27*, 175-180.

Cantani, A., & Micera, M. (2005). Neonatal cow milk sensitization in 143 case-reports: Role of early exposure to cow's milk formula. *European Review for Medical and Pharmacological Sciences*, *9*, 227–230.

Carlson, S. E., Cooke, R. J., Rhodes, P. G., et al. (1991). Long-term feeding of formulas high in linolenic acid and marine oil to very low birth weight infants: Phospholipid fatty acids. *Pediatric Research*, *30*, 404–412.

Centers for Disease Control and Prevention. (2002). *Enterobacter sakazakii* infections associated with the use of powdered formula—Tennessee, 2001. *Morbidity and Mortality Weekly Report*, *51*, 297–300.

Centers for Disease Control and Prevention. (2009). *Cronobacter* species isolation in two infants—New Mexico, 2008. *Morbidity and Mortality Weekly Report, 58*, 1179–1183.

Christensen, R. D., Gordon, P. V., & Besner, G. E. (2010). Can we cut the incidence of necrotizing enterocolitis in half—today? *Fetal and Pediatric Pathology*, *29*, 185–198.

Codispoti, C. D., Levin, L., LeMasters, G. K., Ryan, P., Reponen, T., Villareal, M., Burkle, J., Stanforth, S., Lockey, J. E., Khurana Hershey, G. K., & Bernstein, D. I. (2010). Breast-feeding, aeroallergen sensitization, and environmental exposures during infancy are determinants of childhood allergic rhinitis. *Journal of Allergy and Clinical Immunology*, *125*, 1054–1060.

Corrao, G., Tragnone, A., Caprilli, R., et al. (1998). Risk of inflammatory bowel disease attributable to smoking, oral contraception and breastfeeding in Italy: A nationwide case-control study. Cooperative Investigators of the Italian Group for the Study of the Colon and Rectum (GISC). *International Journal of Epidemiology*, *27*, 397–404.

Crume, T. L., Ogden, L., Maligie, M. B., Sheffield, S., Bischoff, K. J., McDuffie, R., Daniels, S., Hamman, R. F., Norris, J. M., & Dabelea, D. (2011). Long-term impact of neonatal breastfeeding on childhood adiposity and fat distribution among children exposed to diabetes in utero. *Diabetes Care*, *34*, 641–645.

Cunnane, S. C., Francescutti, V., Brenna, J. T., & Crawford, M. A. (2000). Breastfed infants achieve a higher rate of brain and whole body docosahexaenoate accumulation than formula-fed infants not consuming dietary docosahexaenoate. *Lipids*, *35*, 105–111.

Dabard, J., Bridonneau, C., Phillipe, C., et al. (2001). A new lantibiotic produced by a *Ruminococcus gnavus* strain isolated from human feces. *Applied Environmental Microbiology*, *67*, 4111–4118.

Divi, R. L., Hebron, C. C., & Doerge, D. R. (1997). Anti-thyroid isoflavones from soybean: Isolation, characterization, and mechanisms of action. *Biochemical Pharmacology*, *54*, 1087–1096.

Dòrea, J. G. (2009). Breastfeeding is an essential complement to vaccination. *Acta Paediatrica*, *98*, 1244–1250.

Drudy, D., Mullane, N. R., Quinn, T., et al. (2006). *Enterobacter sakazakii*: An emerging pathogen in powdered infant formula. *Clinical Infectious Disease*, *42*, 996–1002.

Duijts, L., Jaddoe, V. W., Hofman, A., & Moll, H. A. (2010). Prolonged and exclusive breastfeeding reduces the risk of infectious diseases in infancy. *Pediatrics*, *126*, e18–e25.

Dusdieker, L. B., Getchell, J. P., Liarakos, T. M., et al. (1994). Nitrate in baby foods: Adding to the nitrate mosaic. *Archives of Pediatric and Adolescent Medicine*, *148*, 490–494.

ESPGHAN Committee on Nutrition, Agostoni, C., Axelsson, I., Goulet, O., Koletzko, B., Michaelsen, K. F., Puntis, J., Rieu, D., Rigo, J., Shamir, R., Szajewska, H., & Turck, D. (2006). Soy protein infant formulae and follow-on formulae: A commentary by the ESPGHAN Committee on Nutrition. *Journal of Pediatric Gastroenterology and Nutrition*, *42*, 352–361.

European Food Safety Authority. (2004). Opinion of the Scientific Panel on Biological Hazards on a request from the Commission related to the microbiological risks in infant formulae and follow-on formulae. *European Food Safety Authority Journal*, *13*, 1–34.

Fein, S. B., & Falci, C. D. (1999). Infant formula preparation, handling, and related practices in the United States. *Journal of the American Dietetic Association*, *99*, 1234–1240.

Fort, P., Moses, N., Fasano, M., Goldberg, T., & Lifshitz, F. (1990). Breast and soy-formula feedings in early infancy and the prevalence of autoimmune thyroid disease in children. *Journal of the American College of Nutrition*, *9*, 164–167.

Fremi-Titulaer, L. W., Cordero, J. F., Haddock, L., et al. (1986). Premature thelarche in Puerto Rico. A search for environmental factors. *American Journal of Diseases of Children*, *140*, 1263–1267.

Goldman, A. S., Chheda, S., & Garofalo, R. (1998). Evolution of immunologic functions of the mammary gland and the postnatal development of immunity. *Pediatric Research*, *43*, 155–162.

González, J., Fernández, M., & García Fragoso, L. (2010). Exclusive breastfeeding reduces asthma in a group of children from the Caguas municipality of Puerto Rico. *Boletín de la Asociación Médica de Puerto Rico*, *102*, 10–12.

Greer, F. R., & Shannon, M. (2005). Infant methemoglobinemia: The role of dietary nitrate in food and water. *Pediatrics*, *116*, 784–786.

Grosse, S. D., Matte, T. D., Schwartz, J., & Jackson, R. J. (2002). Economic gains resulting from the reduction in children's exposure to lead in the United States. *Environmental Health Perspectives*, *110*, 563–569.

Hahn-Zoric, M., Fulconis, F., Minoli, I., et al. (1990). Antibody responses to parenteral and oral vaccines are impaired by conventional and low protein formulas as compared to breastfeeding. *Acta Paediatrica Scandinavica*, *79*, 1137–1142.

Hall, R. T., & Carroll, R. E. (2000, June). Infant feeding. *Pediatrics in Review*, *21*(6), 191–199.

Hanson, L. A. (2004). *Immunobiology of human milk: How breastfeeding protects babies.* Amarillo, TX: Pharmasoft Publishing.

Hanson, L. A., & Korotkova, M. (2002). The role of breastfeeding in prevention of neonatal infection. *Seminars in Neonatology*, *7*, 275–281.

Hart, S., Boylan, L. M., Carroll, S., et al. (2003). Brief report: Breastfed one-week-olds demonstrate superior neurobehavioral organization. *Journal of Pediatric Psychology*, *28*, 529–534.

Hengstermann, S., Mantaring, J. B., 3rd, Sobel, H. L., Borja, V. E., Basilio, J., Iellamo, A. D., & Nyunt, U. S. (2010). Formula feeding is associated with increased hospital admissions due to infections among infants younger than 6 months in Manila, Philippines. *Journal of Human Lactation*, *26*, 19–25.

Hopkins, M. J., Macfarlane, G. T., Furrie, E., Fite, A., & Macfarlane, S. (2005). Characterization of intestinal bacteria in infant stools using real-time PCR and northern hybridization analyses. *FEMS Microbiology Ecology*, *54*, 77–85.

Host, A. (1991). Importance of the first meal on the development of cow's milk allergy and intolerance. *Allergy Proceedings*, *10*, 227–232.

Host, A., & Halken, S. (2005). Primary prevention of food allergy in infants who are at risk. *Current Opinion in Allergy and Clinical Immunology*, *5*, 255–259.

Host, A., Husby, S., & Osterballe, O. (1988). A prospective study of cow's milk allergy in exclusively breastfed infants. *Acta Paediatrica Scandinavia*, *77*, 663-670.

Houlihan, J., & Wiles, R. (1999). *Into the mouths of babes: Bottle-fed infants at risk from atrazine in tap water.* Washington, DC: Environmental Working Group. Retrieved from http://www.ewg.org/report/mouths-babes

Huh, S. Y., Rifas-Shiman, S. L., Taveras, E. M., Oken, E., & Gillman, M. W. (2011). Timing of solid food introduction and risk of obesity in preschool-aged children. *Pediatrics*, *127*, e544–e551.

Inoue, N., Sakashita, R., & Kamegai, T. (1995). Reduction of masseter muscle activity in bottle fed babies. *Early Human Development*, *42*, 185–193.

Institute of Medicine, Committee on the Evaluation of the Addition of Ingredients New to Infant Formula, Food and Nutrition Board. (2004). *Infant formula: Evaluating the safety of new ingredients.* Washington, DC: National Academies Press.

Ip, S., Chung, M., Raman, G., Trikalinos, T. A., & Lau, J. (2009). A summary of the Agency for Healthcare Research and Quality's evidence report on breastfeeding in developed countries. *Breastfeeding Medicine*, *4*(Suppl. 1), S17–30.

Jamieson, E. C., Farquharson, J., Logan, R. W., et al. (1999). Infant cerebellar gray and white matter fatty acids in relation to age and diet. *Lipids*, *34*, 1065–1071.

Jefferson, W. N., & Williams, C. J. (2010, October 15). Circulating levels of genistein in the neonate, apart from dose and route, predict future adverse female reproductive outcomes. *Reproductive Toxicology*. Advance online publication. doi:10.1016/j.reprotox.2010.10.001

Jensen, R. G. (Ed.). (1995). *Handbook of milk composition*. San Diego, CA: Academic Press.

Jing, H., Gilchrist, J. M., Badger, T. M., & Pivik, R. T. (2010). A longitudinal study of differences in electroencephalographic activity among breastfed, milk formula-fed, and soy formula-fed infants during the first year of life. *Early Human Development*, *86*, 119–125.

Kaleita, T. A., Kinsbourne, M., & Menkes, J. H. (1991). A neurobehavioral syndrome after failure to thrive on chloride-deficient formula. *Developmental Medicine and Child Neurology*, *33*, 626–635.

Keating, J., Schears, G. J., & Dodge, P. R. (1991). Oral water intoxication in infants: An American epidemic. *American Journal of Diseases of Children*, *145*, 985–990.

Kleinman, R. E. (Ed.). (2004). *Pediatric nutrition handbook* (5th ed.). Elk Grove Village, IL: Committee on Nutrition, American Academy of Pediatrics.

Koenig, J. S., Davies, A. M., & Thach, B. T. (1990). Coordination of breathing, sucking, and swallowing during bottle feedings in human infants. *Journal of Applied Physiology*, *69*, 1623–1629.

Koletzko, B., Broekaert, I., Demmelmair, H., et al. (2005). Protein intake in the first year of life: A risk factor for later obesity? The EU Childhood Obesity Project. *Advances in Experimental Medicine and Biology*, *569*, 69–79.

Koletzko, S., Sherman, P., Corey, M., et al. (1989). Role of infant feeding practices in development of Crohn's disease in childhood. *British Medical Journal*, *298*, 1617–1618.

Kramer, M. S., Aboud, F., Mironova, E., Vanilovich, I., Platt, R. W., & Matush, L. (2008). Breastfeeding and child cognitive development: New evidence from a large randomized trial. *Archive of General Psychiatry*, *65*(5), 578–584.

Kramer, M. S., & Kakuma, R. (2009). Optimal duration of exclusive breastfeeding (Review). *The Cochrane Library*, no. 4.

Kvaavik, E., Tell, G. S., & Klepp, K. I. (2005). Surveys of Norwegian youth indicated that breastfeeding reduced subsequent risk of obesity. *Journal of Clinical Epidemiology*, *58*, 849–855.

Kwan, M. L., Buffler, P. A., Abrams, B., & Kiley, V. A. (2004). Breastfeeding and the risk of childhood leukemia: A meta-analysis. *Public Health Report*, *119*, 521–535.

Labbok, M., & Krasovec, K. (1990). Toward consistency in breastfeeding definitions. *Studies in Family Planning*, *21*, 226–230.

Laniner-Wolfe, J., Fein, S. B., & Shealy, K. R. (2008). Infant formula-handling education and safety. *Pediatrics*, *122*, S85–S97.

Larkin, M. (1995, April). Estrogen: Friend or foe? *FDA Consumer*, 25–29.

Levy, I., Comarsca, J., Davidovits, M., Klinger, G., Sirota, L., & Linder, N. (2009). Urinary tract infection in preterm infants: The protective role of breastfeeding. *Pediatric Nephrology*, *24*, 527–531.

Lucas, A., Morley, R., Cole, T. J., et al. (1992). Breast milk and subsequent intelligence quotient in children born premature. *Lancet*, *339*, 261–264.

Mathew, O. P. (1991). Breathing patterns of preterm infants during bottle feeding: Role of milk flow. *Journal of Pediatrics*, *119*, 960–965.

McCreadie, R. G. (1997). The Nithsdale schizophrenia surveys 16. Breast feeding and schizophrenia: Preliminary results and hypotheses. *British Journal of Psychiatry*, *170*, 334–337.

McNally, R. J., & Parker, L. (2006). Environmental factors and childhood acute leukemias and lymphomas. *Leukemia and Lymphoma*, *47*(4), 583–598.

Miniello, V. L., Francavilla, R., Brunetti, L., et al. (2008). Primary allergy prevention: Partially or extensively hydrolyzed infant formula? *Minerva Pediatrica, 60,* 1437–1443.

Morelli, L. (2008). Postnatal development of intestinal microflora as influenced by infant nutrition. *Journal of Nutrition, 138,* 1791S-1795S.

Myher, J. J., Kuksis, A., Geher, K., et al. (1996). Stereospecific analysis of triacylglycerols rich in long-chain polyunsaturated fatty acids. *Lipids, 31,* 207–215.

Nelson, C. M., & Innis, S. M. (1999). Plasma lipoprotein fatty acids are altered by the positional distribution of fatty acids in infant formula triacylglycerols and human milk. *American Journal of Clinical Nutrition, 70,* 62–69.

Nollet, L. M. L., & Toldra, F. (2011). *Safety analysis of foods of animal origin.* Boca Raton, FL: CRC Press, Taylor & Francis Group.

Oddy, W. H., Holt, P. G., Sly, P. D., et al. (1999). Association between breastfeeding and asthma in 6-year-old children: Findings of a prospective birth cohort study. *British Medical Journal, 319,* 815–819.

Palmer, B. (1998). The influence of breastfeeding on the development of the oral cavity: A commentary. *Journal of Human Lactation, 14,* 93–98.

Penders, J., Vink, C., Stelma, F. F., Snijders, B., Kummeling, I., van den Brandt, P. A., & Stobberingh, E. E. (2006). Factors influencing the composition of the intestinal microbiota in early infancy. *Pediatrics, 118,* 511–521.

Pettitt, D. J., Forman, M. R., Hanson, R. L., Knowler, W. C., & Bennett, P. H. (1997). Breastfeeding and incidence of non-insulin-dependent diabetes mellitus in Pima Indians. *Lancet, 350,* 166–168.

Pisacane, A., Graziano, L., Mazzarella, G., et al. (1992). Breastfeeding and urinary tract infections. *Journal of Pediatrics, 120,* 87–89.

Rao, M. R., Hediger, M. L., Levine, R. J., et al. (2002). Effect of breastfeeding on cognitive development of infants born small for gestational age. *Acta Paediatrica, 91,* 267–274.

Rowe, S. Y., Rocourt, J. R., Shiferaw, B., et al. (2004). Breastfeeding decreases the risk of sporadic salmonellosis among infants in FoodNet sites. *Clinical Infectious Diseases, 38*(Suppl. 3), S262–S270.

Sabirov, A., Casey, J. R., Murphy, T. F., & Pichichero, M. E. (2009). Breast-feeding is associated with a reduced frequency of acute otitis media and high serum antibody levels against NTHi and outer membrane protein vaccine antigen candidate P6. *Pediatric Research, 66,* 565–570.

Sacker, A., Quigley, M. A., & Kelly, Y. J. (2006). Breastfeeding and developmental delay: Findings from the Millennium Cohort Study. *Pediatrics, 118,* e682–e689.

Sadauskaite-Kuehne, V., Ludvigsson, J., Padaiga, Z., et al. (2004). Longer breastfeeding is an independent protective factor against development of type 1 diabetes mellitus in childhood. *Diabetes/Metabolism Research Reviews, 20,* 150–157.

Scariati, P. D., Grummer-Strawn, L. M., & Fein, S. B. (1997). A longitudinal analysis of infant morbidity and the extent of breastfeeding in the United States. *Pediatrics, 99,* e5.

Schier, J. G., Wolkin, A. F., Valentin-Blasini, L., Belson, M. G., Kieszak, S. M., Rubin, C. S., & Blount, B. C. (2010). Perchlorate exposure from infant formula and comparisons with the perchlorate reference dose. *Journal of Exposure Science and Environmental Epidemiology, 20,* 281–287.

Semple, J. L., Lugowski, S. J., Baines, C. J., et al. (1998). Breast milk contamination and silicone implants: Preliminary results using silicon as a proxy measurement for silicone. *Plastic and Reconstructive Surgery, 102,* 528–533.

Setchell, K. D. R., Zimmer-Nechemias, L., Cai, J., & Heubi, J. E. (1997). Exposure of infants to phyto-estrogens from soy-based infant formula. *Lancet, 350,* 23–27.

Shamir, R. (2009). Nutritional aspects in inflammatory bowel disease. *Journal of Pediatric Gastroenterology and Nutrition*, *48*(Suppl. 2), S86–88.

Shannon, M. W., & Graef, J. W. (1992). Lead intoxication in infancy. *Pediatrics*, *89*, 87–90.

Sheikh, C., & Erickson, P. R. (1996). Evaluation of plaque pH changes following oral rinse with eight infant formulas. *Pediatric Dentistry*, *18*, 200–204.

Shu, X. O., Linet, M. S., Steinbuch, M., et al. (1999). Breastfeeding and the risk of childhood acute leukemia. *Journal of the National Cancer Institute*, *91*, 1765–1772.

Simmer, K. (2003). Longchain polyunsaturated fatty acid supplementation in infants born at term. *Cochrane Database of Systematic Reviews*, *4*, CD000376.

Sørensen, H. J., Mortensen, E. L., Reinisch, J. M., & Mednick, S. A. (2005). Breastfeeding and risk of schizophrenia in the Copenhagen Perinatal Cohort. *Acta Psychiatrica Scandinavica*, *112*(1), 26–29.

Stewart, J. A., Chadwick, V. S., & Murray, A. (2006). Carriage, quantification and predominance of methanogens and sulfate-reducing bacteria in fecal samples. *Letters in Applied Microbiology*, *43*, 58–63.

Straarup, E. M., Lauritzen, L., Faerk, J., et al. (2006). The stereospecific triacylglycerol structures and fatty acid profiles of human milk and infant formulas. *Journal of Pediatric Gastroenterology and Nutrition*, *42*, 293–299.

UNICEF. (1999). *Breastfeeding: Foundation for a healthy future*. New York. Retrieved January 2012 from http://www.unicef.org/publications/files/pub_brochure_en.pdf.

Updegrove, K. (2004). Necrotizing enterocilitis: The evidence for the use of human milk in prevention and treatment. *Journal of Human Lactation*, *20*, 335–339.

U.S. Department of Health and Human Services, Food and Drug Administration, Center for Food Safety and Applied Nutrition. (2006). *Frequently asked questions about FDA's regulation of infant formula*. Guidance for industry. Rockville, MD: Author. Retrieved from http://www.fda.gov/Food/GuidanceComplianceRegulatoryInformation/GuidanceDocuments/InfantFormula/ucm056524.htm

van Odijk, J., Kull, I., Borres, M. P., et al. (2003). Breastfeeding and allergic disease: A multidisciplinary review of the literature (1966–2001) on the mode of early feeding in infancy and its impact on later atopic manifestations. *Allergy*, *58*, 833–843.

Vennemann, M. M., Bajanowski, T., Brinkmann, B., Jorch, G., Yücesan, K., Sauerland, C., Mitchell, E. A. & GeSID Study Group. (2009). Does breastfeeding reduce the risk of sudden infant death syndrome? *Pediatrics*, *123*, e406–e410.

Vennemann, M. M., Findeisen, M., Butterfass-Bahloul, T., et al. (2005). Modifiable risk factors for SIDS in Germany: Results of GeSID. *Acta Paediatrica*, *94*, 655–660.

Viggiano, D., Fasano, D., Monaco, G., & Strohmenger, L. (2004). Breast feeding, bottle feeding, and non-nutritive sucking; effects on occlusion in deciduous dentition. *Archives of Disease in Childhood*, *89*, 1121–1123.

von Kries, R., Koletzko, B., Sauerwald, T., et al. (1999). Breastfeeding and obesity: Cross sectional study. *British Medical Journal*, *319*, 147–150.

Walker, M. (2001). *Selling out mothers and babies: Marketing of breast milk substitutes in the USA*. Weston, MA: National Alliance for Breastfeeding Advocacy.

Williams, C., Birch, E. E., Emmett, P. M., & Northstone, K. (2001). Stereoacuity at age 3.5 y in children born full-term is associated with prenatal and postnatal dietary factors: A report from a population-based cohort study. *American Journal of Clinical Nutrition*, *73*, 316–322.

World Health Organization. (1998). *Complementary feeding of young children in developing countries: A review of current scientific knowledge* (WHO/NUT/98.1). Geneva, Switzerland: Author.

World Health Organization/UNICEF. (2003). *Global strategy for infant and young child feeding.* Geneva, Switzerland: WHO.

Wright, K., Coverston, C., Tiedeman, M., & Abegglen, J. A. (2006). Formula supplemented with docosahexaenoic acid (DHA) and arachidonic acid (ARA): A critical review of research. *Journal for Specialists in Pediatric Nursing, 11,* 100–112.

Young, T. K., Martens, P. J., Taback, S. P., Sellers, E. A. C., Dean, H. J., Cheang, M., & Flett, B. (2002). Type 2 diabetes mellitus in children: Prenatal and early infancy risk factors among Native Canadians. *Archives of Pediatric and Adolescent Medicine, 156,* 651–655.

Zoppi, G., Gasparini, R., Mantovanelli, F., et al. (1983). Diet and antibody response to vaccinations in healthy infants. *Lancet, 2,* 11–14.

CHAPTER 23

Immunology, Infectious Disease, and Allergy Prophylaxis

Linda J. Smith, MPH, IBCLC, FILCA

OBJECTIVES

- Describe the components in human milk that contribute to disease protection and their actions.
- Discuss the role of breastfeeding in the long-term protection against chronic diseases and allergy.
- Identify maternal infectious diseases that are compatible with breastfeeding.
- Describe contraindications to breastfeeding.

INTRODUCTION

The mother serves as the baby's immune system, especially for the first 6 months during exclusive breastfeeding (Hanson, 2002). Breastfeeding and human milk fill an "immunologic gap" between the time when placentally acquired immunity protects the fetus before birth and approximately age 3 to 4 years when the child's own immune system is robustly functional.

Current global recommendations are immediate skin-to-skin contact and breastfeeding immediately after birth (within the first half hour after birth); exclusive breastfeeding for 6 months, followed by breastfeeding with complementary foods for 2 or more years or as long as the mother and child desire. Three important policies underscore this recommendation: the World Health Organization/United Nations Children's Fund's *Global Strategy for Infant and Young Child Feeding* (World Health Organization [WHO], 2003a); a systematic review of the optimum duration of exclusive breastfeeding (Kramer et al., 2004); and the WHO Child Growth Standards (WHO, 2006). Virtually all major health organizations in the world have endorsed and are implementing these recommendations.

There are multiple mechanisms whereby milk components protect the nursling: active attack of pathogens, including inactivation, binding, and destruction; binding nutrients needed by pathogens; creating an inhospitable milieu for pathogen growth and reproduction; and enhancing the growth, activity, effectiveness, and maturation of the infant's own immune system (Goldman, 1993). The mother's secretory immune

(continues)

393

system provides targeted protection against pathogens to which she (or the baby) has been exposed. Sensitized B lymphocytes begin manufacturing targeted secretory immunoglobulin A (SIgA). The lymphocytes and the targeted SIgA migrate to the breast and pass into milk, where they are ingested by the baby and provide additional protection in the infant gut. Milk contains soluble components with immunologic properties and living cells that are immunologically specific (Hanson, 2002; Hanson, 2004; Hanson et al., 2003).

"Non-breastfed human infants experience an acquired immunodeficiency that increases the risk of infections and other diseases. The antimicrobial, anti-inflammatory, and immunomodulating agents in human milk are multi-functional, act synergistically, and compensate for developmental delays in the infant" (Labbok, 2004).

Breastfeeding is strongly protective against allergy, delaying the onset and lessening the symptoms in the child. Dietary prophylaxis during pregnancy and exclusive breastfeeding for 6 months (not 4–6 months as previously recommended; Chantry et al., 2006) have a strongly protective effect on illness prevention. Breastfeeding avoids infant exposure to dietary allergens and slows or prevents absorption of allergens through the gut. Epidemiologic evidence of short- and long-term benefits of breastfeeding to the infant and mother continue to accumulate (Chen et al., 2004; Dewey et al., 1995). Lactation affects the woman's reproductive system, mediates her responses to stress, and reduces risk of several cancers. Breastfeeding protects the baby from numerous infections, improves cognitive and neurological development, and reduces risk of many long-term and chronic diseases and conditions (Loletzko et al., 2000). Delaying breastfeeding increases the risk of neonatal mortality (Edmond et al., 2006). Breastfeeding is rarely contraindicated in cases of maternal infection (Lawrence et al., 2011, pp. 406–473).

I. The Mother Serves as the Baby's Immune System (Hanson, 2000)

A. Prenatal and early postpartum.

1. The placenta passes maternal antibodies to the baby, and this protection persists for several weeks to months. The fetus also breathes and ingests/digests amniotic fluid, which provides significant amounts of protein.

2. Colostrum is exceedingly concentrated with anti-infective properties. Evolutionary evidence suggests that the earliest function of colostrum was to protect the young, with nutrition being a secondary purpose (Goldman et al., 1982; Hennart et al., 1991).

3. Human babies have a proportionally longer duration of colostrum feedings than other mammals do.

B. Actions/features of milk components that protect the infant and the lactating breast.

1. Actively bind to pathogens, thus preventing their passage through the permeable infant gut mucosa. Components are highly targeted to foreign pathogens and ignore the infant's healthy gut flora (Hanson, 2000).
2. Bind and reduce availability of nutrients, vitamins, and/or minerals needed by pathogens.
3. Cellular components directly attack pathogens through phagocytosis.
4. Trigger and enhance development and maturation of infant's own immune system, including the increased effectiveness of immunizations.
5. Support optimal growth and maturation of the infant gut, respiratory, and urogenital tracts.
6. Prevent or reduce inflammation in infant organs and tissues, which protects them from infection.
7. Stimulate infant's immune system: Macrophages and T lymphocytes provide immunologic maturation stimulus through cytokine production (Buescher, 1994; Goldman et al., 1998; Goldman et al., 1997).

C. Secretory immune system (enteromammary and bronchomammary pathways) provides protection against specific organisms to which the mother or infant has been exposed (Hanson, 2002).

1. Mother is exposed to a pathogen by ingestion, inhalation, or other contact, including pathogens that her baby has picked up. The pathogen comes in contact with the mucous membranes in her gut and bronchial tree, triggering an "alarm" in the mother's immune system.
2. T lymphocytes located in the mother's gut (in Peyer patches, or gut-associated lymphoid tissue) and bronchial tree (bronchus-associated lymphoid tissue) notice the new pathogen and pass on the specific message of alarm to nearby B lymphocytes, which immediately begin production of SIgA targeted to that organism.
3. Sensitized B lymphocytes migrate to mother's secretory organs or mucosal surfaces. There they secrete into her blood targeted SIgA, which is transported across the mammary secretory cells and released into the milk. (In addition, more SIgA appears to be synthesized in the mammary glandular cells.)
4. Targeted SIgA appears in milk soon (within hours to days) after maternal exposure to the original pathogen. Some sensitized B lymphocytes also pass into milk and are ingested by the baby and carry on their production of specific SIgA antibodies in the baby's gut.
5. The nursling ingests these targeted antibodies and sensitized live lymphocytes in the next breastfeed. The child may not get sick at all, or the illness is reduced in severity even if the mother becomes ill (Hanson, 2002).

II. Specific Protective Components of Milk (Butte et al., 1984)

A. Cellular components directly attack pathogens, mobilize other defenses, and activate soluble components. Although most live cells in the milk survive and continue to function in the infant gastrointestinal tract, they are usually destroyed by freezing, boiling, and other heat treatments.

    1. Immunologically specific: T lymphocytes, B lymphocytes

    2. Accessory cells: Neutrophils, macrophages, epithelial cells

B. Soluble components have multiple protective functions including binding pathogens, secreting chemical markers, and binding nutrients needed by pathogens.

    1. Immunoglobulins: SIgA, IgE, IgG, IgM

    2. Nonspecific factors: Complement, interferon, bifidus factor, antiviral factors

    3. Carrier proteins: Lactoferrin, transferrin

    4. Enzymes: Lysozyme, lipoprotein lipase, leukocyte enzymes

    5. Cytokines, including interferon and interleukins

    6. Hormones and hormone-like substances: Epidermal growth factor, prostaglandins, relaxin, somatostatin, gonadotropins and ovarian steroids, prolactin, and insulin

C. Anti-inflammatory properties: Human milk lacks initiators of inflammation and destroys pathogens without triggering inflammation.

    1. Specific anti-inflammatory agents: Lactoferrin, SIgA, lysozyme, prostaglandins, oligosaccharides, and epidermal growth factor

D. Interaction of anti-inflammatory and anti-infective factors is synergistic, providing more protection in total than the sum of the parts, thus protecting both the mammary gland and infant from a vast array of pathogens.

E. Immunologic agents are "developmentally delayed" in infancy and are provided by human milk (Labbok, 2004).

    1. Antimicrobial: Lactoferrin, lysozyme, SIgA, memory T cells, antibodies to T-cell-independent antigens

    2. Anti-inflammatory: Lactoferrin, lysozyme, SIgA, interleukin (IL)-10, platelet activating factor acetylhydrolase

    3. Immunomodulatory: SIgA, interferon-gamma (IF-g), IL-8, IL-10

III. Maternal Diseases and Breastfeeding (see also "Acceptable Medical Reasons for Use of Breast-Milk Substitutes" [WHO, 2009])

A. "Breastfeeding is rarely contraindicated in maternal infection. . . . Documenting transmission of infection from mother to infant by breastfeeding requires not only the exclusion of other possible mechanisms of transmission but also the demonstration of the infectious agent in the breast milk and a subsequent clinically significant infection in the infant caused by a plausible infectious process" (Lawrence et al., 2011, pp. 406–473).

B. Standard precautions. "The CDC (Centers for Disease Control and Prevention) does not consider breast milk a body fluid with infectious risks for such policies" (Lawrence et al., 2011, p. 407). (See Appendix B on universal precautions.)

C. Contagious diseases:
  1. Bacterial infections: Most bacteria are blocked.
     a. The mother should be treated and continue breastfeeding.
     b. Maternal Group B streptococcus (GBS) infections are treated prenatally when identified or during the intrapartum period. Acquisition of GBS through breastmilk or breastfeeding is rare. If a breastfed baby develops late-onset GBS, milk is cultured, the mother is treated, and breastfeeding or breastmilk feeding continues. Even highly pathogenic bacteria like syphilis do not survive in human milk. It is currently unknown whether the bacteria causing Lyme disease (Borrelia burgdorferi) survives in infectious form in human milk (Lawrence and Lawrence, 2011).
  2. Viral infections:
     a. Viral fragments for many diseases appear in mother's milk. These are not whole virus particles and do not appear to actually transmit disease. These fragments may act as a "vaccination" against the specific disease (e.g., cytomegalovirus).
     b. Human milk contains specific components active against many viruses, including poliovirus, respiratory syncytial virus, rotavirus, and influenza virus.
     c. Guidelines for breastfeeding or breastmilk feeding when the mother is actively infected with a viral illness at the time the baby is born are published periodically.
        i. See Lawrence et al. (2011) or similar references for treatment protocols for specific illnesses. In most, but not all, cases, breastfeeding can proceed normally. Even if viral fragments occur, the infant generally remains asymptomatic.
        ii. Precautions are necessary when the mother is actively contagious with certain diseases at the time of the baby's birth. For example, the mother with certain strains of influenza including H1N1, active tuberculosis, or chickenpox infection on the day of birth must be isolated from her newborn until she has been treated and/or is not contagious. She can and should provide her milk for her infant because these diseases are not transmitted via breastmilk.
        iii. Active infectious (i.e., herpes) lesions on the breast may require temporary separation of the mother from the baby until the lesions are dried. Careful hand washing, covering other lesions, and avoiding contact of lesions with the baby is necessary.
     d. As of mid-2011, no information is available on risks or benefits of breastfeeding or breastmilk feeding if the mother has a virus that causes highly fatal hemorrhagic fever, such as Ebola or Marburg. Consult current medical references and providers (Lawrence et al., 2011).
     e. "Breastfeeding is even more important when disease exposures are common, and when there are other children or an immune-compromised individual in the household" (Labbok, 2004).

3. Human immunodeficiency virus/acquired immune deficiency syndrome (HIV/AIDS):
   a. As of this writing, mother-to-child transmission of HIV/AIDS appears to occur mainly through direct blood contact at the time of birth or transplacentally in utero. Estimated rates of global mother-to-child transmission range from 15–25% with no interventions and no breastfeeding to 5–20% with breastfeeding "as usual" (WHO, 2010 #48712).
   b. Balancing the risk of transmission through breastfeeding versus the mortality from infectious diseases and malnutrition if the infant is not breastfed is a global goal. In 2010, the calculated incremental additional risk of transmission via breastfeeding is in the range of 4% if antiretroviral medications are not used.
   c. Individual countries and medical associations may have specific policies based on local economic, health, and other conditions. The greatest chance of HIV-free survival is either breastfeeding with antiretroviral (ARV) interventions or avoidance of all breastfeeding.
   d. HIV-1 transmission through breastmilk might be more dependent on the pattern of breastfeeding or potential confounders such as breast disease, cracked nipples, or Candida infection rather than on the total amount or duration of all breastfeeding.
   e. "Infants exclusively breastfed for 3 months or more had no excess risk of HIV transmission over 6 months than those never breastfed" (Coutsoudis et al., 2001; Iliff et al., 2005).
   f. The 2010 WHO principles and recommendations on HIV and infant feeding are as follows:
      i. "When antiretroviral drugs are not immediately available, breastfeeding may still provide infants born to HIV-infected mothers with a greater chance of survival.
      ii. "Mothers who are known to be HIV-infected should be informed about infant feeding alternatives. Skilled counseling and support in appropriate infant feeding practices and ARV interventions to promote HIV-free survival should be available to all pregnant women and mothers.
      iii. "Counseling and support to mothers who are known to be HIV-infected and health messaging to the general population should be carefully delivered to avoid undermining optimal breastfeeding practices among the general population.
      iv. "Mothers who are known to be HIV uninfected or whose HIV status is unknown should be counseled to exclusively breastfeed their infants for the first six months of life and then introduce complementary foods while continuing breastfeeding for 24 months or beyond.
      v. "Mothers whose status is unknown should be offered HIV testing.
      vi. "Mothers who are HIV uninfected should be counselled about ways to prevent HIV infection and about the services that are available such as family planning to help them to remain uninfected.

vii. "Mothers known to be HIV-infected should be provided with lifelong anti-retroviral therapy or antiretroviral prophylaxis interventions to reduce HIV transmission through breastfeeding according to WHO recommendations.

viii. "Mothers known to be HIV-infected (and whose infants are HIV unin-fected or of unknown HIV status) should exclusively breastfeed their infants for the first 6 months of life, introducing appropriate complemen-tary foods thereafter, and continue breastfeeding for the first 12 months of life. Breastfeeding should then only stop once a nutritionally adequate and safe diet without breast milk can be provided.

ix. "Mothers known to be HIV-infected who decide to stop breastfeeding at any time should stop gradually within one month. Mothers or infants who have been receiving ARV prophylaxis should continue prophylaxis for one week after breastfeeding is fully stopped. Stopping breastfeeding abruptly is not advisable."

g. Mothers who are HIV infected and decide not to breastfeed have been offered several options based on the assumption that HIV virus in breastmilk is infec-tious. As of 2011, that assumption has not yet been verified by rigorous research.

   i. Mother's own modified milk, because heat treatment inactivates the virus.

- Institutional pasteurization (Holder pasteurization)
- Home pasteurization by hot water baths, flash heating, Pretoria pas-teurization, or other methods that hold the milk at 60°C for 30 minutes (Hartmann et al., 2006; Israel-Ballard et al., 2005; Jeffery et al., 2000)
- Antimicrobial treatment of the breastfeeding mother with anti-malarial drugs
- Microbicidal treatment of milk with alkyl sulfates
- Banked donor human milk because all banked milk is donated by screened donors and then pasteurized (Human Milk Banking Association of North America, 2011)
- Commercial infant formula
- Homemade formula

h. The lactation consultant's role is to collect and compile current research, resources, and recommendations from the World Health Organization and share these with the mother and her primary care provider(s). She or he may also assist with weaning or other breastfeeding-related issues. The lactation consul-tant does not have a decision-making role in caring for families with this disease.

4. Cross infection:

a. The baby's mouth and mother's breasts are in intimate physical contact many times a day during breastfeeding. Any communicable disease or infection on either the nipple surfaces or in the infant's mouth is quickly transmitted to the other.

b. The dyad needs to be treated simultaneously until both (or all) sites are healthy. Examples: oral thrush and nipple Candida; child with strep throat infects mother's nipple. Breastfeeding should continue during treatments.

c. Standard precautions should be used by all healthcare providers. Concerning human milk:

   i. "Contact with breast milk does not constitute occupational exposure as defined by OSHA [Occupational Health and Safety Administration] standards" (U.S. Department of Labor, 1992).

   ii. "Gloves are not recommended for the routine handling of expressed human milk; but should be worn by health care workers in situations where exposure to breast milk might be frequent or prolonged, for example, in milk banking" (Centers for Disease Control and Prevention [CDC], 2010).

5. Summary of maternal infectious diseases and compatibility with breastfeeding. See **Table 23-1**. Caution: Consult current medical references as new information becomes available. Each situation must be decided individually by the primary care providers. Contraindications to breastfeeding are rare. Updates on newly emerging infectious diseases including influenza H1N1 are available at the following Centers for Disease Control and Prevention page: http://www.cdc.gov/h1n1flu/infantfeeding.htm.

6. Immunizing the breastfeeding mother: Lactating women can be immunized as recommended for other adults (Lawrence et al., 2011, p. 401):

   a. Measles, mumps, rubella, tetanus, diphtheria, influenza, *Streptococcus* pneumoniae, hepatitis A virus, hepatitis B virus, varicella, and may receive Rh immune globulin.

   b. Inactivated polio virus if traveling to a highly endemic area.

   c. No parents of infants are recommended to receive smallpox/cowpox vaccination; if needed, contact precautions must be observed.

   d. For current recommendations, visit "Travel Recommendations for the Nursing Mother" posted by the Centers for Disease Control and Prevention at http://www.cdc.gov/breastfeeding/recommendations/travel_recommendations.htm.

IV. Protective Effects of Breastfeeding on Allergy

A. Milk is species specific. A baby is never allergic to its own mother's milk. The baby and the mother share 50% of the same genetic material. No antibody response to mother's milk has ever been documented. SIgA in milk binds with and prevents transport of dietary allergens until the infant gut is less permeable. This is most important in the early months until the baby begins producing its own SIgA.

B. Breastmilk has multiple effects.

   1. Prevents or avoids the infant's exposure to nonhuman proteins and pathogens

   2. Slows or prevents absorption of antigens through the infant gut

C. Prophylactic management of children with a family history of atopic (allergic) disease.

   1. Allergic disease has a strong hereditary basis.

      a. Forty-seven percent incidence if both parents are allergic

      b. Twenty-nine percent incidence if one parent is allergic

      c. Thirteen percent incidence even if neither parent has a family history of allergy

Table 23-1 Summary of Maternal Infectious Diseases and Compatibility with Breastfeeding

Disease	OK to breastfeed in the United States?*	Condition
Acute infectious disease	Yes	Respiratory, reproductive, GI infections
Active tuberculosis	Yes	If mother is actively infected at birth, separate until after mother has received treatment; milk is still OK.
Hepatitis A	Yes	
Hepatitis B	Yes	After infant receives HBIG, 1st dose before discharge.
Hepatitis C	Yes	If no coinfections (such as HIV).
Herpes simplex	Yes	Except if lesion is on breast where baby would contact; if lesion is on the infant's lips, there is no reason to suspend breastfeeding.
Herpes/cytomegalovirus	Yes	—
Herpes/Epstein-Barr virus	Yes	—
Herpes/Varicella-zoster (chickenpox)	Yes	If mother is actively infected at birth, separate until mother becomes noninfectious; baby can still receive her milk.
Lyme disease	Yes	As soon as mother begins treatment.
Mastitis (infectious)	Yes	Continue or increase breastfeeding; milk stasis will exacerbate the illness.
Toxoplasmosis	Yes	—
Venereal warts	Yes	—
HIV or HTLV-1	NO	*HIV positive—see WHO/UNICEF guidelines.

Source: Adapted from Table 7 in Lawrence, R. (1997). A review of the medical benefits and contraindications to breastfeeding in the United States (Maternal and Child Health Technical Information Bulletin). Arlington, VA: National Center for Education in Maternal and Child Health.

  2. The only effective treatment is to reduce the allergenic load.

  3. Dietary prophylaxis is clearly effective, especially in families with a strong history.

   a. Mothers have been advised to avoid during pregnancy common allergens, especially dairy products, fish, eggs, and peanuts, with mixed results.

   b. Exclusive breastfeeding for about 6 months.

   c. Longer exclusive breastfeeding might be advantageous to the infant with a family history of allergy, although this concept remains controversial.

D. Allergic disease is responsible for one-third of pediatric office visits, one-third of chronic conditions of children younger than age 17 years, and one-third of lost school days as a result of asthma (Lawrence et al., 2011, pp. 614–629). Allergic diseases are strongly linked to artificial feeding, including eczema, asthma, hay fever, gut and respiratory infection, ulcerative colitis, and even sudden death.

E. All nonhuman milks currently available, including hydrolyzed or hypoallergenic products, have been shown to cause anaphylactic reactions in sensitive babies (American Academy of Pediatrics [AAP] Committee on Nutrition, 2000; Ellis et al., 1991; Saylor et al., 1991).

  1. Severe reactions have occurred, even at the "first" exposure. It was discovered that the infants who reacted so strongly had received undocumented feeds of cow's milk formula in a hospital nursery (Host et al., 1988).

  2. Hypoallergenic formulas are not completely nonallergenic; they have the capacity to provoke anaphylactic shock in susceptible infants. Hypoallergenic means that 90% of affected individuals will not be allergic to the product.

  3. "Between 17% and 47% of milk allergic children can have adverse reactions to soy" (Australasian Society of Clinical Immunology and Allergy, 2006). The American Academy of Pediatrics (AAP) does not recommend the use of soy formula when a documented allergy to cow's milk formula exists because soy formula has not been demonstrated to reduce development of atopy in infancy and childhood (AAP Committee on Nutrition, 1998).

F. Food allergies occur in 5.8–6% of children; cow's milk allergy ranges from 0.5–7.5% (Lawrence et al., 2011).

  1. Solid foods introduced before 15 weeks are associated with increased probability of wheezing, respiratory illness, and eczema. Any substance other than mother's own milk can provoke a reaction, and reactions are dose related.

  2. According to the Food Allergy and Anaphylaxis Network (n.d.), the following are eight most common food allergens:

   a. Milk and other dairy products (cow's milk protein)

   b. Eggs

   c. Peanuts

   d. Tree nuts (walnuts, cashews, etc.)

   e. Fish

   f. Shellfish

   g. Soy and soy products (tofu, soy milk, soy nuts, etc.)

   h. Wheat

3. If a mother suspects that her child is having a problem with food allergies or intolerances, and the baby's healthcare provider is dismissive of these concerns, the mother can be advised to ask for a referral to an allergist. Symptoms that would indicate a problem include the following:

   a. Chronic eczema: Long periods of scaly and itchy skin rashes.

   b. Hives often show up as itchy red welts on the surface of the skin.

   c. Chronic unexplained digestive or respiratory problems.

   d. Colic: Chronic, unexplained, excessive crying.

   e. Caution: Anaphylaxis is a severe allergic reaction that can be fatal. Call Emergency Services (9-1-1 in the United States) immediately if you see signs of anaphylaxis: severe hives or hives in conjunction with another reaction, facial swelling, swelling of mouth and throat (constriction of the throat is especially dangerous because as the throat swells shut, the child will stop breathing and turn blue from the lack of oxygen), vomiting, diarrhea, cramping, drop in blood pressure, fainting, death.

4. Gut closure affects allergic sensitization.

   a. Age at which other milks are introduced rather than total breastfeeding length is more closely associated with atopy at 6 years of age.

   b. Arbitrary, inadvertent, or unnecessary cow's milk–based formula supplementation given to susceptible breastfed babies during the first 3 days of life can sensitize these babies and provoke allergic reactions to cow's milk protein later in the first year of life (Walker, 2011, pp. 228–229).

      i. Cow's milk proteins are usually the first foreign antigens encountered by newborn infants in their diet. Intestinal absorption of macromolecules is greatest during the first 2 months of life, which is the critical time period for induction of a specific immune response to dietary antigens. An incomplete mucosal barrier and increased gut permeability are seen in altered immunologic responses.

      ii. For infants prone to developing cow's milk allergy, short exposure to cow's milk–based formula in the hospital or exclusive breastfeeding combined with infrequent intake of small amounts of cow's milk–based formula may stimulate specific IgE antibody production. However, frequent feeding of large volumes of cow's milk–based formula induces development of non-IgE mediated delayed-type hypersensitivity to cow's milk.

      iii. Cow's milk proteins (beta-lactoglobulin) do transfer to human milk, sensitizing predisposed babies to cow's milk (Jakobsson et al., 1985).

      iv. Introduction of cow's milk protein in the first 8 days is a significant risk factor for type 1 diabetes in genetically susceptible populations. The AAP recommends no cow's milk protein for the first year of life if there is a family history of type 1 diabetes (Lawrence et al., 2011, pp. 564–571).

5. Even small allergen exposures (doses) may be sensitizing in allergy-prone people. Prevalence of eczema and food allergy is highest between 1 and 3 years, and respiratory allergy is highest between 5 and 17 years.
   a. Breastfeeding also confers long-term protection against allergic sensitization.
      i. Breastfeeding for longer than 1 month with no other milk supplements offers significant prophylaxis against food allergy at 3 years and respiratory allergy at 17 years (Saarinen et al., 1995).
      ii. Six months of breastfeeding significantly reduces eczema during the first 3 years and at adolescence (Kusunoki et al., 2010; Saarinen et al., 1995).
      iii. Allergic manifestations include recurrent wheezing, elevated IgE levels, eczema, atopic dermatitis, GI symptoms of diarrhea, vomiting, and blood in the stool.
      iv. Exclusive breastfeeding for 6 months is more protective than the former recommendation of exclusive breastfeeding for 4 to 6 months, especially for respiratory tract infections (Kramer et al., 2001).
6. A dose-response relationship exists between the amount of breastmilk as the percentage of the infant's feed, with babies receiving exclusive breastmilk for longer periods of time showing the least amount of short- and long-term disease and allergy. The more breastmilk an infant receives during the first 6 months of life, the less likely that infant is to develop illness or allergy. The largest difference in health outcomes is found in exclusively breastfed compared with exclusively formula-fed children.
7. WHO recommendations for infant feeding, in order of preference (WHO, 2003 #6142), with the most preferred listed first, are as follows:
   a. Direct breastfeeding.
   b. Expressed mother's own milk.
   c. Milk of another woman (wet-nursing or shared nursing).
   d. Pasteurized donor human milk from a milk bank.
   e. Manufactured infant formula:
      i. Animal-based milks (cow milk based)
      ii. Plant-based "milks" (soy based)
   f. Babies who demonstrate an allergic reaction to hydrolyzed formula might need to be fed with elemental or amino acid–derived formulas.

V. Breastfed Infants Have Different Health, Growth, and Developmental Outcomes Than Do Formula-Fed Babies

A. WHO published new growth standards in 2006.
   1. "The World Health Organization is launching new global Child Growth Standards for infants and children up to the age of five. With these new WHO Child Growth Standards it is now possible to show how children should grow. They demonstrate for the first time ever that children born in different regions of the world and given the optimum start in life have the potential to grow and develop to within the same range of height and weight for age" (WHO, 2006).

2. The 2006 WHO Growth Standards are standards (prescriptive: how children *should* grow in optimum conditions) and not references (descriptive: how children *do* grow in certain situations). The data were compiled from six regions of the world.

3. Chapter 31 has more information on the WHO Growth Standards. As of 2011, many nations have adopted these standards as national policy (Grummer-Strawn et al., 2010).

B. Formula-fed babies have an increased risk and incidence of the following (AAP Section on Breastfeeding, 2005; Horta et al., 2007; Ip et al., 2007; Labbok et al., 2004; Scariati et al., 1997):

1. GI disease
   a. Diarrhea: Bacterial, viral, parasitic (Newburg et al., 2005)
   b. Necrotizing enterocolitis

2. Respiratory disease
   a. Otitis media
   b. Upper and lower respiratory infections (Howie et al., 1990)
   c. Wheezing
   d. Asthma (Oddy, 2004)
   e. Allergies (Oddy, 2004; Oddy, 2006; Zieger, 2000)

3. Urinary tract infections

4. Deficient response to childhood immunizations (Hahn-Zoric et al., 1990; Zoppi et al., 1983)

C. Formula-fed babies have a different brain composition than do breastfed babies. Formula-fed babies have half the docosahexaenoic acid (DHA) as do the brains of breastfed infants and can experience the following (Kramer et al., 2008; Lanting et al., 1994; Walker, 2011):

1. Discrepancy in visual acuity

2. Lower IQ

3. Poorer school performance

4. Increased risk for neurological dysfunction (Tanoueet al., 1989)

5. Increased risk for specific language impairment

6. Lower DHA in the gray and white matter of the cerebellum, which coordinates movement and balance

7. Increased risk for multiple sclerosis

References

American Academy of Pediatrics Committee on Nutrition. (1998). Soy protein–based formulas: Recommendations for use in infant feeding. *Pediatrics*, *101*(1), 148–153.

American Academy of Pediatrics Committee on Nutrition. (2000). Hypoallergenic infant formulas. *Pediatrics*, *106*, 346–349.

American Academy of Pediatrics Section on Breastfeeding. (2005). Breastfeeding and the use of human milk. *Pediatrics*, *115*(2), 496–506.

Australasian Society of Clinical Immunology and Allergy. (2006)..Dietary avoidance—soy allergy. Retrieved from http://www.allergy.org.au/ February 5, 2012.

Buescher, E. S. (1994). Host defense mechanisms of human milk and their relations to enteric infections and necrotizing enterocolitis. *Clinical Perinatology*, *21*, 247–262.

Butte, N. F., Goldblum, R. M., Fehl, L. M., et al. (1984). Daily ingestion of immunologic components in human milk during the first four months of life. *Acta Paediatrica Scandinavica*, *73*, 296–301.

Cavataio, F., Iacono, G., Montalto, G., et al. (1996). Clinical and pH-metric characteristics of gastro-oesophageal reflux secondary to cow's milk protein allergy. *Archives of Disease in Childhood*, *75*, 51–56.

Centers for Disease Control and Prevention. (1988). Perspectives in disease prevention and health promotion update: Universal precautions for prevention of transmission of human immunodeficiency virus, hepatitis B virus, and other bloodborne pathogens in health-care settings. *Morbidity and Mortality Weekly Report*, *37*(24), 377–388; updated 1996.

Centers for Disease Control and Prevention. (2010, March). Proper handling and storage of human milk. Retrieved from http://www.cdc.gov/breastfeeding/recommendations/handling_breastmilk.htm

Chantry, C. J., Howard, C. R., & Auinger, P. (2006). Full breastfeeding duration and associated decrease in respiratory tract infection in US children. *Pediatrics*, *117*, 425–432.

Chen, A., & Rogan, W. J. (2004). Breastfeeding and the risk of postneonatal death in the United States. *Pediatrics*, *113*, e435–439.

Coutsoudis, A., Pillay, K., Huhn, L., et al. (2001). Method of feeding and transmission of HIV-1 from mothers to children by 15 months of age: Prospective cohort study from Durban, South Africa. *AIDS*, *15*, 379–387.

Davis, D., & Bell, P. A. (1991). Infant feeding practices and occlusal outcomes: A longitudinal study [Abstract]. *Journal of the Canadian Dental Association*, *57*, 593–594.

Dewey, K. G., Heinig, J., & Nommsen-Rivers, L. (1995). Differences in morbidity between breastfed and formula-fed infants. *Journal of Pediatrics*, *126*, 696–702.

Edmond, K. M., Zandoh, C., Quigley, M. A., et al. (2006). Delayed breastfeeding initiation increases risk of neonatal mortality. *Pediatrics*, *117*, e380–386.

Ellis, M. H., Short, J. A., & Heiner, D. C. (1991). Anaphylaxis after ingestion of a recently introduced hydrolyzed whey protein formula. *Journal of Pediatrics*, *118*(1), 74–77.

Food Allergy and Anaphylaxis Network. (n.d.). Food allergens. Retrieved from http://www.foodallergy.org/section/common-food-allergens1

Goldman, A. S. (1993). The immune system of human milk: Antimicrobial, antiinflammatory and immunomodulating properties. *Pediatric Infectious Disease Journal*, *12*, 664–671.

Goldman, A. S., Cheda, S., & Garofalo, R. (1998). Evolution of immunologic functions of the mammary gland and the postnatal development of immunity. *Pediatric Research*, *43*, 155–162.

Goldman, A. S., Garza, C., Nichols, B. L., & Goldblum, R. M. (1982). Immunologic factors in human milk during the first year of lactation. *Journal of Pediatrics*, *100*, 563–567.

Goldman, A. S., & Goldblum, R. M. (1997). Transfer of maternal leukocytes to the infant by human milk. *Current Topics in Microbiology and Immunology, 222*, 205–213.

Groer, M. W. (2005). Differences between exclusive breastfeeders, formula-feeders, and controls: A study of stress, mood, and endocrine variables. *Biological Research for Nursing, 7*, 106–117.

Grummer-Strawn, L. M., Reinold, C., & Krebs, N. F. (2010). Use of World Health Organization and CDC growth charts for children aged 0-59 months in the United States. *MMWR Recommendations and Reports, 59*(RR-9), 1–15.

Hahn-Zoric, M., Falconis, F., Minoli, I., et al. (1990). Antibody responses to parenteral and oral vaccines are impaired by conventional and low protein formulas as compared to breastfeeding. *Acta Paediatrica Scandinavica, 79*, 1137–1142.

Hanson, L. A. (2000). The mother–offspring dyad and the immune system. *Acta Paediatrica, 89*, 252–258.

Hanson, L. A. (2004a). *Immunobiology of human milk: How breastfeeding protects babies.* Amarillo, TX: Pharmasoft (Hale) Publishing.

Hanson, L. A. (2004b). Protective effects of breastfeeding against urinary tract infection. *Acta Paediatrica, 93*, 154–156.

Hanson, L. A., Ceafalau, L., Mattsby-Baltzer, I., et al. (2000). The mammary gland–infant intestine immunologic dyad. *Advances in Experimental Medicine and Biology, 478*, 65–76.

Hanson, L. A., & Korotkova, M. (2002). The role of breastfeeding in prevention of neonatal infection. *Seminars in Neonatology, 7*, 275–281.

Hanson, L. A., Korotkova, M., Haversen, L., et al. (2002). Breast-feeding, a complex support system for the offspring. *Pediatrics International, 44*, 347–352.

Hanson, L. A., Korotkova, M., Lundin, S., et al. (2003). The transfer of immunity from mother to child. *Annals of the New York Academy of Science, 987*, 199–206.

Hanson, L. A., Silfverdal, S. A., Korotkova, M., et al. (2002). Immune system modulation by human milk. *Advances in Experimental Medicine and Biology, 503*, 99–106.

Hartmann, S. U., Berlin, C. M., & Howett, M. K. (2006). Alternative modified infant-feeding practices to prevent postnatal transmission of human immunodeficiency virus type 1 through breast milk: Past, present, and future. *Journal of Human Lactation, 22*, 75–88; quiz 89–93.

Hasselbalch, H., Jeppesen, D. L., Engelmann, M. D. M., et al. (1996). Decreased thymus size in formula-fed infants compared with breastfed infants. *Acta Paediatrica, 85*, 1029–1032.

Hennart, P. F., Brasseur, D. J., Delogne-Desnoeck, J. B., Dramaix, M. M., & Robyn, C. E. (1991). Lysozyme, lactoferrin, and secretory immunoglobulin A content in breast milk: Influence of duration of lactation, nutrition status, prolactin status, and parity of mother. *American Journal of Clinical Nutrition, 53*(1), 32–39.

Horne, R. S., Parslow, P. M., Ferens, D., Watts, A. M., & Adamson, T. M. (2004). Comparison of evoked arousability in breast and formula fed infants. *Archives of Disease in Childhood, 89*(1), 22–25.

Horta, B. L., Bahl, R., Martinés, J. C., & Victora, C. G. (2007). *Evidence on the long-term effects of breastfeeding: Systematic reviews and meta-analysis.* Geneva, Switzerland: World Health Organization.

Host, A., Husby, S., & Osterballe, O. (1988). A prospective study of cow's milk allergy in exclusively breast-fed infants. Incidence, pathogenetic role of early inadvertent exposure to cow's milk formula, and characterization of bovine milk protein in human milk. *Acta Paediatrica Scandinavica, 77*(5), 663–670.

Howie, P. W., Forsyth, J. S., Ogston, S. A., et al. (1990). Protective effect of breastfeeding against infection. *British Medical Journal, 300*, 11–16.

Human Milk Banking Association of North America. (2011). *Guidelines for the establishment and operation of a donor human milk bank.* Ft. Worth: Human Milk Banking Association of North America.

Iacono, G., Carroccio, A., Vatataio, F., et al. (1996). Gastroesophageal reflux and cow's milk allergy in infants: A prospective study. *Journal of Allergy and Clinical Immunology, 97*, 822–827.

Iliff, P. J., Piwoz, E. G., Tavengwa, N. V., et al. (2005). Early exclusive breastfeeding reduces the risk of postnatal HIV-1 transmission and increases HIV-free survival. *AIDS, 19*, 699–708.

Inoue, N., Sakashita, R., & Kamegai, T. (1995). Reduction of masseter muscle activity in bottle-fed babies. *Early Human Development, 42*, 185–193.

Ip, S., Chung, M., Raman, G., et al. (2007). *Breastfeeding and maternal and infant health outcomes in developed countries.* Rockville, MD: Agency for Healthcare Research and Quality.

Israel-Ballard, K., Chantry, C., Dewey, K., et al. (2005). Viral, nutritional, and bacterial safety of flash-heated and pretoria-pasteurized breast milk to prevent mother-to-child transmission of HIV in resource-poor countries: A pilot study. *Journal of Acquired Immune Deficiency Syndrome, 40*, 175–181.

Jakobsson, I., Lindberg, T., Benediktsson, B., & Hansson, B. G. (1985). Dietary bovine beta-lactoglobulin is transferred to human milk. *Acta Paediatrica Scandinavica, 74*(3), 342–345.

Jeffery, B. S., & Mercer, K. G. (2000). Pretoria pasteurization: A potential method for the reduction of postnatal mother-to-child transmission of the human immunodeficiency virus. *Journal of Tropical Pediatrics, 46*, 219–223.

Koletzko, B., Michaelson, K. F., & Hernell, O. (2000). *Short and long term effects of breastfeeding on child health.* New York, NY: Kluwer Academic/Plenum Publishers.

Kramer, M., Chalmers, B., Hodnett, E., et al. (2001). Promotion of Breastfeeding Intervention Trial (PROBIT): A randomized trial in the Republic of Belarus. *Journal of the American Medical Association, 285*, 413–420.

Kramer, M. S., & Kakuma, R. (2004). The optimal duration of exclusive breastfeeding: A systematic review. *Advances in Experimental Medicine and Biology, 554*, 63–77.

Kramer, M. S., Aboud, F., Mironova, E., Vanilovich, I., Platt, R. W., Matush, L., . . . Shapiro, S. (2008). Breastfeeding and child cognitive development: new evidence from a large randomized trial. *Arch Gen Psychiatry, 65*(5), 578–584.

Kusunoki, T., Morimoto, T., Nishikomori, R., et al. (2010). Breastfeeding and the prevalence of allergic diseases in schoolchildren: Does reverse causation matter? *Pediatric Allergy and Immunology, 21*(1 Pt. 1), 60–66.

Labbok, M. H. (2004). *The immunological secrets of breastfeeding: Implications for policy and practice.* Paper presented at the International Lactation Consultant Association Annual Conference, Scottsdale, AZ.

Labbok, M. H., Clark, D., & Goldman, A. S. (2004). Breastfeeding: Maintaining an irreplaceable immunological resource. *Nature Reviews Immunology, 4*, 565–572.

Labbok, M. H., & Hendershot, G. E. (1987). Does breastfeeding protect against malocclusion? An analysis of the 1981 child health supplement to the National Health Interview Survey. *American Journal of Preventive Medicine, 3*, 227–232.

Lanting, C. E., Fidler, V., Huisman, M., et al. (1994). Neurological differences between 9-year-old children fed breastmilk or formula-milk as babies. *Lancet, 344*, 1319–1322.

Lawrence, R. A, & Lawrence, R. M. (2011). *Breastfeeding: A guide for the medical profession* (7th ed.). Philadelphia, PA: Elsevier/Mosby.

Machida, H. M., Catto Smith, A. G., Gall, D. G., et al. (1994). Allergic colitis in infancy: Clinical and pathologic aspects. *Journal of Pediatric Gastroenterology and Nutrition*, *19*, 22–26.

Newburg, D. S., Ruiz-Palacios, G. M., & Morrow, A. L. (2005). Human milk glycans protect infants against enteric pathogens. *Annual Review of Nutrition*, *25*, 37–58.

Oddy, W. H. (2004). A review of the effects of breastfeeding on respiratory infections, atopy, and childhood asthma. *Journal of Asthma*, *41*, 605–621.

Oddy, W. H., Li, J., Landsborough, L., et al. (2006). The association of maternal overweight and obesity with breastfeeding duration. *Journal of Pediatrics*, *149*, 185–191.

Oddy, W. H., Pal, S., Kusel, M. M., et al. (2006). Atopy, eczema and breast milk fatty acids in a high-risk cohort of children followed from birth to 5 yr. *Pediatric Allergy and Immunology*, *17*, 4–10.

Oddy, W. H., Scott, J. A., Graham, K. I., & Binns, C. W. (2006). Breastfeeding influences on growth and health at one year of age. *Breastfeeding Review*, *14*, 15–23.

Oddy, W. H., Sherriff, J. L., de Klerk, N. H., et al. (2004). The relation of breastfeeding and body mass index to asthma and atopy in children: A prospective cohort study to age 6 years. *American Journal of Public Health*, *94*, 1531–1537.

Saarinen, U. M., & Kajosaari, M. (1995). Breastfeeding as prophylaxis against atopic disease: Prospective follow-up study until 17 years old. *Lancet*, *346*, 1065–1069.

Saylor, J. D., & Bahna, S. L. (1991). Anaphylaxis to casein hydrolysate formula. *Journal of Pediatrics*, *118*(1), 71–74.

Scariati, P. D., Grummer-Strawn, L. M., & Fein, S. B. (1997). A longitudinal analysis of infant morbidity and the extent of breastfeeding in the US. *Pediatrics*, *99*, e5.

Stuebe, A. M., Rich-Edwards, J. W., Willett, W. C., et al. (2005). Duration of lactation and incidence of type 2 diabetes. *Journal of the American Medical Association*, *294*, 2601–2610.

Stuebe, A. M., & Schwarz, E. B. (2010). The risks and benefits of infant feeding practices for women and their children. *Journal of Perinatology, 30*(3), 155–162.

Tanoue, Y., & Oda, S. (1989). Weaning time of children with infantile autism. *Journal of Autism and Developmental Disorders*, *19*, 425–434.

Thior, I., Lockman, S., Smeaton, L. M., et al. (2006). Breastfeeding plus infant zidovudine prophylaxis for 6 months vs formula feeding plus infant zidovudine for 1 month to reduce mother-to-child HIV transmission in Botswana: A randomized trial: The Mashi Study. *Journal of the American Medical Association*, *296*, 794–805.

U.S. Department of Labor. (1992). *Breast milk does not constitute occupational exposure as defined by standard* (Policy Interpretation). Washington, DC: Author. Retrieved from http://www.osha.gov/pls/oshaweb/owadisp.show_document?p_table=INTERPRETATIONS&p_id=20952

Walker, M. (2001). *Selling out mothers and babies: Marketing breastmilk substitutes in the USA*. Weston, MA: NABA REAL.

Walker, M. (2011). *Breastfeeding management for the clinician: Using the evidence* (2nd ed.) Sudbury, MA: Jones and Bartlett.

World Health Organization. (2003a). Global strategy for infant and young child feeding. Geneva, Switzerland: Author. Retrieved from http://www.who.int/nutrition/topics/global_strategy/en/index.html

World Health Organization. (2003b). *HIV and infant feeding: Framework for priority action*. Geneva, Switzerland: Author.

World Health Organization. (2003c). *HIV and infant feeding: Infant feeding options and guidelines for decision-makers*. Geneva, Switzerland: Author.

World Health Organization. (2004). *HIV transmission through breastfeeding: A review of the evidence.* Geneva, Switzerland: Author. Available at: http://www.who.int/nutrition/publications/HIV_IF _Transmission.pdf

World Health Organization. (2006). *WHO child growth standards.* Geneva, Switzerland: Author. Retrieved from http://www.who.int/childgrowth/en

World Health Organization. (2009). *Acceptable medical reasons for use of breast-milk substitutes.* Geneva, Switzerland: Author. Retrieved from http://whqlibdoc.who.int/hq/2009/WHO_FCH _CAH_09.01_eng.pdf

World Health Organization. (2010). *Guidelines on HIV and infant feeding 2010: Principles and recommendations for infant feeding in the context of HIV and a summary of evidence* (pp. 58). Geneva: World Health Organization.

Zieger, R. S. (2000). Dietary aspects of food allergy prevention in infants and children. *Journal of Pediatric Gastroenterology and Nutrition*, *30*, S77–S86.

Zoppi, G., Gasparini, R., Mantovanelli, F., et al. (1983). Diet and antibody response to vaccinations in healthy infants. *Lancet*, *7*, 11–14.

Suggested Reading

Hanson, L. A., Korotkova, M., & Telemo, E. (2003). Breast-feeding, infant formulas, and the immune system. *Annals of Allergy, Asthma, and Immunology*, *90*(6 Suppl. 3), 59–63.

Host, A., & Halken, S. (2004). Hypoallergenic formulas—when, to whom and how long: After more than 15 years we know the right indication! *Allergy*, *59*(Suppl. 78), 45–52.

Host, A., Halken, S., Jacobsen, H. P., Christensen, A. E., Herskind, A. M., & Plesner, K. (2002). Clinical course of cow's milk protein allergy/intolerance and atopic diseases in childhood. *Pediatric Allergy and Immunology*, *13*(Suppl. 15), 23–28.

Montgomery, S. M., Ehlin, A., & Sacker, A. (2006). Breast feeding and resilience against psychosocial stress. *Archives of Disease in Childhood*, *91*, 990–994.

Raisler, J., Alexander, C., & O'Campo, P. (1999). Breastfeeding and infant illness: A dose-response relationship? *American Journal of Public Health*, *89*, 25–30.

CHAPTER 24

Protection Against Chronic Disease for the Breastfed Infant and Lactating Mother

Carol A. Ryan, MSN, IBCLC, FILCA

OBJECTIVES

- List selected chronic diseases that are affected by breastfeeding.
- Discuss long-term outcomes of women who lactate and infants who receive human milk.
- Provide evidence-based support for the World Health Organization (WHO, 2009) and American Academy of Pediatrics (AAP, 2005) recommendations for exclusive breastfeeding for the first 6 months of life and continued breastfeeding to at least 1–2 years of age with the addition of age-appropriate complementary foods as a preventive measure in reducing the incidence of chronic disease in both infants and their mothers.

INTRODUCTION

Both medical research and clinical practice have long acknowledged the immediate and long-term benefits of human milk for the human infant. Longitudinal research has explored and studied breastfed infants into their adulthood. Research findings support many long-term benefits for the world's children when consuming human milk exclusively for 6 months (Kramer et al., 2002; WHO, 2007). This evidence has galvanized the medical community and the general public's support and encouragement of breastfeeding. Some of the most notable and life-sustaining outcomes can be found in studies examining Crohn's disease, ulcerative colitis, types 1 and 2 diabetes, obesity, and some childhood lymphomas and leukemia. Because these diseases can have a devastating impact on the child, his or her family, the community, and the healthcare system, a lactation consultant's working knowledge of these disease entities is essential in both healthcare planning and counseling during the pre- and postnatal periods. Infants who were breastfed demonstrate a reduced incidence of these diseases as lifelong conditions. Those who are not breastfed demonstrate an increased, lifelong incidence of these diseases. Mothers who breastfeed their children have also benefited over their life spans as well with reduced incidences of premenopausal cancers of the breast and ovaries, osteoporosis, hyperlipidemia, and cardiovascular disease. Lactation and breastfeeding significantly affect the short- and long-term benefits for both mothers and their children. There is definitely a reason to feed human milk to human infants. This chapter discusses conditions related to infants and young children in relation to breastfeeding.

I. Asthma and Allergies

A. Healthy newborns present with a low acidic gut pH environment that is sterile, immature, nonimmune, and rich in lactoferrin and bifidobacterium.

B. Heredity and environmental additives in the form of inappropriate first foods distress and enable disease, irritations, and flora and hormonal imbalances within the normal integrity of the maturing infant gut.

C. Decreases in the pathogen-fighting bifidobacterium can predispose infants to allergic disease (Salminen et al., 2005).

D. Human milk precipitates rapid maturation of the infant gut while nonhuman foods do not (Newburg et al., 2007).

E. Susceptible, immature infant guts set the stage for allergies to proteins, especially cow's milk protein (Van Odijk et al., 2003), asthma (Oddy et al., 1999), and atopic dermatitis (Strassburger et al., 2010).

F. Exclusive breastmilk feedings for the first 6 months of life and the avoidance of inappropriate complementary foods, formulas, supplements, or additives before maturation of the infant gut avoids or lessens opportune, long-term asthma and possibly atopy from developing and other long-term illness (Spatz et al., 2011; Strassburger et al., 2010).

II. Crohn's Disease, an Inflammatory Bowel Disease

A. Frequency of the recognition of Crohn's disease by the medical profession has increased because of evidence that suggests this disease is caused by Mycobacterium avium subspecies paratuberculosis similar to the form found in cattle (Stewart et al., 2010; Timms et al., 2011; Uzoigwe et al., 2007).

B. Noted in Western populations with northern European Anglo-Saxon cultures.

C. Found also in developing African American and Hispanic populations.

D. Occurs equally in both sexes.

E. Most common in the Jewish populations.

F. Follows a familial tendency and can overlap with ulcerative colitis.

G. Smoking plays a clear role in Crohn's disease (Rigas et al., 1993).

H. Crohn's disease appears as patchy inflammatory ulcerations on the mucosa of the intestinal wall with a combination of longitudinal and transverse ulcers and intervening mucosal edema.

I. It creates inflammation of the small intestine, most often in the ileum, though it can affect the digestive system from the mouth to the anus.

J. The inflammation can extend into the deepest layers of the intestinal wall.

K. Most common signs and symptoms include diarrhea with abdominal pain, fever, anorexia, weight loss, bleeding, and a right lower quadrant mass or fullness.

L. Children with Crohn's disease can experience delayed development and stunted growth (Calkins et al., 1986).

M. Breastmilk is essential to the development of normal immunologic competence of the intestinal mucosa (Lawrence et al., 2011).

N. Individuals with Crohn's disease are most prevalent in groups with little or no breastfeeding (Kane et al., 2005).

III. Ulcerative Colitis, an Inflammatory Bowel Disease

A. A chronic, nonspecific inflammatory and ulcerative disease arising in the colonic mucosa.

B. Characterized frequently as periods of bloody, mucus-filled diarrhea, and abdominal cramping varying in intensity and duration, and with intermittent exacerbations and remissions (Lawrence et al., 2011).

C. Complications can be life threatening.

D. Can occur in the breastfeeding infant as a result of bovine b-globulin protein in the mother's diet causing severe allergic reactions (Shmerling, 1983).

E. Peak incidences are noted at 15 to 30 years of age, and a smaller peak between ages 50 and 70 years. Most will require surgery (Langholtz, 2010).

F. The disease usually begins in the rectosigmoid area, extending proximally, eventually amassing the whole colon (or the entire large bowel). Included are ulceration and inflammation of the inner rectum and colon linings.

G. Human milk develops normal immunologic competence of the intestinal mucosa, protecting it from adhesion and penetration of bacteria, viruses, and foreign proteins that compromise mucosa integrity and provoke inflammatory responses (Andrew et al., 2009; Klement et al., 2004; Koletzko et al., 1989).

H. Human milk can be therapeutic to a damaged gastrointestinal tract (Howie et al., 1990; Kramer et al., 2001).

IV. Diabetes

A. Type 1 strikes people of all ages with a sudden onset, precipitating a lifelong dependence on an injected or pumped form of insulin (Juvenile Diabetes Research Foundation, 2011).

B. Each year, more than 15,000 children and 15,000 adults, approximately 80 individuals a day, are affected in the United States (Juvenile Diabetes Research Foundation International, 2011).

C. Type 1 is clinically significant because of complications including hyperglycemia (high blood glucose), infinity to diabetic ketoacidosis (coma), infections, nephropathy, atherosclerotic coronary and peripheral disease, neuropathy, and retinopathy (Gerstein, 1994).

D. Type 1 diabetes is caused by a genetically conditioned, immune-mediated, selective destruction of more than 90% of the insulin-secreting pancreatic B cells and can be triggered by an environmental insult, exposure to a toxin, early introduction of bovine milk insulin, or a viral infection (Karjalainen et al., 1992; McKinney et al.,1999; Vaarala, 2002; Vaarala et al., 1999; Young et al., 2002).

E. There may be a 20% increase in risk of type 1 diabetes for children born by cesarean section (Cardwell et al., 2008).

F. Children with diabetes are more likely to have little to no consumption of human milk.

1. Infants who are breastfed at least 4 months are significantly less at risk for type 1 and type 2 diabetes (Ip et al., 2007; Pettitt et al., 1998; Stuebe, 2009; Young et al., 2002; Ziegler et al., 2003).

2. Increased rates of breastfeeding duration are associated with lower rates of type 1 diabetes (Holmberg et al. & ABIS Study Group, 2007; Jarrett, 1984; Malcova et al., 2006; Sadauskaite-Kuehne et al., 2004).

3. Introduction of a cereal before 4 months of age can place an infant at risk for development of type 1 diabetes (Norris et al., 2003).

4. Longer duration of breastfeeding was associated with reduced incidence of type 2 diabetes in young and middle-aged women by improving glucose homeostasis (Knip et al., 2005).

G. Higher weight gain later in life is associated with insulin dependency Johansson et al., 1994).

H. Mechanisms that can lead to a more protective effect by breastfeeding are not well understood.

1. Newly diagnosed children have increased immunoglobulin IgA and IgG antibodies to bovine beta-lactoglobulin (Savilahti et al., 1993).

2. Autoimmune destruction of pancreatic beta cells occurs (Vaarala et al., 1999).

3. Bovine milk is a major environmental trigger (Karjalainen et al., 1992).

4. A specific immune memory can be established at the time of dietary exposure to bovine milk (Wasmuth et al., 2000).

5. The timing of gut closure and presence of digestive enzymes such as trypsin, gastrointestinal (GI) infections, and oral tolerance mechanisms might all be collaborative in initiating an autoimmune response (Goldfarb, 2008; Newburg et al., 2007).

6. Exposure to bovine milk and solid foods before 3 months of age may be particularly important in terms of diabetic risk (Monte et al., 1994; Scott, 1990; Vaarala, 2002; Vaarala et al., 1999).

   a. Infant formula, which contains little to no insulin, causes an increased demand for insulin that can result in an increased beta-cell antigen presentation, and this helps explain the tendency of type 1 and type 2 diabetes to develop during periods of increased insulin demand (Karjalainen et al., 1992; Young et al., 2002).

   b. Breastfeeding less than 2–3 months and early introduction of bovine-based formula can predispose genetically susceptible infants to type 1 diabetes to progressive signs of beta-cell autoimmunity (Kimpimaki et al., 2001; Vaarala, 2002).

7. Insufficient breastfeeding of genetically susceptible newborns might lead to B-cell infections and type 2 diabetes later in life (Lawrence et al., 2011; Taylor et al., 2005).

V. Childhood Cancers

A. Lymphoma, a heterogeneous group of neoplasms arising in the reticuloendothelial and lymphatic systems.

   1. Children with immune deficiencies, regardless of socioeconomic status, have an increased risk for lymphomas resulting from altered immunoregulation (disturbed immune competence), which might contribute to an increased risk of lymphoproliferative disease (Kwan et al., 2004).

   2. A 2005 meta-analysis suggests that "increasing breastfeeding rates from 50% to 100% could prevent at most 5% of childhood lymphomas" (Martin et al., 2005).

B. Hodgkin's disease, a complex cellular immune disorder with chronic infection.

   1. This is a chronic disease with lymphoreticular proliferation of an unknown cause that can present in a localized or disseminated manner.

   2. Hodgkin's disease peaks first around 15 to 34 years of age and then around 60 years of age.

   3. Signs and symptoms vary depending on the disease's progression. Though not necessarily inclusive, the following signs and symptoms can occur: intense pruritis, fever, night sweats, weight loss, lymph node compression, and internal organ obstructions.

   4. Clinical symptoms manifest as the disease progresses from one organ site to another.

   5. Progression rate can range from slow to very aggressive.

   6. Children who were never breastfed or who were breastfed for only a short term have a higher risk of developing Hodgkin's disease—but not non-Hodgkin's lymphoma—than do those who were breastfed for greater or equal to 6 months (Martin et al., 2005).

C. Leukemia: Leukemia is the most common childhood malignancy in Western countries; it accounts for one-third of all cancers occurring in children younger than 15 years of age (Belson et al., 2007).

   1. Breastfeeding duration of 4 months or longer has been associated with a reduction of childhood acute lymphocytic leukemia (Davis et al., 1988; Davis, 1998; Guise et al., 2005; Lawrence et al., 2011; Stuebe, 2009;).

   2. Six months of exclusive breastfeeding decreases risk for developing acute lymphocytic leukemia and acute myelogenous leukemia (Ip et al., 2007).

   3. Specific or nonspecific anti-infectious effects and early immune-stimulating effects of breastmilk might work synergistically or independently to protect children against acute leukemia (Shu et al., 1995, 1999).

VI. Obesity

A. Overweight and obesity in industrialized countries represent the most common nutritional disorder in children and adolescents.

B. Overweight and obesity in children are an ongoing concern worldwide (Centers for Disease Control and Prevention [CDC], Child Obesity Facts, 2011; Grummer-Strawn et al., 2004).

C. A clear dose-dependent effect of the duration of breastfeeding on overweight or obesity prevalence at the time of entry into school is evidence based (Burdett et al., 2006; Dubois & Girard, 2006; Koletzko et al., 2005; Kvaavik et al., 2005; Owen et al., 2005; Stuebe, 2009; Tulldahl et al., 1999; Von Kries et al., 2000).

D. The protectiveness of breastfeeding might have a cell programming effect in reducing overweight conditions and obesity in later life (Dewey, 2003; Gillman et al., 2001; Knip et al., 2005; Plagmann et al., 2005).

E. Infants fed formula have higher plasma concentrations of insulin, which might stimulate fat deposition and development of early adipocytes, or fat cells (Knip et al., 2005).

F. Breastfed babies do not consume as much energy and protein as do formula-fed babies, and this might contribute to a decreased body mass index (BMI) of children and adolescents who were breastfed (Gillman et al., 2001; Weyermann et al., 2006).

G. Weaning foods, behavioral modeling, and exercise are integral to lifelong eating habits and good health.

H. Breastfed babies are leaner than formula-fed babies are at 1 year of age, weighing 1–2 pounds less (Dewey et al., 1993; WHO, 2006).

I. Universally, children grow similarly when their health and basic care needs are optimally met (WHO, 2006). (See Chapter 31, Breastfeeding and Growth: Birth Through Weaning.)

J. Exclusive breastfeeding for 6 months and continued breastfeeding with appropriate weaning and complementary foods contribute to optimal infant and child growth and development (Gartner et al., 2005).

VII. Long-Term Healthcare Considerations for Women Associated with Breastfeeding Duration

A. More than 12 months of lactation provides a reduced risk for hypercholesterolemia, diabetes, hypertension, coronary heart and artery disease at a population level (Schack-Nielsen et al., 2006; Schwarz et al., 2009).

B. Type 2 diabetes in young and middle-aged women who have lactated 12 or more months might be reduced because of improved glucose homeostasis (Knip et al., 2005; Rudnika et al., 2007; Schwarz et al., 2010; Stuebe et al., 2005; Taylor et al., 2005).

C. Breast and ovarian cancer are reduced with long-term lactation in the premenopausal period (Lipworth et al., 2000; Stuebe, Willet et al., 2009; Whittemore, 1994; Zheng et al., 2000).

D. Lower risk for breast cancer is evidenced in premenopausal women, women who have a first birth before 30 years of age, and women who have breastfed cumulatively for a long time (Collaborative Group on Hormonal Factors in Breast Cancer, 2002; DeSilva et al., 2010; Fishman, 2010; Ip et al., 2007; Newton, 1996; Zheng et al., 2001).

E. Hip fractures and osteoporosis are reduced in the postmenopausal period for women who have breastfed their children (Dursun et al., 2006; Turck, 2005).

F. Lactation has no detrimental effects on maternal bone mineral density in postmenopausal age (Lenora et al., 2009; Riordan et al., 2010; Specker et al., 1991).

G. Serum calcium and phosphorous concentrations are greater in lactating than in nonlactating women; lactation also stimulates the greatest increases in fractional calcium absorption and serum calcitriol after weaning (Kalkwarf et al., 1995).

H. Long duration of lactation is associated with a reduced risk of cardiovascular disease in women (Jarvisalo et al., 2009; Martin et al., 2005; Martin et al., 2009; Parikh et al., 2009; Schwarz et al., 2010; Schwarz et al., 2009; Stuebe, Michaels et al., 2009).

I. Cholesterol levels might be improved in adults who were breastfed (Hamosh, 1988; Leon et al., 2009; Martin et al., 2009; Smithers et al., 2010).

J. Obesity is associated with decreased intention to breastfeed, its initiation, and duration (Kulie et al., 2011).

K. The Bellagio Consensus Conference on breastfeeding determined a mother who is breastfeeding and remains amenorrheic has a 98% rate of protection from pregnancy during the first 6 months postpartum if she is fully or nearly fully breastfeeding and has not experienced vaginal bleeding after the 56th postpartum day (Huffman et al., 1994; Short et al., 1991).

L. The lactational amenorrhea method (LAM) is effective in preventing pregnancies, extends the range of contraceptive choices, is cost effective, and is culturally acceptable (Kennedy et al., 1998).

M. The debilitating effects of rheumatoid arthritis can be reduced with 13 months and more of breastfeeding (Karrlson et al., 2004; Pikwer et al., 2009).

N. Exclusive breastfeeding with accompanying lactational amenorrhea has been shown to reduce the risk of postpartum multiple sclerosis relapses (Langer-Gould et al., 2009). Patient relapse episodes and behaviors before and during pregnancy can be predictors of postpartum relapse susceptibility. Therefore, women with a high risk for postpartum relapse can be counseled to forgo breastfeeding (Portaccio et al., 2011). The hormonal effects of lactation do not affect the risk of exacerbation as do the hormonal effect on the mother's immune system (Nelson et al., 1988).

VIII. Conclusion

The short- and long-term health benefits of lactation and breastfeeding can improve maternal and child health outcomes. Healthcare providers, families, communities, and nations need to provide appropriate support systems to increase breastfeeding exclusivity and duration.

References

American Academy of Pediatrics. (2005). Policy statement. Organizational principles to guide and define the child health care system and/or improve the health of all children. Section on Breastfeeding. Breastfeeding and the Use of Human Milk. *Pediatrics, 115*(2).

American Academy of Pediatrics, Work Group on Cow's Milk Protein and Diabetes Mellitus. (1994). Infant feeding practices and their possible relationship to the etiology of diabetes mellitus. *Pediatrics, 94,* 752–755.

Andrew, R. B., Richard, K. R., Michelle, L. W., Gilmour, W. H., Jack, S., & David, C. W. (2009). Systematic review: The role of breastfeeding in the development of pediatric inflammatory bowel disease. *Journal of Pediatrics, 155*(3), 421–426.

Belson, M., Kingsley, B., & Holmes, A. (2007). Risk factors for acute leukemia in children: A review. *Environmental Health Perspectives, 115*(1), 138–145.

Bergstrand, O., & Hellers, G. (1983). Breastfeeding during infancy and later development of Crohn's disease. *Scandinavian Journal of Gastroenterology, 18,* 903.

Borch-Johnsen, K., Joner, G., Mandrup-Poulsen, T., Christy, M., Zachau-Chrsitainsen, B., Kastrup, K., et al. (1984). Relation between breastfeeding and incidence rates of insulin dependent diabetes mellitus. *Lancet, 2,* 1083–1086.

Burdett, H. L., Whitaker, R. C., Hall, W. C., & Daniels, S. R. (2006). Breastfeeding, introduction of complementary foods and adiposity at 5 years of age. *American Journal of Clinical Nutrition, 83,* 550–558.

Calkins, B. M., & Mendeloff, A. I. (1986). Epidemiology of inflammatory bowel disease. *Epidemiology Review, 8,* 60–91.

Cardwell, C. R., Stene, L. C., Joner, G., et al. (2008). Caesarean section is associated with an increased risk of childhood onset type 1 diabetes: A meta-analysis of observational studies. *Diabetologia, 51,* 726–735.

Centers for Disease Control and Prevention. (2009). Breastfeeding report card—United States. Retrieved from http://www.cdc.gov/breastfeeding/data/report_card.htm

Centers for Disease Control and Prevention, Division of Nutrition, Physical Activity, and Obesity, National Center for Disease Prevention and Health Promotion. (2011, August). Breastfeeding among U.S. children born 1999–2006, CDC National Immunization Survey. Retrieved from http://www.cdc.gov/breastfeeding/data/NIS_data/

Centers for Disease Control and Prevention. (2011). Child obesity facts. Retrieved February 6, 2012 at http://www.cdc.gov/healthyyouth/obesity/facts.htm

Chung, M., Raman, G., Trikalinos, T., Lau, J., & Ip, S. (2008). Interventions in primary care to promote breastfeeding: An evidence review for the U.S. Preventive Service Task Force. *Annals of Internal Medicine, 149*(8), 565–582.

Clavano, N. R. (1982). Mode of feeding and its effect on infant mortality and morbidity. *Journal of Tropical Pediatrics, 28,* 287–293.

Collaborative Group on Hormonal Factors in Breast Cancer. (2002). Breast cancer and breastfeeding: Collaborative reanalysis of individual data from 47 epidemiological studies in 30 countries, including 50,302 women with breast cancer and 96,973 without the disease. *Lancet, 360,* 187–195.

Davis, M. K. (1998). Review of the evidence for an association between infant feeding and childhood cancer. *International Journal of Cancer, 11*(Suppl.), 29–33.

Davis, M. K., Savitz, D. A., & Graubard, B. I. (1988). Infant feeding and childhood cancer. *Lancet, 2*(8607), 365–368.

DeSilva, M., Senarath, U., Gunatilake, M., & Lokuhetty, D. (2010). Prolonged breastfeeding reduces risk of breast cancer in Sri Lankan women: A case-control study. *Cancer Epidemiology*, *34*(3), 267–273.

Dewey, K. G. (2003). Is breastfeeding protective of childhood obesity? *Journal of Human Lactation*, *19*(1), 9–18.

Dewey, K. G., Heinig, M. J., Nommsen, L. A., Peerson, J. M., & Lonnerdal, B. (1993). Breastfed infants are leaner than formula-fed infants at one year of age: The DARLING study. *American Journal of Clinical Nutrition*, *57*, 140–145.

Dewey, K. G., Heinig, J., & Nommensen-Rivers, L. A. (1995). Differences in morbidity between breastfed and formula-fed infants. *Journal of Pediatrics*, *126*, 697–702.

Dewey, K. G., Peerson, J. M., Brown, K. H., Krebs, N. F., Michaelsen, K. F., Persson, L. A., et al. (1995). Growth of breastfed infants deviates from current reference data: A pooled analysis of US, Canadian, and European data sets. *Pediatrics*, *96*, 495–503.

Dubois, L., & Girard, M. (2006). Early determinants of overweight at 4.5 years in a population-based longitudinal study. *International Journal of Obesity*, *30*, 610–617.

Dursun, N., Akin, S., Dursun, E., et al. (2006). Influence of duration of total breastfeeding on bone mineral density in a Turkish population: Does the priority of risk factors differ from society to society? *Osteoporosis International*, *17*, 651–655.

Family Health International. (1988). Breastfeeding as a family planning method. *Lancet*, *2*(8621), 1204–1205.

Fishman, A. (2010). The effects of parity, breastfeeding, and infertility treatment on the risk of hereditary breast and ovarian cancer. *International Journal of Gynecological Cancer*, *20*(11, Suppl. 2), S31–S33.

Gartner, L. M., Morton, J., Lawrence, R. A., et al. (2005). Breastfeeding and the use of human milk (American Academy of Pediatric statement). *Pediatrics*, *115*(2), 496–506.

Gerstein, H. C. (1994). Cow's milk exposure and type I diabetes mellitus: A critical overview of the clinical literature. *Diabetes Care*, *17*, 13–18.

Gillman, M. W., Rifas-Shiman, S. L., Camargo, C. A. Jr, Berkey, C. S., Frazier, A. L., Rockett, H. R., Field, A. E., & Colditz, G. A. (2001).Risk of overweight among adolescents who were breastfed as infants. *JAMA*, *285*(19), 2461–2467.

Goldfarb, M. F. (2008). Relation of time of introduction of cow's milk protein to an infant and risk of type 1 diabetes mellitus. *Journal of Proteome Research*, *7*(5), 2165–2167.

Grummer-Strawn, L. M., & Mei, Z. (2004). Does breastfeeding protect against pediatric overweight? Analysis of longitudinal data from the Centers for Disease Control and Prevention Pediatric Nutrition Surveillance System. *Pediatrics*, *113*(2), e81–e86.

Guise, J. M., Austin, D., Morris, C. D. (2005).Review of case-control studies related to breastfeeding and reduced risk of childhood leukemia. *Pediatrics*, *116*(5), e724–e731.

Hamosh, M. (1988). Does infant nutrition affect adiposity and cholesterol levels in adulthood? *Journal of Pediatric Gastroenterology and Nutrition*, *7*, 10.

Holmberg, H., Wahlberg, J., Vaarala, O., Ludvigsson, J., & ABIS Study Group. (2007). Short duration of breastfeeding as a risk factor for beta-cells autoantibodies in 5 year old children from the general population. *British Journal of Nutrition*, *97*, 111–116.

Howie, P. W., Forsyth, J. S., Ogston, S. A., et al. (1990). Protective effect of breastfeeding against infection. *British Medical Journal*, *300*, 11–16.

Huffman, S. L., & Lubbok, M. H. (1994). Breastfeeding in family planning: A help or hindrance. *International Journal of Gynecology and Obstetrics*, *47*(Suppl.), 523–531.

Ip, S., Chung, M., Raman, G., et al. (2007). Breastfeeding and maternal and infant health outcomes in developed countries (AHRQ Publication No. 07-E007). Rockville, MD: Agency for Healthcare Research and Quality. Retrieved from http://www.ahrq.gov/downloads/pub/evidence/pdf/brfout/brfout.pdf

Jarrett, R. J. (1984). Breastfeeding and diabetes. *Lancet*, *2*, 1283.

Jarvisalo, M. J., Hutri-Kahonen, N., Juonala, M., et al. (2009). Breastfeeding in infancy and arterial endothelial function later in life. The Cardiovascular Risk in Young Finns Study. *European Journal of Clinical Nutrition*, *63*(5), 640–645.

Johansson, C., Samuelsson, U., & Ludvigsson, J. (1994). A high weight gain early in life is associated with an increased risk of type I (insulin dependent) diabetes mellitus. *Diabetologia*, *37*, 91–94.

Juvenile Diabetes Research Foundation International. (2011). Annual report. Retrieved February 6, 2012 at http://www.jdrfapps.com/eReport/index.htm

Kalkwarf, H. J., & Specker, B. L. (1995). Bone mineral loss during lactation and recovery after weaning. *Obstetrics and Gynecology*, *86*, 26.

Kane, S., & Lemieux, N. (2005). The role of breastfeeding in postpartum disease activity in women with inflammatory bowel disease. *American Journal of Gastroenterology*, *100*, 102–105.

Karjalainen, J., Martin, J., Knip, M., et al. (1992). A bovine albumin peptide as a possible trigger of insulin dependent diabetes mellitus. *New England Journal of Medicine*, *327*, 302–307.

Karrlson, E. W., Mandl, L. A., Hankinson, S. E., & Grodstein, F. (2004). Do breastfeeding and other reproductive factors influence future risk of rheumatoid arthritis? Results from the Nurses' Health Study. *Arthritis and Rheumatism*, *50*(11), 3458–3467.

Kennedy, K. L., & Kotelchuck, M. (1998). Policy considerations for the introduction and promotion of the lactational amenorrhea method: Advantages and disadvantages of LAM. *Journal of Human Lactation*, *14*(3), 191–203.

Kimpimaki, T., Erkkola, M. Korhonen, S., Kupila, A., Virtanen, S. M., Ilonen, J., et al. (2001). Short term exclusive breastfeeding predisposes young children with increased genetic risk of type 1 diabetes to progressive autoimmunity. *Diabetologia*, *44*, 63–69.

Klement, E., Cohen, R. V., Boxman, J., Joseph, A., & Reif, S. (2004). Breastfeeding and risk of inflammatory bowel disease: a systematic review with meta-analysis. *American Journal of Clinical Nutrition*, *80*(5), 1342–1352.

Knip, M., & Akerblom, H. K. (2005). Early nutrition and later diabetes. *Advances in Experimental Medicine and Biology*, *569*, 142–150.

Koletzko, B., Broekaert, I., Demmelmair, H., et al. (2005). Protein intake in the first year of life: A risk factor for later obesity? The E.U. Childhood Obesity Project. *Advances in Experimental Medicine and Biology*, *569*, 60–79.

Koletzko, S., Sherman, P., Corey, M., et al. (1989). Role of infant feeding practices in development of Crohn's disease in childhood. *British Medical Journal*, *298*, 1617–1618.

Kostraba, J. H., Cruickshanks, K. J., & Lawler-Heavner, J. (1993). Early exposure to cow's milk and solid foods in infancy, genetic predisposition, and risk of IDDM. *Diabetes*, *42*, 288–295.

Kovar, M. G., et al. (1984). Review of the epidemiologic evidence for an association between infant feeding and infant health. *Pediatrics*, *74*, 615–638.

Kramer, M. S., Barr, R. G., Leduc, D. G., et al. (1985). Determinants of weight and adiposity in the first year of life. *Journal of Pediatrics*, *106*, 10.

Kramer, M. S., Chalmers, B., Hodnett, E. D., et al. (2001). Promotion of Breastfeeding Intervention Trial (PROBIT): A randomized trial in the Republic of Belarus. *Journal of the American Medical Association*, *285*(4), 413–420.

Kramer, M. S., & Kakuma, R. (2002). Optimal duration of exclusive breastfeeding. *Cochrane Database of Systematic Reviews*, *1*, CD003517.

Kulie, T., Slattengren, A., Redmer, J., Counts, H., Eglash, A., & Schrager, S. (2011). Obesity and women's health: An evidence-based review. *Journal of the American Board of Family Medicine*, *24*(1), 75–85.

Kvaavik, E., Tell, G. S., & Klepp, K. I. (2005). Surveys of Norwegian youth indicated that breastfeeding reduced subsequent risk of obesity. *Journal of Clinical Epidemiology*, *58*, 849–855.

Kwan, M. L., Buffler, P. A., Abrams, B., & Kiley, V. A. (2004). Breastfeeding and the risk of childhood leukemia: a meta-analysis. *Public Health Reports*, *119*(6), 521–535.

Langer-Gould, A., Huang, S. M., Gupta, R., et al. (2009). Exclusive breastfeeding and the risk of postpartum relapses in women with multiple sclerosis. *Archives of Neurology*, *66*(8), 958–963.

Langholtz, E. (2010). Current trends in inflammatory bowel disease: The natural history. *Therapeutic Advances in Gastroenterology*, *3*(2), 77–86.

Lawrence, R. A., & Lawrence, R. M. (2011). *Breastfeeding: A guide for the medical profession* (7th ed.). St. Louis, MO: Elsevier Mosby.

Lenora, J., Lekamwassam, S., & Karlsson, M. K. (2009). Effects of multiparity and prolonged breast-feeding on maternal bone mineral density: A community-based cross-sectional study. *BMC Women's Health*, *9*, 19.

Leon, D. A., & Ronalds, G. (2009). Breastfeeding influences on later life. *Advances in Experimental Biology*, *639*, 153–166.

Lipworth, L., Bailey, L. R., & Trichopoulos, D. (2000). History of breastfeeding in relation to breast cancer risk: A review of the epidemiologic literature. *Journal of the National Cancer Institute*, *92*(4), 302–312.

Malcova H., Sumnik, Z., Drevinek. P., Venhacova, J., Lebl, J., & Cinek, O. (2006). Absence of breast-feeding is associated with the risk of type 1 diabetes: a case-control study in a population with rapidly increasing incidence. *European Journal of Pediatrics*, *165*(2), 114–149.

Martin, R. M., & Davey Smith, G. (2009). Does having been breastfed in infancy influence lipid profile in later life? A review of the literature. *Advances in Experimental Medicine and Biology*, *646*, 41–50.

Martin, R. M., Ebrahim, S., Griffin, M., et al. (2005). Breastfeeding and atherosclerosis: Intima-media thickness and plaques at 65-year follow-up of the Boyd-Orr cohort. *Arteriosclerosis, Thrombosis, and Vascular Biology*, *25*(7), 1482–1488.

Mathur, G. P., Gupta, N., Mathur, S., Gupta, V., Pradhan, S., Dwivedi, J. N., et al. (1993). Breastfeeding and childhood cancer. *Indian Pediatrics*, *30*, 651–657.

Mayer, E. J., Hamman, R. F., Gay, E. C., et al. (1988). Reduced risk of IDDM among breastfed children: The Colorado IDDM Registry. *Diabetes*, *37*, 1625.

McKinney, P. A., Parslow, R., Gurney, K. A., et al. (1999). Perinatal and neonatal determinants of childhood Type I diabetes. A case-control study in Yorkshire, UK. *Diabetes Care*, *22*(6), 928–932.

Monte, W. D., Johnston, C. S., & Roll, L. E. (1994). Bovine serum albumin detected in infant formula is a possible trigger for insulin dependent diabetes mellitus. *Journal of the American Dietetic Association*, *94*, 314–316.

Nelson, L. M., Franklin, G. M., & Jones, M. C. (1988). Risk of multiple sclerosis exacerbation during pregnancy and breastfeeding. *Journal of the American Medical Association*, *259*(23), 3441–3443.

Newburg, D. S., & Walker, W. A. (2007). Protection of the neonate by the innate immune system of developing gut and of human milk. *Pediatric Research*, *61*, 2–8.

Newton, E. R. (1996). Does breastfeeding protect women from breast cancer? *ABM News and Views, 2*(2), 1.

Norris, J. M., Barriga, K., Klingensmith, G.., et al. (2003). Timing of initial cereal exposure in infancy and risk of islet autoimmunity. *Journal of the American Medical Association, 290*(13), 1713–1720.

Oddy, W. H., Holt, P. G., Sly, P. D., et al. (1999). Association between breastfeeding and asthma in 6 year old children: Findings of a prospective birth cohort study. *British Medical Journal, 319*, 815–819.

Owen, C. G., Martin, R. M., Whincup, P. H., et al. (2005). Effect of infant feeding on the risk of obesity across the life course: A quantitative review of published evidence. *Pediatrics, 115*, 1367–1377.

Parikh, N. I., Hwang, S. J., Inglesson, E., et al. (2009). Breastfeeding in infancy and adult cardiovascular disease risk factors. *American Journal of Medicine, 122*(7), 656–663, e1.

Pettitt, D. J., Forman, M. R., Hanson, R. L., et al. (1997). Breastfeeding and incidence of non-insulin dependent diabetes mellitus in Pima Indians. *Lancet, 350*(9072), 166–168.

Pettitt, D. J., & Knowler, W. C. (1998). Long-term effects of the intrauterine environment, birth weight, and breastfeeding in Pima Indians. *Diabetes Care, 21*(Suppl. 2), B138–141.

Pikwer, M., Bergstrom, U., Nilsson, J. A., Jacobsson, L., Berglund, G., & Turesson, C. (2009). Breastfeeding, but not use of oral contraceptives, is associated with reduced risk of rheumatoid arthritis. *Annals of the Rheumatic Diseases, 68*(4), 514–518.

Plagmann, A., & Harter, T. (2005). Breastfeeding and the risk of obesity and metabolic diseases in the child. *Metabolic Syndrome and Related Disorders, 3*(3), 222–232.

Portaccio, E., Ghezzi, A., Hakiki, B., et al. (2011). Breastfeeding not related to postpartum relapses in multiple sclerosis. *Neurology, 77*(2), 145–150.

Porter, R. S., & Kaplan, J. L. (Eds.). (2011). *Merck manual of diagnosis and therapy* (19th ed.). Rathway, NJ: Merck Research Laboratories.

Rigas, A., Rigas, B. & Glasserman, M. (1993). Breastfeeding and maternal smoking in the etiology of Crohn's disease and ulcerative colitis in childhood. *Annals of Epidemiology, 3*, 387–392.

Riordan, J., & Wambach, K. (Eds.). (2010). *Breastfeeding and human lactation* (4th ed.). Sudbury, MA: Jones and Bartlett.

Rudnicka, A. R., Owen, C. G., & Strachan, D. P. (2007). The effect of breastfeeding and cardiorespiratory risk factors in adult life. *Pediatrics, 719*, e1107–e1115.

Sadauskaite-Kuehne, V., Ludvigsson, J., Padaiga, Z., et al. (2004). Longer breastfeeding is an independent protective factor against development of type 1 diabetes mellitus in childhood. *Diabetes/Metabolism Research and Reviews, 20*, 150–157.

Salminen, S. J., Gueimonde, J., & Isolauri, E. (2005). Probiotics that modify disease risk. *Journal of Nutrition, 135*, 1294–1298.

Samuelson, U., Johansson, C., & Ludvigsson, J. (1988). Breastfeeding seems to play a marginal role in the prevention of insulin dependent diabetes mellitus (IDDM) among breastfed children. *Diabetes, 37*, 1625–1632.

Savilahti, E., Saukkonen, T. T., Virtala, E. T., et al. (1993). Increased levels of cow's milk and beta-lactoglobulin antibodies in young children with newly diagnosed IDDM. *Diabetes Care, 16*, 984–989.

Schack-Nielsen, L., Mølgaard, C., Larsen, D., Martyn, C., & Michaelsen, K. F. (2005). Arterial stiffness in 10-year-old children: Current and early determinants. *British Journal of Nutrition, 9*(6), 1004–1011.

Schack-Nielsen, L., & Michaelsen, K. F. (2006). Breast feeding and future health. *Current Opinion in Clinical Nutrition and Metabolic Care, 9* (3), 289–296.

Schwarz, E. B., Brown, J. S., Creasman, J. M., Stuebe, A. M., McClure, C. K., Van Den Eeden, S. K., & Thom, D. (2010). Lactation and maternal risk of type 2 diabetes: A population based study. *American Journal of Medicine, 123*(9), 863.

Schwarz, E. B., McClure, C. K., Tepper, P. G., Thurston, R., Janssen, I., Matthews, K. A., & Sutton-Tyrrell, K. (2010). Lactation and maternal measures of subclinical cardiovascular disease. *Obstetrics and Gynecology, 115*(1), 41–48.

Schwarz, E. B., Ray, R. M., Stuebe, A. M., Allison, M. A., Ness, R. B., Freiberg, M. S., & Cauley, J. A. (2009). Duration of lactation and risk factors for maternal cardiovascular disease. *Obstetrics and Gynecology, 113*(5), 974–982.

Scott, F. W. (1990). Cow milk and insulin dependent diabetes mellitus: Is there a relationship? *American Journal of Clinical Nutrition, 51*, 489–491.

Shmerling, D. H. (1983). Dietary protein induced colitis in breastfed infants. *Journal of Pediatrics, 103*, 500.

Short, R. V., Lewis, P. R., Renfree, M. B., & Shaw, G. (1991). Contraceptive effects of extended lactational amenorrhea: Beyond the Bellagio Consensus. *Lancet, 337*(8743), 715–717.

Shu, X. O., Clemens, J., Zheng, W., et al. (1995). Infant breastfeeding and the risk of childhood lymphoma and leukaemia. *International Journal of Epidemiology, 24*, 27–32.

Shu, X. O., Linet, M., Steinbuch, M., et al. (1999). Breastfeeding and risk of childhood acute leukemia. *Journal of the National Cancer Institute, 91*, 1765–1772.

Smithers, L., & McIntyre, E. (2010). Impact of breastfeeding—translating recent evidence for practice. *Australian Family Physician, 39*(10), 757–760.

Spatz, D. L., & Lessen, R. (2011). *The risks of not breastfeeding.* Morrisville, NC: International Lactation Consultant Association.

Specker, B. L., Tsang, R. C., & Ho, M. L. (1991). Changes in calcium homeostasis over the first year postpartum: Effect of lactation and weaning. *Obstetrics and Gynecology, 78*(1), 56–62.

Stewart, L. C., Day, A. S., Pearson, J., et al. (2010). SLC 11A1 polymorphisms in inflammatory bowel disease and Mycobacterium avium subspecies paratuberculosis status. *World Journal of Gastroenterology, 16*(45), 5727–5731.

Strassburger, S. Z., Vitolo, M. R., Bortolini, G. A., Pitrez, P. M., Jones, M. H., & Stein, R. T. (2010). Nutritional errors in the first months of life and their association with asthma and atopy in preschool children. *Journal of Pediatrics* (Rio J), *86*(5), 391–399.

Stuebe, A. M. (2009). The risks of not breastfeeding for mothers and infants. *Reviews in Obstetrics and Gynecology, 2*(4), 222–231.

Stuebe, A. M., Michaels, K. B., Willett, W. C., Manson, J. E., Rexrode, K., & Rich-Edwards, J. W. (2009). Duration of lactation and incidence of myocardial infarction in middle to late adulthood. *American Journal of Obstetrics and Gynecology, 200*(2), 138.e1–138.e8.

Stuebe, A. M., Rich-Edwards, J. U., Willett, W. C., Manson, J. E., & Michels, J. E. (2005). Duration of lactation and incidence of type 2 diabetes. *Journal of the American Medical Association, 294*(20), 2601–2610.

Stuebe, A. M., Willet, W. C., Xue, F., & Michels, K. B. (2009). Lactation and incidence of premenopausal breast cancer: A longitudinal study. *Archives of Internal Medicine, 169*(15), 1364–1371.

Suskind, V., Green, A., Cain, C., et al. (1997). Breastfeeding, menopause, and epithelial ovarian cancer in young women. *Epidemiology, 8*, 188.

Taylor, J. S., Kacmer, J. E., Nothnagle, M., & Lawrence, R. A. (2005). A systematic review of the literature associating breastfeeding with type 2 diabetes and gestational diabetes. *Journal of the American College of Nutrition, 24*(5), 320–326.

Timms, V. J., Gehringer, M. M., Mitchell, H. M., Das Kalopoulos, G., & Neilon, B. A. (2011). How accurately can we detect Mycobacterium avium subsp. Paratuberculosis infection? *Journal of Microbiological Methods, 85*(1), 1–8. Advance online publication.

Tulldahl, J., Pettersson, K., Andersson, S. W., & Hulthen, L. (1999). Mode of infant feeding and achieved growth in adolescence: Early feeding patterns in relation to growth and body composition in adolescence. *Obesity Research, 7*, 431–437.

Turck, D. (2005). Comité de nutrition de la Société française de pédiatrie. Breast feeding: health benefits for child and mother. *Archives de pediatrie, 12*(Suppl. 3), S145-S165.

Uzoigwe, J. C., Khaitas, M. L., & Gibbs, P. S. (2007). Epidemiological evidence for Mycobacterium avium subspecies paratuberculosis as a cause for Crohn's disease. *Epidemiology and Infection, 135*(7), 1057–1068.

Vaarala, O. (2002). The gut immune system and type 1 diabetes. *Annals of the New York Academy of Science, 958*, 39–46.

Vaarala, O., Knip, M., Paronen, J., et al. (1999). Cow's milk formula feeding induces primary immunization to insulin in infants at genetic risk for type 1 diabetes. *Diabetes, 48*(7), 1389–1394.

Van Odijk, J., Kull, I., Borres, M. P., et al. (2003). Breastfeeding and allergic disease: A multidisciplinary review of the literature (1996–2001) on the mode of early feeding in infancy and its impact on later atopic manifestations. *Allergy, 58*, 833–843.

Virtanen, S. M., Rasanen, L., Aro, A., et al. (1991). Infant feeding in Finnish children less than seven years of age with newly diagnosed IDDM. Childhood Diabetes in Finland Study Group. *Diabetes Care, 14*(5), 415.

Von Kries, R., Koletzko, B., Sauerwald, T., et al. (1999). Breastfeeding and obesity: Cross sectional study. *British Medical Journal, 313*, 147–150.

Von Kries, R., Koletzko, B., Sauerwald, T., et al. (2000). Does breastfeeding protect against childhood obesity? *Advances in Experimental Medicine and Biology, 478*, 29–39.

Wasmuth, H. E., & Kolb, H. (2000). Cow's milk and immune-mediated diabetes. *Proceedings of the Nutrition Society, 59*(4), 573–579.

Weyermann, M., Rothenbacher, D., & Brenner, H. (2006). Duration of breastfeeding and risk of overweight in childhood: A prospective birth cohort study from Germany. *International Journal of Obesity, 30*, 1281–1287.

Whittemore, A. S. (1994). Characteristics relating to ovarian cancer risk: Implications for prevention and detection. *Gynecologic Oncology, 55*(3, Pt. 2), S15.

Whorwell, P. J., Hodstack, G., Whorwell, G. M., & Wright, R. (1979). Bottle-feeding, early gastroenteritis, and inflammatory bowel disease. *British Journal of Medicine, 1*, 382.

World Health Organization, UNICEF. (2007). *Planning guide for national implementation of the global strategy for infant and young child feeding.* Geneva, Switzerland: WHO.

World Health Organization. (2006). *Child growth standards: Methods and development.* Geneva, Switzerland: Author.

World Health Organization. (2009). *Infant and young child feeding: Model chapter for textbooks for medical students and allied health professionals.* Geneva, Switzerland: Author.

World Health Organization Multicentre Growth Reference Study Group. (2006). Assessment of differences in linear growth among populations in the WHO Multicentre Reference Study, *Acta Pædiatrica, 450*(Suppl.), 56–65.

Young, T. K., Martens, P. J., Taback, S. P., et al. (2002). Type 2 diabetes mellitus in children. *Archives of Pediatric and Adolescent Medicine, 156*, 651–655.

Zheng, T., Holford, T. R., Mayne, S. T., Owens, P. H., Zhang, Y., Zhang, B., et al. (2001). Lactation and breast cancer risk: A case-control study in Connecticut. *British Journal of Cancer, 84*, 1472–1476.

Ziegler, A., Schmid, S., Huber, D., et al. (2003). Early infant feeding and the risk of developing type 1 diabetes associated antibodies. *Journal of the American Medical Association, 290*, 1721–1728.

Suggested Reading

Andrew, N., & Harvey, K. (2011). Infant feeding choices: Experience, self-identity and lifestyle. *Maternal and Child Nutrition, 7*(1), 48–60.

Archabald, K., Lundsberg, L., Triche, E., Norwitz, E., & Illuzzi, J. (2011). Women's prenatal concerns regarding breastfeeding: Are they being addressed? *Journal of Midwifery and Women's Health, 56*(1), 2–7.

Blyth, R., Creedy, D. K., Dennis, C. L., Moyle, W., Pratt, J., & DeVries, S. M. (2002). Effect of maternal confidence on breastfeeding duration: An application of breastfeeding self-efficacy theory. *Birth, 29*(4), 278–284.

Clifford, J., & McIntyre, E. (2008). Who supports breastfeeding? *Breastfeeding Review, 16*(2), 9–19.

Craig, H. J., & Dietsch, E. (2010). "Too scary to think about": First time mothers' perceptions of the usefulness of antenatal breastfeeding education. *Women and Birth, 23*(4), 160–165.

Declercq, E., Labbok, M. H., Sakala, C., & O'Hara, M. (2009). Hospital practices and women's likelihood of fulfilling their intention to exclusively breastfeed. *American Journal of Public Health, 99*(5), 929–935.

Hauck, Y. L., Fenwick, J., Dhallwal, S. S., Butt, J., & Schmied, V. (2011). The association between women's perceptions of professional support and problems experienced on breastfeeding cessation: A western Australian study. *Journal of Human Lactation, 27*(1), 49–57.

Mickens, A. D., Modeste, N., Montgomery, S., & Taylor, M. (2009). Peer support and breastfeeding intentions among black WIC participants. *Journal of Human Lactation, 25*(2), 157–162.

CHAPTER 25
Lactational Pharmacology

Thomas W. Hale, RPh, PhD, and Frank J. Nice, RPh, DPA, CPHP

OBJECTIVES

- Determine the need for medication.
- Minimize infant drug exposure.
- Describe the entry of medications into human milk.
- Evaluate the breastfeeding infant.
- Evaluate use of prescription, over-the counter, and herbal medications.

INTRODUCTION

Safely using medications in breastfeeding mothers requires a certain basic knowledge of how drugs enter breastmilk, which drugs are of potential risk, and factors that might increase or decrease the infant's sensitivity to the medication. The amount of drug entering breastmilk is largely determined by its maternal plasma kinetics, protein binding, lipid solubility, molecular mass, and other factors. The use of these kinetic parameters makes determining the risks of medications much less difficult, particularly with newer medications. Although there are many exceptions, in general, less than 1% of the maternal dose ultimately finds its way into the milk (and subsequently, to the baby). Also, the infant's daily dose (from ingested breastmilk), adjusted for the infant's weight, can be compared to the mother's weight-adjusted daily dose (relative infant dose = RID). If the infant's weight-adjusted dose is less than 10% of the mother's, the drug is generally considered safe for the infant.

I. Determine the Need for Medication

A. Withhold the drug.
   1. Avoid the use of nonessential medications by enlisting the mother's cooperation. If you don't need it, don't use it.
   2. Some medications are only minimally effective and might not be necessary.
   3. If a medication is not efficacious, then its use might not be advisable.
   4. Some medications such as herbals, dietary supplements, and megadoses of vitamins are not really necessary; thus, their risks might outweigh the benefits of their use.

B. Try nondrug therapies.
1. Instead of analgesics: Relaxation techniques, massage, warm baths
2. Instead of cough, cold, or allergy products: Saline nose drops, cool mist, steam
3. Instead of antiasthmatics: Avoid known allergens, particularly animals
4. Instead of antacids: Eat small meals, sleep with head propped, avoid head-bending activities, avoid gas-forming foods
5. Instead of laxatives: Eat high-fiber cereal, prunes; drink hot liquids with breakfast and more water throughout the day
6. Instead of antidiarrheals: Discontinue solid foods for 12 to 24 hours, and increase fluid intake; eat toast/saltine crackers
C. Delay therapy.
1. Mothers who are ready to wean the infant might be able to delay elective drug therapy or elective surgery.
2. Mothers could wait several months before undergoing therapy, such as for a toenail fungus, or a cosmetic surgical procedure.
3. This does not mean delaying therapy for depression or mania or other serious diseases. The mother's health always takes precedence.

II. Minimize Infant Drug Exposure

A. Choose drugs that pass poorly into milk.
1. Within some drug classes, there are large differences among class members in drug distribution into milk.
B. Choose more breastfeeding-compatible dosage forms.
1. Take the lowest recommended dose, avoid extra-strength and long-acting preparations, avoid combination ingredient products.
C. Choose an alternative route of administration.
1. Local application of drugs to the affected maternal site can minimize drug concentrations in milk and subsequently the infant's dose.
D. Avoid breastfeeding at times of peak drug concentrations in milk.
1. Breastfeeding before a dose is given might avoid the peak drug concentrations in milk that occur approximately 1 to 3 hours after an oral dose.
2. This works only for drugs with short half-lives.
3. This will not work well for antidepressants and anticonvulsants because they have long half-lives.
4. Assume prolonged-release products are long-half-life products.
E. E. Administer the drug before the infant's longest sleep period.
1. This minimizes the infant's dose and is useful for long-acting drugs that can be given once daily.
2. Again, this works only for short-half-life products or those administered only occasionally. A short half-life is a few hours.

F. Temporarily withhold breastfeeding.
   1. Depending on the estimated length of drug therapy, nursing can be temporarily withheld.
   2. Mothers might be able to express a sufficient quantity of milk beforehand for use during therapy. The pharmacokinetics of the drug must be examined to determine when the resumption of breastfeeding is advisable.
   3. Mothers must express milk regularly during therapy to maintain milk production.
G. Discontinue breastfeeding.
   A few drugs are simply too toxic to allow breastfeeding to continue.

III. Maternal Factors That Affect Drug Transfer

A. Dose of medication
   1. Determine the postpartum interval. If the mother is 2–4 days postpartum, the dose the infant receives is minimal because the volume of colostrum is minimal (30–60 mL/day). If the mother is 12 or more months postpartum, her volume of milk is generally lower, and hence the dose of the drug is lower. Also the infant's metabolism becomes highly functional at 9–12 months and infants can handle small loads of drugs via milk.
   2. Is the dose of the medication greater or lesser than the normal range? If excessively high, use caution in recommending breastfeeding.
   3. How is the plasma level of the medication changed by the dose used in the mother? (For example, if a mother is using 25,000 units of vitamin A, that is significantly more risky than a 5,000-unit dose.)
   4. Is the medication formulation a rapid or sustained-release product?
      a. How does this medication change the mother's plasma levels and the risk to the infant?
      b. Sustained-release drugs should be considered as if they are long-half-life drugs.
   5. When is the medication dosed, and how does the dosing interval affect plasma levels and milk levels?
      a. If a mother takes a medication at night and does not breastfeed until the morning, this situation is significantly different from when she breastfeeds every 2 hours.
   6. Is the dose of medication absorbed orally by the mother?
      a. Thus, what are her plasma levels? Are they high or really low?
      b. Plasma levels are generally in equilibrium with the milk at all times.
      c. Higher plasma levels generally mean higher milk levels.
   7. Most asthma medications are used via inhalation; thus, maternal plasma levels of the medication are virtually nil and are not likely to produce milk levels at all.
   8. Plasma levels of most topical and ophthalmic preparations are virtually nil and are not likely to produce milk levels at all.

IV. Entry of Drugs into Human Milk

   A. The amount of drug excreted into milk depends on a number of factors.
      1. The lipid solubility of the drug.
      2. The acid dissociation constant of the drug, more commonly called the pKa, determines how polar the drug is as a function of pH and how well it can exit the milk compartment.
      3. The molecular size of the drug.
      4. The blood level attained in the maternal circulation.
      5. The maternal volume of distribution of the drug.
      6. Protein binding in the maternal circulation.
      7. Oral bioavailability in the infant and mother.
      8. The half-life in the maternal and infant plasma compartments.
   B. Although this description is somewhat simplistic for a sophisticated and somewhat obscure system, these pharmacokinetic terms provide a reasonably complete system for evaluating drug penetration into milk and the degree of exposure of the infant.

V. Drug Entry into the Milk Compartment

   A. Drugs enter the breastmilk primarily by diffusion driven by equilibrium forces between the maternal plasma compartment and the maternal milk compartment.
      1. Medications enter the milk by transferring from the maternal plasma, through the capillary walls, past the alveolar epithelium, and into the milk compartment.
      2. During the first 4 days postpartum, large gaps exist between alveolar cells.
      3. These gaps might permit enhanced drug entry into human milk during the colostral period, but the absolute amount of the drug in the milk might still be quite low (see **Figure 25-1**).

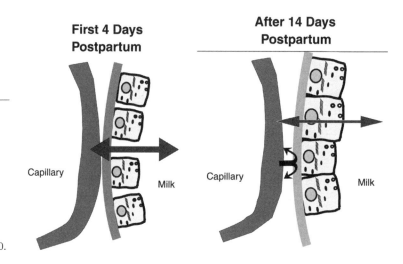

Figure 25-1

Alveolar cell gaps during the colostral phase and 4 days postpartum.

Source: Courtesy Thomas Hale, *Medications and Mothers' Milk*, 2010.

4. After 4 to 6 days, the alveolar cells enlarge—shutting off many of the intercellular gaps—and the amount of drug entry into the milk is reduced.

5. Because the alveolar epithelium has rather tight junctions, most drugs must dissolve through the bilayer membranes of the alveolar cells before they can enter milk.

6. Dissolving through the bilayer lipid membranes is difficult for most medications, particularly for drugs that are ionic or polar.

7. The more lipid soluble a drug, the greater the capability of the drug to penetrate into the milk.

8. Drugs that are active in the central nervous system (CNS) generally attain higher levels in the milk compartment simply because their chemistry is ideal for entry.

9. Drugs in the maternal plasma compartment are in complete equilibrium with the milk compartment; there might be more or less in the milk compartment, but they are still in equilibrium.

10. Several drug pumping systems exist in the alveolar cells, one of which is most important.
    a. For example, iodine has a rather high milk/plasma ratio and is readily pumped into the milk compartment.
    b. Therefore, prolonged or high doses of iodine salts should be avoided. This includes oral intake of iodine, such as from seaweed and potassium iodide tablets, or the vaginal use of povidone iodide (Betadine).
    c. Any form of radioactive iodine (I-131, I-125, I-123) should be avoided while breastfeeding and can be extraordinarily dangerous to the breastfed infant.

11. Many electrolytes (such as sodium chloride, magnesium) are tightly controlled by the alveolar cell; even high maternal levels might not produce significant changes in milk-electrolyte composition.

B. Protein binding and its effect on drug levels in milk
   1. As a general rule, most drugs are transported in blood bound to plasma albumin, which is a large-molecular-weight protein that resides in the plasma.
   2. The more the drug is bound to plasma protein, the less that is free in the plasma compartment to enter into various other compartments, particularly the milk compartment.
   3. As the percentage of drug binding increases, the level of the drug in the milk decreases.
   4. Drugs that have high protein binding should be chosen to attempt to reduce milk levels.

C. Lipid solubility
   1. As a general rule, the more lipid soluble a drug, the higher the milk levels.
   2. The more polar or water soluble a drug, the less the milk levels will be.
   3. Although it is hard to determine the lipid solubility of most compounds, a good rule is that if the drug readily enters the brain compartment (CNS), then it is more likely to enter the milk.

4. A drug that is active in the brain should be more closely scrutinized than one that is not active. Examples of these types of drugs include those used to treat depression and epilepsy, psychotherapeutic drugs, and narcotic analgesics.

D. Half-life of the medication

1. Elimination half-life of the medication generally describes the time interval that is required after administration of the medication until one-half of the drug is eliminated from the body.

2. It is better to choose drugs that have shorter half-lives because the length of exposure of the infant to the medication (via milk) is generally reduced.

3. Milk levels during the day will generally be lower if the maternal peak is avoided by waiting several half-lives to breastfeed the infant.

4. Long-half-life drugs might have a tendency to build up in an infant.
   a. In many instances, the half-life of the medication might be much longer in a newborn infant than in the adult.

5. Prolonged exposure to long-half-life medications might lead to increasing plasma levels of the medication in the infant (refer to the drug fluoxetine [Prozac] as an example).

6. In essence, long-half-life medications really become a problem only if they are ingested by the mother over a long period because the infant builds up higher and higher plasma levels of the medications.
   a. Acute use of long-half-life medications is not typically a problem.

7. Long-half-life medications cannot always be avoided.
   a. In these instances, become aware of the clinical dose provided to the infant via milk.
   b. If this dose is still low, then accumulation is not as likely to occur in the infant.

8. A general guideline is that it takes approximately five half-lives before a drug is completely eliminated from the system.

E. Bioavailability

1. Bioavailability of a medication is a measure of how much medication reaches the plasma of that individual.

2. There are not a lot of studies of bioavailability of drugs in pediatric patients, but it is generally thought that bioavailability does not differ greatly from that of an adult.

3. Measured as a percentage, a drug that has 50% bioavailability generally means that only 50% of the medication administered actually reaches the plasma compartment of the mother or infant.

4. Drugs that have poor bioavailability fail to reach the plasma compartment for a variety of reasons.
   a. They are sequestered in the liver and cannot exit.
   b. They are destroyed in the gut (proteins, peptides, aminoglycosides, etc.).
   c. They are not absorbed in the small intestine (vancomycin).
   d. They are metabolized in the gut wall (domperidone).

5. The drug that has the lowest bioavailability should be chosen for breastfeeding mothers because it will greatly reduce the exposure of the infant to the medication.

F. Molecular size of the medication (mass is measured in Daltons [D])

1. In general, the larger the molecular size of the medication, the less likely it is to enter into the milk compartment.

a. Although most medications administered will reach the milk compartment, those with large molecular weights (>900 D) are virtually excluded from the milk compartment.

2. Drugs that have huge molecular sizes (25,000–200,000 D) are virtually excluded from milk in clinically relevant amounts.

3. Some commonly used drugs that have huge molecular sizes include heparin, insulin, interferons, and low-molecular-weight heparins.

G. Milk/plasma ratio

1. Scientifically, the milk/plasma ratio is a useful tool to evaluate the relative concentration of medication in the maternal plasma compared to the maternal milk compartment.

2. Drugs with high milk/plasma ratio enter milk easily, whereas drugs with low milk/plasma ratios are less attracted to the milk compartment.

a. Unless both levels (plasma and milk) are known in the specific patient, the milk/plasma ratio might not indicate the true risk of using the medication.

3. In the case where a medication has a high milk/plasma ratio, it might, or might not, be hazardous for the infant. For example, iodine has a very efficient pump (16- to 25-fold), and excessive levels of iodine can occur in breastmilk, thus endangering the infant. Ranitidine has a 6-fold pump, but because its plasma levels are so low, its absolute dose in milk is still quite low.

4. Unless a great deal is known about the maternal plasma level, the milk/plasma ratio might give the clinician the wrong impression.

5. The most realistic measure of exposure to medication is the relative infant dose (RID). The RID is the dose of medication (milligrams per kilogram per day) provided to the infant via milk divided by the maternal dose in milligrams per kilogram per day. This provides the clinician with a good estimate of the percentage of maternal dose that enters milk. If the RID is less than 10%, the drug is generally considered safe.

VI. Evaluating the Infant

A. Assume that the preterm infant is more susceptible to maternal drugs.

1. Although many medications are often used in these situations, increased attentiveness to the risks is warranted.

2. Using a medication in an 8-month-old infant is significantly less risky than with a preterm infant or even a full-term newborn.

B. Always ask about the health and well-being of the infant.

C. What medication(s) is the infant ingesting?
  1. Drug–drug interactions might occur between medications that the mother is ingesting and medications that the infant is ingesting.
D. Sedating medications should be avoided.
  1. These include diazepam-like drugs (such as Valium), barbiturates, and older antihistamines, particularly in infants who have apnea or who are susceptible to sudden infant death syndrome.
  2. However, their use in acute, one-time situations is significantly less problematic.
E. Over-the-counter (OTC) medications (see **Tables 25-1** and **25-2**):
  1. OTC medications and herbals are also drugs.
  2. Many mothers self-medicate without consulting a healthcare professional.
  3. Mothers should avoid medications that are labeled as extra strength, maximum strength, or long acting.
    a. Usually, the lowest possible dose is recommended and is marked or labeled as regular strength.
  4. Mothers should avoid (if possible) medications that contain a variety of ingredients
F. Minimizing the effect of maternal medication on the infant.
  1. Avoid the use of long-acting forms of medications; the infant might have difficulty excreting the medication because detoxification by an immature infant's liver is required.
  2. Doses can be scheduled so that the minimum amount of drug enters the milk; medications can be taken right before or right after a breastfeeding.
  3. Infants should be watched for unusual or adverse signs or symptoms, such as a change in feeding patterns, level of alertness, or sleeping patterns; fussiness; rash; and bowel changes.
  4. Drugs should be chosen that produce the lowest level in milk.
G. Radioactive drugs:
  1. Administration of any radiopharmaceutical will result in at least some excretion of radioactivity in milk.
    a. The amount and time course of excretion varies among radiopharmaceuticals.
    b. Interruption of breastfeeding depends on the total radioactivity present in milk, the drug's overall risk, and its radioactive half-life.
    c. The ideal method is to assay the breastmilk for radioactivity and resume breastfeeding when levels are safe. However, this is practically impossible in most instances.
    d. The most accurate evaluation of the risk and time to interrupt breastfeeding is provided by the U.S. Nuclear Regulatory Commission in Hale's (2010) *Medications and Mothers' Milk*.

Table 25-1 Common Over-the-Counter Medications

Analgesics

Acetaminophen 325 mg—Y

Acetaminophen 500 mg—N

Actron (ketoprofen)—Y

Advil (ibuprofen)—Y

Aleve (naproxen)—Y

Alka-Seltzer Effervescent Antacid and Pain Reliever (aspirin, sodium bicarbonate)—N

Anacin (aspirin, caffeine)—N

Anacin Maximum Strength (aspirin, caffeine)—N

Anacin-3 Regular Strength (acetaminophen)—Y

Anacin-3 Maximum Strength (acetaminophen)—N

Anodynos (aspirin, salicylamide, caffeine)—N

Arthritis Pain Formula (aspirin, aluminum-magnesium hydroxide)—N

Arthritis Foundation (ibuprofen)—Y

Arthritis Foundation Aspirin Free (acetaminophen)—N

Arthritis Foundation Nighttime (acetaminophen, diphenhydramine)—N

Arthritis Foundation Safety Coated Aspirin (aspirin)—N

Arthropan (choline salicylate)—N

Ascriptin Arthritis Pain (aspirin, aluminum-magnesium hydroxide, calcium carbonate)—N

Ascriptin Regular Strength (aspirin, aluminum-magnesium hydroxide, calcium carbonate)—N

Aspercin (aspirin)—N

Aspercin Extra (aspirin)—N

Aspergum (aspirin)—N

Aspermin (aspirin)—N

Aspirin 81 mg—N

Aspirin 325 mg—N

Aspirin 500 mg—N

Aspirin Free Pain Relief (acetaminophen)—Y

Azo-Diac (phenazopyridine)—Y

Azo-Standard (phenazopyridine)—Y

Backache Caplets (magnesium salicylate)—N

Back-Quell (aspirin, ephedrine sulfate, atropine sulfate)—N

Bayer Adult Low Strength (aspirin)—N

Bayer Arthritis Extra Strength (aspirin)—N

Bayer Aspirin (aspirin)—N

Bayer Aspirin Extra Strength (aspirin)—N

Bayer Regular Strength (aspirin)—N

Bayer Plus Extra Strength (aspirin)—N

Bayer PM Aspirin Plus Sleep Aid (aspirin, diphenhydramine)—N

BC Arthritis Strength (aspirin, salicylamide, caffeine)—N

BC Powder (aspirin, salicylamide, caffeine)—N

Bromo-Seltzer (acetaminophen, sodium bicarbonate, citric acid)—N

Bufferin Analgesic Tablets (aspirin)—N

Bufferin Arthritis Strength (aspirin)—N

Bufferin Extra-Strength (aspirin)—N

Cope (aspirin, caffeine, aluminum-magnesium hydroxide)—N

Datril Extra Strength Non-Aspirin (acetaminophen)—N

Doan's Extra Strength (magnesium salicylate)—N

Doan's PM Extra Strength (magnesium salicylate, diphenhydramine)—N

Doan's Regular Strength (magnesium salicylate)—N

Dynafed EX (acetaminophen)—N

Dynafed IB (ibuprofen)—Y

Dyspel (acetaminophen, ephedrine sulfate, atropine sulfate)—N

(continues)

Note: Y = usually safe when breastfeeding; Y* = usually safe when breastfeeding, monitor infant for drowsiness; Y** = usually safe when breastfeeding, monitor for decreased milk production, mother should drink extra fluids; Y*** = use of loperamide should not exceed two days; N = avoid when breastfeeding; N* = less than 150 mg two to three times a day has no apparent effect on breastfeeding infant. Probably better to drink a cup of coffee than to take the drug; X* = consultation with a physician is highly recommended prior to use.

Table 25-1 Common Over-the-Counter Medications (continued)

Analgesics (continued)

Ecotrin Low, Regular, or Maximum Strength (aspirin)—N

Emagrin (aspirin, caffeine, salicylamide)—N

Empirin Aspirin (aspirin)—N

Empirin Free (acetaminophen, caffeine)—N

Excedrin Aspirin Free (acetaminophen, caffeine)—N

Excedrin Extra Strength (acetaminophen, aspirin, caffeine)—N

Excedrin PM (acetaminophen, diphenhydramine)—N

Feverall Adult Strength Suppository (acetaminophen)—Y

Goody's Extra Strength (acetaminophen, aspirin, caffeine)—N

Goody's Extra Strength Headache (acetaminophen, aspirin, caffeine)—N

Haltran (ibuprofen)—Y

Healthprin Brand Aspirin (aspirin)—N

Heartline (aspirin)—N

Ibuprohm (ibuprofen)—Y

Legatrin (acetaminophen, diphenhydramine)—N

Midol IB Cramp Relief Formula (ibuprofen)—Y

Midol Menstrual Maximum Strength (acetaminophen, caffeine, pyrilamine)—N

Midol Menstrual Regular Strength Multisymptom Formula (acetaminophen, pyrilamine)—N

Midol PMS Maximum Strength (acetaminophen, pamabrom, pyrilamine)—N

Midol Teen Maximum Strength (acetaminophen, pamabrom)—N

Mobigesic (magnesium salicylate, phenyltoloxamine)—N

Momentum (magnesium salicylate)—N

Motrin IB (ibuprofen)—Y

Nuprin (ibuprofen)—Y

Orudis KT (ketoprofen)—Y

P-A-C (aspirin, caffeine)—N

Panadol Maximum Strength (acetaminophen)—N

Percogesic (acetaminophen, phenyltoloxamine)—N

Premsyn PMS (acetaminophen, pamabrom, pyrilamine)—N

Prodium (phenazopyridine)—Y

Re-Azo (phenazopyridine)—Y

St. Joseph Adult Aspirin (aspirin)—N

Stanback AF Extra Strength Powder (acetaminophen)—N

Stanback Original Formula Powder (aspirin, salicylamide, caffeine)—N

Supac (acetaminophen, aspirin, calcium gluconate, caffeine)—N

Tapanol Extra Strength (acetaminophen)—N

Tempra (acetaminophen)—Y

Tempra Quicklet (acetaminophen)—Y

Tylenol Arthritis Extended Relief (acetaminophen)—N

Tylenol Extra Strength (acetaminophen)—N

Tylenol PM (acetaminophen, diphenhydramine)—N

Tylenol Regular Strength (acetaminophen)—Y

Ultraprin (ibuprofen)—Y

Unisom with Pain Relief Nighttime (acetaminophen, diphenhydramine)—N

Uristat (phenazopyridine)—Y

UroFemme (phenazopyridine)—Y

Valorin (acetaminophen)—Y

Valorin Extra (acetaminophen)—N

Valorin Super (acetaminophen, caffeine)—N

Valprin (ibuprofen)—Y

Vanquish (aspirin, acetaminophen, caffeine, aluminum-magnesium hydroxide)—N

XS Hangover Relief (acetaminophen, calcium citrate, magnesium trisilicate, calcium carbonate, caffeine)—N

Cough, Cold, Allergy Preparations

Actifed (tripolidine, pseudoephedrine)—Y*, Y**

Actifed Allergy Daytime (pseudoephedrine)—Y**

Actifed Allergy Nighttime (pesudoephedrine, diphenhydramine)—Y**

Actifed Plus (acetaminophen, pseudoephedrine, tripolidine)—N

Actifed Sinus Daytime (acetaminophen, pseudoephedrine)—N

Actifed Sinus Nighttime (acetaminophen, pseudoephedrine, diphenhydramine)—N

Advil Cold and Sinus (ibuprofen, pseudoephedrine)—N

Alcomed 2-60 (dexbrompheniramine, pseudoephedrine)—Y*, Y**

Alka-Seltzer Plus Cold & Cough Medicine (aspirin, chlorpheniramine, phenylpropanolamine, dextromethorphan)—N

Alka-Seltzer Plus Cold & Cough Medicine Liqui-Gels (aspirin, chlorpheniramine, phenylpropanolamine, dextromethorphan)—N

Alka-Seltzer Plus Cold & Flu Medicine (acetaminophen, dextromethorphan, phenylpropanolamine, chlorpheniramine)—N

Alka-Seltzer Plus Cold & Flu Medicine Liqui-Gels (acetaminophen, dextromethorphan, phenylpropanolamine, chlorpheniramine)—N

Alka-Seltzer Plus Cold Medicine (aspirin, chlorpheniramine, pseudoephedrine, acetaminophen)—N

Alka-Seltzer Plus Cold Medicine Liqui-Gels (aspirin, chlorpheniramine, pseudoephedrine, acetaminophen)—N

Alka-Seltzer Plus Cold & Sinus Medicine (aspirin, phenylpropanolamine)—N

Alka-Seltzer Plus Cold & Sinus Medicine Liqui-Gels (pseudoephedrine, acetaminophen)—N

Alka-Seltzer Plus Night-Time Cold Medicine (aspirin, phenylpropanolamine)—N

Alka-Seltzer Plus Night-Time Cold Medicine Liqui-Gels (dextromethorphan, doxylamine, pseudoephedrine, acetaminophen)—N

Allerest Headache Strength (acetaminophen, chlorpheniramine, pseudoephedrine)—N

Allerest Maximum Strength (chlorpheniramine, pseudoephedrine)—Y*, Y**

Allerest No Drowsiness (acetaminophen, pseudoephedrine)—N

Allerest Sinus Pain Formula (acetaminophen, pseudoephedrine)—N

Allerest 12 Hour (chlorpheniramine, phenylpropanolamine)—N

Bayer Select Sinus Pain Relief Formula (acetaminophen, pseudoephedrine)—N

BC Allergy Sinus Cold Powder (aspirin, phenylpropanolamine, chlorpheniramine)—N

BC Sinus Cold Powder (aspirin, phenylpropanolamine)—N

Benadryl Allergy/Congestion (diphenhydramine, pseudoephedrine)—Y*, Y**

Benadryl Allergy/Cold (diphenhydramine, pseudoephedrine, acetaminophen)—N

Benadryl Allergy Liquid or Dye-Free Liquid (diphenhydramine)—Y*

Benadryl Allergy Sinus Headache Caplets & Gelcaps (diphenhydramine, pseudoephedrine, acetaminophen)—N

Benadryl Allergy Ultratab Tablets, Ultratab Kapseals, Chewables, or Dye-Free Liqui-Gels (diphenhydramine)—Y*

Benylin Adult Formula (dextromethorphan)—Y*

Denylin Cough Syrup (diphenhydramine)—Y*

Benylin Expectorant (dextromethorphan, guaifenesin)—Y*

Benylin Multisymptom (guaifenesin, pseudoephedrine, dextromethorphan)—N

Buckley's Mixture (dextromethorphan, ammonium carbonate, camphor, balsam, glycerin, menthol, pine needle oil)—N

Cerose DM (dextromethorphan, chlorpheniramine, phenylephrine, alcohol 2.4%)—N

Cheracol-D (dextromethorphan, guaifenesin)—Y*

Cheracol Plus (phenylpropanolamine, dextromethorphan, chlorpheniramine)—N

Cheracol Sinus (dexbrompheniramine, pseudoephedrine)—N

Chlor-Trimeton 4-Hour Allergy (chlorpheniramine)—Y*

Chlor-Trimeton 4-Hour Allergy/ Decongestant (chlorpheniramine, pseudoephedrine)—Y*, Y**

(continues)

Table 25-1 Common Over-the-Counter Medications (continued)

Cough, Cold, Allergy Preparations (continued)

Chlor-Trimeton 8- and 12-Hour Allergy (chlorpheniramine)—N

Chlor-Trimeton 12-Hour Allergy/Decongestant (chlorpheniramine, pseudoephedrine)—N

CoADVIL (ibuprofen, pseudoephedrine)—N

COMTREX Deep Chest Cold and Congestion Relief (acetaminophen, guaifenesin, phenyl-propanolamine, dextromethorphan)—N

COMTREX Maximum Strength Multi-Symptom Acute Head Cold & Sinus Pressure Relief (acetaminophen, brompheniramine, pseudoephedrine)—N

COMTREX Maximum Strength Multi-Symptom Cold & Cough Relief Caplet or Tablet (acetaminophen, pseudoephedrine, chlorpheniramine, dextromethorphan)—N

COMTREX Maximum Strength Multi-Symptom Cold & Cough Relief Liquid (acetaminophen, pseudoephedrine, chlorpheniramine, dextromethorphan)—N

COMTREX Maximum Strength Multi-Symptom Cold & Cough Relief Liqui-Gels (acetaminophen, phenylpropanolamine, chlorpheniramine, dextromethorphan)—N

Contac Severe Cold & Flu (phenylpropanolamine, chlorpheniramine, acetaminophen, dextromethorphan)—N

Contac 12-Hour Caplets (phenylpropanolamine, chlorpheniramine)—N

Contac 12-Hour Capsules (phenylpropanolamine, chlorpheniramine)—N

Coricidin D Decongestant (acetaminophen, chlorpheniramine, phenylpropanolamine)—N

Coricidin HBP Cold & Flu (acetaminophen, chlorpheniramine)—N

Coricidin HBP Cough & Cold (chlorpheniramine, dextromethorphan)—N

Coricidin HBP Nighttime Cold & Cough Liquid (acetaminophen, diphenhydramine)—N

Delsym Cough Formula (dextromethorphan)—N

Dimetapp Cold & Allergy Chewable Tablets or Quick Dissolving Tablets (brompheniramine, phenylpropanolamine)—N

Dimetapp Cold & Cough Liqui-Gels (brompheniramine, phenylpropanolamine, dextromethorphan)—N

Dimetapp Cold and Fever Suspension (acetaminophen, pseudoephedrine, brompheniramine)—N

Dimetapp DM Elixir (brompheniramine, phenyl-propanolamine, dextromethorphan)—N

Dimetapp Elixir (brompheniramine, phenylpropanolamine)—N

Dimetapp Extentabs (brompheniramine, phenylpropanolamine)—N

Dimetapp Tablets and Liqui-Gels (brompheniramine, phenylpropanolamine)—N

Dristan (phenylephrine, chlorpheniramine, acetaminophen)—N

Dristan Maximum Strength (pseudoephedrine, acetaminophen)—N

Drixoral Allergy/Sinus (pseudoephedrine, dexbrompheniramine, acetaminophen)—N

Drixoral Cold & Allergy (pseudoephedrine, dexbrompheniramine)—N

Drixoral Cold & Flu (acetaminophen, dexbrompheniramine, pseudoephedrine)—N

Drixoral Nasal Decongestant (pseudoephedrine)—N

Efidac-24 (pseudoephedrine)—N

Expressin 400 (guaifenesin, pseudoephedrine)—Y**

4-Way Cold Tablets (acetaminophen, phenylpropanolamine, chlorpheniramine)—N

Guaifed (guaifenesin, pseudoephedrine)—Y**

Guaitab (guaifenesin, pseudoephedrine)—Y**

Hyland's Cough Syrup with Honey (ipecac, potassium antimony tartrate)—N

Hyland's C-Plus Cold Tablets (herbs, potassium iodide)—N

Isoclor Timesule (chlorpheniramine, phenylpropanolamine)—N

Isohist 2.0 (dexbrompheniramine)—Y*

Motrin IB Sinus Pain Reliever (ibuprofen, pseudoephedrine)—N

Nasalcrom A Tablets (chlorpheniramine)—Y*

Nasalcrom CA Caplets (pseudoephedrine, acetaminophen)—N

Novahistine (chlorpheniramine, phenylephrine)—Y*, Y**

Novahistine-DMX (dextromethorphan, guaifenesin, pseudoephedrine)—N

Oscillococcinum Pellets (herbs)—N

Pertussin DM Extra Strength (dextromethorphan)—N

Pyrroxate (chlorpheniramine, phenylpropanolamine, acetaminophen)—N

Robitussin (guaifenesin)—Y

Robitussin-CF (guaifenesin, phenylpropanolamine, dextromethorphan)—N

Robitussin-DM (guaifenesin, dextromethorphan)—Y*

Robitussin-PE (guaifenesin, pseudoephedrine)—Y**

Robitussin Cold—Cold, Cough, & Flu Liqui-Gels (acetaminophen, guaifenesin, pseudoephedrine, dextromethorphan)—N

Robitussin Cold—Night-Time Liqui-Gels (acetaminophen, pseudoephedrine, dextromethorphan)—N

Robitussin Cold—Severe Congestion Liqui-Gels (guaifenesin, pseudoephedrine)—Y**

Ryna Liquid (chlorpheniramine, pseudoephedrine)—Y*, Y**

Ryna-C Liquid (codeine)—N

Ryna-CX Liquid (codeine, pseudoephedrine, guaifenesin)—N

Scot-Tussin DM (dextromethorphan, chlorpheniramine)—N

Scot-Tussin Expectorant (guaifenesin)—Y

Scot-Tussin Sugar Free, Alcohol Free Expectorant (guaifenesin)—Y

Scot-Tussin Sugar-Free Allergy Relief Formula (diphenhydramine)—Y*

Scot-Tussin Sugar-Free DM (dextromethorphan, chlorpheniramine)—N

Sinarest No Drowsiness (acetaminophen, pseudoephedrine)—N

Sinarest Regular and Extra Strength (acetaminophen, chlorpheniramine, phenylpropanolamine)—N

Sine-Aid Maximum Strength Sinus Medication (acetaminophen, pseudoephedrine)—N

Sine-Off No Drowsiness Formula (acetaminophen, pseudoephedrine)—N

Sine-Off Sinus Medicine (chlorpheniramine, pseudoephedrine, acetaminophen)—N

Singlet (pseudoephedrine, chlorpheniramine, acetaminophen)—N

Sinutab Non-Drying Liquid Caps (pseudoephedrine, guaifenesin)—Y**

Sinutab Sinus Allergy Medication Maximum Strength (acetaminophen, chlorpheniramine, pseudoephedrine)—N

Sudafed Cold & Allergy Tablets (chlorpheniramine, pseudoephedrine)—Y*, Y**

Sudafed Cold & Cough Liquid Caps (acetaminophen, guaifenesin, pseudoephedrine, dextromethorphan)—N

Sudafed Cold & Sinus Liquid Caps (acetaminophen, pseudoephedrine)—N

Sudafed Nasal Decongestant (pseudoephedrine)—Y**

Sudafed Non-Drying Sinus Liquid Caps (guaifenesin, pseudoephedrine)—Y**

Sudafed Severe Cold Formula (acetaminophen, pseudoephedrine, dextromethorphan)—N

Sudafed Sinus (acetaminophen, pseudoephedrine)—N

Sudafed 12-Hour Tablets (pseudoephedrine)—N

Sudafed 24-Hour Tablets (pseudoephedrine)—N

Suppressin DM (dextromethorphan, guaifenesin)—Y*

TAVIST Allergy Tablets (clemastine)—Y*

TAVIST-D Caplets or Tablets (clemastine, phenylpropanolamine)—N

TAVIST Sinus Caplets or Gelcaps (acetaminophen, pseudoephedrine)—N

Theraflu Flu and Cold Medicine (acetaminophen, pseudoephedrine, chlorpheniramine)—N

Theraflu Maximum Strength Flu, Cold and Cough Medicine (acetaminophen, dextromethorphan, pseudoephedrine, chlorpheniramine)—N

Theraflu Maximum Strength Flu and Cold Medicine (acetaminophen, pseudoephedrine, chlorpheniramine)—N

(continues)

Table 25-1 Common Over-the-Counter Medications (continued)

Cough, Cold, Allergy Preparations (continued)

Theraflu Maximum Strength Nighttime (acetaminophen, pseudoephedrine, chlorpheniramine)—N

Theraflu Maximum Strength Non-Drowsy (acetaminophen, pseudoephedrine, dextromethorphan)—N

Triaminic AM Cough and Decongestant (pseudo-ephedrine, dextromethorphan)—N

Triaminic AM Decongestant (pseudoephedrine)—Y*

Triaminic Cold & Allergy Softchews (pseu-doephedrine, dextromethorpham, chlorpheniramine)—Y*, Y**

Triaminic Cold & Cough Softchews (pseu-doephedrine, dextromethorphan, chlorpheniramine)—N

Triaminic DM Syrup (phenylpropanolamine, dextromethorphan)—N

Triaminic Expectorant (guaifenesin, phenylpropanolamine)—N

Triaminic Night Time (pseudoephedrine, dextro-methorphan, chlorpheniramine)—N

Triaminic Severe Cold & Fever (acetamino-phen, pseudoephedrine, dextromethorphan, chlorpheniramine)—N

Triaminic Sore Throat (acetaminophen, dextromethorphan)—N

Triaminic Syrup (phenylpropanolamine, chlorpheniramine)—N

Triaminic Throat Pain & Cough Softch-ews (acetaminophen, pseudoephedrine, dextromethorphan)—N

Triaminicin Tablets (acetaminophen, phenylpro-panolamine, chlorpheniramine)—N

Triaminicol Cold & Cough (phenylpropanolamine, dextromethorphan, chlorpheniramine)—N

Tylenol Allergy Sinus Maximum Strength (acetaminophen, chlorpheniramine, pseudoephedrine)—N

Tylenol Allergy Sinus NightTime Maximum Strength (acetaminophen, pseudoephedrine, diphenhydramine)—N

Tylenol Cold Medication Multi-Symptom Formula (acetaminophen, chlorpheniramine, pseudoephedrine, dextromethorphan)—N

Tylenol Cold Medication No Drowsiness Formula (acetaminophen, pseudoephedrine, dextromethorphan)—N

Tylenol Cold Multi-Symptom Severe Congestion (acetaminophen, dextromethorphan, guaifen-esin, pseudoephedrine)—N

Tylenol Flu NightTime Maximum Strength Gelcap (acetaminophen, diphenhydramine, pseudoephedrine)—N

Tylenol Flu NightTime Maximum Strength Hot Medication (acetaminophen, diphenhydr-amine, pseudoephedrine)—N

Tylenol Flu NightTime Maximum Strength Liquid (acetaminophen, dextromethorphan, doxyl-amine, pseudoephedrine)—N

Tylenol Severe Allergy (acetaminophen, diphenhydramine)—N

Tylenol Sinus Maximum Strength (acetamino-phen, pseudoephedrine)—N

Tylenol Sinus NightTime Maximum Strength (acetaminophen, doxylamine, pseudoephedrine)—N

Ursinus (pseudoephedrine, aspirin)—N

Vicks DayQuil LiquiCaps, Liquid (pseudoephed-rine, acetaminophen, dextromethorphan)—N

Vicks DayQuil Sinus Pressure & Pain Relief (ibuprofen, pseudoephedrine)—N

Vicks 44 Cough Relief (dextromethorphan, alcohol 5%)—Y*

Vicks 44D Cough & Head Congestion Relief (dex-tromethorphan, pseudoephedrine, alcohol 5%)—N

Vicks 44E Cough & Chest Congestion Relief (dextromethorphan, guaifenesin, alcohol 5%)—Y*

Vicks 44M Cough, Cold & Flu Relief (dextro-methorphan, pseudoephedrine, chlorphenira-mine, acetaminophen, alcohol 10%)—N

Vicks NyQuil Liquid (doxylamine, destrometho-rphan, acetaminophen, pseudoephedrine, alcohol 10%)—N

Cough and Cold Lozenges and Sprays

Celestial Seasonings Soothers Herbal Throat Drops (menthol, pectin)—Y

Cepacol Maximum Strength Sore Throat Lozenges (menthol, cetylpyridinium, benzocaine)—Y

Cepacol Maximum Strength Sore Throat Spray (dyclonine, cetylpyridinium)—Y

Cepacol Regular Strength Sore Throat Lozenges (menthol, cetylpyridinium)—Y

Cepastat Cherry Lozenges (phenol, menthol)—N

Cepastat Extra Strength Lozenges (phenol, menthol eucalyptus oil)—N

Cepastat Lozenges (phenol)—N

Cheracol Sore Throat Spray (phenol)—N

Halls Mentho-Lyptus Drops (menthol)—Y

Halls Plus Cough Suppressant Drops (menthol, pectin)—Y

HOLD Lozenges (dextromethorphan)—Y*

Listerine Lozenges (hexylresorcinol)—N

N'ICE Lozenges (menthol)—Y

Robitussin Cough Drops (menthol, pectin, eucalyptus)—Y

Scot-Tussin Sugar-Free Cough Chasers (dextromethorphan)—Y*

Sucrets 4-Hour Cough Suppressant Lozenges (menthol, dextromethorphan)—Y*

Sucrets Maximum Strength lozenges (dyclonine)—Y

Sucrets Regular Strength (hexylresorcinol)—N

Sucrets Regular Strength Vapor (dyclonine)—Y

Vicks Chloraseptic Lozenges (benzocaine, menthol)—Y

Vicks Cough Drops (menthol)—Y

Nasal Preparations

Afrin Allergy Spray (phenylephrine)—Y**

Afrin Extra Moisturizing Spray (oxymetazoline)—Y**

Afrin Moisturizing Saline Mist (sodium chloride)—Y

Afrin Original Spray, Nose Drops and Pump Mist (soxymetazoline)—Y**

Afrin Saline Mist with Eucalyptol and Menthol (Sodium chloride)—Y

Afrin Severe Congestion Spray (oxymetazoline)—Y**

Afrin Sinus Nasal Spray (oxymetazoline)—Y**

Alconefrin (phenylephrine)—Y**

AYR Saline Mist and Drops (sodium chloride)—Y

Benzedres Inhaler (propylhedrine)—N

Cheracol Spray (oxymetazoline)—Y**

Dristan Long Lasting Spray (oxymetazoline)—Y**

Dristan Spray (phenylephrine, pheniramine)—N

Duration 12-Hour Spray (oxymetazoline)—Y**

4-Way Fast Acting Nasal Spray (phenylephrine)—Y**

4-Way Long Acting Spray (oxymetazoline)—Y**

4-Way Saline Moisturizing Mist (sodium chloride)—Y

HuMIST Saline (sodium chloride)—Y

Little Noses Saline (sodium chloride)—Y

Nasalcrom Nasal Spray (cromolyn sodium)—Y

Nasal Moist Gel (aloe vera)—Y

Nasal Moist Solution (sodium chloride)—Y

Neo-Synephrine Drops (phenylephrine)—Y**

Neo-Synephrine Extra Strength Drops (phenylephrine)—Y**

Neo-Synephrine Mild, Regular, and Extra Strength Spray (phenylephrine)—Y**

Neo-Synephrine 12-Hour Extra Moisturizing Spray (oxymetazoline)—Y**

Neo-Synephrine 12-Hour Spray (oxymetazoline)—Y**

Nose Better Natural Mist (glycerin, sodium chloride)—Y

Nostril Nasal Decongestant (phenylephrine)—Y**

NTZ Spray and Drops (oxymetazoline)—Y**

(continues)

Table 25-1 Common Over-the-Counter Medications (continued)

Nasal Preparations (continued)

Ocean Nasal Mist (sodium chloride)—Y

Otrivin Nasal Drops and Spray (xylometazoline)—N

Pretz (glycerin)—Y

Priviner Nasal Spray and Solution (naphazoline)—N

St. Joseph Nasal Decongestant (phenylephrine)—Y**

Salinex Nasal Mist and Drops (sodium chloride)—Y

Vicks Sinex Nasal Spray and Ultra Fine Mist (phenylephrine, camphor, eucalyptol, menthol)—N

Vicks Vapor Inhaler (leumetamfetamine, menthol, camphor)—N

Asthma Preparations

Asthmahaler (epinephrine)—x

Asthmanephrin (racepinephrine)—x

Bronkaid Caplets (ephedrine, guaifenesin, theophylline)—x

Bronkaid Mist (epinephrine)—x

Bronkoelixir (ephedrine, guaifenesin, theophylline, phenobarbital)—x

Primatene Mist (epinephrine)—x

Antacids and Digestive Aids

Alka-Mints (calcium carbonate)—Y

Alka-Seltzer (aspirin, sodium bicarbonate)—N

Alka-Seltzer Extra Strength (aspirin, sodium bicarbonate)—N

Alka-Seltzer Gas Relief (simethicone)—Y

Alka-Seltzer Gold (sodium, potassium bicarbonate)—N

Alkets/Alkets Extra Strengh (calcium carbonate)—Y

Almora (magnesium gluconate)—Y

AlternaGEL (aluminum hydroxide)—Y

Alu-Cap (aluminum hydroxide)—Y

Aludrox (aluminum-magnesium hydroxide)—Y

Alu-Tab (aluminum hydroxide)—Y

Amitone (calcium carbonate)—Y

Amphogel (aluminum hydroxide)—Y

Axid AR (nizatidine)—Y

Basaljel (aluminum carbonate)—Y

Beano (enzymes, sorbitol)—Y

BeSure (food enzymes)—Y

Chooz Antacid Gum (calcium carbonate)—Y

Citrocarbonate (sodium bicarbonate-citrate)—N

Creamalin (aluminum-magnesium hydroxide)—Y

Dairy Ease (lactase)—Y

DDS-Acidophilus (lactobacillus acidophilus)—Y

Dicarbosil (calcium carbonate)

DiGel (simethicone, calcium carbonate, magnesium hydroxide)—Y

Eno (sodium tartrate-citrate)—N

Gas-X (simethicone)—Y

Gas-X Extra Strength (simethicone)—Y

Gaviscon Extra Strength (aluminum hydroxide, magnesium carbonate)—Y

Gaviscon Regular Strength Liquid (aluminum hydroxide, magnesium carbonate)—Y

Gaviscon Regular Strength Tablets (aluminum hydroxide, magnesium trisilicate)—Y

Gaviscon-2 (aluminum hydroxide, magnesium trisilicate, sodium bicarbonate)—N

Gelusil (aluminum-magnesium hydroxide, simethicone)—Y

Kudrox (simethicone, aluminum-magnesium hydroxide)—Y

Lactaid Original, Extra Strength, and Ultra (lactase)—Y

Lactinex (lactobacillus culture)—Y

Lactrase (lactase)—Y

Maalox Anti-Gas (simethicone)—Y

Maalox Anti-Gas Extra Strength (simethicone)—Y

Antacids and Digestive Aids (continued)

Maalox Heartburn Relief (aluminum hydroxide, magnesium-calcium carbonate, potassium bicarbonate)—N

Maalox Magnesia and Alumina Oral Susp. (magnesium-aluminum hydroxide)—Y

Maalox Maximum Strength (magnesium-aluminum hydroxide, simethicone)—Y

Maalox Quick Dissolve Tablets (calcium carbonate)—Y

Marblen (magnesium-calcium carbonate)—Y

Mylanta AR (famotidine)—Y

Mylanta Fast-Acting (aluminum-magnesium hydroxide, simethicone)—Y

Mylanta Maximum Strength (aluminum-magnesium hydroxide, simethicone)—Y

Mylanta Supreme (calcium carbonate, magnesium hydroxide)—Y

Mylanta Tablets and Gelcaps (calcium carbonate, magnesium hydroxide)—Y

Nephrox (aluminum hydroxide)—Y

Pepcid AC (famotidine)—Y

Pepto-Bismol Original (bismuth subsalicylate)—N

Pepto-Bismol Maximum Strength (bismuth subsalicylate)—N

Phazyme-125 Softgels (simethicone)—Y

Phazyme-166 Maximum Strength (simethicone)—Y

Phillips Milk of Magnesia (magnesium hydroxide)—Y

Riopan (magaldrate)—Y

Riopan Plus (magaldrate, simethicone)—Y

Riopan Plus 2 (magaldrate, simethicone)—Y

Rolaids (calcium carbonate, magnesium hydroxide)—Y

Sodium Bicarbonate (sodium bicarbonate)—N

Tagamet HB (cimetidine)—Y

Tempo (calcium carbonate, aluminum-magnesium hydroxide)—Y

Titralac (calcium carbonate)—Y

Titralac Extra Strength (calcium carbonate)—Y

Titralac Plus Antacid (calcium carbonate, simethicone)—Y

Tums E-X Antacid (calcium carbonate)—Y

Tums Regular (calcium carbonate)—Y

Tums ULTRA Antacid (calcium carbonate)—Y

Zantac 75 (ranitidine)—Y

Laxatives, Stool Softeners

Bisacodyl—N

Cascara Sagrada—Y

Ceo-Two Evacuant Suppository (sodium bicarbonate, potassium bitartrate)—Y

Citrucel (methylcellulose)—Y

Colace (docusate)—Y

Correctol Laxative (bisacodyl)—N

Correctol Stool Softener (docusate)—Y

Dialose (docusate)—Y

Doxidan (casanthranol, docusate)—N

Dulcolax Tablets and Suppositories (bisacodyl)—N

Effer-Syllium (psyllium)—Y

Emulsoil (caster oil)—N

Epsom Salt (magnesium sulfate)—Y

Evac-Q-Kwik (bisacodyl)—N

Ex-Lax Chocolate or Regular (sennosides)—Y

Ex-Lax Maximum (sennosides)—N

Fiberall (psyllium)—Y

Fibercon (calcium polycarbophil)—Y

Fiber Naturale (methylcellulose)—Y

Fleet Enema Regular (sodium biphosphate, phosphate)—Y

Fleet Laxative (bisacodyl)—N

Garfield's Tea (senna)—Y

Gentlax S (senna concentrate, docusate)—N

Gentle Nature (sennosides)—Y

Glycerin Suppositories—Y

Haley's M-O (magnesium hydroxide, mineral oil)—N

Herb-Lax (senna)—Y

Hydrocil (psyllium)—Y

(continues)

Table 25-1 Common Over-the-Counter Medications (continued)

Laxatives, Stool Softeners (continued)

Innerclean Herbal (senna, psyllium)—N

Kellogg's Tasteless Castor Oil (castor oil)—N

Kondremul (mineral oil)—N

Konsyl Fiber (polycarbophil)—Y

Konsyl Powder (psyllium)—Y

Maalox Daily Fiber (psyllium)—Y

Maltsupex (barley malt extract)—Y

Metamucil (psyllium)—Y

Milkinol (mineral oil)—N

Mitrolan (polycarbophil)—Y

Mylanta Natural Fiber Supplement (psyllium)—Y

Nature's Remedy Tablets (cascara sagrada, aloe)—N

Neoloid (castor oil)—N

Perdiem Fiber (psyllium)—Y

Perdiem Overnight Relief (psyllium, senna)—N

Peri-Colace (casanthranol, docusate)—N

Phillips Gelcaps (docusate)—Y

Phillips Milk of Magnesia (magnesium hydroxide)—Y

Phospho-Soda (sodium phosphate)—Y

Purge Concentrate (castor oil)—N

Regulace (casanthranol, docusate)—N

Regulax SS (docusate)—Y

Regutol (docusate)—Y

Senokot (sennosides)—Y

Senokot-S (sennosides, docusate)—N

SenokotXTRA (sennosides)—N

Surfak (docusate)—Y

Syllact (psyllium)—Y

Anti-Diarrheal Preparations

Dairy Ease (lactase)—Y

Diar Aid (loperamide)—Y***

Diarrid (loperamide)—Y***

Diasorb (attapulgite)—Y

Donnagel (attapulgite)—Y

Equalactin (polycarbophil)—Y

Hylant's Diarrex (arsenicum, podophyllum, phos-

phorus, mercurius)—N

Imodium A-D (loperamide)—Y***

Imodium Advanced (loperamide, simethicone)—Y***

Kao-Paverin (kaolin, pectin)—Y

Paopectate (attapulgite)—Y

Pepto-Bismol (bismuth subsalicylate)—N

Rheaban (attapulgite)—Y

Nausea and Vomiting, Motion Sickness Preparation

Benadryl (diphenhydramine)—Y*

Bonine (meclizine)—N

Calm-X (dimenhydrinate)—Y*

Dramamine (dimenhydrinate)—Y*

Dramamine Less Drowsy (meclizine)—N

Emetrol (phosphorated carbohydrates)—Y

Pepto-Bismol (bismuth subsalicylate)—N

Nauzene (diphenhydramine)—Y*

Triptone (dimenhydrinate)—Y*

Hemorrhoidal Preparations

Americaine (benzocaine)—Y

Anusol HC-Ointment (hydrocortisone)—Y

Anusol Ointment (pramoxine, mineral oil, zinc oxide)—Y

Anusol Suppositories (starch)—Y

Balneol (mineral oil, lanolin oil)—Y

Calmol 4 (zinc oxide, cocoa butter)—Y

Fleet Medicated Wipes (witch hazel)—Y

Fleet Pain-Relief (pramoxine)—Y

Hemorrhoidal Preparations (continued)

Hemorid for Women (pramoxine, phenylephrine)—Y

Hydrosal Hemorrhoidal (benzyl alcohol, ephedrine, zinc oxide)—Y

Nupercainal (dibucaine)—Y

Nupercainal Anti-Itch Cream (hydrocortisone)—Y

Nupercainal Suppositories (cocoa butter, zinc oxide)—Y

Pazo (benzocaine, ephedrine, zinc oxide, camphor)—Y

Peterson's Ointment (phenol, camphor)—Y

Preparation H Hydrocortisone Cream (hydrocortisone)—Y

Preparation H Ointment, Suppositories, and Cream (phenylephrine, shark liver oil)—Y

Procto Foam Non-Steroid (pramoxine)—Y

Rectacaine Ointment (petrolatum, shark liver oil, mineral oil)—Y

Rectacaine Suppositories (phenylephrine)—Y

Tronolane Cream (pramoxine)—Y

Tronothane Hydrochloride (pramoxine, glycerin)—Y

Tronolane Suppository (zinc oxide)—Y

Tucks Pads (witch hazel)—Y

Wyanoids (cocoa butter, shark liver oil, glycerin)—Y

Sleep Preparations

Alka-Seltzer PM Pain Reliever & Sleep Aid Medicine (aspirin, diphenhydramine)—N

Anacin PM Aspirin Free (acetaminophen, diphenhydramine)—N

Bayer PM Extra Strength Aspirin Plus Sleep Aid (aspirin, diphenhydramine)—N

Benadryl (diphenhydramine)—Y*

Compoz (diphenhydramine)—Y*

Doan's PM Extra Strength (magnesium salicylate, diphenhydramine)—N

Dormarex and Dormarex 2 (diphenhydramine)—Y*

Dormin (diphenhydramine)—Y*

Excedrin PM (acetaminophen, diphenhydramine)—N

Goody's PM (acetaminophen, diphenhydramine)—N

Legatrim PM (diphenhydramine, acetaminophen)—N

Melatonex (melatonin)—N

Melatonin (melatonin)—N

Melatonin (pyridoxine, melatonin)—N

Melatonin Lozenge (melatonin, xylitol)—N

Melatonin PM Dual Release (calcium, vitamin B6, magnesium, niacin, melatonin, xylitol)—N

Midol PM Night Time Formula (diphenhydramine, acetaminophen)—N

Nervine Nightime Sleep Aid (diphenhydramine)—Y*

Nite Gel (doxylamine, acetaminophen, pseudoephedrine, dextromethorphan)—N

Nytol Natural (ignatia amara, aconitum radix)—N

Nytol Quickcaps and Quickgels (diphenhydramine)—Y*

Restyn 76 (diphenhydramine)—Y*

Sleep-Ettes D (diphenhydramine)—Y*

Sleep-Eze 3 (diphenhydramine)—Y*

Sleepinal (diphenhydramine)—Y*

Sleepiness (diphenhydramine)—Y*

Sleep Rite (diphenhydramine)—Y*

Snooze Fast (diphenhydramine)—Y*

Sominex Original (diphenhydramine)—Y*

Sominex Pain Relief Formula (diphenhydramine, acetaminophen)—N

Tranquil (diphenhydramine)—Y*

Tranquil Plus (diphenhydramine, acetaminophen)—N

Unisom Maximum Strength (diphenhydramine)—Y*

Unisom with Pain Relief (acetaminophen, diphenhydramine)—N

Stimulants

No Doz (caffeine 200 mg)—N*

Vivarin (caffeine 200 mg)—N*

Table 25-2 Herbal Preparations Contraindicated in Breastfeeding Mothers and Their Recommended Alternatives

Herb	Typical Use	Recommended Alternative
—	Possible Galactagogues	Blessed Thistle*, Chaste Tree Fruit*, Fennel*, Fenugreek*, Garlic, Goat's Rue, Milk Thistle*
—	Minor Galactagogues	Alfalfa*, Anise*, Borage*, Caraway, Coriander*, Dandelion*, Dill, Fennel*, Hops, Marshmallow Root*, Oat Straw, Red Clover, Red Raspberry*, Stinging Nettle*, Vervain
Comfrey	Analgesics	Bugleweed*,**
Feverfew, Gordolobo Yerba Tea, Mistletoe	Anti-Inflammatory/Headache (Migraine) Agents	Evening Primrose Oil*
Coltsfoot, Margosa Oil	Anti-Infectives/Cough, Cold, and Allergy Products	Echinacea, Elder Flower
Ephedra	Anti-Asthmatic Preparations	—
Aloes, Buckthorn, Cascara Sagrada, Licorice, Peppermint and Caraway Oil, Rhubarb, Sage	Gastrointestinal Agents	Chamomile, Flaxseed, Psyllium Seed (Blonde), Senna*
—	Nausea and Vomiting Preparations	Ginger
Hawthorn	Lipid Lowering Agents	Soy Lecithin
Bearberry, Germander, Petasites, Uva Ursi	Diuretics/Urinary Tract Infection Preparations	Cranberry*, Goldenrod
—	Thrush Agents	Grapefruit Seed*
Blue Cohosh, Pennyroyal Oil	Hormonal Imbalance	—
Indian Snakeroot, Jin Bu Huan, Kava Kava, Skullcap	Anti-Anxiety Agents	Passionflower*, St. John's Wort*, Valerian*
Angelica Root, Dong Quai, Ginseng Root, Mate Tea	Stimulants	Ginkgo Biloba*, Siberian Ginseng
—	Sleep Aid Preparations	Melatonin
—	Antioxidants	Grape Seed*
Bilberry	Eye Health Products	—

* Monitor nursling for potential side effects
** May decrease prolactin level

2. Basically, three options exist in a radiopharmaceutical/breastfeeding situation:
   a. Discontinue breastfeeding.
      i. Breastfeeding should probably be discontinued following the use of radioactive I^{131} because of the enhanced risk of thyroid carcinoma in the infant.
      ii. This also might require extended (or complete) interruptions when the dose of radioiodine is quite high.
   b. Interrupt breastfeeding for a period of five to seven radioactive half-lives.
      i. Milk can be expressed and stored for use during interruptions.
      ii. Milk must be regularly expressed during interruptions to maintain milk supply.
      iii. Milk can be stored for five to seven half-lives and be safely used after exposure to most radioactive compounds.
   c. Do not interrupt breastfeeding.
      i. None to only brief interruptions are required with some radiopharmaceuticals, such as Technetium-99 products. Again, please consult Hale's (2010) *Medications and Mothers' Milk*.
3. The Office of Nuclear Regulatory Research's guide and the guidelines from the American College of Radiology contain instructions and recommendations on the use of radiopharmaceuticals during breastfeeding. In addition, objective mathematically derived guidelines for the administration of radiopharmaceuticals in nursing mothers have been developed (Hale, 2010).

VII. Resources for the Lactation Consultant

A. InfantRisk Center of the Texas Tech University Health Sciences Center: www.infantrisk.com
B. InfantRisk Center mobile applications: www.infantrisk.com/mobile
C. Texas Tech University Health Sciences Center recommendations for radiocontrast agents: www.infantrisk.com/content/recommendations-radiocontrast-agents
D. U.S. Library of Medicine Drugs and Lactation Database (LactMed): http://toxnet.nlm.nih.gov/cgi-bin/sis/htmlgen?LACT

References

American Academy of Pediatrics Committee on Drugs. (1994). The transfer of drugs and other chemicals into human milk. *Pediatrics, 13*, 137–150.

Anderson, P. O. (1991). Drug use during breast-feeding. *Clinical Pharmacy, 10*, 594–624.

Briggs, G., Freeman, R., & Yaffe, S. (1998). *Drugs in pregnancy and lactation: A reference guide to fetal and neonatal risk* (5th ed.; pp. 72–73, 217, 222, 407–408, 548, 661–662, 958–959). Baltimore: Williams & Wilkins.

Britt, R., & Pasero, C. (1999). Using analgesics during breastfeeding. *American Journal of Nursing, 99*, 20.

Committee on Drugs, American Academy of Pediatrics. (1983). The transfer of drugs and other chemicals into human breast milk. *Pediatrics, 72*, 375–383.

Courtney, T., Shaw, R., Cedar, E., et al. (1988). Excretion of famotidine in breast milk. *British Journal of Pharmacology*, *26*, 639P.

Covington, T., & Pau, A. (1985). Oxymetazoline. *American Pharmacy, NS25*, 21–26.

Davies, H., Clark, J., Dalton, K., & Edwards, O. (1989). Insulin requirements of diabetic women who breastfeed. *BMJ*, *298*, 1357–1358.

Egan, P. C., Marx, C. M., Heyl, P. S., et al. (1984). Saccharin concentration in mature human milk. *Drug Intelligence & Clinical Pharmacy*, *18*, 511.

Figueroa-Quintanilla, D., Lindo, E., Sack, B., et al. (1993). A controlled trial of bismuth subsalicylate in infants with acute watery diarrheal disease. *New England Journal of Medicine*, *328*, 1653–1658.

Findlay, J., DeAngelis, R., Kearney, M., et al. (1981). Analgesic drugs in breast milk and plasma. *Clinical Pharmacology & Therapeutics*, *29*, 625–633.

Hagemann, T. (1998). Gastrointestinal medications and breastfeeding. *Journal of Human Lactation*, *14*, 259–262.

Hale, T. (2010). *Medications and mothers' milk: A manual of lactational pharmacology* (14th ed.). Amarillo, TX: Hale Publishing.

Hornby, P., & Abrahams, T. (1996). Pulmonary pharmacology. *Clinical Obstetrics and Gynecology*, *39*, 17–35.

Juszczak, M., & Stempniak, B. (1997). The effect of melatonin on suckling-induced oxytocin and prolactin release in the rat. *Brain Research Bulletin*, *44*, 253–258.

Kanfer, I., Dowse, R., & Vuma, V. (1993). Pharmacokinetics of oral decongestants. *Pharmacotherapy*, *13*, 116S–128S.

Kearns, G., McConnell, R., Trang, J., & Lkuza, R. (1985). Appearance of ranitidine in breast milk following multiple dosing. *Clinical Pharmacy*, *4*, 322–324.

Kok, T. H., Taitz, L. S., Bennett, M. J., et al. (1982). Drowsiness due to clemastine transmitted in breast milk. *Lancet*, *1*, 914–915.

Meny, R. G., Naumburg, E. G., Alger, L. S. et al. (1993). Codeine and the breastfed neonate. *Journal of Human Lactation*, *9*, 237–240.

Nice, F. J. (1992). Breastfeeding and OTC medications. *Pharmacy Times*, *58*, 114–124, 126–127.

Nice, F. J. (2011). *Nonprescription drugs for the breastfeeding mother* (2nd ed.). Amarillo, TX: Hale Publishing.

Nikodem, V. C, & Hofmeyr, G. J. (1992). Secretion of the antidiarrhoeal agent loperamide oxide in breast milk. *European Journal of Clinical Pharmacology*, *42*, 695–696.

Obermeyer, B., Bergstrom, R., Callaghan, J., et al. (1990). Secretion of nizatidine into human breast milk after single and multiple dosing. *Clinical Pharmacology & Therapeutics*, *47*, 724–730.

Oo, C., Kuhn, R., Desai, N., & McNamara, P. (1995). Active transport of cimetidine into human milk. *Clinical Pharmacology & Therapeutics*, *58*, 548–555.

Rathmell, J. P., Viscomi, C. M., & Ashburn, M. A. (1997). Management of nonobstetric pain during pregnancy and lactation. *Anesthesia & Analgesia*, *85*, 1074–1087.

Redetzki, H. M. (1981). Alcohol. In J. T. Wilson (Ed.), *Drugs in breast milk* (pp. 46–49). Balgowlah, Australia: ADIS Health Science Press.

Ryu, J. (1985). Effect of maternal caffeine consumption on heart rate and sleep time of breast-fed infants. *Developmental Pharmacology and Therapeutics*, *8*, 355–363.

Scariati, P., Grummer-Strawn, L., & Fein, S. (1997). A longitudinal analysis of infant morbidity and the extent of breastfeeding in the United States. *Pediatrics*, *99*, E5.

Somogyi, A., & Gugler, R. (1979). Cimetidine excreation into breast milk. *British Journal of Clinical Pharmacology*, *7*, 627–629.

Stegink, L. D., Filer, L. J., & Baker, G. L. (1979). Plasma, erythrocyte, and human milk levels of free amino acids in lactating women administered aspartame or lactose. *Journal of Nutrition*, *109*, 2173–2181.

Stewart, J. J. (1981). Gastrointestinal drugs. In J. T. Wilson (Ed.), *Drugs in breast milk* (pp. 65–71). Balgowlah, Australia: ADIS Health Science Press.

Stoukides, C. (1993). Topical medications and breastfeeding. *Journal of Human Lactation*, *9*, 185–187.

Wilkes, D. (1998, December 9). The international perspective on the OTC market. *IMS Health Self Medication/OTC Bulletin*.

Yurchak, A. M., & Jusko, W. J. (1976). Theophylline secretion into breast milk. *Pediatrics, 57*, 518–520.

Suggested Reading

American Academy of Pediatrics Committee on Drugs. (2001). The transfer of drugs and other chemicals into human milk. *Pediatrics*, *108*(3), 776–789. Retrieved from http://aappolicy. aappublications.org/cgi/content/full/pediatrics%3b108/3/776

Briggs, G. G., Freeman, R. K., & Yaffe, S. J. (2011). *Drugs in pregnancy and lactation: A reference guide to fetal and neonatal risk* (9th ed.). Philadelphia, PA: Williams & Wilkins.

Hale, T. (2010). *Clinical therapy in breastfeeding mothers.* Amarillo, TX: Pharmasoft Publishing.

Lawrence, R. A., & Lawrence, R. M. (2011). *Breastfeeding: A guide for the medical profession* (7th ed.). St. Louis, MO: Mosby.

Nice, F. J., DeEugenio, D., DiMino, T. A., et al. (2004). Medications and breast-feeding: A guide for pharmacists, pharmacy technicians, and other healthcare professionals, Part I. *Journal of Pharmacy Technology*, *20*, 17–27.

Nice, F. J., DeEugenio, D., DiMino, T. A., et al. (2004). Medications and breast-feeding: A guide for pharmacists, pharmacy technicians, and other healthcare professionals, Part II. *Journal of Pharmacy Technology*, *20*, 85–95.

Nice, F. J., DeEugenio, D., DiMino, T. A., et al. (2004). Medications and breast-feeding: A guide for pharmacists, pharmacy technicians, and other healthcare professionals, Part III. *Journal of Pharmacy Technology*, *20*, 165–177.

Nice, F. J., & Luo, A. C. (2012). Medications and breast-feeding: Current concepts. *Journal of the American Pharmacists Association*, *52*, 86-94.

CHAPTER 26
Lactation Toxicology

Teresa Baker, MD, and Thomas W. Hale, RPh, PhD

OBJECTIVES

- Discuss the issue of environmental chemicals in human milk.
- Discuss recreational and illegal drug use in lactating women.

INTRODUCTION

The first step in trying to establish whether a toxin will enter the breastmilk compartment is to understand the properties that guide the transfer of a drug from the maternal plasma into the milk compartment. Molecular weight, pKa (the acid dissociation constant of the drug), and lipophilicity are some of the characteristics known to govern the transfer into breastmilk.

For any drug or toxin to enter into the milk compartment that drug or toxin must meet the following conditions (Hale, 2010):

1. Attain a high concentration within the maternal plasma compartment
2. Be small in size (molecular weight less than 500 Daltons [D])
3. Be unbound to plasma protein, for the most part
4. Pass into the brain easily

Children and nursing babies are at higher risk for toxic exposures because they have a higher consumption of air per body weight, higher consumption of food per body weight, breathing zones that are close to the ground where toxic residues settle in dust, and higher gastrointestinal absorption of heavy metal and other toxicants. Neonates especially have immature glomerular and hepatic functions (Sudak et al., 2007).

I. Air Pollutants

A. Asbestos: A mineral fiber used in manufacturing and building construction and as a flame retardant.

    1. The U.S. Environmental Protection Agency (EPA) has banned several asbestos products, and manufacturers have also voluntarily limited asbestos production because of its association with long-term abdominal, chest, and lung cancers.

        • Asbestos is most commonly found in older homes, paints, and floor tiles. Elevated concentrations of airborne asbestos can occur after asbestos-containing material has been disturbed (such as by cutting, sanding, or other remodeling activities; (Agency, 2012).

    2. No studies indicate that asbestos transfers into human milk. This transfer would be virtually impossible. It is likely that environmental exposure to both mother and infant is the burden of the exposure.

B. Carbon monoxide (CO): An odorless, colorless, and tasteless toxic gas.

    1. At low levels of exposure CO causes mild effects that include headache, dizziness, nausea, and fatigue. At high concentrations, CO is deadly because of the formation of carboxyhemoglobin in the blood, which inhibits oxygen intake (EPA, 2011).

    2. Unvented kerosene and gas space heaters, leaking chimneys and furnaces, gas water heaters, wood stoves, gas stove generators, and automobile exhaust are the leading sources of CO in the home.

    3. Average levels in homes without gas stoves vary from 0.5 to 5 parts per million (ppm). Levels near properly adjusted gas stoves are usually 5–15 ppm. Levels near poorly adjusted stoves may be 30 ppm or higher.

    4. The U.S. Occupational Safety and Health Administration (OSHA) has set the permissible exposure limit for CO at 50 ppm of air (55 mg/m^3) as an 8-hour time-weighted average. The U.S. National Institute of Occupational Safety and Health has established a recommended exposure limit for CO of 35 ppm (40 mg/m^3) as an 8-hour time-weighted average.

    5. Carbon monoxide binds avidly to hemoglobin and would be excluded from the milk compartment. Although no studies confirm the transfer of CO into the breastmilk compartment, this transfer would be unlikely to take place. Thus, environmental exposure to environmental carbon monoxide by both mother and infant is the burden of exposure, not via breastmilk.

C. Nitrous oxide: A gas that produces significant analgesia and some anesthesia. It is rapidly eliminated from the body as a result of rapid exchange (less than 1 minute) with nitrogen via the pulmonary alveoli (Adriani, 1983).

    1. Because of poor lipid solubility, uptake by adipose tissue is relatively poor, and only insignificant traces of nitrous oxide circulate in the blood after discontinuing the gas.

2. There are no data on the entry of nitrous oxide into human milk; however, it would be minimal to nil. Chronic exposure, such as in dental care workers, could cause some elevated risk to the unborn fetus (Adriani, 1983).

3. Because of its rapid clearance, the use of nitrous oxide in breastfeeding mothers should not pose any problem for breastfeeding.

D. Radon: An odorless, tasteless, and invisible gas produced by the decay of naturally occurring uranium in soil and water. Radon is ubiquitous and found in outdoor and indoor air.

1. It is a proven carcinogen with documented cases of lung cancer in humans.

2. Air pressure inside the home is usually lower than pressure in the soil around the home foundation; therefore, radon enters the home through foundation cracks and other openings. Thus far, there is no evidence that children are at greater risk of lung cancer than are adults (EPA, 2010).

3. The EPA recommends homes be sealed if the radon level is 4 pCi/L (picocuries per liter) or more. The average radon concentration in the indoor air of U.S. homes is about 1.3 pCi/L. The average concentration of radon in outdoor air is 0.4 pCi/L.

4. Radon could potentially enter milk, but the greater hazard to the infant is from environmental (air) exposure in the home.

II. Volatile Air Compounds

A. Benzene, perchloroethylene emissions (dry cleaning materials, methylene chloride (paint thinners/adhesive removers/aerosol sprays): Very little is known on the transfer of volatile organic compounds into human milk.

1. The extent of bioaccumulation depends on the level of exposure, the length of time during which exposure occurs, and the time period between exposure events. More data are needed before anyone can comment on exposure of the nursing mother to these compounds (Fisher, 1997).

2. Kim et al., (2007) observed that the infant dose from inhalation exceeded that from milk ingestion by approximately 25- to 135-fold. They state that in general the indoor air levels were more closely related to the infant dose, which implies that air control strategies would be best because they have the advantage of reducing infant inhalation and reducing any ingestion exposure (Kim et al., 2007).

B. Formaldehyde: Exposure in laboratory or embalming environments is strictly controlled by general regulations to a permissible level of 2 ppm. At exposure of 1-4 ppm formaldehyde is a strong mucous membrane irritant, producing burning and lacrimation (Ellenhorn, 1978).

1. Formaldehyde is rapidly destroyed by plasma and tissue enzymes. It is very unlikely that any would enter human milk following environmental exposures. However, acute intoxication following high oral or inhaled doses could lead to significant levels of maternal plasma formic acid, which could enter milk.

2. No data suggest untoward side effects in nursing infants as a result of mild to minimal environmental exposure of the mother to formaldehyde (Hale, 2010).

3. Mothers should reduce overall exposure to a minimum, if possible, and follow OSHA guidelines to control environmental exposure. The transfer of intact formaldehyde into human milk is highly unlikely.

III. Heavy Metals

A. Zinc: An essential element required for enzyme function within cells.

   1. Recommended Daily Allowance for adults is 12–15 mg/day. Average oral dose of supplements is 25–50 mg/day. Doses used for treatment of cold symptoms averaged 13.3 mg to be taken every 2 hours.
   2. Zinc sulfate should not be used.
   3. Absorption of dietary zinc is nearly twice as high during lactation as before conception. In 13 women studied, the preconception absorption of zinc was 14% and during lactation, 25%. (Fung, 1997).
   4. Zinc absorption in infants from human milk is high, averaging 41%. Minimal daily requirements of zinc in full-term infants vary from 0.3 to 0.5 mg/kg/day.
   5. Daily ingesting of zinc from breastmilk has been estimated to be 0.35 mg/kg/day and declines over the first 17 weeks of life because older neonates require less zinc as a result of slower growth rates.
   6. Supplementation with 25–50 mg/day is probably safe. Excessive doses are discouraged because of the enhanced absorption mechanism present in neonates and the breast. Another author shows that zinc levels in breastmilk are independent of maternal plasma zinc concentrations or dietary zinc intake (Krebs, 1995).
   7. Recent data on intranasal application of zinc has shown profound damage to the olfactory cells and significant loss of smell (Lim et al., 2009). Do not use intranasal zinc.

B. Lead: Under normal circumstances, levels of 2–5 μg/L are found in milk from mothers.

   1. Lead is an environmental pollutant. It serves no useful purpose in the body and tends to accumulate in the body's bony structure as a function of environmental exposure. Because of the rapid development of the nervous system, children are particularly sensitive to elevated levels.
   2. Lead apparently transfers into human milk at a rate proportional to maternal blood levels, but the absolute degree of transfer is controversial.
   3. Studies of lead levels in milk vary enormously and probably reflect the enormous difficulty in measuring lead in milk.
   4. In mothers who have previously been exposed to high-lead environments, the greatest chance of lead toxicity is with the first pregnancy. The mother's blood lead levels are highest postpartum because lead becomes mobilized during lactation and enters milk.
   5. A baby's greatest chance of exposure is in utero because intestinal absorption of lead from milk is low (Manton et al., 2009).
   6. One study evaluated lead transfer into human milk in a population of women with an average blood lead of 45 μg/dL. The average level of lead in milk was

2.47 µg/dL. Using these parameters, the average intake in an infant would be 8.1 µg/kg/day. The daily permissible level by the World Health Organization (WHO) is 5 µg/kg/day.

7. Mothers contaminated with lead should not breastfeed their infants until they have undergone chelation therapy to reduce maternal lead levels.

8. In a larger study of Shanghai mothers (n = 165), the transfer of lead to the fetus was highly correlated with maternal blood lead levels. Levels of lead in cord blood and breastmilk increased as a function of lead levels in the maternal blood with a coefficient of correlation of 0.714 and 0.353, respectively.

9. The average concentration of lead in breastmilk for 12 occupationally exposed women was 52.7 µg/L, which was almost 12 times higher than that for the occupationally nonexposed population (4.43 µg/L). These data suggest that lead levels in milk pose a potential health hazard to the breastfed infant, but only in mothers with high plasma lead levels (Li et al., 2000).

10. Lead exposure of military personnel on firing ranges has been questioned. Lead levels in frequent target shooters are known to be elevated as a result of exposure to lead from unjacketed bullets and lead in primers. Breastfeeding mothers should avoid confined, unventilated ranges, but brief exposure to military firing in well-ventilated areas with jacketed bullets is probably safe. Individuals should avoid dust in such areas, such as from sweeping or cleaning fire ranges (Gelberg, 2009).

11. In the last decade, the permissible blood lead level in children, according to the Centers for Disease Control and Prevention (CDC), has dropped from 25 to less than 10 µg/dL. Lead poisoning is known to significantly alter IQ and neurobehavioral development, particularly in infants.

12. Infants receiving breastmilk from mothers with high lead levels should be closely monitored. Both mother and infant might require chelation, and the infant might need to be weaned to formula.

C. Mercury: Levels of 1.4–1.7 µg/L are found in milk from mothers under normal circumstances.

1. Mercury is an environmental contaminant that is available in multiple salt forms. Mercury poisoning produces encephalopathy, acute renal failure, severe gastrointestinal necrosis, and numerous other systemic toxicities.

2. Elemental mercury, the form found in thermometers, is poorly absorbed orally (0.01%) but completely absorbed via inhalation (>80%) (Woff, 1983).

3. Inorganic mercury causes most forms of mercury poisoning and is available in mercury disk batteries (7–15% orally bioavailable).

4. Organic mercury is readily absorbed (methylmercury fungicides, phenyl mercury), 90% orally.

5. Mercury transfers into human milk with a milk/plasma ratio that varies according to the form of mercury. Pickin et al. (2000) reports that in the United States 100 unexposed women had 0.9 µg/L total mercury in their milk (Pickin et al., 2000).

6. Concentrations of mercury in human milk are generally much higher in populations that ingest large quantities of fish. Oskarsson et al. (1990) suggests in

a study of Swedish women that the exposure of the infant to mercury from breastmilk was less than 0.3 μg/kg/day. This exposure is only one-half the tolerable daily intake for adults recommended by the WHO (Oskarsson et al., 1990).

7. A total of five studies generally conclude that although mercury dental amalgams (fillings) can increase the transfer of mercury to the infant, most transfer occurs in utero. The replacement of amalgam fillings should, if possible, be postponed until after pregnancy and breastfeeding because the removal of amalgam fillings while breastfeeding could potentially increase the transfer of mercury to the breastfed infant and largely depends on the precautions taken by the dentist (Ramirez et al., 2000).

8. The transfer of mercury into human milk is transiently high at birth and then drops significantly at 2 months. Although methylmercury has been removed from virtually all pediatric immunizations in the United States, this has not occurred in other countries. In infants receiving three doses of hepatitis B vaccine and three DTP (diphtheria, tetanus toxoids, and pertussis vaccine adsorbed USP) vaccines during the first 6 months of life, the exposure to methylmercury was 25 μg for each vaccine. Mercury levels in the infant's hair increased 446% during these 6 months, whereas maternal hair mercury decreased 57%. This provides evidence that the extra mercury exposure is caused by the vaccination rather than maternal milk.

D. Cadmium: Exists ubiquitously in the environment.

1. Cadmium is found in breastmilk at concentrations of less than 1 μg/L under normal conditions, but mothers who are exposed environmentally or occupationally can have higher levels in their breastmilk.

2. Cadmium interacts with essential elements such as zinc, copper, iron, and calcium. In particular, cadmium interferes with calcium and vitamin D metabolism in the bone, kidney, and intestine.

3. Calcium absorption is decreased by competition with cadmium in the intestine, and more calcium is released from maternal bone and transferred to the neonate by lactation (Ohta et al., 2002).

E. Aluminum: Commonly used in antacid preparations such as Maalox.

1. Under usual conditions, absorption of aluminum from the gastrointestinal (GI) tract is extremely low and thus aluminum should not be present in breastmilk. Fruit juices, citrates, ascorbate, and lactate can increase the absorption of aluminum hydroxide (Domingo, 1995).

2. Aluminum toxicity can occur in patients with renal impairment. Long-term therapy can also interfere with other medications as a result of changes in the gastric pH, absorption, or binding to drugs and changes in the urine pH.

3. Pregnant or breastfeeding mothers should avoid extensive or daily use of aluminum-containing antacids.

IV. Pesticides

A. Organochlorines (DDT): Lipophilic and their presence in human milk and blood have been documented in India as well as other countries.

    1. One study of an agriculturally contaminated area in India showed that the level of total organochlorine pesticides in blood ranged from 3.3 to 6.2 mg/L while in milk it ranged from 3.9 to 4.6 mg/L (Kumar et al., 2005).

    2. Without doubt, lipophilic organochlorine pesticides can accumulate in maternal adipose tissue and transfer readily to a breastfeeding infant. Mothers heavily contaminated with DDT should not breastfeed.

B. DEET (N, N-diethyl-meta-toluamide): The active ingredient in many insect repellents.

    1. One-third of the U.S. population is exposed to DEET annually. Formulations for direct use on humans range from 4–100% DEET.

    2. The EPA has established that, if used as directed, DEET formulations do not present a health concern to humans.

    3. DEET is not to be applied to the hands or eyes or near the mouths of young children, and DEET products are not to be used under clothing.

    4. DEET was specifically studied in children and has been approved by the EPA for use on children with no age restriction and no restriction on the percentage of DEET.

    5. The CDC support these findings and report that Lyme disease (tick borne) is a much larger risk to humans than exposure to DEET.

    6. It is considered safe for a breastfeeding mother to use DEET-containing products on her clothing, but she must specifically avoid any contact with her breasts or areas that the infant's mouth might contact.

C. Permethrin: The most widely used pesticide for both residential and industrial purposes.

    1. Permethrin alters the normal biochemistry and physiology of nerve membrane sodium channels in insects. It has been associated with two reproducible benign tumor types (lung and liver).

    2. The EPA states that on balance the benefits of permethrin outweigh any risks.

    3. It is the most widely used mosquito repellant in the United States. It is also used in almost all treatments for lice that are available on the market.

    4. The advantage of the permethrin class is that these pesticides show very little mammalian toxicity and have very short environmental half-lives.

    5. Currently, there is a large EPA-funded trial that studies the transfer of permethrin products to infants through environmental exposure as well as via breastmilk.

V. Beauty Aids and Cosmetics

When used as directed, these products pose a low toxicity risk (Caraccio et al., 2007). Most unintentional cosmetic ingestions are by children. Hair straighteners and nail glue removers are the chemicals with the greatest potential for harm. There are no studies available to prove whether these substances enter the breastmilk compartment.

  A. Hair products: Toxic if directly ingested by a child.
  B. Colognes/perfumes: These products contain ethanol. If applied to the skin, little is absorbed transcutaneously.
  C. Nail care products:
    1. Nail polish removers: These products contain acetone, acetonitrile, or ethanol. Can be very toxic if directly ingested by a child. Little or none is absorbed transcutaneously by a lactating woman.

VI. Radioactive Compounds

  A. Iodine: Radioactive iodine concentrates in the thyroid gland as well as in breastmilk, and if ingested by an infant, it can suppress the infant's thyroid function or increase the risk of future thyroid carcinomas (Hale, 2010).
    1. Radioactive iodine is clinically used to diagnose thyroid malignancy and ablate or destroy the thyroid gland.
    2. Following ingestion, radioactive iodine concentrates in the thyroid and lactating tissues. It is estimated that 27.9% of total radioactivity is secreted via breastmilk (Robinson et al., 1994).
    3. Two potential half-lives exist for radioactive iodine.
      a. One is the radioactive half-life, which is solely dependent on radioactive decay of the molecule.
      b. Second is the biological half-life, which is often briefer and is the half-life of the iodine molecule itself in the human being. This is mostly influenced by elimination via the kidneys and other routes (Hale, 2010). The biological or effective half-life might be shorter as a result of excretion in urine, feces, and milk (Palmer, 1979). Holding the infant close to the breast or thyroid gland for long periods of time may expose the infant to gamma irradiation, and parents should consult with the radiologist concerning exposure of the infant.
    4. Because radioactivity decays at a set rate, milk can be stored in the freezer for at least 8–10 half-lives and then fed to the infant without problem. The entire radioactivity will be gone (Hale, 2010). Because radiation can be emitted during the storage period, it would be best to store the radioactive milk in a freezer located in a garage. If not possible, people should avoid frequent contact with the contents. Emitted radiation will not damage stored food. Infants can be exposed both from transfer of the isotope into human milk and by close contact with the mother directly through the skin. Mothers should not sleep with partners or infants for 3–23 nights, depending on dose, and should stay a minimum of 6 feet away during the majority of this time. This is not to say

that brief contact to change a diaper or similar activity is hazardous, just that mothers should avoid continuous close contact. Check the InfantRisk Center (www.infantrisk.com) for close contact and other recommendations about radioisotopes.

5. I^{131}: The radioactive half-life of I^{131} is 8.1 days. (Dydek, 1988). Dydek reviewed the transfer of both tracer and ablation doses of I^{131} and found that if the tracer doses are kept minimal (0.1 μCi or 3.7 kBq), breastfeeding could resume as early as the 8th day. However if larger tracer doses are used, nursing could not resume until 46 days following therapy (Dydek, 1988).

6. I^{125}: The radioactive half-life of I^{125} is 60.2 days. If this product is used, in general the recommendation is to discontinue breastfeeding.

7. I^{123}: The radioactive half-life of I^{123} is 13.2 hours. Following the use of less than 2 mCi of I^{123}, the patient should be advised to express milk for 12–24 hours. Milk can be saved and used after five to seven half-lives (approximately 3–4 days). A table on the use of radioisotopes in breastfeeding mothers is available (Hale, 2010).

B. Thallium (TI^{201}): The radioactive half-life of Thallium is 73.1 hours. Breastfeeding mothers should interrupt breastfeeding for a minimum of 48 hours if less than 3 mCi are used. However, to avoid all exposure to this radioisotope, withdraw the infant for up to 2 weeks. Expressed milk can be saved and used after 21 days.

C. Gallium^{67}: The radioactive half-life of gallium is 78.3 hours. It is recommended to interrupt breastfeeding for more than 3 weeks for a dose of 4 mCi[1]. Expressed milk can be saved and used after one month.

D. Technetium^{99}: The radioactive half-life of technetium is 6.02 hours. With a very short half-life the risk to the infant is small, but it is still recommended that a mother wait 12–24 hours to breastfeed her infant after receiving technetium. Milk expressed during the interruption can be saved and used after 24–42 hours.

VII. Persistent Organic Pollutants

Persistent organic pollutants are chemicals manufactured for either a specific purpose or produced as a by-product of incinerated waste. These emissions have deposited into the air, soil, and water and from there they find their way into the food chain.

A. Humans accumulate these chemicals over time, collecting what is referred to as the lifetime body burden (Nickerson, 2006).

B. The transfer of these pollutants into human milk is of interest because of their affinity for deposition in fat, and potentially milk fat. When consumed, they concentrate in adipose tissue. Because of their very long half-life they can accumulate with age and level of exposure.

C. Humans excrete these pollutants slowly through stool; however, when a woman initiates lactation, her fat stores are mobilized more efficiently and the pollutants stored in adipose tissue are mobilized as well. The concentrations of these pollutants can be 10 times higher in breastmilk lipids than in lipids of ordinary food (Kreuzer et al., 1997).

D. Some have estimated that maternal PCB/dioxin body burden decreases as much as 20–70% during 6 months of exclusive breastfeeding (Kreuzer et al., 1997). The majority of the transfer occurs while a woman nurses her first infant, and transfer decreases with each subsequent child.

E. Very few studies of the effect of exposure of neonates to these pollutants exist.

F. Perinatal exposure to PCBs and DDE did not seem to affect pubertal development based on Tanner staging and onset of menses (Gladen et al., 1988). Neurodevelopment studies have been conducted, but are not definitive.

G. It is estimated that the overall body burden of these substances (of breastfed vs. formula-fed infants) eventually equalizes by the age of 10 years (Kreuzer et al., 1997). Despite the high levels of PCB and dioxins transferred via breastmilk, breastfeeding seemed to have a beneficial effect on neurological status compared to formula feeding (Koopman-Esseboom et al., 1994; Patadin et al., 1999).

H. The World Health Organization states: "The advantages of breastfeeding far outweigh the potential risks from environmental pollutants. Taking into account breastfeeding's short- and long-term health benefits for infants and mothers, WHO recommends breastfeeding in all but extreme circumstances."

I. Polychlorinated biphenyls (PCBs; banned in the United States in 1979): These are present in electrical and heat transfer equipment, hydraulics, plastics, rubber, pigments, dyes, and carbonless copy paper.

   1. In industrialized nations, where manufacturing is a large industry, PCBs are probably the most widespread chemical contaminant in human milk.

   2. The levels of PCBs in the breastmilk of Europeans and North Americans are generally higher than those of women in nonindustrialized nations.

   3. In one study of 246 children in Michigan, the serum PCB level in formula-fed children was 0.3 ± 0.7 ng/mL compared with 5.1 ± 3.9 ng/mL in children who were breastfed for at least 6 months (Kreuzer, 1997).

   4. Postnatal exposure via breastfeeding is the principal determinant of body burden levels in early childhood, is significantly correlated with maternal levels, and is based on the length and dose of breastfeeding (Jacobsen et al., 1990; Karmaus et al., 2001; Kreuzer et al., 1997).

J. Dioxins (polychlorinated dibenzodioxins, polychlorinated dibenzodifurans, polychlorinated biphenyls, polybrominated biphenyls, polybrominated diphenyl ethers): Dioxins are a by-product of combustion of chlorinated compounds. The half-life of dioxins in adults is 4.2–5.6 years (Smith, 1999).

   1. One study of 8,132 U.S. residents stratified by age, region, and gender noted that infants and older children had substantially higher polybrominated diphenyl ether (PBDE) concentrations. The study indicated that higher PBDE concentration in infants is primarily the result of maternal transfer in breastmilk (Toms et al., 2008).

   2. Levels of dioxins are consistently higher in industrialized countries (LaKind et al., 2009). The main source of environmental exposure of dioxins is through food of animal origin, such as meat, dairy products, and fish (Papke, 1998).

K. Organochloride pesticides (DDT and DDE): These pesticides were banned in the United States in 1972. Levels of DDT and DDE in human milk have decreased in areas where cessation of use has occurred (Smith, 1999).

VIII. Nonpersistent Organic Pollutants

A. Phthalates and diethylhexyl phthalate (DEHP): These are high-production-volume chemicals used as plasticizers of polyvinyl chloride in the manufacture of a wide variety of consumer goods (building products, car products, clothing, food packaging, children's products) and medical devices made of polyvinyl chloride, particularly intravenous (IV) bags and IV lines.

  1. The public can be exposed to DEHP by ingesting food, drink, or dust contaminated with DEHP-containing materials. Estimates are that the general population of the United States is exposed to DEHP in the range of 1–30 µg/kg/day.

  2. There is significant concern that certain intensive medical treatments of male infants can result in DEHP exposure levels that adversely affect development of the male reproductive tract. There is also concern for adverse effects on development of the reproductive tract in male offspring of pregnant and breastfeeding women undergoing certain medical procedures that can result in exposure to high levels of DEHP ("NTP-CERHR Monograph on the Potential Human Reproductive and Developmental Effects of Di (Ethylhexyl) Phthalate (DEHP)," 2006). There is concern for effects of DEHP exposure on development of the male reproductive tract of infants less than 1 year of age. Oral exposure to products made with DEHP can have similar effects. Dietary intake and certain medical treatments may lead to DEHP exposure that may be higher than for the general population.

  3. One review of 33 lactating women in North Carolina suggests that phthalate metabolites were most frequently detected in urine of lactating women and less often detected in serum, milk, or saliva (Hines et al., 2009).

B. Bisphenol A (BPA): Bisphenol A is a high-production-volume chemical used in manufacturing polycarbonate plastics and epoxy resins used in food packaging and many plastic products. It is a monomer used in manufacturing most or all polycarbonate plastics, the majority of epoxy resins, and certain other products such as flame retardants.

  1. Public concern led industry to move toward non-BPA-based materials in such products as baby bottles, cups, and spoons and adult drinking bottles.

  2. There is general agreement that BPA has estrogenic and dopaminergic activity and might alter reproductive and neurobehavioral development. In animal studies, levels greater than 50 mg/kg/day delayed puberty in male and female rats. Levels greater than 235 mg/kg/day caused reduced fetal birth weight and effects on testes of male rats. Greater than 500 mg/kg/day decreased fertility in mice, altered estrous cycling in female rats, and reduced survival of fetuses. There is significant controversy concerning effects seen at lower doses in animals (less than 1 mg/kg/day), which is relevant to humans. The concern led

Canada to take precautionary action to restrict BPA exposures of infants and young children.

3. However, many of the studies remain contradictory. Ryan compared BPA with the oral contraceptive ethinyl estradiol (EE) and found that low in utero doses of EE affected sexual differentiation in female rats, but low in utero doses of BPA produced no such effects (Ryan et al., 2010). In other studies, in male rats exposed to in utero EE, BPA produced no effects (Howdeshell et al., 2008). However, Newbold et al. (2009) reports that prenatal exposure to BPA in mice led to adverse effects on the female reproductive tract later in life.

4. BPA has been found in human biological samples (serum, breastmilk, urine, fetal blood, and umbilical cord blood).

5. Many scientific groups have studied BPA and offer mixed recommendations mainly because there is such uncertainty with regard to actual risk at very low doses.

6. Breastfeeding is largely protective of BPA exposure for the neonate because of the lack of exposure to plastic nipples or bottles that might contain BPA (Agency, 2010)

IX. Silicone (Implants and in Formula)

Silicone transfer to breastmilk was studied in one group of 15 breastfeeding mothers with bilateral silicone breast implants (Semple et al., 1998).

A. Silicone levels were measured in breastmilk, whole blood, cow's milk, and 26 brands of infant formula. In a comparison of implanted women to controls, mean silicone levels were not significantly different in breastmilk (55.45 ± 35 and 51.05 ± 31 ng/mL, respectively) or in blood (79.29 ± 87 and 103.76 ± 112 ng/mL, respectively). Mean silicone levels measured in store-bought cow's milk was 708.94 ng/mL and that for 26 brands of commercially available infant formula was 4,402.5 ng/mL. The authors concluded that silicone levels in breastmilk and blood are similar in lactating women with silicone implants as compared with control women.

B. These studies show that silicone levels are 10 times higher in cow's milk and even higher in infant formulas.

C. It is not known for certain if ingestion of leaking silicone by a nursing infant is hazardous to breastfed infants. Although one article was published showing esophageal strictures, it was subsequently recalled by the author.

D. Silicone by nature is extremely inert and is unlikely to be absorbed in the GI tract by a nursing infant, although good studies are lacking.

E. Silicone is a ubiquitous substance, found in all foods and liquids (Hale, 2010).

X. Anthrax (*Bacillus anthracis*)

Anthrax is caused by a Gram-positive, spore-forming bacterium *Bacillus anthracis*.

A. The most common forms of the disease are inhaled, oral, and cutaneous.

B. The CDC recently published guidelines for treating exposed breastfeeding mothers (CDC, 2012). Treating an infected woman with appropriate antibiotic therapy is the most prudent option. The CDC website includes the most current recommendations. Thus far, all of the anthrax strains released by bioterrorists have been sensitive to ciprofloxacin, doxycycline, and the penicillin family. In breastfeeding women, amoxicillin (80 mg/kg/d in three divided doses) is an option for antimicrobial prophylaxis when B. anthracis is known to be penicillin-susceptible and no contraindication to maternal amoxicillin use is indicated. The American Academy of Pediatrics also considers ciprofloxacin and tetracyclines (which include doxycycline) to be usually compatible with breastfeeding because the amount of either drug absorbed by infants is small, but little is known about the safety of long-term use. Until culture-sensitivity tests have been completed, the breastfeeding mother should be treated with ciprofloxacin (ofloxacin or levofloxacin are alternates) or doxycycline (< 3 weeks). Because of possible dental staining following prolonged exposure, this author does not suggest long-term use (60 days) of doxycycline in a breastfeeding mother. The CDC offers several alternative antibiotics such as rifampin, vancomycin, imipenem, clindamycin, and clarithromycin in those patients with allergic conditions. Because of the risks posed by infection with anthrax, mothers who test positive for this infection should probably not breastfeed their infants until after treatment and testing negative for this species.

XI. Vaccines

A. Measles, mumps, rubella: Generally considered safe in breastfeeding mothers.

B. Yellow fever: Some hazard, but safer than disease.

C. Hepatitis A: Considered safe in breastfeeding mothers.

D. Hepatitis B: Considered safe in breastfeeding mothers.

E. Diphtheria, pertussis, tetanus: Generally considered safe in breastfeeding mothers.

F. Influenza intranasal (FluMist): Probably safe, but not recommended. Use injectable formulations instead.

G. Influenza injectable: Generally considered safe in breastfeeding mothers.

H. Varicella: Generally considered safe in breastfeeding mothers.

I. Human papillomavirus (HPV; Gardasil): Generally considered safe in breastfeeding mothers.

XII. Recreational Drugs/Drugs of Abuse

A. Tobacco

1. "Mothers who smoke are encouraged to quit, however, breast milk remains the recommended food for a baby even if the mother smokes. Although nicotine may be present in the milk of a mother who smokes, there are no reports of adverse effects on the infant due to breastfeeding. Secondary smoke is a separate concern regarding the child's long-term health." (CDC Website)

2. The American Academy of Pediatrics does not consider maternal smoking an absolute contraindication to breastfeeding though smoking should be strongly

discouraged particularly due to secondary exposure and increased risk of SIDS and respiratory allergy (AAP, 2012).

3. Bachour and colleagues (2012) reported that smoking was associated with a 26% decrease in milk lipids, a 12% decrease in milk protein, and a slower infant growth rate. Infants whose mothers smoke need careful follow-up and frequent weight checks. These infants may need more frequent feeding.

4. One study reported that the incidence of acute respiratory illness is higher among artificially fed infants with smoking mothers as compared with breastfed infants of smoking mother (Woodward, 1990). "It may be that breastfeeding and smoking is less detrimental to the child than bottle-feeding and smoking." Other studies confirm this protective effect of breastfeeding (Nafstad, 1996; Chatzimichael et al., 2007; Kuiper et al., 2007).

5. Woodard et al studied breastfeeding infants of mothers actively smoking tobacco. They measured urine cotinine levels in 101 infants aged 3 months and found a linear dose response between mothers smoking rate and infant urine cotinine level. Secondhand smoke did not increase the urine cotinine level in the infant's urine (Woodward et al., 1986).

6. Yilmaz et al. studied the protective effect of lactation on infants who were exposed to second hand smoke thus increasing their risk of growth restriction, respiratory tract infections and otitis media. The authors proved that breastfeeding decreased the rate of infection by 5.4% (Yilmaz et al., 2009).

7. Becker et al. studied 507 infants and found that urinary cotinine levels during the first 2 weeks of life were significantly increased in infants whose mothers smoked. Urinary cotinine levels were 5 times higher in breastfed infants whose mothers smoked than in those whose mothers smoked but did not breastfeed (Becker et al., 1999).

8. Dahlstrom et al. found that postnatal exposure to nicotine via breast milk influenced autonomic cardiovascular control in infants. In a separate study he found a very close correlation between nicotine in mothers' plasma and milk after smoking (Dahlstrom et al., 2008; Dahlstrom et al., 1990).

9. Ilett et al. compared 15 lactating women who were smokers who participated in a trial of nicotine patch to assist in smoking cessation. They found that nicotine and cotinine concentrations in milk were not significantly different between smoking (mean of 17 cigarettes per day) and the 21-mg/d patch. There was a significant downward trend in absolute infant dose from smoking or use of 21 mg patch through to the 14 mg and the 7 mg patch. They concluded that the absolute infant dose of nicotine and its metabolite cotinine decreases by about 70% from when subjects were smoking or using the 21 mg patch to when they were using the 7 mg patch (Ilett et al., 2003).

B. Alcohol
   1. Alcohol transfers into milk readily, with an average milk/plasma ratio of about 1.0.
   2. The absolute amount of alcohol transferred into milk is generally low and is a function of the maternal level.

3. In a study of 12 breastfeeding mothers who ingested 0.3 g/kg of ethanol in orange juice, the mean maximum concentration of ethanol in milk was 320 mg/L (Mennella, 2001).

4. In another group of five women who consumed 0.4 grams/kg at one setting, milk and maternal plasma levels were similar. Levels of alcohol in milk averaged 0.44 g/L at peak and fell to 0.09 g/L at 180 minutes (da-Silva et al., 1993).

5. Excess levels of alcohol in infants may lead to drowsiness, deep sleep, weakness and decreased linear growth in infants. Maternal blood alcohol levels must attain 300 mg/dL before significant side effects are reported in the infant.

6. Avoid breastfeeding during and for at least 2 hours for each drink after drinking moderate levels of alcohol. Heavy drinkers should wait longer.

C. Marijuana

1. Cannabis should not be used during pregnancy or breastfeeding. Delta-9-tetrahydrocannabinol (THC) transfers and concentrates in the mother's milk and is absorbed and metabolized by the nursing infant) (Astley et al., 1990).

2. THC is stored in the fat tissues for long periods (weeks to months)

3. Small to moderate secretion into breastmilk has been documented. In one mother who consumed marijuana once daily, milk levels were reportedly 105 µg/L (Perez-Reyes et al., 1982).

4. In another mother who consumed marijuana 7-8 times daily, milk levels of THC were 340 µg/L (Perez-Reyes et al., 1982).

5. Analysis of breastmilk in a chronic heavy user revealed an eightfold accumulation of THC in breastmilk compared to plasma.

6. Sixty-eight breastfed infants exposed to marijuana were studied at one year and compared to nonexposed infants. Those exposed appeared to have motor development delays (Astley et al., 1990).

7. Mothers should be advised to not use marijuana while pregnant or breastfeeding.

D. Heroin/Methadone

1. Heroin is diacetyl-morphine (diamorphine), a pro-drug that is rapidly converted by plasma cholinesterases to 6-acetylmorphine and more slowly to morphine.

2. Heroin, as is morphine, is known to transfer into breastmilk.

3. Addicts of heroin may use extraordinarily large doses of heroin, and at such doses, it is likely to be very dangerous for a breastfed infant.

4. Heavily dependent users should probably be advised against breastfeeding and their infants converted to formula.

5. Methadone is a potent and very long-acting opiate analgesic. It is primarily used to prevent withdrawal in opiate addiction.

   a. Jansson et al. studied four pairs of methadone-maintained women who were breastfeeding beyond the neonatal period and found that concentrations of methadone in blood and breast milk were low and recommended that breastfeeding be allowed for some methadone-maintained women (Jansson et al., 2008).

    b. The Motherrisk Team in Canada also states that for women using methadone for treatment of opioid dependence, the benefits of breastfeeding generally outweigh any theoretical minimal risks (Glatstein et al., 2008).

    c. In one study of 10 women receiving methadone 10-80 mg/day, the average milk/plasma ratio was 0.83. Due to the variable doses used, the milk concentrations ranged from 0.05 mg/L in one patient receiving 10 mg/day, to 0.57 mg/L in a patient receiving 80 mg/day (Blinick et al., 1975).

    d. One infant death has been reported in a breastfeeding mother receiving maintenance methadone therapy although it is not clear that the only source of methadone to this infant was from breastmilk (Smialek et al., 1977).

    e. In an excellent study eight mother/infant pairs ingesting from 40 to 105 mg/day methadone, the average (AUC) concentration of R-methadone and S-methadone enantiomers varied from 42-259 µg/L and 26-126 µg/L respectively. The relative infant dose was estimated to be 2.8% of the maternal dose. Interestingly, there was little difference in methadone milk levels in immature and mature milk (Begg et al., 2001).

E. Cocaine/Amphetamines

  1. Cocaine is a potent central nervous system stimulant.

  2. Adverse effects of cocaine ingestion include agitation, nervousness, restlessness, euphoria, hallucinations, tremors, tonic-clonic seizures and myocardial arrhythmias.

  3. Pharmacologic effects of cocaine are relatively brief (20-30 min) due to a short half-life of 50 minutes and redistribution out of the brain.

  4. Urine samples can be positive for cocaine metabolites for up to 7 days or longer in adults, although these metabolites are inactive.

  5. Breastfeeding infants will likewise have positive urine screens for cocaine for even longer periods.

  6. Significant secretion into breastmilk is suspected with a probable high milk/plasma ratio.

  7. There is one case report of a mother who used cocaine 3 days before delivery, reported a milk level 6 days later of 8 ng/mL. The authors propose that if this mother consumed 0.5 g of cocaine, then the infant would have likely received 0.48 mg of cocaine, or 1.62% of the maternal dose per kilogram (Sarkar et al., 2005).

  8. In another study of 11 mothers who admitted to cocaine use in pregnancy cocaine was detected in six milk samples. The highest cocaine concentration found was over 12 µg/mL (Winecker et al., 2001).

  9. Topical application to nipples is extremely dangerous and is definitely contraindicated. (Chaney, Franke, & Wadlington, 1988)

  10. Breastfeeding mothers should avoid cocaine absolutely. For those individuals who have ingested cocaine, a minimum pump and discard period of 24 hours is recommended for clearance.

  11. Use of cocaine is strongly discouraged in breastfeeding.

12. There are conflicting reports about how much cocaine transfers to the infant after maternal exposure to cocaine. Chasnoff, Winecker, and Sarkar have all published case reports with varying degree of drug transfer (Chasnoff et al., 1987; Sarkar, et al., 2005; Winecker et al., 2001)
13. All infants exposed who tested positive in urine samples were symptomatic.
14. Methylamphetamines and amphetamine have been studied in a few case reports.
     a. Bartu et al. conducted two such cases and found that there is significant entry of these drugs into human breast milk (Bartu et al., 2009).
     b. Breastfeeding should be withheld for at least 48 hours after recreational amphetamine use (Bartu et al., 2009).
  F. Hallucinogens
     1. There are no human studies on this subject.
     2. Kaufman et al. describe the presence of phencyclidine (PCP) in the breastmilk of a young drug abuser (Kaufman et al., 1983).
     3. Nicholas et al. published a study of 10 lactating mice and found that PCP crossed rapidly into breast milk and reached concentrations that were 10 times that of plasma (Nicholas et al., 1982).

References

Adriani, J. (1983). General anesthetics. In L. M. Haddad & J. F. Winchester (Eds.), *Clinical management of poisoning and drug overdose* (2d ed., pp. 762–763). Toronto: W.B. Saunders Company.

Agency, E. P. (2012). Where can i find asbestos and when can it be a problem? Retrieved from http://www.epa.gov/asbestos/pubs/ashome.html.

Agency, E. P. (2010). Impacts of life-stage exposures to BPA and phthalates on growth and development. *bpa_action_plan.pdf*. Retrieved from http://www.epa.gov

American Academy of Pediatrics Section on Breastfeeding. Breastfeeding and the use of human milk. Pediatrics. Published online Feb 27, 2012. Retrieved from http://pediatrics.aappublications.org/content/early/2012/02/22/peds.2011-3552

Astley, S. J., & Little, R. E. (1990). Maternal marijuana use during lactation and infant development at one year. *Neurotoxicology and teratology, 12*(2), 161–168.

Bachour, P., Yafawi, R., Jaber, F., Choueiri, E., Abdel-Razzak, Z. (2012). Effects of smoking, mother's age, body mass index, and parity number on lipid, protein and secretory immunoglobulin A concentrations of human milk. *Breastfeeding Medicine*, December 2011 (advance online publication).

Bartu, A., Dusci, L. J., & Ilett, K. F. (2009). Transfer of methylamphetamine and amphetamine into breast milk following recreational use of methylamphetamine. *British Journal of Clinical Pharmacology, 67*(4), 455-459. doi: 10.1111/j.1365-2125.2009.03366.x

Becker, A. B., Manfreda, J., Ferguson, A. C., Dimich-Ward, H., Watson, W. T., & Chan-Yeung, M. (1999). Breast-feeding and environmental tobacco smoke exposure. *Archives of Pediatrics & Adolescent Medicine, 153*(7), 689–691.

Begg, E. J., Malpas, T. J., Hackett, L. P., & Ilett, K. F. (2001). Distribution of R- and S-methadone into human milk during multiple, medium to high oral dosing. *British Journal of Clinical Pharmacology, 52*(6), 681–685.

Blinick, G., Inturrisi, C. E., Jerez, E., & Wallach, R. C. (1975). Methadone assays in pregnant women and progeny. *American Journal of Obstetrics and Gynecology, 121*(5), 617–621.

Caraccio, T. R., & McFee, R. B. (2007). Cosmetics and toilet articles. In M. W. Shannon, S. W. Borron, & M. J. Burns (Eds.), *Haddad and Winchester's clinical management of poisoning and drug overdose* (4th ed., pp. 1–18). Philadelphia, PA: Saunders Elsevier.

CDC. (2012). What should a breastfeeding woman do if she has been exposed to Anthrax? Retrieved from http://www.cdc.gov/breastfeeding/disease/anthrax.htm

Centers for Disease Control and Prevention. (2011). Breastfeeding and tobacco use. Retrieved from http://www.cdc.gov/breastfeeding/disease/tobacco.htm

Chaney, N. E., Franke, J., & Wadlington, W. B. (1988). Cocaine convulsions in a breast-feeding baby. *Journal of Pediatrics, 112*(1), 134–135.

Chasnoff, I. J., Lewis, D. E., & Squires, L. (1987). Cocaine intoxication in a breast-fed infant. *Pediatrics, 80*(6), 836–838.

Chatzimichael A, Tsalkidis A, Cassimos D et al. (2007). The role of breastfeeding and passive smoking on the development of severe bronchiolitis in infants. *Minerva Pediatrics, 59*(3), 199–206.

Dahlstrom, A., Ebersjo, C., & Lundell, B. (2008). Nicotine in breast milk influences heart rate variability in the infant. *Acta Paediatrica, 97*(8), 1075-1079. doi: 10.1111/j.1651-2227.2008.00785.x

Dahlstrom, A., Lundell, B., Curvall, M., & Thapper, L. (1990). Nicotine and cotinine concentrations in the nursing mother and her infant. *Acta Paediatrica Scandinavica, 79*(2), 142–147.

da-Silva, V. A., Malheiros, L. R., Moraes-Santos, A. R., Barzano, M. A., & McLean, A. E. (1993). Ethanol pharmacokinetics in lactating women. *Brazilian Journal of Medical and Biological Research, 26*(10), 1097–1103.

Domingo, J. L. (1995). Reproductive and developmental toxicity of aluminum: A review. *Neurotoxicology and Teratology, 17*(4), 515–521.

Dydek, G. B. (1988). Human breast milk excretion of iodine following diagnostic and therapeutic administration to a lactating patient with Graves' disease. *Journal of Nuclear Medicine, 29*(3), 407–410.

Ellenhorn, M. (1978). Medical toxicology: A primer for the medicolegal age. *Clinical Toxicology, 13*(4), 439–462.

Environmental Protection Agency. (2010). Consumer's guide to radon reduction. Retrieved from http://www.epa.gov/radon/pubs/consguid.html

Environmental Protection Agency. (2011). Indoor air: Carbon monoxide (CO). Retrieved from http://www.epa.gov/iaq/co.html

Fisher, J., Bankston, L., Greene, R., & Gearhart, J. (1997). Lactational transfer of volatile chemicals in breast milk. *American Industrial Hygiene Association Journal, 58*(6), 425–431.

Fung, E. B. (1997). Zinc absorption in women during pregnancy and lactation: A longitudinal study. *American Journal of Clinical Nutrition, 66*(1), 80–88.

Gelberg, K. H. (2009). Lead exposure among target shooters. *Archives of Environmental and Occupational Health, 64*(2), 115–120.

Gladen, B. R., Rogan, W. J., Hardy, P., Thullen, J., Tingelstad, J., & Tully, M. (1988). Development after exposure to polychlorinated biphenyls and dichlorodiphenyl transplacentally and through human milk. *Journal of Pediatrics, 113*, 991–995.

Glatstein, M. M., Garcia-Bournissen, F., Finkelstein, Y., & Koren, G. (2008). Methadone exposure during lactation. *Canadian Family Physician/Medecin de famille canadien, 54*(12), 1689–1690.

Hale, T. W. (2010). *Medications and mothers' milk* (14th ed.). Amarillo, TX: Hale Publishing.

Hines, E. C., Silva, M. J., Medola, P., & Fenton, S. E. (2009). Concentrations of phthalate metabolites in milk, urine, saliva, and serum of lactating North Caolina women. *Environmental Health Perspectives, 117*(1), 86–92.

Howdeshell, K. F., Lambright, C. R., Wilson, V. S., Ryan, B. C., & Gray, L. E. (2008). Gestational and lactational exposure to ethinyl estradiol, but not bisphenol A, decreases androgen-dependent reproductive organ weights and epididymal sperm abundance in the male Long-Evans hooded rat. *Toxicological Sciences, 102*(2), 371–382.

Ilett, K. F., Hale, T. W., Page-Sharp, M., Kristensen, J. H., Kohan, R., & Hackett, L. P. (2003). Use of nicotine patches in breast-feeding mothers: transfer of nicotine and cotinine into human milk. *Clinical Pharmacology and Therapeutics, 74*(6), 516–524. doi: 10.1016/j.clpt.2003.08.003

Jacobsen, J. J., & Humphrey, H. E. B. (1990). Effects of in utero exposure to polychlorinated biphenyls and related contaminants on cognitive functioning in young children. *Journal of Pediatrics, 116*, 38–45.

Jansson, L. M., Choo, R., Velez, M. L., Harrow, C., Schroeder, J. R., Shakleya, D. M., & Huestis, M. A. (2008). Methadone maintenance and breastfeeding in the neonatal period. *Pediatrics, 121*(1), 106–114. doi: 10.1542/peds.2007-1182

Karmaus, W. D., Kruse, H., Witten, J., & Osiua, N. (2001). Early childhood determinants of organochlorine concentrations in school age children. *Pediatric Research, 50*, 331–336.

Kaufman, K. R., Petrucha, R. A., Pitts, F. N., Jr., & Weekes, M. E. (1983). PCP in amniotic fluid and breast milk: case report. *Journal of Clinical Psychiatry, 44*(7), 269–270.

Kim, S. R., Halden, R. U., & Buckley, T. J. (2007). Volatile organic compounds in human milk: Methods and measurements. *Environmental Science and Technology, 41*(5), 1662–1667.

Koopman-Esseboom, C. M., Weisglas-Kuperus, N., Lutkeschipholt, I. J., et al. (1994). Effects of dioxins and polychlorinated biphenyls on thyroid hormone status of pregnant women and their infants. *Pediatric Research, 36*, 468–473.

Krebs, N. R., Hartley, S., Robertson, A. D., & Hambridge, K. M. (1995). Zinc supplementation during lactation: Effects on maternal status and milk zinc concentrations. *American Journal of Clinical Nutrition, 61*(5), 1030–1036.

Kreuzer, P. C., Baur, C., Kessler, W., Papke, O., & Greim, H. (1997). Tetrachlorodibenzo-p-dioxin (TCDD) and congeners in infants. A toxicokinetic model of human lifetime body burden by TCDD with special emphasis on its uptake by nutrition. *Archives of Toxicology, 71*, 383–400.

Kuiper, S., Muris, J. W., & Dompeling, E. (2007). Interactive effect of family history and environmental factors on respiratory tract-related morbidity in infancy. *Journal of Allergy Clinicians Immunology, 120*(2), 388–395.

Kumar, A., Baroth, A., Soni, I., Bhatnagar, P., & John, P. J. (2005). Organochlorine pesticide residues in milk and blood of women from Anupgarh, Rajasthan, India. *Environmental Monitoring and Assessment, 116*, 1–7.

LaKind, J. B., Sjödin, A., Turner, W., Wang, R. Y., Needham, L. L., Paul, I. M., Stokes, J. L., Naiman, D. Q., & Patterson, D. G., Jr. (2009). Do human milk concentrations of persistent organic chemicals really decline during lactation? Chemical concentrations during lactation and milk/serum partitioning. *Environmental Health Perspectives, 117*(10), 1625–1631.

Li, P. H., Wang, Q. Y., Gu, L. Y., & Wang, Y. L. (2000). Transfer of lead via placenta and breast milk in human. *Biomedical and Environmental Sciences, 13*(2), 85–89.

Lim, J. H., Davis, G. E., Wang, Z., Li, V., Wu, Y., Rue, T. C., & Storm, D. R. (2009). Zicam-induced damage to mouse and human nasal tissue. *PLoS One, 4*(10), e7647.

Manton, W. A., Stanek, K. L., Kuntzelman, D., Reese, Y. R., & Kuehnemann, T. J. (2009). Release of lead from bone in pregnancy and lactation. *Environmental Research, 92*, 139–151.

Mennella, J. A. (2001). Regulation of milk intake after exposure to alcohol in mothers' milk. *Alcoholism, Clinical and Experimental Research, 25*(4), 590–593.

Nafstad, P. (1996). Breastfeeding, maternal smoking and lower respiratory tract infections. *European Respiratory Journal, 9*, 2623–2629.

Newbold, R. J., & Padilla-Banks, E. (2009). Prenatal exposure to bisphenol A at environmentally relevant doses adversely affects the murine female reproductive tract later in life. *Environmental Health Perspectives, 117*(6), 879–885.

Nicholas, J. M., Lipshitz, J., & Schreiber, E. C. (1982). Phencyclidine: Its transfer across the placenta as well as into breast milk. *American Journal of Obstetrics and Gynecology, 143*(2), 143–146.

Nickerson, K. (2006). Environmental contaminants in breast milk. *American College of Nurse-Midwives, 51*(1), 26–34.

Ohta, H. I., & Seki, Y. (2002). Effects of cadmium intake on bone metabolism of mothers during pregnancy and lactation. *Tohoku Journal of Experimental Medicine, 196*(1), 33–42.

Oskarsson, A. S., Skerfving, S., Hallen, I. P., Ohlin, B., & Lagerkvist, B. J. (1990). Total and inorganic mercury in breast milk in relation to fish consumption and amalgam in lactating women. *Archives of Environmenatl Health, 51*(3), 234–241.

Palmer, K. (1979). Excretion of 1251 in breast milk following administration of labelled fibrinogen. *British Journal of Radiology, 52*(620), 672–673.

Papke, O. (1998). PCDD/PCDF: Human background data for Germany, a 10-year experience. *Environmental Health Perspectives, 106*(Suppl. 2), 723–731.

Patadin, S. L., Mulder, P. G. H., Boersma, E. R., Sauer, P. J. J., & Weisglas-Kuperus, N. (1999). Effects of environmental exposure to polychlorinated biphenyls and dioxins on cognitive abilities in Dutch children at 42 months of age. *Journal of Pediatrics, 134*, 33–41.

Perez-Reyes, M., & Wall, M. E. (1982). Presence of delta9-tetrahydrocannabinol in human milk. *New England Journal of Medicine, 307*(13), 819–820. doi: 10.1056/NEJM198209233071311

Pickin, R. B., Filer, L. J., & Reynolds, W. A. (2000). Mercury in human maternal and cord blood, placenta, and milk. *Pediatrics, 106*(4), 774–781.

Ramirez, G. C., Pagulayan, O., Ostrea, E., & Dalisay, C. (2000). The Tagum study 1: Analysis and clinical correlates of mercury in maternal and cord blood, breast milk, meconium, and infant's hair. *Pediatrics, 106*(4), 774–781.

Robinson, P. B., Campbell, A., Henson, P., Surveyor, I., & Young, P. R. (1994). Iodine in breast milk following therapy for thyroid carcinoma. *Journal of Nuclear Medicine, 35*(11), 1797–1801.

Ryan, B. C. H., Crofton, K. M., & Gray, L. E., Jr. (2010). In utero and lactational exposure to bisphenol A, in contrast to ethinyl estradiol, does not alter sexually dimorphic behavior, puberty, fertility and anatomy of female LE rats. *Toxicological Sciences, 114*(1), 133–148.

Sarkar, M., Djulus, J., & Koren, G. (2005). When a cocaine-using mother wishes to breastfeed: proposed guidelines. *Therapeutic Drug Monitoring, 27*(1), 1–2.

Semple, J. L., Baines, C. J., Smith, D. C., & McHugh, A. (1998). Breast milk contamination and silicone implant: Preliminary results using silicon as proxy measurement for silicone. *Plastic and Reconstrive Surgery, 102*(2), 528–533.

Smialek, J. E., Monforte, J. R., Aronow, R., & Spitz, W. U. (1977). Methadone deaths in children. A continuing problem. *JAMA: Journal of the American Medical Association, 238*(23), 2516–2517.

Smith, D. (1999). Worldwide trends in DDT levels in human breast milk. *International Journal of Epidemiology, 28,* 179–188.

Sudak, N., & Harvie, J. (2007). Reducing toxic exposures. In D. Rakel (Ed.), *Integrative medicine* (2nd ed., pp. 1–3). Philadelphia, PA: Saunders.

Toms, L. M., Harden, F., Paepke, O., Hobson, P., Ryan, J. J., & Mueller, J. F. (2008). Higher accumulation of polybrominated diphenyl ethers in infants than in adults. *Environmental Science and Technology, 42*(19), 7510–7515.

Winecker, R. E., Goldberger, B. A., Tebbett, I. R., Behnke, M., Eyler, F. D., Karlix, J. L., . . . Bertholf, R. L. (2001). Detection of cocaine and its metabolites in breast milk. *Journal of Forensic Sciences, 46*(5), 1221–1223.

Woodward, A. (1990). Acute respiratory illness in Adelaide children: breast feeding modifies the effect of passive smoking. *Journal of Epidemiology and Community Health, 44,* 224–30.

Woodward, A., Grgurinovich, N., & Ryan, P. (1986). Breast feeding and smoking hygiene: major influences on cotinine in urine of smokers' infants. *Journal of Epidemiology and Community Health, 40*(4), 309–315.

Yilmaz, G., Hizli, S., Karacan, C., Yurdakok, K., Coskun, T., & Dilmen, U. (2009). Effect of passive smoking on growth and infection rates of breast-fed and non-breast-fed infants. *Pediatrics International: Official Journal of the Japan Pediatric Society, 51*(3), 352–358. doi: 10.1111/j.1442-200X.2008.02757.x

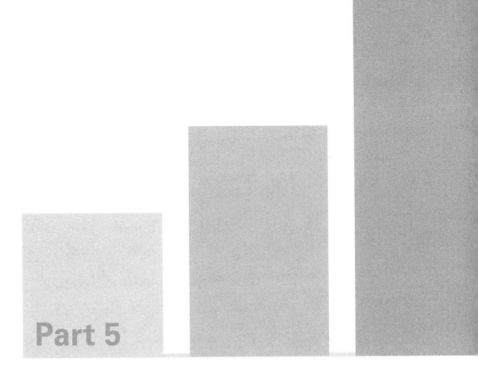

Part 5

Breastfeeding Technique

CHAPTER 27
Assessment of Infant Oral Anatomy

Barbara Wilson-Clay, BSEd, IBCLC, FILCA

OBJECTIVES

- Identify key aspects of assessment of infant orofacial structures and oral motor functions.
- Identify abnormal infant oral anatomy and discuss its effect on breastfeeding.
- List the oral feeding reflexes and describe their abnormal presentations.
- Discuss coordination of the suck-swallow-breathe (SSB) triad and its importance in breastfeeding.
- Discuss the issue of the "fit" between the infant's oral anatomy and the mother's breast.

INTRODUCTION

This chapter provides an overview of the structures and function of the face and mouth that influence feeding behavior and later dentition, speech, and appearance. An understanding of normal appearance and function helps identify abnormal presentations so that clinicians can develop timely, evidence-based interventions for at-risk dyads (Bosma, 1977; Genna, 2008; Lawrence et al., 2011; Merkel-Piccini et al., 2003; Ogg, 1975).

I. Overview

A. Oral assessment of the breastfeeding infant begins after global assessments have been made during which the lactation consultant (LC) observes the infant's tone and color, state behavior, side-to-side symmetry, and respiration. Oral assessment then focuses on the following items:
  1. Observation of the infant's orofacial anatomy
     a. Lips, cheeks, jaws, tongue, palate, and nasal passages
  2. Identification of abnormal infant oral anatomy and consideration of how it might contribute to dysfunctional feeding behavior

3. Observation of infant feeding reflexes and their abnormal presentations
   a. Review the rooting reflex, the sucking reflex (including absent suck, weak suck, and uncoordinated suck), the swallowing reflex, the gag reflex, and the cough reflex.
   b. Describe nutritive suck (NS) and nonnutritive suck (NNS; Mizuno & Ueda, 2006).
4. Observation of the effectiveness of feeding (coordination of the suck-swallow-breathe triad; Bamford et al., 1992)
5. Observation of the "fit" between the infant's mouth and the mother's nipple

II. Anatomy of the Infant's Oral Cavity

A. Importance
   1. Feeding, respiration, dentition, and speech are influenced by the anatomy of the mouth.
   2. The tone and functioning of the muscles of the face, neck, and trunk affect feeding.
   3. Some aspects of oral anatomy change with maturation and growth or can be surgically corrected (Bosma, 1977).
   4. Sometimes orofacial structures change as the infant recovers from minor injury (for example, bruising during birth or trauma related to instrument delivery) (Caughey et al., 2005).
   5. Orofacial structure and function can be impaired by injury ((Smith et al., 1981), congenital malformation, neurological deficits, prematurity, or illness.
      a. Impairment can negatively affect breastfeeding.
      b. The presence of these factors in a case signal the need for more focused assessment and might identify a dyad in need of greater lactation support (Genna, 2008; Ogg, 1975; Wolf et al., 1992).
B. Lips (Morris, 1977; Ogg, 1975; Wolf et al., 1992)
   1. The infant uses the lips to draw in the nipple and stabilize it in the mouth.
   2. Lips are normally intact, with no evidence of a cleft, and appear mobile, well defined, and expressive.
   3. The lips flange and seal smoothly around the breast during breastfeeding.
   4. Abnormal presentations:
      a. Weak lip tone
         i. Hypotonic lip tone results in weak ability of the lips to seal around the breast. This can impair the amount of suction that the infant can generate. Because the infant keeps losing the seal and having to re-form it, the work of feeding increases. Feeding becomes inefficient and tiring, resulting in reduced infant intake.
         ii. Weak lip seal can result in a loss of liquid during feeding (milk spilling).
         iii. Weak lip tone reflects poor motor/muscular control of the lips and might be revealed as intermittent breaks in suction (smacking sounds).

      iv. Low muscle tone or weakness (owing to prematurity, muscular weakness, or illness) creates stamina deficits that impair the baby's ability to maintain lip seal. Ideally, an entire feeding is observed to detect stamina-related problems that might occur only late in the feeding, increasing risk of fatigue aspiration.

    b. Abnormal tongue movements and abnormally wide jaw excursions can cause breaks in lip seal. Although not directly involving the lips, these problems can affect lip seal.

    c. Tight labial frenum (a growth of the tissue that attaches the upper lip to the upper gum):

      i. Classified (similar to tongue-tie) as a minor midline congenital defect, a tight labial frenum can affect dentition and formation of dental caries (Kotlow, 2010).

      ii. The forward attached frenum creates a gap between the front teeth.

      iii. If the upper labial frenum is nonelastic, it can contribute to lip retraction during breastfeeding. The retracted lips can cause friction trauma that damages the mother's nipples. The inability to flange the upper lip normally was reported in one case as a factor contributing to breastfeeding difficulty (Wiessinger et al., 1995).

    d. Excessive lip tone:

      i. Hypertonic lip tone or reliance on increased lip activity to hold the breast in the mouth might reflect neurological abnormality or injury of the tongue, jaws, or facial nerves (Smith et al., 1981).

      ii. If tongue or jaw function is impaired, or facial nerves are injured, the baby might compensate by using increased lip activity to hold onto the breast.

    e. "Purse string lips" inhibit the ability of the infant to open the lips to allow objects into the mouth.

      i. They are also revealed as a pulling up at the corners of the mouth and increased tension around the lips.

      ii. Hypertonic lips can be a marker for neurological involvement (Wilson-Clay et al., 2005).

    f. Cleft lip:

      i. A relatively common congenital midline defect generally repaired in the early postpartum.

      ii. Although disfiguring, cleft lip does not significantly interfere with successful breastfeeding (Garcez et al., 2005).

5. Assessment of the lips:

    a. Visually assess a feeding (ideally an entire feeding) to observe whether the infant can seal the lips smoothly around the breast and maintain the seal during feeding without evidence of early fatigue.

    b. Observe the shape of the lips. A bow-shaped upper lip with a well-defined philtrum generally indicates normal lip tone.

    c. Observe for the presence of a tight upper labial frenum.

d. Listen for breaks in the seal while the infant feeds.

e. Observe for lip retraction and lip tremors.

f. Observe for leaking milk (during both breast and alternative feeding).

g. Apply gentle digital pressure against the lips; some resistance to this pressure should be felt.

h. Note uncommon events:
   i. In infants younger than 3 months of age, drooling is associated with weak control of swallowing (even of the infant's own saliva) or can reveal pharyngeal or esophageal obstruction (Riordan, 2005).
   ii. Observe the baby while crying for signs of neonatal asymmetric crying facies—a relatively common condition (1 per 160 live births) marked by asymmetrical lip movement seen only when the baby cries (Sapin et al., 2005).

i. Identify the presence of sucking blisters.
   i. Sucking blisters are caused by friction abrasion resulting from retracted lips during breastfeeding (or by a tight upper labial frenum that restricts upper lip flanging).

6. Methods of assisting when the feeding problem results from structural abnormalities or abnormal tone of the lips:

a. Use firm pressure stimulus (tapping, stretching) of the lips prior to feeding to improve tone and strengthen lip seal (Alper et al.,1996).

b. Insert a clean finger or a round, somewhat firm pacifier and partially pull it out of the baby's mouth to induce the baby to pull it back. This exercises and strengthens the ability of the lips to grip objects.

c. Mimic "open wide" mouth positions to encourage the infant to imitate lip movement.

d. Observe the infant for stress cues when engaging in these activities and discontinue when the infant becomes fatigued.

e. Teach the mother of an infant with a cleft lip to use a finger or breast tissue to seal the cleft.

f. Refer to speech-language pathologists or occupational therapists for assessment and remediation.
   i. Communicate with cleft lip/palate teams to facilitate support for human milk feeds.

g. Share research that documents the fact that postoperative breastfeeding after cleft lip repair is safe and results in better weight gain than does bottle-feeding (Darzi et al., 1996; Weatherly-White et al., 1987).

h. Demonstrate to the mother how to use her fingertip to gently pull back on the skin above the baby's upper lip to correct lip retraction. The mother can manually flange the lip as often as needed, especially if lip retraction causes nipple pain. Refer to appropriate specialists for evaluation if a tight labial frenum appears to require release to facilitate breastfeeding.

i. Reassure parents that lip tone typically improves as the infant matures and grows. This tends to be the case even if the underlying cause is an enduring neurological disorder or is related to a structural abnormality.

C. Cheeks (Genna, 2008; Wolf et al., 1992)

1. Facial tone influences oral function.

   a. Subcutaneous fat deposits in the cheeks help provide structural support for infant oral and pharyngeal activity.

   b. Fat pads give the baby a "puffy cheek" appearance and should be visible for 6 to 8 months (Wolf et al., 1992).

2. Poorly developed fat pads (owing to prematurity or low birth weight) and thin cheeks affect facial tone.

   a. Low or weak tone can cause the infant to experience difficulty in creating and sustaining adequate levels of suction.

3. Abnormal presentation of the cheeks:

   a. Weak cheek tone/thin cheeks

      i. Facial hypotonia (low tone) and weakness contribute to poor cheek stability.

      ii. The cheeks influence lip seal; low facial tone makes it harder for the infant to use the lips normally.

      iii. Thin cheeks mean that the infant's intraoral space is larger than would normally be the case. The infant must therefore create a larger vacuum to generate and sustain suction, so the work of feeding is increased. The infant can fatigue early before finishing feedings.

4. Assessment of the cheeks (Wilson-Clay et al., 2005; Wolf et al., 1992):

   a. Digitally assess the subcutaneous fat deposits in the cheeks by placing a gloved finger inside the infant's mouth and a thumb on the outside of the cheek to sense the thickness of the fat pads.

      i. Performing this examination on a number of babies gives the examiner the awareness that dimensions of fat pads vary, but in babies with thin cheeks, the fingers almost touch.

   b. Observe the shape of the cheeks at rest and during feeding.

      i. Identify deep creases under the infant's eyes as a marker for thin cheeks.

   c. If the cheeks are weak, thin, or unstable, they will collapse while sucking. Identify cheek collapsing (revealed by dimpling).

   d. Observe the duration of feeds for infant fatigue.

      i. Early discontinuation of feeds owing to fatigue is a risk factor for poor infant intake and poor stimulation of milk production. (Test weights are confirmatory; Sachs et al., 2002).

5. Methods of assisting when feeding problems or slow growth result from thin cheeks or low facial muscle tone (Wilson-Clay et al., 2005):

   a. Use external counterpressure applied to the cheeks during feeding (the so-called Dancer's hand technique) to improve cheek stability (Danner, 1992; Wilson-Clay et al., 2005, p. 175, Figs. 357–358).

    b. Supplement (ideally with own mother's milk) to improve infant growth. As the fat pads develop in the cheeks, facial stability will improve, contributing to improvement in breastfeeding ability.

D. Jaws (Palmer, 1993; Wilson-Clay et al., 2005; Wolf et al., 1992)

    1. The jaws provide stability for the movements of the tongue, lips, and cheeks.

    2. Some degree of mandibular retrognathia (receding lower jaw) is characteristic in infants. Dramatic forward growth usually occurs during the first 4 months of life (Ranley, 1998).

    3. Normal jaw movements are neither too wide nor too narrow during feeding; opening and closing motions are smooth, graded, and regular.

    4. Preterm infants often have jaw instability owing to immature muscles and low muscle tone (which is characteristic for preterm babies; Palmer, 1993).

    5. Abnormal presentations of the jaw:

        a. Micrognathia: An abnormally receding chin that can be familial, is associated with chromosomal disorders, or can result from intrauterine positioning that prevents the jaw from growing forward (as in certain breech presentations)

            i. Severe micrognathia positions the tongue posteriorly, where it can obstruct the airway as in Pierre Robin syndrome (Bull et al., 1990).

            ii. A receding jaw can contribute to sore nipples unless the infant's head is tipped back in a slightly extended position to bring the chin closer to the breast.

            iii. Jaw asymmetry contributes to poor jaw function and unstable feeding, including inability to breastfeed. It can be caused by birth injury, asymmetrical muscle tone (i.e., torticollis), injury, paralysis, breech position, or structural deformity (Wall et al., 2006). Note how the face of the infant in **Figure 27-1** droops to the right. Her jaw asymmetry and low facial tone contributed to inefficient feeding and failure to thrive.

        b. Abnormally wide jaw excursions

            i. Poor grading of the jaw movements can cause breaks in the seal formed at the breast, resulting in loss of suction and increased work of feeding. Intake may be decreased.

        c. Jaw clenching

            i. Sometimes infants clench their jaws as a strategy to manage rapid milk flow. If clenching to manage milk flow is ruled out, jaw clench or thrusting generally reflects hypertonia. It also can be a compensatory action resulting from weakness in another area (for example, poor tongue function or low lip tone that forces the baby to overuse the jaws to hold in the nipple). Clenching contributes to sore nipples/breasts.

    6. Assessment of the jaws:

        a. Observe for asymmetry.

        b. Identify micrognathia.

        c. Observe breastfeeding to identify jaw grading, clenching, or tremors.

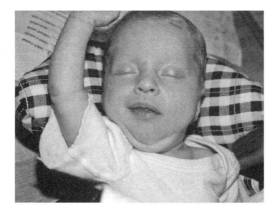

Figure 27-1 Facial asymmetry and low facial tone.

Source: Reproduced with permission from Barbara Wilson-Clay.

    d. Insert a gloved (pinkie, or "little") finger in the corner of the infant's mouth between the gum pads.

        i. Count the number of reflexive bites (chews) elicited.

        ii. The infant should respond with approximately 10 little chews on each side.

        iii. Observe for difficulty producing these reflexive bites or for infant stress cues during this assessment.

        iv. Weakness of the jaw is revealed by inability to perform the activity (Palmer, 1993).

  7. Methods of assisting when the feeding problem relates to abnormalities, weakness, or injury involving the jaws:

    a. Provide external jaw support with a finger placed under the bony part of the lower jaw to control and stabilize the distance of jaw excursions.

    b. Hip flexion and stabilization of the infant's trunk facilitates stable feeding (Redstone et al., 2004).

    c. For a minute or so at each feeding time, exercise the jaws (using the same assessment method described previously to elicit an increased number of reflexive bites). Avoid stressing the infant.

    d. Position the infant carefully and maintain head extension as a strategy for bringing the lower jaw closer to the breast.

    e. Refer the infant for physical therapy, occupational therapy, or infant massage if issues relating to abnormal muscular tension impinge on jaw activity.

    f. Work carefully to identify feeding positions that emphasize postural stability. Side-lying feeding positions are useful.

E. Tongue (Palmer, 1993; Wolf et al., 1992)

  1. Normally soft, thin, and mobile, with a rounded tip and good tone. The infant uses the tongue with the lips to draw in the nipple.

  2. Assists the lips in helping to seal the oral cavity. When the infant cheek is pulled back, a small section of cupped tongue is visible at the corners of the mouth during breastfeeding.

3. In relation to the hard tissue of the mouth, the rest position of the tongue shapes the structures around it. Therefore, the tongue affects dentition and speech (Merkel-Piccini et al., 2003).

4. Ramsay's work (2004a) suggests that suction is the primary mechanism of milk extraction during breastfeeding, although other lactation physiologists describe a dynamic interplay between suction and positive pressure from the tongue. Whatever mechanism is found to predominate, the tone and mobility of the tongue is critical to milk removal.

5. The tongue must be able to lift freely and thin the mother's nipple against the hard palate so that with each subsequent drop of the tongue, there is an adequate enlargement of the oral cavity to create negative pressure (Ramsay, Langton, et al., 2004).

6. The tongue forms a central groove that provides a channel that organizes the bolus of milk for safe swallowing.

7. The tongue tip extends over the lower gum ridge, providing a degree of padding during breastfeeding that helps protect the mother's nipples.

8. When the tongue moves improperly, the baby cannot suck, swallow, or breathe efficiently. The work of feeding increases in such instances, putting the baby at risk for early discontinuation of feeds and limited intake; there is also a risk of poor breast emptying.

9. Limitations in the mobility or strength of the tongue require the infant to use compensatory activities to feed. Compensations might involve increased jaw activity (clenching) or lip retraction. The mother may describe the suck as "strong" when actually it is weak. It is the baby's compensations that often damage the nipples.

10. Abnormal presentations of the tongue:

    a. Ankyloglossia (tongue-tie)

        i. A congenital midline anomaly in which the bottom of the tongue is attached to the floor of the mouth by a membrane (the lingual frenulum) that limits the range of motion of the tongue (Fernando, 1998; Lalakea et al., 2003; Messner et al., 2000).

        ii. Typically there is a "heart shaped" appearance to the tongue tip; however, one variety of tongue-tie consists of a nonelastic posterior adhesion of the tongue to the floor of the mouth. This is more difficult to visualize, but healthcare providers should be aware of the extent to which it can interfere with breastfeeding (Coryllos et al., 2004; Hong et al., 2010).

        iii. Incidence of ankyloglossia ranges between 0.02% and 5% of infants, occurring more commonly in males. Typically, it is an isolated anatomic variation and can run in families. It appears with increased frequency in association with various congenital syndromes (Flinck et al., 1994; Lalakea et al., 2003; Ricke et al., 2005).

        iv. Some infants can breastfeed without difficulty (Messner et al., 2000).

      v. May affect maternal comfort during breastfeeding, and may impair effective milk removal with resultant ill effect on milk production and risk of failure to thrive in the infant (Ballard et al., 2004; Forlenza et al., 2010; Neifert, 1999; Powers, 1999).

     vi. Either frenotomy (simple release achieved by clipping the lingual frenulum) or frenulectomy/frenuloplasty (resectioning of the tongue) is curative and changes the sucking dynamics of the breastfeeding infant (Ramsay, Langton, et al., 2004).

       (a) Frenotomy is often performed without anesthesia as an office procedure and has a high satisfaction rate and few complications (Amir et al., 2005).

       (b) Frenulectomy and frenuloplasty are more involved surgical procedures with a longer recovery period but appear to be successful in remediating significant ankyloglossia (Ballard et al., 2004).

  b. A bunched or retracted tongue

    i. May be caused by abnormally high muscle tone or by ankyloglossia

  c. Tongue protrusion

    i. May result from abnormal tongue development (large tongue) or low muscle tone (as in Down syndrome). Tongue protrusion contributes to poor coordination of sucking and swallowing.

  d. Tongue-tip elevation

    i. Tongue-tip elevation can make insertion of the nipple frustrating and difficult.

    ii. Touch to the tongue tip results in reflexive tongue extrusion, causing the baby to keep pushing objects out of the mouth.

  e. Tongue asymmetry

    i. Tongue asymmetry can result from injury (such as forceps trauma that damages the nerves controlling the tongue) (Smith et al., 1981).

    ii. Also may be associated with syndromic conditions.

11. Assessment of the tongue:

  a. Sometimes poor infant head position during feeding negatively influences tongue position. Correct the feeding position before evaluating the tongue during feeding.

  b. Visual assessment identifies the shape and position of the tongue and rules out tongue-tie and other abnormal presentations.

  c. Digital exam consists of gentle pressure with a clean, gloved fingertip to the surface of the tongue at midsection. There should be some resistance and the examiner should sense the tongue pressing up against the finger.

  d. Insertion of a finger should elicit sealing and sucking. The lactation consultant should sense the tongue cupping around the finger. The examiner must be careful not to insert the finger too deeply (to avoid triggering a gag reflex).

    e. While the infant is breastfeeding, gently pull the breast away from the cheek and observe the corners of the lips. The side of the tongue should be visible, helping the lips form the seal that preserves suction.

    f. Listen for breaks in seal (revealed by smacking noises).

        i. A weak tongue can interfere with maintaining a seal at breast.

        ii. A normal infant who is struggling with rapid milk flow may deliberately break the seal at breast (with resultant smacking noises).

        iii. In a compromised infant, such sounds often mean that the jaw has dropped so far that the tongue has lost contact with the breast.

        iv. Too-wide jaw excursions and frequent loss of seal usually result in poor milk transfer.

    g. Observe the ability of the infant to lift the tongue past the midline of the mouth with the mouth open wide.

        i. The tongue should lift to the palate.

        ii. Limited lift reveals ankyloglossia, even without the sign of an obviously forward-placed lingual frenulum (Coryllos et al., 2004).

    h. Observe tongue extension by tapping the tongue tip to elicit tongue protrusion.

        i. Can the infant extend the tongue beyond the gum, and ideally the lower lip line? Inhibition of extension may reveal ankyloglossia.

    i. Can the infant lateralize the tongue?

        i. This is another assessment of mobility.

        ii. The tongue should seek the examiner's finger as it moves from side to side.

        iii. Limited lateralization may reveal ankyloglossia.

12. Methods of assisting when the feeding problem results from dysfunction or anomalies of the tongue:

    a. The same exercises that can be used to strengthen the lips can assist in exercising a weak tongue.

    b. Short, frequent feedings allow the baby recovery time if the tongue gets tired.

    c. Positioning the baby with the head in extension brings the lower jaw close in to the breast.

        i. Reducing the distance a short or restricted tongue must reach (to extend over the lower gum ridge) can help protect the nipples from trauma.

    d. Inform the mother of ways to manage nipple trauma (topical cleansing of open cuts, alternating pumping with breastfeeding, etc.).

    e. Refer infant to the pediatrician; family practice doctor; pediatric ear, nose, and throat (ENT) specialist; or to a pediatric dentist for evaluation for release of ankyloglossia.

    f. Occupational therapy or speech and language therapy can facilitate improved function if the tongue is injured, affected by paralysis, recovering from frenuloplasty, or is weak owing to a syndromic condition.

g. Reassure parents that although some infants feed well immediately following simple clips of a tongue-tie, other infants may not breastfeed well until the tongue fully heals.

h. Supplement with pumped milk if needed to stabilize infant growth and protect milk production with pumping as long as necessary.

F. Assessment of the palates (Cleft Palate Foundation, 2006; Glenny et al., 2004; Goldman, 1993; Gorski et al., 1994; Kogo et al., 1997; Paradise et al., 1994; Snyder, 1997; Turner et al., 2001; Wilson-Clay et al., 2005; Wolf et al.,1992)

1. The shape of the palates can be influenced by hereditary and genetic factors or result from circumstances that prevent the normal shaping of the hard palate by the tongue during gestation (such as ankyloglossia or breech position).

   a. **Figure 27-2** shows an infant after a simple frenotomy to clip a forward-placed lingual frenulum. However, baby still demonstrates limited ability to lift the tongue to the upper gum ridge (Coryllos et al., 2004).

   b. Note bubble shape of the hard palate that has resulted from ankyloglossia.

2. Hard palate:

   a. The bony hard palate opposes the tongue, helping to compress the nipple and maintain nipple position in the mouth.

   b. It should be intact with no evidence of a cleft.

   c. The slope should be moderate and smooth and should approximate the shape of the tongue (Merkel-Piccini et al., 2003).

   d. Small, round, white cysts (Epstein's pearls; **Figure 27-3**) are often observed along the ridge of the hard palate (also the gums, where they may be identified as teeth). Although sometimes also mistaken for oral thrush, these cysts are benign, resolve around 2 months of age, and do not interfere with feeding (Riordan, 2005).

3. Soft palate:

   a. The soft palate is a muscle that works with the tongue to create a posterior seal of the oral cavity, permitting the creation of suction.

   b. It should be intact and elevate during swallowing.

4. Abnormal presentations of the hard and soft palates:

   a. Abnormalities of the palate make breastfeeding difficult (Lawrence et al., 2011).

   b. Familial high-arched, grooved, or bubble-shaped hard palate makes it difficult for the infant to properly position the nipple and to compress it with the tongue.

   c. Long periods of intubation or syndromic conditions such as Down or Turner syndrome can create grooves in the hard palate, and this may contribute to the higher incidence of breastfeeding problems experienced in these populations of infants (Lawrence et al., 2011). Later, food or other chewed objects can become trapped in the channel or bubble (Rovet, 1995).

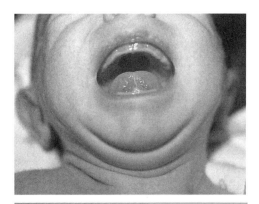

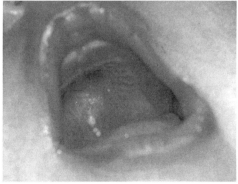

Figure 27-2 Bubble palate (note limited tongue elevation).

Source: Reproduced with permission from Wilson-Clay, Barbara, & Hoover, Kay. (2008). *The breastfeeding atlas*. Austin, TX: LactNews Press.

Figure 27-3 Epstein's Pearls on the palate (sometimes mistaken for thrush).

Source: Reproduced with permission from Wilson-Clay, Barbara, & Hoover, Kay. (2008). *The breastfeeding atlas*. Austin, TX: LactNews Press.

 5. Cleft palate:
   a. A common congenital midline defect with an incidence of 1 in 600–800 births. Clefts are more common in Native Americans, Maoris, and Chinese.
   b. Clefts can be unilateral or bilateral and are classified as partial or incomplete, or complete.
      i. A partial or incomplete cleft is isolated.
      ii. A complete cleft extends from the lip to the soft palate and may also involve the nose.
   c. Regardless of the size, clefts of the hard or soft palate make it difficult or impossible for the infant to fully breastfeed because the baby is unable to seal the oral cavity to generate suction, which negatively affects infant growth and milk production.
   d. Some infants with wide palatal clefts have additional swallowing problems owing to problems with intraoral muscular movements. There is no palatal back guard for tongue movements (Lawrence et al., 2011).
   e. Palatal obturators are a prosthetic device that can increase feeding efficiency in infants with clefts (Kogo et al., 1997; Turner et al., 2001). Masarei et al. (2007) reported that such presurgical devices did not improve feeding efficiency. Consequently, in regions where bottle-feeding is safer owing to access to clean water for washing up and refrigeration, obturators are seldom used. In case reports from the developing world, improved early feeding ability is mentioned as a rationale for the use of palatal prostheses (Radojicic et al., 2009; Sultana et al., 2011). Additionally, use of palatal devices with the most severe types of alveolar and palatal clefts appears to evoke growth of the palate, reducing the area requiring surgical closure and enhancing outcomes (Tomita et al., 2010).

f. An infant with a cleft may feed constantly, mostly sleeping at breast. Intake must be empirically assessed with test weights on an accurate scale, and growth should be carefully monitored. Infants with cleft defects require careful growth monitoring because they are at increased risk for failure to thrive as the result of underlying increased metabolic need (Lawrence et al., 2011).

g. Feeding tube devices and specially designed bottles can assist, but considerable experimentation is often needed to find a method of feeding that ensures adequate growth. Feedings are slow and often stressful, owing to aspiration (Glenny et al., 2004).

h. Submucosal clefts:

   i. Defects of the closure of the shelves of the hard palate are difficult to identify, owing to the presence of a layer of skin that has grown over the cleft.

   ii. Shining a light on the palate reveals a translucent area on the palate that identifies a submucosal cleft (that is, one can see the cleft under the skin).

i. A family history of cleft lip or cleft lip and palate should cue the lactation consultant to examine the palate more carefully.

6. Weak soft palate:

   a. Because the palate is a muscle, generalized low muscle tone (resulting from prematurity or a syndromic condition) can affect soft palate function.

   b. Poor infant stamina can influence soft palate function. As the infant tires and loses muscle control, the soft palate fails to work with the tongue to effectively seal off the mouth as the baby swallows and breathes.

   c. Adversely affects control of safe swallowing, creating an increased risk of choking known as fatigue aspiration (Wolf et al., 1992).

7. Assessment of the hard and soft palates:

   a. Visual assessment of the palates should identify intact structures and the presence of an uvula.

   b. Bifid (forked) uvula or absent uvula reveals abnormal formation of the soft palate (that is, a cleft of the soft palate).

   c. With a gloved finger, gently slide a fingertip along the hard palate starting just behind the upper gum ridge.

      i. Assess the slope of the hard palate for bony prominences, clefts, or abnormally prominent rugae (ridges).

   d. Observe a feeding and elicit information regarding nasal regurgitation. Nasal regurgitation of milk or excessive nasal stuffiness might reveal a weak soft palate seal (or, more rarely, the presence of a submucosal cleft; Morris, 1977).

8. Methods of assisting when the feeding problem results from abnormalities of the hard and/or soft palates:

   a. Feeding problems related to the abnormal formation of the palates are difficult to correct.

   b. Cleft defects can be corrected surgically at various ages.

   c. Monitor infant intake carefully and supplement with mother's pumped milk or banked milk; the incidence of chronic otitis media (a risk for infants with cleft defects) is reduced when infants are exclusively human-milk fed (Paradise et al., 1994).

    d. Help the mother position the baby for breastfeeding in upright positions such as the seated straddle. Demonstrate chin support to stabilize the latch. Teach breast compression as a method of expressing milk into the baby's mouth (Mohrbacher et al., 2003).

    e. Assist the mother in finding a method of alternative feeding that is effective and does not stress the infant (Wilson-Clay, 2005).

    f. Teach the mother to observe for infant stress cues that will help her feed in a manner that protects the baby from developing feeding aversions (Abadie et al., 2001).

    g. Protect the milk supply by establishing an appropriate pumping schedule.

    h. Refer to appropriate specialists, including cleft palate teams.

G. Nasal passages (Alper et al., 1996; Bosma, 1977; Wilson-Clay, 2005; Wilson-Clay et al., 2005; Wolf et al., 1992)

    1. Although infants typically are nose breathers, they can adapt to mouth breathing if the nasal passages are occluded.

    2. If nasal breathing is impaired, the infant will resist feeding, owing to his or her need to protect mouth breathing.

    3. Nasal congestion (in the absence of symptoms of respiratory illness) can reveal dried accumulations of milk aspirated during feedings.

    4. Nasal stuffiness can be the result of fluid aspirated during reflux episodes.

    5. Abnormal presentations of the nasal passages:

        a. Rarely, abnormally small nasal openings are observed.

            i. Choanal atresia is a congenital condition in which the openings of one or both of the nasal cavities are partially or completely blocked by a bony or membranous occlusion.

        b. Facial bruising (resulting from birth trauma or instrument-assisted delivery) can create swelling of the nose and impair breathing.

    6. Assessing the nasal passages:

        a. The nasal passages should be visually assessed if the infant's breathing sounds congested or if the infant struggles and pulls away gasping while being fed.

        b. Elicit information about birth trauma, instrument-assisted delivery, bruising, nasal regurgitation, and so forth.

    7. Methods to assist an infant with feeding problems related to the nasal passages:

        a. Baby-strength saline nose drops can be useful to help clear the nasal passages. Bulb syringes used to extract nasal debris can increase internal swelling.

        b. Employ external pacing methods during feeding to protect respiratory stability (Wilson-Clay, 2005).

        c. Refer the infant to the primary medical care provider or pediatric ENT specialist for further assessment if a problem related to the nasal passages interferes with feeding.

III. Infant Feeding Reflexes

A. Rooting reflex (Wolf et al., 1992)

1. Helps the baby to locate the nipple.
2. It is stimulated by touch to any part of the head.
   a. Pushing on the head during latch-on can distract the baby from turning toward the nipple.
3. It is present at birth and extinguishes between 2 and 4 months of age, although it can persist longer in breastfed infants.
4. An absent or diminished rooting reflex can signal poor tactile receptivity or poor neural integration.
5. If excessive, a hypersensitive (hyperreactive) rooting reflex can interfere with latching on.
   a. Possible management strategies to assist might include decreasing the other stimuli in the environment, avoiding touching the infant's head, feeding when the infant is sleepy and less aware.

B. Sucking reflex (Premji et al., 2000; Wolf et al., 1992)

1. Observed in utero as early as 15 to 18 weeks gestation.
2. Categorized into two modes: nutritive sucking (NS) and nonnutritive sucking (NNS) (Mizuno et al., 2006). (See also Chapter 18, Anatomy and Physiology of Infant Suckling.)
   a. NS can be effective or ineffective.
3. It is stimulated by pressure (and perhaps chemical receptors) along the tongue and stroking near the junctions of the hard and soft palates.
4. Some infants can sustain effective feeding at 34 to 35 weeks gestational age for brief periods of time. However, preterm infants are at risk for fatigue during feeding and for hospital readmittance secondary to poor feeding (Kramer et al., 2000).
5. Inadequate breast emptying owing to a weakly sucking infant creates a risk of rapid, early downregulation of milk production (Kent et al., 1999).
6. When a weakly sucking infant is identified, careful infant growth monitoring is required.
   a. The infant might require supplementation (ideally with own mother's pumped hindmilk).
   b. Protect the milk supply with pumping (Alper et al., 1996; Hill et al., 2001; Kavanaugh et al., 1995; Scanlon et al., 2002; Valentine et al., 1994).
7. Absent or diminished sucking might indicate central nervous system (CNS) immaturity, prematurity, delayed maturation, CNS maldevelopment (various trisomies), prenatal CNS insults (drugs in labor, asphyxia, trauma), or systemic congenital problems (heart disease, sepsis, infant hypothyroidism) (McBride et al., 1987).
8. A weak suck might indicate CNS abnormalities associated with hypotonia, medullary lesions, myasthenia gravis or botulism, or abnormalities of the muscles resulting in weak oral and buccal (cheek) musculature (McBride et al., 1987).

9. Discoordinated sucking is marked by a mistiming of normal movements or is marked by interference by hyperactive reflexes.
   a. It can result from asphyxia, perinatal cerebral insults, and CNS maldevelopment (McBride et al., 1987).
10. Nutritive sucking (NS) (Alper et al., 1996; Palmer, 1993; Wolf et al., 1992):
    a. NS is organized into a series of sucking bursts and pauses and occurs solely in the presence of oral fluid.
    b. Because breathing must be interspersed with swallowing, the sucking rate is slower during NS than it is during NNS. The breathing rate increases during pauses between sucking bursts (Geddes et al., 2006).
    c. New technologies will hopefully better elucidate the SSB relationships more accurately (Geddes et al., 2006).
    d. It is useful to count sucking bursts.
       i. Infants who are unable to sustain long bursts (taking fewer than 10 SSBs per burst) manifest weak or immature sucking (Bamford et al., 1992; Palmer et al., 1993).
    e. If short sucking bursts result from prematurity, maturation that occurs around 36–38 weeks will begin a process that normalizes the stability of sucking (Palmer et al., 1993).
    f. Other sucking problems (described earlier) can prove enduring and more difficult to resolve.
11. Nonnutritive sucking (NNS) (Alper et al., 1996; Palmer et al., 1993)
    a. NNS is not the same thing as ineffective suck; it is simply sucking that occurs for reasons other than feeding, that is, to stimulate the milk ejection reflex, to regulate state, to manage pain (Gray et al., 2002; Mizuno et al., 2006; Premji et al., 2000).
    b. NNS is characterized by fast, shallow sucks, and with more sucking than swallowing.
    c. Swallowing is infrequent and consists primarily of swallowing saliva or pooled milk.
    d. There is typically a 6–8 sucks: 1 swallow ratio in NNS.
C. Swallowing reflex (Wolf et al., 1992)
   1. Develops early in fetal life (12–14 weeks gestation).
   2. Triggered by the delivery of a bolus of fluid to the back of the tongue.
   3. Also triggered by chemical receptors in the tongue.
   4. Abnormalities of the tongue and palate can create problems with swallowing that can lead to a risk of aspiration.
   5. Swallowing dysfunction can result in poor weight gain and aversive feeding responses.
   6. Reflux is classified as a swallowing disorder.
      a. Although most infants experience some degree of reflux, serious cases can create significant problems for the infant.

b. Because the infant begins to associate eating with pain, feeding aversion can result.

c. The baby with severe reflux might self-limit intake, contributing to a diagnosis of failure to thrive.

d. Respiratory illness might also be present, owing to aspiration of ascending fluids that cause inflammation of the airways and nasal passages.

D. Gag reflex (Morris, 1977)

1. The function of the gag reflex is to protect the airway from large objects.

a. The gag is generally triggered by pressure to the rear of the tongue but can be stimulated at a more shallow depth in the mouths of young infants (Wolf et al., 1992).

2. The gag reflex can be hyperactive.

3. Constant activation by long nipples or invasive procedures can create feeding aversion.

4. Observe the infant during latch for gagging.

5. Gentle digital exam with a gloved finger can identify a gag reflex that is triggered by shallow oral penetration.

a. Infants with easily triggered gag reflexes might simply be immature, or they might require occupational therapy to facilitate acceptance of objects in the mouth.

E. Cough reflex (Wolf et al., 1992)

1. Protects against the aspiration of fluids into the airways.

2. May be immature in preterm and even in some term newborns.

3. The immature response to fluids in the airways is apnea (breath-holding) followed by attempts to swallow with a delayed cough.

4. Silent aspiration, which is prolonged apnea and aspiration of fluids without the signal of coughing, can occur in immature infants (Law-Morstatt et al., 2003).

5. Coughing during feeding is generally in response to aspiration of descending fluids.

6. Coughing between feedings might be in response to aspirating ascending fluids (reflux).

IV. Coordination of the Suck-Swallow-Breathe Triad

A. Feeding evaluation must consider all three aspects of the SSB triad (Glass et al., 1994).

B. Sucking, swallowing, and breathing are functionally and anatomically interrelated (overlapping function of cranial nerves and structures).

C. Observation of feeds in compromised infants should include observation of the entire feed to permit identification of fatigue, loss of rhythmicity, evidence of respiratory distress, color changes, and so on (Alper et al., 1996; Wolf et al., 1992).

D. Dysrhythmic sucking and poor coordination of SSB are common even in term infants during the first few days of life (Bamford et al., 1992).

1. Observe feedings for:

a. Stridor: A raspy, respiratory noise heard on inspiration (as with laryngo-malacia) or on expiration (as with tracheomalacia) caused by narrowing or obstruction of the airway.

b. Wheezing: A high-pitched noise occurring during exhalation (caused by airway constriction resulting from inflammation or reactive airway disease caused by silent microaspiration during feeding).

c. Apnea during feeding: Periodic breath-holding while attempting to manage swallows (Law-Morstatt et al., 2003).

d. Fatigue during feeding: Falling asleep too early during a feeding as the result of the infant being unable to accomplish the work of feeding or owing to stress.

e. Poor intake: Test weights on reliable scales are critical when assessing the intake of the unstable feeder (Sachs et al., 2002; Scanlon et al., 2002).

f. Poor growth: Newborn infant weight loss of more than 8% and failure to promptly recover birth weight are markers for suboptimal infant feeding behavior. Prompt, careful lactation assessment is required (Dewey et al., 2003).

g. Feeding aversion: Can result owing to aspiration, respiratory compromise, choking, reflux, or sensory-based problems (Palmer et al., 1993).

V. The "Fit" Between the Infant's Oral Anatomy and Maternal Breast/Nipple Anatomy

The effect of maternal breast variations has the potential to affect breastfeeding. Infants of mothers with flat or inverted nipples or with large breasts and/or nipples require closer growth monitoring (Gunther, 1955; Neifert, 1999; Vazirinejad et al., 2009; Wilson-Clay et al., 2005).

A. The breastfeeding mother and baby form a dyad.

B. Evaluation involves the assessment of both.

C. The diameter, consistency, length, elasticity, and shape of the maternal nipple might or might not be a good fit with the baby's mouth. See Chapter 15: Maternal Breastfeeding Anatomy.

1. Certain configurations of breasts/nipples might be more or less easy for infants with certain oral anomalies.

a. A mother with soft, elastic breast tissue might be able to use her breast tissue to plug a cleft lip.

b. A mother with taut breast tissue might not be able to assist her infant in this way.

References

Abadie, V., Andre, A., Zaouche, A., et al. (2001). Early feeding resistance: A possible consequence of neonatal oro-esophageal dyskinesia. *Acta Pediatrica*, *90*, 738–745.

Alper, M., & Manno, S. (1996). Dysphagia in infants and children with oral-motor deficits: Assessment and management. *Seminars in Speech and Language*, *17*, 283–305, 309.

Amir, L., James, J., & Beatty, J. (2005). Review of tongue-tie release at a tertiary maternity hospital. *Journal of Pediatric and Child Health*, *41*, 243–245.

Ballard, J., Auer, C., & Khoury, J. C. (2004). Ankyloglossia: Assessment, incidence, and effect of frenuloplasty on the breastfeeding dyad. *Pediatrics*, *110*, e63.

Bamford, O., Taciak, V., & Gewolb, I. H. (1992). The relationship between rhythmic swallowing and breastfeeding during suckle feeding in term neonates. *Pediatric Research*, *31*(6), 619–624.

Bosma, J. (1977). Structure and function of the infant oral and pharyngeal mechanisms. In J. Wilson (Ed.), *Oral-motor function and dysfunction in children* (pp. 25–28, 39, 52, 69). Chapel Hill, NC: University of North Carolina at Chapel Hill.

Bull, M., & Givan, D. (1990). Improved outcome in Pierre Robin sequence: Effect of multidisciplinary evaluation and management. *Pediatrics*, *86*, 294–301.

Caughey, A., Sandberg, P., Zlatnik, M., et al. (2005). Forceps compared with vacuum: Rates of neonatal and maternal morbidity. *Obstetrics and Gynecology*, *106*, 908–912.

Cleft Palate Foundation. (2006). Booklets and fact sheets. Pittsburgh, PA: Author. Retrieved from http://cleftline.org/what_we_do/publications

Coryllos, E., Genna, C., & Salloum, A. (2004, Summer). Congenital tongue-tie and its impact on breastfeeding. *Breastfeeding: Best for Baby and Mother*, 1–6. Retrieved from http://www.tongue-tie.org/Congenital-Tongue-Tie-and-its-Impact-on-Breastfeeding.html

Danner, S. C. (1992). Breastfeeding the neurologically impaired infant. *NAACOG's Clinical Issues in Perinatal and Women's Health Nursing*, *3*, 640–646.

Darzi, M., Chowdri, N., & Bhat, A. (1996). Breast feeding or spoon feeding after cleft lip repair: A prospective, randomized study. *British Journal of Plastic Surgery*, *49*, 24–26.

Dewey, K., Nommsen-Rivers, L., & Heinig, M. J. (2003). Risk factors for suboptimal infant breastfeeding behavior, delayed onset of lactation, and excess neonatal weight loss. *Pediatrics*, *112*, 607–619.

Fernando, C. (1998). *Tongue tie: From confusion to clarity*. Sydney, Australia: Tandem Publications.

Flinck, A., Paludan, A., Matsson, L., et al. (1994). Oral findings in a group of Swedish children. *International Journal of Paediatric Dentistry*, *2*, 67–73.

Forlenza, G., Paradise Black, N., McNamara, E., et al. (2010). Ankyloglossia, exclusive breastfeeding, and failure to thrive. *Pediatrics*, *125*(6), e1500–e1504.

Garcez, L., & Giugliani, E. (2005). Population-based study on the practice of breastfeeding in children born with cleft lip and palate. *Cleft Palate-Craniofacial Journal*, *42*(6), 687–693.

Geddes, D., McClellen, H., Kent, J., et al. (2006, September 22–26). *Patterns of respiration in infants during breastfeeding*. Paper presented at the 13th International Conference of the International Society for Research in Human Milk and Lactation (ISRHML), Niagara-on-the-Lake, Ontario, Canada.

Genna, C. W. (2008). *Supporting sucking skills in breastfeeding infants*. Sudbury, MA: Jones and Bartlett.

Glass, R., & Wolf, L. (1994). Incoordination of sucking, swallowing, and breathing as an etiology for breastfeeding difficulties. *Journal of Human Lactation*, *10*, 185–189.

Glenny, A., Hooper, L., Shaw, W., et al. (2004). Feeding interventions for growth and development in infants with cleft lip, cleft palate or cleft lip and palate. *Cochrane Database of Systematic Reviews, 3,* CD003315.

Goldman, A. (1993). The immune system of human milk: Antimicrobial, anti-inflammatory and immunomodulating properties. *Pediatric Infectious Disease Journal, 12,* 664–671.

Gorski, S., Adams, K., Birch, P. H., et al. (1994). Linkage analysis of X-linked cleft palate and ankyloglossia in Manitoba Mennonite and British Columbia native kindreds. *Human Genetics, 94,* 141–148.

Gray, L., Miller, L., Philipp, B., et al. (2002). Breastfeeding is analgesic in healthy newborns. *Pediatrics, 109,* 590–593.

Gunther, M. (1955). Instinct and the nursing couple. *Lancet, 1,* 575–578.

Hill, P., Aldag, J., & Chatterton, R. (2001). Initiation and frequency of pumping and milk production on non-nursing preterm infants. *Journal of Human Lactation, 17*(1), 9–13.

Hong, O., Lago, D., Seargeant, J., et al. (2010). Defining ankyloglossia: A case series of anterior and posterior tongue ties. *International Journal of Pediatric Otorhinolaryngology, 74*(9), 1003–10006.

Jones, N. (2005). The protective effects of breastfeeding for infants of depressed mothers. *Breastfeeding Abstracts, 24,* 19–20.

Kavanaugh, K., Mead, L., Meier, P., et al. (1995). Getting enough: Mothers' concerns about breastfeeding a preterm infant after discharge. *Journal of Obstetric, Gynecologic, and Neonatal Nursing, 24,* 23–32.

Kent, J., Mitoulas, L., Cox, D., et al. (1999). Breast volume and milk production during extended lactation. *Experimental Physiology, 84,* 435–447.

Kogo, M., Okada, G., Ishii, S., et al. (1997). Breast feeding for cleft lip and palate patients, using the Hotz-type plate. *Cleft Palate-Craniofacial Journal, 34*(4), 351–353.

Kotlow, L. A. (2010). The influence of the maxillary frenum on the development and pattern of dental caries on anterior teeth in breastfeeding infants: Prevention, diagnosis, and treatment. *Journal of Human Lactation, 26*(3), 304–308.

Kramer, M., Demissie, K., Yang, H., et al. (2000). The contribution of mild- and moderate preterm birth to infant mortality. *Journal of the American Medical Association, 284,* 843–849.

Lalakea, M., & Messner, A. (2003). Ankyloglossia: Does it matter? *Pediatric Clinics of North America, 50,* 381–397.

Law-Morstatt, L., Judd, D., Snyder, P., et al. (2003). Pacing as a treatment technique for transitional sucking patterns. *Journal of Perinatology, 23,* 483–488.

Lawrence, R. A., & Lawrence, R. M. (2011). *Breastfeeding: A guide for the medical profession.* Maryland Heights, MO: Elsevier Mosby

Masarei, A. G., Wade, A., Mars, M., et al. (2007). A randomized control trial investigating the effect of presurgical orthopedics on feeding in infants with cleft lip and/or palate. *Cleft Palate-Craniofacial Journal, 44*(2), 182–193.

McBride, M., & Danner, S. (1987). Sucking disorders in neurologically impaired infants: Assessment and facilitation of breastfeeding. *Clinics in Perinatology, 14,* 109–130.

Merkel-Piccini, R., & Rosenfeld-Johnson, S. (2003). Connections between tongue placement and dental alignment. *ADVANCE for Speech-Language Pathologists and Audiologists, 13,* 9.

Messner, A., Lalakea, L., Aby, J., et al. (2000). Ankyloglossia: Incidence and associated feeding difficulties. *Archives of Otolaryngology—Head and Neck Surgery, 126,* 36–39.

Mizuno, K., & Ueda, A. (2006). Changes in sucking performance from nonnutritive sucking to nutritive sucking during breast- and bottle-feeding. *Pediatric Research, 59*(5), 728–731.

Mohrbacher, N., & Stock, J. (2003). *The breastfeeding answer book* (3rd ed.). Schaumburg, IL: La Leche League International.

Morris, S. (1977). A glossary of terms describing the feeding process. In J. Wilson (Ed.), *Oral-motor function and dysfunction in children* (p. 160). Chapel Hill, NC: University of North Carolina at Chapel Hill.

Neifert, M. (1999). Clinical aspects of lactation. *Clinical Perinatology, 26*, 282–283.

Neifert, M., Lawrence, R., & Seacat, J. (1995). Nipple confusion: Toward a formal definition. *Journal of Pediatrics, 126*, S125–S129.

Ogg, L. (1975). Oral-pharyngeal development and evaluation. *Physical Therapy, 55*, 235–241.

Palmer, M. (1993). Identification and management of the transitional suck pattern in premature infants. *Journal of Perinatal and Neonatal Nursing, 7*, 66–75.

Paradise, J., Elster, B., & Tan, L. (1994). Evidence in infants with cleft palate that breast milk protects against otitis media. *Pediatrics, 94*, 853–860.

Powers, N. (1999). Slow weight gain and low milk supply in the breastfeeding dyad. *Clinics in Perinatology, 26*(2), 399–430.

Premji, S., & Paes, B. (2000). Gastrointestinal function and growth in premature infants: Is non-nutritive sucking vital? *Journal of Perinatology, 1*, 46–53.

Radojicic, J., Tanic, T., & Blazej, Z. (2009). Application of palatal RB obturator in babies with isolate palatal cleft (article in Serbian). *Vojinosanit Pregl, 66*(11), 914–919.

Ramsay, D., Langton, D., Gollow, I., et al. (2004). Ultrasound imaging of the effect of frenulotomy on breastfeeding infants with ankyloglossia [Abstract]. *Proceedings of the 12th International Conference of the International Society for Research in Human Milk and Lactation*, Queens College, Cambridge, England.

Ramsay, D., Mitoulas, L., Kent, J., et al. (2004). Ultrasound imaging of the sucking mechanics of the breastfeeding infant [Abstract]. *Proceedings of the 12th International Conference of the International Society for Research in Human Milk and Lactation*, Queens College, Cambridge, England.

Ranley, D. (1998). Early orofacial development. *Journal of Clinical Pediatric Dentistry, 22*, 267–275.

Redstone, F., & West, J. (2004). The importance of postural control for feeding. *Pediatric Nursing, 30*, 97–100.

Ricke, L., Baker, N., Madlon-Kay, D., et al. (2005). Newborn tongue-tie: Prevalence and effect on breastfeeding. *Journal of the American Board of Family Practitioners, 18*, 1–7.

Riordan, J. (2005). *Breastfeeding and human lactation* (3rd ed.). Sudbury, MA: Jones and Bartlett.

Rovet, J. (Ed.). (1995). *Turner syndrome across the lifespan*. Markham, Ontario, Canada: Kelin Graphics.

Sachs, M., & Oddie, S. (2002). Breastfeeding—weighing in the balance: Reappraising the role of weighing babies in the early days. *MIDIRS Midwifery Digest, 12*, 296–300.

Sapin, S., Miller, A., & Bass, H. (2005). Neonatal asymmetric crying facies: A new look at an old problem. *Clinical Pediatrics, 44*(2), 109–119.

Scanlon, K., Alexander, M., Serdula, M., et al. (2002). Assessment of infant feeding: The validity of measuring milk intake. *Nutrition Reviews, 60*(8), 235–251.

Smith, J., Crumley, R., & Harker, L. (1981). Facial paralysis in the newborn. *Otolaryngology—Head and Neck Surgery, 89*, 1021–1024.

Snyder, J. (1997). Bubble palate and failure to thrive: A case report. *Journal of Human Lactation, 13*, 139–143.

Sultana, A., Rahman, M. M., Rahman, M. M., et al. (2011). A feeding aid prosthesis for a preterm baby with cleft lip and palate. *Mymensingh Medical Journal, 20*(1), 22–27.

Tomita, Y., Juroda, S., Nakanishi, H., et al. (2010). Severity of alveolar cleft affects prognosis of infant orthopedics in complete unilateral cleft lip and palate: three-dimensional evaluation from cheiloplasty to palatoplasty. *Journal of Craniofacial Surgery, 21*(5), 1503–1507.

Turner, L., Jacobsen, C., Humenczuk, M., et al. (2001). The effects of lactation education and a prosthetic obturator appliance on feeding efficiency in infants with cleft lip and palate. *Cleft Palate-Craniofacial Journal, 38*(5), 519–524.

Valentine, C., Hurst, N., & Schanler, R. (1994). Hindmilk improves weight gain in low-birth-weight infants fed human milk. *Journal of Pediatric Gastroenterology and Nutrition, 18*(4), 474–477.

Vazirinejad, R., Darakhshan, S., Esmaeili, A., et al. (2009). The effect of maternal breast variations on neonatal weight gain in the first seven days of life. *International Breastfeeding Journal, 4*, 13. doi:10.1186/1746-4358-4-13

Wall, V., & Glass, R. (2006). Mandibular asymmetry and breastfeeding problems: Experience from 11 cases. *Journal of Human Lactation, 22*, 328–334.

Weatherly-White, R., Kuehn, D., Mirrett, P., et al. (1987). Early repair and breast-feeding for infants with cleft lip. *Plastic and Reconstructive Surgery, 79*, 879–885.

Wiessinger, D., & Miller, M. (1995). Breastfeeding difficulties as a result of tight lingual and labial frena: A case report. *Journal of Human Lactation, 11*, 313–316.

Wilson-Clay, B. (1996). Clinical use of nipple shields. *Journal of Human Lactation, 12*, 279–285.

Wilson-Clay, B. (2005). *External pacing techniques: Protecting respiratory stability during feeding* (Pharmasoft Publishing Independent Study Module). Amarillo, TX: Pharmasoft Publishing.

Wilson-Clay, B., & Hoover, K. (2008). *The breastfeeding atlas.* Austin, TX: LactNews Press.

Wolf, L., & Glass, R. (1992). *Feeding and swallowing disorders in infancy.* Tucson, AZ: Therapy Skill Builders.

CHAPTER 28
Guidelines for Facilitating and Assessing Breastfeeding

Marie Davis, RN, IBCLC

OBJECTIVES

- Identify two factors that will aid the baby in his or her transition to extrauterine life.
- Give at least two examples of physiologic and psychological benefits to the mother and baby related to early first contact.
- Identify at least two routine hospital procedures that disrupt the normal first attachment needs of both mother and baby.
- State one rationale for skin-to-skin (STS) contact between the mother and the neonate.
- List key positioning components for mother-led and infant-led attachment.
- Describe the components of proper latch-on.
- List the signs of milk transfer and swallowing.
- Describe three criteria for assessing sufficient milk intake.
- Document a breastfeeding assessment.

INTRODUCTION

The establishment of lactation begins with the separation of the placenta. A mother's breastfeeding experience can be "profoundly affected by what happens during the first hours after birth" (Newman et al., 2000a, p. 43). Birth interventions that disrupt the natural interaction between the mother and the infant in the immediate postpartum period can affect long-term breastfeeding success and should be avoided. The lactation consultant might not be present for the first mother–infant breastfeeding contact. However, she or he can educate parents and medical providers about how critical this first step is toward successful breastfeeding and how to handle it safely and effectively.

The lactation consultation draws from a foundation in the scientific, cultural/ social, and psychological disciplines to formulate a plan of care to support and encourage mothers to successfully meet their breastfeeding goals. They are able to perform a comprehensive assessment that includes general physiologic and psychosocial health of mother and infant, positioning, latch-on, and milk transfer (International Lactation

(continues)

Consultant Association [ILCA], 2005b). Recommendations for continuing care of the breastfeeding dyad are made that integrate evidence-based practices/treatments and the cultural, psychosocial, and nutritional aspects of breastfeeding. Lactation consultants use the principles of family-centered care while maintaining a collaborative, supportive relationship with clients. The lactation consultant must also document the assessment and recommendations in the medical record to communicate the assessment and plan of care to other healthcare providers (International Board of Lactation Consultant Examiners [IBLCE], 2010).

I. Facilitating Breastfeeding in a Perinatal Setting

A. Encourage parents to have a labor support person and written birth and feeding plans (Coates & Riordan, 2010) before hospital admission.

  1. Continuous support of the mother in labor has been shown to have positive effects on birth, bonding, and breastfeeding success (Hodnett et al., 2011; Kennell et al., 1991; Langer et al., 1998; Morhason-Bello et al., 2009; Perez, 1998).

    a. A combination of doula support and female family support appears to be the most effective in a positive birth experience (Rosen, 2004).

    b. Doula support is a powerful force intrapartum (Berg et al., 2006)

      i. Reduces medical costs: Reduces the need for medical interventions including Pitocin (oxytocin injection), epidural anesthesia, and cesarean sections (Gordon et al., 1999; Kennell et al., 1991)

      ii. Shortened labors (averaging slightly less than 6 hours for the first-time mother).

      iii. Postpartum doula facilitates breastfeeding (Bonaro et al., 2004; Kroeger et al., 2004).

B. Limit the use of labor interventions.

  1. Artificial rupture of membranes.

  2. Induction and augmentation (Pitocin/prostaglandins).

  3. Routine fluid loading during labor and postpartum:

    a. Excessive intravenous (IV) fluids: Large amounts of IV fluids (especially with the addition of Pitocin) increase the risk of maternal fluid retention, an edematous areola, and an inflated infant birth weight.

    b. Infant diuresis of the excess fluid might be misconstrued as abnormal weight loss (Chantry, Nommsen-Rivers, Peerson, Cohen, & Dewey, 2010; Cotterman, 2004; Merry et al., 2000; Walker, 2009).

  4. Analgesics: Mothers who have been medicated during labor are more likely to leave the hospital without having established breastfeeding.

    a. Medications can depress the efficacy of early suckling, interfere with state and motor control, and disturb or delay important newborn behaviors such as breast-seeking, latch-on, and suckling that stimulate the mother's breast

(Jordan et al., 2009; Lieberman, Lang, et al., (2000); Perlman, 1999; Petrova et al., 2001; Phillip et al., 1999; Ransjo-Arvidson et al., 2001; Walker, 1997).

   b. Narcotics, barbiturates can sedate the baby.

   c. Epidural analgesia: Increases the risk of maternal intrapartum fever, leading to separation, septic workup for the baby, and the use of antibiotics (Dashe et al., 1999; Gross et al., 2002; Leighton et al., 2002; Lieberman et al., 1997; Lieberman et al., 2002; Negishi et al., 2001; Torvaldsen et al., 2006).

      i. In mothers who develop a fever from the epidural, babies have an increased risk of seizures (Lieberman, Fichenwald, Mathur, et al., 2000).

      ii. Mothers who have epidurals spend less time with their baby during the hospital stay (Sepkoski et al., 2005).

  5. Routine episiotomy: Can be extremely painful for 10 days or more, making it more difficult to attain a comfortable breastfeeding position (Stainton et al., 1999).

  6. Limit the need for instrument-assisted delivery by facilitating more natural birthing positions.

   a. Vacuum extraction and the use of forceps: Increases the risk for intracranial hemorrhage and subdural hematoma, which are serious and can be fatal (Food and Drug Administration [FDA], 1998; Towner et al., 1999).

   b. Infants delivered by vacuum extraction might have impaired suckling reflexes, delaying successful breastfeeding initiation (Hall et al., 2002; Vestermark et al., 1991).

   c. The infant might have some head pain in the first few days after birth from head compression that can be exaggerated by instrument-assisted delivery.

C. Delay, minimize, or eliminate neonatal and postpartum procedures that interfere with first contact; stress on the neonate from procedures can result in sensory overload and cause the baby to temporarily shut down to reorganize his or her nervous system (Bystrova et al., 2007; Karl, 2004).

  1. Minimize suctioning.

   a. Bulb suctioning of the mouth and/or nares can cause physical injury and/or nasal edema and stuffiness, making latch-on and breathing difficult.

   b. Routine suctioning of gastric contents can be harmful for healthy term newborns (Kiremitci et al., 2011).

      i. Can result in injury to the oropharynx

      ii. Can cause retching/vomiting

      iii. Can cause physiologic changes, such as increased blood pressure, changes in heart rate, and electrolyte imbalance

   c. Disrupts prefeeding behavior or cueing (Widstrom et al., 1987).

   d. Can affect the baby's desire to latch on for several days as a result of pain/injury to the oropharynx; baby might demonstrate oral defensiveness (American Academy of Pediatrics [AAP], 2005).

e. In situations where intubation, visualization, and deep suctioning of the trachea and bronchial tree below the vocal cords are required because of possible meconium aspiration, suctioning should be done as gently as possible.

2. Delay bathing to prevent the loss of amniotic fluid odors and thermal losses (with resultant hypoglycemia), until at least after the initial bonding period.
   a. The vernix should be allowed to soak into the skin to lubricate and protect it.
   b. The baby recognizes his or her mother by oral, tactile, and olfactory modes (Marlier et al., 1997).
   c. Odors play an important role in the mediation of an infant's early behavior (Varendi et al., 1998).
      i. The baby learns the smell of amniotic fluid in utero and shows a preference for objects that are coated with amniotic fluid (Schaal et al., 2004; Varendi et al., 2001).
      ii. This preference changes to a preference for the smell of the mother's milk 4 or 5 days after birth.
   d. Dry the infant except for the hands and forearms; leaving some amniotic fluids on the hands and forearms; amniotic fluid transferred to the mother's breast when the baby is placed on the mother's chest can be beneficial for latching on (Mennella et al., 2001).
   e. Some hospitals now delay the infant bath for at least 24 hours or until after hospital discharge (BFHI listserv communication, 2011).
      i. Medical indications for giving the bath immediately include maternal HIV and hepatitis B or C.

3. Delay giving eye treatments, which can cause blepharospasm (prevents the infant from opening the eyes); the mother has a high emotional need for eye-to-eye contact with the infant immediately after birth.

4. Delay vitamin K injection until after first contact.

5. Delay painful procedures such as circumcision until the baby has had several effective feedings.

D. Keep the mother and infant together after birth; separation of the mother and the infant after birth has been shown to interfere with breastfeeding and bonding.
   1. "The most appropriate position for the healthy full term newborn is in close body contact with the mother" (Christensson et al., 1995).
      a. Provide for skin-to-skin (STS) contact (also called kangaroo care), with the mother immediately after birth and for the first few hours after birth (Anderson et al., 2003).
      b. STS also has been shown to assist preterm infants (34–36 weeks gestation) with recovering from birth-related fatigue (Lawn et al., 2010; Ludington-Hoe et al., 1999).
      c. STS contact has been shown to help the infant regulate his or her body temperature, breathing, and heart rate faster than radiant warmers and incubators (Chiu et al., 2005; Walters et al., 2007).

        d. If contact with the mother is not possible because of cesarean delivery or maternal condition, then STS contact with the father should be provided (Christensson, 1996).

    2. Babies may be genetically encoded against separation from their mothers; when separated, babies display "separation distress calls" (crying that occurs in pulses) that stops upon reunion (Christensson et al., 1995; Michelsson et al., 1996).

E. Immediately post birth:

    1. First contact should occur as soon as possible after birth, usually within the first hour (AAP, 2005; World Health Organization [WHO] & UNICEF, 2009).

    2. Mother and baby are in a heightened state of readiness (Riordan, 2010).

    3. Quiet alert state can last up to 2 hours after birth; after which the baby may sleep for as long as 24 hours (Riordan, 2010).

    4. The mother might need reassurance if she is concerned because the infant does not breastfeed as vigorously as expected.

    5. The role of the lactation consultant, nurse, or healthcare provider is one of quiet observer.

F. Encourage parents and healthcare providers to recognize and facilitate the baby's reflexes for self-attachment.

    1. Healthy infants should be given the opportunity to show hunger and optimal reflexes and attach to the areola by himself or herself (Lawrence et al., 2011).

    2. Mothers who initiate breastfeeding within an hour of birth breastfeed longer than those who have delayed contact (Mikiel-Kostyra et al., 2002; Nakao et al., 2008).

    3. Most babies from unmedicated births will self-attach and suckle correctly in fewer than 50 minutes (Righard et al., 1990).

        a. If left undisturbed with the mother, the baby responds with an unlearned pattern of attachment; the process is innate (Righard et al., 1990).

        b. When a baby self-attaches, he or she will attach correctly to the areola and not to the nipple alone (Righard et al., 1990).

    4. Infants have been observed to engage in a sequence of behaviors that begins immediately after birth and terminates with grasping the nipple, suckling, and then falling asleep.

        a. When crying immediately after birth stops, infants might have a short period of relaxation after which they become more alert. They demonstrate the following behaviors:

          i. An awakening phase

          ii. An active phase with movements of limbs, rooting activity, and looking at the mother's face

          iii. A crawling phase with soliciting sounds

          iv. A familiarization phase with licking of the areola

          v. A suckling phase

          vi. A sleeping phase

        b. Inborn breastfeeding reflexes might be somewhat depressed at birth, possibly because of a depressed sensory system.

    c. It is hypothesized that when the infant is given the option to peacefully go through the nine behavioral phases—cry, relaxation, awakening, activity, crawling, resting, familiarization, suckling, and sleeping—when skin to skin with its mother this results in early optimal self-regulation and successful attachment to the breast (Widström et al., 2011).

    d. Licking movements precede and follow the rooting reflex in alert infants.

    e. The tongue is placed on the floor of the mouth during this distinct rooting.

    f. "Mouth and lip-smacking movements begin, and the infant begins to drool. The baby then begins to move forward slowly, starts to turn the head from side to side, and opens the mouth widely upon nearing the nipple. After several attempts, the lips latch on to the areola and not the nipple" (Kennell et al., 1998, p. 6).

5. If separated from the mother, the baby's initial suckling attempts are disturbed (AAP, 2005).

6. Delayed gratification of the early sucking reflex might make it more difficult for the infant to suckle later on (Riordan, 2010).

7. Human imprinting: "Comfort sucking and formation of nipple preference are genetically determined behaviors for imprinting on the mother's nipple" (Lawrence et al., 2011, pp. 223–224; Mohrbacher et al., 2003, p. 83).

8. Self-attachment reflexes appear to last beyond the newborn period (Colson, 2005a, 2005b; Colson et al., 2008).

G. Physiologic effects of first contact:

1. For the human female, the window of time in the first few hours after delivery is the sensitive period for bonding (Lawrence et al., 2011).

2. Contact between the mother and the infant brings about a number of bioactive processes that are interconnected and mutually dependent (Hamosh, 2001).

    a. Maternal hormonal release of progesterone, oxytocin, and prolactin is believed to be responsible for many mothering behaviors. (See **Table 28-1**.)

    b. Stimulates the release of gastrointestinal hormones such as insulin, cholecystokinin, somatostatin, and gastrin.

    c. Other supporting hormones are released that alter gut hormones in mother and infant, coordinating their metabolisms (Kennell et al., 1998).

    d. Facilitates infant adaptation to the new nonsterile environment.

        i. Infant's skin, respiratory tract, and gastrointestinal tract are colonized with maternal body flora, which tend to be nonpathogenic microorganisms and immunological factors, such as secretory immunoglobulin A (sIgA).

        ii. The mother's normal body flora colonizes her baby's body, but only if she is the first person to hold the baby rather than a nurse, physician, or others (Lauwers et al., 2010).

    e. Swallowing colostrum causes digestive peristalsis.

        i. Encourages early passing of the bilirubin-laden meconium, reducing neonatal jaundice.

        ii. Meconium is the first medium for Lactobacillus bifidus, which is introduced through colostrum.

Table 28-1 Hormones

Hormone	Maternal	Neonate
Prolactin	Often called "the milk-making hormone."	Present in milk; might be soothing/calming to the baby. Biologically potent and absorbed by the infant; affects intestinal fluid and electrolyte absorption as well as sodium, potassium, and calcium in the newborn (Lawrence Ft Lawrence, 2005; Riordan, 2005).
	"Mothering hormone" hormone of love."	
	The amount is proportional to the amount of nipple stimulation Released in pulses directly related to nipple stimulation. postpartum bleeding.	
Oxytocin It is appropriate to optimize mother-infant interaction at this highest point of oxytocin by facilitating infant suckling (Kennell a Klaus, 1998, p. 8; Lawrence a Lawrence, 2005, p. 249).	Induces uterine contractions, expels placenta, prevents excessive bleeding. Known as the "cuddle hormone" (Lauwers a Swisher, 2005), Associated with maternal bonding Helps mold maternal behavior. Oxytocin targets myoepithelial cells in the breast, but also disperses into a closed system within the brain, bathing the area that is responsible for social preferences and affiliative behavior. Oxytocin deficiency has been reported with epidural block. Opiates can inhibit the sucking-induced oxytocin release. (Lindow et al., 1999) Causes the mother to feel relaxed or sedated and calmer. Increases skin temperature (flushing). Increases thirst.	Oxytocin contained in the mother's milk is destroyed in the baby's stomach. The oxytocin found in neonatal serum is produced by the baby Whether oxytocin has a physiological effect on the neonatal gut or other systems is unknown (Lawrence a Lawrence, 2005).
Other supporting hormones Hormones released by vagal signals alter gut hormones in mother and infant, coordinating their metabolisms (Kennell a Klaus, 1998).	High levels of endorphins in response to pain in the mother pass on to the baby in her breastmilk.	Endorphins help make the transition easier for the baby, facilitating relaxation and calm. May assist with overcoming birth stress Cortisol: Aids in pancreatic growth of the infant and controls the transport of fluids and salt to the infant's gastrointestinal tract Catecholaminein the baby insure the baby is alert.

3. Early mother–infant contact has profound emotional effects (Newman et al., 2005a, p. 44).

    a. Mother: Boosts mothering confidence

    b. Baby: Calms, relaxes, and stops crying

4. The infant should not be left alone in bed with a mother or any other individual who has been heavily medicated or is extremely sleepy.

    a. The infant should remain STS on mother's chest, covered with a light blanket.

    b. The infant should not be placed in a bed, sofa, or chair next to the mother if she is drowsy or asleep.

    c. Assign an alert support person to be observant of infant safety.

H. Subsequent feedings in a perinatal setting (Henderson et al., 2001):

1. Provide for mother's physical and emotional (psychological) comfort.

    a. Structure the environment.

        i. For privacy: assess the mother's comfort with visitors and family. If indicated, ask them to leave and return after the feeding.

        ii. Eliminate environmental distractions to facilitate a quiet environment (e.g., regulate room temperature, turn off telephone, television).

    b. Give pain medication prior to feedings if necessary.

    c. The mother should wash her hands.

    d. Washing the nipples and areolae are unnecessary.

I. Care of the mother and infant when the infant refuses to or is unable to latch on:

1. Preserve and protect milk production when the infant is unable to latch on. (See also section on preterm infants.)

    a. Some infants are unwilling to nurse or suck poorly following birth.

    b. There can be multiple causes including labor medications, birth trauma, vigorous suctioning, or anomalies of the face, neck, or mouth.

    c. During the first 24 hours of life, the infant must recover from the rigors of labor and birth.

    d. In most cases, the passage of time corrects the problem.

2. If the normal healthy newborn has not latched or nursed effectively after the first 24 hours, stimulation of the breasts and milk removal is crucial to establishing a milk supply.

    Note: For the mother of a preterm infant, stimulation of milk production should begin within 6 hours of delivery or sooner, if she is physically able to do so.

3. Expression of colostrum provides nourishment for the infant who will not latch and results in increased milk production.

    a. Early removal of colostrum from the breast is associated with a better prognosis for successful lactation (Neville et al., 2001).

    b. Frequent stimulation increases milk volume (DeCarvalho et al., 1983) and prevents engorgement, which can further delay latch-on.

4. Manual expression is recommended during lactogenesis I (Morton et al., 2009).

a. Colostrum does not express easily because it is thick and low volume.

b. Warmth, massage, and gravity assist with the flow of colostrum.

5. Use appropriately sized containers for collection of colostrum.

a. Mother might express only a few drops at first.

b. Colostrum might stick to containers or breast pump parts and become inaccessible (Yerge-Cole, 2010).

6. Instruct the mother in proper storage and labeling of human milk.

7. All expressed colostrum or mother's milk should be fed to the baby by an alternative method if possible (ABM Protocol 3; Academy of Breastfeeding Medicine Protocol Committee, 2009).

8. Once milk volume increases, the combination of breast pump suction, breast compression, and hand expression (called "hands-on-pumping") has been found effective in maintaining the milk supply (Morton et al., 2009).

9. If the healthy newborn infant has not latched or fed effectively after the first 24 hours, instruct the mother in ways to address the situation (ABM Protocol 3; Academy of Breastfeeding Medicine Protocol Committee, 2009); American Academy of Pediatrics Section on Breastfeeding, 2009).

a. Encourage skin-to-skin contact to facilitate self-attachment reflexes.

b. Instruct parents to watch closely for feeding cues.

c. Attempt to breastfeed during quiet, alert times, whenever the infant shows interest or at least every 3–4 hours.

d. Avoid activities immediately prior to a feeding that can disrupt attachment reflexes (e.g., diaper changing, bathing, changing clothing).

e. Encourage the mother to massage her breasts and hand express colostrum onto her nipple or into the baby's mouth during feeding attempts.

f. Encourage patience, practice, and persistence.

10. If the baby continues to feed poorly, establish a routine for milk expression.

a. The frequency and duration of milk expression directly correspond to the amount of milk produced (Hill et al., 2005).

b. Assist in obtaining an effective breast pump for use until the baby can latch and nurse effectively.

c. The mother should express her milk at least eight times per 24 hours.

d. She should express for approximately 10–15 minutes until milk flow stops, and then massage the breasts and manually express any additional milk (Morton et al., 2009).

e. Explain the importance of not missing an expression session during the night.

11. Depending on the clinical situation, it might be appropriate to delay discharge of the couplet to provide further breastfeeding support (Academy of Breastfeeding Medicine Protocol Committee, 2010).

12. A follow-up visit or contact should be scheduled within 24 hours of discharge. For a chart of guidelines on interventions for the infant who is not latching, go to www.go.jblearning.com/corecurriculum.

II. Key Points for Teaching the Mother Positioning and Latch-on Techniques

A. Proper maternal and infant positioning facilitates successful breastfeeding (Maffei et al., 2004; Mohrbacher et al., 2005; Morton, 1992). See **Table 28-2** and **Figures 28-1** through **28-5**.

1. Effective positioning and attachment facilitate milk transfer, minimize nipple trauma, and increase the duration of breastfeeding (Tully et al., 2005).

2. Numerous options and variations exist for positioning and can be adapted to each mother–baby couplet.

3. Mothers do not need to know all of these positions, and their positioning preference should be respected.

4. The primary purpose of positioning is the mother's comfort, with the infant in an optimal position for latch-on.

    a. Positioning of the infant at breast is key to effective latch and milk transfer.

    b. There is no single "right" position for breastfeeding; mothers should choose what works best for them and their infants.

    c. Biological nurturing (laidback breastfeeding), infant-led attachment, or ventral positioning suggest the newborn is an abdominal feeder who displays antigravity reflexes, aiding latch-on (Colson, 2005; Colson et al., 2008; Smilie, 2007).

        i. Breastfeeding initiation appears to be innate for both mother and baby, not learned, as previously believed.

        ii. Baby is preprogrammed with reflexive skills geared toward attachment.

        iii. Neonatal reflexes are best stimulated when the mother is in a semireclined posture.

        iv. Baby self-attaches with little or no assistance from the mother. (See the section "E. Immediately post birth" earlier in this chapter.)

        v. This technique is especially helpful if the mother has had difficulty with latch-on.

    d. Encourage the mother to try different positions until she finds one that is comfortable for her and her baby.

        i. Positioning of the mother for feedings should not become so cumbersome or complicated that it results in emotional distress for her or her baby or delays feeding.

        ii. Mothers often cite "too many rules" as a reason for early breastfeeding cessation.

B. Positions for mother-led attachment include key points for mother and infant.

1. Maternal:

    a. The mother is in a comfortable position.

    b. Her body is in good alignment with the baby, supported in such a way that the weight of the infant does not cause fatigue.

    c. She brings baby to breast, rather than breast to baby.

Table 28-2 Review of Basic Positions for Breastfeeding

Position	Uses	Points	Disadvantages/Cautions
MOTHER SEATED			
Laid-back breastfeeding, or Biological Nurturing (**Figure 28-1**)	Encourages baby's natural breastfeeding instincts. Works well with mother's who have been struggling with latch-on	The mother "leans back" well supported in a bed or large recliner—not flat, but comfortably "leaning back." Baby is dressed in a diaper only. The baby is on placed on the mother's chest with the cheek near the mother's bare breast—baby's chest to mother's chest The baby's body rests entirely on the mother. Baby is allowed to self attach	Mother's worry that baby could fall off
Madonna or Cradle Hold (**Figure 28-2**)	Most commonly used position. Feels the most natural to the mother	The baby lies across the mother's forearm on the side that the mother will be using for the feeding. The baby's head is either in the bend of the mother's elbow or midway down her forearm, whichever results in the best positioning. Keeping her arm level, the mother holds the baby's buttocks with her hand. The baby's lower arm can be placed around the mother's back or tucked down along next to his or her body. The baby's legs can be wrapped around the mother's waist if needed to bring the baby closer to the breast. Baby's entire body should be facing the mother; chest-to-chest rather than chest-to-ceiling. Infant's mouth should be with the level mother's nipple. Pillow(s) needed to support the baby's body in mother's lap, helps prevent downward drift. Pillow(s) for the mother's back and arm as needed.	Offers the least amount of control over the infant's head. Difficult to achieve good sitting position in hospital bed; use chair if possible. Requires sitting; episiotomy, cesarean incision or hemorrhoids make sitting a less desirable position. Mothers tend to hunch over taking the breast to the baby Mother's arm or breast, infant's arm may be in the way. Baby can drift downward putting pressure on the breast, which may alter the latch, or pull the breast out of the baby's mouth.

(continues)

Table 28-2 Review of Basic Positions for Breastfeeding (continued)

Position	Uses	Points	Disadvantages/Cautions
MOTHER SEATED			
Clutch or Football Hold **(Figure 28-3)**	Often preferred when a new mother is having difficulty with latch-on. Improves the mother's view of her nipple and areola and of the baby's mouth. Helpful after cesarean birth Helpful for women with especially large breasts	Baby lays next to the mother at breast level Baby can be placed next to the mother with baby's hips flexed, baby's bottom against the back of the chair/couch/bed, the feet aiming toward the ceiling. Or the baby lays on his or her side with the entire body turned toward the mother (wrapped around her side) Baby's arms can be placed across his or her chest or around the breast Mother's arm is under the infant's back with the hand at the base of the baby's head Pillows needed beside the mother and to support her arm.	Often difficult in hospital bed Gives the mother better control of the infant's head. Pressure on the infant's feet can trigger arching and the stepping reflex. Pressure on the occipital area of the infant's head can cause arching May be suffocation hazard if the mother is has received medication that makes her drowsy.
Elevated Clutch Hold	Same advantages as clutch hold Helps stabilize the infant's body Mother can slide her pelvis forward, sitting more on the sacrum and not the perineum so she is in a reclined position. May be the optimal position for stimulating the baby's innate breastfeeding behaviours	The baby is "seated" in an upright position with the baby's bottom on pillow(s), hips flexed (legs tucked up) with the knees flexed so baby's entire body faces the mother. Infant's arms can be folded across the chest, tucked under or to the sides of the mother's breast. Mother's arm supports baby's back, her hand placed at the at the at the nape of the baby's neck (the base of the baby's head) A pillow supporting her lower back Encourage mother to lean back	
Cross-Cradle Hold **(Figure 28-4)**	Principles are the same as for the cradle hold. Also used for preterm infants.	The baby lies across the forearm of the opposite arm from the breast being used for the feeding (e.g. the left arm for the right breast). The baby's head is held just below the ears at the nape of the neck. The breast is supported with the hand on the same side as the breast to be used for the feeding.	Be sure that infant is chest-to-chest rather than chest-to-ceiling

Use folded receiving blanket behind infant to maintain chest-to-chest position.

Mother's body should be at a slight angle to the mattress, leaning backward just a bit against a pillow.

MOTHER LAYING DOWN

Side Lying (**Figure 28-4**)	Mothers may experience less fatigue if breastfeeding while lying down. Some mothers express concern over the number of pillows or that side lying is too cumbersome for them to arrange by themselves.	With the mother on her side, place a pillow behind her upper back and have her roll toward the pillow (pillow stabilizes the mother's position) The baby is placed on the bed, turned toward the breast. The mother can use her arm to hold the infant in position. The breast is held by the mother's upper hand.	May be suffocation hazard due to the number of pillows needed to maintain the position comfortably May be suffocation hazard if the mother is has received medication that makes her drowsy. Lying completely at a 90 degree angle to the bed, will make it difficult for baby to latch-on. The breast may be turned into bed in such a way that the nipple and areola are inaccessible to the baby.
Australian or Posture Feeding (Prone Oblique)	May be needed if the mother has complications from an epidural or spinal. Used for mothers who have a forceful milk ejection reflex that is overwhelming the baby. Also used for babies who: a. Bite or retract their tongue; helps the jaw and tongue move down and forward. b. Have upper airway disorders such as tracheomalacia and laryngomalacia.	The baby is placed on his or her abdomen across the mother's chest with the mother lying flat on her back. Not an optimum position for breastfeeding. The weight of the infant against her breast might be painful. The infant's face might become buried in the breast.	The mother might need to support the baby's forehead with the heel of her hand to prevent the baby's head from falling forward. Care must be taken that the breasts are adequately drained when using this position.

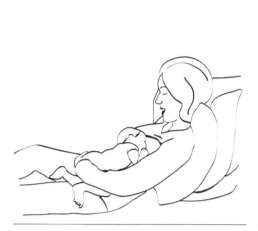

Figure 28-1 Laidback breastfeeding, or biological nurturing.

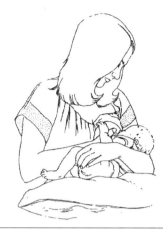

Figure 28-2 Madonna or cradle hold.

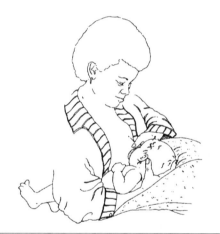

Figure 28-3 Clutch or football hold.

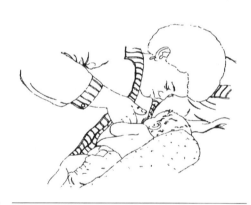

Figure 28-4 Cross-cradle hold.

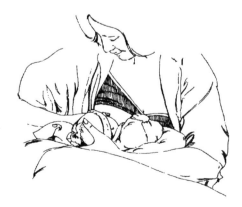

Figure 28-5 Side-lying position.

    d. Her hand is placed at the base of the baby's head to avoid pressure against the back of the baby's head (occipital area) because this action causes the baby to arch away from the breast.

    e. The baby's head is supported so that the neck is neither extended nor flexed (chin to chest).

2. Infant:

    a. The baby is in position to readily access the mother's breast.

    b. The nose and mouth are aligned with the nipple and areola.

    c. The body is level, slightly flexed, and well supported.

    d. The limbs are tucked in toward the baby's body to prevent flailing.

    e. The baby faces the mother's body with his or her ear, shoulder, and hip in a straight line.

C. Positioning for infant-led attachment (Colson, 2010):

1. Mother in a semireclining position

2. Baby placed on his or her stomach between the breasts

3. Baby self-attaches with little or no assistance from the mother except what might be needed to prevent falling

D. Breast support:

1. Hand and finger placement

    a. The mother should support the weight of the breast to prevent the baby from pulling down on the nipple or losing the latch.

    b. Neonates do not have enough oral strength to maintain their position on a heavy breast.

    c. Fingers need to be far enough back to allow full access to the mother's areola.

       i. Many women grasp the breast with the thumb well up on the breast but the fingers too close to the areola on the underside of the breast.

       ii. The mother cannot easily see her finger position on the breast.

       iii. Suggest that the mother practice holding her breast in front of a mirror.

    d. Large-breasted women may benefit from a rolled washcloth or towel placed under the breast to elevate it.

    e. Small-breasted women might not need to support the breast, but to help direct the breast, they might need to place the heel of the hand against their chest rather than beneath the breast so that the infant's access is not obstructed by the hand.

2. C-hold (thumb on top of the breast with all four fingers below) works well for most mothers.

3. The scissors hold (breast grasped between the index and middle fingers) might work for some mothers as long as the fingers are well away from the areola.

4. The dancer hold (breast grasped from below, the hand in a U shape, with the baby's chin resting in the fleshy part between the thumb and index finger) might be needed for preterm infants or for infants who have poor jaw support or control.

5. The sandwich analogy: The mother sandwiches the breast with thumb and fingers while pushing back toward the chest wall (Wiessinger, 1998).

   a. Elongates and narrows the areola, which enables the baby to latch on more easily.

   b. May be helpful for large-breasted women.

   c. Ensure that mother's fingers are parallel to baby's lips to facilitate a deep, areolar latch.

E. Latching: Good attachment can prevent many breastfeeding problems such as nipple pain/trauma and breast engorgement (Blair et al., 2003).

F. The ideal is infant-led attachment. The following steps are for those mothers and infants who need some assistance with the latch process.

   1. It is important to stress that a baby should never be forced to the breast.

      a. Pushing, shoving, or holding the baby into the breast is counterproductive.

      b. Traumatizing for both mother and infant.

      c. A crying infant is disorganized and may not latch on until calm.

   2. Optimal infant behavioral state for latch-on ranges from slightly drowsy to active alert. The quiet alert state is ideal. (See the section titled "E. Assess behavioral state of the baby before and after feeding" in section III, "The Lactation Consultant's Assessment," later in this chapter.)

      a. Encourage mother to breastfeed any time her baby exhibits feeding cues.

      b. Baby displays cues even before awakening.

         i. At first, baby might wiggle, toss and turn, or be restless in sleep.

         ii. Might begin to root toward hand and even attempt to suckle it or anything near the mouth.

      c. If early cues are ignored, the baby begins to fuss and eventually becomes disorganized (Marasco et al., 1999).

   3. Brush the lips lightly with the nipple to elicit the rooting reflex.

      a. The mother should do this by gently moving her breast up and down.

      b. Caution the mother to keep her fingers away from the baby's mouth.

         i. Some mothers are tempted to pry the mouth open with the index finger.

         ii. Touching the baby's mouth or chin can cause clamping (bite reflex).

         iii. Some babies respond with a better gape if the upper lip is stimulated.

   4. Wait for baby's mouth to be open wide, with tongue at the floor of the mouth.

      a. A crying baby might open the mouth wide, but the tongue is often at the roof of the mouth.

      b. Verbal and visual cues given to the baby, such as the mother saying "open" and opening her own mouth wide, can assist with latch-on.

      c. The baby will open his or her mouth slightly at first, drop the head back slightly, and then gape and move toward the breast.

5. As the baby moves toward the breast with a wide-open mouth, the mother should quickly pull the baby into the breast.
   a. Avoid the rapid arm movement technique because this action often startles the baby and is counterproductive.
   b. The baby's chin should touch the breast first, with both the chin and the tip of the nose touching the breast.
   c. The baby's mouth should be brought up and over the areola with the baby leading with his or her chin.
6. Concerns over the infant's nose and ability to breathe:
   a. Infants are obligate nose breathers; the normal healthy neonate will not continue to nurse if he or she cannot breathe.
   b. The tip of the infant's nose is firm and pointed upward, placing the nares at the sides, which allows baby to breathe even when close to the breast.
   c. Mother should be able to see the tip of the infant's nose.
   d. Many mothers naturally push into the breast to keep it away from the baby's nose.
      i. May alter the latch-on by pulling the breast out of the baby's mouth.
      ii. May be a cause for nipple pain and/or plugged ducts.
      iii. If the mother cannot see the baby's nose, she should alter the baby's body position or the position of her hand.
         (a) Raising the infant's bottom half so that it is more level with the head can clear the nose.
         (b) Wrapping the baby's legs around the mother's waist (pulling the baby in closer to mom's body) might also work.
         (c) Lifting up slightly from underneath the breast can clear the nose.
G. Infant mouth position on the breast:
   1. The breast is not placed into the baby's mouth; the baby draws the breast into his or her mouth.
   2. Opinions differ as to the position of the baby's mouth on the areola.
      a. Some say centered.
      b. Some say asymmetrical, with the lower jaw covering more of the areola than the upper jaw (Newman et al., 2000).
      c. The most important factors are maternal comfort, areolar latch, and good milk transfer.
   3. When latched on, the baby's mouth should be wide open.
      a. Some say an angle of 130° to 150° at the corner of the mouth (Hoover, 1996).
   4. The baby's cheeks should not dimple inward with suckling.
      a. Can indicate that the tongue is held behind the lower gum and that the baby is sucking, as if from a straw.
      b. Can indicate a tight lingual frenulum.

    c. Both lips should be flared outward.

        i. Common for baby to have the upper lip curled in.

        ii. The mother should gently roll the upper lip out or relatch if this occurs.

        iii. Tight labial (maxillary) frenulum can keep the upper or lower lip from rolling outward and can be a later risk factor in development of dental caries (Kotlow, 2010; Wiessinger et al., 1995).

    d. The nipple and approximately one-fourth of the areola (about 0.5 inch) should be in the mouth; it is not necessary for the baby to draw the entire areola into his or her mouth.

  H. Signs of milk transfer (swallowing) during lactogenesis II:

    1. Puff of air from the nose.

    2. "Ca" sound from the throat.

    3. Deeper jaw excursion preceding each swallow.

    4. Slight movement can be seen just in front of the ear near the temporal region of the face.

    5. Can hear the swallow with a stethoscope placed on the baby's throat.

    6. Top of the areola moves inward toward baby's mouth.

III. The Lactation Consultant's Assessment (Tully et al., 2006; Walker, 1989a, 1989b)

A number of tools are used to assess and document various aspects of breastfeeding. The validity and reliability of some tools have been studied, which shows advantages and disadvantages of each (Adams et al., 1997; Jenks, 1991; Riordan, 1998; Riordan et al., 2001; Riordan et al., 1997; Schlomer et al., 1999). The lactation consultant should use or develop an assessment tool that assists in a comprehensive consultation. (See **Table 28-3**.)

  A. If in private practice, the lactation consultant obtains signed consent from the mother before the consultation.

  B. Lactation history:

    1. Accurate and complete history taking are especially important for the lactation consultant (Dewey et al., 2003).

      a. Breastfeeding difficulties can be a manifestation or symptom of another problem or illness.

      b. The lactation consultant cannot form a hypothesis or plan of care if the data collected are incomplete.

    2. History taking is done by means of obtaining both subjective and objective data.

      a. Subjective data are based on the interpretation of the facts, feelings, or events, by the person relating the history. Under most circumstances, these type of data cannot be verified.

      b. Objective data are verifiable, based on direct observation or measurement, as in the following examples:

        i. Evaluation of the infant in relation to feeding ability (weight, gestational age, skin color, bilirubin or blood glucose level, presence of cephalohematoma, etc.)

Table 28-3 Breastfeeding Assessment Tools

Systematic Assessment of the Infant at Breast [SAIB] (Shrago & Bocar, 1990	**Infant Breastfeeding Assessment Tool** (Matthews, 1988).
1. Assesses the mechanics of positioning, latch-on, and swallowing. 2. Validity and reliability have not been thoroughly studied.	1. Looks at the readiness to feed. 2. Lacks a measurable criterion for swallowing or milk transfer.
L-A-T-C-H (Jensen, Wallace, Et Kelsay, 1994)	**Mother-Baby Assessment Scale** [MBA] (Mulford, 1992).
1. Evaluates the amount of help a mother needs to physically breastfeed. 2. Does not clearly evaluate the latch-on component.	Has a strong evaluation component of the mother's developing skills in both recognizing when it is time to feed the baby and how to feed the baby.
Potential Early Breast Feeding Problem Tool (Kearney, Cronenwett, Et Barrett, 1990).	**Maternal Breast Feeding Evaluation Scale** (Leff, Jeffries, Gagne, 1994).
1. Has 23 questions that use a four-point Likert scale. 2. Developed to determine which breastfeeding problems are rated highest among breastfeeding mothers. 3. The higher the score, the more breastfeeding problems occurred.	1. Consists of three subscales: maternal enjoyment/role attainment, infant satisfactions/growth, and lifestyle/maternal body image. 2. Designed to measure positive and negative aspects of breastfeeding that mothers have identified as important in defining successful lactation.
Mother-Baby Assessment Scale [MBA] (Mulford, 1992).	**Latch-on and Positioning Parameters** (LAT_tm) (Cadwell 2004)
Has a strong evaluation component of the mother's developing skills in both recognizing when it is time to feed the baby and how to feed the baby.	The LAT incorporates assessment parameters mentioned in the breastfeeding literature as well as suggested corrective interventions designed to optimize latch-on and positioning

    ii. Evaluation of the mother in relation to lactation risk factors (breast size, nipple shape/protractility, presence of swelling or erythema, surgical scars, etc.)

    iii. Observation of positioning, latch-on, suckling, infant behavioral state post feed

3. History and current conditions obtained verbally from the mother (and from the written medical record, if available) should include:

    a. Previous breastfeeding experience.

        i. Has the mother breastfed previous children? If so, for how long?

        ii. Did she have nipple pain/trauma or other problems?

        iii. When and reason for weaning.

b. Previous breastfeeding education (classes, reading, videos, etc.).

c. Cultural influences.

d. Assess the mother's concerns regarding modesty.

e. Who functions as her support system?

f. Intrapartum:

   i. What type of labor medications (if any) did she receive? Some can cause sedation or poor responsiveness in the infant (Kroeger & Smith, 2004; Walker, 1997).

   ii. Did she have a vaginal delivery?

     (a) Episiotomy pain influences the mother's comfort and position.

     (b) Assisted delivery (were vacuum extraction or forceps used?).

   iii. Did she have a cesarean delivery?

     (a) Type and location of incision.

     (b) Pain might limit her early positions.

     (c) Cesarean delivery is a risk factor for delayed lactogenesis II.

   iv. What type of medications did she have following labor for subsequent pain control?

     (a) Is she currently taking pain medication?

       (i) Response to pain medications is highly individualized.

       (ii) During the early postpartum period incisional pain, from an episiotomy or cesarean section, can interfere with mother's ability to comfortably feed her infant and can inhibit milk ejection reflex.

       (iii) An analgesic taken 20 minutes prior to a feeding can increase maternal comfort level so that she can focus on her infant.

       (iv) Narcotic pain medications might sedate her and potentially her baby.

       Note: If the mother is sedated or she has low muscle tone (e.g., as a side effect of magnesium sulfate administration), the baby should not be left in bed with her without continuous supervision by an unimpaired individual.

   v. Is she taking any regular medications, vitamins, nutritional supplements, and/or herbs?

g. Are there any complications from childbirth?

   i. Extension of episiotomy or tears.

   ii. Bladder, cervical, uterine, rectal, or perineal problems.

   iii. Fever, infection.

   iv. Level and location of any pain.

h. What are her limitations?

   i. Physical

   ii. Psychological/social

- Feelings of inadequacy
- Lack of self-confidence
- Sensitivity to comments and criticism

- Is she taking medications for depression?
- Overwhelmed
- Fatigued
    iii. Medical
  i. Environmental concerns.
    i. What support will she have at home?
    ii. Will she be working outside the home?
C. Assessment
  1. Condition of breasts and nipples
    a. Size and shape of breasts.
    b. The direction that the nipple points influences where the baby's mouth is placed.
    c. Breast fullness or engorgement.
    d. Anomalies (tubular, asymmetric).
    e. Condition of the nipples and areola:
      i. Everted, flat, retracted/inverted.
      ii. Edematous areola from intravenous fluids can flatten a normal nipple as it is enveloped with swollen areolar tissue.
    f. Nipple anomalies, supernumerary nipples with or without auxiliary breast tissue.
  2. General condition of the infant (Thureen et al., 1999)
    a. Did the baby have any difficulties after birth? "Increased weight loss, hypoglycemia, infrequent nursing, or maternal reports of poor feeding are predictive of early problems." (Dann, 2005)
    b. Current weight (Vazirinejad et al., 2009):
      i. Steady weight gain (approximately 1 oz per day after lactogenesis II occurs) confirms nutritional intake.
      ii. Increasing weight loss indicates a feeding problem might be present.
    c. Color of skin: Jaundice, a visible yellowing of the skin, occurs in more than 50% of newborns (AAP, Subcommittee on Hyperbilirubinemia, 2004; Brown et al., 1993).
    d. Obvious physical anomalies. (See Chapter 27, Assessment of Infant Oral Anatomy.)
D. Current intake and output patterns (Academy of Breastfeeding Medicine Protocol Committee, 2009; Arizona Healthy Mothers, Healthy Babies Coalition Breastfeeding Task Force, 1989).
  1. Has the baby received any formula or other liquids? (bottles, pacifiers)
  2. How many voids and stools in a 24 hour day, color and consistency of stool.
    a. Voids:
      i. First 5 days: The baby should have a minimum of one void multiplied by day of age and a minimum of one stool per day.
      ii. By the 5th day of life:
        (a) Minimum of six voids with light yellow to clear urine per 24 hours.
        (b) Appearance of urate crystals after 4 days of age suggests dehydration (Neifert et al., 1986, p. 35).
        (c) Changes in voiding pattern are a late sign of poor intake.

   b. Stools:
      i. Failure of the baby to pass meconium and convert to normal breastfed stools by 5 days of age or infrequent stools is highly suggestive of inadequate intake.
      ii. Yellow, liquid, or curdy stools should follow most feedings during the first month of life.
      iii. After 6 weeks of age, it is not uncommon for the entirely breastfed infant to go several days between stools, as long as appropriate weight gain continues.
      iv. Infrequent or small, hard stools can indicate malnutrition.
E. Assess behavioral state of the baby before and after feeding (Karl, 2004).
   1. Deep sleep: Limp extremities, no body movement, placid face, quiet breathing, cannot be easily aroused.
   2. Light or active sleep: Resistance in extremities when moved, mouthing or suckling motions, facial grimaces, more easily awakened, more likely to remain awake if disturbed; if left undisturbed, will easily fall back asleep.
   3. Drowsy: Eyes open and close intermittently, might make sounds (murmur or whisper), might yawn and stretch.
   4. Quiet alert: Looks around; interacts with environment, body still and watchful, breathing even and regular. Excellent time for breastfeeding.
   5. Active alert: Moves extremities, wide eyed, irregular breathing, more sensitive to discomfort (wet diaper or excessive stimulation).
   6. Crying: Agitated, disorganized, needs comforting. Poor state to attempt breastfeeding.
F. Systematic evaluation of a nursing session
   1. Assess the mother and infant's positioning.
   2. Assess for effective latch:
      a. Wide open mouth
      b. Flared lips
      c. Chin touching the breast
   3. Maternal comfort:
      a. Continuation of nipple pain indicates an incorrect latch even if the infant is swallowing milk.
      b. Only the mother can confirm a good latch based on her personal comfort.
   4. Assess the mother for signs of milk ejection reflex (milk release).
      a. Breast softening while feeding
      b. Relaxation or drowsiness
      c. Thirst
      d. Uterine contractions or increased lochia flow during or after feeding
      e. Milk leaking from opposite breast while feeding

 5. Assess the infant for signs of milk transfer.
   a. Sustained rhythmic suck-swallow-breathe pattern with periodic pauses
   b. Audible swallowing
   c. Relaxed arms and hands
   d. Moist mouth
 6. The lactation consultant corrects positioning and latch-on techniques only as needed.
   a. The lactation consultant:
      i. Avoids "take over" behavior
      ii. Avoids positioning and latching the baby for the mother
      iii. Avoids pushing on the back of the baby's head
      iv. Avoids compressing the mother's areola
      v. Avoids inserting the areola into the baby's mouth
   b. The latch-on process is facilitated so that the mother learns to this do herself.
G. Following a breastfeeding:
 1. Assess nipple appearance immediately after feeding.
   a. The nipple comes out of the infant's mouth round and of equal color with the areola and shows no evidence of trauma.
   b. Note any abnormal nipple shape, blisters, and/or blanching.
   c. Note any continued nipple or breast pain.
 2. The mother appears relaxed.
 3. The mother reports the absence of shoulder, neck, or back pain.
 4. The baby is calm, satiated, and relaxed. Note any irritability and/or fussiness.
H. Implement an appropriate clinical strategy for any interventions.
 1. Observe a return demonstration of skills learned by mother.
 2. The mother verbalizes confidence in positioning herself and her infant.
 3. Address the mother's main concerns promptly.
   a. Perceived insufficient milk is a common maternal concern and reason for supplementing with formula.
   b. Unresolved painful breastfeeding leads to premature weaning.
 4. Give written instructions to mother for ongoing self-care.
I. Document the consultation.
 1. If inpatient, document in mother and infant's medical record.
 2. If outpatient, document in structured lactation consult form (see samples at www.go.jblearning.com/corecurriculum).
J. Arrange for follow-up care.
 1. In-person follow-up within a reasonable amount of time
 2. Telephone follow-up if appropriate
K. Consult with another healthcare provider as needed.
 1. Immediate contact of the medical provider where warranted.
 2. Provide a written report to the mother and baby's healthcare provider (ILCA, 2005b).

References

Academy of Breastfeeding Medicine Protocol Committee. (2009). Academy of Breastfeeding Medicine clinical protocol #3: Hospital guidelines for the use of supplementary feedings in the healthy term breastfed neonate, revised 2009. *Breastfeeding Medicine*, *4*(3), 175–182.

Academy of Breastfeeding Medicine Protocol Committee. (2010). Academy of Breastfeeding Medicine clinical protocol #7: Model breastfeeding policy (revision 2010). *Breastfeeding Medicine*, *5*(4), 173–177.

Adams, D., & Hewell, S. D. (1997). Maternal and professional assessment of breastfeeding. *Journal of Human Lactation*, *13*, 279–283.

American Academy of Pediatrics. (2005). Breastfeeding and the use of human milk. *Pediatrics*, *115*, 496–506. Retrieved from http://pediatrics.aappublications.org/content/115/2/496.full

American Academy of Pediatrics Section on Breastfeeding. (2009). *Sample hospital policy on breastfeeding for newborns*. Elk Grove Village, IL: American Academy of Pediatrics.

American Academy of Pediatrics, Subcommittee on Hyperbilirubinemia. (2004). Management of hyperbilirubinemia in the newborn infant 35 or more weeks gestation. *Pediatrics*, *114*(1), 297–316.

Anderson, G. C., Moore, E., Hepworth, J., & Bergman, N. (2003). Early skin-to-skin contact for mothers and their healthy newborn infants. *Cochrane Database of Systematic Reviews*, *2*, CD003519.

Arizona Healthy Mothers, Healthy Babies Coalition Breastfeeding Task Force. (1989). *Model breastfeeding hospital policy and breastfeeding education protocol manual*. Tucson, AZ: Nutrition Council of Arizona Breastfeeding Advocates.

Becker, G. E., McCormick, F. M., & Renfrew, M. J. (2008, October 8). Methods of milk expression for lactating women. *Cochrane Database of Systematic Reviews*, *4*, CD006170. Retrieved from http://www2.cochrane.org/reviews/en/ab006170.html

Berg, M., & Terstad, A. (2006). Swedish women's experiences of doula support during childbirth. *Midwifery*, *22*, 330–338.

Biancuzzo, M. (2002). *Breastfeeding the newborn: Clinical strategies for nurses* (2nd ed.). St. Louis, MO: Mosby.

Blair, A., Cadwell, K., Turner-Maffei, C., & Brimdyr, K. (2003). The relationship between positioning, the breastfeeding dynamic, the latching process and pain in breastfeeding mothers with sore nipples. *Breastfeeding Review*, *11*(2), 5–10.

Bonaro, D., & Pascali, M. K. (2004). Continuous female companionship during childbirth: A crucial resource in times of stress or calm. *Journal of Midwifery and Women's Health, 49*(Suppl. 1), 19–27.

Brown, L. P., Arnold, L., Allison, D., Klein, M. E., & Jacobsen, B. (1993). Incidence and pattern of jaundice in healthy breast-fed infants during the first month of life. *Nursing Research*, *42*(2), 106–110.

Bystrova, K., Widström, A.-M., Matthiesen, A.-S., Ransjö-Arvidson, A,-B., Welles-Nyström, B., Vorontsov, I., & Uvnäs-Moberg, K. (2007). Early lactation performance in primiparous and multiparous women in relation to different maternity home practices. A randomised trial in St. Petersburg. *International Breastfeeding Journal*, *2*, 9. Retrieved from http://www.internationalbreastfeedingjournal.com/content/2/1/9

Cadwell, K., Turner-Maffei, C., Blair, A., Brimdyr, K., McInerney, & Z. M. (2004). Pain reduction and treatment of sore nipples in nursing mothers. *Journal of Perinatal Education*, *13*(1), 29–35.

Cadwell, K., Turner-Maffei, C., O'Connor, B., & Blair, A. (2002). *Maternal and infant assessment for breastfeeding. and human lactation: A guide for the practitioner*. Sudbury, MA: Jones and Bartlett.

Chantry, C. J., Nommsen-Rivers, L. A., Peerson, J. M., Cohen, R. J., & Dewey, K. G. (2011). Excess weight loss in first-born breastfed newborns relates to maternal intrapartum fluid balance. *Pediatrics, 127*(1), e171–179

Chiu, S. H., Anderson, G. C., & Burkhammer, M. D. (2005). Newborn temperature during skin-skin breastfeeding in couples having breastfeeding difficulties. *Birth, 32*, 115–121.

Christensson, K. (1996). Fathers can effectively achieve heat conservation in healthy newborn. *Acta Paediatrica, 85*(11), 1354–1360.

Christensson, K., Cabrera, T., Christensson, E., et al. (1995). Separation distress call in the human neonate in the absence of maternal body contact. *Acta Paediatrica, 84*,468–473.

Coates, M., & Riordan, J. (Eds.). (2010). *Breastfeeding and human lactation* (4th ed.). Sudbury, MA: Jones and Bartlett.

Colson, S. (2005a). Maternal breastfeeding positions: Have we got it right? *Practising Midwife, 8*(11), 29–32.

Colson, S.(2005b). Maternal breastfeeding positions: Have we got it right? *Practising Midwife, 8*(10), 24–27.

Colson, S. (2010, Fall). What happens to breastfeeding when mother lie back? Clinical applications of biological nurturing. *Clinical Lactation. Journal of the US Lactation Consultant Association, 1.*

Colson, S. D., Meek, J., & Hawdon, J. M. (2008). Optimal positions triggering primitive neonatal reflexes stimulating breastfeeding. *Early Human Development, 84*(7), 441–449.

Cotterman, K. J. (2004). Reverse pressure softening: A simple tool to prepare areola for easier latching during engorgement. *Journal of Human Lactation, 20*, 227–237.

Dann, M. H. (2005). The lactation consult: Problem solving teaching and support for the breastfeeding family. *Journal of Pediatric Health Care, 19*(1), 12–16. Retrieved from http://www.medscape.com/viewarticle/498609_4

Dashe, J. S., Rogers, B. B., Mclntire, D. D., & Leveno, K. J. (1999). Epidural analgesia and intrapartum fever: Placental findings. *Obstetrics and Gynecology, 93*, 341–344.

Davies, B., Edwards, N., Ploeg, J., & Virani, T. (2008). Insights about the process and impact of implementing nursing guidelines on delivery of care in hospitals and community settings. *BMC Health Services Research, 8*, 29. Retrieved from http://www.biomedcentral.com/1472-6963/8/29

DeCarvalho, M., Robertson, S., Friedman, A., & Klaus, M. (1983). Effect of frequent breast feeding in early milk production and infant weight gain. *Pediatrics, 71*, 307–311.

Dewey, K. G., Nommsen-Rivers, L. A., Heinig, M. J., & Cohen, R. J. (2003). Risk factors for suboptimal infant breastfeeding behavior, delayed onset of lactation, and excess neonatal weight loss. *Pediatrics, 112*, 607–619.

Fletcher, D., & Harris, H. (2000). The implementation of the HOT (hands off technique) program at the Royal Women's Hospital. *Breastfeeding Review, 8*, 19–23.

Food and Drug Administration. (1998, May 21). FDA public health warning: Need for caution when using vacuum assisted delivery devices. Retrieved from http://www.fda.gov/MedicalDevices/Safety/AlertsandNotices/PublicHealthNotifications/UCM062295

Furman, L., Minich, N., & Hack, M. (2002). Correlates of lactation in mothers of very low birth weight infants [Abstract]. *Pediatrics, 109*, 695–696. Retrieved from http://www.pediatrics.org/cgi/content/full/109/4/e57

Gordon, N. P., Walton, D., McAdam, E., et al. (1999). Effects of providing hospital-based doulas in health maintenance organization hospitals. *Obstetrics and Gynecology, 93*, 422–426.

Grajeda, R., & Pérez-Escamilla, R. (2002). Stress during labor and delivery is associated with delayed onset of lactation among urban Guatemalan women. *Journal of Nutrition, 132,* 3055–3060.

Gross, J. B., Cohen, A. P., Lang, J. M., et al. (2002). Differences in systemic opioid use do not explain increased fever incidence in patients receiving epidural analgesia. *Anesthesiology, 97,* 157–161.

Hall, R. T., Mercer, A. M., Teasley, S. L., et al. (2002). A breastfeeding assessment score to evaluate the risk for cessation of breastfeeding by 7 to 10 days of age. *Journal of Pediatrics, 141,* 659–664.

Hamosh, M. (2001). Bioactive factors in human milk. *Pediatric Clinics of North America, 48*(1), 69–86.

Henderson, A., Stamp, G., & Pincombe, J. (2001). Postpartum positioning and attachment education for increasing breastfeeding: A randomized trial. *Birth, 28*(4), 236–242.

Henrikson, M. (1990). A policy for supplementary/complementary feedings for breastfed newborn infants. *Journal of Human Lactation, 6*(1), 11–14.

Hill, P. D., Aldag, J. C., & Chatterton, R. T. (1999). Effects of pumping style on milk production in mothers of non-nursing preterm infants. *Journal of Human Lactation, 15,* 209–216.

Hill, P. D., Aldag, J. C., Chatterton, R. T., & Zinaman, M. (2005). Primary and secondary mediators' influence on milk output in lactating mothers of preterm and term infants. *Journal of Human Lactation, 21,* 138–150.

Hodnett, E. D., Gates, S., Hofmeyr, G. J., Sakala, C., & Weston, J. (2011). Continuous support for women during childbirth. *Cochrane Database of Systematic Reviews, 2,* CD003766. doi:10.1002/14651858.CD003766.pub3

Hoover, K. (1996). Visual assessment of the baby's wide open mouth. *Journal of Human Lactation, 12,* 9.

Hoover, K. (2000). Latch-on difficulties: A clinical observation. *Journal of Human Lactation, 16*(1), 6.

Hopkinson, J. M., Schanler, R. J., & Garza, C. (1988). Milk production by mothers of premature infants. *Pediatrics, 81,* 815–820.

Ingram, J., Johnson, D., & Greenwood, R. (2002). Breastfeeding in Bristol: Teaching good positioning, and support from fathers and families. *Midwifery, 18*(2), 87–101.

International Board of Lactation Consultant Examiners (IBLCE). (2010). Clinical competencies for the practice of International Board Certified Lactation Consultants (IBCLCs). Retrieved from http://www.iblce.org/upload/downloads/ClinicalCompetencies.pdf

International Lactation Consultant Association. (2005a). *Clinical guidelines for the establishment of exclusive breastfeeding* (2nd ed.). Rockville, MD: Maternal and Child Health Bureau.

International Lactation Consultant Association. (2005b). Standards of practice for International Board certified lactation consultants. Retrieved from http://www.ilca.org

Jenks, M. A. (1991). Latch assessment in the hospital nursery. *Journal of Human Lactation, 7,*19–20.

Jensen, D., Wallace, S., & Kelsay, P. (1994). L-A-T-C-H: A breastfeeding charting system and documentation tool. *Journal of Obstetric, Gynecologic, and Neonatal Nursing, 23,* 27–32.

Jordan, S., Emery, S., Watkins, A., Evans, J., Storey, M., & Morgan, G. (2009). Associations of drugs routinely given in labour with breastfeeding at 48 hours: Analysis of the Cardiff Births Survey. *BJOG, 116,* 1622–1632.

Karl, D. J. (2004). Using principles of newborn behavioral state organization to facilitate breastfeeding. *American Journal of Maternal and Child Nursing, 29,* 292–298.

Kearney, M., Cronenwett, L., & Barrett, J. (1990). Breastfeeding problems in the first week postpartum. *Nursing Review, 39,* 90–95.

Kennell, J., Klaus, M., McGrath, S., & Robertson, S. (1991). Continuous emotional support during labor in a U.S. hospital. A randomized controlled trial. *Journal of the American Medical Association, 256,* 2197–2201.

Kennell, J. H., & Klaus, M. H. (1998). Bonding: Recent observations that alter perinatal care. *Pediatrics Review, 19*, 4–12.

Kiremitci, S., Tuzun, F., Yesilirmak, D. C., Kumral, A., Duman, N., & Ozkan, H. (2011). Is gastric aspiration needed for newborn management in delivery room? *Resuscitation, 82*(1), 40–44. Retrieved from http://www.ncbi.nlm.nih.gov/pubmed/20951491

Klaus, M., & Klaus, P. (1998). *Your amazing newborn*. Reading, MA: Perseus Books.

Kroeger, M., & Smith, L. (2004). *Impact of birthing practices on breastfeeding: Protecting the mother–baby continuum* (2nd ed.). Sudbury, MA: Jones and Bartlett.

Langer, A., Compero, L., Garcia, C., & Reynoso, S. (1998). Effects of psychosocial support during labor and childbirth on breastfeeding, medical interventions, and mothers' well-being in a Mexican public hospital: A randomized clinical trial. *British Journal of Obstetrics and Gynaecology, 105*,1056–1063.

Lauwers, J., & Swisher, A. (2010). *Counseling the nursing mother: A lactation consultant's guide* (5th ed.). Sudbury, MA: Jones and Bartlett.

Lawn, J. E., Mwansa-Kambafwile, J., Horta, B. L., Barros, F. C., & Cousens, S. (2010). "Kangaroo mother care" to prevent neonatal deaths due to preterm birth complications. *International Journal of Epidemiology, 39*, i144–i154.

Lawrence, R. A., & Lawrence, R. M. (2011). *Breastfeeding: A guide for the medical profession* (7th ed.). New York, NY: Mosby.

Leff, E., Jeffries, S., & Gagne, M. (1994). The development of the maternal breastfeeding evaluation scale. *Journal of Human Lactation, 10*, 105–111.

Leighton, B. L., & Halpern, S. H. (2002). The effects of epidural analgesia on labor, maternal, and neonatal outcomes: A systematic review. *American Journal of Obstetrics and Gynecology, 186*(5 Suppl. Nature), S69–S77.

Lewallen, L. P. (2006). A review of instruments used to predict early breastfeeding attrition. *Journal of Perinatal Education, 15*(1), 26–41.

Lieberman, E., Fichenwald, E., Mathur, G., et al. (2000). Intrapartum fever and unexplained seizures in term infants. *Pediatrics, 106*, 983–988.

Lieberman, E., Lang, J., Richardson, D. K., et al. (2000). Intrapartum maternal fever and neonatal outcome. *Pediatrics, 105*, 813.

Lieberman, F., Lang, J. M., Frigoletto, F., Jr., et al. (1997). Epidural analgesia, intrapartum fever, and neonatal sepsis evaluation. *Pediatrics, 99*, 415–419.

Lieberman, F., & O'Donoghue, C. (2002). Unintended effects of epidural analgesia during labor: A systemic review. *American Journal of Obstetrics and Gynecology, 186*(5 Suppl. Nature), 531–568.

Lothian, J. A. (2005). The birth of a breastfeeding baby and mother. *Journal of Perinatal Education, 14*(1), 42–45. Retrieved from http://www.ncbi.nlm.nih.gov/pmc/articles/PMC1595228/

Ludington-Hoe, S. M., Anderson, G. C., Simpson, S., et al. (1999). Birth-related fatigue in 34–36 week preterm neonates: Rapid recovery with very early Kangaroo (skin-to-skin) care. *Journal of Obstetric, Gynecologic, and Neonatal Nursing, 28*, 94–103.

Maffei, C., Blair, A., Brimdyr, K., & McInerney, Z. M. (2004). Pain reduction and treatment of sore nipples in nursing mothers. *Journal of Perinatal Education, 13*(1), 29-35

Marasco, L., & Barger, J. (1999). Examining the evidence for cue feeding of breastfed infants. *Breastfeeding Abstracts*, June 1999. Retrieved from http://www.ezzo.info/Aney/cuefeeding.pdf

Marlier, L., Schaal, B., & Soussignan, R. (1997). Orientation responses to biological odours in the human newborn. Initial pattern and postnatal plasticity. *Comptes Rendus de l'Académie des Sciences* III, *320*, 999–1005.

Matthews, M. K. (1988). Developing an instrument to assess infant breastfeeding behavior in the early neonatal period. *Midwifery*, *4*, 154–165.

Mennella, J. A., Jagnow, C. P., & Beauchamp, G. K. (2001). Prenatal and postnatal flavor learning by human infants. *Pediatrics*, *107*, e88. Retrieved from http://www.ncbi.nlm.nih.gov/pubmed/11389286

Merry, H., & Montgomery, A. (2000). Do breastfed babies whose mothers have had labor epidurals lose more weight in the first 24 hours of life? Annual Meeting Abstracts. *Academy of Breastfeeding Medicine News and Views*, *6*, 21.

Michelsson, K., Christensesson, K., Rothganger, H., & Winberg, J. (1996). Crying in separated and nonseparated newborns: Sound spectrographic analysis. *Acta Paediatrica*, *85*, 471–475.

Mikiel-Kostyra, K., Mazur, J., & Boltruszko, I. (2002). Effect of early skin-to-skin contact after delivery on duration of breastfeeding: A prospective cohort study. *Acta Paediatrica*, *91*, 1301–1306.

Minchin, M. (1989). Positioning for breastfeeding. *Birth*, *16*, 67–73.

Mohrbacher, N., & Kendall-Tackett, K. (2005). *Breastfeeding made simple: Seven natural laws for nursing mothers*. Oakland, CA: Harbinger Books.

Mohrbacher, N., & Stock, J. (2003). *The breastfeeding answer book* (rev. ed.). Schaumburg, IL: La Leche League International.

Morhason-Bello, I. O., Adedokun, B. O., & Ojengbede, O. A. (2009). Social support during childbirth as a catalyst for early breastfeeding initiation for first-time Nigerian mothers. *International Breastfeeding Journal*, *4*, 16. Retrieved from http://www.internationalbreastfeedingjournal.com/content/4/1/16

Morton, J., Hall, J. Y., Wong, R. J., Thairu, L., Benitz, W. E., & Rhine, W. D. (2009). Combining hand techniques with electric pumping increases milk production in mothers of preterm infants. *Journal of Perinatology*, *29*(11), 757–764. Advance online publication..

Morton, J. A. (1992). Ineffective suckling: A possible consequence of obstructive positioning. *Journal of Human Lactation*, *8*(2), 83–85.

Mulford, C. (1992). The Mother-Baby Assessment (MBA): An "Apgar score" for breastfeeding. *Journal of Human Lactation*, *8*, 79–82.

Nakao, Y., Moji, K., Honda, S., & Oishi, K. (2008). Initiation of breastfeeding within 120 minutes after birth is associated with breastfeeding at four months among Japanese women: A self-administered questionnaire survey. *International Breastfeeding Journal*, *3*, 1. Retrieved from http://www.internationalbreastfeedingjournal.com/content/3/1/1

Negishi, C., Lenhardt, R., Ozaki, M., et al. (2001). Opioids inhibit febrile responses in humans, whereas epidural analgesia does not: An explanation for hyperthermia during epidural analgesia. *Anesthesiology*, *94*, 218–222.

Neifert, M., & Seacat, J. (1986). A guide to successful breast-feeding. *Contemporary Pediatrics*, *3*, 26–40.

Neville, M. C., & Morton, J. (2001). Physiology and endocrine changes underlying human lactogenesis II. *Journal of Nutrition*, *131*, 3005S–3008S.

Newman, J., & Pitman, T. (2000a). *Dr. Jack Newman's guide to breastfeeding*. Toronto, Canada: Harper Collins.

Newman, J., & Pitman, T. (2000b). *The ultimate breastfeeding book of answers*. Roseville, CA: Prima.

Perez, P. G. (1998). Labor support to promote vaginal delivery. *Baby Care Forum*, *1*, 3.

Perlman, J. M. (1999). Maternal fever and neonatal depression: Preliminary observations. *Clinical Pediatrics (Phila)*, *38*, 287–291.

Petrova, A., Demissie, K., Rhoads, G. G., et al. (2001). Association of maternal fever during labor with neonatal and infant morbidity and mortality. *Obstetrics and Gynecology*, *98*, 20–27.

Philip, J., Alexander, J. M., Sharma, S. K., et al. (1999). Epidural analgesia during labor and maternal fever. *Anesthesiology*, *90*, 1271–1275.

Powers, N. G., & Slusser, W. (1997). Breastfeeding update 2: Clinical lactation management. *Pediatrics Review*, *18*, 147–161.

Ransjo-Arvidson, A.-B., Matthiesen, A.-S., Lilja, G., et al. (2001). Maternal analgesia during labor disturbs newborn behavior: Effects on breastfeeding, temperature and crying. *Birth*, *28*, 512.

Renfrew, M., Fisher, C., & Arms, S. (2000). *Breastfeeding: Getting breastfeeding right for you* (rev. ed.). Berkeley, CA: Celestial Arts.

Righard, L., & Alade, M. O. (1990). Effect of delivery room routines on success of first breastfeed. *Lancet*, *336*, 1105–1107.

Righard, L., & Alade, M. O. (1992). Sucking technique and its effect on success of breastfeeding. *Birth*, *19*(4), 185–189.

Riordan, J. (1998, December). Predicting breastfeeding problems. *AWHONN Lifelines*, 31–33.

Riordan, J., Bibb, D., Miller, M., & Rawlins, T. (2001). Predicting breastfeeding duration using the LATCH breastfeeding assessment tool. *Journal of Human Lactation*, *17*, 20–23.

Riordan, J. M., & Koehn, M. (1997). Reliability and validity testing of three breastfeeding assessment tools. *Journal of Obstetric, Gynecologic, and Neonatal Nursing*, *26*, 181–187.

Rosen, P. (2004). Supporting women in labor: Analysis of different types of caregivers. *Journal of Midwifery and Women's Health*, *49*, 24–31.

Schaal, B., Hummel, I., & Soussignan, R. (2004). Olfaction in the fetal and premature infant: functional status and clinical implications. *Clinical Perinatology*, *31*, vi–vii, 261–285.

Schlomer, J. A., Kemmerer, J., & Twiss, J. J. (1999). Evaluating the association of two breastfeeding assessment tools with breastfeeding problems and breastfeeding satisfaction. *Journal of Human Lactation*, *15*, 35–39.

Sepkoski, C., Lester, B. M., Ostbeimer, G. W., & Brazelton, T. B. (2005). Neonatal effects of maternal epidurals. *Developmental Medicine and Child Neurology*, *36*, 375–376.

Shrago, L., & Bocar, D. (1990). The infant's contribution to breastfeeding. *Journal of Obstetric, Gynecologic, and Neonatal Nursing*, *19*, 209–215.

Smillie, C. M. (2007). How infants learn to feed: A neurobehavioral model. In C. W. Genna (Ed.), *Supporting sucking skills in breastfeeding infants* (pp. 79–95). Sudbury, MA: Jones and Bartlett.

Stainton, C., Edwards, S., Jones, B., & Switonski, C. (1999). The nature of maternal postnatal pain. *Journal of Perinatal Education*, *8*(2), 1–10.

Thureen, P., Deacon, J., O'Neill, P., & Hernandez, J. (Eds.). (1999). Assessment and care of the well newborn. Philadelphia, PA: W. B. Saunders.

Torvaldsen, S., Roberts, C. L., Simpson, J. M., Thompson, J. F., & Ellwood, D. A. (2006). Intrapartum epidural analgesia and breastfeeding: A prospective cohort study. *International Breastfeeding Journal*, *1*, 24. Retrieved from http://www.internationalbreastfeedingjournal.com/content/1/1/24

Towner, D., Castro, M. A., Eby-Wilkins, E., & Hilbert, W. M. (1999). Effect of mode of delivery in nulliparous women on neonatal intracranial injury. *New England Journal of Medicine*, *341*, 1709–1714.

Tully, M. & Overfield, M. (2006). Breastfeeding counseling guide (2nd ed.). Raleigh, NC: Lactation Consultants of North Carolina.

Varendi, H., Christensson, K., Winberg, J., & Porter, R. H. (1998). Soothing effect of amniotic fluid smell in newborn infants. *Early Human Development*, *51*, 47–55.

Varendi, H., & Porter, R. H. (2001). Breast odor as the only maternal stimulus elicits crawling towards the odour source. *Acta Paediatrica*, *90*, 372–375.

Vazirinejad, R., Darakhshan, S., Esmaeili, A., & Hadadian, S. (2009). The effect of maternal breast variations on neonatal weight gain in the first seven days of life. *International Breastfeeding Journal*, *4*, 13. Retrieved from http://www.internationalbreastfeedingjournal.com/content/4/1/13

Vestermark, V., Hogdall, C. K., Birch, M., et al. (1991). Influence of the mode of delivery on initiation of breast-feeding. *European Journal of Obstetrics, Gynecology, and Reproductive Biology*, *38*, 33–38.

Walker, M. (1989a). Functional assessment of infant feeding patterns. *Birth*, *16*(3), 140–147.

Walker, M. (1989b). Management of selected early breastfeeding problems seen in clinical practice. *Birth*, *16*(3), 148–158.

Walker, M. (1997). Do labor medications affect breastfeeding? *Journal of Human Lactation*, *13*, 131–137.

Walker, M. (2009). *Breastfeeding management for the clinician: Using the evidence* (2nd ed.). Sudbury, MA: Jones and Bartlett.

Walters, M. W., Boggs, K. M., Ludington-Hoe, S., Price, K. M., & Morrison, B. (2007). Kangaroo care at birth for full term infants: A pilot study. *MCN: American Journal of Maternal and Child Nursing*, *32*(6), 375–381.

Widström, A. M., Lilja, G., Aaltomaa-Michalias, P., Dahllöf, A., Lintula, M., & Nissen, E. (2011). Newborn behaviour to locate the breast when skin-to-skin: A possible method for enabling early self-regulation. *Acta Paediatrica*, *100*(1), 79–85.

Widström, A. M., Ransiö-Arvidson, A. B., Christensson, K., Matthiesen, A.-S., Winberg, J., & Uvnäs-Moberg, K. (1987). Gastric suction in healthy newborn infants: Effects on circulation and developing feeding behaviour. *Acta Pædiatrica Scandinavica*, *76*, 566–572.

Wiessinger, D. (1998). A breastfeeding teaching tool using a sandwich analogy. *Journal of Human Lactation*, *14*(1), 51–56.

Wiessinger, D., & Miller, M. (1995). Breastfeeding difficulties as a result of tight lingual and labial frena: A case report. *Journal of Human Lactation*, *11*, 313–316.

World Health Organization & UNICEF. (2009). *Baby-friendly hospital initiative: Revised, updated and expanded for integrative care*. Retrieved from http://www.who.int/nutrition/publications/infantfeeding/9789241594950/

Yerge-Cole, G. (2010). Collecting every drop. *Journal of Human Lactation*, *26*, 10.

Suggested Reading

American Academy of Pediatrics. (n.d.). Breastfeeding residency curriculum. Retrieved from http://www2.aap.org/breastfeeding/curriculum/

Morton, J. (n.d.). *Hand expression of breast milk* [video]. Retrieved from http://newborns.stanford.edu/Breastfeeding/HandExpression.html.

CHAPTER 29
Breastfeeding a Preterm Infant

Mary Grace Lanese, RN, BSN, IBCLC, and Melissa Cross, RN, IBCLC

OBJECTIVES

- Understand problems associated with prematurity and their effects on the establishment of breastfeeding.
- Understand the nutritional needs of the preterm infant and the importance of human milk.
- Understand the importance of the use of donor human milk if mother's own milk is not available.
- List the scientific basis for breastfeeding the preterm infant.
- Describe how maturation influences suckling, swallowing, and breathing coordination and the impact on the preterm infant's ability to breastfeed.
- List characteristics of preterm and late preterm infants that challenge successful breastfeeding.
- Understand the importance of kangaroo care to parents, infants, and establishing successful breastfeeding.
- Describe the importance of a developmentally sensitive environment in the intensive care nursery.
- Describe a discharge feeding plan for the preterm infant.

INTRODUCTION

Establishing breastfeeding for a preterm infant can be a challenge. Problems include how to provide adequate nutrients the infant can absorb and utilize in amounts that promote optimal growth and development without causing unnecessary stress to the immature infant. Mother's own breastmilk is the most appropriate milk to provide adequate nutrition as well as protection from disease and infections. In all regions of the world, infants not fed mother's own breastmilk have an increased morbidity and mortality rate. If mother's own milk is not available, donor milk is the next most appropriate option.

Support and appropriate management in establishing and maintaining milk production when the infant is unable to initiate breastfeeding are critical to a successful outcome. The lactation consultant must take into consideration the special needs of

(continues)

the preterm infant and incorporate into these knowledge of the physiological process of breastfeeding the healthy term infant. Ideally, the lactation consultant is a member of a multidisciplinary collaborative team that, in addition to parents, also includes nurses, physicians, nutritionists, occupational therapists, massage therapists, social workers, developmental specialists, and discharge planners. Lactation support must be a team effort that is research based and comprehensive. Breastfeeding the preterm infant requires commitment of maternal time and energy, and nurturing support and compassion from the healthcare team.

An important factor affecting breastfeeding success is maternal morbidity. Many mothers experience a complicated pregnancy, possibly including illness, prolonged bed rest, and cesarean birth. They also may lack breastfeeding knowledge. Social and economic factors of the parents and gestational age, weight, and morbidity of the infant are other factors that affect successful breastfeeding. As a result of improved technology, the age of viability has improved so that infants of gestational age as early as 23 to 24 weeks are surviving. This situation presents a unique set of hurdles in achieving optimal short-term nutrition and long-term physical and cognitive development. Mothers of preterm infants experience challenges that are unique to the preterm situation in addition to the stress that is involved in a life event that has an uncertain outcome.

I. Definition of a Preterm Infant

   A. Birth prior to 37th week of gestation.
   B. Weight:
      1. Less than 2,500 g is referred to as low birth weight.
      2. Less than 1,500 g is referred to as very low birth weight (VLBW).
      3. Less than 1,250 g is often referred to as extremely low birth weight (ELBW).
   C. Gestational age and weight are assessed together to determine whether the infant is small for gestational age as a result of intrauterine growth retardation, appropriate for gestational age, or large for gestational age.
   D. Each preterm infant is unique in development and required care; a 35-week preterm infant who was born at 24 weeks is developmentally different from a preterm infant born at 35 weeks.

II. Hospital Obstacles to Breastfeeding the Preterm Infant

   A. Inconsistent or incorrect information
      1. Information should be based on research and not personal experience or opinion.
      2. Mothers can be confused by the same information being said in different ways; scripting can help. Scripting is a prepared statement followed by all to explain something. For example: Breastfeed your baby at least every 3 hours versus breastfeed your baby at least eight times a day. These statements are the same but might be viewed by some mothers as different and inconsistent. Therefore,

pick one phrase and use it consistently in all education materials and teaching opportunities with mothers.

B. Lack of family-centered developmental care philosophy that actively involves parents in the care of their infant (Huppertze et al., 2005)

C. Lack of private space for nursing or pumping

D. Lack of proper equipment

E. Lack of acknowledgment of the value of human milk

F. Pressure for early discharge

III. Needs of the Preterm Infant to Facilitate Normal Growth and Development

A. Respiratory rate within normal range and stable.

B. Maintain blood sugar above 2.5 mM/L (40 mg/dL).

C. Maintain body temperature within normal range.

D. Adequate nutrition unique to each infant:

    1. The metabolized energy requirement varies according to gestational age, weight, and wellness of the preterm; it can vary from 109 to 140 kcal/kg/day.

    2. Feedings for a 2,000-g and more than 32 weeks at birth preterm infant usually vary only in volume and frequency from the full-term infant.

E. Regular kangaroo care skin-to-skin contact with parents, daily, if possible (Anderson, 2003).

IV. Needs of Mother and Father Who Have a Preterm Infant

A. It is common for the mother of the preterm infant to be ill as a result of complications of the pregnancy or labor. The mother may require special medical considerations.

B. Mothers should be provided with information to make an informed decision regarding breastfeeding and/or providing human milk for their infants.

    1. Withholding information in attempts to avoid making mothers feel guilty if they choose not to breastfeed or provide milk denies women the right to make decisions based on factual information (Miracle et al., 2004).

    2. Mothers are highly influenced by the advice of professionals who care for the infant, feeling thankful for (not coerced by) their guidance and even resentful if misinformed about formula being equally acceptable (Miracle et al., 2004).

C. Support and education on parenting a preterm infant.

D. Facilitating parental infant care in the nursery.

E. Establishment and maintenance of lactation by regular, frequent milk expression:

    1. Milk expression and breastfeeding can be highly significant for the mother.

        a. These two actions are contributions to the infant's care that only the mother can make.

        b. They represent a normalization of an abnormal event.

        c. Breastfeeding is a caregiving behavior that does not have to be forfeited because of the preterm birth.

F. A knowledge of the appropriate storage conditions of expressed milk (Human Milk Bank Association of North America, 2011).

G. Open visiting/accommodations for parents with their infant:

    1. Parents have a need for close physical contact with their infant, such as early and frequent kangaroo care.

        a. Skin-to-skin care is associated with increased mounts of milk, longer duration of breastfeeding, and breastfeeding success (Furman et al., 2002).

H. Skilled health professionals knowledgeable about breastfeeding management are an important element of the support of the mother in her goal to breastfeed.

    1. The mother and healthcare team should establish a breastfeeding plan.

    2. Mother's breastfeeding plan should be regularly reviewed to ensure that it reflects the infant's current state of development.

I. Mothers have identified five positive outcomes or rewards from their preterm breastfeeding experience and have concluded that the rewards outweigh the efforts (Kavanaugh et al., 1997).

    1. The health benefits of breastmilk

    2. Knowing that they gave their infants the best possible start in life

    3. Enjoyment of the physical closeness and the perception that their infant preferred breastfeeding to bottle-feeding

    4. Knowing that they made a unique contribution to the infant's care

    5. Belief and experience that breastfeeding was more convenient

V. Common Conditions Associated with Prematurity and Their Effects on Breastfeeding

A. Respiratory distress syndrome: Severe impairment of respiratory function in a preterm newborn, caused by immaturity of the lungs.

B. Necrotizing enterocolitis (NEC): A potentially fatal inflammation with cell death in the lining of the intestines.

    1. Breastmilk-fed infants have a reduced evidence of necrotizing enterocolitis (Guthrie et al., 2003; Henderson et al., 2007; Thompson et al., 2011).

C. Hyperbilirubinemia.

D. Intracranial hemorrhage.

E. Hypoglycemia.

F. Bronchopulmonary dysplasia: Iatrogenic chronic lung disease that develops in preterm infants after a period of positive pressure ventilation.

G. The optimal growth of preterm infants.

H. All of the preceding conditions and their treatments usually result in prolonged separation of the preterm infant and the mother, resulting in the delay and/or interruption of breastfeeding.

VI. Advantages of Human Milk for Preterm Infants

A. Mother's own milk is the optimal milk for the preterm infant.
   1. Morbidity and mortality rates increase significantly when the infant is not fed human milk (Schanler, 2001, 2011).
   2. Preterm infants who are fed human milk accrue immune system enhancement, gastrointestinal (GI) maturation, and nutrient availability (Schanler, 2011;).
   3. If mother's own milk is not available, fortified donor human milk or preterm formula are options (Wight et al., 2008; Ziegler et al. & the "Food For Thought" Exploratory Group NIC/Q 2005, 2007). **Figure 29-1** is an example of a lactation consultant placing donor human milk in storage. (See Chapter 36: Donor Human Milk Banking.)

B. Achievement of greater enteral feeding tolerance and more rapid advancement to full enteral feeds.
   1. Physiological amino acids and fatty acid profiles enhance the digestion and absorption of these nutrients.
   2. Low renal solute load.

C. Gastric emptying time in a formula-fed preterm infant can be up to twice the time of a breastmilk-fed infant (51 vs. 25 min; Van den Driessche et al., 1999).

D. Contains active enzymes (such as lipase, amylase, and lysozyme) that are lacking in the underdeveloped intestine or intestinal system and provide trophic factors that hasten the maturation of the preterm intestinal system (Lawrence et al., 2010).

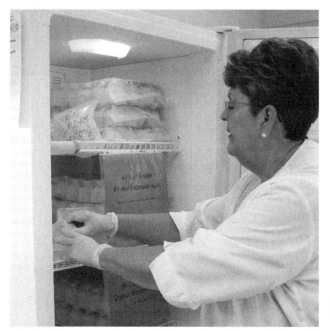

Figure 29-1

E. Reduced risk of allergy in atopic families (American Academy of Pediatrics [AAP], 2005; Saarinen et al., 1995).

F. Weight gain of not only fat and water, but also bone and other tissue.

G. Optimal development of visual acuity and retinal health (Schanler, 2011).

H. Cognitive and neurodevelopmental outcomes are enhanced, with preterm infants who have been fed breastmilk showing higher IQs (Lucas et al., 1992; Vohr et al., 2006).

    1. Long-chain polyunsaturated fatty acids present in breastmilk but not in many formulas are considered to be closely linked to this outcome (Lucas et al., 1992; Vohr et al., 2006).

I. Protection from environmental pathogens (Schanler, 2011).

    1. Particularly important in a special care nursery with invasive treatments and many staff members handling the infant.

J. Preterm human milk is optimally suited to the maturation of systems, immunological requirements, and growth of the preterm infant.

    1. Human milk is a medicine for both the infant and the mother: the milk for the infant, and the provision of it for the mother (Wight et al., 2008).

VII. Components of Preterm Human Milk

A. When compared to full-term breastmilk, preterm milk has higher concentrations of calories, lipids, high nitrogen protein, sodium, chloride, potassium, iron, and magnesium (Gross et al., 1980; Lawrence et al., 2010).

B. Calcium and phosphorus are the most commonly lacking macrominerals (Polberger et al., 1993).

C. The addition of extra nutrients, vitamins, and minerals is needed for the VLBW infant.

D. Preterm human milk is optimal for the preterm infant because of his or her limited renal concentrating and diluting capacities, a large surface area in relation to weight, and insensible water loss.

E. The milk of mothers of preterm infants matures to the level of term milk at about 4 to 6 weeks.

F. Research confirms that human milk with appropriate fortification for the very low birth weight infant is the standard of care (AAP, 2005; Wight et al., 2008; Ziegler et al., 2007).

VIII. Nutritional Considerations and Optimal Growth of Preterm Infants

A. Optimal growth is typically based on the growth curve that would have been followed if the preterm infant had remained in utero.

    1. This target can be achieved more easily in infants who have higher gestational ages.

    2. The ELBW infant has a high energy requirement but limited volume tolerance, so intake might be restricted.

B. Early enteral feedings (EEF) of breastmilk before the infant is actually ready to be fed by mouth are sometimes used to prime the gut (Wight et al., 2008).

    1. EEF are variously referred to as trickle feeds, trophic feeds, or GI priming feeds: 0.5–1 mL bolus via nasogastric tube every 3 or 6 hours (McClure et al., 2000).

    2. EEF are based on the concept that GI hormones are absent in the gut of infants who have never been fed.

    3. Trophic feeds facilitate protective gut flora, improve bowel emptying of meconium, and decrease morbidity and mortality from NEC.

    4. More mature motor patterns in the gut are seen with these small feeds (Schanler, Shulman et al., 1999a).

    5. If infusion pumps are used for feeding, the syringe should be tilted upward at a 25° to 45° angle so that the lipids rise to the Luer of the syringe and are infused first.

C. Many guidelines for the progression of preterm infant feeding exist throughout the world.

    1. Practices depend on the level and availability of technology within each country and within each individual nursery.

    2. Many nurseries are implementing kangaroo care, which reduces or changes the need for extensive policies for initiating and maintaining breastfeeding in the preterm infant.

IX. Fortification of Human Milk

A. Human milk can be fortified with commercial fortifiers that include cow's milk–based protein, electrolytes, and a number of vitamins and minerals (Schanler, 1996).

B. Human milk can be fortified with specific nutrients, such as calcium and phosphorus.

C. Fortification is usually begun after full feeding is established and discontinued before discharge from the intensive or special care unit.

D. Using the hindmilk portion of expressed milk (lacto-engineering) as a concentrated source of lipids provides a high-calorie, low-volume, low-osmolaric, readily absorbable supplement (Kirsten et al., 1999).

E. Hindmilk and commercial fortifiers are used for different purposes.

    1. Commercial fortifiers are used to supplement essential nutrients.

    2. Hindmilk provides a concentrated source of lipids and calories and can be used to increase caloric intake if mother's milk production is in excess of infant's needs (Wight et al., 2008).

F. Lacto-engineering can further refine and tailor the milk to a specific infant's needs (Meier et al., 1996). More research is needed on fortification in conjunction with the long-term use of hindmilk.

G. A mother's milk can be analyzed using specialized testing techniques available in some clinical settings. The results can be used to determine the needs for fortification for the infant.

H. The lipid and caloric content of breastmilk can be estimated by creamatocrit (Griffin et al., 2000).

    1. Creamatocrit is determined by centrifuging a small milk specimen in a capillary tube, separating the lipid portion, and then measuring the content as a percentage of total milk volume (Meier et al., 1996).

X. Issues Associated with Fortification of Human Milk

A. Significantly slower gastric emptying times and, therefore, implications for feeding intolerance (Ewer et al., 1996).

B. Neutralizing effect of some of the anti-infective (lactoferrin) properties of human milk (Quan et al., 1994).

C. May increase the risk of infection.

D. Incomplete absorption of additives such as medium chain triglyceride oil.

E. Increased osmolarity of fortified milk increasing the morbidity from GI disease.

F. Some nutrient loss can occur through enteral feeding tubes.

   1. Lipids can adhere to the lumen of a feeding tube and not reach the infant; this is more common when giving continuous enteral feeds.

   2. The greatest lipid losses occur with continuous slow infusions; therefore, bolus feedings (intermittent gavage) are recommended when possible.

G. Fortification might influence short-term outcomes (such as weight gain and bone mineralization), but long-term growth and development outcomes have not been shown to be enhanced (Lucas et al., 1999).

   1. Bone mineral content of 8- to 12-year-old children who are born preterm and are fed breastmilk is as high or higher than children who are born at term (Lucas et al., 1999).

H. The use of powdered fortifiers is controversial and requires surveillance and additional research (Schanler, 1996).

   1. Powdered fortifiers and powdered preterm formulas are not sterile.

   2. The U.S. Food and Drug Administration (FDA), European Food Safety Authority, and the Centers for Disease Control and Prevention (CDC) have issued guidelines stating that powdered formulas should not be used in preterm or immunocompromised infants (CDC, 2002; U.S. Food and Drug Administration, 2002).

I. An alternative for powdered fortification is the use of liquid fortifiers.

   1. Often used in a 1:1 ratio with human milk, resulting in a reduction of human milk intake

   2. May be used when the volume of available human milk is inadequate

J. Increasingly, hospitals are using pasteurized, fortified donor human milk when available. If mother's own milk is not immediately available, the clinician should consider the use of pasteurized, donor human milk, which has most of the properties of fresh human milk (immunoglobulins, growth and developmental hormones, enzymes, anti-inflammatory factors, etc.), is sterile, and reduces NEC while improving feeding tolerance (Lucas et al., 1990; Wight et al., 2008; Ziegler et al., 2007; Ziegler et al., 2002).

XI. Scientific Basis for Breastfeeding a Preterm Infant

A. No scientific evidence justifies delaying or discouraging the initiation of breastfeeding of preterm infants because the infants are unable to bottle-feed.

1. Strong evidence shows that delaying initiation of direct breastfeeding until after hospital discharge or discouraging it completely leads to premature weaning and/or suboptimal breastmilk intake (Buckley et al., 2006; Callen et al., 2005).

2. Until recently, it was widely assumed that breastfeeding was more tiring and bottle-feeding was less work; consequently, preterm infants were required to demonstrate the ability to consistently bottle-feed before being introduced to breastfeeding.

3. It would seem prudent for clinicians to identify newborns at risk for nipple confusion and to minimize the use of bottles in such babies (Neifert et al., 2011).

4. Early breastfeeding has been shown to be less stressful to a preterm infant than is bottle-feeding (Meier et al., 1987).

5. Bottle-feeding has been shown to produce adverse and undesirable physiological and biochemical changes in small infants, including hypoxia, apnea, bradycardia, oxygen desaturation, hypercarbia, reduced minute and tidal volume hypothermia, and irregular breathing frequency (Chen et al., 2000).

6. Bottle-feeding when a mother's goal is to breastfeed undermines her efforts at expressing and supplying her breastmilk for her infant.

XII. Maturation and Influences on Sucking, Swallowing, and Breathing Coordination

A. The ability of an infant to breastfeed depends on the suck, swallow, and breathing coordination of the innate reflexes.

1. Esophageal peristalsis and swallowing have been seen in the fetus as early as 11 weeks of gestation.

2. Sucking has been described between 18 and 24 weeks.

3. Lactase, a brush border intestinal enzyme that digests lactose, is present at 24 weeks.

4. Lingual and gastric lipases are detectable at 26 weeks.

5. The gag reflex is seen in preterm infants at 26 to 27 weeks.

6. Rooting is seen around 32 weeks.

7. The coordination of suck, swallow, and breathe actions is seen at 32 to 35 weeks.

8. Some infants as young as 28 weeks are able to lick expressed milk from the mother's nipple.

9. At 28 to 30 weeks, some oral feeding might be possible at the breast.

10. From 32 to 34 weeks, some infants might be able to take a complete breastfeed once or twice a day (Wolf et al., 1992).

11. From 35 weeks onward, efficient breastfeeding that maintains adequate growth is possible (Wolf et al., 1992).

12. Some characteristics of preterm infants that challenge successful breastfeeding:
    a. Weak, immature, disorganized suck
    b. A lack of coordination between sucking, swallowing, and breathing
    c. Diminished stamina
    d. Low muscle tone
13. Immature suck pattern:
    a. Three to five sucks per burst
    b. A pause of equal duration, often detaching from the breast
14. Transitional suck pattern (Palmer, 1993):
    a. Six to 10 sucks per burst
    b. A pause of equal duration with occasional detaching
    c. An apneic episode can follow longer suck bursts
15. Mature suck pattern:
    a. Ten to 30 sucks per burst
    b. Brief pauses
    c. Suck/swallow in a 1:1 ratio
16. Disorganized sucking is a lack of rhythm of the total sucking activity.
17. Dysfunctional sucking is the interruption of the feeding process by abnormal movements of the tongue and jaw.
B. Nonnutritive sucking (NNS; sucking without significant intake of milk)
    1. Some characteristics:
       a. Can be observed from 18 weeks gestation
       b. Rate of two sucks per second
       c. Weak, uncoordinated flutter sucking
       d. Absence of swallow
    2. Advantages of NNS:
       a. Reduces the length of hospital stay (Schanler, Hurst et al., 1999).
       b. When the infant is provided NNS opportunities during gavage feedings, the infant associates the act of sucking with the pleasurable feeling of a full stomach.
       c. NNS opportunities are sometimes provided by the mother's softened, drained breast or a pacifier.
    3. When possible, it is advantageous for NNS to occur at the mother's "empty" breast during gavage feeding.
       a. To avoid imprinting on an artificial nipple
       b. To begin developing early breastfeeding skills (suck, swallow, and breathe coordination)
       c. To increase maternal milk production
       d. To increase maternal involvement in infant care

XIII. Kangaroo Care (Skin-to-Skin)

A. Can begin when infant is stable, but still intubated (Gale et al., 1993).

B. Infant and parent maintain skin-to-skin contact.

   1. Infant is naked except for diaper.
   2. Infant is held mostly upright and snuggled between mother's breasts or against father's bare chest.
   3. Infant's back is covered:
       a. Inside parent's shirt
       b. With parent's hand
       c. With clothing
       d. With a blanket

C. Benefits of kangaroo care to infant (Anderson, 2003; World Health Organization [WHO], 2003):

   1. Stable heart rate (De Leeuw et al., 1991; Ludington-Hoe et al., 2004)
   2. More regular breathing
       a. A 75% decrease in apneic episodes (De Leeuw et al., 1991; Ludington-Hoe et al., 2004).
   3. Improved oxygen saturation levels (Acolet et al., 1989)
   4. No cold stress, more temperature stability(Acolet et al., 1989)
   5. Longer periods of sleep (Ludington-Hoe et al., 1995)
   6. More rapid weight gain (Charpak et al., 2001)
   7. Less caloric expenditures (Ludington-Hoe et al., 1995)
   8. More rapid brain development (Feldman et al., 2002)
   9. Reduction of "purposeless" activity (flailing of arms and legs)
   10. Decreased crying (Ludington-Hoe et al., 2002)
   11. Longer periods of alertness
   12. More successful breastfeeding episodes (Whitlaw et al., 1988)
   13. Increased breastfeeding duration (Hurst et al., 1997; Whitlaw et al., 1988)
   14. Earlier hospital discharge (Charpak et al., 2001)

D. Benefits of kangaroo care to parents (WHO, 2003):

   1. Increased bonding because of increased serum oxytocin levels (Uvnas-Moberg et al., 1996).
   2. Promotes confidence in the parents' caregiving (Affonso et al., 1989).
   3. Parents feel more in control.
   4. Relief of parental stress over having an infant in the intensive care nursery (Boyd, 2004).
   5. Increased maternal milk production (Mohrbacher et al., 2003).
   6. Significantly reduced cost resulting from decreased length of stay (Charpak et al., 2001).
   7. Earlier discharge from hospital.

E. Early breastfeeding practice can be a component of kangaroo care, with skin-to-skin care gradually transitioning to breastfeeding (Anderson, 2003; WHO, 2003).

XIV. Developmental Care

A. Neonatal individualized developmental care can be incorporated into practice in all intensive or special care nurseries.

1. It is based on the positive development of the five senses: sight, hearing, taste, touch, and smell (Als et al., 2004).

B. Some benefits of a developmentally sensitive environment include:

1. Greater parental involvement and nurturing care
2. More time for adequate rest for infant, which promotes brain development
3. Prevention of overstimulation
   a. Reduced heart rate
   b. Reduced need for oxygen
4. Earlier removal from ventilator
5. Earlier initiation of breastfeeding
6. Better weight gain (Charpak et al., 2001; Ludington-Hoe et al., 1996)
7. Reduction in rates of infection (Charpak et al., 2001)
8. Shorter hospital stays (Charpak et al., 2001)
9. Improved medical and neurodevelopmental outcomes (Gupta, 2001)

C. Following are examples of an environmentally sensitive special care nursery (Als, 1996; NIDCAP, 1996):

1. Lights below 60 foot-candles (Committee to Establish Recommended Standards for Newborn ICU Design, 1999).
2. Blanket-covering isolette low enough to protect eyes.
3. Day and night rhythmicity (Mirmiran et al., 2000).
4. Cluster care across disciplines, allowing for longer sleep periods.
5. Controlled noise levels:
   a. Less than 50 decibels (AAP, 1997; AAP & American College of Obstetricians and Gynecologists [ACOG], 2002).
   b. Voice level, particularly at shift change.
   c. Ensure quiet trash removal.
   d. Ensure quiet closing of isolette doors.
   e. Ensure quiet monitor/vent alarms.
   f. Ensure that telephone rings are not disruptive.
6. Positioning infant to promote feelings of security (that is, side and foot rolls to provide borders for infant to lie or push against).
7. Hand containment—preferably done by parent.
   a. Gentle pressure on infant's back or chest with opened hand helps infant to organize himself or herself.
8. Support infant with blankets and rolls while supine or prone.
9. Midline flexion and containment.
10. Provide boundaries.

11. When infant is lying prone, wet fist with breastmilk and position it near nose and mouth (Sullivan et al., 1998).

12. Use of breastmilk for oral care helps the infant identify his or her mother's smell and the taste of her milk.

13. Preterm infants have a keen sense of smell and usually respond to human milk by extending the tongue to taste milk and then opening mouth.
    a. Once infant is comfortably positioned at the breast, the mother can express a drop of milk that remains on the tip of her nipple for the infant to smell and then taste.
    b. Preterm infants are slow to respond to stimuli, so the mother should be patient.

14. Sucking pressures are lower in preterm infants, increasing the difficulty in transferring milk.
    a. Goal of early feedings is to allow the infant to gradually increase breastfeeding skill and stamina, which comes with time and patience.
    b. Focusing on weight or milk transfer too early can undermine mother's confidence and put breastfeeding at risk.

15. Breastfeeding is a developmental skill and will happen when an infant is neurobehaviorally ready.

16. Encourage continual skin-to-skin/kangaroo care when mother/parents are present.

17. Appropriate pain management.

18. Massage therapy (Als et al., 2004; Lindrea & Stainton, 2000).

XV. Readiness to Breastfeed

A. Readiness to breastfeed depends on the individual infant's cues (Nyqvist & Ewald, 1999).

   1. Traditionally, infants needed to be of a certain weight or gestational age before attempts were made at the breast; these criteria had no scientific basis. There are no universally agreed-upon criteria for when to initiate feedings at the breast.

   2. The literature supports the observations that infants vary considerably in ability to consume measurable amounts of milk at the breast and require an individualized approach to initial feeding readiness.

   3. Baby-led breastfeeding assessment:
      a. **Table 29-1** is an example of an infant-led feeding assessment that meets the infant's individual needs while not missing opportunities for oral feedings. The feeding plan is based on the score of the infant's individual development level. Prior to each feeding, the infant can be assessed for readiness to orally feed.

   4. The transition to the breast can be gradual, with daily kangaroo care advancing to limited periods of sucking on a partially drained breast, if necessary.

   5. Numerous protocols are used to transition the infant to the breast; whereas some use bottles in the absence of the mother, many protocols currently use

Table 29-1 Baby-Led Breastfeeding Assessment

Observation	Score	Feeding Technique
Drowsy, alert, or fussy prior to care. Rooting and/or hands to mouth/sucks on fingers and thumb. Good tone.	1	Attempt breastfeeding
Drowsy or alert once handled. Some rooting or sucks finger(s). Adequate tone.	2	
Briefly alert with care. No hunger cues. No change in tone.	3	Place infant skin-to-skin with mother for 20 minutes.
Sleeping throughout care. No hunger cues. No change in tone.	4	If no change, begin N/G feeding. If score improves to 1 or 2, above.
Needs increased O_2 with care. Apnea and/or bradycardia with care. Tachypnea over base line with care.	5	N/G feeding only

gavage feeding or cup feeding in the mother's absence (Kliethermas et al., 1999; Lang et al., 1994; Valentine et al., 1995).

B. Positions for breastfeeding the preterm infant:

1. The preterm infant's head is heavy in relation to the weak neck musculature that is supposed to support it.

    a. Failure to provide suitable head and jaw stability can result in the infant not effectively latching on to the breast, tiring too quickly, biting the nipple to maintain latch, or frequently slipping off the breast.

    b. The preterm infant usually benefits from positions that provide extra support for the head and torso.

2. Two positions that work well with the preterm are the cross-cradle hold and the football hold.

3. To bring the chin into the breast first, the head can be supported by the mother's fingers and the shoulders by the palm of her hand, giving support to the infant's head, neck, and torso, but not bringing the nose in first.

    a. Bringing the chin in first when the infant opens his or her mouth increases the success of effective latch. The breast is then well supported with the mother's opposite hand in a U hold, with the mother being careful to push into the breast rather than pinch the fingers together (**Figure 29-2**).

    b. It is helpful to hold the breast throughout the feeding so that there is less stress and weight on the infant's jaw.

    c. The preterm infant might have difficulty opening his or her mouth wide enough to latch properly.

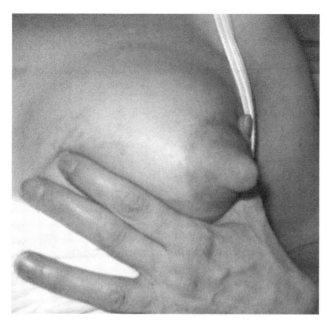

Figure 29-2
Position for breastfeeding the preterm infant.

Source: Used with permission.

    4. The infant's entire head can be encircled by the mother's hand, or she can use the dancer hand position for jaw stability.

        a. This position can be particularly helpful with larger preterm infants and neurologically impaired infants, but less so when breastfeeding the small preterm. (See Chapter 38, Congenital Anomalies, Neurologic Involvement, and Birth Trauma.)

C. Intake of milk while breastfeeding:

    1. Intake can be estimated by the use of test weights (also known as pre- and post-feed weights) if accuracy is paramount. Test weights are helpful in situations where decisions must be made regarding the amounts of supplement, determination of milk transfer problems, or simple reassurance to the mother or staff (Meier et al., 1996).

    2. Mother's milk supply also plays a part in assessing infant intake.

        a. When determining amount of supplement needed, it is helpful to know status of mother's milk supply.

        b. Low milk supply dictates greater amount of supplement.

    3. Daily weights or weights every second day are used as the infant begins taking more milk at the breast and the supplement is decreased.

    4. Preterm infants often do not demonstrate a predictable, cue-based feeding pattern until close to their corrected term age.

    5. Intake-related problems can also be helped by the use of a tube feeding device at the breast that delivers additional milk as the infant suckles at the breast. (See Chapter 34, Breastfeeding Devices and Equipment.)

6. Indications for use of a tube feeding device at the breast:
   a. An infant who latches on to the breast but exerts low sucking pressures.
   b. Lack of sucking rhythm.
   c. Mother's request to supplement at breast. Some mothers want to see the amount of infant intake; others prefer the supplement be given at the breast rather than using an alternative feeding device.
   d. Mother who has a limited milk supply.
   e. Impaired milk ejection reflex.
7. When limited intake is a result of the infant's inability to draw in enough of the nipple/areola (or if the areola is puffy or the nipple very large in relation to the infant's mouth), a thin nipple shield has been successfully used on a temporary basis until the infant is capable of forming a teat by himself or herself (Meier et al., 2000).
8. One of the major concerns of mothers of preterm infants relates to whether the infant is consuming adequate volumes of milk when breastfeeding (Kavanaugh et al., 1995).
   a. Milk transfer depends on milk supply, milk ejection, and infant sucking.
      i. If sucking is immature, then interventions can be targeted toward optimizing milk production and milk ejection to compensate for weak or immature sucking patterns.
      ii. The infant should thoroughly soften the first breast before being placed on the other side.
   b. Mothers might perceive that their infant is not taking the majority of the milk available.
   c. Infants might slip off the breast, fall asleep at the breast, or simply stop feeding.
   d. Immature feeding patterns are gradually replaced with more mature patterns as the infant nears his or her term-corrected age.

XVI. Establishing Full Breastfeeding

A. Phase one: Initiate lactation by the expression and collection of breastmilk.
   1. Lactation should be initiated by hand expression or use of a breast pump as early as possible and within 6 hours of birth. (See Chapter 33, Milk Expression, Storage, and Handling.)
   2. Hand expression can be used effectively where mechanical expression is not practical or possible (Stanford School of Medicine Newborn Nursery at LPCH, n.d.).
   3. Mothers should plan to hand express or pump 8 to 12 times each 24 hours for the first 7 to 10 days for optimal milk yield. This plan might change to fewer sessions if the level of production is maintained. A combination of pumping and hand expression can significantly increase milk production (Stanford School of Medicine Newborn Nursery at LPCH, n.d.).
   4. This plan should yield 800 to 1,000 mL of milk daily by days 7 to 10.
   5. An abundant milk supply at this point greatly reduces the risk of insufficient milk later (Hill et al., 205).

6. A 50% breastmilk oversupply provides a cushion.
   a. If the milk production drops for any reason, saved milk can be fractionated to provide hindmilk supplements.
   b. An oversupply aids the infant with an easy flow of milk from a full breast.
7. Mothers might find that massaging and compressing each breast during expression contributes to increased milk yields, more thorough draining of the breast, and higher fat content of the expressed milk (Foda et al., 2004).
8. Mothers can plan to use a hospital-grade electric breast pump with double collection kits, if available. (See Chapter 34, Breastfeeding Devices and Equipment.)
9. Simultaneous milk expression can increase prolactin levels, increase milk yield, and reduce the time spent pumping.
10. Mother's milk should be fed to preterm infants immediately after it is pumped, when possible. Fresh breastmilk is preferable for preterm infants (Jones et al., 2006).
11. Previously frozen colostrum can be given first before fresh breastmilk if the infant cannot be fed enterally for the first few days.
    a. Colostrum coats the immature porous intestine and reduces the absorption of harmful bacteria and food antigens.
12. Fresh breastmilk can be refrigerated 24 to 48 hours before use (Jones et al., 2006).
13. Breastmilk can be frozen for later use; it should be used in the order it was expressed. Frozen milk can be used up to 24 hours after thawing.
14. Low milk volume is a common problem, especially if the infant cannot breastfeed for several weeks or if the infant was born extremely early; a number of possible interventions have proven helpful (Clavey, 1996). (See Chapter 42, Insufficient Milk Supply.)
    a. Frequent kangaroo care.
    b. Encourage the infant to suckle at the emptied breast.
    c. Pump during or right after skin-to-skin contact (Ehrenkranz et al., 1986).
    d. Pump at the infant's bedside.
    e. Medications can increase milk supply in some mothers.
       i. Metoclopramide (Budd et al., 1993), known to produce side effects in some women.
       ii. Domperidone (da Silva et al., 2001).
       iii. The use of oxytocin nasal spray has been used to stimulate the milk ejection reflex (Ruis et al., 1981). However, a recent randomized, controlled trial (Fewtrell et al., 2006) shows no significant difference in milk collection with the use of oxytocin nasal spray.
    f. Acupuncture (Clavey, 1996).
    g. Human growth hormone (Gunn et al., 1996).
       i. Shown to increase breastmilk volume with no adverse effects seen in mothers or infants
       ii. Not widely used because of expense

B. Phase two: Introduce the infant to the breast.
  1. Will require continued gavage feedings of expressed breastmilk in the beginning.
  2. Maintenance of milk supply by expression.
  3. Scheduled feeds every 3 hours are typically required until the infant is mature enough to begin cue-based feeding.
  4. Cue-based feeding frequency can gradually increase to every 2 hours (Saunders et al., 1991).
  5. Combine breastfeeds and supplemental feedings until the infant is mature enough to sustain all feeding at the breast.
C. Phase three: Optimize early feedings.
  1. Optimal positioning and attachment of the infant.
    a. Football (clutch) hold, cross-cradle hold, and use of the dancer hand position with larger preterm infants
  2. Continue frequent kangaroo care.
D. Phase four: Transition to full cue-based breastfeeding.
  1. Healthcare team assesses the readiness to transition to full breastfeeding. (See the section titled "XV. Readiness to Breastfeed" earlier in this chapter.)
  2. Will occur over time with most infants able to achieve cue-based feeding by the time they are term equivalent.
  3. Infant shows signs of demand sucking.
  4. Able to sustain full breastfeeding on demand and gain adequate weight.
  5. Awake and alert at feeding times.
  6. Sucking on fist.
  7. Mouthing.
  8. Able to sustain a full breastfeed.
  9. Stamina to fully breastfeed on demand and gain adequate weight.
E. Several sample feeding protocols have been published.
  1. Feeding regimens
    a. Six-step feeding strategy for preterm infants (Valentine et al., 1995).
      i. Infants begin 10 to 20 mL/kg/day of expressed breastmilk (oral-gastric, bolus, or continuous drip by using an automated syringe pump) and are progressed daily at the same rate (if tolerated) to the goal of 150 mL/kg/day of expressed breastmilk. During this time period, infants are transitioning off parenteral nutrition.
      ii. Once the infant is receiving 150 mL/kg/day, a powdered human milk fortifier is added at two packets per 100 mL of expressed breastmilk (EBM); after 24 hours of tolerance, this amount is increased to four packets per 100 mL of EBM.
      iii. If infant growth falters (less than 15 g/kg/day), then the volume of fortified human milk is increased to 160 to 180 mL/kg/day. Other clinical

factors associated with slow growth are first ruled out (for example, aci-dosis or anemia).

    iv. If growth remains 15 g/kg/day, use fortified hindmilk at 180 mL/kg/day and fortify as earlier.

    v. If growth falters, the infant is supplemented with corn oil 0.5 mL every 3 hours given as a bolus rather than mixed with the milk.

    vi. If growth falters, four feedings are replaced with premature formula, and four fortified breastmilk feeds are continued.

2. Transition to breastfeeding

    a. Transitioning preterm infants with nasogastric tube supplementation: Increased likelihood of breastfeeding (Kliethermas et al., 1999)

        i. Supplementation provided through an indwelling 3.5 French nasogas-tric tube when the mother is not available to breastfeed or if additional supplemental feedings are required.

        ii. Daily weights, with supplements reduced gradually as the infant consis-tently meets or surpasses the expected weight gain of 20 to 30 g/day.

        iii. Nasogastric tube removed 24 to 48 hours prior to discharge with supple-ments given if needed by cup.

        iv. Definitions of latch and breastfeeding abilities:

- *Breastfeeds well.*
  - (a) Good latch-on with a wide-open mouth and lips flanged.
  - (b) Areola drawn in with sucking.
  - (c) Tongue is down and cupped; infant retains a vacuum when the forehead is gently pushed away from the breast.
  - (d) No dimpling of infant's cheeks.
  - (e) Long draws with rhythmical sucking and audible swallowing.
  - (f) Mother requires minimal help with positioning and latch-on.
  - (g) Breastfeeding is greater than or equal to 5 to 8 minutes.
- *Breastfeeds fairly.*
  - (a) Occasional latch-on.
  - (b) Short sucks, fewer long draws, infrequent audible swallowing, mother requires help with positioning.
  - (c) Time of active suckling is less than 5 minutes.
- *Breastfeeds poorly.*
  - (a) Some rooting or licking movements.
  - (b) No latch-on.
  - (c) Mother requires assistance with positioning.

XVII. Discharge Planning

A. Parents require a detailed plan of caring/parenting their preterm infant after discharge.

1. Ongoing care and information should include the following (Academy of Breastfeeding Medicine Protocol Committee, 2004):

   a. Signs that the infant is getting enough breastmilk; weight checks; test weights if necessary; diaper counts of wet diapers and bowel movements.

   b. Expected feeding patterns; at least eight feeds per 24 hours with only one prolonged sleep period of up to 5 hours, maximum; cues that indicate the infant is ready to feed.

   c. Continued milk expression until the infant is fully established at the breast, with adequate weight gain and no need for supplemental feedings.

   d. Mothers usually need to continue milk expression after the infant has been discharged; expression might be needed after each feeding or only a few times each day, depending on the number of supplemental feedings.

   e. Experts recommend that the mother produce about 50% more milk than the infant needs at discharge because the increased volume helps the milk flow freely in the presence of a weaker suck.

   f. Proper use of supplemental feeding devices, when appropriate.

      i. Cup.

      ii. Feeding tube at breast.

      iii. Supervision of the use of a nipple shield.

      iv. Close follow-up should continue as progress is made toward full breastfeeding.

2. If parents choose to bottle-feed human milk during the infant's hospitalization, a lactation consultant can help transition the infant to the breast before or after discharge.

3. The lactation consultant should conduct postdischarge telephone follow-up (Elliott et al., 1998).

4. Parents should be provided information about the availability of support services after discharge.

   a. Primary healthcare provider

   b. International Board Certified Lactation Consultants

   c. Health professional who has expertise in breastfeeding preterm infants (e.g., specially trained midwives, doulas, and peer counselors; Elliott et al., 1998)

   d. Community support groups

   e. Social services

   f. La Leche League International

   g. U.S. Department of Agriculture's Supplemental Nutrition System for Women, Infants, and Children

XVIII. The Late Preterm Infant

The term *late preterm* applies to infants born at gestational ages between 34 weeks and 0/7 days, and 36 weeks and 6/7 days (Academy of Breastfeeding Medicine Protocol Committee, 2011; Engle, 2006; Raju et al., 2006). The incidence of late preterm births has been reported to be on the increase for the following reasons:

- Increase in maternal age, obesity and diabetes, poor nutrition, smoking, alcohol use, and assisted reproductive technology births resulting in multiple deliveries (Goldenberg, Culhane, Iams, & Romero, 2008; Hamilton et al., 2010; Schieve et al., 2004)
- Increased obstetrical surveillance that detects maternal and fetal condition, which results in medically indicated birth (i.e., induction of labor or cesarean delivery) (Goldenberg et al., 2008; Hamilton et al., 2010; Schieve et al., 2004)
- Late preterm infants require particular surveillance while hospitalized and following their discharge to home until they have demonstrated they can gain weight and grow consistently.
- Late preterm infants are particularly vulnerable because they might look full term and weigh nearly the same as some full-term infants. They, however, are at increased risk for hypoglycemia, hypothermia, respiratory morbidity, apnea, severe hyperbilirubinemia, dehydration, feeding difficulties, prolonged artificial milk supplementation, weight loss, and hospital readmission.

A. Birth
1. Because of the wide range from 34 weeks to 36-6/7 weeks of gestation these infants require an individualized plan of care that depends on their gestational age and their capabilities.
2. The infant's gestational age and stability often determine whether the infant is cared for in the intensive care nursery (ICN) or the well-baby nursery.
   a. If the infant is cared for in the ICN, care often parallels that of the preterm infant.
   b. A nasogastric (NG) tube might be inserted, the infant placed in an isolette, and blood glucose, temperature, heart rate, and oxygen saturation monitored.
3. If the infant is stable, he or she should be put to mother's chest skin to skin immediately after birth.
   a. The infant can be dried and Apgar scoring can take place during this skin-to-skin time.
   b. A warm blanket can cover both mother and baby and a hat can be placed on the baby's head.
4. Extended skin-to-skin contact keeps the infant warm, prevents crying, and allows for frequent feedings, all of which help prevent hypoglycemia and hypothermia (Bergman et al., 2004).
   a. Infants interact more with their mothers, are more likely to breastfeed and to breastfeed longer, and show better cardiorespiratory stability if they have early skin-to-skin contact (Moore et al., 2003).

5. Avoiding or delaying disruptive procedures (e.g., excessive handling, unnecessary suctioning, administration of vitamin K, eye prophylaxis, and hepatitis B vaccine) minimizes thermal and metabolic stress, improves initial feeding behavior, and enhances early parent–infant interaction immediately after birth.
   a. Bathing should be delayed (Black, 2001; Voucher & Wight, 2007).

B. Positioning infant at breast
   1. Mothers should be helped to position the infant at breast to prevent excessive flexion of the baby's neck and trunk.
      a. The cross-cradle hold works well. (See Chapter 28: Guidelines for Facilitating and Assessing Breastfeeding, for more information on positions.)
      b. When positioning the infant in the football hold care should be taken so that the weight of the breast is not on the infant's chest.
   2. The late preterm infant can have decreased muscle tone and might not be able to maintain a latch at the breast and maintain and sustain strong enough sucking to transfer milk.
      a. Use of the dancer hold for support of the breast and chin can help the infant with jaw stability.
      b. The use of an ultrathin silicone nipple shield can be considered if latch is difficult, cannot be sustained, or there is evidence of ineffective milk transfer (Meier et al., 2000).
   3. Because late preterm infants tend to be sleepier than full-term infants, they might need awakening every 2 to 3 hours for feeding attempts (California Perinatal Quality Care Collaborative [CPQCC], 2007, p. 6).
   4. Provision should be made for close observation and assessment of the infant at breast at least twice daily by two different skilled lactation professionals (Academy of Breastfeeding Medicine Protocol Committee, 2011).
      a. Determination of milk transfer is essential.
      b. The use of a breastfeeding assessment tool such as LATCH, IBFAT can be helpful. (See Chapter 28.)
      c. Close daily monitoring of urinary and stool patterns is important.
      d. If the amount of milk transfer and nursing effectiveness are in question, the occasional use of test weights can be helpful.
   5. Unless the late preterm infant is nursing effectively every 2 to 3 hours (determined by skilled evaluation and documentation) the mother should be instructed to initiate breast expression.
      a. Milk expression is most efficient with a combination of hand expression and electric pump (Morton, 2009).
      b. If milk expression with a breast pump does not yield sufficient colostrum, hand expression after pumping can increase milk collection.
   6. Continual skin-to-skin contact can facilitate feeding and breastmilk production (CPQCC, 2009).

7. When supplementing, an alternate feeding method such as supplementing at breast or cup feeding can avoid the infant becoming habituated to the bottle (Howard et al., 1999; Howard et al., 2003; Lanese, 2011; Marinelli et al., 2001).

   a. If the infant tires easily, an NG tube can be inserted (Meier et al., 1987).

8. If supplementation is indicated, mother's own milk is the first best choice followed by pasteurized donor milk, then infant formula until mother's supply is adequate.

9. The quantities of supplementation after breastfeeding should be small: 5 to 10 mL per feeding on day 1 and 10–30 mL per feeding thereafter (Academy of Breastfeeding Medicine Protocol Committee, 2011).

10. When supplementation is necessary, small amounts should continue until the infant can transfer appropriate amounts of milk while breastfeeding and mother's milk is sufficient for the infant to gain weight.

11. Mother should continue milk expression until her infant demonstrates the ability to sustain breastfeeding at least eight times each 24 hours and shows appropriate weight gain over time.

12. Parents of the late preterm infant should be included in their infant's plan of care and can be taught to participate fully in their infant's care.

C. Discharge

1. Discharge planning with parents should begin at birth.

   a. Particularly when the late preterm infant is cared for in a well-baby nursery, anticipatory guidance to parents and staff should include a discussion that the late preterm infant is not a full-term baby and discharge home might not be within the expected 36–48 hours after birth.

2. Every effort should be made to keep infant and mother together during the hospital stay.

   a. The mother can be offered rooming-in to be with her infant after her discharge. When the infant is ready they can be sent home simultaneously.

3. Discharge readiness: Breastfeeding well, or in combination with appropriate supplementation by alternate feeding method, that demonstrates stable weight or increasing weight.

   a. Evidence mother's milk supply is becoming established

   b. Ability to maintain normal temperature in an open crib

   c. Bilirubin stable or decreasing

4. Discharge strategies:

   a. Parents can demonstrate comfort with alternate feeding methods if use is necessary.

   b. Mother feels confident with breastfeeding.

   c. Follow-up visit with healthcare provider scheduled within 24–48 hours of discharge and then weekly until infant is exclusively breastfeeding (AAP, 2005).

   d. Postdischarge feeding plan developed with family, lactation consultants, and healthcare provider (Walker, 2009).

   e. Include a feeding log that documents number of feedings, urinary output, and stooling pattern.

   f. Lactation Warm Line phone number.

   g. Referral to postdischarge lactation support group.

References

Academy of Breastfeeding Medicine Protocol Committee. (2004, September). *ABM clinical protocol no. 12: Transitioning the breastfeeding/breastmilk-fed premature infant from neonatal intensive care unit to home*. Retrieved from http://www.bfmed.org/Resources/Download.aspx?filename =Protocol_12.pdf

Academy of Breastfeeding Medicine Protocol Committee. (2011, June). ABM clinical protocol no. 10: Breastfeeding the late preterm infant (3407 to 366/7 weeks gestation). *Breastfeeding Medicine*, *6*(3), 151–156.

Acolet, D., Sleath, K., & Whitelaw, A. (1989). Oxygenation, heart rate and temperature in very low birthweight infants during skin-to-skin contact with their mothers. *Acta Paediatrica Scandinavica*, *78*, 189–193.

Affonso, D., Wahlberg, V., & Persson, V. (1989). Exploration of mother's reactions to the kangaroo method of prematurity care. *Neonatal Network*, *7*, 43–51.

Als, H. (1996). Program Guide Newborn Individualized Developmental Care and Assessment Program (NIDCAP): An education and training program for health care professionals. Boston: National NIDCAP Training Center, Harvard Medical School, Children's Hospital.

Als, H., Duffy, F. H., McAnulty, G. B., et al. (2004). Early experience alters brain function and structure. *Pediatrics*, *114*, 1738–1739.

American Academy of Pediatrics. (1997). Noise: A hazard for the fetus and newborn. *Pediatrics*, *100*, 724–727.

American Academy of Pediatrics. (2005). Policy statement: Breast feeding and the use of human milk. *Pediatrics*, *115*, 496–506.

American Academy of Pediatrics & American College of Obstetricians and Gynecologists. (2002). *Guidelines for perinatal care* (5th ed.). Elk Grove Village, IL; Author.

Anderson, G. C. (2003). Mother–newborn contact in a randomized trial of kangaroo (skin-to-skin) care. *Journal of Obstetric, Gynecologic, and Neonatal Nursing*, *2*, 604–611.

Arslanoglu S, Zeigler EE, Moro GE, J Perinat Med 2010 Jul: 38 (4) 347-51.

Bergman, N. J., Linley, L. L., & Fawcus, S. R. (2004). Randomized controlled trial of skin to skin contact from birth versus conventional incubator for physiological stabilization in 1200 to 2199 gram newborns. *Acta Paediatrica*, *93*, 779–785.

Black, L. (2001). Incorporating breastfeeding care into daily newborn rounds and pediatric office practice. *Pediatric Clinics of North America*, *48*(2), 299–319.

Boyd, S. (2004). Within these walls: Moderating parental stress in the neonatal intensive care unit. *Journal of Neonatal Nursing*, *10*, 80–84.

Buckley, K., & Charles, G. E. (2006). Benefits and challenges to transitioning preterm infants to at-breast feeding. *International Breastfeeding Journal*, *1*, 13.

Budd, S. C., Erdman, S. H., Long, D. M., Trombley, S. K., & Udall, J. N., Jr. (1993). Improved lactation with Metoclopramide, a case report. *Clinical Pediatrics (Phila)*, *32*, 53–57.

California Perinatal Quality Care Collaborative (CPQCC). (2007). Quality improvement toolkit. Retrieved from http://www.CPQCC.org/quality_improvement/qi_toolkits

California Perinatal Quality Care Collaborative (CPQCC). (2008). Quality improvement toolkit. Retrieved from http://www.CPQCC.org/quality_improvement/qi_toolkits

Callen, J., Pinelli, J., Atkinson, S., & Saigal, S. (2005). Qualitative analysis of barriers to breastfeeding in very low birth weight infants in the hospital and post discharge. *Advances in Neonatal Care*, *5*, 93–103.

Centers for Disease Control (CDC), US Food and Drug Administration 2002

Charpak, N., Ruiz-Pelaez, J. G., Figueroa de, C. Z., & Charpak, Y. (2001). A randomized, controlled trial of kangaroo mother care: Results of a follow-up at one year of corrected age. *Pediatrics, 108*, 1072–1079.

Chen, C.-H., Wang, T.-M., Chang, H.-M., & Chi, C.-S. (2000). The effect of breast- and bottle-feeding on oxygen saturation and body temperature in preterm infants. *Journal of Human Lactation, 16*, 21–27.

Clavey, S. (1996). The use of acupuncture for the treatment of insufficient lactation. *American Journal of Acupuncture, 24*, 35–46.

Committee to Establish Recommended Standards for Newborn ICU Design. (1999). Recommended standards for newborn ICU design small. *Journal of Perinatology, 19*, S1–S12.

da Silva, O. P., Knopport, D. C., Angelini, M. M., & Forret, P. A. (2001). Effect of domperidone on milk production in mothers of premature newborns; a randomized, double-blind, placebo-controlled trial. *Canadian Medical Association Journal, 164*, 17–21.

De Leeuw, R., Collin, E. M., Dunnebbier, E. A., & Mirmiran, M. (1991). Physiologic effects of kangaroo care in very small preterm infants. *Biology of the Neonate, 59*, 149–155.

Ehrenkranz, R. A., & Ackerman, B. A. (1986). Metoclopramide effect on faltering milk production by mothers of premature infants. *Pediatrics, 78*, 614–620.

Elliott, S., & Reimer, C. (1998). Postdischarge telephone follow-up program for breastfeeding preterm infants discharged from a special care nursery. *Neonatal Network, 17*, 41–45.

Engle, W. A. (2006). Recommendation for the definition of "late preterm" (near term) and the birth weight–gestational age classification system. *Seminars in Perinatology, 30*(1), 2–7.

Ewer, A. K., & Yu, V. Y. (1996). Gastric emptying in preterm infants: The effect of breast milk fortifier. *Acta Paediatrica, 85*, 1112–1115.

Feldman, R., Eidelman, A., Sirota, L., & Weller, A. (2002). Comparison of skin-to-skin (Kangaroo) and traditional care: Parenting outcomes and preterm infant development. *Pediatrics, 110*, 16–26.

Fewtrell, M. S., Loh, K. L., Blake, A., et al. (2006). Randomised, double blind trial of oxytocin nasal spray in mothers expressing breast milk for preterm infants. *Archives of Disease in Childhood: Fetal and Neonatal Edition, 91*, F169–F174.

Foda, M. I., Kawashima, T., Nakamura, S., et al. (2004). Composition of milk obtained from unmassaged versus massaged breasts of lactating mothers. *Journal of Pediatric Gastroenterology and Nutrition, 38*, 477–478.

Furman, L., Minich, N., & Hack, M. (2002). Correlates of lactation in mothers of very low birth weight infants. *Pediatrics, 109*, e57.

Gale, G., Franck, L., & Lund, C. (1993). Skin-to-skin (Kangaroo) holding of the intubated premature infant. *Neonatal Network, 12*, 49–57.

Goldenberg, R. L., Culhane, J. F., Iams, J. D., & Romero, R. (2008). Epidemiology and causes of preterm birth. *Lancet, 371*, 75.

Griffin, T. L., Meier, P. P., Bradford, L. P., et al. (2000). Mother's performing creamatocrit measures in the NICU: Accuracy, reactions, and cost. *Journal of Obstetric, Gynecologic, and Neonatal Nursing, 29*, 249–257.

Gross, S. J., David, R. J., Bauman, L., et al. (1980). Nutritional composition of milk from mothers delivering preterm and at term. *Journal of Pediatrics, 96*, 641–644.

Gunn, A. J., Gunn, T. R., Rabone, D. L., et al. (1996). Growth hormone increases breast milk volumes in mothers of preterm infants. *Pediatrics, 98*, 279–282.

Gupta, G. (2001). NICU environment and the neonate. *Journal of Neonatalogy, 15*(4), 7–15.

Guthrie, J. O., Gordon, P. V., Thomas, V., & Thorp, J. A. (2003). Necrotizing enterocolitis among neonates in the United States. *Journal of Perinatalogy, 23*(4), 278–285.

Hamilton, B. E., Martin, J. A., Ventura, S. J., et al. (2010). Birth: Final data for 2007. *National Vital Statistics Report, 58*, 24. Retrieved from http://www.cdc.gov/nchs/data/nvsr/nvsr58/nvsr58_24.pdf

Henderson, G., Graig, F., Brocklehurst, P., & McGuire, W. (2007). Enteral feeding regimens and necrotising enterocolitis in preterm infants: Multi center case-control study. *Archives of Disease in Childhood: Fetal and Neonatal Edition, 94*, F120–F123. doi:10.1136/adc.2007.119560

Hill, P. D., Aldag, J. C., Chatterton, R. T., & Zinamann, M. (2005). Primary and secondary mediators' influence on milk output in lactating mothers and preterm infants. *Journal of Human Lactation, 21*, 138–150.

Howard, C. R., de Blieck, E. A., Hoopen, C. B., et al. (1999). Physiological stability of newborns during cup and bottle feeding. *Pediatrics, 104*, 1204–1207.

Howard, C. R., Howard, F. M., Lanphear, B., et al. (2003). Randomized clinical trial of pacifier use and bottle-feeding or cup feeding and their effect on breastfeeding. *Pediatrics, 111*, 511–518.

Human Milk Bank Association of North America. (2011). 2011 best practice for expressing, storing and handling human milk in hospitals, homes, and child care settings (3rd ed.). Available at https://www.hmbana.org/publications-buy-online.

Huppertze, C., Gharavi, B., Schott, C., & Linderkamp, O. (2005). Individual development care based on Newborn Individualized Developmental Care and Assessment Program (NIDCAP). *Kinderkrankenschwester, 9*, 359–364.

Hurst, N. M., Valentine, C. J., Renfro, L., et al. (1997). Skin-to-skin holding in the neonatal intensive care unit influences maternal milk volume. *Journal of Perinatology, 17*, 213–217.

Jones, F., & Tully, M. R. (2006). *Best practices for expressing, storing and handling human milk in hospital, homes and child care settings*. Raleigh, NC: Human Milk Bank Association of North America.

Kavanaugh, K., Mead, L., Meier, P., & Mangurten, H. H. (1995). Getting enough: Mothers' concerns about breastfeeding a preterm infant after discharge. *Journal of Obstetric, Gynecologic, and Neonatal Nursing, 24*, 23–32.

Kavanaugh, K., Meier, P., Zimmerman, B., & Mead, L. (1997). The rewards outweigh the efforts: Breastfeeding outcomes for mothers of preterm infants. *Journal of Human Lactation, 13*, 15–21.

Kirsten, D., & Bradford, L. (1999). Hindmilk feedings. *Neonatal Network, 18*, 68–70.

Kliethermas, P., Cross, M. L., Lanese, M. G., et al. (1999). Transitioning preterm infants with nasogastric tube supplementation: Increased likelihood of breastfeeding. *Journal of Obstetric, Gynecologic, and Neonatal Nursing, 28*, 264–273.

Lanese, M. G. (2011). Cup feeding—a useful tool. *Journal of Human Lactation, 27*(1), 12.

Lang, S., Lawrence, C. J., & Orme, R. L. (1994). Cup feeding: An alternative method of infant feeding. *Archives of Disease in Childhood, 71*, 365–369.

Lawrence, R. A., & Lawrence, R. M. (2010). *Breastfeeding: A guide for the medical profession* (7th ed.). Philadelphia, PA: Mosby-Elsevier.

Lindrea, K. B., & Stainton, M. C. (2000). A case study of infant massage outcomes. *MCN: The American Journal of Maternal/Child Nursing, 25*, 95–99.

Lucas, A., & Cole, T. J. (1990, December). Breast milk and neonatal necrotizing enterocolitis. *Lancet, 336*, 1519–1523.

Lucas, A., Fewtrell, M. S., Morley, R., et al. (1999). Randomized outcome trial of human milk fortification and developmental outcome in preterm infants. *American Journal of Clinical Nutrition, 64*, 142–151.

Lucas, A., Morley, R., Cole, T. J., Lister, G., & Leeson-Payne, C. (1998). Breastmilk and subsequent intelligence quotient in children born preterm. *Lancet, 339*, 261–264.

Ludington-Hoe, S. M., Cong, X., & Hashemi, F. (2002). Infant crying: Nature, physiologic consequences, and select intervention. *Neonatal Network, 21*, 29–36.

Ludington-Hoe, S. M., & Kasper, C. E. (1995). A physiologic method of monitoring preterm infants during kangaroo care. *Journal of Nursing Management, 3*, 13–29.

Ludington-Hoe, S. M., & Swinth, J. Y. (1996). Developmental aspects of kangaroo care. *Journal of Obstetric, Gynecologic, and Neonatal Nursing, 25*, 691–703.

Ludington-Hoe, S. M., Swinth, J. V., Thompson, C., & Hadeed, A. J. (2004). Randomized controlled trial of kangaroo care: Cardiorespiratory and thermal effects on healthy preterm infants. *Neonatal Network, 23*, 39–48.

Marinelli, K. A., Burke, G. S., & Doss, V. L. (2001). A comparison of the safety of cup feedings and bottle feedings in premature infants whose mothers intend to breastfeed. *Journal of Perinatology, 21*, 350–355.

McClure, R. J., & Newell, S. J. (2000). Randomized control study of clinical outcome following trophic feeding. *Archives of Disease in Childhood: Fetal and Neonatal Edition, 82*, F29–F33.

Meier, P., & Anderson, G. C. (1987). Responses of small preterm infants to bottle- and breast-feeding. *MCN: The American Journal of Maternal/Child Nursing, 12*, 97–105.

Meier, P. P., & Brown, L. P. (1996). State of the science: Breastfeeding for mothers and low birth weight infants. *Nursing Clinics of North America, 31*, 351–365.

Meier, P. P., Brown, L. P., Hurst, N. M., et al. (2000). Nipple shields for preterm infants: Effect on milk transfer and duration of breastfeeding. *Journal of Human Lactation, 16*, 106–114.

Meier, P. P., Engstrom, J. L., Fleming, B. A., et al. (1996). Estimating intake of hospitalized preterm infants who breastfeed. *Journal of Human Lactation, 12*, 21–26.

Mikiel-Kostyra, K., Mazur, J., & Boltruszko, I. (2002). Effect of early skin-to-skin contact after delivery on duration of breastfeeding: A prospective cohort study. *Acta Paediatrics, 91*, 1301–1306.

Miracle, D. J., Meier, P. P., & Bennett, P. A. (2004). Mother's decision to change from formula to mothers' milk for very-low-birth-weight infants. *Journal of Obstetric, Gynecologic, and Neonatal Nursing, 33*, 692–703.

Mirmiran, M., & Arigagno, A. (2000). Influence of light in the NICU on the development of circadian rhythms in preterm infants. *Seminars in Perinatology, 24*, 247–257.

Mohrbacher, N., & Stock, J. (2003). The breastfeeding answer book (pp. 285–287), Schaumburg, IL: LaLeche League International.

Moore, E. R., Anderson, G. C., & Bergman, N. (2003). Early skin to skin contact for mothers and their healthy new born infant. *Cochrane Database of Systematic Reviews, 2*, CDOO3519. doi:10.1002/14651858.CD003519.pub2

Morton, J., Hall, J. Y., Wong, R. J., & Thairu, L. (2009). *Journal of Perinatology, 29*, 757–764.

Neifert, M., Lawrence, R., & Seacat, J. (2011). Nipple confusion: Toward a formal definition. *Journal of Pediatrics, 126*(6), S125–129.

Nyqvist, K., Sjödén, P-O., & Ewald, U. (1999). The development of preterm infants breastfeeding behavior. *Early Human Development, 55*, 247–264.

Palmer, M. M. (1993). Identification and management of the transitional suck pattern in premature infants. *Journal of Perinatal and Neonatal Nursing, 7*, 66–75.

Polberger, S., & Lonnerdal, B. (1993). Simple and rapid macronutrient analysis of human milk for individualized fortification: Basis for improved nutritional management of very-low-birth-weight infants? *Journal of Pediatric Gastroenterology and Nutrition, 17*, 283–290.

Quan, R., Yang, C., Rubinstein, S., et al. (1994, June). The effect of nutritional additives on anti-infective factors in human milk. *Clinical Pediatrics*, 325–328.

Raju, T. N., Higgins, R. D., Stark, A. R., & Leveno, K. J. (2006). Optimizing care and outcome for late preterm (near-term) infants: A summary of the workshop sponsored by the National Institute of Child Health and Human Development. *Pediatrics, 118*(3), 1207–1214.

Ruis, H., Rolland, R., Doesburg, W., et al. (1981). Oxytocin enhances onset of lactation among mothers delivering prematurely. *British Medical Journal, 283*, 340–342.

Saarinen, U. M., & Kajosaari, M. (1995). Breastfeeding as prophylaxis against atopic disease: Prospective follow-up study until seventeen years old. *Lancet, 346*, 1065–1069.

Saunders, R. B., Friedman, C. B., & Stramoski, P. R. (1991). Feeding preterm infants: Schedule or demand? *Journal of Obstetric, Gynecologic, and Neonatal Nursing, 20*, 212–218.

Schanler, R. J. (1996). Human milk fortification for premature infants. *American Journal of Clinical Nutrition, 64*, 249–250.

Schanler, R. J. (2001). Human milk for premature infants. *Pediatric Clinics of North America, 48*, 207–219.

Schanler, R. J. (2011). Outcomes of human milk-fed premature infants. *Seminar in Perinatology, 35*, 29–33.

Schanler, R. J., Hurst, N. M., & Lau, C. (1999). The use of human milk and breastfeeding in premature infants. *Clinical Perinatology, 26*, 379–398.

Schanler, R. J., Shulman, R. J., Lau, C., et al. (1999a). Feeding strategies for premature infants: Randomized trial of gastrointestinal priming and tube feeding method. *Pediatrics, 103*, 434–439.

Schanler, R. J., Shulman, R. J., & Lau, C. (1999b). Feeding strategies for premature infants: Beneficial outcomes of feeding fortified human milk versus preterm formula. *Pediatrics, 103*, 1150–1157.

Schieve, L. A., Ferre, C., Peterson, H. B., et al. (2004). Perinatal outcome among singleton infants conceived through assisted reproductive technology in the United States. *Obstetrics and Gynecology, 103*, 1144.

Stanford School of Medicine Newborn Nursery at LPCH. (n.d.). Getting started with breastfeeding [Videos]. Retrieved from http://newborns.stanford.edu/Breastfeeding/

Stutte, P. C., Bowles, B. C., & Morman, G. Y. (1988). The effects of breast massage on volume and fat content of human milk. *Genesis, 10*, 22–25.

Sullivan, R. M., & Toubas, P. (1998). Clinical usefulness of maternal odor in newborns: Mouthing and feeding preparatory responses. *Biology of the Neonate, 74*, 402–408.

Thompson, A., Bizzarro, M., Yu, S., Diefenbach, K., Simpson, B. J., & Moss, R. L. (2011, March 24). Risk factors for necrotizing enterocolitis totalis: A case-control study. *Journal of Perinatology*. Advance online publication.

U.S. Food and Drug Administration. (2002). Health professionals letter on Enterobacter sakazakii infections associated with use of powdered (dry) infant formulas in neonatal intensive care units. Retrieved from http://www.FDA.gov/food/foodsafety/product-specificinformation/infantformula/alertssafetyinformation/ucm111299.htm

Uvnas-Moberg, K., & Eriksonn, M. (1996). Breastfeeding: Physiological endocrine and behavioral adaptation caused by oxytocin and local neurogenic activity in the nipple and mammary gland. *Acta Paediatrica Scandinavica, 85*, 523–530.

Valentine, C. J., & Hurst, N. M. (1995). A six-step feeding strategy for preterm infants. *Journal of Human Lactation, 11*, 7–8.

Van den Driessche, M., Peeters, K., Marien, P., et al. (1999). Gastric emptying in formula-fed and breast-fed infants measured with the 13C-octanoic acid breath test. *Journal of Pediatric Gastroenterology and Nutrition, 29*, 46–51.

Vohr, B., Poindexter, B. B., & Dusick, A. M. (2006). Beneficial effects of breast milk in the neonatal intensive care unit on development outcome of extremely low birth weight infants at eighteen months of age. *Pediatrics, 118E*, 115–123.

Walker, M. (2009). *Breastfeeding the late preterm infant*. Amarillo, TX: Hale Publishing.

Whitlaw, A., Heisterkanp, G., Sleath, K., et al. (1988). Skin-to-skin contact for very low birth weight infants and their mothers. *Archives of Disease in Childhood, 63*, 1377–1381.

Wight, N. E., Morton, J. A., & Kim, J. H. (2008). *Best medicine: Human milk in the NICU*. Amarillo, TX: Hale Publishing.

Wolf, L. S., & Glass, R. P. (1992). *Feeding and swallowing disorders in infancy: Assessment and management*. Tucson, AZ: Therapy Skill Builders.

World Health Organization. (2003). *Kangaroo mother care: A practical guide*. Geneva, Switzerland: Author.

Ziegler, E. E., Pantoja, A., & the "Food For Thought" Exploratory Group NIC/Q 2005. (2007). Vermont Oxford network, tools for improvement series.

Suggested Reading

Affonso, D., Bosque, E., Wahlberg, V., & Brady, J. P. (1993). Reconciliation and healing for mothers through skin-to-skin contact provided in an American tertiary-level intensive care nursery. *Neonatal Network, 12*, 25–32.

Als, H., & Gilkerson, L. (1995). Developmentally supportive care in the neonatal intensive care unit. *Zero to Three, 15*, 2–10.

Anderson, G. C. (1991). Current knowledge about skin-to-skin (Kangaroo) care for preterm infants. *Journal of Perinatology, 11*, 216–226.

Becker, P. T., Grunwald, P. C., Moorman, J., & Stuhr, S. (1993). Effects of developmental care on behavioral organization in very-low-birth-weight infants. *Nursing Research, 42*, 214–220.

Bell, E. H., Geyer, J., & Jones, L. (1995). A structured intervention improves breastfeeding success for ill or preterm infants. *MCN: The American Journal of Maternal/Child Nursing, 20*, 309–314.

Bier, J. B., Ferguson, A., Anderson, L., et al. (1993). Breast-feeding of very low birth weight infants. *Journal of Pediatrics, 123*, 773–779.

Bier, J. B., Ferguson, A. E., Morales, Y., et al. (1996). Comparison of skin-to-skin contact with standard contact in low birth weight infants who are breastfed. *Archives of Pediatric and Adolescent Medicine, 150*, 1265–1269.

Bowles, B. C., Stutte, P. C., & Hensley, J. H. (1988). Alternate massage in breastfeeding. *Genesis, 9*, 5–9, 17.

Charpak, N., Ruiz-Pelaez, J. G., Charpak, Y, Rey-Martinez, Kangaroo mother program: An alternative way of caring for low birth weight infants? One year mortality in a two cohort study. *Pediatrics, 94*, 804–810.

Durand, R., Hodges, S., LaRock, S., et al. (1997, March/April). The effect of skin-to-skin breastfeeding in the immediate recovery period on newborn thermoregulation and blood glucose values. *Neonatal Intensive Care*, 23–27.

Feher, S. D. K., Berger, L. R., Johnson, J. D., & Wilde, J. B. (1989). Increasing breast milk production for premature infants with a relaxation/imagery audiotape. *Pediatrics*, *83*, 57–60.

Glass, R. P., & Wolf, L. S. (1994). A global perspective on feeding assessment in the neonatal intensive care unit. *American Journal of Occupational Therapy*, *48*, 514–526.

Goldman, A. S., Chheda, S., Keeney, S. E., et al. (1994). Immunologic protection of the premature newborn by human milk. *Seminars in Perinatology*, *18*, 495–501.

Gupta, A., Khanna, K., & Chattree, S. (1999). Cup feeding: An alternative to bottle feeding in a neonatal intensive care unit. *Journal of Tropical Pediatrics*, *45*, 108–110.

Hamosh, M. (1994). Digestion in the premature infant: The effects of human milk. *Seminars in Perinatology*, *18*, 485–494.

Hill, P. D., & Aldag, J. C. (2006). Milk volume on day 4, and income predictive of lactation adequacy at 6 weeks of mothers of preterm infants. *Journal of Perinatal and Neonatal Nursing*, *19*, 273–282.

Hill, P. D., Andersen, J. L., & Ledbetter, R. J. (1995). Delayed initiation of breast-feeding the preterm infant. *Journal of Perinatal and Neonatal Nursing*, *9*, 10–20.

Hill, P. D., Brown, L. P., & Harker, T. L. (1995). Initiation and frequency of breast expression in breastfeeding mothers of LBW and VLBW infants. *Nursing Research*, *44*, 352–355.

Lang, S. (1997). *Breastfeeding special care infants*. Philadelphia, PA: W. B. Saunders.

Law, H. (2001). The use of comforting touch and massage to reduce stress for preterm infants in the neonatal intensive care unit. *Newborn and Infant Nursing*, *1*, 235–241.

Ludington, S. (1993). *Kangaroo care: The best you can do for your preterm infant*. New York, NY: Bantam Books.

Ludington, S. M. (1990). Energy conversion during skin-to-skin contact between premature infants and their mothers. *Heart and Lung*, *19*, 445–451.

Meier, P. (1988). Bottle- and breast-feeding: Effects on transcutaneous oxygen pressure and temperature in preterm infants. *Nursing Research*, *37*, 36–41.

Mennella, J. A., & Beauchamp, G. K. (1996). The human infants' response to vanilla flavors in mother's milk and formula. *Infant Behavior and Development*, *19*, 13–19.

Nyqvist, K. H., Ewald, U., & Sjödén, P. O. (1996). Supporting a preterm infant's behavior during breastfeeding: A case report. *Journal of Human Lactation*, *12*, 221–228.

Nyqvist, K. H., Rubertsson, C., Ewald, U., et al. (1996). Development of the preterm infant breastfeeding behavior scale (PIBBS): A study of nurse–mother agreement. *Journal of Human Lactation*, *12*, 207–219.

Nyqvist, K. H., Sjödén, P. O., & Ewald, U. (1994). Mothers' advice about facilitating breastfeeding in a neonatal intensive care unit. *Journal of Human Lactation*, *10*, 237–243.

Nyqvist, K. H., Sjödén, P.-O., & Ewald, U. (1999). The development of preterm infants' breastfeeding behavior. *Early Human Development*, *55*, 247–264.

Valentine, C. J., Hurst, N. M., & Schanler, R. J. (1994). Hindmilk improves weight gain in low-birth-weight infants fed human milk. *Journal of Pediatric Gastroenterology and Nutrition*, *18*, 474–477.

CHAPTER 30
Breastfeeding Twins and Higher Multiple-Birth Infants/Toddlers

M. Karen Kerkhoff Gromada, MSN, IBCLC, FILCA

OBJECTIVES

- Discuss the antenatal, intrapartum, and postnatal conditions and events that often affect the initiation of breastfeeding and lactation with twin and higher multiple births.
- Describe strategies for initiating and coordinating breastfeeding with multiple-birth neonates.
- Identify physiological and psychosocial factors that often affect breastfeeding duration with multiple-birth infants and children.

INTRODUCTION

When providing breastfeeding/lactation care to women who have multiple-birth children, the lactation consultant may assume the following:

- Single-infant pregnancy and birth are the norms for *Homo sapiens*. As such, multiple-birth infants/children strain maternal physical and emotional reserves. This strain extends to the breastfeeding relationship(s).
- Each multiple-birth infant (child) and his or her mother have the same right to the breastfeeding relationship and the normal physical and psychosocial advantages breastfeeding and lactation offer each infant (child) and mother.
- Breastfeeding initiation and duration with multiples are affected by more than an ability to replicate appropriate breastfeeding mechanics or typical lactation management strategies with two or more infants or children.
- Infant or maternal complications present at birth often affect breastfeeding initiation and can have long-lasting effects on breastfeeding duration or the feeding pattern with one or more of the multiple infants.
- Coordinating the breastfeeding of two or more infants with varying abilities to breastfeed effectively or differing but normal feeding patterns and styles might be perceived by a mother as breastfeeding problems rather than an aspect of the reality of having multiple infants or children.

(continues)

- Many older infant and toddler multiples engage in interactive behaviors during breastfeeding that can affect maternal coping and perception of the breastfeeding relationship.
- Women breastfeeding and/or human-milk-feeding multiple newborns, infants, or children are likely to need increased and specialized breastfeeding and lactation support and reinforcement.

I. Increased Multiple-Birth Rates

A. Incidence of twin and higher multiple births in Western cultures. Statistics cited are for the United States, but most industrial nations report similar increases in multiple births (Australian Bureau of Statistics, 2010; D'Addato, 2007; Martin et al., 2011; Statistics Canada, Minister of Industry, 2009). See **Figure 30-1**.

   1. Twins: 76% increase from 1980 to 2009

      a. 1980: Twins resulted in 1.89 per 100 births

      b. 2009: Twins resulted in 3.33 per 100 births

   2. Higher multiples (triplets/+): More than 400% increase from 1980 until peaking in 1998

      a. 2009: 153.5 per 100,000 births resulted in higher multiples; this number is approximately 20% lower than in 1998.

      b. 1980: 37 per 100,000 births resulted in triplets or higher multiples.

   3. Many European and other industrialized nations are noting decreases over the last several years in the percentage of multiple births, which are related to changes in assisted reproductive technology (ART) implementation (Cook et al., 2011; de Mouzon et al., 2010; Wang et al., 2008).

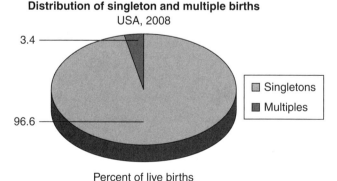

Distribution of singleton and multiple births
USA, 2008

3.4

96.6

- Singletons
- Multiples

Percent of live births

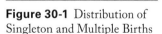

Figure 30-1 Distribution of Singleton and Multiple Births

Source: National Center for Health Statistics, final natality data. Retrieved April 2, 2011, from www.marchofdimes.com/peristats.

B. Factors associated with the increased incidence of multiple births are mainly related to the use of fertility-enhancing treatments (Bowers et al., 2006; Cook et al., 2011; de Mouzon et al., 2010; Martin et al., 2010).

1. Ovulatory induction (OI) medications or controlled ovarian stimulation (COH) using injectable fertility-enhancing medications to increase ova (eggs) growth and development.

2. ART, including intrauterine insemination (IUI), in vitro fertilization (IVF), intracytoplasmic sperm injection (ICSI).

3. Increased twinning related to reproductive technologies mostly increases the incidence of dizygotic (DZ/fraternal) multiples—fertilization of two or more separate ova by separate sperm.

   a. Older maternal age with childbearing has also affected the dizygotic twinning rate.

   b. ART also is associated with increased risk for monozygotic twinning (MZ/identical) and, therefore, a greater likelihood for the development of a monochorionic (MC; single, shared) placenta.

II. The Right to the Mother–Infant Breastfeeding Relationship

A. Breastfeeding, human milk, and lactation offer species-specific physical and psychosocial advantages for the human infant and lactating woman (Ip et al., 2007; León-Cava et al., 2002; Stuebe, 2009)

1. Other animal or plant species-derived infant milk poses risks for each infant in a set of multiples and for their mother (McNeil et al., 2010; Stuebe, 2009).

   a. The increased risks with multiple births increase the importance of providing species-specific milk and can potentiate the risks of nonhuman infant milks for multiple-birth infants.

2. Multiple-birth infants and their mothers have the same right to the breastfeeding relationship, human milk, and lactation as does the single-birth infant and mother (Gromada, 2007; Leonard, 2000, 2003; Leonard et al., 2006; Multiple Births Foundation [MBF], 2011).

   a. Women expecting multiples deserve factual information if they are to make informed infant-feeding decisions.

   b. Multiple births are at more risk for complications that can affect initiation and maintenance of breastfeeding and lactation.

3. Breastfeeding and providing human milk for multiple infants requires health professional, family, and social network education and support that has been adapted specifically for multiple-birth families (Damato et al., 2005a; Gromada, 2007; Lederman et al., 2006; Leonard, 2000, 2003; Leonard et al., 2006; MBF, 2011; Ooki, 2008; Östlund et al., 2010; Welsh, 2011; Yokoyama et al., 2004)

   a. Mothers report they were discouraged from breastfeeding their multiple-birth infants by health professionals for reasons based on assumption or anecdote rather than evidence.

   b. Health professional lack of knowledge regarding breastfeeding multiples can affect a mother's confidence to initiate or continue breastfeeding and/or expressing her milk, thereby affecting breastfeeding initiation and duration.

III. Multiple Pregnancy Factors Affecting the Initiation of Breastfeeding

A. Breastfeeding initiation rate

   1. Mothers of multiples (MOMs) initiate or intend breastfeeding/lactation at rates similar to or higher than women with single-birth infants (Damato et al., 2005b; Geraghty, Pinney et al., 2004; Mothers of Supertwins, 2007; Ooki, 2008; Östlund et al., 2010; Yokoyama et al., 2006)

      a. Twin initiation rates: Reports range from 64% to 89.4%.

      b. Triplets/+ initiation rates: Reports range from 55% to 86%.

      c. Most researchers did not distinguish between direct breastfeeding and the feeding of expressed human milk of multiples, or between full and partial breastfeeding/human-milk-feeding.

   2. The demographics of women using ART to achieve pregnancy—increased maternal age, education, socioeconomic status—are associated with populations that initiate breastfeeding at higher rates.

      a. Ooki (2008) found that women older than 35 years were less likely to breast-feed their twins.

B. Risk factors of multiple pregnancy/birth (See **Figures 30-2** through **30-6**).

   1. Infant factors affecting breastfeeding initiation include an increased incidence of the following:

      a. Preterm birth (less than 37 completed weeks gestation) or very preterm (less than 32 weeks). For example, in the United States in 2009 following are the average lengths of gestation (Martin et al., 2011):

         i. Single-infant pregnancy was 38.7 weeks with 10.4% born at < 37 weeks, of which 1.6% were < 32 weeks.

         ii. Twin pregnancy was 35.3 weeks with 58.8% born at < 37 weeks, of which 11.4% were <32 weeks.

         iii. Triplet pregnancy was 31.9 weeks with 94.4% born at < 37 weeks, of which 36.8% were < 32 weeks.

         iv. Quadruplet pregnancy was 29.5 weeks with 98.3% born at < 37 weeks, of which 64.5% were < 32 weeks.

         v. Quintuplet (or greater) pregnancy was 26.6 weeks with 96.3% born at < 37 weeks, of which 95% were < 32 weeks.

         vi. Statistics vary but the increased percentage of preterm birth for multiples is similar for other industrialized nations with wide variation among European nations from 42.2% (Republic of Ireland) to 68.4% (Austria) (Blondel et al., 2006).

         vii. Multiples account for 3.33% of all U.S. births but comprise 17% of all preterm and 23% of very preterm infants.

         viii. Multiples also account for < 3% of live births in most European nations yet are responsible for up to 20% of the preterm rate in many of those nations (EURO-PERISTAT Project, 2008).

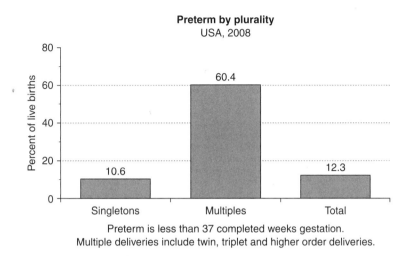

Figure 30-2 Preterm by Plurality

Source: National Center for Health Statistics, final natality data. Retrieved April 2, 2011, from www.marchofdimes.com/peristats.

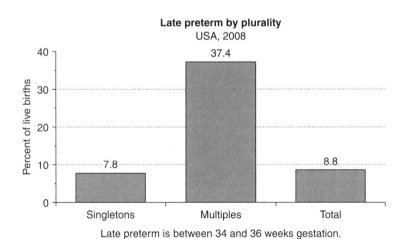

Figure 30-3 Late Preterm by Plurality

Source: National Center for Health Statistics, final natality data. Retrieved April 2, 2011, from www.marchofdimes.com/peristats.

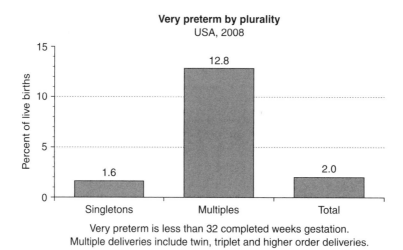

Figure 30-4 Very Preterm by Plurality

Source: National Center for Health Statistics, final natality data. Retrieved April 2, 2011, from www.marchofdimes.com/peristats.

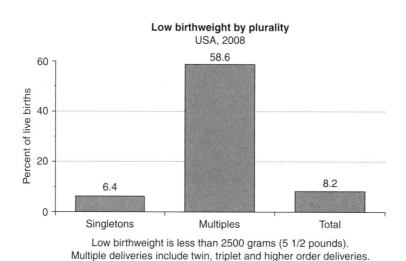

Figure 30-5 Low Birthweight by Plurality

Source: National Center for Health Statistics, final natality data. Retrieved April 2, 2011, from www. marchofdimes.com/peristats.

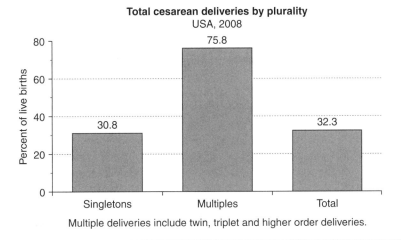

Figure 30-6 Total Cesarean Deliveries by Plurality

Source: National Center for Health Statistics, final natality data. Retrieved April 2, 2011, from www.marchofdimes.com/peristats.

    b. Monochorionic (MC) "shared" placenta is associated only with monozygotic (MZ) twinning, also referred to as identical twins. An MC placenta results when there is a split of one egg (ovum) fertilized by one sperm after uterine implantation (American College of Obstetricians and Gynecologists [ACOG], 2004; Bowers et al., 2006).

      i. Of MZ twins, 30% are dichorionic (DC with separate placentas) as a result of zygotic split before uterine implantation; 65–69% are MC but diamniotic (DA—having separate amniotic sacs); 1% are monoamniotic (MA—having a single, shared amniotic sac) as well as MC (referred to as MA/MC or MoMo).

        (a) Without more intensive ultrasound surveillance or elective preterm delivery, MoMo is associated with a 40–70% mortality rate mainly because of umbilical cord entanglement.

      ii. Approximately 15% of MC twins develop twin-to-twin transfusion syndrome (TTTS) related to the type or severity of the vascular connection(s) or communication(s) within an MC placenta.

        (a) One MZ twin acts as a blood donor to the other recipient twin.

        (b) Grave complications can occur for both the smaller, anemic donor twin and the larger, plethoric, hypervolemic recipient twin.

      iii. Cord anomalies or insertion deviations are more common with MC placentation.

c. Intrauterine growth restriction (IUGR)/fetal growth restriction (FGR) is related to one or more of the following (ACOG, 2004; Bowers et al., 2006):

    i. Decreasing fetal growth curves beginning at approximately 32 weeks for twins, 29–30 weeks for triplets, and 27 weeks for higher multiples

    ii. Discordant growth (15–25% decrease in fetal weight of smaller twin compared to larger twin) generally related to placental development or cord anomalies, especially for MC MZ twins

      (a) May be a normal variation for dizychotic (DZ—resulting from the fertilization of two or more eggs [ova] and two or more sperm) multiples with genetic differences for size

    iii. Twin-to-twin transfusion syndrome (TTTS), resulting in growth restriction for the donor twin (described earlier)

d. Low birth weight (LBW; < 5 lb, 8 oz or 2,500 g) and very low birth weight (VLBW; < 3 lb, 3 oz or 1,500 g). For example, in the United States in 2009, average birth weights (ABW) were as follows (Martin et al., 2011):

    i. Single infant: 7 lb, 4.26 oz, or 3,296 g (6.4% LBW; of these 1.1% VLBW).

    ii. Twins: 5 lb, 2.2 oz, or 2,336 g (56.6% LBW; of these 9.9% VLBW).

    iii. Triplets: 3 lb, 10.5 oz, or 1,660 g (95.1 % LBW; of these 35% VLBW).

    iv. Quadruplets: 2 lb, 13.53 oz, or 1,291 g (98.6% LBW; of these 68.1% VLBW).

    v. Quintuplets/+: 2 lb, 3.3 oz, or 1,002 g (94.6% LBW; of these 86.5% VLBW).

    vi. Multiple births: 3.33% of all live births but approximately 24% of all LBW and 26% of VLBW infants.

    vii. Statistics vary but are similar for other industrialized nations (EURO-PERISTAT Project, 2008; Laws et al., 2010).

e. Increased incidence of congenital or pregnancy-related anomalies, such as cardiac or digestive system defects; brain or central nervous system defects (Down syndrome, developmental delays, cerebral palsy); musculoskeletal defects of the head and neck (e.g., clefts, torticollis, jaw asymmetry), and lower extremity defects (e.g., hip dislocation, club foot) (Glinianaia et al., 2008; Pharoah et al., 2009; Tang et al., 2006).

    i. Singletons overall: 2.4%

    ii. Multiples overall: 4.06%

    iii. Higher for MZ multiples: 6.3% versus DZ multiples: 3.4%

    iv. There is a 46% increased risk of anomalies for a multiple-birth infant compared with a single-born infant.

    v. A congenital anomaly for one or more of multiple-birth infants can also affect breastfeeding or ongoing milk expression because of the effect of maternal coping or maternal–infant attachment formation, time management, and related ongoing special healthcare appointments/procedures (Gromada, 2007).

f. Infant mortality by plurality in the United States in 2006 (Mathews et al., 2010):

    i. Single births: 5.87/1,000 live births.

    ii. Multiple births: 30.07/1,000 live births.

      iii. Infant mortality is higher in the United States than in many industrialized nations.

      iv. Multiple births are 3% of all live births but 15% of overall infant mortality.

      v. Death of one or more multiples can affect breastfeeding because of the effect of related maternal grieving process on maternal–infants attachment formation, ongoing milk expression, and a transition to direct breastfeeding for the surviving multiple(s) (Gromada et al., 2005; Hanrahan, 2000; Pector, 2004)

  2. Maternal factors affecting breastfeeding initiation (ACOG, 2004; Bowers et al., 2006)—increased incidence:

    a. Pregnancy-induced hypertension (PIH) (may be referred to as preeclampsia or toxemia): 2.6 times higher

      i. Symptoms are often more severe or present with more advanced symptoms.

      ii. Progression to a more serious variation of PIH HELLP syndrome, which is characterized by hemolysis (breakdown of red blood cells), elevated liver enzymes, and low platelets (blood clotting factor), is more common with multiple pregnancy.

    b. Gestational diabetes mellitus (GDM): 1.8 times higher per each additional fetus

    c. Anemia: 21–36%; two to three times higher than for single-infant pregnancy

    d. Perinatal hemorrhage: Affects 1.2% of single-infant pregnancies but 6% of twin, 12% of triplet, and 21% of quadruplet pregnancies and is generally related to:

      i. Antenatal or intrapartum placental conditions; for example, previa, abruption

      ii. Postnatal uterine atony

    e. Surgical delivery in the United States in 2006: 72.9% of twin births; 93.9% triplet/+ births compared with 29.6% of single births (Centers for Disease Control and Prevention [CDC], 2009)

    f. Certain maternal health conditions that are also associated with the increased use of fertility-enhancing treatments/ART, which may result in lower milk production (West et al., 2009)

    g. Perinatal mood disorders, including depression and anxiety, and post-traumatic response to "high-risk" perinatal care/treatments or complications (Choi et al., 2009; Gromada et al., 2005)

C. Effect of infant or maternal complications on breastfeeding initiation (Beck, 2002a; Choi et al., 2009; Damato et al., 2005b; Gromada, 2007; Gromada et al., 2005; Leonard, 2000; Maloni, 2010; MBF, 2011)

  1. Depletion of maternal physical and psychological/emotional reserves during the early postpartum period

    a. Physical recuperation from multiple pregnancy, birth, and postpartum complications can conflict with ability to care for two or more newborns.

    b. Perinatal mood disorders can interfere with responding to individual infants' cues.

  2. Delayed initiation of breastfeeding or compensatory milk expression

  3. Delayed or lower milk production

IV. Prenatal Preparation

A. Infant-feeding decision

1. Reinforce research and case study evidence that demonstrate most women can produce enough milk for two or more newborns through infancy and into toddlerhood (Berlin, 2007; Leonard, 2000; Mead et al., 1992; Saint et al., 1986).

2. Discuss advantages and disadvantages pertinent to the breastfeeding of two or more newborns/infants for exclusive and partial breastfeeding/human-milk-feeding (Damato et al., 2005b; Gromada, 2010; Gromada et al., 2005; Leonard et al., 2006; MBF, 2011)

   a. Advantages (focusing on multiples-specific)

      i. Less risk of infection related to multiples:

         (a) More "at-risk" infants at birth with effects that can extend into later infancy/childhood

         (b) Likely to "share" any contagious illnesses

      ii. Breastfeeding ensures mother–babies contact many times in 24 hours, which in turn "forces" mothers to stop, sit, and focus on one or more babies.

      iii. Many mothers say breastfeeding enhances individual attachments with multiple infants.

      iv. Allows mother to invest time in babies rather than in obtaining supplies, preparation (sometimes of different artificial infant milks [AIM] for different multiples), and cleanup.

      v. Easier to feed two simultaneously.

   b. Disadvantages (focuses on multiples specific)

      i. Breastfeeding is perceived as more time intensive with multiple infants:

         (a) The idea that "no one can help"

         (b) Maternal concerns about sleep deprivation

      ii. Initiation often involves milk expression and the use of a breast pump, including related expenses.

         (a) The combination of infant care plus frequent, ongoing milk expression while trying to transition two or more newborns to direct breastfeeding feels overwhelming and a "burden" for many women.

         (b) May intensify with a maternal return to employed position.

3. Develop situation-based short- and long-term breastfeeding goals with multiple infants (Gromada, 2007, 2010).

   a. Direct breastfeeding and/or milk expression, depending on length of gestation, infant and/or maternal complications, and so forth.

   b. Full or partial breastfeeding/breastmilk-feeding.

   c. Breastfeeding duration: Literature indicates women have breastfed one or more of a set of multiples into the toddler period (Auer et al., 1998; Gromada, 2007; Poulson, 2009; Szucs et al., 2009a).

   d. Individual goals might be affected by maternal perceptions of caring for two or more infants (Leonard et al., 2006).

4. Provide anticipatory guidance for issues affecting breastfeeding/lactation initiation. For example:

    a. Improving infant outcomes regarding increased gestational age at birth and increased birth weights

        i. Multiple-birth newborn outcomes are associated with a maternal pregnancy weight gain of 37 to 54 lb (17.3–24.5 kg) (for average BMI) for twins; higher amount for triplets/+ (Fox et al., 2010; Gromada, 2007; Institute of Medicine & National Research Council, 2009).

        ii. Avoidance of "routine" surgical delivery via expectant management of multiple pregnancy (Childbirth Connection, 2011).

    b. Developing a plan for early initiation and the management of early breastfeeding or milk expression related to individual infant condition or maternal complications (Gromada, 2007; Leonard, 2003; Leonard et al., 2006; MBF, 2011)

5. Discuss maximizing milk production and related adaptation or options for multiple (2/+) well, surrogate, adopted, preterm, or physically compromised infants.

    a. Encourage early, frequent colostrum/milk removal via effective direct breastfeeding and milk expression if needed.

    b. Discuss options for obtaining donor human milk if there is insufficient maternal milk production (Szucs et al., 2009a, 2009b).

    c. Discuss that induced lactation and at least partial breastfeeding are possible in surrogate and adoptive situations (Szucs et al., 2010).

V. Initiating Breastfeeding

A. Healthy, full/late preterm twins and triplets (Gromada, 2007; Gromada et al., 1998; Leonard et al., 2006) (Also see Chapter 28: Guidelines for Facilitating and Assessing Breastfeeding; and Chapter 29: Breastfeeding a Preterm Infant.)

1. Implement immediate mother–infant skin contact with each newborn to allow for individual infant-led breastfeeding within 60–90 minutes of birth.

2. Encourage rooming-in (or modified rooming-in) for frequent, "cued" breastfeeding of each newborn. (See the following "Maternal complications.")

3. Encourage individual rather than simultaneous feedings until at least one multiple is assessed for consistent, effective breastfeeding behaviors.

    a. Introduction of simultaneous feeding depends on infants' abilities to latch and demonstrate appropriate suckling behaviors.

    b. This can vary within hours to weeks and occasionally months of birth.

4. Provide appropriate discharge planning that includes the following:

    a. Coordinating breastfeeding (discussed later) and other infant care

    b. Distinguishing breastfeeding issues from "two or more infants" issues

    c. Identifying support systems—physical, such as household help, emotional, and breastfeeding support

B. Maternal complications

    1. Direct breastfeeding (Gromada, 2007; Gromada et al., 1998)

        a. Encourage a round-the-clock, supportive assistant (partner, relative, friend) to help with infants' care and breastfeeding care—for positioning infants, holding an infant in place if needed, and so forth.

    2. Implement effective milk removal via breastfeeding or milk expression more than or equal to eight times in 24 hours if direct breastfeeding is not yet feasible.

        a. Assess whether mother is able to accomplish milk expression herself or needs the help of a caregiver.

            i. Assist mother or express the mother's milk for her until she is able to do so.

            ii. Instruct a family caregiver in how to assist the mother or express her milk until she is able to do so.

C. Preterm or sick twins/higher-order multiples

    1. Establish lactation for two or more newborns via milk expression (Gromada, 2007; MBF, 2011).

        a. Encourage frequent kangaroo care (skin-to-skin contact) of mother with each baby.

        b. Develop a realistic breastfeeding/milk expression plan with multiples. This may differ from a plan for a mother expressing for a single infant. (See Chapter 33: Milk Expression, Storage, and Handling.)

        c. Initiate milk expression as soon as possible following birth and initially for more than pumping sessions per 24 hours.

            i. "Hands-on" techniques in combination with the use of a hospital-grade electric breast pump can influence later volumes obtained and time required to obtain milk (Morton et al., 2009).

            ii. Breast pump suction pattern during the immediate postpartum can influence later volumes obtained and time required to obtain milk (Meier et al., 2011).

        d. Encourage the use of a hospital-grade electric pump with a double collection kit for postdischarge pumping sessions until all multiples to breastfeed effectively.

        e. Offer pumping session options that enhance production yet save time (West et al., 2008). For example:

            i. Continued hands-on techniques (breast massage, reverse pressure softening [RPS], intermittent manual expression) in combination with the hospital-grade electric breast pump (Morton et al., 2009)

            ii. Cluster-pumping sessions (10 minutes pumping, 10 minutes off, repeat three or four times) (Cannon et al., 2007)

            iii. Hands-free devices (bustier, bra, etc.)

            iv. Pump one breast while simultaneously breastfeeding a baby (assumes the ability of at least one multiple to breastfeed effectively) (Gromada, 2010)

2. Transitioning two or more preterm or sick neonates to breastfeeding (Gromada, 2007; MBF, 2011)

    a. Develop a realistic plan for multiples—inclusion of various feeding aids or devices may differ from a plan for a mother transitioning a single infant to direct breastfeeding.

    b. Assess and intervene based on varying individual infant ability (Nyqvist, 2002; Pineda, 2011).

        i. Encourage continued kangaroo care and maternal positioning for laid-back breastfeeding, which is more likely to facilitate individual infant progress to direct breastfeeding.

        ii. Expect infants to progress at different paces—each multiple is a different individual.

        iii. Mother, family members, and care providers often treat the "unit" of multiples:

            (a) Expect all to be ready to transition to breastfeeding at the same time.

            (b) May fail to recognize when one more is ready to move to effective breastfeeding.

    c. Expect a learning curve for breastfeeding. Maternal patience and persistence are needed as two or more preterm or sick newborns (of differing abilities) learn to breastfeed effectively.

        i. Household assistance provides time for mother and babies to "practice" breastfeeding.

        ii. Maternal confidence can affect the timing of the transition process.

    d. One or more preterm or compromised multiples can be prescribed additional calories or nutrients for varying lengths of time for several months to a year of age.

3. Plan for neonatal intensive care unit or special care unit (NICU/SCN) discharge (Gromada, 2007; MBF, 2011). Provide anticipatory guidance and follow-up resources for:

    a. Staggered homecoming in which one baby is discharged home prior to other(s) who remain in the NICU. This can affect bonding processes, frequency of pumping, time available for "practice" breastfeedings, and so forth.

    b. Parental anxiety related to assuming care and related concerns with the growth and development of two or more preterm or sick newborns.

    c. Coping with differing breastfeeding learning curves for individual infants while maintaining adequate milk removal.

VI. Maternal Postpartum Biopsychosocial Issues Affecting Breastfeeding Duration with Multiples

A. Duration of breastfeeding or human-milk-feeding

1. Term multiples are breastfed or human-milk-fed longer than preterm multiples are, but both breastfeed/human-milk-feed for less time than singletons do (Damato et al., 2005a; Geraghty, Pinney et al., 2004; Mothers of Supertwins, 2007; Östlund et al., 2010).

2. Research indicates that mothers either continue to breastfeed/human-milk-feed all or wean all at approximately the same time, indicating duration is unrelated to individual infant need or ability (Geraghty, Khoury, et al., 2004, 2005).

3. Most common reasons cited for discontinuing any breastfeeding/human-milk-feeding are as follows:

   a. Maternal: Primiparity; inadequate production; role strain, including return to work; lack of support by family or other social networks; time management issues, including pumping as an ongoing "burden" (Damato et al., 2005b; Flidel-Rimon et al., 2006; Leonard, 2003; Östlund et al., 2010; Yokoyama et al., 2004)

   b. Infants: Difficulties with the mechanics of breastfeeding; prematurity; small size; health issues (Auer et al., 1998; Ooki, 2008; Yokoyama et al., 2004)

B. Physiological conditions related to depleted maternal reserves (Gromada, 2007; Gromada et al., 2005; Gromada et al., 1998; MBF, 2011)

1. Potential for negative impact on milk production related to certain physiological conditions often associated with use of fertility-enhancing treatments/ART (West et al., 2008)

   a. Assess first for adequate, effective/thorough milk removal

2. Sequelae related to the physiological stress of a multiple pregnancy; complications or interventions/treatments to prolong the pregnancy may affect maternal coping

3. Recovery from surgical birth (See **Figure 30-7**.)

4. Profound sleep deprivation related to frequent interruptions for multiples' care and feeding

C. Mental-emotional conditions more frequent after multiple pregnancy (Academy of Breastfeeding Medicine Protocol Committee, 2011; Beck, 2002a, 2002b; Gromada, 2007; Gromada et al., 2005; Leonard, 2000; Yokoyama et al., 2004)

1. Chronic feeling of being overwhelmed or isolated.

   a. Unrealistic expectations for the maternal role with multiple infants

   b. Scope of infant needs and care tasks

   c. Lack of physical or emotional support systems

2. Incidence of postpartum mood disorders (PPMD) is two to three times higher in mothers of multiples (Choi et al., 2009; Gromada et al., 2005).

    a. Use *caution* when considering the use of a galactogogue if an increased risk of "depressed mood" is a side effect of a medication or herbal preparation.

3. High-risk pregnancy/birth and NICU experience can be associated with symptoms similar to posttraumatic stress disorder (PTSD) (Maloni, 2010).

D. Mother–infant(s) attachment—a different process (Beck, 2002b; Gromada, 2007)

    1. Common variations (Gromada, 2007)

        a. Unit attachment: Initial feelings of attachment are for the set of babies as a whole.

        b. Flip-flop attachment: Alternating focus of attention on one infant at a time, but the focus does change from one baby to another.

        c. Preferential attachment: Persistent, deeper attachment for a particular baby; presents emotional risks for all babies.

    2. Differentiation: Parental comparisons of multiples' physical and behavioral traits

        a. Desire to treat infants as separate yet also treat all equally.

        b. "Equal" treatment can result in ignoring individual infants' approaches to feeding, including feeding cues, number of feedings, and duration of feedings.

            i. Type of twinning/zygosity can affect infants' behavioral approaches to feeding (Gromada, 2007; Gromada et al., 1998; Ooki, 2008)

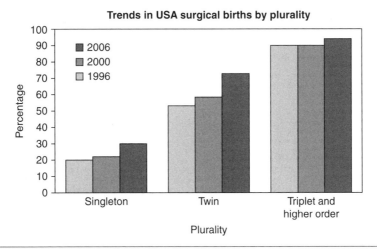

Figure 30-7 Trends in USA Surgical Births by Plurality

Source: CDC (2009).

VII. Maintaining Breastfeeding

A. Coordinating breastfeeding related to two or more individual infant feeding patterns (Gromada, 2007; Gromada et al., 2005; MBF, 2011).

1. Individual variations related to within normal variations in breastfeeding patterns—typical number and length of feedings per 24 hours

2. Individual outcome measures related to within normal limits of urine/stool outputs and weight gains

   a. Coordinate 24-hour feeding charts by clearly marking for each infant or using a different color paper for each infant's chart.

   b. Assess adequate or inadequate outcomes for individual breastfeeding ability/effectiveness of the milk transfer.

B. Feeding rotation (once effective breastfeeding is assessed for each multiple): Any option works if based on individual infants' cues (Gromada, 2007; MBF, 2011). Following are rotation options:

1. Alternate breasts and babies with each feeding—less favored option by mothers

2. Alternate breasts and babies every 24 hours (more often if a mother has an odd number of multiples)—option favored by many mothers of multiples

3. Assign each multiple a specific breast (assuming adequate function of both breasts)

   a. Benefits

      i. Increase breast self-regulation by two individual infants, which may:

         (a) Enhance the ability to suckle effectively for one/more infants

         (b) Decrease infant's consequences of "overactive" milk ejection reflex (OAMER) or gastroesophageal reflux disorder (GERD)

      ii. May facilitate breastfeeding for a multiple with certain positional anomalies, such as torticollis

      iii. Minimizes cross-contamination during certain infective conditions, such as thrush

   b. Risks

      i. May affect milk production if ineffective breastfeeding of one multiple is missed

      ii. May affect one infant's intake/growth if one breast is less "capable" of full milk production

      iii. Infant refusal to feed on the opposite breast if one breast cannot be suckled for any reason; problematic because of increased risk of nursing strike with multiples

      iv. Significant difference in maternal breast size (temporary)

C. Individual/separate versus simultaneous feeding (Flidel-Rimon et al., 2006; Gromada, 2007; Gromada et al., 1998; La Leche League International, 2009; MBF, 2011)

1. Affected by infants' suckling abilities or feeding styles and maternal choice.

2. Rationale for simultaneous feeding:
   a. Saves maternal time and may facilitate development of a routine
   b. Theoretical increase in milk production
      i. Many mothers report their multiples breastfeed separately for most/all feeds yet they had no problem with milk production.
      ii. Probably related to cue-based breastfeeding for each infant.
   c. Effective breastfeeding of one infant can enhance breastfeeding in another by one triggering the milk ejection reflex (MER) for the other.
3. Most MOMs combine simultaneous with separate feedings.
4. Pillows as needed for support/"extra arms":
   a. Household bed or sofa pillows
   b. Larger, deeper commercial nursing pillow designed to support two babies, one at each breast
5. Positions for simultaneous feeding (see **Figure 30-8**):
   a. Double laidback/prone (variation = double alongside)
   b. Double clutch/double football/double underarm (variation = double perpendicular)
   c. Double cradle or crisscross cradle (variation = V-hold)
   d. Cradle/clutch combination; also called layered or parallel hold
   e. Double straddle (variation = double upright; baby held or seated on one of mother's thighs facing a breast)

D. Maternal comfort (Gromada, 2007)
   1. Because of the increased time spent breastfeeding multiple infants, many mothers create a nursing station consisting of:
      a. A wide, padded chair or sofa such as an upholstered rocker/recliner
      b. A nearby table with snacks, beverages, portable telephone, remote controls, and so on within easy reach
      c. Convenient location—the room where the mother spends most of her time
   2. Nutrition (maternal): Effective breastfeeding/lactation for multiples should result in a natural increase in maternal hunger and thirst.
      a. Need strategies for eating while breastfeeding; for example, keeping one-handed snacks and a sports mug with water on the "nursing station" table.
      b. Hydration needs vary, so mothers should drink to thirst and produce pale, yellow urine.
         i. May caution mothers that "busy-ness" with multiple infants' care may result in ignoring personal thirst cues
      c. Suppressed/minimal/lack of appetite in a breastfeeding mother of multiples might be a symptom of inadequate milk production or a postpartum mood disorder (PPMD).

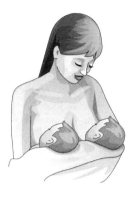

Figure 30-8a
Combination
Cradle-Football/
Layered/Parallel Hold

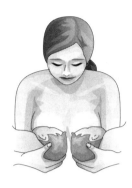

Figure 30-8b
Double-Football/
Double-Clutch Hold

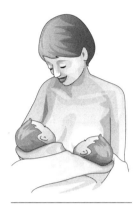

Figure 30-8c
Criss-Cross/
Double Cradle Hold

E. Developing a routine: Routine versus schedule—flexible versus rigid (Gromada, 2007; Gromada et al., 2005)

1. Cultural pressure affects notion of strict scheduling of infant care tasks.

   a. Parental knowledge deficit related to newborn/infant emotional development, need for close contact, and possible variations/differences for the individuals within the set.

   b. Many MOMs report they need or that others "insist" a strict schedule is needed to cope with multiples.

      i. Maternal desire for control (when other aspects can seem out of control).

      ii. An ability to anticipate infants' care/feeding needs appears to increase with each additional multiple infant in set.

2. Profound sleep deprivation/recovery from multiple pregnancy and birth:

   a. Many groups for parents of multiples encourage "sleep training" methods that can interfere with individual infant needs and effective, cue-based breastfeeding.

3. Strategies that support breastfeeding and better meet maternal and individual infant needs (Gromada, 2007; Leonard et al., 2006; MBF, 2011):

   a. Discuss realistic expectations for young infants and the individual infant temperaments/behavioral patterns.

   b. Wake a second infant to feed with or immediately after another; day and/or night.

      i. Risk of inadequate feeding of one or more babies related to ignoring an individual infant's need for more or longer feedings or a need for more contact.

ii. Consider occasional to daily use of EBM for one or more multiples to meet maternal need for a few hours of uninterrupted sleep.
Caution: Related to impact of any sudden change regarding several hours without milk removal for a woman with increased milk production, for example, increased potential for plugged duct(s), mastitis

c. Co-sleeping options to increase maternal sleep—proximal sleeping and safer bedsharing (Ball, 2007; Gromada, 2007; Hutchison et al., 2010; Leonard et al., 2006):

i. Co-bedding (shared sleep) of twins in one crib/cot: Associated with more mother–infants proximity during sleep and more synchronous sleep by infants.

ii. Co-bedding is a common sleep strategy; the younger the multiples, the more likely to be used as a strategy.

iii. Safer co-bedding strategies should be addressed with mothers of multiples.

VIII. Ongoing Breastfeeding Difficulties

(Also refer to chapters specific to difficulty.)

A. Infant-related difficulties: Cited most commonly as associated with early cessation of breastfeeding by mothers of multiples (Damato et al., 2005b;

B. Gromada, 2007; MBF, 2011)

1. Ongoing latch-on or suckling difficulty of one baby can affect breastfeeding for all.
   a. Limited maternal time/energy to work with affected multiple(s).
   b. Limited time for compensatory milk expression related to decreased milk removal by the affected infant(s).
   c. Lack of effective milk removal results in down-regulation of milk production.

2. Inadequate weight gain of one or more multiples:
   a. Real/actual: Consistent inadequate outputs or poor gain
   b. Perceived: Genetic or intrauterine-related slower but within normal limits growth/gain of one or more
      i. Postnatal growth and development for multiple infants may be associated with their individual prenatal growth and should be considered with weight gain assessment (Monset-Couchard et al., 2004).
      ii. Growth curves can be tracked on formula-fed infant-based growth charts.

3. Ongoing fortification of breastfeeding/human-milk-feeding prescribed for one/more infant(s): Interferes with transition to direct exclusive breastfeeding when desired.

C. Maternal-related difficulties (Beck, 2002b; Damato et al., 2005b; Geraghty, Khoury et al., 2004; Geraghty, Pinney, et al., 2004; Gromada, 2007; MBF, 2011)

    1. Milk sufficiency: Cited most often for early cessation of breastfeeding multiples

        a. Real/actual is related to

            i. Maternal sequelae of pregnancy/birth complications or an underlying maternal condition (possibly related to preconception fertility issues or related to greater physical demands of multiple pregnancy, birth or postpartum)

            ii. Delayed, infrequent, or insufficient milk removal resulting from inadequately "scheduled" or ineffective breastfeeding/milk expression

        b. Perceived: Confusion resulting from an increase in the total number of daily breastfeedings or from variation in the infants' breastfeeding patterns; difficulty differentiating one infant from another

        c. Intervention: Increased compensatory milk expression to establish/increase/maintain milk production, which can require temporarily limiting time at breast for any multiple affected by ineffective breastfeeding

            i. A mother is more likely to feel confident and continue breastfeeding efforts with improved milk production.

            ii. The infant's ability at the breast usually improves with time/maturity; adequate milk removal is crucial for improving/maintaining milk production until that occurs.

    2. Nipple or breast pain

        a. Increased likelihood of nipple pain or damage results from the increased risk of ineffective breastfeeding related to the increase of preterm and near-term birth for multiples.

        b. Infant-related complications and maternal surgical birth are more likely to result in antibiotic use and development of fungal infection that may spread to a mother's nipples and areolas.

        c. Delayed or missed feedings combined with increased milk production and/or decreased maternal resistance for illness can have a greater impact on the maternal system.

            i. Milk stasis can lead more quickly to engorgement, a plugged duct, or mastitis if a breastfeeding is postponed or missed.

        d. There is less time to consistently implement suggested interventions for sore/damaged nipples related to the number of infants requiring care.

    3. Long-term pumping and a return to work have also been cited as related to weaning at 6 months or younger for mothers of multiples.

IX. Full/Exclusive or Partial Breastfeeding and Human-Milk-Feeding Options for Multiples

A. Descriptions (Gromada, 2007; MBF, 2011)

    1. Full/exclusive breastfeeding: All feeding is directly at breast.

        a. Achieved for weeks to months with two to four multiples

        b. Subjective reports in the press of exclusive breastfeeding by higher multiples

2. Partial breastfeeding: Some feeding occurs directly at breast and some via an alternative infant feeding method.
   a. Common practice when caring for multiple newborns/infants.
   b. Varies from occasional "topping off" to regular, scheduled supplementary feedings that replace one or more direct breastfeedings.
   c. Partial breastfeeding can include the use of expressed breast milk (EBM), artificial infant milk (AIM), or a combination.
3. Full/exclusive or partial human-milk-feeding: Feeding of expressed breastmilk for all/some feedings via an alternative feeding method.
4. Amount of full/exclusive versus partial breastfeeding and/or human-milk-feeding can vary for individual members among the set.
   a. Individual infant abilities or anomalies can affect feeding method.
   b. Evidence indicates amount of breastfeeding/human milk per multiple tends to be similar over time (Geraghty, Khoury et al., 2004, 2005).

B. Implementation of full/exclusive versus partial breastfeeding or breast-milk-feeding options (Gromada, 2007; Leonard, 2000; Leonard et al., 2006; MBF, 2011)
   1. Any option can be used with one/more/all multiple(s) at any time during lactation.
   2. Any option can be used for the short or long term.
      a. MOMs have moved from human-milk-feeding to full/exclusive or partial direct breastfeeding.
      b. With direct breastfeeding, MOMs have moved from:
         i. Full/exclusive to partial breastfeeding
         ii. Partial to full/exclusive breastfeeding
      c. Movement within feeding options generally depends on complex interaction between or among maternal personal and environmental factors, including changing infants' needs.
   3. Factors involved in maternal decision making often include the following:
      a. Effect of ongoing infant or maternal physical conditions affecting breast-feeding or lactation
      b. Psychosocial issues related to the care of two or more newborns/infants
      c. Choice to continue to breastfeed (or express) for at least some feedings versus complete cessation

C. Factors associated with partial breastfeeding (Gromada, 2007; Ip et al., 2007; León-Cava et al., 2002; MBF, 2011; Ooki, 2008)
   1. Benefits (actual or perceived):
      a. Ensures adequate infant nutrition (when intake is of concern for one or more infants).
      b. Help with one/more infants' feedings.
      c. Some breastfeeding/human milk is better than no breastfeeding/human milk related to milk properties and maternal–infant(s) attachment (Flidel-Rimon et al., 2006).

2. Risks (actual) associated with implementing partial breastfeeding/ human-milk-feeding:

    a. Lower or decreasing milk production related to less time for transitioning infants to breast for increased pumping sessions

    b. Increased infant preference for an alternative feeding method yet less time to work with/help any infant at breast as a result of caring for two or more infants

    c. Increased infant infectious illnesses related to less than full/exclusive breastfeeding/human-milk-feeding

3. Maintaining milk production when implementing partial breastfeeding:

    a. Maintain effective milk removal at least 8–12 times per 24 hours.

    b. Minimize use of supplementary (replacement of breastfeeding) feedings; for example, "top off" or complement with small amount after a breastfeeding rather than supplement/replace an entire feeding.

    c. Supplement one or more on an as need (prn) basis; for example, a maternal need for several hours of uninterrupted sleep with breastfeeding or pumping immediately before/after.

    d. Avoid alternating feeding methods every other feeding.

        i. Equals all the work of both methods

        ii. May work if a full-time helper is available to handle alternative feedings

X. Breastfeeding Older Infant and Toddler Multiples

A. Supplementary vitamins (other than vitamin D) or minerals, including iron (Gromada, 2007)

    1. Provision should be based on the individual infant screening outcomes:

        a. Pediatric associations recommend 400 IU of vitamin D for breastfed infants in North America.

    2. Preterm birth or other intrauterine conditions, such as anemia in TTTS donor, can affect need for additional trace minerals.

B. Introducing solid foods (Gromada, 2007; MBF, 2011)

    1. Provide anticipatory guidance related to the encouragement MOMs often receive for the early introduction of solid foods (or EBM or AIM thickened with rice carbohydrate).

        a. Mothers might perceive that solid food or thickened feedings lengthen the time between feedings for increased nighttime sleep.

        b. Preterm multiples' gastrointestinal tracts are less mature.

           i. Often less ready for early introduction of solids.

           ii. Increased likelihood of GERD. Weigh benefits and risks of thickened supplementary feedings, especially if such feedings interfere with direct breastfeeding.

2. Individual multiples are likely to demonstrate readiness for solid food introduction at different times, especially DZ multiples.
   a. Anticipatory guidance should address individual infant readiness to address a parental tendency to treat multiples alike or equal, which can result in the introduction of solid food to both/all at once whether both/all indicate readiness.

C. Common behaviors associated with breastfeeding older infant/toddler multiples that differ from a single infant/toddler (Gromada, 2007) (See **Figures 30-9** through **30-10**.)
   1. Increased nursing strikes noted in mid- to later infancy (etiology unknown), possibly related to:
      a. Inadvertent delays getting a cueing baby to breast or purposeful "scheduling" of breastfeeding resulting from the increased care needs of two or more
      b. Increased use of alternative feedings for one/more in a set of multiples related to:
         i. Partial breastfeeding at home for any reason
         ii. Mother–babies separation resulting from mother's return to an employed position
   2. Increased biting during breastfeeding possibly related to simultaneous feeding and less ability to monitor for signs indicating an onset of biting.
   3. Increased interaction between multiples during breastfeeding.
      a. Playful to more aggressive behaviors—often includes an escalation of poking, pushing, punching behaviors
      b. Strategy to diminish behavior quickly—consistent, calm halt to breastfeeding when interactions interfere with maternal or the other multiple's comfort; may be brief and mother should repeat as needed
   4. "Jealous" breastfeeding: Need of one multiple to breastfeed results in a demand by the other(s) to breastfeed without an apparent need associated.
      a. "Demand" is related only to the breastfeeding of another.
      b. Can be a frequent occurrence by one/both/all and often influences weaning style.

D. Approach to weaning (Gromada, 2007)
   1. Individual baby-led/child-led weaning: May occur weeks, months, or years apart for different members of a set of multiples.
   2. Mother-encouraged, baby-led weaning: Imposition of some type of limit(s) on breastfeeding, such as time or place related to breastfeeding near the end of or after the first year and often in response to:
      a. Multiples' physical interactions while at the breast
      b. Ongoing maternal sleep deprivation

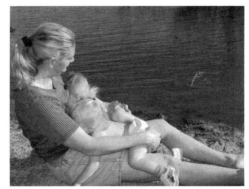

Figure 30-9 Breastfeeding Toddlers

Source: Copyright © karengromada.com, 2012; reprinted with permission.

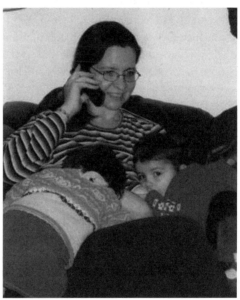

Figure 30-10 Multitasking while Breastfeeding Toddlers

Source: Copyright © karengromada.com, 2012; reprinted with permission.

3. Mother-led weaning: A purposeful decrease in the number of breastfeedings by the mother; often related to maternal feelings of being overwhelmed by multiple infants'/toddlers' behaviors during breastfeeding or sleep, and interactions at other times
   a. Gradual: Purposeful decrease in breastfeeding with acceleration based on personal or multiples' responses to decreased breastfeeding
      i. Mother may delay or slow process if decreased breastfeeding reaches physically or emotionally comfortable level for herself or her multiples.
   b. Abrupt: Sudden, complete cessation of breastfeeding
      i. Gradual weaning may become acceptable to mother to try once she is informed of the implications of abrupt weaning for herself or her infants/ toddlers.

E. Timing of older infant, toddler, or child breastfeeding cessation (Gromada, 2007)
  1. Early (10–12 months), abrupt baby-led weaning is slightly more common with multiples; may affect one or more of multiple infants.
     a. Assess to distinguish from "nursing strike."
  2. Some researchers have noted more of a decrease in MOM milk production compared to women with single infants between 9 and 12 months (Saint et al., 1986).
     a. Not clear whether decreases were related more to physiological or behavioral factors
  3. Many MOMs have breastfed their multiples for well over 1 year.
     a. Continued breastfeeding may or may not be part of a mother's breastfeeding goal (Poulson, 2009).
     b. Often, continued breastfeeding involves all multiples in a set, but it might continue for one or more of a set if one or more stops breastfeeding before the other or others.
     c. MOMs have reported one or more of a set breastfeeding for 4–5 years.

References

Academy of Breastfeeding Medicine Protocol Committee (2011). ABM clinical protocol no. 9: Use of galactogogues in initiating or augmenting the rate of maternal milk secretion (First Revision January 2011). *Breastfeeding Medicine, 6*(1), 41–49. Retrieved from http://www.bfmed.org/Media/Files/Protocols/Protocol%209%20-%20English%201st%20Rev.%20Jan%202011.pdf

American College of Obstetricians and Gynecologists. (2004). Multiple gestation: Complicated twin, triplet, and high-order multifetal pregnancy (ACOG Practice Bulletin No. 56). *Obstetrics and Gynecology, 104*(4), 869–883. Retrieved from https://www.smfm.org/attachedfilesPubs/ACOG%20SMFM%20joint%20practice%20bulletin%20Multiple%20gestation%202004.pdf

Auer, C., & Gromada, K. (1998). A case report of breastfeeding quadruplets: Factors perceived as affecting breastfeeding. *Journal of Human Lactation, 14*(2), 135–141.

Australian Bureau of Statistics. (2010). *Births, Australia, 2009.* Cat. no. 3301.0. Sydney, NSW: Commonwealth of Australia. Retrieved from http://www.ausstats.abs.gov.au/Ausstats/subscriber.nsf/0/10BEDC49AFCACC1FCA2577CF000DF7AB/$File/33010_2009.pdf

Ball, H. L. (2007). Together or apart? A behavioural and psychological investigation of sleeping arrangements for twin babies. *Midwifery, 23*(4), 404–412.

Beck, C. T. (2002a). Releasing the pause button: Mothering twins during the first year of life. *Qualitative Health Research, 12*(5), 593–608.

Beck, C. T. (2002b). Mothering multiples: A meta-synthesis of qualitative research. *MCN: The American Journal of Maternal Child Nursing, 27*(4), 214–221.

Berlin, C. (2007). "Exclusive" breastfeeding of quadruplets. *Breastfeeding Medicine, 2*(2), 125–126.

Blondel, B. , Macfarlane, A., Gissler, M., Breart, G., Zeitlin, J., & PERISTAT Study Group. (2006). Preterm birth and multiple pregnancy in European countries participating in the PERISTAT project. *BJOG, 113*(5), 528–535. Retrieved from http://onlinelibrary.wiley.com/doi/10.1111/j.1471-0528.2006.00923.x/pdf

Bowers, N., & Gromada, K. K. (2006). *Care of the multiple-birth family: Pregnancy and birth* (Rev. ed., nursing module). White Plains, NY: March of Dimes.

Cannon, A., Jacobson, H., & Morgan, B. (2007). *Living with chronic low milk supply: A basic guide.* MOBI Motherhood International. Retrieved from http://www.mobimotherhood.org/MM/article-lms.aspx

Centers for Disease Control and Prevention. (2009). Quick stats: Percentage of live births by cesarean delivery, by plurality—United States, 1996, 2000, and 2006. *Morbidity and Mortality Weekly Report, 58*(19), 542. Retrieved from http://www.cdc.gov/mmwr/preview/mmwrhtml/mm5819a9.htm

Childbirth Connection. (2011). *Options: C-section.* New York, NY: Author. Retrieved from http://www.childbirthconnection.org/article.asp?ck=10167

Choi, Y., Bishal, D., & Minkovitz, C. S. (2009). Multiple births are a risk factor for postpartum maternal depressive symptoms. *Pediatrics, 123*(4), 1147–1154. Retrieved from http://pediatrics.aappublications.org/cgi/content/full/123/4/1147

Cook, J. L., Collins, J., Buckett, W., Racowsky, C., Hughes, E., & Jarvi, K. (2011). Assisted reproductive technology-related multiple births: Canada in an international context. *Journal of Obstetrics and Gynaecology Canada, 33*(2), 159–167. Retrieved from http://www.sogc.org/jogc/abstracts/full/201102_HealthPolicy_1.pdf

D'Addato, A. V. (2007). Secular trends in twinning rates. *Journal of Biosocial Science, 39*(1), 147–151.

Damato, E. G., Dowling, D. A., Madigan, E. A., & Thanattherakul, C. (2005a). Duration of breastfeeding for mothers of twins. *Journal of Obstetric, Gynecologic, and Neonatal Nursing, 34*(2), 201–209.

Damato, E. G., Dowling, D. A., Standing, T. S., & Schuster, S. D. (2005b). Explanation for the cessation of breastfeeding in mothers of twins. *Journal of Human Lactation, 21*(3), 296–304.

de Mouzon, J., Goossens, V., & Bhattacharya, J. A. (2010). Assisted reproductive technology in Europe, 2006: Results generated from European registers by ESHRE. *Human Reproduction, 25*(8), 1851–1862. Retrieved from http://humrep.oxfordjournals.org/content/25/8/1851.full

EURO-PERISTAT Project. (2008). *European perinatal health report.* Paris, France: Author. Retrieved from http://www.europeristat.com/bm.doc/european-perinatal-health-report.pdf

Flidel-Rimon, O., & Shinwell, E. S. (2006). Breast feeding twins and high multiples. *Archives of Disease in Childhood: Fetal and Neonatal Edition, 91*(5), F377–F380. Retrieved from http://www.ncbi.nlm.nih.gov/pmc/articles/PMC2672857/pdf/F377.pdf

Fox, N. S., Rebarber, A., Roman, A. S., Klauser, C. K., Peress, D., & Saltzman, D. H. (2010). Weight gain in twin pregnancies and adverse outcomes: Examining the 2009 Institute of Medicine guidelines. *Obstetrics and Gynecology, 116*(1), 100–106. Retrieved from http://journals.lww.com/greenjournal/Fulltext/2010/07000/Weight_Gain_in_Twin_Pregnancies_and_Adverse.17.aspx#

Geraghty, S. R., Khoury, J. C., & Kalkwarf, H. J. (2004). Comparison of feeding among multiple birth infants. *Twin Research, 7*(6), 542–547.

Geraghty, S. R., Khoury, J. C., & Kalkwarf, H. J. (2005). Human milk pumping rates of mothers of singletons and mothers of multiples. *Journal of Human Lactation, 21*(4), 413–420.

Geraghty, S. R., Pinney, S. M., Sethurman, G., Roy-Chaudhury, A., & Kalkwarf, H. J. (2004). Breast milk feeding rates of mothers of multiples compared to mothers of singletons. *Ambulatory Pediatrics, 4*(3), 226–231.

Glinianaia, S. V., Rankin, J., & Wright, C. (2008). Congenital anomalies in twins: A register-based study. *Human Reproduction, 23*(6), 1306–1311. Retrieved from http://humrep.oxfordjournals.org/content/23/6/1306.full

Gromada, K. (2010). ILCA's inside track a resource for breastfeeding mothers: Twins. *Journal of Human Lactation, 26*(3), 331–332.

Gromada, K. K. (2007). *Mothering multiples: Breastfeeding and caring for twins or more* (rev. ed.). Schaumburg, IL: La Leche League International.

Gromada, K. K., & Bowers, N. (2005). *Care of the multiple-birth family: Birth through early infancy* (Rev. ed., nursing module). White Plains, NY: March of Dimes.

Gromada, K. K., & Spangler, A. (1998). Breastfeeding twins and higher-order multiples. *Journal of Obstetric, Gynecologic, and Neonatal Nursing, 27*(4), 441–449.

Hanrahan, J. (2000). Breastfeeding after the loss of a multiple. *Leaven, 36*(5), 12. Retrieved from http://www.llli.org/llleaderweb/lv/lvoctnov00p102.html

Hutchison, B. L., Stewart, A. W., & Mitchell, E. A. (2010). The prevalence of cobedding and SIDS-related child care practices in twins. *European Journal of Pediatrics, 169*(12), 1477–1485.

Institute of Medicine & National Research Council. (2009). *Weight gain during pregnancy: Reexamining the guidelines.* Washington, DC: National Academies Press. Retrieved from http://www.nap.edu/catalog.php?record_id=12584#toc

Ip, S., Chung, M., Raman, G., Chew, P., Magula, N., DeVine, D., Trikalinos, T., & Lau, J. (2007). *Breastfeeding and maternal and infant health outcomes in developed countries* (Evidence Report/ Technology Assessment No. 153, AHRQ Publication No. 07-E007). Rockville, MD: Agency for Healthcare Research and Quality. Retrieved from http://www.ahrq.gov/downloads/pub/ evidence/pdf/brfout/brfout.pdf

La Leche League International. (2009). *Tips for breastfeeding twins* (Information sheet no. 10237). Schaumburg, IL: Author.

Laws, P. J., Li, Z., & Sullivan, E. A. (2010). *Australia's mothers and babies 2008* (Perinatal statistics series no. 24, Cat. no. PER 50). Canberra, Australia: AIHW. Retrieved from www.aihw.gov.au/ WorkArea/DownloadAsset.aspx?id=6442472762

Lederman, S., & Hopkinson, J. (2006). Response to Geraghty et al regarding the use of pumps and breastfeeding (Letters to the editor). *Journal of Human Lactation, 22*(4), 387.

Leonard, L. G. (2000). Breastfeeding triplets: The at-home experience. *Public Health Nursing, 17*(3), 211–221.

Leonard, L. G. (2003). Breastfeeding rights of multiple birth families and guidelines for health professionals. *Twin Research, 6*(1), 34–45.

Leonard, L. G., & Denton, J. (2006). Preparation for parenting multiple birth children. *Early Human Development, 82*(6), 371–378. Retrieved from http://www.multiplebirthscanada.org/ english/documents/Preparationforparentingmultiplebirthchildren.pdf

León-Cava, N., Lutter, C., Ross, J., & Martin, L (2002). *Quantifying the benefits of breastfeeding: A summary of the evidence* (PAHO ref no. HPN/66/2). Washington, DC: Pan American Health Organization. Retrieved from http://www.linkagesproject.org/media/publications/Technical %20Reports/BOB.pdf

Maloni, J. A. (2010). Antepartum bed rest for pregnancy complications: Efficacy and safety for preventing preterm birth. *Biological Research for Nursing, 12*(2), 106–124.

Martin, J. A., Hamilton, B. E. & Osterman, M. J. K. (2012). Three decades of twin births in the United States, 1980-2009. *NCHS Data Brief*, no. 80. Hyattsville, MD: National Center for Health Statistics. Retrieved from http://www.cdc.gov/nchs/data/databriefs/db80.pdf.

Martin, J. A., Hamilton, B. E., & Ventura, S. J. (2011). Births: Final data for 2009. *National Vital Statistics Report, 60*(1). Retrieved from http://www.cdc.gov/nchs/data/nvsr/nvsr60/nvsr60_01.pdf.

Mathews, T. J., & MacDorman, M. F. (2010). Infant mortality statistics from the 2006 period linked birth/infant death data set. *National Vital Statistics Report, 58*(17). Hyattsville, MD: National Center for Health Statistics. Retrieved from http://www.cdc.gov/nchs/data/nvsr/nvsr58/nvsr58_17.pdf

McNeil, M. E., Labbok, M. H., & Abrahams, S. W. (2010). What are the risks associated with formula feeding? A re-analysis and review. *Birth, 37*(1), 50–58. Retrieved from http://onlinelibrary.wiley.com/doi/10.1111/j.1523-536X.2009.00378.x/full

Mead, L., Chuffo, R., Lawlor-Klean, P., & Meier, P. (1992). Breastfeeding success with preterm quadruplets. *Journal of Obstetric, Gynecologic, and Neonatal Nursing, 21*(3), 221–227.

Meier, P. P., Engstrom, J. L., Janes, J. E., Jegier, B. J., & Loera, F. (2011). Breast pump suction patterns that mimic the human infant during breastfeeding: Greater milk output in less time spent pumping for breast pump-dependent mothers with premature infants. *Journal of Perinatology*. Advance publication online.

Monset-Couchard, M., de Bethmann, O., & Relier, J.-P. (2004). Long term outcome of small versus appropriate size for gestational age co-twins/triplets. *Archives of Disease in Childhood: Fetal and Neonatal Edition, 89*(4), F310–314. Retrieved from http://www.ncbi.nlm.nih.gov/pmc/articles/PMC1721732/pdf/v089p0F310.pdf

Morton, J., Hall, J. Y., Wong, R. J., Thairu, L., Benitz, W. E., & Rhine, W. D. (2009). Combining hand techniques with electric pumping increases milk production in mothers of preterm infants. *Journal of Perinatology 29*(11), 757–764.

Mothers of Supertwins. (2007). *Supertwins statistics: Breastfeeding*. Retrieved from http://www.mostonline.org/facts_breastfeeding.htm

Multiple Births Foundation. (2011). *Guidance for health professionals on feeding twins, triplets and higher order multiples*. London, England: Author. Retrieved from http://www.multiplebirths.org.uk/MBF_Professionals_Final.pdf

Nyqvist, K. H. (2002). Breast-feeding in preterm twins: Development of feeding behavior and milk intake during hospital stay and related caregiving practices. *Journal of Pediatric Nursing, 17*(4), 246–256.

Ooki, S. (2008). Breast-feeding rates and related maternal and infants' obstetric factors in Japanese twins. *Environmental Health and Preventive Medicine, 13*(4), 187–197.

Östlund, A., Nordström, M., Dykes, F., & Flacking, R. (2010). Breastfeeding in preterm and term twins—maternal factors associated with early cessation: A population-based study. *Journal of Human Lactation, 26*(3), 327–329.

Pector, E. A. (2004). How bereaved multiple-birth parents cope with hospitalization, homecoming, disposition for deceased, and attachment to survivors. *Journal of Perinatology, 24*(11), 714–722. Retrieved from http://www.nature.com/jp/journal/v24/n11/full/7211170a.html

Pharoah, P. O. D., & Dundar, Y. (2009). Monozygotic twinning, cerebral palsy and congenital anomalies. *Human Reproduction Update, 15*(6), 239–248. Retrieved from http://humupd.oxfordjournals.org/content/15/6/639.long

Pineda, E. (2011). Direct breast-feeding in the neonatal intensive care unit: Is it important? *Journal of Perinatology 31*(8), 540–545.

Poulson, M. (2009). Breastfeeding toddler twins. *New Beginnings, 30*(5-6), 14–15. Retrieved from http://viewer.zmags.com/publication/445c4023#/445c4023/16

Rasmussen, K. M., & Yaktine, A. L. (Eds.). (2009). Weight gain during pregnancy: Reexamining the guidelines. Washington, DC: National Academies Press. Retrieved from http://www.nap.edu/catalog.php?record_id=12584#toc

Saint, L., Maggiore, P., & Hartmann, P. (1986). Yield and nutrient content of milk in eight women breast-feeding twins and one woman breast-feeding triplets. *British Journal of Nutrition, 56*(1), 49–58. Retrieved from http://journals.cambridge.org/download.php?file=%2FBJN%2FBJN56_01%2FS0007114586000855a.pdf&code=0547b8c4f3a0fb384579326df0a7aa58

Statistics Canada, Minister of Industry. (2009). *Births 2007* (Catalogue no. 84F0210X). Ottawa, Ontario: Author. Retrieved from http://dsp-psd.pwgsc.gc.ca/collection_2009/statcan/84F0210X/84f0210x2007000-eng.pdf

Stuebe, A. (2009). The risks of not breastfeeding for mothers and infants. *Reviews in Obstetrics and Gynecology, 2*(4), 222–231. Retrieved from http://www.ncbi.nlm.nih.gov/pmc/articles/PMC2812877/?tool=pubmed

Szucs, K. A., Axline, S. E., & Rosenman, M. B. (2009a). Quintuplets and a mother's determination to provide human milk: It takes a village to raise a baby—how about five? *Journal of Human Lactation, 25*(1), 79–84.

Szucs, K. A., Axline, S. E., & Rosenman, M. B. (2009b). The quintuplets receiving human milk: An update. *Journal of Human Lactation, 25*(3), 269.

Szucs, K. A., Axline, S. E., & Rosenman, M. B. (2010). Induced lactation and exclusive breast milk feeding of adopted premature twins. *Journal of Human Lactation, 26*(3), 309–313.

Tang, Y., Ma, C.-X., Cui, W., Chang, V., Ariet, M., Morse, S. B., Resnick, M. B., & Roth, J. (2006). The risk of birth defects in multiple births: A population-based study. *Maternal and Child Health Journal, 10*(1), 75–81. Retrieved from http://mch.peds.ufl.edu/recent_pubs/tang_risk_of_birth_defects_in_multiple_births.pdf

Wang, Y. A., Dean, J. H., Badgery-Parker, T., & Sullivan, E. A. (2008). *Assisted reproduction technology in Australia and New Zealand 2006* (Assisted Reproduction Technology series no. 12, AIHW cat. no. PER 43). Sydney, Australia: AIHW National Perinatal Statistics Unit. Retrieved from http://www.preru.unsw.edu.au/PRERUWeb.nsf/resources/ART_2005_06/$file/art12.pdf

Welsh, S. R. (2011). Breastfeeding twins with confidence. *New Beginnings, 36*(3), 7. Retrieved from http://viewer.zmags.com/publication/946b8eeb#/946b8eeb/8

West, D., & Marasco, L. (2008). *The breastfeeding mother's guide to making more milk*. New York, NY: McGraw-Hill.

Yokoyama, Y., & Ooki, S. (2004). Breast-feeding and bottle-feeding of twins, triplets and higher order multiple births. *Nihon Koshu Eisei Zasshi, 51*(11), 969–974.

Yokoyama, Y., Wada, S., Sugimoto, M., Katayama, M., Saito, M., & Sono, J. (2006). Breastfeeding rates among singletons, twins and triplets in Japan: A population-based study. *Twin Research & Human Genetics, 9*(2), 298–302.

CHAPTER 31
Breastfeeding and Growth: Birth Through Weaning

Nancy Mohrbacher, IBCLC, FILCA

OBJECTIVES

- Identify how close body contact and feeding positions after birth affect infant stability and breastfeeding.
- Discuss normal growth in the full-term breastfeeding baby and compare differences in growth when babies are not breastfed.
- Explain how culture, infant stomach size, and mothers' breast storage capacity can affect breastfeeding patterns.
- Recognize how breastfeeding behaviors change during the first 12 months and beyond as a result of normal growth and development.
- Identify recommendations for breastfeeding duration and compare them to the natural age of weaning.
- Describe safe and gentle weaning strategies for families who choose to end breastfeeding prior to their child's natural readiness to wean.

INTRODUCTION

Expectations of breastfeeding behavior are influenced by culture, and a wide range of breastfeeding behaviors and weaning ages are considered normal at different times and in different places. At one end of the spectrum, it is culturally normal to breastfeed several times per hour round the clock for the first 2 years of life among the Kung of Africa, one of the world's last hunter-gatherer societies (Stuart-Macadam, 1995). This culture also expects frequent and intense breastfeeding for the first 3 to 4 years of life. At the other end of the spectrum is the modern-day United States, where cultural beliefs about breastfeeding are influenced by bottle-feeding norms. During the first few months of life, babies in the United States are generally expected to breastfeed at regular intervals of no less than 2 to 3 hours. In this culture, as babies age, the intervals between breastfeedings are expected to increase. When babies indicate they want to breastfeed more often than these cultural expectations, mothers are often encouraged to supplement with formula. Complete weaning is generally expected by about 1 year of age.

I. Close Mother–Baby Body Contact After Birth Stabilizes Baby and Releases Reflexes That Can Facilitate Early Breastfeeding

  A. Healthy babies are born with reflexes that can help them move to the breast and breastfeed.

    1. After birth, healthy newborns in a ventral position on mother's semireclined body follow a predictable series of behaviors that move them to the breast, stimulate oxytocin release in the mother (Matthieson et al., 2001; Widstrom et al., 2011), and lead to breastfeeding, usually about an hour after birth (**Table 31-1**).

    2. If a mother receives specific pain medications during labor or mother and baby are separated before the first breastfeeding, these reflexes may be temporarily suppressed in some newborns (Righard et al., 1990; Wiklund et al., 2009).

  B. Babies separated from their mothers during the early newborn period are at greater risk for unstable body functions and feeding problems.

    1. Newborns separated from their mothers exhibit the "protest-despair" response that also occurs in other infant mammals.

      a. During this response, the newborn first emits a distinctive "separation distress" cry (Christensson et al., 1995).

      b. If separation continues, levels of stress hormones rise and body functions such as temperature, blood sugar, breathing, and heart rate may become unstable (Christensson et al., 1992).

      c. If the newborn's cry is not responded to and separation continues, the baby's physiology changes to "despair mode," slowing digestion and growth to increase odds of survival (Bergman, 2008).

    2. Continuous contact between mother and baby is associated with fewer feeding problems, less crying, and more stable body functions (Christensson et al., 1992).

Table 31-1 Predictable Newborn Behaviors After Birth

Time (minutes)	Behavior
6	Opens eyes
11	Massages the breast
12	Hand to mouth
21	Rooting
25	Moistened hand to breast
27	Tongue stretches and licks nipple
80	Breastfeeding

Source: Adapted from Matthieson, A., Ransjo-Arvidson, A., Nissen, E., & Uvnäs-Moberg, K. (2001). Postpartum maternal oxytocin release by newborns: Effects of infant hand massage and sucking. *Birth, 28*, 12–19.

3. The longer mother and baby are in skin-to-skin contact during the first 3 hours after birth, the more likely they are to be exclusively breastfeeding at hospital discharge (Bramson et al., 2010).

C. The feeding position used influences whether the baby's reflexes make early breastfeeding easier or act as barriers to breastfeeding.

1. During the early weeks in upright or side-lying breastfeeding positions, gravity pulls baby's body away from mother and baby's reflexes, such as arm and leg cycling, can act as barriers to breastfeeding (Colson, 2010).

2. Research indicates that during the early weeks human newborns might feed best in ventral positions (**Figure 31-1**) because in these positions gravity works in harmony with babies' reflexes (Colson et al., 2008).

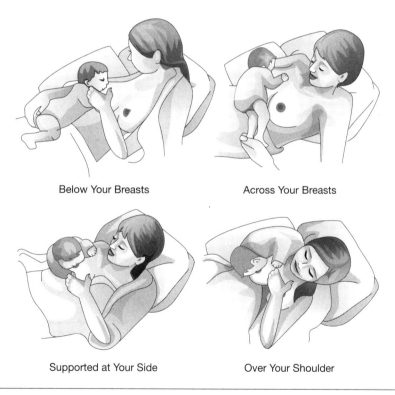

Below Your Breasts   Across Your Breasts

Supported at Your Side   Over Your Shoulder

Figure 31-1 Examples of ventral positions

Source: © Nancy Mohrbacher, IBCLC, FILCA; www.NancyMohrbacher.com

3. Babies' reflexes are hardy and long lasting and can be released for months and possibly years after birth to help transition babies to the breast or overcome breastfeeding problems (Smilie, 2008).

4. When mothers breastfeed in semireclined, "laidback" breastfeeding positions, they have one or both hands free and research has found that during spontaneous interactions with their babies many mothers instinctively trigger the right reflexes in their babies at the right time (Colson et al., 2008).

II. Mammalian Biology and Cultural Anthropology Indicate That Continuous Contact and Frequent Feedings Are Normative for Human Babies

A. Mammalian species fall into four broad categories, with maturity at birth and milk composition (especially fat and protein content) determining biologically normal feeding frequency (Kirsten et al., 2001).

1. Cache mammals (such as deer, seals, and rabbits) are born most mature; mothers can leave their newborns for 12 or more hours before returning to feed because their milks have the highest fat and protein content.

2. Follow mammals (such as giraffes and cows) are less mature at birth; newborns follow the mothers to feed at shorter intervals because their milks have a lower fat and protein content than the milks of cache mammals.

3. Nest mammals (such as dogs and cats) are still less mature at birth; mothers return to their litter to feed more often because their milks have lower fat and protein content than follow mammals' milks.

4. Carry mammals (such as marsupials, primates, and humans) are the least mature at birth; the young maintain continuous contact with the mother's body throughout infancy and feed around the clock because their mothers' milks have the lowest fat and protein content (human milk is among the lowest in this category of mammal).

B. In hunter-gatherer societies, which comprise more than 99% of human existence, mothers breastfeed their babies several times each hour around the clock for the first several years of life, indicating that frequent, round-the-clock feedings is likely the human norm (Stuart-Macadam, 1995).

III. Growth Curves for Breastfed Babies Differ from Babies Fed Nonhuman Milks

A. In 2006, the World Health Organization (WHO) published its child growth standards based on primary growth data from 8,500 children from six ethnically and culturally diverse countries, using breastfed children as the normative model for growth and development (WHO Multicentre Growth Reference Study Group, 2006b).

1. Previous growth charts did not control for differences in feeding method and provided a basis for comparison only.

2. The current standards set international benchmarks and serve as guidelines for how all children should grow.

3. Mothers who participated in the study that led to these standards breastfed optimally, did not smoke, and added healthy complementary foods to their baby's diet between 4 and 6 months, the recommended age at the time of the study.

B. Breastfed babies are leaner than babies fed nonhuman milks from 4 to 12 months, and boys gain weight slightly faster than girls do (**Figures 31-2** and **31-3**).

   1. Using the 2006 growth standards, more children will be considered overweight than with previous charts.

   2. In comparison to the previous growth references, when the 2006 growth standards are used, from birth to 6 months more children will be considered underweight, and from 6 to 12 months fewer children will be considered underweight.

C. Growth in length varies by sex, with boys growing slightly faster than girls do (**Figures 31-4** and **31-5**), and occurs in spurts rather than continuously (Lampl et al., 1992).

D. Included in these data are internationally valid windows of achievement for gross motor milestones (**Figure 31-6**).

IV. Breastfeeding Patterns During Infancy Vary by Cultural Expectations, Infant Stomach Size, Mother's Breast Storage Capacity, and Time of Day

A. Cultural expectations influence breastfeeding patterns.

   1. In some traditional cultures, babies breastfeed intensely—as often as several times each hour—day and night for 3 to 4 years (Stuart-Macadam, 1995).

      a. In these cultures, mothers keep their babies against their bodies as they work, and babies have ready access to the breast at all times.

      b. Intense breastfeeding is considered normal and desirable.

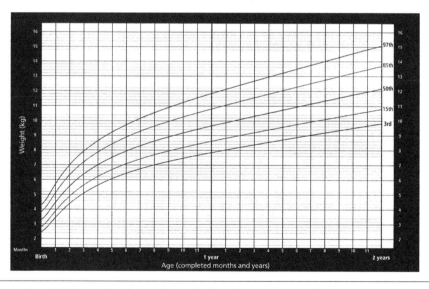

Figure 31-2 WHO weight-for-age boys, birth to 2 years (percentiles)

Source: WHO Multicentre Growth Reference Study Group. (2006b). WHO child growth standards. Geneva, Switzerland: World Health Organization.. Web site: http://www.who.int/childgrowth/en.

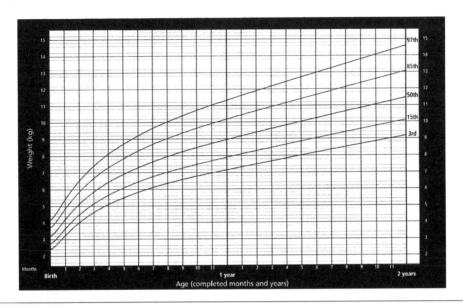

Figure 31-3 WHO weight-for-age girls, birth to 2 years (percentiles)

Source: WHO Multicentre Growth Reference Study Group. (2006b). WHO child growth standards. Geneva, Switzerland: World Health Organization.

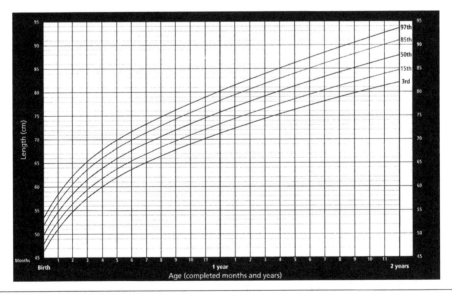

Figure 31-4 WHO length-for-age boys, birth to 2 years (percentiles)

Source: WHO Multicentre Growth Reference Study Group. (2006b). WHO child growth standards. Geneva, Switzerland: World Health Organization.

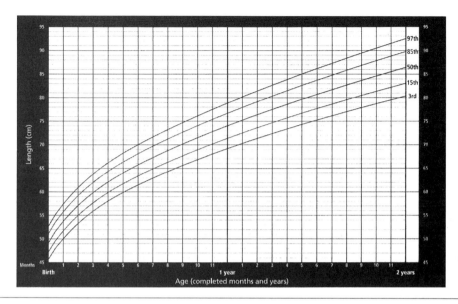

Figure 31-5 WHO length-for-age girls, birth to 2 years (percentiles)

Source: WHO Multicentre Growth Reference Study Group. (2006b). WHO child growth standards. Geneva, Switzerland: World Health Organization.

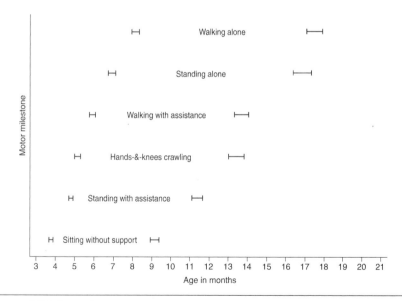

Figure 31-6 WHO windows of achievement for six gross milestones.

Source: WHO Multicentre Growth Reference Study Group. (2006b). WHO child growth standards. Geneva, Switzerland: World Health Organization. Web site: http://www.who.int/childgrowth/en.

2. In many Western cultures, mothers are expected to regulate breastfeeding by the clock.
    a. Mothers are told to encourage babies—even newborns—to breastfeed at set intervals of no less than 2 to 3 hours.
    b. The use of breast substitutes, such as pacifiers/dummies and bottles, is common and encouraged.
    c. Separation of mothers and babies is considered normal and desirable, and mothers are encouraged to schedule time away from their babies.
    d. Work is usually distinct from home life, and most mothers leave their babies with a caregiver to do their work in another location.
    e. Many babies are expected to self-soothe, sleep alone, and be weaned within the first year.
B. A baby's age and stomach size determine in part how much milk is taken at each feeding, which affects how many times per day a baby needs to breastfeed to thrive.
    1. A breastfed baby's daily milk consumption varies by age until about 1 month (Butte et al., 2002).
        a. On the first day, on average a breastfed baby consumes about 30 mL/day.
        b. At about 1 week, average intake has increased to about 300 to 450 mL/day.
        c. By about 1 month, a breastfed baby consumes about 750 to 1,050 mL/day.
        d. Daily milk intake stays relatively stable from 1 to 6 months.
        e. When solid foods are introduced at around 6 months, the volume of mother's milk consumed decreases because solid food replaces some milk in a baby's diet (Islam et al., 2006).
    2. During the first day of life, a newborn's stomach does not expand as it does later (Zangen et al., 2001); its capacity increases during the first month of life and by 1 month, a breastfed baby averages 60 to 120 mL per feeding (Kent et al., 2006). Common hospital practices encourage overfeeding of all newborns, both breast-fed and formula fed, because of misconceptions about physiologically appropriate volume of intake in the first few days of life. The average reported intakes of healthy breastfed newborns are (Academy of Breastfeeding Medicine [ABM] Protocol Committee, 2009):
        a. During the first 24 hours, average intake per feeding is 2–10 mL.
        b. From 24–48 hours, average intake per feeding is 5–15 mL.
        c. From 48–72 hours, average intake per feeding is 15–30 mL.
        d. By 72–96 hours, average intake per feeding is 30–60 mL.
C. Mother's breast storage capacity (the maximum volume of milk consumed by the baby at a feeding over the course of a day) affects the amount of milk a baby has access to at a feeding (Kent, 2007).
    1. Mothers with a large breast storage capacity have more milk available at each feeding, which in some cultures can have a profound effect on breastfeeding patterns.
        a. The baby might always be satisfied with one breast per feeding.
        b. The baby might feed fewer times per day than average but gain weight at an average or above-average rate.

      c. The baby might feed less often at night at an earlier age than an average baby.

    2. Mothers with a small breast storage capacity can produce plenty of milk overall, but their babies can have a very different breastfeeding pattern.

      a. The baby might need to breastfeed more times per day to get the same amount of milk.

      b. The baby might always want both breasts at a feeding.

      c. The baby might need to feed often at night throughout infancy and beyond.

  D. Time of day also can influence breastfeeding patterns, especially in Western cultures where babies are expected to feed at regular intervals.

    1. It is common for babies in Western cultures to breastfeed less often during morning hours.

    2. It is common for babies in Western cultures to breastfeed more often or even continuously during the evening.

V. As Babies Grow and Mature, Breastfeeding Behaviors Change

  A. Irrespective of cultural expectations, babies tend to breastfeed long and often during the first 40 days postpartum.

    1. Newborns in Western cultures breastfeed on average 20 to 40 minutes per feeding, with their feeding times tending to shorten with practice and maturity.

    2. During the first 6 weeks or so, many babies breastfeed at least 8 to 12 times per day and "cluster" their feedings together, especially during the evening.

  B. After 6 weeks, many babies in Western cultures spend less time breastfeeding (Mohrbacher, 2010).

    1. Feeding length tends to shorten from about 20 to 40 minutes on average during the newborn period to about 15 to 20 minutes later.

    2. If mother's breast storage capacity allows, number of feedings may decrease as a baby's stomach size increases and he or she can hold more milk (WHO Multicentre Growth Reference Study Group, 2006a).

  C. Babies might return to intense breastfeeding to adjust their mothers' milk production as needed, which is sometimes referred to as growth spurts that often occur around 2 to 3 weeks, 6 weeks, and again at 3 months.

  D. Beginning at around 3 months, babies who were previously content to breastfeed without interruption now become easily distracted from the breast by activities going on around them (Mohrbacher, 2010).

    1. Mothers are sometimes concerned about this change in breastfeeding and worry about whether their babies are getting enough milk (Rempel, 2004).

      a. During this developmental phase, many babies breastfeed longer and drain the breast more fully at night.

      b. If a mother wants to encourage more consistent breastfeeding during the day, she can try breastfeeding in a darkened room with fewer distractions. Usually babies outgrow this distractible phase, so this is a temporary situation.

    c. If a mother has other children, avoiding distractions during the day can be difficult.
  2. Even with distractions during breastfeeding, as long as a mother allows baby ready access to the breast, a baby can get the milk needed by breastfeeding more often or longer at other times.
E. As babies begin to teethe and teeth appear, they might bear down on the breast during feedings to help relieve gum soreness, causing nipple pain or trauma.
  1. To prevent this, suggest the mother give her baby something cold to chew on to numb the gums before breastfeeding, such as a cold wet cloth.
  2. If the baby is taking other foods, the mother might choose to provide cold or frozen foods before breastfeeding.
F. As a baby learns to crawl and then walk, he or she can become even more distracted during breastfeeding, especially during daylight hours, and might begin to take more milk at night.

VI. A Minimum of 1 Year (American Academy of Pediatrics [AAP] Work Group on Breastfeeding, 2012) to 2 Years or More (WHO, 2001) of Breastfeeding Is Recommended, with Solid Foods Added at About 6 Months of Age

A. Exclusive breastfeeding is recommended for the first 6 months of life (Kramer et al., 2002; WHO, 2001)
B. Recommendations for minimum duration of breastfeeding are based on a large body of research linking shorter duration of breastfeeding to increased incidence for the child of many health problems later in life, including obesity, diabetes, childhood cancers, allergies, inflammatory bowel diseases, and others (AAP Work Group on Breastfeeding, 2005; Ip et al., 2007).
C. Women who do not breastfeed or who breastfeed for shorter durations are at increased risk for breast cancer, ovarian cancer, type 2 diabetes, and other health problems (AAP Work Group on Breastfeeding, 2005; Ip et al., 2007).

VII. When Weaning Age Is Considered Independent of Culture, the Human Norm Has Been Calculated at Between 2.5 and 7 Years (Dettwyler, 1995; Figure 31-7)

A. Weaning before age 3 years is associated with a greater incidence of morbidity and mortality (Molbak et al., 1994).
B. Breastfeeding is the natural outlet for a child's sucking urge until this urge is outgrown.
  1. In some cultures, this desire to suck is satisfied with breast substitutes, such as pacifiers/dummies or bottles.
  2. No breastfeeding and early weaning are associated with an increased incidence of oral malformations (Carrascoza et al., 2006; Kobayashi et al., 2010).
C. No matter what the child's age, the sucking and skin-to-skin of breastfeeding release oxytocin in mother and child (Uvnäs-Moberg, 2003), which is associated with:
  1. Enhanced maternal–infant attachment
  2. Easier transition to sleep for both mother and child
  3. Greater calm during times of crisis or upset

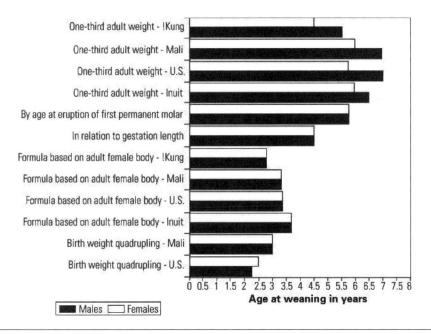

Figure 31-7 Natural age at weaning according to technique used.

Source: Dettwyler, K. (1995). A time to wean: The hominid blueprint for the natural age of weaning in modern human populations. In P. Stuart-Macadam & K. Dettwyler (Eds.), *Breastfeeding: Biocultural perspectives* (pp. 39-73). New York: Aldine de Gruyter.

VIII. Clinical Breastfeeding Challenges from 6 to 12 Months and Beyond

A. Candidiasis and mastitis (breast inflammation sometimes referred to as plugged ducts or breast infections) can occur any time during the course of breastfeeding.

B. Some situations are unique to the mother of an older breastfeeding baby and child.

   1. Return of menstruation

      a. For most women who exclusively breastfeed for the first 6 months, add solid foods gradually, and continue to breastfeed at night, menstruation is delayed, often for as long as 1 to 2 years (Labbok, 2007).

      b. Some mothers report that right before their menstrual cycle or during its first day or two their babies are reluctant to breastfeed or refuse the breast.

      c. Some women report slowing milk production around their menstrual cycle, with production increasing after a day or two of frequent breastfeeding.

      d. Some women feel nipple pain or tenderness during their menstrual cycle each month.

   2. New pregnancy

      a. Research indicates that 74% of breastfeeding women experience nipple pain during pregnancy (Mead et al., 1967).

      b. Mature milk reverts to colostrum at about 4 to 5 months of pregnancy.

    c. Abrupt weaning by the baby or child is possible during pregnancy, as is the desire to continue breastfeeding.

    d. Some children wean during the pregnancy but resume breastfeeding after the birth of the baby.

  3. Nursing strikes (Mohrbacher, 2010)

    a. Sudden refusal to breastfeed can occur after a period of uneventful breastfeeding.

    b. Common causes include otitis media, nasal congestion, unusual separation of mother and baby, a negative emotional encounter (often associated with a bite), frequent use of bottles and/or pacifiers, low milk production; sometimes the cause is unknown.

    c. This problem is almost always temporary and can be resolved with frequent skin-to-skin contact without pressure to breastfeed, attempting breastfeeding while baby is asleep or half asleep, and elimination of artificial nipples.

    d. Illness should always be ruled out as a cause.

    e. Mothers can feel this as a personal rejection.

    f. Suggest the mother express her milk as often as her baby was breastfeeding to preserve her milk production until the baby accepts the breast again and offer the expressed milk to the baby in a cup.

IX. The Lactation Consultant Should Be Prepared to Offer Help to a Family Who Chooses to Wean Before the Child Is Developmentally Ready

  A. Examine own beliefs regarding appropriate age of weaning.

  B. Assist the family in viewing breastfeeding within the context of the child's normal development.

  C. Discuss their feelings and reasons for wanting to wean.

    1. In cultures or families where breastfeeding an older baby or child is viewed with disapproval, social pressure can influence parents' decision to wean.

    2. If their goals for weaning are unlikely to be met (that is, the child will become more independent or start sleeping more at night), be sure to inform them that weaning might not accomplish the goals.

    3. Depending on the reason for weaning (that is, the mother feels "touched out"), it can be appropriate to suggest a partial rather than a full weaning.

    4. If a medical issue is involved, encourage the parents to get a second opinion.

  D. Provide specific strategies for gradual weaning that are consistent with the age of the child and the parents' cultural beliefs.

    1. If possible, abrupt or sudden weaning should be avoided because it increases the mother's risk of severe pain and mastitis.

    2. When weaning a baby younger than 12 months, discuss weaning issues specific to this age range.

      a. An appropriate substitute for human milk needs to be chosen, which should be done in consultation with the baby's healthcare provider.

b. Discuss feeding method; in countries where bottles are not safe, a young baby might need to be fed the substitute milk by cup or spoon.

c. Babies older than 6 to 8 months might be able to take all their liquid from a cup.

d. To allow her milk production to slow gradually and comfortably, suggest the mother substitute one daily breastfeeding with a feeding of the substitute milk and then wait 2 to 3 days before eliminating another breastfeeding, repeating this process until the mother has weaned from all feedings at the breast.

e. If at any time during weaning a mother's breasts feel uncomfortably full, suggest she express just enough milk to make herself comfortable, which will prevent pain and decrease risk of mastitis.

3. When weaning a baby older than 12 months, discuss issues specific to the older child (Mohrbacher, 2010).

a. A child needs more food to offset the loss of human milk in the diet, but these can be foods from the family table.

b. For weaning to be a positive transition, explain that the older baby or child considers breastfeeding more than just a feeding method; it also provides closeness, comfort, and mother's attention.

c. There are many time-tested strategies for helping the older baby or child make this a gentle transition (Mohrbacher et al., 2010).

    i. Don't offer the breast, but don't refuse if the child asks.

    ii. Change daily routines so that the child asks to breastfeed less, which (depending on the child) might mean getting away from home more or staying home more.

    iii. Have the mother's partner take a more active role by getting up with the child at night and getting up with the child and providing breakfast in the morning.

    iv. Offer other foods and drinks before the child usually asks to breastfeed to decrease hunger and thirst.

    v. Avoid the place where breastfeeding usually occurs.

    vi. Breastfeed when asked, but for a shorter time than usual.

    vii. Postpone breastfeeding.

    viii. Bargaining can sometimes be used with an older child, but only with a child old enough to understand the meaning of a promise.

d. Encourage the family to use those strategies that work well for their child and avoid those that don't.

References

Academy of Breastfeeding Medicine Protocol Committee. (2009). ABM clinical protocol no. 3: Hospital guidelines for the use of supplementary feedings in the healthy term breastfed neonate, revised 2009. *Breastfeeding Medicine, 4*(3), 175–182.

American Academy of Pediatrics Work Group on Breastfeeding. (2012). Breastfeeding and the use of human milk. *Pediatrics, 29*(8), e827–e841.

Bergman, N. (2008). Breastfeeding and perinatal neuroscience. In C. W. Genna (Ed.), *Supporting sucking skills in breastfeeding infants* (pp. 43–56). Sudbury, MA: Jones and Bartlett.

Bramson, L., Lee, J. W., Moore, E., Montgomery, S. Neish, C., Bahjri, K., & Melcher, C. L. (2010). Effect of early skin-to-skin mother-infant contact during the first 3 hours following birth on exclusive breastfeeding during the maternity hospital stay. *Journal of Human Lactation, 26,* 130–137.

Butte, N. F., Lopez-Alarcon, M. G., & Garza, C. (2002). *Nutrient adequacy of exclusive breastfeeding for the term infant during the first six months of life.* Geneva, Switzerland: World Health Organization. Retrieved from http://whqlibdoc.who.int/publications/9241562110.pdf

Carrascoza, K. C., Possobon R. de F., Tomita, L. M., & Moraes, A. B. (2006). Consequences of bottle-feeding to the oral facial development of initially breastfed children. *Jornal de Pediatria, 82*(5), 395–397.

Christensson, K., Cabrera, T., Christensson, E., Uvnas-Moberg, K., & Winberg, J. (1995). Separation distress call in the human neonate in the absence of maternal body contact. *Acta Paediatrica, 84*(5), 468–473.

Christensson, K., Siles, C., Moreno, L., Belaustequi, A., De La Fuenta, P., Lagercrantz, H., Puyol, P., & Winberg, J. (1992). Temperature, metabolic adaptation and crying in healthy full term newborns cared for skin to skin or in a cot. *Acta Paediatrica, 81*(6–7), 488–493.

Colson, S. (2010). *An introduction to biological nurturing: New angles on breastfeeding.* Amarillo, TX: Hale Publishing.

Colson, S. D., Meek, J. H., & Hawdon, J. (2008). Optimal positions for the release of primitive neonatal reflexes stimulating breastfeeding. *Early Human Development, 84*(7), 441–449.

Dettwyler, K. (1995). A time to wean: The hominid blueprint for the natural age of weaning in modern human populations. In P. Stuart-Macadam & K. Dettwyler (Eds.), *Breastfeeding: Biocultural perspectives* (pp. 39–73). New York, NY: Aldine de Gruyter.

Ip, S., Chung, M., Raman, G., Chew, P., Magula, N., DeVine, D., Trikalinos, T., & Laur, J. (2007). *Breastfeeding and maternal and infant health outcomes in developed countries* (Evidence Reports/ Technology Assessments, No. 153, Report 07-E007). Rockville, MD: Agency for Healthcare and Research Quality.

Islam, M. M., Peerson, J. M., Ahmed, T., Dewey, K. G., & Brown, K. H. (2006). Effects of varied energy density of complementary foods on breast-milk intakes and total energy consumption by healthy, breastfed Bangladeshi children. *American Journal of Clinical Nutrition, 83*(4), 851–858.

Kent, J., Mitoulas, L., Cregan, M., Ramsay, D., Doherty, D., & Hartmann, P. E. (2006). Volume and frequency of breastfeedings and fat content of breast milk throughout the day. *Pediatrics, 117,* 387–395.

Kent, J. C. (2007). How breastfeeding works. *Journal of Midwifery and Women's Health, 52*(6), 564–570.

Kirsten, G. F., Bergman, N. J., & Hann, F. M. (2001). Kangaroo mother care in the nursery. *Pediatric Clinics of North America, 48*(2), 443–452.

Kobayashi, H. M., Scavone, H., Jr., Ferreira, R. I., & Garib, D. G. (2010). Relationship between breastfeeding duration and prevalence of posterior crossbite in the deciduous dentition. *American Journal of Orthodontics and Dentofacial Orthopedics, 137*(1), 54–58.

Kramer, M. S., & Kakuma, R. (2002). Optimal duration of exclusive breastfeeding. *Cochrane Database of Systematic Reviews, 1,* CD003517. doi:10.1002/14651858.CD003517

Labbok, M. (2007). Breastfeeding, birth spacing, and family planning. In T. Hale & P. E. Hartmann (Eds.), *Hale & Hartmann's textbook of human lactation* (pp. 305–318). Amarillo, TX: Hale Publishing.

Lampl, M., Velduis, J., & Johnson, M. (1992). Saltation and stasis: A model of human growth. *Science, 258,* 801–803.

Matthieson, A., Ransjo-Arvidson, A., Nissen, E., & Uvnäs-Moberg, K. (2001). Postpartum maternal oxytocin release by newborns: Effects of infant hand massage and sucking. *Birth, 28,* 13–19.

Mead, M., & Newton, N. (1967). Cultural patterning of perinatal behavior. In S. Richardson & A. Guttmacher (Eds.), *Childbearing: Its social and psychological aspects* (pp. 142–242). Baltimore, MD: Williams & Wilkins.

Mohrbacher, N. (2010). *Breastfeeding answers made simple: A guide for helping mothers.* Amarillo, TX: Hale Publishing.

Mohrbacher, N., & Kendall-Tackett, K. (2010). *Breastfeeding made simple: Seven natural laws for nursing mothers* (2nd ed.). Oakland, CA: New Harbinger Publications.

Molbak, K., Gottschau A., Aaby P., Hojlyng, L., Ingholt, N., & Da Silva, A. P. (1994). Prolonged breastfeeding, diarrhoeal disease, and survival of children in Guinea-Bissau. *British Medical Journal, 308,* 1403–1406.

Newton, N., & Theotokatos, M. (1979). Breastfeeding during pregnancy in 503 women: Does a psychobiological weaning mechanism exist in humans? *Emotion and Reproduction, 20B,* 845–849.

Rempel, L. A. (2004). Factors influencing the breastfeeding decisions of long-term breastfeeders. *Journal of Human Lactation, 20*(3), 306–318.

Righard, L., & Alade, M. (1990). Effects of delivery room routines on success of first breast-feed. *Lancet, 336,* 1105–1107.

Smilie, C. (2008). How babies learn to feed: A neurobehavioral model. In C. W. Genna (Ed.), *Supporting sucking skills in breastfeeding infants* (pp. 79–95). Sudbury, MA: Jones and Bartlett.

Stuart-Macadam, P. (1995). Breastfeeding in prehistory. In P. Stuart-Macadam & K. Dettwyler (Eds.), *Breastfeeding: Biocultural perspectives* (pp. 75–99). New York, NY: Aldine de Gruyter.

Uvnäs-Moberg, K. (2003). *The oxytocin factor: Tapping the hormone of calm, love, and healing.* Cambridge, MA: De Capo Press.

Widstrom, A.-M., Lilja, G., Aaltomaa-Michalia, P., Dahllof, A., & Nissen, E. (2011). Newborn behavior to locate the breast when skin-to-skin: A possible method for enabling early self-regulation. *Acta Pediatrica, 100,* 79–85.

Wiklund, I., Norman, M., Uvnas-Moberg, K., Ransjo-Arvidson, A. B., & Andolf, E. (2009). Epidural anesthesia: Breast-feeding success and related factors. *Midwifery, 25,* e31–e38.

World Health Organization. (2001). *The optimal duration of exclusive breastfeeding: Report of an expert consultation.* Geneva, Switzerland: Author.

World Health Organization Multicentre Growth Reference Study Group. (2006a). Breastfeeding in the WHO Multicentre Growth Reference Study. *Acta Paediatrica, 95*(Suppl. 450), 16–26.

World Health Organization Multicentre Growth Reference Study Group. (2006b). *The WHO child growth standards.* Geneva, Switzerland: Author. Retrieved from http://www.who.int/childgrowth/en/

Zangen, S., Di Lorenzo, C., Zangen, T., Mertz, H., Schwankovsky, L., & Hyman, P. E. (2001). Rapid maturation of gastric relaxation in newborn infants. *Pediatric Research, 50,* 629–632.

CHAPTER 32
Breastfeeding Mothers with Disabilities

Noreen Siebenaler, MSN, RN, IBCLC, and Judi Rogers, OTR/L

OBJECTIVES

- List five maternal disabilities that can create barriers to successful breastfeeding.
- State two methods of assisting or adaptations that are most appropriate for each disability.
- Discuss four reasons why women with physical, sight, or hearing disabilities often find breastfeeding easier than bottle-feeding.
- List three community services for breastfeeding mothers with physical, sight, or hearing disabilities.

INTRODUCTION

As increasing numbers of women with physical and sensory disabilities are choosing to become mothers lactation consultants will need to learn how to work effectively with mothers who have a variety of needs surrounding disabilities. Many professionals have not seen anyone with a disability take care of and breastfeed a baby, and it can be difficult to imagine how they might manage. Some mothers with disabilities have been able to breastfeed successfully as well as take care of their babies even without proper equipment support. Having appropriate equipment and support can make breastfeeding and baby care more successful.

Additionally, people with and without physical disabilities can have learning difficulties. When working with a mother with a disability who seems to have difficulty grasping information, try to give small pieces of information separately and check for understanding before giving more information. A small percentage of people with cerebral palsy (CP) have some learning difficulties; however, do not confuse people who have speech involvement with people who have learning difficulties. People with CP and multiple sclerosis (MS) who have speech involvement have their tongue and mouth muscles affected by their disability. MS is another disability that can cause some learning difficulties such as short-term memory loss or slowed processing of information.

A part of developing skills as a professional is to expand the perception you have of breastfeeding women to include women with disabilities. When working with mothers

(continues)

who have disabilities, it is important to remember that they are no different from other mothers who want to breastfeed. Be respectful when asking questions; explain exactly what you need to know and why.

Women with disabilities who want to breastfeed do not always have support from their families and friends. Family members may think breastfeeding will drain the mother of her limited energy or that it will be too physically demanding. One mother, with a neuromuscular disability, explaining why breastfeeding was so important to her, said, "This is the only thing I can do for my baby that no one else can do" (Rogers, 2005).

In general, it is rare for medical researchers to include people with disabilities in their studies. If a study concerns a congenital disability, it is not replicated. Most studies involve MS or arthritis, and more research is needed.

Medication needs to be evaluated for safety while a mother is breastfeeding because many women are prescribed medication to manage their disabilities. The main authority for medications in lactation is Dr. Thomas Hale. Lactation consultants can contact his Infant Risk Center at 1-806-352-2519. Another resource is Lawrence and Lawrence Lactation Study Center in Rochester, New York, at 1-585- 275-0088.

The Organization of Teratology Information Specialists (OTIS) is a nonprofit organization made up of individual teratology information services located throughout the United States and Canada. The goal is the elimination of preventable birth defects through the promotion of healthy pregnancies. Contact information is 1-866-626-6847 and www.otispregnancy.org.

The following are general guidelines for lactation consultants to use in practice:

1. Women who have been physically disabled for a long time are usually very knowledgeable about their abilities and limitations. Involve them in decision making. Ask for their opinions (Mohrbacher et al., 2007).

2. Help mothers find comfortable feeding positions, such as laidback or reclined, and use supportive breastfeeding pillows as appropriate.

3. Assist the mother in locating other types of supportive equipment such as adaptable pumps and bras that make breastfeeding easier.

4. Use creativity in problem solving, involve supportive family members, promote coordination of services that enhance the mother's abilities, and locate appropriate community and internet resources.

5. This might be the first time the mother has handled a baby.

I. Repetitive Stress Disorders

A. Carpal tunnel syndrome

1. Etiology and symptoms

a. A painful disorder of the wrist and hand where the median nerve is compressed, causing part of the wrist and hand to have parasthesia (numbness, tingling, and weakness).

       b. Swelling from irritated tendons narrows the carpel tunnel and causes the median nerve to be compressed.

       c. More common in women, especially during pregnancy.

       d. During pregnancy, the hormone relaxin loosens connections between tendons, which can result in pressure on the median nerve.

       e. Compression of the median nerve causes weakness, pain with opposition of the thumb as well as burning, tingling, or aching that radiates to the forearm and shoulder joint. Pain is intermittent or constant and often is most intense at night.

  2. Diagnosis

       a. By physical exam, electromyography (EMG), and magnetic resonance imaging (MRI)

  3. Treatment

       a. A splint can help diminish the pain.

       b. See the section on treatment for De Quervain's tendonitis, which follows.

B. De Quervain's tendonitis

  1. Etiology and symptoms

       a. Also called new mother's tendonitis. Pain and inflammation are caused by an irritation of two tendons at a point where they run through a very tight channel on the thumb side of the wrist.

       b. The irritation at the base of the thumb can cause difficulty in turning the wrist and gripping.

       c. Repetitive stress disorder may be present as a work-related injury prior to childbirth.

       d. "Aggravated by radial and ulnar deviation activity. It is important to cease aggravating activity. In the mother's case alternate lifting and breast-feeding holding positions need to be adopted. The breastfeeding mother is more susceptible to aggravation of the condition due to hormonal effects on soft tissues" (Connolly et al., 2003).

       e. Maintaining the wrist in a flexed position after latching can cause this tendonitis.

  2. Diagnosis

       a. To diagnose de Quervain's doctors often confirm the following:

          i. Tenderness when pressure is applied on the thumb side of the wrist.

         ii. Positive results on a Finkelstein test. The Finkelstein test consists of the patient bending the thumb across the palm and bending the fingers down over the thumb. Then, the patient bends the wrist toward the little finger. If this causes pain on the thumb side of the wrist, the test is considered positive.

  3. Treatment (carpal tunnel and De Quervain's tendonitis)

       a. Anti-inflammatory medications, oral analgesics, ice or cool packs to relieve symptoms. Most anti-inflammatory medications are compatible with breastfeeding.

      b. Steroids are commonly given.

      c. Wrist splint can minimize pressure on the nerves; keeps the wrist straight at night to minimize pain; also forearm splint for carpal tunnel.

      d. Change repetitive work activities, resting affected area for 2 weeks if possible.

      e. Physical therapy exercise and ultrasound over affected areas to strengthen and reduce swelling.

      f. Surgical intervention is occasionally needed to relieve symptoms.

C. Thoracic outlet syndrome (TOS)

    1. Etiology and symptoms

      a. A group of distinct disorders that result in compressions of nerves and blood vessels in the brachial plexus, a network of nerves that extends from the base of the neck to the axilla and conducts signals from the shoulder, arm, and hand.

      b. Many physical and occupational therapists believe TOS is caused by injury to the nerves in the brachial plexus.

      c. The main symptom of this disorder is pain. Shoulder and elbow pain can radiate to the little finger and ring finger.

      d. Abnormal burning or prickling sensations may be felt in the arms or hands.

      e. TOS is often caused by repetitive activities or by a hyperextension injury.

    2. Diagnosed by physical exam, EMG, and MRI

    3. Treatment

      a. Physical therapy:

        i. Can strengthen surrounding muscles of the shoulder

        ii. Can stretch muscles in the arm and shoulder as well as the scalenes in the neck

      b. Postural exercises help with standing and sitting straighter, which reduces pressure on nerves and blood vessels, relieving pain.

      c. Ergonomic assessment of work environment to avoid strenuous activities.

      d. Anti-inflammatory medications and oral analgesics, most of which are compatible with breastfeeding.

D. Possible effect on breastfeeding of repetitive stress disorders

    1. Difficulties with picking up the baby, positioning baby, moving the baby at the breast or between breasts, and burping the baby because of pain that affects wrist and hand movements

    2. Limited ability to use two hands to assist baby with latch-on

    3. Reduced finger dexterity to open and close bra

E. Methods of assisting

    1. Use firm breastfeeding pillows that go around mother's waist and bring baby up to breast level, thus keeping the baby's weight off mother's arms, wrists, and hands.

    2. Use football or clutch positions using pillows to hold baby so that mother does not have to use arms, wrists, and hands when breastfeeding.

    3. Breastfeed one breast per feeding.

    4. Latch on using one hand and without bending wrists (**Figure 32-1**).

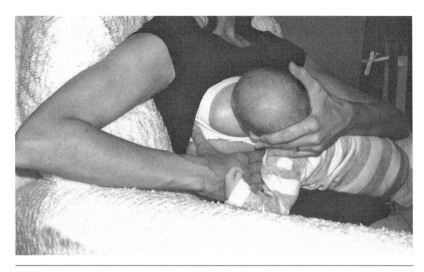

Figure 32-1 Latch on without bending wrists.

5. Roll a small towel for under breast to eliminate a need for hand support.
6. Mothers with TOS often find a side-lying position too painful because of compression of thoracic nerves. A 45° supine position, also called laidback breastfeeding, might be the most effective and least painful for nighttime feedings. (See Chapter 28: Guidelines for Facilitating and Assessing Breastfeeding for information on positions.)
7. Slings can make breastfeeding easier for mothers with carpal tunnel and tendonitis because babies can breastfeed in slings with less wrist and hand movement.
8. Women with TOS will have increasing pain and related symptoms if they use small electric breast pumps that vibrate. Some small electric pump designs have proven to be easier for mothers with arm or hand pain. Hospital-grade automatic cycling pumps or other higher level nonvibrating pumps are most appropriate.
9. Hands-free pumping bras and devices that hold pump pieces in place during pumping without using hands prevent symptoms of repetitive stress and are available in stores and on Internet sites.
10. Breastfeeding a baby without appropriate aids and techniques can increase pain for women who have repetitive stress disorders such as carpal tunnel, tendonitis, or thoracic outlet syndrome (TOS). Some women with these specific disabilities and situations may find that partial breastfeeding minimizes pain (Carthy et al., 1990).

II. Multiple Sclerosis

A. Etiology and symptoms

   1. MS usually appears between the ages of 20 and 40 years.

      a. It has a variety of symptoms that vary over time.

      b. It may not be diagnosed until years after the first symptoms occur because the symptoms are variable and confusing.

      c. Symptoms of MS can be sensory (visual problems, numbness and/or tingling in hands and feet).

      d. There can be limitations in movement to one or all four extremities as well as limitations to fine motor skills, speech, and central body movement.

      e. There are four subtypes:
         * *Relapsing-Remitting (RR):* Most common, begins as a series of attacks followed by complete or partial remissions as the symptoms mysteriously lessen, only to return later after a period of stability.
         * *Primary-Progressive (PP):* Characterized by a gradual clinical decline in function, with no distinct remissions. There may be temporary plateaus or minor relief from symptoms.
         * *Secondary-Progressive (SP):* Begins with a relapsing-remitting course followed by a later primary-progressive course.
         * *Progressive-Relapsing (PR):* In rare cases, patients may have a progressive-relapsing (PR) course in which the disease becomes progressively worse, with acute attacks flaring up along the way.
            Primary-progressive, secondary-progressive, and progressive-relapsing are sometimes lumped together and called chronic progressive multiple sclerosis.

   2. Symptoms are caused by demyelinization (reduction of the myelin sheaths covering nerves).

      a. Myelin sheaths help with nerve conduction.

      b. Remission of symptoms results when the glial scar forms over the myelin sheath, repairing the sheath.

   3. Causes of MS are not completely understood. It is an autoimmune disorder in which a person's antibodies attack the myelin sheath covering the nerves.

   4. Depression is often associated with MS.

B. Diagnosis

   1. Physical exam, symptom history, MRI, and spinal tap

      a. A greater than normal amount of protein in cerebrospinal fluid is characteristic of MS.

      b. The diagnosis is difficult to make because many other conditions affect the nervous system and produce similar symptoms.

C. Treatment

   1. Corticosteroids and other medications are used both to treat symptoms such as bladder, bowel, and visual disturbances and to slow the progression.

2. Treatment goals include maintaining mobility and providing adaptations needed during exacerbations.

3. All medications should be evaluated for their passage into breastmilk and any effect they may have on the baby (Hale, 2010).

D. Possible effects on breastfeeding

1. Symptoms of MS are more likely to exacerbate during the postpartum period (Lorenzi et al., 2002).

2. A preliminary study showed an association between increased breastfeeding and decreased postpartum exacerbations (Gulick et al., 2002).

3. Upper extremities can be affected, causing difficulty with picking up, holding, and latching on (see **Figure 32-2**).

4. If the baby breastfeeds easily, a mother may find breastfeeding easier than bottle-feeding (Adelson, 2003).

5. Some mothers may find the first weeks of breastfeeding and motherhood stressful and tiring and may consider partial breastfeeding (Eggum, 2001). Ensure that the mother has adequate social supports to help with stress and fatigue. If the mother chooses to supplement, give appropriate information to the mother.

III. Cerebral Palsy

A. Etiology and symptoms

1. Cerebral palsy (CP) involves damage to the motor area of the brain. Damage may occur prenatally, during birth or the postpartum period, or in infancy/childhood.

2. Limitations involve one to four limbs, trunk, and speech. When one side is affected, it is called hemiplegia; both legs affected is diplegia, three limbs affected is triplegia, four limbs affected is quadriplegia (or tetraplegia).

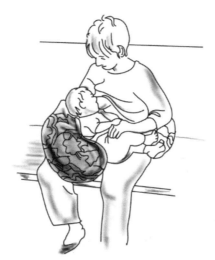

Figure 32-2 Supportive position for mothers with MS.

3. Classifications of cerebral palsy:
   a. Athetoid CP is characterized by involuntary, irregular, slow movements of the affected body part.
   b. Spastic CP is characterized by increased muscle tone that results in the affected limb being stiffly held, making it hard to move the limb.
   c. Ataxic CP is characterized by a wide-based, unsteady gait and often reduced manual dexterity.
   d. Types of CP are distinguished by muscle tone and pattern of movement.
B. Diagnosis
   1. Usually occurs during infancy
   2. Based on symptoms, delays in developmental milestones, and MRI
C. Treatment
   1. Physical therapists and occupational therapists can help with increasing and maintaining ability to function.
   2. All medications should be evaluated for their passage into breastmilk and any effect they may have on the baby (Hale, 2010). "Generally, if the baby is over two months old, the number of medications the mom can take is pretty wide. Very rarely are medications considered incompatible with breastfeeding after a baby turns 2 months" (S. Alvarado, personal communication, June 14, 2011).
D. Possible effects on breastfeeding
   1. Limited upper extremity functioning resulting from hemiplegia, triplegia, or quadriplegia. This results in difficulty with positioning on the less involved or nonaffected side, plus difficulty switching baby from the affected side to the nonaffected side.
   2. Upper extremities can be affected, causing difficulty with picking up or holding the baby as well as latching on and burping.

IV. Spinal Cord Injury

A. Etiology and symptoms
   1. Spinal cord injury (SCI) refers to irreversible damage to the spinal cord caused by trauma or tumor.
      a. The spinal cord is a bundle of nerves inside the vertebral column that carries messages between the brain and the rest of the body.
      b. Nerves from the cord come out at each vertebra, and the vertebral level is where the extent of injury is determined.
      c. Neck vertebrae are C1 to C7; injuries at this level affect all four limbs (quadriplegia).
   2. Injury to the spinal cord usually causes both loss of movement (paralysis) and loss of sensation. There can also be movement with loss of sensation or sensation with loss of movement.
   3. Thoracic vertebrae are located on the upper and mid back.
      a. Vertebrae are numbered T1 to T12. Injury between T1 and T8 causes high paraplegia in which trunk control is affected.

4. Injury to the lumbar-level vertebrae affects leg movement and sensation; injury to the sacral level affects groin, leg, and toe movement.

5. The level of injury determines the level of function lost.

   a. The higher the injury, the more functions are lost.

   b. Breathing is affected if the injury is above C4.

6. An SCI at T6 or above places people at risk for autonomic dysreflexia, a condition caused by noxious or painful stimuli to the sympathetic system that cause increased blood pressure.

   a. A noxious stimulus can include an extended bladder, labor and delivery, nipple pain, or breast pain.

   b. Some symptoms of dysreflexia, such as headaches, sweating, goose bumps, and fluctuations of blood pressure, if unresolved, can result in stroke (Walker, 2009).

B. Diagnosis made by computed tomography (CT) scan, MRI, and myelography

C. Treatment

1. Treatment involves physical therapy and occupational therapy to increase functional abilities (Herman, 2002).

D. Possible effects on breastfeeding

1. A reduction in milk production may be seen as soon as 3 to 5 days after birth and as late as 6 weeks postpartum in a mother with an injury at T4 (Rogers, 2005).

   a. Colostrum does not seem to be affected.

   b. Reduced milk production may be caused by the lack of sensation at the nipples and the decreased sympathetic nervous system feedback to the pituitary, resulting in decreased prolactin secretion (Halbert, 1998; Walker, 2009).

2. In a woman who has an SCI below the T6 level, milk production is not affected (Rogers, 2005).

3. Breastfeeding can create pain causing dysreflexia. Nausea, anxiety, sweating, and goose bumps below the level of the SCI are the first symptoms of dysreflexia.

4. Possible limited ability to hold, position for breastfeeding, lift, or burp the baby.

V. Rheumatoid Arthritis

A. Etiology and symptoms

1. Rheumatoid arthritis (RA) is defined as an inflammatory condition of the joints, characterized by pain and swelling, fatigue, stiffness especially in the morning, pain associated with prolonged sitting, weakness, flu-like symptoms, and muscle pain, including a low-grade fever. A loss of appetite may be present as well as depression, weight loss, anemia, cold and/or sweaty hands and feet (Andersen et al., 2005).

   a. A chronic, destructive, sometimes deforming autoimmune collagen disease most commonly beginning in the joints of the hands and wrists.

   b. Results in a symmetric inflammation of the synovium (fluid surrounding joints) and swelling of joints.

    c. Joint involvement is usually symmetrical, meaning that if a joint hurts on the left hand, the same joint hurts on the right hand.

    d. Effects of RA can vary from person to person. There is growing evidence that RA is not one disease but may be several different diseases with the same symptoms (Brennan et al., 1994).

  2. Exacerbations and remissions are common.

    a. Remission often occurs during pregnancy (Jacobsson et al., 2003).

    b. Exacerbations are likely to occur during the postpartum period.

    c. Karlson showed that women who breastfed for a cumulative total of 13–24 months had a 20% reduction in risk for development of RA and those breastfeeding for at least 24 months during their childbearing years had a total risk reduction of 50% (Karlson et al., 2004).

  3. Stress aggravates RA and increases symptoms.

B. Treatment

  1. In severe pain, intra-articular injections of corticosteroids may give relief.

  2. Patients are advised to avoid situations known to cause anxiety, worry, fatigue, and other stressors.

  3. Treatment includes sufficient rest, exercise to maintain joint function, medications for the relief of pain and to reduce inflammation, orthopedic interventions to prevent deformities, and dietitian-guided weight loss if needed.

  4. Medications used to decrease pain and inflammation are usually compatible with breastfeeding.

    a. Steroids are commonly given.

  5. Hale (2010) recommends expressing and discarding mother's milk for a minimum of 4 days when methotrexate therapy is used.

C. Diagnosis

  1. Lab tests can verify and differentiate between arthritis and other diseases.

D. Possible effects on breastfeeding

  1. Mothers need additional rest resulting from the sometimes overwhelming fatigue, stiffness, and pain that occur postpartum.

VI. Systemic Lupus Erythematosus

A. Etiology and symptoms

  1. Similar to rheumatoid arthritis

  2. Systemic lupus erythematosus (SLE) is an autoimmune disorder that is a systemic disease, affecting many organ systems.

  3. Causes a variety of symptoms and different combinations of symptoms.

  4. Many people experience remissions of symptoms.

  5. Because the symptoms of lupus vary from one person to another, the treatment of the disease is tailored to the specific problems that arise in each person. In many cases, the best approach to treating lupus is with a healthcare team.

  6. The most common problems are pain and swelling in the joints and kidney damage.

7. Other problems include fever, fatigue, weakness, skin rashes, sensitivity to sunlight, headaches, and muscle aches.

8. If the brain is affected, seizures, personality changes, or emotional depression may result.

B. Diagnosis

1. The diagnosis of lupus is based on a combination of physical symptoms and laboratory results. For most people, it is not a one-time diagnosis. Often it is a diagnosis that evolves over time toward more certainty that a person does or does not meet the criteria for a diagnosis of lupus.

C. Treatment

1. There are many categories of drugs for the treatment of lupus. Of all these drugs, only a few are approved specifically for lupus by the Food and Drug Administration (FDA): corticosteroids, including prednisone, prednisolone, methylprednisolone, and hydrocortisone; the antimalarial hydroxychloroquine; and aspirin.

2. Many medications are used to treat the symptoms of lupus.

    a. Most medications are compatible with breastfeeding. Refer to Hale (2010) or the Lactation Study Center for specific drug information.

D. Possible effects on breastfeeding

1. Preeclampsia. About 2 in 10 pregnant women with lupus get preeclampsia.

2. Close to half of women with lupus deliver prematurely.

3. If breastfeeding becomes too demanding physically, the mother may consider partial breastfeeding. Expressing milk to be used later also might help.

4. Worsening of symptoms often affects baby care activities such as diapering.

5. Some women find it hard to readjust to the pain of SLE after delivery.

VII. Myasthenia Gravis

A. Etiology and symptoms

1. Chronic autoimmune disease causing weakness in voluntary muscles throughout the body.

2. Antibodies interfere with messages sent from nerve endings to muscles.

3. There are three types of myasthenia gravis (MG): a hereditary type that may cause the baby to have a weakened suck, a type with ocular involvement, and a third type with generalized involvement.

4. Those with generalized involvement comprise 85–90% of MG patients.

    a. This type also involves voluntary muscles that control movement, eyelids, chewing, swallowing, coughing, and facial expression.

    b. Involuntary muscles that can be affected are those that control eye movement, eyelids, chewing, swallowing, coughing, and facial expressions.

5. There is usually no pain experienced with this form of autoimmune disease.

6. When breathing muscles are affected, myasthenic crisis may occur and respiratory support may be needed. Usually there are progressive warning signs before a crisis, and it is more likely to occur when difficulty with swallowing and talking have been present.

7. Remission of symptoms is common and can last for long periods of time.

B. Diagnosis

   1. Medical history, physical and neurological exam

   2. Assessment for impairment of eye movements or muscle weakness without any changes in ability to feel things

   3. Tests for muscle responsiveness and blood tests for the presence of immune molecules or acetylcholine receptors

   4. Nerve conduction tests:

      a. The most current information can be found on the National Institutes of Health website (see Internet Resources at the end of this text).

C. Treatment

   1. Medications used to treat MG help improve neuromuscular transmission and increase muscle strength. Immunosuppressive drugs may be used to improve muscle strength by suppressing the production of abnormal antibodies.

   2. Thymectomy, surgical removal of the thymus gland, helps reduce symptoms in more than 70% of affected persons and may provide a cure in some cases.

D. Possible effects on breastfeeding

   1. Weakness and fatigue of arm and neck muscles can result in difficulty with positioning and attachment.

   2. Fatigue associated with specific muscle groups increases the need for rest periods.

VIII. Methods of Assisting MD, MS, CP, SCI, RA SLE (Lupus), and MG

A. Women may be unable to hold and position their babies for breastfeeding without proper equipment, even when using biological nurturing positioning techniques. They often have more difficulty breastfeeding outside of their homes because of their possible need for physical support such as having a nursing pillow available.

B. If partial breastfeeding is indicated because of the mother's exacerbations, and/or fatigue/stress, provide information on maintaining adequate milk production (Wade et al., 1999).

C. Trying out different breastfeeding pillows allows a mother to determine which one works best for her.

   1. The pillow should hold the baby at breast level and keep the weight of the baby on the pillow and off the mother's arms.

   2. A pillow that attaches around the waist ensures stability for baby and mother.

D. Increase the mother's knowledge of different breastfeeding positions so that she can find which positions are easiest and most comfortable for her.

E. Encourage and assist the mother to try different positions while lying down. This can help fatigue issues and nighttime feedings.

   1. Lying on the affected side is helpful so that the mother can use her unaffected arm.

   2. A 45° supine position (laidback breastfeeding) also may be helpful for breastfeeding the baby.

   3. When it is difficult to hold a baby, a baby sling might help with holding and positioning the infant for breastfeeding (**Figures 32-3** and **32-4**).

F. Use of a lifting harness, after the baby is a month old, also can help with changing baby's position and burping (see Internet Resources).

G. Breastfeeding on one side per feeding may be easier.

H. Mothers with limited hand and wrist movement can use the latch-on and positioning suggestions listed for repetitive stress disorders.

I. Place a rolled cloth diaper or small cloth towel under the mother's breast so that she does not have to use her hand to hold her breast while feeding.

J. Clothing may need to be adapted to make breastfeeding easier for the mother.

   1. A breastfeeding top or jacket allows easy access and keeps the mother's stiff shoulders warm.

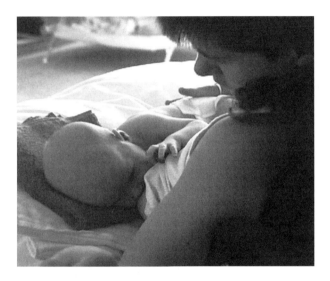

Figure 32-3 A good position for mother and baby.

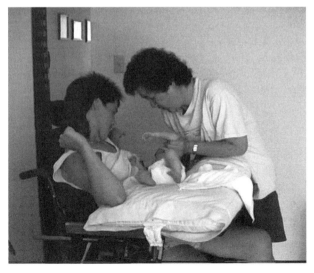

Figure 32-4 Assisting with breastfeeding by attendant.

    2. Holes can be cut in a bra to expose the areola and nipple.

    3. This provides breast support while feeding and helps to position the breast for easier latch-on.

    4. Hands-free pumping bras may vary from extremely effective to minimally effective.

        a. For some women with hand and wrist limitations, this may be the only way they can pump independently or without pain.

  K. Avoid nipple pain by teaching the mother how to position and latch her baby correctly.

  L. Women need to be aware of possible pain associated with breastfeeding, such as the pain of engorgement, mastitis, and nipple pain, so that they can minimize the pain, prevent it, or seek treatment early.

    1. Breastfeeding pain can trigger increased spasticity in women with a variety of disabilities.

  M. Support team:

    1. If the mother has a personal care attendant (PCA), the mother may choose to ask the PCA to help her with breastfeeding.

    2. Family or friends also may help with positioning, latch-on, and burping.

    3. The lactation consultant can show the support team how to assist with positioning and attachment.

  N. Discuss with the mother and determine which baby care activities are most important to her.

    1. Her choice may be determined by her need to conserve energy for the more enjoyable tasks such as feeding and playing with her baby as well as a desire for her spouse or partner to do some of the baby care tasks (Rogers et al., 2004).

  O. Adaptive baby care equipment and advice are available to mothers (see Internet Resources).

  P. Help the mother articulate her needs and what type of help she would like.

    1. It is important to take her family dynamics into consideration.

    2. If there is difficulty in matching the mother's needs with the family's desire to help, recommend a consult with a family therapist.

  Q. Discuss with the mother any adjustments that are necessary to adapt her environment to facilitate breastfeeding, such as breastfeeding in a wheelchair or wheelchair access to the baby's crib (Coates et al., 2010).

IX. Visual Disability

  A. According to 2006 WHO estimates, about 314 million people are visually impaired, 45 million of who are blind. More than 82% of all blind people are 50 years of age or older. (WHO 2007)

    1. Females in every region of the world have significantly higher risk of visual impairment than men, mostly due to longer life expectancy and lack of access to services in poorer societies.

B. The legally blind person has a visual acuity of 20/200 or less meaning he/she will be able to see at 20 feet or less what a fully sighted person can see at 200 feet.(Good Mojab, 1999).

C. Total blindness means a visual acuity of 3/60 or a corresponding visual field loss to less than 10 degrees. (WHO 2007)

D. Blindness or partial sight is most often caused by eye diseases or refractive errors (WHO 2007).

E. Some partially blind individuals see only shadows or have fluctuating vision. They may see better during the day and be totally blind at night or may be very light sensitive.

F. Diagnosis

    1. Diagnosis of visual impairment occurs through an eye exam by an optometrist.

      a. A more thorough visual evaluation by an ophthalmologist follows, which includes a functional vision assessment.

G. Methods of assisting

    1. Breastfeeding may be easier because there are no bottles to prepare and clean.

    2. Ask the mother what she can see because many mothers have partial vision.

    3. Turn visual demonstrations into verbal descriptions.

    4. A football hold allows easy access to the baby's face so that a mother can feel how the baby's jaw is moving during sucking.

    5. A baby sling gives a mother the ability to use both hands for latch by using the index finger (Braille finger) to locate the baby's nose and lips.

    6. Cradle, cross-cradle, or laidback positioning may give better "tummy to tummy" orientation with the baby's body.

    7. Refer to experienced breastfeeding mothers who are partially sighted or blind.

    8. Resources for blind mothers: Braille communications and audiotapes for partially sighted or blind mothers are available from La Leche League International (Martin, 1992).

X. Hearing Loss and/or Deafness

A. Etiology and symptoms

    1. Deafness may result from prenatal exposure to various conditions such as rubella, cytomegalovirus, hereditary conditions, premature birth, congenital conditions, or medical conditions.

B. Diagnosis

    1. Diagnosis of deafness occurs through audiologic screening at a hospital or doctor's office or through newborn hearing screenings.

C. Methods of assisting

    1. Sign language as a communication method to accompany one-to-one breastfeeding assistance for mothers with hearing impairment may be available at the mother's clinic, hospital, or in the community (Bowles, 1991).

a. In the United States, healthcare organizations are required to provide sign language interpreters for patients with hearing impairments (Office of Minority Health, 2007).

2. Deaf mothers communicate in a variety of ways. Ask what they prefer: speaking, writing, signing, or e-mail (Bykowski, 1994).

3. Vibration pagers for deaf mothers have different vibrations for different sounds so that a pager can vibrate a certain way when a baby cries (see Internet Resources).

4. The most effective teaching methods for deaf mothers may be video, written materials, and recommended websites.

5. Telephone systems specifically designed for deaf individuals are easily available for home use. Mothers can use these systems to call lactation consultants when questions or problems arise.

Note: Some of the material in this chapter was developed under Through the Looking Glass funding from the U.S. Department of Education, National Institute on Disability and Rehabilitation Research (#H133A04001). The content and opinions do not necessarily represent the policy of NIDRR nor should anyone assume endorsement by the Federal Government.

References

Adelson, R. (2003). MS and pregnancy: The main event. *Inside MS, 21*(2).

Andersen, K., Novak, P., & Keith, J. (2005). *Mosby's medical, nursing, and allied health dictionary* (6th ed., pp. 1421–1422). St. Louis, MO: Mosby Yearbook.

Begum, M. (2001, February/March). Breastfeeding with multiple sclerosis. *Association of Women's Health, Obstetric and Neonatal Nursing (AWHONN) Lifelines*, 37–40.

Bowles, B. C. (1991). Breastfeeding consultation in sign language. *Journal of Human Lactation*, 7(1), 21.

Brennan, P., Ollier, B., Worthington, J., et al. (1996). Are both genetic and reproductive associations with rheumatoid arthritis linked to prolactin? *Lancet, 348*, 106–109.

Brennan, P., & Silman, A. (1994). Breastfeeding and the onset of rheumatoid arthritis. *Arthritis and Rheumatism, 37*, 808–813.

Bykowski, N. (1994, May–June). Helping mothers who are deaf or hard of hearing. *Leaven*, 45–46.

Carthy, E., Conine, T. A., & Hall, L. (1990). Comprehensive health promotion for the pregnant woman who is disabled. *Journal of Nurse-Midwifery, 35*, 133–142.

Coates, M., & Riordan, J. (2010). Baby guidelines for physically disabled breastfeeding mothers. In J. Riordan & K. Wambach (Eds.), *Breastfeeding and human lactation* (4th ed., pp. 472–475). Sudbury, MA: Jones and Bartlett.

Connolly, B., & Prosser, R. (2003). *Rehabilitation of the hand and upper limb*. Sydney, Australia: Butterworth Heinemann.

Good Mojab, C. (1999). Helping the visually impaired or blind mother breastfeed. *Leaven, 35*, 51–56.

Gulick, E., & Halper, J. (2002). Influence of feeding method on postpartum relapse of mothers with MS. *International Journal of MS Care, 4*, 183–191.

Halbert, L. (1998). Breastfeeding in the woman with a compromised nervous system. *Journal of Human Lactation, 14*, 327–331.

Hale, T. (2010). *Medications and mother's milk* (14th ed.). Amarillo, TX: Hale Publishing.

Herman, A. (2002). Challenges and solutions for parents with disabilities. *Spinal network* (3rd ed., pp. 365–368). Horsham, PA: Leonard Media Group.

Jacobsson, L. T. H., Jacobsson, M. E., Askling, J., & Knowler, W. C. (2003). Perinatal characteristics and risk of rheumatoid arthritis. *British Medical Journal, 326*, 1068–1069.

Karlson, E. W., Mandl, L. A., Hankinson, S. E., & Grodstein, F. (2004). Do breastfeeding and other reproductive factors influence future risk of rheumatoid arthritis? Results from the Nurses' Health Study. *Arthritis and Rheumatism, 50*, 3458–3467.

Lorenzi, A., & Ford, H. (2002). Multiple sclerosis and pregnancy. *Postgraduate Medical Journal, 78*, 460–464.

Martin, C. D. (1992). La Leche League and the mother who is blind. *Leaven, 5*, 67–68.

Mohrbacher, N., & Stock, J. (2007). Chronic illness or physical limitations. *The breastfeeding answer book* (6th ed., pp. 557–569). Schaumburg, IL: La Leche League International.

Office of Minority Health. (2007). National standards on culturally and linguistically appropriate services (CLAS). Retrieved from http://www.minorityhealth.hhs.gov/templates/browse. aspx?lvl=2&lvlid=15

Rogers, J. (2005). *The disabled woman's guide to pregnancy and birth*. New York, NY: Demos Medical Publishing.

Rogers, J., Tuleja, C., & Vensand, K. (2004). Baby care preparation. In S. Welner & F. Haselstine (Eds.), *Welner's guide to the care of women with disabilities* (p. 171). Philadelphia, PA: Lippincott Williams & Wilkins.

Wade, M., Foster, N., Cullen, L., et al. (1999). Breast and bottle-feeding for mothers with arthritis and other physical disabilities. *Professional Care of the Mother Child, 9*, 35–38.

Walker, M. (2009). *Breastfeeding management for the clinician: Using the evidence* (2nd ed.). Sudbury, MA: Jones and Bartlett.

Internet Resources

Through the Looking Glass (TLG). A community nonprofit organization formed in 1982 as a resource center for families in which one or more members have a disability. TLG's mission is to create, demonstrate, and encourage resources and model early intervention services that are health promoting and empowering. TLG consults with parents and professionals nationally and internationally. Adaptive baby care equipment including lifting harnesses and advice for mothers is available. Available at www.lookingglass.org.

Arthritis

Arthritis Foundation. Search diseases center. Available at www.arthritis.org.

Brennen, P. (1994, June). Breastfeeding and the onset of rheumatoid arthritis. *Arthritis and Rheumatism, 37*(6). Available at http://onlinelibrary.wiley.com/doi/10.1002/art.1780370605/abstract.

CBS News. Healthwatch. *Breastfeeding Fights Arthritis*. Available at www.cbsnews.com/stories/2004/11/04/health/webmd/main653734.shtml.

Web MD. Search *rheumatoid arthritis*. Available at www.webmd.com.

Carpal Tunnel

National Institute of Neurological Disorders and Stroke. Search *carpel tunnel syndrome*. Available at www.ninds.nih.gov.

Hearing Impairment

Deaf Counseling, Advocacy, and Referral Agency. Available at www.dcara.org.

HEAR-MORE Co. Sonic Alert Bed Vibrator D/C Auxiliary Jack. Available at www.hearmore.com/store/prodList.asp?idstore=1.

National Association of the Deaf (NAD). Available at www.nad.org.

Lupus

Lupus Foundation of America. (n.d.). About lupus. Available at www.lupus.org/webmodules/webarticlesnet/templates/new_learntreating.aspx?articleid=2245&zoneid=525.

Multiple Sclerosis

International Multiple Sclerosis Support Foundation, Jean Sumption, founder. A website of physicians with MS. Available at www.msnews.org.

Med TV Health Information Brought to Life. Available at http://multiple-sclerosis.emedtv.com/multiple-sclerosis/types-of-multiple-sclerosis.html.

Multiple Sclerosis Association of America. Available at www.msaa.com.

Multiple Sclerosis Foundation. Available at www.msfacts.org.

Myasthenia Gravis

Children's Hospital of the King's Daughters. (n.d.). Myasthenia gravis. Available at www.chkd.org/healthlibrary/Content.aspx?pageid=P02612.

Cooper University Hospital. (n.d.). Myasthenia gravis. Available at www.cooperhealth.org/content/greystone_17601.

Minami, J. (2000). Fitting breastfeeding into your life. *Leaven*, *36*(10), 5. Available at www.llli.org/llleaderweb/lv/lvfebmar00p5.html.

Spinal Cord Injury

Benzel, E. C. (2009). Spinal cord injury (SCI): Aftermath and diagnosis. Spine Universe. Available at http://www.Spineuniverse.com/displayarticle.php/ article1445.html.

Medline Plus. Available at www.nlm.nih.gov/medlineplus/spinalcordinjuries.html.

National Spinal Cord Injury Association. Available at www.spinalcord.org.

Thoracic Outlet Syndrome

National Institute of Neurological Disorders and Stroke. Search *thoracic outlet syndrome*. Available at www.ninds.nih.gov.

Visual Disability

American Council of the Blind. Available at www.acb.org.

American Foundation for the Blind. Available at www.afb.org.

La Leche League International. Audiotapes and Braille. Available at www.lalecheleague.org.

CHAPTER 33
Milk Expression, Storage, and Handling

Rebecca Mannel, BS, IBCLC, FILCA
Revised by Marsha Walker, RN, IBCLC

OBJECTIVES

- Describe indications and methods for expression of human milk.
- Discuss the types and action of available mechanical pumps.
- Describe the techniques of hand and mechanical expression.
- Discuss current guidelines for storage and handling of human milk.

INTRODUCTION

At some time during the course of lactation, many women may choose or need to express their milk. Whether to initiate, maintain, or increase milk production, the removal of a mother's milk from her breasts either by hand or mechanical breast pump is a learned technique. Women benefit from clear instructions and guidelines on how to express milk in an efficient manner and of a sufficient quantity to meet their individual needs. Expressed milk needs to be handled and stored in a safe manner to ensure that the milk remains usable in a variety of situations.

I. Mothers May Choose or Need to Express Milk for a Number of Reasons

A. To increase the milk supply

B. To stimulate lactogenesis II when breastfeeding initiation is delayed because of separation of baby and mother

C. To supply milk if her baby is ill, preterm, or hospitalized and cannot breastfeed directly or effectively

D. To prevent or relieve breast engorgement

E. To have milk available if she leaves the baby with another caregiver

F. To provide her baby with milk while she is at work or at school

G. To maintain or increase milk production when:
   1. Breastfeeding is interrupted because of travel, maternal hospitalization, or maternal use of medications contraindicated during lactation.

2. Milk production has decreased as a result of infrequent feedings or inadequate milk removal.

3. A mother chooses to provide only expressed milk to her baby rather than directly breastfeed.

H. To contribute to a milk bank

II. Hand Expression of Human Milk

A. The most common form of milk expression throughout the world

1. No equipment or electricity is required.

2. Hands are always available.

3. No cost to mother.

4. Every mother should learn how to hand express her milk (AAP, 2009).

5. All hospital maternity nursing staff should be trained in teaching mothers hand expression (AAP 2009).

B. Reasons to express milk by hand (in addition to the preceding)

1. To soften the areola to make it easier for baby to latch on

2. To elicit the milk ejection reflex prior to breastfeeding or pumping

3. During breastfeeding to increase milk transfer, especially with a sleepy or preterm baby to keep them suckling (Walker, 2010)

4. For more effective collection of colostrum in the first three days postpartum (Flaherman, et al., 2011; Ohyama et al., 2010)

5. In combination with use of an electric pump to increase milk production, for mothers who are exclusively pumping (Morton et al., 2009)

6. If the nipples are sore or macerated and the use of a pump will exacerbate the tissue damage

7. In emergencies if no electricity or breast pump is available

8. Where breast pumps are unaffordable

9. Where unfavorable sanitation conditions preclude the adequate cleaning of pump parts

III. Mechanical Expression of Human Milk

A. Mechanical devices for expressing milk have been used for centuries (Walker, 2010).

1. Some cost involved to purchase.

2. May require electricity.

3. Replacement parts may be needed at times.

4. Minimal to no regulations for breast pumps exist in most countries.

a. In the United States, pumps are regulated by the Food and Drug Administration (FDA) for safety. Adverse events are reported to the FDA (www.fda.gov/MedicalDevices/default.htm).

B. Reasons to express milk with a breast pump:

1. See section I.

2. Can be easier, less tiring than hand expression.
    a. Mothers with physical impairments may be unable to hand express.
3. Can be faster than hand expression.
    a. Several types allow for simultaneous pumping of both breasts.
    b. Employed mothers with limited break times may find a high-efficiency electric breast pump more suitable to their needs and limitations.
4. Can collect more milk.
    a. Mothers often collect more milk with mechanical expression than with hand expression (Paul et al., 1996; Slusher et al., 2007).
    b. Mothers collect more milk with simultaneous pumping (Auerbach, 1990; Jones et al., 2001).
5. Can be more comfortable.
    a. Mothers with severely engorged breasts may find hand expression too painful.
6. Some sexual abuse survivors may tolerate mechanical pumping over hand expression or direct breastfeeding (Lauwers et al., 2010; Riordan et al., 2010).

IV. Factors to Consider in Choosing Type of Pump

A. Age of baby
B. Condition of the baby
C. Condition of the mother
D. Reason/need for pumping
E. Availability and affordability
F. Efficacy and comfort
G. Ease of use and cleaning
H. Availability of replacement parts/service
I. Safety
    1. The rubber bulb or "bicycle horn" type manual pumps should be avoided because of the great potential for bacterial contamination of milk as well as nipple pain and damage (Foxman et al., 2002; Lawrence et al., 2010).
    2. Electric or battery-operated pumps that maintain constant negative pressure are more likely to cause nipple/breast trauma (Egnell, 1956; Lawrence et al., 2010).
    3. Many mothers use a borrowed breast pump or one that has previously been used by another mother (Clemons et al., 2010), which is a potentially risky practice.
        a. *Many* single-user pumps are open systems and may not have any protective barrier to prevent cross-contamination from multiple users.
        b. A borrowed pump can be ineffective or break, necessitating the purchase of a replacement pump.
        c. Because pumps have a limited lifetime, some mothers who borrow or purchase previously used pumps may put their milk supply at risk because the device cannot operate at its optimum. The motor may be worn down and cannot generate enough vacuum to be effective.

d. Multiple use of single-user devices typically invalidates the manufacturer's warranty.

e. In the United States, the FDA regulates breast pumps as Class II medical devices and provides guidance on previously used breast pumps. (See www.fda.gov/MedicalDevices/ProductsandMedicalProcedures/HomeHealthandConsumer/ConsumerProducts/BreastPumps/ucm061939.htm for more information.)

J. Price

1. Some mothers may have difficulty affording a suitable pump for their needs.

2. Inexpensive pumps may not be suitable for long-term or frequent pumping.

3. In the United States, breast pumps can be purchased using a flexible spending account.

4. Some hospitals, agencies, and the Women, Infants, and Children's program (WIC) may lend pumps to mothers.

V. Action: How Milk Is Removed from the Breast

A. Infants use a combination of suction and compression to remove milk from the breast (Geddes et al., 2008). Pumps use suction only in a cyclic pattern (Zoppou et al., 1997b).

B. When milk flow is low, infants suckle faster. When milk flow is high, infants suckle slower. Average suckling rate is 74 cycles/minute with a range of 36 to 126 cycles/minute (Bowen-Jones et al., 1982).

C. Negative pressure generated by infant suckling averages 50 to 155 mm Hg with a maximum of 241 mm Hg (Prieto et al., 1996).

D. Effective pumps create a vacuum that forms a pressure gradient. Under the higher pressure of the milk ejection reflex, milk flows or is "pushed out" to the lower pressure of the milk collection container.

E. Effective pumps do not suck, pull, or pump milk out of the breast.

F. Effectively nursing infants can transfer more milk from the breast than the mother who is pumping (Chapman et al., 2001; Zoppou et al., 1997a).

G. A few pumps also use compression.

H. Pump settings can be varied on most of the electric pumps. Both the cycling characteristics and amount of vacuum can be adjusted for comfort, as well as for efficiency. Mothers should adjust the settings for maximal milk output.

I. Mothers should start out pumping on the lower vacuum settings and gradually increase to use the maximum amount of vacuum that they are comfortable with (Kent et al., 2008).

VI. Manual or Hand Pumps

A. Advantages

1. Affordable; least expensive type of pump.

2. Available; easily found in most communities.

3. Portable; no electricity or batteries required.

4. Most are easy to use and easy to clean.

5. Some can be adapted for use on electric pumps.

B. Disadvantages

    1. Inconsistent or inadequate suction levels.

    2. Most require sequential pumping rather than simultaneous.

    3. Longer pumping sessions (15–20 minutes/breast).

    4. User fatigue.

    5. Not recommended for frequent, full-time use (such as working mother or mother of preterm, hospitalized infant).

C. Types/action

    1. Squeeze-handle pumps

        a. Vacuum is generated when the mother squeezes and releases a handle.

        b. Some have adjustable vacuum.

        c. Some have adjustable cycling.

        d. Parts need to be disassembled for adequate cleaning.

VII. Battery-Operated Pumps

A. Advantages

    1. Portable:

        a. No electricity required.

        b. Batteries are available in most communities.

        c. Rechargeable batteries are an option, although they may decrease pump efficiency.

    2. Easy to use:

        a. Requires only one hand

        b. No user fatigue

    3. Some can be adapted for use on larger, electric pumps.

    4. Some mothers buy two and use for simultaneous pumping.

    5. Some are designed for simultaneous pumping.

    6. Most have adjustable vacuum.

    7. Most accept an A/C adapter and can be plugged into an electrical outlet when desired.

B. Disadvantages

    1. Require replacement of batteries, which can be frequent depending on how much the mother is pumping.

    2. Several types require manual release of the vacuum during the pumping cycle; nipple trauma can occur with prolonged vacuum (Egnell, 1956).

    3. Vacuum in some pumps takes up to 30 seconds to reach the appropriate level. Time for recovery of the vacuum following release varies from brand to brand and can limit the number of cycles to 6 per minute, which is below acceptable ranges.

    4. As batteries deteriorate, the vacuum recovery time lengthens. Some types of batteries are not as effective as others.

5. Maximum vacuum can continue decreasing after each release during the pumping session.
6. Not recommended for mothers pumping for preterm/hospitalized infants.

C. Types/action
1. The batteries/electricity power a small motor that generates a vacuum.
2. A/C adapters save on battery life and allow motor to achieve maximum cycling of vacuum.

VIII. Electric Pumps

A. Advantages
1. Often available in hospitals for mothers of preterm or sick infants.
   a. Some communities have these pumps available for rental.
   b. Some insurance companies cover the cost of rental for mothers of hospitalized infants.
      i. Some hospitals provide pumps for mothers to use after discharge while their baby is still a patient.
      ii. In the United States, breast pumps can be purchased with funds from a mother's flexible spending account.
   c. A prescription for breastmilk from the baby's physician might be required to secure the rental and to extend it for use after the baby is discharged.
2. Some employers make these pumps available to their employees who return to work and continue breastfeeding.
3. Most allow for simultaneous pumping of both breasts.
4. No user fatigue.
5. Shorter pumping sessions (10–15 minutes total for simultaneous pumping).
6. Most have adjustable vacuum.
7. Some have automatic cycling that approaches physiological suckling (Mitoulas et al., 2002a).
8. Recommended for mothers who are pumping for preterm/hospitalized infants (that is, daily use).

B. Disadvantages
1. Least affordable type of pump.
2. May not be readily available in some communities.
3. Electricity is required. Some have accessory adapter for use in automobiles; some can operate with batteries.
4. Several types require manual release of the vacuum during the pumping cycle (semiautomatic cycling); nipple trauma can occur with prolonged vacuum (Egnell, 1956).

C. Types/action
   1. Semiautomatic pumps
      a. Require manual release of the vacuum during the pumping cycle.
         i. The mother typically has to cover a hole in the flange base to create the vacuum.
      b. Most mothers need practice to find the technique of vacuum release/cycling that facilitates effective milk removal.
      c. Smallest and least expensive of the electric pumps.
   2. Automatic pumps
      a. Hospital-grade
         i. Designed for use by many mothers; each mother has a personal collection kit to prevent cross-contamination.
         ii. Some have automatic cycling that approaches physiological suckling (Mitoulas et al., 2002a).
         iii. Mothers of preterm infants more likely to achieve full milk supply (Hill et al., 2005a, 2006).
      b. Personal use
         i. Designed for daily use by one mother for one or more infants.
         ii. Some have automatic cycling that approaches physiological suckling (Mitoulas et al., 2002a).
         iii. Bacterial contamination may occur when loaned/given to other mothers.
         iv. Motor may wear out when loaned/given to other mothers.

IX. Techniques of Milk Expression: General Guidelines

A. Milk can be expressed into any type of container, such as a bottle, cup, glass, jar, or bowl. It helps if the container has a wide opening.
B. Frequency of milk expression depends on the reason for expression.
   1. For occasional expressing, pump during, after, or between feedings, whichever gives the best results.
   2. Express as many times as required to obtain the amount of milk needed to use or store.
   3. Many mothers tend to express more milk first thing in the morning because of higher residual volumes of milk (Riordan et al., 2010).
   4. For employed mothers, expressing may be needed on a regular basis for at least the number of breastfeeds that are missed.
   5. To increase a low milk supply, the mother can express after each feeding. Mothers who are supplementing with expressed human milk and/or formula should express at least each time baby receives a supplemental feeding.
      i. Morton and colleagues (2009) demonstrated that in pump-dependent mothers of preterm babies, those who used hand expression greater than five times per day, as well as using an electric pump five times per day during the first 3 days postpartum, produced significantly larger volumes of milk than mothers who used only an electric pump.

ii. Massaging each breast while using an electric breast pump significantly increased the amount of milk pumped at each session (Morton et al., 2007).

6. For preterm or ill babies, the mother should begin expressing milk as early as possible within the first 24 hours and 8 to 10 times each 24 hours thereafter (Hill et al., 1999, 2001, 2005b).

7. For engorgement, she can express for a few minutes to soften the breasts before she breastfeeds and express after she breastfeeds if she still feels full or uncomfortable (International Lactation Consultant Association [ILCA], 2005).

C. Eliciting milk ejection reflex (milk release).

1. An infant on average takes 54 seconds to elicit the milk ejection reflex while a breast pump can take up to 4 minutes (Kent et al., 2003; Mitoulas et al., 2002b).

2. Some women have difficulty with their milk release when trying to express their milk.

a. Embarrassment, tension, fear of failure, pain, fatigue, and anxiety may block the neurochemical pathways required for milk ejection (Walker, 2010).

3. Some women are successful having their baby nurse and stimulate the milk release before pumping or hand expressing.

4. Applying warm compresses, taking a warm shower, thinking about baby, looking at a picture of baby, and/or relaxation techniques help some women elicit the milk ejection reflex.

5. Gentle nipple stimulation (avoid pulling or squeezing) can stimulate oxytocin release (Rojansky et al., 2001; Summers, 1997).

6. Breast massage is widely recognized to stimulate milk release.

7. Holding baby skin to skin (including during hospitalization) can stimulate oxytocin release (Uvnäs-Moberg et al., 2005).

8. A randomized, controlled trial showed no significant difference in milk amounts with the use of oxytocin nasal spray; however, it may assist those mothers with inhibited milk release (Fewtrell et al., 2006).

D. Breast massage.

1. Stimulates oxytocin release, which controls milk ejection reflex (Matthiesen et al., 2001).

2. Increases milk collection and thus milk production (Jones et al., 2001).

3. Improves composition of human milk by increasing gross energy and lipid content (Foda et al., 2004).

4. Various methods (Okeya, Oketani) are widely promoted in Japan (Foda et al., 2004; Kyo, 1982).

5. Adds external pressure, which increases pressure gradient in the breast, facilitating milk flow to negative pressure area of the pump or milk collection container (Walker, 2010).

6. Can be done in different ways, with the mother deciding which method works best for her.

   a. Hold the breast with one or both hands (depending on the size of the breast) so that the thumbs are on top of the breast and the fingers beneath it. Gently compress the breast between the fingers and thumbs, rotating fingers and thumbs around the breast.

   b. Use fingertips to massage in small circles all around the breast. This circular motion can cover some of the harder-to-reach areas on the underside of the breast and under the arms.

X. Hand Expression

A. Always wash hands before expressing milk.

B. Cup the breast with the thumb and forefingers directly opposite each other without touching the nipple or areola (depending on the extent of the areola). Push back into the chest wall and then forward in a rhythmical movement to massage the breast. Repeat this action, rotating around the breast, being careful to massage forward and not pinch or squeeze (Glynn et al., 2005).

C. Another method that some mothers find helpful is to hold the breast so that the thumb is on the top margin of the areola and the other four fingers are cupping the breast from underneath, with the little finger touching the rib.

   1. To express milk, she will start a wave-like motion from her little finger, pushing gently into the breast followed by the fourth finger, then the third, then the index finger while the thumb compresses from above.

   2. She can perform this action a few times and rotate the hand position so that all areas of the breast are reached.

   3. When she is finished on the first breast, she will continue on the second one.

   4. To obtain more milk, she can return to the first breast again, alternating back and forth to take advantage of the several milk ejection reflexes.

D. Avoid squeezing, rubbing, or pulling breast tissue.

E. Thorough milk removal and softening of the breast may take 20 to 30 minutes.

XI. Mechanical Expression

A. Follow manufacturer's instructions on assembly, use, and cleaning for specific types of pumps.

   1. Ensure that mother understands mechanism for vacuum release.

B. Wash hands before any milk expression.

C. Assemble collection equipment; ensure cleanliness.

   1. Washing equipment in the dishwasher or with hot soapy water is usually sufficient to keep it clean.

   2. All parts that come in contact with the milk should be washed after each use.

D. Some pumps come with various types of inserts that can be placed inside the flange (cone-shaped part that is placed over the nipple/areola) for a better fit.

E. Many pumps come with variable-sized flanges to accommodate larger nipples.

    1. The mother should use a flange that "fits" her nipple: the nipple should move freely back and forth in the "tunnel" or straight shaft of the flange and should not pinch, chafe, or rub during pumping. Flange diameters range from 21 mm to 40 mm.

    2. Pumping can cause areolar edema (Wilson-Clay et al., 2008).

    3. Continued pumping with a flange that is too tight will cause nipple pain/trauma and reduction of milk supply (Meier et al., 2004).

    4. More than half of mothers who are pumping for preterm/hospitalized infants may require flanges with diameters that are greater than 24 mm (Meier et al., 2004).

    5. Indications for use of a larger flange include the following:

       • Nipple rubs or sticks.

       • Nipple does not move freely after 5 minutes.

       • Not all of nipple fits into nipple tunnel.

       • Mother experiences pain.

       • Nipple tip becomes sore or blistered.

       • Areas of the breast are not well drained.

       • Ring of sloughed skin seen on inside of flange.

       • Base of nipple blanches while pumping.

F. The flange should be centered over the nipple and areola during pumping.

G. Some mothers massage breasts before and during pumping for optimal milk collection.

    1. If using a double collection kit, the flanges can be held in place with the forearm to free the other hand for breast massage.

    2. Some women secure the flanges to their bra to free one or both hands for breast massage.

    3. Some women express both breasts twice following breast massage.

H. Set the pump on the lowest suction setting, increasing it as needed. The mother should feel firm, nonpainful tugging.

    1. Pumps that allow the mother to adjust the suction and cycling should initially be set on lower suction with faster cycling. Once milk release has occurred, the suction can be increased and cycling decreased to more closely mimic physiological suckling (Mitoulas et al., 2002b).

I. Duration of pumping session.

    1. Mothers who are pumping occasionally may pump until they have collected the desired quantity of milk.

    2. Mothers who are pumping for preterm/hospitalized infants or to increase milk production should pump until the milk stops flowing.

J. Mothers who are using a manual pump may choose to prop their arm on a pillow, table, or wide chair arm if their arm gets tired.

XII. Expected Milk Volumes (Hill et al., 2005a)

A. Refer to **Table 33-1** for data on expected milk output.

B. Mothers produce 30 to 100 mL of milk in the first 24 hours (ILCA, 2005).

C. The average of milk output at postpartum days 6 and 7 is predictive of milk output at postpartum week 6.

D. Adequate milk volume is defined as greater than 500 mL/day at postpartum week 6. (See **Table 33-1**.)

   1. Preterm mothers are encouraged to produce more than average (750–1,000 mL/day) by postpartum day 14 to ensure adequate milk production and facilitate infant transition to direct breastfeeding before hospital discharge. (See Chapter 29, Breastfeeding a Preterm Infant.)

   2. Milk production less than 500 mL/day by postpartum day 14 is a marker for inadequate long-term milk production (Hill et al., 1999).

XIII. Common Problems

A. Pain with pumping

   1. Check flange fit.

      a. Change to wider diameter flange if chafing/pinching nipple (**Figure 33-1**).

      b. Nipples swell during pumping (Wilson-Clay et al., 2008).

   2. Check vacuum/suction levels of pump.

      a. Reduce suction level.

   3. Check cycling of pump.

      a. Instruct mother how to release suction consistently during milk expression if her pump does not automatically cycle.

   4. Check duration of pumping sessions.

      a. "Marathon" sessions (45–60 minutes) do not increase milk production.

      b. Instruct mother to pump until the milk stops flowing.

   5. Consider possible infection of the breast or nipple.

      a. Inadequate breast draining leads to milk stasis, a risk factor for mastitis.

      b. Nipple trauma is a risk factor for candidiasis and mastitis (Academy of Breastfeeding Medicine Protocol Committee, 2008; Foxman et al., 2002).

Table 33-1 Expected Milk Output (mL/day)

	Week 1	Week 6 (days 6 and 7 average)
Term, Breastfeeding	511 ±209	663 ±218
Preterm, Expressing	463 ±388	541 ±461

Source: Data are from Hill et al., 2005a.

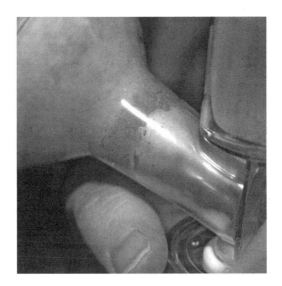

Figure 33-1 Poor flange fit.

Source: Wilson-Clay, B., & Hoover K. (2005). *The breastfeeding atlas. Austin, TX: LactNews Press.*

6. Consider changing to a different brand/type of pump.
    a. Breast pump adverse events are likely underreported to the FDA in the United States (Brown et al., 2005).
        i. Most commonly reported adverse events for electric breast pumps were pain/soreness, need for medical intervention, and breast tissue damage.
        ii. Most frequently reported adverse events for manual breast pumps were breast tissue damage and infection.
B. Dwindling or decreasing milk collection
    1. Preterm mothers who are expressing milk have a 2.8 times higher risk of having an inadequate milk supply than term mothers who are breastfeeding (Hill et al., 2005a). See **Table 33-1**.
    2. Many mothers who return to work struggle to maintain an adequate milk supply (Chezem et al., 1998; Hills-Bonczyk et al., 1993).
        a. Pumping every 45–120 minutes on days off for several periods of time during the day is called "power pumping," "cluster pumping," or "super pumping."
        b. A modification of this is when a mother pumps for as long as it takes to elicit the first milk ejection reflex and removes the milk made available during the time the milk ducts stay dilated. Up to 45% of the milk available in the breast is released during the first milk ejection (Ramsay et al., 2006). This may be no longer than a 5-minute period. The mother can pump again in 15 minutes or so to once more take advantage of the first and largest milk ejection reflex of a pumping session. She may cluster this pattern for perhaps an hour several times a day during her days off.
    3. **Table 33-2** lists strategies to increase milk production when expressing milk.

Table 33-2 Dwindling Milk Supply

Assess Expression Technique for Possible Causes of Faltering Milk Supply	Additional Strategies If Pumping Regularly with Effective Pump
Duration of expression/pumping	Expressing while holding/touching baby (skin to skin) at least once a day
Adequacy of breast emptying	Breast massage with expression
Frequency of expression/pumping	Conscious relaxation or visualization
Type of pump	Pumping for 2 minutes beyond milk flow
Maternal medication use	Medication/herbs prescribed by physician to increase prolactin levels

Source: Data are from HMBANA et al., 2006.

4. For more information on specific situations related to low milk production, refer to the following chapters:
   a. Insufficient milk production, Chapter 42
   b. Induced lactation/relactation, Chapter 35
   c. Preterm/hospitalized infants, Chapter 29

XIV. Guidelines for Storage and Handling of Human Milk

A. Storage of human milk for the hospitalized infant (Human Milk Banking Association of North America [HMBANA], Jones et al., 2006)
   1. Milk should be stored in clean, hard-sided containers that are food-grade clean.
      a. Polypropylene or polybutylene plastic or glass with leak-proof lids.
      b. Fill containers three-quarters full.
      c. Label with child/mother's name, hospital ID number, date/time of expression.
      d. Milk from each breast at a pumping session can be put in the same container; avoid combining milk from different pumping sessions to minimize contamination.
      e. Human milk does not require biohazard labeling (Centers for Disease Control and Prevention [CDC], 1994).
   2. **Table 33-3** shows a list of milk storage guidelines.
      a. Although HMBANA guidelines state that fresh, expressed human milk can be stored for up to 7 days in the refrigerator, many hospital policies recommend 48 hours for the hospitalized infant.
B. Storage of human milk for the healthy infant at home or in child care settings (HMBANA et al., 2006)
   1. Refer to **Table 33-4** for milk storage guidelines for the healthy infant.

Table 33-3 Milk Storage Guidelines for the Hospitalized Infant

Method	Hospitalized Infant
Room Temperature [77°F or 25°C] (best to refrigerate immediately)	< 4 hours
Refrigerator [39°F or 4°C] (fresh expressed)	up to 7 days
Insulated cooler with frozen gel packs [59°F or 15°C] (transported milk)	< 24 hours
Completely thawed and placed in refrigerator [39°F or 4°C]	< 24 hours
Previously frozen, brought to room temperature [77°F or 25°C]	< 4 hours
Freezer Compartment (1-door refrigerator)	Not Recommended
Freezer Compartment [23°F or 25°C] (2-door refrigerator) *not in door	< 3 months
Deep Freezer [24°F or 220°C]	< 6 months

Source: Data are from HMBANA et al., 2006.

Table 33-4 Milk Storage Guidelines for the Healthy Infant

Method	Healthy Infant
Room Temperature [77°F or 25°C]	< 6 hours
Refrigerator [39°F or 4°C] (fresh expressed)	< 8 days
Insulated cooler with frozen gel packs [59°F or 15°C] (transported milk)	< 24 hours
Completely thawed and placed in refrigerator [39°F or 4°C]	< 24 hours
Freezer Compartment (1-door refrigerator)	2 weeks
Freezer Compartment [23°F or 25°C] (2-door refrigerator) *not in door	< 6 months
Deep Freezer [24°F or 220°C]	< 12 months

Source: Data are from HMBANA et al., 2006; Williams-Arnold, 2000.

2. Expressed milk can be stored in glass or plastic baby bottles; clean food storage containers with tight-fitting, solid lids; disposable feeding bottle liners and mother's milk bags.
  a. Double bagging is recommended to protect the milk because some plastic bags/bottle liners can tear easily.
  b. Fill containers three-quarters full.
  c. Label with child/mother's name; date/time of expression.
  d. Chill freshly expressed milk before adding it to already refrigerated or frozen milk.
  e. Freeze milk in small amounts of 2 to 4 oz (60–120 mL) to avoid waste and speed thawing.
  f. Human milk does not require biohazard labeling (CDC, 1994).
C. Handling expressed human milk (HMBANA et al., 2006)
  1. Hospitalized infants
    a. Sample hospital policy at www.go.jblearning.com/corecurriculum.
  2. Healthy infants
    a. Use any freshly pumped milk if available. Otherwise, use milk with oldest storage date first.
    b. Milk can be thawed quickly in a container of warm water (not to exceed 37°C or 98.6°F); ensure water does not touch lid.
    c. Milk can be thawed slowly in the refrigerator or at room temperature. If thawing at room temperature, monitor milk and refrigerate before it is completely thawed, while ice crystals are still present.
    d. Warm milk for feeding by putting container in warm water or holding under running water.
    e. Never microwave human milk, either to defrost it or to warm it.
      i. Microwaving liquids creates hot spots that might burn the baby.
      ii. Microwaving human milk destroys sIgA and other immune components.
    f. If thawed milk has a soapy odor/taste that bothers the baby, the milk can be scalded prior to storing.
      i. Heat milk to ~180°F (82°C) or until small bubbles form around edge of pan; chill quickly and store until use.
      ii. Some mothers have high lipase levels; scalding the milk will inactivate the lipase.
      iii. Milk with soapy odor/taste is not harmful to the baby.

References

Academy of Breastfeeding Medicine Protocol Committee. (2008). *ABM clinical protocol no. 4: Mastitis. Revision May 2008*. Retrieved from http://www.bfmed.org/Media/Files/Protocols/protocol_4mastitis.pdf.

American Academy of Pediatrics. (2009). *Sample Hospital Breastfeeding Policy for Newborns.*

Auerbach, K. G. (1990). Sequential and simultaneous breast pumping: A comparison. *International Journal of Nursing Studies, 27,* 257–265.

Bowen-Jones, A., Thompson, C., & Drewett, R. F. (1982). Milk flow and sucking rates during breast-feeding. *Developmental Medicine and Child Neurology, 24,* 626–633.

Brown, S. L., Bright, R. A., Dwyer, D. E., & Foxman, B. (2005). Breast pump adverse events: Reports to the food and drug administration. *Journal of Human Lactation, 21,* 169–174.

Centers for Disease Control and Prevention. (1994). *Guidelines for preventing transmission of human immunodeficiency virus through transplantation of human tissue and organs. Morbidity and Mortality Weekly Report, 43*(RR-8), 1–17.

Chapman, D. J., Young, S., Ferris, A. M., & Perez-Escamilla, R. (2001). Impact of breast pumping on lactogenesis stage II after cesarean delivery: A randomized clinical trial. *Pediatrics, 107,* E94.

Chezem, J., Friesen, C., Montgomery, P., et al. (1998). Lactation duration: Influences of human milk replacements and formula samples on women planning postpartum employment. *Journal of Obstetric, Gynecologic, and Neonatal Nursing, 27,* 646–651.

Clemons, S. N., & Amir, L. H. (2010). Breastfeeding women's experience of expressing: A descriptive study. *Journal of Human Lactation, 26,* 258–265.

Coates, M., & Riordan, J. (2010). *Breastfeeding and human lactation* (4th ed.). Sudbury, MA: Jones and Bartlett.

Egnell, E. (1956). The mechanics of different methods of emptying the female breast. *Journal of the Swedish Medical Association, 40,* 1–8.

Fewtrell, M. S., Loh, K. L., Blake, A., et al. (2006). Randomised, double blind trial of oxytocin nasal spray in mothers expressing breast milk for preterm infants. *Archives of Disease in Childhood: Fetal and Neonatal Edition, 91,* F169–F174.

Flaherman, V. J., et al. (2011). Randomised trial comparing hand expression with breast pumping for mothers of term newborns feeding poorly. *Arch Dis Child Fetal Neonatal Ed,* doi:10.1136/F2 of 6 adc.2010.209213.

Foda, M. I., Kawashima, T., Nakamura, S., et al. (2004). Composition of milk obtained from unmassaged versus massaged breasts of lactating mothers. *Journal of Pediatric Gastroenterology and Nutrition, 38,* 484–487.

Foxman, B., D'Arcy, H., Gillespie, B., et al. (2002). Lactation mastitis: Occurrence and medical management among 946 breastfeeding women in the United States. *American Journal of Epidemiology, 155,* 103–114.

Geddes, D. T., Kent, J. C., Mitoulas, L. R., & Hartmann, P. E. (2008). Tongue movement and intra-oral vacuum in breastfeeding infants. *Early Human Development, 84,* 471–477.

Glynn, L., & Goosen, L. (2005). Manual expression of breast milk. *Journal of Human Lactation, 21,* 184–185.

Hill, P. D., Aldag, J. C., & Chatterton, R. T. (1999). Effects of pumping style on milk production in mothers of non-nursing preterm infants. *Journal of Human Lactation, 15,* 209–216.

Hill, P. D., Aldag, J. C., & Chatterton, R. T. (2001). Initiation and frequency of pumping and milk production in mothers of non-nursing preterm infants. *Journal of Human Lactation, 17,* 9–13.

Hill, P. D., Aldag, J. C., Chatterton, R. T., & Zinaman, M. (2005a). Comparison of milk output between mothers of preterm and term infants: The first 6 weeks after birth. *Journal of Human Lactation*, *21*, 22–30.

Hill, P. D., Aldag, J. C., Chatterton, R. T., & Zinaman, M. (2005b). Primary and secondary mediators' influence on milk output in lactating mothers of preterm and term infants. *Journal of Human Lactation*, *21*, 138–150.

Hill, P. D., Aldag, J. C., Demirtas, H., Zinaman, M., & Chatterton, R. T. (2006). Mood states and milk output in lactating mothers of preterm and term infants. *Journal of Human Lactation*, *22*(3), 305–314.

Hills-Bonczyk, S. G., Avery, M. D., Savik, K., et al. (1993). Women's experiences with combining breast-feeding and employment. *Journal of Nurse-Midwifery*, *38*, 257–266.

Human Milk Banking Association of North America, Jones, F., & Tully, M. R. (2006). *Best practice for expressing, storing and handling human milk in hospitals, homes and child care settings.* Raleigh, NC: HMBANA.

International Lactation Consultant Association. (2005). *Clinical guidelines for the establishment of exclusive breastfeeding.* Washington, DC: U.S. Department of Health and Human Services, Maternal/Child Health Bureau.

Jones, E., Dimmock, P., & Spencer, S. (2001). A randomised controlled trial to compare methods of milk expression after preterm delivery. *Archives of Disease in Childhood: Fetal and Neonatal Edition*, *85*, F91–F95.

Kent, J. C., Mitoulas, L. R., Cregan, M. D., et al. (2008). Importance of vacuum for breastmilk expression. *Breastfeeding Medicine*, *3*, 11–19.

Kent, J. C., Ramsay, D. T., Doherty, D., et al. (2003). Response of breasts to different stimulation patterns of an electric breast pump. *Journal of Human Lactation*, *19*, 179–186, quiz 87–88, 218.

Kyo, T. (1982). Observation on initiation of breast feeding: The relationship between Okeya's method of breast massage and the quantity of milk secretion. *Josanpu Zasshi*, *36*, 548–549. [in Japanese]

Lauwers, J., & Swisher, A. (2010). *Counseling the nursing mother* (5th ed.). Sudbury, MA: Jones and Bartlett.

Lawrence, R. A., & Lawrence, T. (2010). *Breastfeeding: A guide for the medical profession* (7th ed.). Maryland Heights, MO: Elsevier Mosby.

Matthiesen, A. S., Ransjo-Arvidson, A. B., Nissen, E., & Uvnäs-Moberg, K. (2001). Postpartum maternal oxytocin release by newborns: Effects of infant hand massage and sucking. *Birth*, *28*, 13–19.

Meier, P. P., Motykowski, J. E., & Zuleger, J. L. (2004). Choosing a correctly-fitted breastshield for milk expression. *Medela Messenger*, *21*, 1, 8–9.

Mitoulas, L. R., Lai, C. T., Gurrin, L. C., et al. (2002a). Effect of vacuum profile on breast milk expression using an electric breast pump. *Journal of Human Lactation*, *18*, 353–360.

Mitoulas, L. R., Lai, C. T., Gurrin, L. C., et al. (2002b). Efficacy of breast milk expression using an electric breast pump. *Journal of Human Lactation*, *18*, 344–352.

Morton, J., Hall, J. Y., Thairu, L., et al. (2007). Breast massage maximizes milk volumes of pump-dependent mothers [Abstract]. Retrieved from http://www.abstracts2view.com/pasall/view.php?nu=PAS07L1_32.

Morton, J., Hall, J. Y., Wong, R. J., Thairu, L., Benitz, W. E., & Rhine, W. D. (2009). Combining hand techniques with electric pumping increases milk production in mothers of preterm infants. *Journal of Perinatology*, *29*, 757–764.

Ohyama, M., Watabe, H., & Hayasaka, Y. (2010). Manual expression and electric breast pumping in the first 48 h after delivery. *Pediatrics International, 52*, 39–43.

Paul, V. K., Singh, M., Deorari, A. K., et al. (1996). Manual and pump methods of expression of breast milk. *Indian Journal of Pediatrics, 63*, 87–92.

Prieto, C. R., Cardenas, H., Salvatierra, A. M., et al. (1996). Sucking pressure and its relationship to milk transfer during breastfeeding in humans. *Journal of Reproduction and Fertility, 108*, 69–74.

Ramsay, D.T., Mitoulas, L.R., Kent, J.C., Cregan, M.D., Doherty, D.A., Larsson, M., Hartmann, P.E. (2006). Milk flow rates can be used to identify and investigate milk ejection in women expressing breast milk using an electric breast pump. *Breastfeeding Medicine*, 1, 14-23.

Riordan, J., & Wambach, K. (2010). *Breastfeeding and human lactation* (4th ed.). Sudbury, MA: Jones and Bartlett.

Rojansky, N., Tsafrir, A., Ophir, E., & Ezra, Y. (2001). Induction of labor in breech presentation. *International Journal of Gynaecology and Obstetrics, 74*, 151–156.

Slusher, T., Slusher, I. L., Biomdo, M., Bode-Thomas, F., Curtis, B. A., & Meier, P. (2007). Electric breast pump use increases maternal milk volume in African nurseries. *Journal of Tropical Pediatrics, 53*, 125–130.

Summers, L. (1997). Methods of cervical ripening and labor induction. *Journal of Nurse-Midwifery, 42*, 71–85.

Uvnäs-Moberg, K., & Petersson, M. (2005). Oxytocin, a mediator of anti-stress, well-being, social interaction, growth and healing. *Zeitschrift fur Psychosomatische Medizin und Psychotherapie, 51*, 57–80. Review. [in Swedish]

Walker, M. (2010). Breast pumps and other technologies. In J. Riordan & K. Wambach (Eds.), *Breastfeeding and human lactation* (4th ed., pp. 379-424). Sudbury, MA: Jones and Bartlett.

Williams-Arnold, L. D. (2000). *Human milk storage for healthy infants and children*. Sandwich, MA: Health Education Associates.

Wilson-Clay, B., & Hoover, K. (2008). *The breastfeeding atlas* (3rd ed.). Austin, TX: LactNews Press.

Zoppou, C., Barry, S. I., & Mercer, G. N. (1997a). Comparing breastfeeding and breast pumps using a computer model. *Journal of Human Lactation, 13*, 195–202.

Zoppou, C., Barry, S. I., & Mercer, G. N. (1997b). Dynamics of human milk extraction: A comparative study of breast feeding and breast pumping. *Bulletin of Mathematical Biology, 59*, 953–973.

Suggested Reading

Academy of Breastfeeding Medicine. (2004). *ABM clinical protocol no. 8: Human milk storage information for home use for healthy full term infants*. Retrieved from http://www.bfmed.org/Media/Files/Protocols/Protocol%208%20-%20English%20revised%202010.pdf

Biancuzzo, M. (1999). Selecting pumps for breastfeeding mothers. *Journal of Obstetric, Gynecologic, and Neonatal Nursing, 28*, 417–426.

Bowles, B. C., Stutte, P. C., & Hensley, J. H. (1987–1988). New benefits from an old technique: Alternate massage in breastfeeding. *Genesis, 9*, 5–9, 17.

Daly, S. E., & Hartmann, P. E. (1995). Infant demand and milk supply. Part I. Infant demand and milk production in lactating women. *Journal of Human Lactation, 11*, 21–25.

Daly, S. E., Kent, J. C., Huynh, D. Q., et al. (1992). The determination of short-term breast volume changes and the rate of synthesis of human milk using computerized breast measurement. *Experimental Physiology, 77*, 79–87.

Daly, S. E. J., & Hartmann, P. E. (1995). Infant demand and milk supply. Part 2: The short-term control of milk synthesis in lactating women. *Journal of Human Lactation*, *11*, 27–37.

Daly, S. E. J., Owens, R. A., & Hartmann, P. E. (1993). The short-term synthesis and infant regulated removal of milk in lactating women. *Experimental Physiology*, *78*, 209–220.

Groh-Wargo, S., Toth, A., Mahoney, K., et al. (1995). The utility of a bilateral breast pumping system for mothers of premature infants. *Neonatal Network*, *14*, 31–35.

Hill, P. D., & Aldag, J. C. (2005). Milk volume on day 4 and income predictive of lactation adequacy at 6 weeks of mothers of nonnursing preterm infants. *Journal of Perinatal and Neonatal Nursing*, *19*, 273–282.

Hill, P. D., Aldag, J. C., & Chatterton, R. T. (1999). Breastfeeding experience and milk weight in lactating mothers pumping for preterm infants. *Birth*, *26*, 233–238.

Hill, P. D., Brown, L. P., & Harker, T. L. (1995). Initiation and frequency of breast expression in breastfeeding mothers of LBW and VLBW infants. *Nursing Research*, *44*, 352–355.

Hurst, N. M., Valentine, C. J., Renfro, L., et al. (1997). Skin-to-skin holding in the neonatal intensive care unit influences maternal milk volume. *Journal of Perinatology*, *17*, 213–217.

Stutte, P. C., Bowles, B. C., & Morman, G. Y. (1988). The effects of breast massage on volume and fat content of human milk. *Genesis*, *10*, 22–25.

Walker, M. (2010). *Breastfeeding management for the clinician: Using the evidence*. Sudbury, MA: Jones and Bartlett.

Woolridge, M. W. (1986). The anatomy of infant sucking. *Midwifery*, *2*, 164–171.

Zinaman, M. J., Hughes, V., Queenan, J. T., et al. (1992). Acute prolactin and oxytocin responses and milk yield to infant suckling and artificial methods of expression in lactating women. *Pediatrics*, *89*, 437–440.

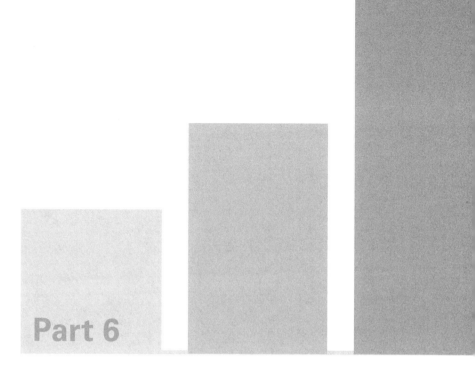

Part 6

Breastfeeding Technology

CHAPTER 34
Breastfeeding Devices and Equipment

Vergie I. Hughes, MS, IBCLC, FILCA

OBJECTIVES

- Choose the appropriate breastfeeding aids to remedy specific breastfeeding problems.
- List two advantages and two drawbacks of each specific aid.
- Describe the appropriate use of the aid.

INTRODUCTION

When mothers experience discomfort while breastfeeding or encounter infants who have difficulty latching on to the breast or gaining weight, interventions might be necessary to correct the problem. The role of the lactation consultant is to identify potential causes of the problem and to offer intervention options to remedy the situation. Often, refining the mother's technique (positioning, latch-on, breastfeeding frequency and duration, etc.) is the first strategy toward solving a number of problems. When additional intervention is needed, specific devices and equipment might be helpful. The goal is to establish or return the mother and baby to direct breastfeeding as soon as possible.

I. Nipple Shields

A. A device placed over the nipple and areola on which the baby sucks; considered a short-term solution until the baby can be transferred to the breast.

    1. Types not recommended (Wilson-Clay et al. 2008):

        a. Thick rubber or latex shields: Can reduce milk transfer (Auerbach, 1990; Lawrence et al., 2011, Woolridge et al., 1980)

        b. Plastic or glass base with a bottle-like nipple attached

    2. Types recommended (Wilson-Clay et al., 2008):

        a. Thin silicone.

        b. One type covers the entire areola.

        c. One type has partial coverage of the areola with the upper portion cut away to allow the infant's nose to touch the mother's skin and smell the areola.

        d. May have ribs on inner surface.

3. Sizes (vary with manufacturer) (Riordan et al., 2010; Wilson-Clay et al. 2008).
   a. Height of nipple portion 0.75 inch to 0.875 inch (19 to 22 millimeters)
   b. Width of nipple portion at base 0.625 inch to 1 inch (15.7 to 25.4 millimeters)
4. Holes in tip.
5. Shields have from one to five holes; milk flows best through nipple shields that have multiple holes (Nicholson, 1993).

B. Uses. Although nipple shields are not always fully successful, they can be useful in a variety of situations (Barger, 1997; Clum et al., 1996; Frantz, 2000; Marriott, 1997; Walker, 2011; Wilson-Clay et al., 2008), including the following:

1. The infant is unable to latch on because of flat or inverted nipples (Drazen, 1998; Elliott, 1996; Powers et al., 2004).
2. The baby is unable to open his or her mouth wide enough to achieve a deep latch.
3. The baby is unable to draw the nipple/areola into his or her mouth (Meier et al., 2000; Powers et al., 2004; Wight et al., 2008).
4. The mother has an overactive letdown reflex or oversupply where the baby has difficulty handling the flow (Mohrbacher et al., 2003; Powers et al., 2004; Wilson-Clay et al., 2008).
5. The mother's nipples/areola are very sore, damaged, or infected (Brigham, 1996; Drazen, 1998; Powers et al., 2004; Riordan et al., 2010).
6. The baby has a weak, disorganized, or dysfunctional suck (Isaacson, 2006; Marmet et al., 2000; Powers et al., 2004; Watson-Genna, 2008; Wilson-Clay, 1996).
7. There is nipple confusion and/or breast refusal (Powers et al., 2004; Wilson-Clay, 1996; Woodworth et al., 1996).
8. Can be helpful in some circumstances when the baby has certain congenital conditions (cleft palate, Pierre-Robin syndrome, short frenulum) (Powers et al., 2004; Wilson-Clay et al., 2008).
9. Can be helpful with upper airway problems such as laryngomalacia and tracheomalacia (Walker, 2011).
10. Mother is considering premature weaning (Walker, 2011).

C. Advantages:
1. May give immediate results.
2. Provides shape to a flat or inverted nipple.
3. Helps stretch and improve the elasticity of a flat or inverted nipple when the baby sucks strongly over the shield (Wilson-Clay et al., 2008).
4. Reinforces a wide-open mouth position at the breast (Wilson-Clay et al., 2008).
5. Can reduce pain experienced by the mother (Walker, 2011).
6. May help keep the baby at the breast during remediation of the problem (Brigham, 1996).
7. Prolactin levels seem unaffected by the use of the thin silicone shields (Amatayakul et al., 1987; Chertok et al., 2006).
8. Little or no reduction of milk transfer using thin silicone shield (Chertok et al., 2006; Jackson et al., 1987).

9. Increases milk intake at the breast for some preterm infants (Meier et al., 2000; Wight, 2008).
10. No difference in weight gain over 2 months with and without shield (Chertok, 2009).
11. Can prevent premature weaning (Chertok et al., 2006; Wilson-Clay, 1997).
D. Disadvantages:
   1. Thick rubber shields, bottle-like nipples, and thick latex shields have the capability to reduce milk transfer (Auerbach, 1990; Woolridge et al., 1980).
   2. Inner ribbed protrusions (if present) can cause discomfort and pain.
   3. Complementary feedings may be needed to compensate until milk transfer improves.
   4. Use of a breast pump after feedings with the shield may be necessary to initiate and/or maintain an optimal milk supply.
   5. Infant may become dependent on the shield (DeNicola, 1986; Hunter, 1999; Johnson, 1997; Newman, 1997).
   6. Latex shields carry the risk of inducing a latex allergy in the mother and/or infant.
   7. Providers may overrely on the shield to solve problems (Newman et al., 2006).
E. Some institutions require a written consent for the use of nipple shields that outlines the concerns with use and the importance of follow-up with a lactation professional (Lactation Education Consultants, 1996; Riordan et al., 2010).
F. When a nipple shield is used during the period when the mother's milk is still coming in, the mother should use a breast pump four to six times per day to establish her milk supply. Monitor the baby's weight and output. Pumping can be slowly discontinued once supply is well established (Riordan et al., 2010).
G. Sizing the nipple shield (Wilson-Clay et al., 2008):
   1. First, size the shield to the infant's mouth.
      a. The teat height should not exceed the length of the infant's mouth from the lips to the junction of the hard and soft palates.
      b. If the height of the teat is greater than this width, the probability increases that the infant's gum ridges will rest beyond where the tongue should begin to exert its peristaltic motion. If this situation happens, the nipple and areola might not be drawn into the teat shaft far enough for compression by the infant's tongue, which will reduce the milk transfer.
      c. In some babies, this excessive length can trigger a gag reflex and an aversion to feeding. In these cases, Wilson-Clay and Hoover (2008) recommend using the shortest available teat with the height under 2 cm.
   2. Second, consider the size of the mother's nipple.
      a. Some small shields are not wide enough at the base to accommodate larger nipples. Wide bases might be too large for some babies who have small mouths. Compromise to find the best fit for both mother and infant.
   3. When sizing a shield for use with a tongue-tie infant, select the largest size that the baby's mouth will accommodate (Watson-Genna, 2008).

H. To apply the nipple shield, roll the shield back about one-third of the length of the nipple shank and apply to the breast, unrolling the shield onto the nipple and areola (Watson-Genna, 2009; Wilson-Clay et al., 2008).
   1. To ensure the shield remains in place during the feeding:
      a. Moisten the areolar portion of the shield.
      b. Apply small amount of a sticky breast cream.
      c. Warm the shield under hot running water prior to application.
   2. Suggestions to place the mother's nipple deeper into the nipple shank (Mohrbacher et al., 2003; Wilson-Clay et al., 2008):
      a. May stretch the area near the base of the shank with the fingers and release when placed over the nipple.
      b. The baby can pull the nipple even farther into the shield after several minutes of vigorous sucking.
   3. If the mother feels pain through the nipple shield, either the nipple is not deeply positioned into the shield or the shield is too small for the nipple.
I. The shield may be prefilled with fluid to give the infant a faster reward (Watson-Genna, 2008, 2009).
J. Present the nipple shield to the infant as you would a breast nipple, touching the philtrum first to stimulate a wide latch-on (Watson-Genna, 2009).
K. A feeding tube can be used in conjunction with a nipple shield to temporarily increase milk flow (Mohrbacher et al., 2003; Riordan et al., 2010; Walker, 2011; Wilson-Clay, 1996; Wilson-Clay et al., 2008).
   1. Tube placed outside the shield
      a. Nipple keeps good fit inside the shield.
   2. Tube placed inside the shield
      a. Easy for mother to position both in infant's mouth.
      b. May lose suction.
      c. Baby swallows more air.
      d. Mom feels less "pulling."
L. The shield can be removed once vigorous sucking is achieved and the infant quickly can be placed directly on the mother's breast before the nipple/areola loses its shape (Mohrbacher et al., 2003; Wilson-Clay et al., 2008).
M. Assess milk transfer (Watson-Genna, 2009).
   1. Test weights.
   2. Assess suck:swallow ratio.
   3. Milk observed in tip of shield.
N. Weaning from the shield:
   1. Start the feeding with the shield, and then remove it. If the baby will not latch, replace the shield and try at the next feeding (Walker, 2011).
   2. Avoid cutting pieces off the tip of the shield in an attempt to wean the baby from it; blunt uncomfortable edges might remain (Mohrbacher et al., 2003).
   3. Attempt to latch the baby at breast when the breast is full or soft depending on infant's ability to latch (Watson-Genna, 2009).

4. Attempt to latch the infant to breast when sleepy, full, or hungry.

O. Follow-up with a lactation consultant is essential.

P. Have been used long term in some situations (Brigham, 1996).

Q. Typical problems of small preterm infants at the breast include failure to latch on, sucking for insufficient length of time, immature feeding behaviors, falling asleep as soon as he or she is positioned at the breast, and repeated slipping off the nipple.

    1. Preterm infants might need to rely on a shield for longer periods of time (2–3 weeks or until term-corrected age) (Meier et al., 2000).

    2. Shields have been demonstrated to increase the volume of milk transfer (Meier et al., 2000).

    3. Weigh the baby before and after a feeding with an electronic scale capable of measuring differences of 1–2 grams (Brigham, 1996).

    4. Monitor output and weight often.

II. Breast Shells

A. A two-piece plastic device consisting of a dome or cup and a concave backing contoured to fit the shape of the breast; held in place over the nipple/areola by the mother's bra (Frantz, 2000). Not in common use because of lack of evidence of effectiveness (Riordan et al., 2010).

B. Types for flat or inverted nipples:

    1. Designed to evert a flat nipple; the part in contact with the breast has a small opening that is just large enough for the nipple to protrude through.

    2. The pressure on the areola was thought to break adhesions that were anchoring the nipple to the base of the areola (Otte, 1975; Riordan et al., 2010).

    3. The dome has one or more air vents to enable air to circulate around the nipple.

    4. Some brands are constructed with flexible silicone backs.

C. Types for sore nipples:

    1. Most brands have an optional back with a much larger opening to keep the bra off the nipple and enable air to circulate.

    2. Some brands have a cotton liner that surrounds the backing for a comfortable fit.

    3. Some shells have an absorbent cotton pad that is placed in the bottom of the shell under the areola to absorb leaked milk.

D. Uses:

    1. To evert flat or inverted nipples either prenatally or postpartum

    2. To collect leaking milk

    3. To relieve engorgement

    4. For protection of painful, tender nipples

E. Advantages:

    1. May assist flat or inverted nipples to protrude (Mohrbacher et al., 2003)

    2. May protect painful nipples by preventing chafing caused by clothing, bra, and so forth (Brent et al., 1998)

    3. May encourage milk to leak and help relieve engorgement

    4. Drip milk should not be fed to the baby (Lawrence, 1999; Mohrbacher et al., 2003).

F. Disadvantages:
   1. Theoretical risk of stimulating preterm labor contractions. Discuss with mother's healthcare provider. May be used in healthy pregnancy with no threat of preterm labor.
   2. Often not effective in everting a flat or retracted nipple (Alexander et al., 1992; MAIN Trial Collaborative Group, 1994; Riordan et al., 2010; Wilson-Clay et al., 2008).
   3. Might cause irritation to the nipple or areola either from contact with the skin or from moisture buildup in the shell and the resulting skin breakdown.
   4. Drip milk can leak out of some shells when the mother leans over.
   5. Some shells are obvious under the bra.
   6. The bra might need to be a cup size larger to accommodate the shell.
   7. May cause plugged ducts and mastitis (Mohrbacher et al. 2003).
   8. Women who have fibrocystic breasts might experience discomfort from the constant pressure.
   9. Research on effectiveness of breast shells is limited and insufficient to base treatment decisions.
   10. Prenatal use of shells may discourage women from attempting to breastfeed (Alexander et al., 1992).
   11. May increase risk of infection from poor hygiene (Fetherston, 1998).
G. Techniques for use:
   1. Center the opening of the shell over the nipple and apply the bra to hold it in place.
   2. Apply a cotton liner if appropriate.
   3. Wear them for gradually longer periods of time during the day.
   4. Shells should be removed for naps and at bedtime because duct obstruction can occur.
   5. In hot weather or if moisture builds up, remove them, allow the breast to dry, and reapply.

III. Nipple Everters

Limited or no research is available on this category of devices at this time (Riordan et al., 2010; Watson-Genna, 2009).

A. Types:
   1. A syringe-like device that is placed over the nipple; the plunger is gently pulled to apply suction to the nipple.
      a. Commercially available syringe (Evert-it) has a soft, flexible areolar cone (Watson-Genna, 2009).
   2. Thimble-shaped dome (Nipplette) placed over the nipple prenatally, suction is generated by pulling on syringe and sealing off the dome (McGeorge, 1994; Watson-Genna, 2009).
      a. Follow manufacturer's instructions for safe use.

3. Thimble-shaped dome (SuppleCup) placed over the nipple.

    a. Squeeze to apply and pull nipple out; wear for several hours daily or prior to feedings (Watson-Genna, 2009).

    b. Apply lanolin for better adherence.

4. Small bulb syringe device (Latch-assist).

    a. Pull nipple out prior to feedings (Watson-Genna, 2009).

    b. Difficult to clean after use.

5. Noncommercial device can be made from a 10- or 20-milliliter syringe (Arsenault, 1997; Kesaree et al., 1993; Watson-Genna, 2009).

    a. The end of the barrel is cut off where the needle attaches to form a hollow tube.

    b. The plunger is inserted into the cut end, leaving the smooth side to be placed over the nipple.

    c. There is legal concern over adapting medical equipment to a purpose for which it was not intended.

B. Uses:

1. Evert a flat or retracted nipple in the prenatal or postpartum period

2. Form a nipple to make latch-on easier for a baby who is having difficulty grasping and holding the nipple

C. Advantages:

1. Simple, low-cost technique to aid in latch-on and nipple erection (Kesaree et al., 1993).

2. Mother can control to her level of comfort.

D. Disadvantages:

1. If used too vigorously or incorrectly, has the potential to cause pain or skin damage.

2. The nipple might not remain everted long enough for the baby to achieve latch-on.

3. There is no evidence to demonstrate the effectiveness of these devices.

E. Technique:

1. The mother applies the suction to the nipple and gently pulls back on the plunger to her level of comfort and holds the nipple everted for about 30 seconds (Kesaree et al., 1993).

F. She performs this action prior to each breastfeeding and can repeat between feedings if desired.

G. Rubber band placed at base of nipple (Chakrabarti et al., 2011):

1. Apply nipple everter and rubber band prior to feeding.

2. May cause pain; baby can get rubber band into mouth.

IV. Gel Dressings

Three-dimensional networks of cross-linked hydrophilic polymers that are insoluble in water and absorb fluids (Watson-Genna, 2009)

A. Gel dressings promote moist wound healing and are used for nipples that have cracks, fissures, and deep wounds (Cable et al., 1998; Cable et al., 1997; Dodd et al., 2003; Wilson, 2001).

   1. Absorb excess drainage
   2. Maintain a moist wound surface that enables epidermal cells to migrate across the wound
   3. Provide thermal insulation for improved blood flow
   4. Protect the wound from bacterial invasion or trauma

B. Types (Watson-Genna, 2009):

   1. Glycerin-based
   2. Water-based
   3. Available in gel, gauze, and precut sheet forms

C. Uses:

   1. Used on nipples for superficial or partial thickness wounds to enhance the healing process (Walker, 2011)

D. Advantages:

   1. Provides instant soothing relief of nipple pain (Dodd et al., 2003)
   2. Speeds wound granulation and healing; prevents scab formation
   3. Can be reused for several days
   4. Nonadherent
   5. Oxygen permeable
   6. Maintains a clean, moist environment
   7. Comfortable and flexible
   8. May reduce bacterial skin infections (Brent et al., 1998; Dodd et al., 2003)

E. Disadvantages:

   1. Might macerate periwound skin.
   2. Some brands have minimal absorption.
   3. Water-based products can dry out rapidly when exposed to air.
   4. Have the potential in certain situations to contribute to yeast, bacterial overgrowth, or mastitis (Zeimer et al., 1995).
      a. Dressings should not be applied in the presence of a known wound infection.
      b. Wound should be inspected frequently for presence of infection and reported to physician.
   5. Mixed reviews in the research show that it may not be more effective than other treatments
   6. If the mother forgets that the gel dressing is in place and/or has cut it very small, the baby can suck it into the mouth and choke on it.
   7. Can be expensive.

F. Technique for use (Watson-Genna, 2009):
   1. Wash hands before handling.
   2. The dressing should be cut about one-fourth to one-half inch larger than the wound.
   3. Some dressings are manufactured specifically for nipple care and are small and round, not requiring cutting.
   4. Remove the backing to the dressing and apply the gel side to the wound.
   5. The dressing is removed before nursing and placed on a clean surface, gel side up or in manufacturer's protective covering.
   6. The dressing can be chilled and reapplied following each feeding.
   7. The breast does not need to be washed prior to nursing.
   8. Rinsing the breast with plain water before and after feedings may reduce the incidence of infections (Wilson-Clay et al., 2008).
   9. May not be tolerated by mothers with nipple vasospasm.
   10. If the dressing becomes stuck, flood with ample water to loosen.
   11. Follow manufacturer's directions.
      a. Water-based dressing may be rinsed.
      b. Glycerin-based dressings should not be rinsed.
      c. Discard and apply new dressing according to manufacturer's instructions.
G. Creams (cosmetic, nonmedicated):
   1. Creams have been used to soothe and/or "treat" sore nipples for hundreds of years; most creams have a soothing effect but do not prevent or cure nipple pain. Instruction in breastfeeding technique is more effective (Frantz, 2000; Hewat et al., 1987; Moreland-Schultz, 2005; Morse, 1989a, 1989b; Pugh et al., 1996; Riordan et al., 2010).
   2. Types:
      a. Purified lanolin or lanolin-predominant creams.
         i. Modified lanolin generally has the lowest level of free alcohol and appears to be free of pesticides.
      b. Peppermint water (Melli et al., 2007).
      c. Honey-based topical cream (Watson-Genna, 2009).
      d. Some creams have questionable ingredients and are not recommended:
         i. Vitamin E oil, cocoa butter, Bag Balm, vitamins A and D ointment, Vaseline, baby oil
   3. Uses:
      a. Reduce nipple pain (especially when used with breast shells).
      b. Create a moist wound healing environment (Hinman et al., 1963; Huml, 1995, 1999).
      c. Lanolin used with breast shells reduces and promotes healing (Brent et al., 1998).
      d. May be used in women with vasospasm (Watson-Genna, 2009).

4. Advantages:
   a. Can speed healing process (Huml, 1995; Pugh et al., 1996; Spangler et al., 1993).
   b. Might reduce pain and have a soothing effect.
   c. Widely available and inexpensive.
   d. Most do not need to be washed off prior to feedings.
   e. Might serve to lubricate dry skin and protect it from maceration.
5. Disadvantages:
   a. Some products might need to be washed off before each feeding. This wiping off can remove moisture from the skin, create further damage, and slow wound healing.
   b. Some combination creams have ingredients that could provoke an allergy in the infant, such as peanut oil.
   c. Some have petroleum bases and other ingredients that could irritate nipple skin.
   d. Lanolin should have the lowest possible free alcohol content to avoid aggravating a wool allergy in susceptible mothers.
   e. Research does not support the use of any types of creams over good positioning and latch-on instruction (Cadwell et al., 2004; Mohammadzadeh et al., 2005; Tait, 2000).

V. Droppers

A plastic or glass tube with a squeeze bulb at one end. Little research is available on the use of droppers.

A. Types:
   1. May be made completely of soft plastic; some are glass with a rubber bulb; some are small, child size.
B. Uses:
   1. Provide milk incentives at the breast to achieve latch-on.
      a. Finger-feed to take the edge off hunger before attempting latch-on.
   2. Complementary feeding when breastmilk intake is not sufficient.
   3. Temporary aid to improve suck organization.
C. Advantages:
   1. Avoids the use of artificial nipples.
   2. Inexpensive and widely available.
   3. Easy to use and teach parents.
   4. Quick way for baby to receive small amounts of milk while learning to breastfeed.
   5. Baby may be more eager to breastfeed because sucking needs are not met.
D. Disadvantages:
   1. Can be difficult to clean.
   2. Must be continually refilled.

   3. Baby does not learn to suck unless the dropper is used in conjunction with finger feeding.
   4. Sucking on the dropper alone will not teach correct sucking patterns.
   5. Time consuming and messy (Wight, 2008).
   6. Research on use of droppers for supplementation is very limited.
   E. Technique (Marmet et al., 1984; Mohrbacher et al., 2003; Ross, 1987):
   1. If using with a finger, place the filled dropper along the side of the finger as the baby draws the finger into his or her mouth.
   2. Allow the baby to suck the milk out of the dropper. If the baby is unable to perform this task, one or two drops can be placed on the baby's tongue to initiate swallowing and sucking.
   3. Milk should not be squirted into the baby's mouth.
   F. A dropper can be placed into the corner of the baby's mouth while latching on to the breast; one or two drops of milk can then be placed on the tongue to initiate a swallow followed by a suck.
   1. The infant must be alert, not sleepy, and have a functioning swallow reflex.

VI. Spoons (Jones, 1998; Mohrbacher et al., 2003; Wilson-Clay et al., 2008)

   A. Types
   1. Teaspoon, tablespoon, plastic spoon, medicine spoon with a hollow handle, commercially available spoon-shaped device attached to a milk reservoir
   B. Uses
   1. Feed the baby when breastfeeding is interrupted (Darzi et al., 1996)
   2. Complementary feeding when breastfeeding is not sufficient
   3. Feed the baby colostrum that has been hand-expressed or pumped to complement the early feedings and prevent hypoglycemia
   4. Prime the baby for feeding at the breast
   C. Advantages
   1. Avoids the use of artificial nipples
   2. Can be used as a temporary aid to initiate milk intake for the baby who has not yet latched on
   3. Inexpensive and easily available
   4. Easy to use and clean
   5. Baby may be more eager to breastfeed because sucking needs are not met
   6. Can be used to administer small volumes (such as colostrum) efficiently
   D. Disadvantages
   1. Must be continually refilled.
   2. Does not teach the baby to suck at the breast.
   3. Fluid in the mouth is not associated with sucking.
   4. Does not correct improper sucking patterns.
   5. Research to support spoon feeding is limited.

E. Technique
1. Position the baby in a semiupright position.
2. Place the spoon just inside the infant's lips over the tongue.
3. Allow the infant to pace the feeding by sipping or lapping.
4. Avoid pouring the milk into the baby's mouth.
5. The baby should be alert with a functioning swallow reflex.

VII. Cups (Academy of Breastfeeding Medicine [ABM], 2007; Armstrong, 1987; Biancuzzo, 1997; Cloherty et al., 2005; Davis et al., 1948; Fredeen, 1948; Jones, 1998; Kuehl, 1997; Lang, 1994; Mohrbacher et al., 2003; Musoke, 1990; Newman, 1990; Wilson-Clay et al., 2008)

A. Types
1. 1-ounce (28–30 milliliters) medicine cups, plastic small drinking cups
2. Small cups with an extended lip or edge to control the flow of milk
3. Flexible silicone cups with a restricted outlet
4. Paladai—a small pitcher-shaped device from India
B. Uses
1. Feed the infant when breastfeeding is interrupted.
2. Complementary feeding when breastfeeding is not sufficient.
3. Used with both term and preterm infants to avoid bottle nipple preference.
4. The mother is unavailable to breastfeed.
C. Advantages (Collins et al., 2004; Gupta et al., 1999; Howard, de Blieck et al., 1999; Howard et al., 2003; Kuehl, 1997; Lang, 1994; Mosley et al., 2001; Rocha et al., 2002)
1. Avoids the use of artificial nipples.
2. Inexpensive and widely available.
3. Easy to use and to teach parents to use.
4. Reduces the incidence of bottle-feeding-associated apnea and bradycardia in preterm infants (Marinelli et al., 2001).
5. Noninvasive alternative to gavage feeding; reduces the risk of esophageal perforation and oral aversion (Lang et al., 1994).
6. Baby may be more eager to breastfeed because sucking needs are not met.
7. A quick way to supplement or complement breastfeeding.
8. Physiological stability.
9. Good weight gain.
10. Promotes breastfeeding in preterm infants. The baby is fed by cup when the mother is not present to breastfeed (Kuehl, 1997).
11. Increases the likelihood late preterm or premature infant will be fully breastfed at hospital discharge (Collins et al., 2004; Abouelfettoh et al., 2008; Wight, 2008).
12. Reduces nipple confusion (Huang et al., 2009).
13. Does not hyperstimulate the buccinators muscle as bottle-feeding does (Gomes et al., 2006).

D. Disadvantages (Dowling et al., 2002; Thorley, 1997)

1. The cup must be frequently refilled.
2. The baby can dribble much milk, reducing intake.
   a. Using a paladai gives greater control and reduces the amount of spilled milk (Malhotra et al., 1999).
   b. If measuring intake is critical, the bib can be weighed before and after feeding to determine the volume lost.
3. The baby does not learn to suck; therefore, cups might delay return to the breast.
4. The infant, parents, or healthcare providers can become dependent on the cup.
5. Risk of aspiration (similar to that of bottle-feeding) if cup feeding is performed improperly.
6. May delay hospital discharge of preterm infant (Collins et al., 2004).
7. Paladai showed more spillage and stress cues than bottle-feeding did (Aloysius et al., 2007).

E. Technique (Biancuzzo, 2002; Healow, 1995; Kuehl, 1997; Lang et al., 1994; Mohrbacher et al., 2003; Wilson-Clay et al., 2008)

1. The baby should be in a calm, alert state (not sleepy).
2. Position the baby in a nearly upright position, wrapped so that his or her hands do not bump the cup.
3. Fill the cup about half full.
4. Place the rim of the cup on the baby's lower lip with the cup tilted just to the point of the milk coming into contact with the upper lip.
5. Do not apply pressure to the lower lip.
6. Let the baby pace the feeding by sipping or lapping at the milk (Lang, 1994; Mizuno et al., 2005; Rocha et al., 2002).
7. Do not pour the milk into the baby's mouth. Do not overwhelm the infant with milk.
8. Leave the cup in the same position during the baby's pauses so that the baby does not need to continually reorganize oral conformation.
9. Refill as needed.

VIII. Syringes (Marmet et al., 1984; Mohrbacher et al., 2003; Riordan, 2005; Ross, 1987; Watson-Genna, 2008)

A. Types

1. 10-milliliter to 50-milliliter capacity; used with a 5 French gavage tube or tubing from butterfly needle (needle removed) (Edgehouse et al., 1990; Walker, 2011; Watson-Genna, 2009).
2. Periodontal syringe, 10-milliliter capacity with a curved tip.
3. Regular syringes (without the needle) are usually not used because the infant might have difficulty forming a complete seal.

B. Uses
  1. To provide an incentive at the breast to encourage latch-on, to initiate suckling, or to aid in sustaining the suckling once started
  2. To provide complementary or supplementary feeding while the infant simultaneously sucks on a caregiver's finger

C. Advantages (Marmet et al., 1984; Riordan, 2005)
  1. Avoids the use of artificial nipples and keeps the baby at the breast
  2. Might help improve uncoordinated mouth and tongue movements
  3. Provides a source of milk flow that will work to regulate the suck
  4. Easy to teach parents to do

D. Disadvantages
  1. Supplies might not be widely available.
  2. More intrusive.
  3. Infant can become dependent on the method.
  4. Infant might demonstrate poor jaw excursion while sucking on an adult finger.
  5. Some periodontal syringes have a rough tip that could irritate the baby's mouth.
  6. Some have legal concerns about using equipment for a purpose that it was not intended.
  7. Research to support syringe feeding is limited.

E. Technique (Mohrbacher et al., 2003; Oddy et al., 2003; Ross, 1987; Walker, 2011; Wilson-Clay, 2008)
  1. At the breast, insert the tip of the syringe (or feeding tube) just inside the infant's lips at the corner of his or her mouth.
  2. Give a small bolus of milk (0.25–0.5 milliliter) when the infant sucks.
     a. Rate initially: Suck: bolus: suck: bolus.
     b. When infant is sucking well, the pattern will be "suck, suck, bolus: suck, suck, bolus" or "suck, suck, suck, bolus: suck, suck, suck, bolus."
  3. On the finger, place the infant in a semiupright position in the caregiver's arms or in an inclined infant seat.
  4. Parents can use a washed finger; the healthcare provider should wash his or her hands and use a finger cot.
  5. Use the finger that is closest in size to the circumference of the mother's nipple.
  6. Introduce the finger into the infant's mouth pad up, enabling the baby to pull the finger back to the junction of the hard and soft palates.
  7. If the infant resists, withdraw the finger slightly, pause until he or she is comfortable, and then proceed.
  8. Place the syringe or tubing next to the finger, making sure that it is positioned so that it will not poke the infant.
  9. As the infant sucks, reward correct suckling motions with a small bolus of milk.
  10. Use the rate of suck:bolus to entice a reluctant feeder, allowing the infant to gradually suck the milk from the device.
  11. Once sustained sucking is achieved, slow rate to suck, suck, suck, bolus.

12. Time frame is about 15 to 20 minutes.

13. If this technique is being used to prime the baby for the breast, place the baby at the breast when he or she demonstrates a sucking rhythm.

14. If the baby stops for more than 10 to 20 seconds, arouse the baby.

15. If the tongue lies behind the lower gum ridge, apply slight pressure to the back of the tongue to stroke it forward over the lower gum ridge.

IX. Tube Feeding Devices

Commercially available devices usually consist of a reservoir or container for milk, with one or two thin flexible lengths of tubing attached. The container for milk can be a syringe, a bottle clipped to the shoulder area, a bottle suspended on a cord around the mother's neck, a plastic bag, or a bottle with a regular artificial nipple through which the tubing is threaded. The container might have one or two thin lengths of flexible tubing. Follow the manufacturer's instructions for using larger or smaller tubing sizes.

A. Tubing is usually attached by tape to the mother's nipple/areola or to the finger of the feeder.

B. Uses (Newman et al., 2006; Watson-Genna, 2009):

1. To provide complementary feeding to an infant at the breast for low milk supply, inefficient suckling, slow weight gain, adoptive nursing, relactation, preterm infant, or for neurologically affected infants.

2. The tubing can also be attached to a finger for others to feed the baby or to prime the baby for going to the breast.

C. Advantages (Borucki, 2005; Mohrbacher et al., 2003; Riordan, 2005; Wilson-Clay et al., 2008):

1. Avoids the use of artificial nipples.

2. Might help improve sucking organization and patterns.

3. Enables delivery of supplements if needed while preserving the breastfeeding.

4. Increasing the flow rate at the breast may encourage a reluctant infant to breastfeed.

D. Disadvantages (Hughes, 2010; Sealy, 1996):

1. More intrusive and complex technique to learn and to repeat many times per day; may be rejected by mothers.

2. Supplies might not be widely available.

3. Cost.

4. Infant can become dependent on the method.

5. Infant can learn to prefer faster flow rate at breast.

6. The infant might exhibit shallow jaw excursions while sucking on an adult finger.

7. Time consuming to clean the equipment after each use.

8. Some mothers find it awkward at first to get both the tubing and the nipple into the infant's mouth.

9. If the milk container is positioned too low or the tubing is kinked, the infant might not receive milk.

10. If the milk container is too high, the infant may receive milk without sucking.

11. Some mothers might be allergic to the tape that is used to secure the tubing in place at the breast; consider paper tape or nonallergenic tapes or dressings.

12. Do not allow the infant to suck on the tubing like a straw without the nipple also in her or his mouth.

13. There is little published research on the efficacy of feeding tube devices. Manufacturers are the source of information.

E. Technique (Benakappa, 2002; Hughes, 2010; Jones, 1998; Newman, 1990; Newman et al., 2006; Walker, 2011; Watson-Genna, 2008; Wilson-Clay et al., 2008):

1. Tube feeding on a finger proceeds in a similar manner as with the syringe feeding (described earlier).

2. When used at the breast, the milk reservoir can be elevated or lowered to achieve control over the milk flow speed and placed so that the top of the fluid is level with the mother's nipples; the milk should flow only when the baby sucks.

3. The baby should take both the nipple and areola and the tubing into his or her mouth.

4. Tape the tubing so that it enters the infant's mouth in the corner or under the mother's nipple over the infant's tongue (preferred).

5. Position the tube so that it will not extend beyond the nipple tip when positioned in the infant's mouth.

6. To increase the flow for small or weaker babies, lower the container. If the device has two tubes, open the other tube as a vent or use both tubes on one breast, or raise the device higher or use both tubes on one breast.

7. If the device has a choice of tubing sizes, use the largest size for a preterm baby, a disorganized infant, or one who needs an easier flow; advance the baby to the smaller sizes as sucking improves (Wilson-Clay et al., 2008).

8. Babies need close follow-up for frequent weight checks and to be weaned off the device as soon as possible.

X. Haberman Feeder

A specialized feeding bottle with a valve and teat mechanism to adjust the milk flow to prevent overwhelming or flooding the baby with milk. Three lines on the bottle correspond to three flow rates.

A. Uses
1. Severe feeding problems, such as Down syndrome, cleft lip/palate, neurological dysfunction, disorganized sucking, preterm infants, cardiac defects, cystic fibrosis (Riordan & et al., 2010; Trenouth et al., 1996; Watson-Genna, 2008)

B. Advantages (Mohrbacher et al., 2003; Riordan, 2005; Ross, 1987; Wilson-Clay et al., 2008)
1. May be effective with an infant who is otherwise difficult to feed.

2. If the baby cannot nurse at all or needs assistance, the bottle can be squeezed to release a limited volume of milk.

3. The smaller feeder has a shorter teat for smaller babies.

4. Can be used as a quicker means of complementary or supplementary feeding.

C. Disadvantages

1. Exposes the infant to an artificial nipple.

2. Might promote a shallow latch-on when the infant goes to the breast.

3. Might be difficult to obtain.

4. Cost.

5. Little research exists regarding the efficacy of Haberman feeders; the manufacturer is the source of information.

D. Technique (Watson-Genna, 2008)

1. Place the nipple onto the infant's upper lip or philtrum or lay across lips resting on philtrum. Allow infant to draw it into the mouth if capable.

2. Pull back on the nipple gently if the baby has a shallow gag reflex or to help the baby to start sucking.

3. Teat may be squeezed to assist milk flow in infants who have weak suck or are unable to achieve seal.

4. Rotate the nipple to adjust the rate of flow to meet the needs and capability of the baby. Rotate the feeder to achieve a 1:1:1 (suck:swallow:breathe) ratio. Follow any particular guidance/instructions for babies with cleft palates.

XI. Pacifiers (Dummies)

A wide variety of shapes of pacifiers are manufactured but generally consist of a nipple-shaped tip, a wide guard that rests on the infant's lips, and a handle. Used by 50–80% of mothers (Riordan et al., 2010).

A. Uses

1. Treat delayed swallowing.

2. In nonorally fed infants, pacifiers help maintain oral motor patterns and tactile response that will be necessary to transition to feeding at the breast (Barros et al., 1995; Engebretson et al., 1997).

3. Meets high sucking needs.

4. Frequently used in United States to calm a fussy baby in the absence of the mother.

5. Nonnutritive sucking practice for premature infant (Pinelli et al., 2002; Wight, 2008).

6. Reduce pain during painful procedures (Boyle et al., 2006; Curtis et al., 2007; Mathai et al., 2006; Phillips et al., 2005).

7. Pacifier use may be a marker for other breastfeeding difficulties (O'Connor et al., 2009).

B. Advantages (Cockburn et al., 1996; Measel et al., 1979; Medoff-Cooper et al., 1995; Riordan, 2005; Victora et al., 1993; Watson-Genna, 2008; Wilson-Clay et al., 2008)
   1. Enables sucking activity for an infant who might otherwise overfeed (Riordan et al., 2010).
   2. Might quiet a crying baby in the absence of the mother.
   3. May reduce pain in preterm infants (Pinelli et al., 2002).
   4. Nonnutritive sucking in the preterm infant might help in more rapid transition to oral feeding (Drosten, 1997; Gill et al., 1988; Kinneer et al., 1994).
   5. Pacifier use when infants are laid down to sleep has been associated with reduced incidence of sudden infant death syndrome in infants older than 1 month of age (American Academy of Pediatrics [AAP], 2005; Hauck et al., 2005). However, this finding needs further study, and pacifier use continues to be open to debate (Mitchell et al., 2006).
   6. May be used while infant is being fed by tube feeding to associate sucking and stomach fullness.
C. Disadvantages (Aarts et al., 1999; Drane, 1996; Hill et al., 1997; Howard, Howard et al., 1999; Neimela et al., 1995; Newman et al., 2000; North et al., 1999; Righard, 1998; Righard et al., 1997; Schubiger et al., 1997; Vogel et al., 2001; Wilson-Clay et al., 2008)
   1. Exposes an infant to an artificial nipple.
   2. Displaces sucking from the breast.
   3. Might cause drowsiness in the baby and missed feedings.
   4. Increased incidence of otitis media.
   5. Vector for continued fungal infection.
   6. May cause shorter breastfeeding duration (Abdun-Nur et al., 2010; Benis, 2002; Victora et al., 1997; Victora et al., 1993).
   7. Might see increased rates of malocclusion and dental problems (Peres et al., 2007).
   8. Increases the risk for latex allergy (Venuta et al., 1999).
   9. Pacifiers with balls on the tip enable the baby to maintain the pacifier in the mouth with a weak lick–suck motion, rather than functional sucking activity (Ferrante et al., 2006).
   10. Orthodontic pacifiers might flatten the central grooving of the tongue.
D. Technique
   1. Pacifiers should be used with caution.
   2. Nonorally fed infants might benefit from sucking on a number of differently shaped pacifiers to avoid becoming accustomed to only one shape.
   3. Pacifiers should be avoided until after the first month of life when breastfeeding is well established (AAP, 2005).
   4. Pacifiers should be discontinued after 6 months of life to reduce ear infections (Sexton et al., 2009).

XII. Artificial Nipples

A. Bottle nipples come in a wide range of shapes and sizes. No artificial bottle nipple precisely mimics the dynamic qualities of the human breast (Ardran et al., 1958; Coats, 1990; Davis et al., 1948; Glover et al., 1990; Henrison, 1990; Jones, 1998; Matthew, 1991, 1998; Nowak et al., 1994, 1995; Riordan, 2005; Turgeon-O'Brien et al., 1996; Weber et al., 1986; Woolridge, 1986).

    1. Artificial nipples are made from silicone, rubber, or latex.

    2. Numerous sizes and shapes are available.

    3. Round, cross-section nipples tend to be straight and gradually taper to a flared base.

    4. Orthodontic nipples have bulblike ends and narrow necks.

    5. Some have a very wide base to encourage the baby to keep the mouth open wider.

    6. Artificial nipples do not elongate in the mouth as the human breast does.

    7. Types of openings:

       a. Holes.

       b. Crosscuts.

       c. Crosscut nipples do not enable milk to drip from them, but compression on them removes fluid.

    8. Hole size is one of the major determinants of flow rate.

       a. Nipples have high, medium, and low flow rates depending on the number of holes and the size of the holes. Hole diameter can vary from nipple to nipple from the same manufacturer.

       b. Some nipples have the hole on the top rather than the tip to avoid milk squirting down the infant's throat.

B. Advantages

    1. Ease and speed of feedings.

    2. Some artificial nipples are used in special situations to assist infants in learning sucking patterns (Kassing, 2002; Medoff-Cooper, 2004).

    3. Easily obtained.

    4. Useful when parents reject alternative feeding methods (Wilson-Clay et al., 2008)

C. Disadvantages (see **Table 34-1**)

    1. Infant might learn to prefer the bottle nipple (Newman, 1990; Righard 1998; Stein, 1990).

    2. Flow might be faster than with breastfeeding and is especially likely during the first few days postpartum, so baby becomes accustomed to a quick delivery of milk.

    3. Fast flow can contribute to apnea and bradycardia in preterm or stressed infants (Wilson-Clay et al., 2008).

    4. Shape is different and consistency is firmer, potentially causing the infant to prefer the stronger stimulus of the artificial nipple (Neifert et al., 1995; Newman, 1990).

    5. Encourages the baby to close his or her mouth, not open wide, and even bite on the narrowed neck of some of the nipples.

Table 34-1 Comparison of Bottle- and Breastfeeding

Bottle-feeding	Breastfeeding
Firm nipple	Soft, amorphous shaped nipple
Inelastic nipple	Nipple elongates during sucking
Flow begins instantly	Flow is delayed until the milk ejection reflex occurs
Flow is very fast	Flow is slow, faster during the milk ejection reflex
Feeding is very quick	Feeding a newborn may take 30 to 45 minutes
Sucking on bottle is suction/vacuum	Suckling at breast is peristaltic tongue movement
Tongue is humped in back of mouth	Tongue is forward cupped around the nipple

Source: Adapted from Woolridge, 1986; Weber, Wooldridge, & Baum, 1986; Medoff-Cooper, 2004; Medoff-Cooper et al., 1995; Ardran et al., 1958; Jones, 1998; Wilson-Clay et al., 2008; Riordan, 2005; Walker, 2011.

6. Orthodontic nipples cause a "squash and fill" type of sucking, remove the central grooving of the tongue, and enable the infant to close the mouth tightly around the nipple (McBride et al., 1987; Wilson-Clay et al., 2008).

7. Long nipples might trigger a gag reflex in some babies.

8. Can contribute to latex allergy.

9. Weakens the strength of the suck; reduces the strength of the masseter muscle (Inoue et al., 1995; Sakashita et al., 1996).

10. Muscles involved in breastfeeding are either immobilized, overactive, or malpositioned during bottle-feeding, which can contribute to abnormal dental and facial development in the child (Palmer, 1998).

11. Bottle-feeding has been positively correlated with finger sucking, which can deform the palate and contribute to malocclusion (Palmer, 1998).

12. Risk of aspiration from a too-fast flow (Wilson-Clay et al., 2008).

13. May shorten the duration of breastfeeding (Cronenwett et al., 1992; Kurinij & Shiono, 1991; Righard, 1998; Schubiger et al., 1997; Wright et al., 1996).

14. Infants may not self-regulate volume, leading to obesity (Li et al., 2010).

D. Technique (sometimes called paced bottle-feeding; Coats, 1991; Kassing, 2002; Noble et al., 1997; Wilson-Clay et al., 2008)

1. Select a nipple with a long shank, wide base, and slow flow of milk.

2. Position the infant nearly upright in caregiver's arms (not infant seat).

3. Tickle the infant's lips with the nipple and allow the baby to draw the nipple into the mouth him- or herself.

4. Position the bottle horizontally with just enough angle to keep fluid in the nipple tip.

5. Mother holds infant with cheek to her breast.

6. Position the bottle so the infant's jaws are over the wide base.

7. Observe for signs of a milk flow that is too fast or too slow and for stress cues (Wilson-Clay et al., 2008).

8. Pace the feeding to approximately the same suck:swallow ratio as a breastfeeding. If the infant drinks too quickly or does not breathe within three to five sucks, tip the bottle down or remove the bottle to allow a short break (Law-Morstatt et al., 2003).

9. If the bottle is removed, wait for the infant's cues (seeking, open mouth) before replacing it.

10. May squeeze the nipple before inverting the bottle; this creates a small amount of suction that slows the flow.

11. Switch sides halfway through the feeding.

12. During pacing, the bottle can be removed from the infant's mouth and rested on the philtrum until infant shows readiness. Or it can be lowered so that there is no fluid in the nipple until the infant shows readiness, then it can be raised again (Wilson-Clay et al., 2008).

13. Return infant to breast. If the baby resists, feed with bottle near breast, offer the bottle, then the breast; if infant refuses, use the bottle again. Continue until infant takes breast (Watson-Genna, 2008).

XIII. Infant Scale

An infant scale that can measure weight changes within 2 grams is appropriate for use with a breastfeeding baby to determine intake (Haase et al., 2009; Meier et al., 1990, 1994, 1996). Other researchers question the accuracy of test weights (Savenije et al., 2006).

A. Uses

1. Determine breastmilk intake at a feeding session.

2. Determine infant weight gain/loss over time.

3. Milk consumed at the breast can be used to determine whether supplementation is necessary (Wilson-Clay et al., 2008).

4. Information can contribute to decision to discharge preterm infant from the hospital.

B. Advantages

1. Weight gain in grams is equal to volume consumed (Meier et al., 1994).

2. Measures small weight increases (Meier et al., 1994).

3. More accurate than observation of a breastfeeding session by a trained observer (Meier et al., 1994, 1996; Wight, 2008).

4. Reassuring to mothers of preterm infants of adequate intake (Hurst et al., 2004) but not related to maternal confidence and competence scores (Hall et al., 2002).

C. Disadvantages

    1. Cost of the scale

    2. Must use digital scale, not mechanical or balance scale (Meier et al., 1990)

    3. Possibility of error caused by tubing or wires attached to infant

D. Technique (Spatz, 2004)

    1. Place scale on a flat surface and ensure the leveling bubble is centered.

    2. Periodically check the accuracy of the scale with a reference weight.

    3. If the scale is used by many infants, clean it first with disinfectant solution.

    4. When weighing an infant, ensure that all parameters are the same for the before-feeding weight and the after-feeding weight: use the same clothing, same diaper, same tubing, and wires if the infant is attached to medical equipment.

    5. Do not drape blankets or clothing over the scale that could affect its accuracy.

    6. Disconnect any tubing or wires that are safe to temporarily disconnect. Any leads or tubing attached to the baby can be weighed with the baby. Any tubing that cannot be safely disconnected should be marked with tape so that the exact amount of tubing is weighed both times.

      a. Do not lift tubing or leads during weighing because this leads to error.

    7. Obtain prefeed weight, two times for accuracy.

    8. Remove the infant for feeding.

    9. Reweigh the infant after each breast, or at the end of the feeding, two times for accuracy.

    10. Determine the weight gain.

References

Aarts, C., Hornell, A., Kylberg, E., et al. (1999). Breastfeeding patterns in relation to thumb sucking and pacifier use. *Pediatrics, 104*, e50. Retrieved from http://www.pediatrics.org/cgi/content/full/104/4/e50

Abdun-Nur, D., & Abdun-Nur, K. (2010). Do pacifiers reduce the risk of sudden infant death syndrome? *American Family Physician, 1*(5), 456.

Abouelfettoh, A. M., Dowling, D. A., Dabash, S. A., et al. (2008). Cup versus bottle feeding for hospitalized late preterm infants in Egypt: A quasi-experimental study. *International Breastfeeding Journal, 3*, 27.

Academy of Breastfeeding Medicine. (2009). Hospital guidelines for the use of supplementary feedings in the healthy term breastfed neonate. Retrieved from http://www.bfmed.org/Media/Files/Protocols/Protocol%203%20English%20Supplementation.pdf

Alexander, J. M., Grant, A. M., & Campbell, M. J. (1992). Randomized controlled trial of breast shells and Hoffman's exercises for inverted and non-protractile nipples. *British Medical Journal, 304*, 1030–1032.

Aloysius, A., & Hickson, M. (2007). Evaluation of paladai cup feeding in breast-fed preterm infants compared with bottle feeding. *Early Human Development, 83*(9), 619–621.

Amatayakul, K., Vutyavanich, T., Tanthayaphinat, O., et al. (1987). Serum prolactin and cortisol levels after sucking for varying periods of time and the effect of a nipple shield. *Acta Obstetricia et Gynecologica Scandinavica, 66*, 47–51.

American Academy of Pediatrics. (2005). Policy statement. The changing concept of sudden infant death syndrome: Diagnostic coding shifts, controversies regarding the sleeping environment and new variables to consider in reducing risk. *Pediatrics, 115,* 1245–1253.

Ardran, G. M., Kemp, F. H., & Lind, J. (1958). A cineradiographic study of bottle feeding. *British Journal of Radiology, 31,* 11–22.

Armstrong, H. (1987). Feeding low birth weight babies: Advances in Kenya. *Journal of Human Lactation, 3,* 34–37.

Arsenault, G. (1997). Using a disposable syringe to treat inverted nipples. *Canadian Family Physician, 43,* 1517–1518.

Auerbach, K. G. (1990). The effect of nipple shields on maternal milk volume. *Journal of Obstetric, Gynecologic, and Neonatal Nursing, 19,* 419–427.

Barger, C. (1997). Nipple shields: LCs not looking for quick fix. *Journal of Human Lactation, 13,* 193–194.

Barros, F. C., Victoria, C. G., Semer, T. C., et al. (1995). Use of pacifiers is associated with decreased breastfeeding duration. *Pediatrics, 95,* 497–499.

Benakappa, A. (2002). A new lact-aid technique. *Indian Pediatrics, 39,* 1169.

Benis, M. M. (2002). Are pacifiers associated with early weaning from breastfeeding? *Advances in Neonatal Care, 2(5),* 259–266.

Biancuzzo, M. (1997). Creating and implementing a protocol for cup feeding. *Mother and Baby Journal, 2,* 27–33.

Biancuzzo, M. (2002). *Breastfeeding the newborn: Clinical strategies for nurses* (2nd ed.). St. Louis, MO: Mosby.

Bodley, V., & Powers, D. (1996). Long-term nipple shield use—a positive perspective. *Journal of Human Lactation, 12,* 301–304.

Borucki, L. C. (2005). Breastfeeding mothers' experiences using a supplemental feeding tube device: Finding an alternative. *Journal of Human Lactation, 21*(4), 429–439.

Boyle, E. M., Freer, Y., Khan-Orakzai, Z., et al. (2006). Sucrose and non-nutritive sucking for the relief of pain in screening for retinopathy of prematurity: A randomized controlled trial. *Archives of Disease in Childhood: Fetal and Neonatal Edition, 91*(3), F166–168.

Brent, N., Rudy, S. J., Redd, B., et al. (1998). Sore nipples in breast-feeding women: A clinical trial of wound dressings vs conventional care. *Archives of Pediatric and Adolescent Med*icine, *152*(11), 1077–1082.

Brigham, M. (1996). Mother's reports of the outcome of nipple shield use. *Journal of Human Lactation, 12,* 91–97.

Brown, S. H., Alexander, J., & Thomas, P. (1999). Feeding outcome in breast-fed term babies supplemented by cup or bottle. *Midwifery, 15*(2), 92–96.

Brown, S. J. (2003). Nipple shields—never a good thing? *Practising Midwife, 6,* 42.

Buchko, B., Pugh, L., Bishop, B., et al. (1993). Comfort measures for breastfeeding, primiparous women. *Journal of Obstetric, Gynecologic, and Neonatal Nursing, 23,* 1.

Cable, B. (2001). Hydrogel dressings. *Journal of Human Lactation, 17*(4), 295.

Cable, B., & Davis, J. (1998). Hydrogel dressings not to be used on infected tissue [Abstract]. *Journal of Human Lactation, 14,* 205.

Cable, B., Stewart, M., & Davis, J. (1997). Nipple wound care: A new approach to an old problem. *Journal of Human Lactation, 13,* 313–318.

Cadwell, K., Turner-Maffei, C., Blair, A., et al. (2004). Pain reduction and treatment of sore nipples in nursing mothers. *Journal of Perinatal Education, 13*(1), 29–35.

Centuori, S., Burmaz, T., Ronfani, L., et al. (1999). Nipple care, sore nipples, and breastfeeding: A randomized trial. *Journal of Human Lactation, 15*(2), 125–130.

Charkrabarti, K., & Basu, S. (2011). Management of flat or inverted nipples with simple rubber bands. *Breastfeeding Medicine, 6*, 215–219.

Chertok, I. R. (2009). Reexamination of ultra-thin nipple shield use, infant growth and maternal satisfaction. *Journal of Clinical Nursing, 18*(21), 2949–2955.

Chertok, I. R., Schneider, J., & Blackburn, S. (2006). A pilot study of maternal and term infant outcomes associated with ultrathin nipple shield use. *Journal of Obstetric, Gynecologic, and Neonatal Nursing, 35*, 265–272.

Cloherty, M., Alexander, J., Holloway, I., et al. (2005). The cup-versus-bottle debate: A theme from an ethnographic study of the supplementation of breastfed infants in hospital in the United Kingdom. *Journal of Human Lactation, 21*, 151–162.

Clum, D., & Primomo, J. (1996). Use of a silicone nipple shield with premature infants. *Journal of Human Lactation, 12*, 287–290.

Coats, M. M. (1990). Bottle-feeding like a breastfeeder: An option to consider. *Journal of Human Lactation, 6*, 10–11.

Coats, M. M. (1991). Learning at the conference [Abstract]. *Journal of Human Lactation, 7*(4), 174.

Cockburn, F., Tappin, D., & Stone, D. (1996). Breastfeeding, dummy use, and adult intelligence. *Lancet, 347*, 1765–1766.

Collins, C. T., Makrides, M., Gillis, J., et al. (2008). Avoidance of bottles during the establishment of breast feeds in preterm infants. *Cochrane Database of Systematic Reviews, 8*(4), CD005252.

Collins, C. T., Ryan, P., Crowther, C. A., et al. (2004). Effect of bottles, cups, and dummies on breast feeding in preterm infants: A randomised controlled trial. *British Medical Journal, 329*(7459), 193–198.

Cronenwett, L., Stukel, T., Kearney, M., et al. (1992). Single daily bottle use in the early weeks postpartum and breastfeeding outcomes. *Pediatrics, 90*, 760–766.

Curtis, S. J., Jou, H., Ali, S., et al. (2007). A randomized controlled trial of sucrose and/or pacifier as analgesia for infants receiving venipuncture in a pediatric emergency department. *BMC Pediatrics, 18*(7), 27.

Darzi, M. A., Chowdri, N. A., & Bhat, A. N. (1996). Breast feeding or spoon feeding after cleft lip repair: A prospective, randomized study. *British Journal of Plastic Surgery, 49*, 24–26.

Davanzo, R., Travan, L., & Brovedani, P. (2010). Practical strategies for promoting breastfeeding in neonatal intensive care. *Minerva Pediatrics, 62*(3 Suppl. 1), 205–206.

Davis, G. (2001). Safety of hydrogel dressings. *Journal of Human Lactation, 17*(2), 117.

Davis, H. V., Sears, R. R., Miller, H. C., et al. (1948). Effects of cup, bottle, and breastfeeding on oral activities of newborn infants. *Pediatrics, 2*, 549–558.

DeNicola, M. (1986). One case of nipple shield addiction. *Journal of Human Lactation, 2*, 28–30.

Dodd, V., & Chalmers, C. (2003). Comparing the use of hydrogel dressing to lanolin ointment with lactation mothers. *Journal of Obstetric, Gynecologic, and Neonatal Nursing, 32*, 486–494.

Dowling, D. A., Meier, P. P., DiFiore, J., et al. (2002). Cup-feeding for preterm infants: Mechanics and safety. *Journal of Human Lactation, 18*, 13–20.

Drane, D. (1996). The effect of use of dummies and teats on orofacial development. *Breastfeeding Review, 4*, 59–64.

Drazen, P. (1998). Taking nipple shields out of the closet. *Birth Issues, 7*, 41–49.

Drosten, F. (1997). Pacifiers in the NICU: A lactation consultant's view. *Neonatal Network, 16*, 47, 50.

Edgehouse, L., & Radzyminski, S. G. (1990). A device for supplementing breastfeeding. *American Journal of Maternal and Child Nursing, 15*, 34–35.

Elliott, C. (1996). Using a silicone nipple shield to assist a baby unable to latch. *Journal of Human Lactation, 12*(4), 309–313.

Engebretson, J., & Wardell, D. W. (1997). Development of a pacifier for low-birth-weight infants' nonnutritive sucking. *Journal of Obstetric, Gynecologic, and Neonatal Nursing, 26*, 660–664.

Ferrante, A., Silvestri, R., & Montinaro, C. (2006). The importance of choosing the right feeding aids to maintain breast-feeding after interruption. *International Journal of Orofacial Myology, 32*, 58–67.

Fetherston, C. (1998). Risk factors for lactation mastitis. *Journal of Human Lactation, 14*(2), 101–109.

Flint, A., New, K., & Davies, M. W. (2007). Cup feeding versus other forms of supplemental enteral feeding for newborn infants unable to fully breastfeed. *Cochrane Database of Systematic Reviews, 18*(2), CD005092.

Frantz, K. (2000). *Breastfeeding product guide.* Sunland, CA: Geddes Productions.

Fredeen, R. C. (1948). Cup feeding of newborn infants. *Pediatrics, 2*, 544–548.

Fucile, S., Gisel, E., Schanler, R. J., & Lau, C. (2009). A controlled-flow vacuum-free bottle system enhances preterm infants' nutritive sucking skills. *Dysphagia, 24*(2), 145–151.

Gill, N., Behnke, M. L., Conlon, M., et al. (1988). Effect of nonnutritive sucking on behavioral state in preterm infants before feeding. *Nursing Research, 37*, 347–350.

Glover, J., & Sandilands, M. (1990). Supplementation of breastfeeding infants and weight loss in hospital. *Journal of Human Lactation, 6*, 163–166.

Gomes, C. F., Trezza, E. M., Murade, E. C., et al. (2006). Surface electromyography of facial muscles during natural and artificial feeding of infants. *Journal of Pediatrics (Rio J), 82*(2), 103–109.

Gupta, A., Khanna, K., & Chattree, S. (1999). Cup feeding: An alternative to bottle feeding in a neonatal intensive care unit. *Journal of Tropical Pediatrics, 45*, 108–110.

Haase, B., Barreira, J., Murphy, P. K., et al. (2009). The development of an accurate test weighing technique for preterm and high-risk hospitalized infants. *Breastfeeding Medicine, 4*(3), 151–156.

Hall, W. A., Shearer, K., Mogan, J., & Berkowitz, J. (2002). Weighing preterm infants before and after breastfeeding: Does it increase maternal confidence and competence? *MCN American Journal of Maternal and Child Nursing, 27*, 318–326.

Hauck, F. R., Omojokun, O. O., & Siadaty, M. S. (2005). Do pacifiers reduce the risk of sudden infant death syndrome? A meta-analysis. *Pediatrics, 116*, 716–723.

Healow, L. K. (1995). Finger-feeding a preemie. *Midwifery Today, 33*, 9.

Henrison, M. A. (1990). Policy for supplementary/complementary feedings for breastfed newborn infants. *Journal of Human Lactation, 6*, 1–14.

Hewat, R. J., & Ellis, D. J. (1987). A comparison of the effectiveness of two methods of nipple care. *Birth, 14*, 41–45.

Hill, P. D., Humenick, S. S., Brennan, M. L., et al. (1997). Does early supplementation affect long-term breastfeeding? *Clinical Pediatrics, 36*, 345–350.

Hinman, C. D., & Maibach, H. (1963). Effect of air exposure and occlusion on experimental human skin wounds. *Nature, 200*, 377–388.

Howard, C. R., de Blieck, E. A., ten Hoopen, C. B., et al. (1999). Physiologic stability of newborns during cup- and bottle-feeding. *Pediatrics, 104*, 1204–1207.

Howard, C. R., Howard, F. M., Lanphear, B., et al. (1999). The effects of early pacifier use on breastfeeding duration. *Pediatrics*, *103*, e33.

Howard, C. R., Howard, F. M., Lanphear, B., et al. (2003). Randomized clinical trial of pacifier use and bottle-feeding or cupfeeding and their effect on breastfeeding. *Pediatrics*, *111*, 511–518.

Huang, Y. Y., Gau, M. L., Huang, C. M., & Lee, J. T. (2009). Supplementation with cup-feeding as a substitute for bottle-feeding to promote breastfeeding. *Chang Gung Medical Journal*, *32*(4), 423–431.

Huang, Y. Y., & Huang, C. M. (2006). Nipple confusion and breastfeeding: A literature review. *Hu Li Za Zhi*, *53*(2), 73–79.

Hughes, V. (2010). *Alternative feeding methods*. Fairfax, VA: Lactation Education Resources.

Huml, S. (1995, April). Cracked nipples in the breastfeeding mother. Looking at an old problem in a new way. *Advance for Nurse Practitioners*.

Huml, S. (1999). Sore nipples: A new look at an old problem through the eyes of a dermatologist. *Practising Midwife*, *2*, 28–31.

Hunter, H. H. (1999). Nipple shields. A tool that needs handling with care. *Practising Midwife*, *2*, 48–52.

Hurst, N. M., Meier, P. P., Engstrom, J. L., & Myatt, A. (2004). Mothers performing in-home measurement of milk intake during breastfeeding of their preterm infants: Maternal reactions and feeding outcomes. *Journal of Human Lactation*, *20*, 178–187.

Inoue, N., Sakashita, R., & Kamegai, T. (1995). Reduction in masseter muscle activity in bottle-fed babies. *Early Human Development*, *42*, 185–193.

Isaacson, L. J. (2006). Steps to successfully breastfeed the premature infant. *Neonatal Network*, *25*, 77–86.

Jackson, D., Woolridge, M., Imong, S. M., et al. (1987). The automatic sampling shield: A device for sampling suckled breastmilk. *Early Human Development*, *15*, 295–306.

Jackson, J. M., & Mourino, A. P. (1999). Pacifier use and otitis media in infants twelve months of age or younger. *Pediatric Dentistry*, *21*, 256–261.

Johnson, S. M. (1997). Further caution re: Nipple shields. *Journal of Human Lactation*, *13*, 101.

Jones, B. (1998). Choosing a supplementation method. *Journal of Human Lactation*, *14*, 245–246.

Kassing, D. (2002). Bottle-feeding as a tool to reinforce breastfeeding. *Journal of Human Lactation*, *18*(1), 56–60.

Kesaree, N., Banapurmath, C. R., Banapurmath, S., & Shamanur, K. (1993). Treatment of inverted nipples using a disposable syringe. *Journal of Human Lactation*, *9*, 27–29.

Kinneer, M., & Beachy, P. (1994). Nipple feeding premature infants in the neonatal intensive-care unit: Factors and decisions. *Journal of Obstetric, Gynecologic, and Neonatal Nursing*, *23*, 105–112.

Kuehl, J. (1997). Cup-feeding the newborn: What you should know. *Journal of Perinatal and Neonatal Nursing*, *11*, 56–60.

Kurinij, N., & Shiono, P. (1991). Early formula supplementation of breastfeeding. *Pediatrics*, *88*, 745–750.

Lactation Education Consultants. (1996). *Consent to use nipple shield*. Wheaton, IL: Author.

Lang, S. (1994). Cup-feeding: An alternative method. *Midwives Chronicle and Nursing Notes*, *107*, 171–176.

Lang, S. (2002). *Breastfeeding special care babies* (2nd ed.). London, England: Baillière Tindall.

Lang, S., Lawrence, C. J., & Orme, R. L. (1994). Cup feeding: An alternative method of infant feeding. *Archives of Disease in Childhood*, *71*, 365–369.

Lanses, M. G. (2011). Cup feeding—a valuable tool. *Journal of Human Lactation*, *27*(1), 12–13.

Lavergne, N. (1997). Does application of tea bags to sore nipples while breastfeeding provide effective relief? *Journal of Obstetric, Gynecologic, and Neonatal Nursing*, *26*(1), 53–58.

Law-Morstatt, L., Judd, D., Snyder, P., et al. (2003). Pacing as a treatment technique for transitional sucking patterns. *Journal of Perinatology, 23*, 483–488.

Lawrence, R. A. (1999). Storage of human milk and the influence of procedures on immunological components of human milk. *Acta Paediatrica, 88*(Suppl. 430), 14–18.

Lawrence, R. A., & Lawrence, T. (2011). *Breastfeeding: A guide for the medical profession* (7th ed.). Philadelphia, PA: Mosby.

Lennon, I., & Lewis, B. (1987). Effect of early complementary feeds on lactation failure. *Breastfeeding Review, 11*, 25–26.

Leslie, A., & Marlow, N. (2006). Non-pharmacological pain relief. *Seminars in Fetal and Neonatal Medicine, 11*(4), 246–250.

Li, R., Fein, S. B., & Grummer-Strawn, L. M. (2010). Do infants fed from bottles lack self-regulation of milk intake compared with directly breastfed infants? *Pediatrics, 125*(6), e1386–1393.

MAIN Trial Collaborative Group. (1994). Preparing for breast feeding: Treatment of inverted and non-protractile nipples in pregnancy. *Midwifery, 10*(4), 200–214.

Malhotra, N., Vishwimbaran, I., Sundaram, K. R., & Narayanan, I. (1999). A controlled trial of alternative methods of oral feeding in neonates. *Early Human Development, 54*, 29–38.

Marinelli, K. A., Burke, G. S., & Dodd, V. L. (2001). A comparison of the safety of cup feedings and bottle feedings in premature infants whose mothers intend to breastfeed. *Journal of Perinatology, 21*(6), 350–355.

Marmet, C., & Shell, E. (1984). Training neonates to suck correctly. *American Journal of Maternal and Child Nursing, 9*, 401–407.

Marmet, C., Shell, E., & Aldana, S. (2000). Assessing infant suck dysfunction: Case management. *Journal of Human Lactation, 16*, 332–336.

Marriott, M. (1997). Nipple shields used successfully. *Journal of Human Lactation, 13*, 12.

Mathai, S., Natrajan, N., & Rajalakshmi, N. R. (2006). A comparative study of nonpharmacological methods to reduce pain in neonates. *Indian Pediatrics, 43*(12), 1070–1075.

Matthew, O. P. (1991). Science of bottle feeding. *Journal of Pediatrics, 114*, 511–519.

Matthew, O. P. (1998). Nipple units for newborn infants: A functional comparison. *Pediatrics, 81*, 688–691.

McBride, M. C., & Danner, S. C. (1987). Sucking disorders in neurologically impaired infants: Assessment and facilitation of breastfeeding. *Clinical Perinatology, 14*, 190–130.

McGeorge, D. D. (1994). The "Niplette": An instrument for the non-surgical correction of inverted nipples. *British Journal of Plastic Surgery, 47*, 46–49.

McInnes, R. J., & Chambers, J. (2008). Infants admitted to neonatal units—interventions to improve breastfeeding outcomes: A systematic review 1990–2007. *Maternal and Child Nutrition, 4*(4), 235–263.

McKechnie, A. C., & Eglash, A. (2010). Nipple shields: A review of the literature. *Breastfeeding Medicine, 5*, 309–314.

Measel, C. P., & Anderson, G. C. (1979). Nonnutritive sucking during tube feeding: Effect on clinical course in premature infants. *Journal of Obstetric, Gynecologic, and Neonatal Nursing, 8*, 265–272.

Medoff-Cooper, B. (2004). Nutritive sucking research from clinical questions to research answers. *Journal of Perinatal and Neonatal Nursing, 19*, 265–272.

Medoff-Cooper, B., & Ray, W. (1995). Neonatal sucking behaviors. *Image: Journal of Nursing Scholarship, 27*, 195–199.

Meier, P. P., Brown, L. P., Hurst, N. M., et al. (2000). Nipple shields for preterm infants: Effect on milk transfer and duration of breastfeeding. *Journal of Human Lactation, 16*, 106–114.

Meier, P. P., Engstrom, J. L., Crichton, C. L., et al. (1994). A new scale for in-home test-weighing for mothers of preterm and high risk infants. *Journal of Human Lactation, 10*, 163–168.

Meier, P. P., Engstrom, J. L., Fleming, B. A., et al. (1996). Estimating milk intake of hospitalized preterm infants who breastfeed. *Journal of Human Lactation, 12*, 21–26.

Meier, P. P., Lysakowski, T. Y., Engstrom, J. L., et al. (1990). The accuracy of test weighing for preterm infants. *Journal of Pediatric Gastroenterology and Nutrition, 10*, 62–65.

Melli, M. S., Rashidi, M. R., Delazar, A., et al. (2007). Effect of peppermint water on prevention of nipple cracks in lactating primiparous women: A randomized controlled trial. *International Breastfeeding Journal, 2*, 7.

Melli, M. S., Rashidi, M. R., Nokhoodchi, A., et al. (2007). A randomized trial of peppermint gel, lanolin ointment, and placebo gel to prevent nipple crack in primiparous breastfeeding women. *Medical Science Monitor, 13*(9), CR406–411.

Mitchell, E. A., Blair, P. S., & L'Hoir, M. P. (2006). Should pacifiers be recommended to prevent sudden infant death syndrome? *Pediatrics, 117*(5), 1755–1758.

Mizuno, K., & Kani, K. (2005). Sipping/lapping is a safe alternative feeding method to suckling for preterm infants. *Acta Paediatrica, 94*, 574–580.

Mohammadzadeh, A., Farhat, A., & Esmaeily, H. (2005). The effect of breast milk and lanolin on sore nipples. *Saudi Medical Journal, 26*(8), 1231–1234.

Mohrbacher, N., & Stock, J. (2003). *The breastfeeding answer book* (3rd ed.). Schaumburg, IL: La Leche League.

Moreland-Schultz, K., & Hill, P. D. (2005). Prevention of and therapies for nipple pain: A systematic review. *Journal of Obstetric, Gynecologic, and Neonatal Nursing, 34*(4), 428–437.

Morse, J. (1988a). The hazards of lanolin. *Maternal and Child Nursing, 14*, 204.

Morse, J. (1989b). Lanolin recommended to breastfeeding mothers to prevent nipple discomfort and pain. *Birth, 16*, 35.

Mosley, C., Whittle, C., & Hicks, C. (2001). A pilot study to assess the viability of a randomized controlled trial of methods of supplementary feeding of breast-fed pre-term babies. *Midwifery, 17*, 150–157.

Musoke, R. N. (1990). Breastfeeding promotion: Feeding the low birth weight infant. *International Journal of Obstetrics and Gynecology, 31*(Suppl. 1), 67–68.

Neifert, M., Lawrence, R., & Seacat, J. (1995). Nipple confusion: Toward a formal definition. *Journal of Pediatrics, 126*, S125–S129.

Neimela, M., Uhari, M., & Mottonen, M. (1995). A pacifier increases the risk of recurrent acute otitis media in children in day care centers. *Pediatrics, 96*, 884–888.

Newman, J. (1990). Breastfeeding problems associated with the early introduction of bottles and pacifiers. *Journal of Human Lactation, 6*, 59–63.

Newman, J. (1997). Caution regarding nipple shields. *Journal of Human Lactation, 13*, 12–13.

Newman, J. (1998). Using a lactation aid. Retrieved from http://www.obgyn.net/pregnancy-birth/pregnancy-birth.asp?page=/pregnancy-birth/articles/bf_newman5_0599

Newman, J., & Pitman, T. (2000). *Dr. Jack Newman's guide to breastfeeding*. Toronto, Canada: Harper Collins.

Newman, J., & Pitman, T. (2006). *The latch and other keys to breastfeeding success*. Amarillo, TX: Hale Publishing.

Nicholson, W. L. (1993). The use of nipple shields by breastfeeding women. *Journal of the Australian College of Midwives, 6*, 18–24.

Noble, R., & Bovey, A. (1997). Therapeutic teat use for babies who breastfeed poorly. *Breastfeeding Review, 5*, 37–42.

North, K., Fleming, P., Golding, J., et al. (1999). Pacifier use and morbidity in the first six months of life. *Pediatrics, 103*, e34.

Nowak, A. J., Smith, W. L., & Erenberg, A. (1994). Imaging evaluation of artificial nipples during bottle feeding. *Archives of Pediatric and Adolescent Medicine, 148*, 40–42.

Nowak, A. J., Smith, W. L., & Erenberg, A. (1995). Imaging evaluation of breastfeeding and bottle feeding systems. *Journal of Pediatrics, 126*, S130–S134.

O'Connor, N. R., Tanabe, K. O., Siadaty, M. S., et al. (2009). Pacifiers and breastfeeding: A systematic review. *Archives of Pediatric and Adolescent Medicine, 163*(4), 378–382.

Oddy, W. H., & Glenn, K. (2003). Implementing the Baby Friendly Hospital Initiative: The role of finger feeding. *Breastfeeding Review, 11*, 5–10.

Otte, M. J. (1975). Correcting inverted nipples—an aid to breastfeeding. *American Journal of Nursing, 3*, 454–456.

Palmer, B. (1998). The influence of breastfeeding on the development of the oral cavity: A commentary. *Journal of Human Lactation, 14*, 93–98.

Peres, K. G., Barros, A. J., Peres, M. A., et al. (2007). Effects of breastfeeding and sucking habits on malocclusion in a birth cohort study. *Revista de Saúde Pública, 41*(3), 343–350.

Phillips, R. M., Chantry, C. J., & Gallagher, M. P. (2005). Analgesic effects of breast-feeding or pacifier use with maternal holding in term infants. *Ambulatory Pediatrics, 5*(6), 359–364.

Pinelli, J., Symington, A., & Ciliska, D. (2002). Nonnutritive sucking in high-risk infants: Benign intervention or legitimate therapy? *Journal of Obstetric, Gynecologic, and Neonatal Nursing, 31*, 582–591.

Powers, D., & Tapia, V. (2004). Women's experiences using a nipple shield. *Journal of Human Lactation, 20*, 327–333.

Pugh, L. C., Buchko, B. L., Bishop, B. A., et al. (1996). A comparison of topical agents to relieve nipple pain and enhance breastfeeding. *Birth, 23*, 88–93.

Righard, L. (1998). Are breastfeeding problems related to incorrect breastfeeding technique and the use of pacifiers and bottles? *Birth, 25*, 40–44.

Righard, L., & Alade, M. O. (1997). Breastfeeding and the use of pacifiers. *Birth, 24*, 116–120.

Riordan, J., & Wambach, K. (2010). *Breastfeeding and human lactation* (4th ed.). Sudbury, MA: Jones and Bartlett.

Rocha, N., Martinez, F., & Jorge, S. (2002). Cup or bottle for preterm infants: Effect on oxygen saturation, weight gain and breastfeeding. *Journal of Human Lactation, 18*, 132–137.

Ross, M. (1987). Back to the breast: Retraining infant suckling patterns. In *The lactation consultant series*. Garden City Park, NY: Avery Publishing Group.

Sakashita, R., Kamegai, T., & Inoue, N. (1996). Masseter muscle activity in bottle feeding with the chewing type bottle teat: Evidence from electromyographs. *Early Human Development, 45*, 83–92.

Savenije, O. E. M., & Brand, P. L. P. (2006). Accuracy and precision of test weighing to assess milk intake in newborn infants. *Archives of Disease in Childhood: Fetal and Neonatal Edition, 91*(5), F330–F332.

Scheel, C. E., Schanler, R. J., & Lau, C. (2005). Does the choice of bottle nipple affect the oral feeding performance of very-low-birthweight (VLBW) infants? *Acta Paediatrica, 94*(9), 1266–1272.

Schubiger, G., Schwarz, U., & Tonz, O. (1997). UNICEF/WHO Baby-Friendly Hospital Initiative: Does the use of bottles and pacifiers in the neonatal nursery prevent successful breastfeeding. *European Journal of Pediatrics, 156*, 874–877.

Sealy, C. N. (1996). Rethinking the use of nipple shields. *Journal of Human Lactation, 12*, 29–30.

Sexton, S., & Natale, R. (2009). Risks and benefits of pacifiers. *American Family Physician, 79*(8), 681–685.

Spangler, A., & Hildebrandt, H. (1993). The effect of modified lanolin on nipple pain/damage during the first 10 days of breastfeeding. *International Journal of Childbirth Education, 8*, 15–18.

Spatz, D. (2004). Ten steps for promoting and protecting breastfeeding for vulnerable infants. *Journal of Perinatal and Neonatal Nursing, 18*, 385–396.

Stein, M. J. (1990). Breastfeeding the premature infant: A protocol without bottles. *Journal of Human Lactation, 6*, 167–170.

Tait, P. (2000). Nipple pain in breastfeeding women: Causes, treatment and prevention strategies. *Journal of Midwifery and Women's Health, 45*(3), 2000.

Thorley, V. (1997). Cup feeding: Problems created by incorrect use. *Journal of Human Lactation, 13*, 54–55.

Trenouth, M. J., & Campbell, A. N. (1996). Questionnaire evaluation of feeding methods for cleft lip and palate neonates. *International Journal of Paediatric Dentistry, 6*, 241–244.

Turgeon-O'Brien, H., Lachapelle, D., Gragnon, P. F., et al. (1996). Nutritive and non-nutritive sucking habits: A review. *ASDC Journal of Dentistry for Children, 63*, 321–327.

Venuta, A., Bertolani, P., Pepe, P., et al. (1999). Do pacifiers cause latex allergy? *Allergy, 54*, 1007.

Victora, C. G., Behague, D. P., Barros, F. C., et al. (1997). Pacifier use and short breastfeeding duration: Cause, consequence, or coincidence? *Pediatrics, 99*(3), 445–453.

Victora, C., Tomasi, E., Olinto, M., & Barros, F. (1993). Use of pacifiers and breastfeeding duration. *Lancet, 341*, 404–406.

Vogel, A. M., Hutchison, B. L., & Mitchell, E. A. (2001). The impact of pacifier use on breastfeeding: A prospective cohort study. *Journal of Paediatric and Child Health, 37*, 58–63.

Walker, M. (1990). Breastfeeding premature babies. In *The lactation consultant series*. Schaumburg, IL: La Leche League.

Walker, M. (2010). *Breastfeeding management for the clinician: Using the evidence*. Sudbury, MA: Jones and Bartlett.

Watson-Genna, C. (2008). *Supporting sucking skills in breastfeeding infants*. Sudbury, MA: Jones and Bartlett.

Watson-Genna, C. (2009). *Selecting and using breastfeeding tools*. Amarillo, TX: Hale Publishing.

Weber, R., Woolridge, M. W., & Baum, J. D. (1986). An ultrasonographic study of the organization of sucking and swallowing by newborn infants. *Developmental Medicine and Child Neurology, 28*, 19–24.

Wight, N. E. (1998). Cup-feeding. ABM news and views. *Academy of Breastfeeding Medicine, 4*, 1–5.

Wight, N. E. (2008). *Best medicine: Human milk in the NICU*. Amarillo, TX: Hale Publishing.

Wilson, P. D. (2001). Hydrogel dressing for treatment of sore nipples during early lactation: Should we be promoting these products? *Journal of Human Lactation, 17*(4), 295–297.

Wilson-Clay, B. (1996). Clinical use of silicone nipple shields. *Journal of Human Lactation, 12*, 655–658.

Wilson-Clay, B. (1997a). Comment on "Nipple shields: Just another tool." *Journal of Human Lactation, 12*, 279–285.

Wilson-Clay, B. (1997b). Nipple shields: Just another tool. *Journal of Human Lactation, 13*(3), 194.

Wilson-Clay, B., & Hoover, K. (2008). *The breastfeeding atlas* (4th ed.). Austin, TX: LactNews Press.

Wolf, L. S., & Glass, R. P. (1992). *Feeding and swallowing disorders in infancy*. Tucson, AZ: Therapy Skill Builders.

Woodworth, M., & Frank, E. (1996). Transitioning to the breast at six weeks: Use of a nipple shield. *Journal of Human Lactation, 12*, 305–307.

Woolridge, M. W. (1986). The "anatomy" of infant sucking. *Midwifery, 2*, 164–171.

Woolridge, M. W., Baum, J. D., & Drewett, R. F. (1980). Effect of a traditional and of a new nipple shield on sucking patterns and milk flow. *Early Human Development, 4*, 57–64.

Wright, A., Rice, S., & Wells, S. (1996). Changing hospital practices to increase the duration of breastfeeding. *Pediatrics, 97*, 669–675.

Zeimer, M., Cooper, D. M., & Pigeon, J. G. (1995). Evaluation of a dressing to reduce nipple pain and improve nipple skin condition in breastfeeding women. *Nursing Research, 44*, 347–351.

Zempsky, W. T., & Cravero, J. P. (2004). Relief of pain and anxiety in pediatric patients in emergency medical systems. *Pediatrics, 114*(5), 1348–1356.

CHAPTER 35
Induced Lactation and Relactation

Virginia Thorley, PhD, IBCLC, FILCA

OBJECTIVES

- Define induced lactation and relactation.
- Discuss the historical basis and cultural issues of induced lactation and relactation.
- List indications for inducing lactation and for relactation.
- Describe infant-related factors that influence the outcome of induced lactation.
- Describe the hormonal and physiological changes required for lactation to occur nonpuerperally.
- Describe physical and nonpharmaceutical actions that can assist in inducing lactation and relactation.
- List medications prescribed to induce lactation and/or relactate and levels of evidence.
- Describe nonpharmaceutical substances traditionally used as galactogogues and the level of evidence for their efficacy.
- Describe management of induced lactation and relactation.

INTRODUCTION

Breast development and maturation during pregnancy are the usual precursors to lactation. However, both the historical and contemporary literature demonstrate that a woman can produce milk without the preparatory effect of pregnancy and birth, that is, nonpuerperally. After breast and nipple stimulation is commenced, many women experience breast fullness and tenderness. Induced lactation and relactation have occurred and continue to occur with unknown prevalence in indigenous societies (Basedow, 1925; Kramer, 1995; Nemba, 1994; Slome, 1956; Wieschhoff, 1940), in developing countries (Abejide et al., 1997; Banapurmath et al., 1993b; Brown, 1977; De et al., 2002; Kesaree, 1993), and also in the developed world (Australian Breastfeeding Association [ABA], 2004; Auerbach et al., 1980, 1981; Boyle, 1993; Hormann, 1977; Phillips, 1993; Raphael, 1973; Scantlebury, 1923). Nonpuerperal lactation has also been described in animals, both female and male, in response to suckling (Anon., 1845; Archer, 1990; Creel et al., 1991).

(continues)

Where the society or the family has a strong breastfeeding culture, relactation is part of lactation, with some women resuming lactation after a gap for a number of reasons (Datta et al., 1993; Marquis et al., 1998; Phillips, 1993; Thorley, 1997). Indeed, Mobbs et al. (1971) considered nonpuerperal lactation to be a normal physiological response of the breasts to suckling. Interest in induced lactation and relactation appears to have paralleled the increased interest in breastfeeding in developed countries. Where breastfeeding is accepted as the norm, the normal course of lactation in individual women might differ from the stereotype of exclusive breastfeeding, followed sequentially by mixed feeding and weaning. Breastfeeding can follow a number of other patterns (**Table 35-1**), with the first weaning followed by one of more episodes of partial or exclusive breastfeeding (Datta et al., 1993; Marquis et al., 1998; Phillips, 1993).

Table 35-1 Patterns in Human Lactation

Pattern	Type
EBF □ MF □ W	(1)
MF □ W	(2)
MF □ EBF □ MF □ W	(3)
EBF □ MF □ W^n □ MF □ W	(4)
EBF □ MF □ W □ MF □ W	(5)
EBF □ MF □ EBF □ MF □ W	(5)
MF □ W □ MF □ EBF □ MF □ W	(5)
MF □ W □ MF □ W	(5)
NBF □ MF □ EBF □ MF □ W	(6)
NBF □ MF □ W	(6)

Abbreviations: EBF, exclusive breastfeeding; MF, mixed feeding/part breastfeeding; W, weaned; NBF, never breastfed.

(1) Classic physiological breastfeeding pattern after delivery of an infant.

(2) Initial difficulties followed by weaning.

(3) Progression to classic pattern after initial difficulties.

(4) Data from pattern observed by Marquis et al., 1998, with one or more temporary weanings (W^n), followed by relactation.

(5) Other patterns involving relactation (space prevents every variation of these patterns being tabulated here).

(6) Two patterns associated with both adoptive breastfeeding and establishing breastfeeding for the mother's biological child who was not initially breastfed.

I. Definitions

    A. *Induced lactation:* The purposeful stimulation of lactation where it was previously absent, usually in the absence of a pregnancy in the months immediately prior to the induction of lactation (nonpuerperally). The term also includes adoptive breast-feeding where a woman who is not breastfeeding induces lactation, whether or not she has ever breastfed in the past (Thorley, 2010; Waletzky et al., 1976).

    B. *Relactation:* Properly, relactation means induced lactation in a mother who has previously breastfed the index baby (that is, reversing weaning), but the term also is used where a mother induces lactation for a biological child she has never breastfed following the suppression of lactation postpartum. The term is loosely used as a generic term for any type of induced lactation (Thorley, 2010). Some authors include reversing a significant decrease or a lag in breastmilk production in their definition of relactation (de Aquino et al., 2009; Lakhkar et al., 1999; Seema et al., 1997).

    C. *Nursing:* Used here to mean breastfeeding.

    D. *Mother:* Used here as any woman inducing lactation, whether she is the biological, adoptive, or foster mother.

II. Physiological Mechanisms

    A. The hormonal influences on the development of secretory tissue in the breast during a pregnancy and the events triggered by the delivery of the placenta are described elsewhere in this text.

    B. In the absence of a pregnancy, mammary stimulation triggers the release of prolactin and facilitates proliferation of secretory tissue, enabling milk secretion to occur (World Health Organization [WHO], 2009).

    C. Suckling or expression, or other nipple stimulation, stimulates prolactin secretion and the release of oxytocin (Hill et al., 1996; Hormann et al., 1998; Zinaman et al., 1992).

    D. It is milk removal that enables milk secretion to continue.

    E. Confidence-building is important to the release of oxytocin by the posterior pituitary, a process that can be inhibited by stress.

    F. Oxytocin release can become a conditioned response (Hill, Chatterton, & Aldag, 1999).

    G. Clinical indications:

        1. Induced lactation and relactation are recommended in humanitarian emergency situations, such as after natural disasters, warfare, or civil strife (ILCA, 2011; WHO, 2009).

        2. Induced lactation has been practiced in most cultures and for a variety of reasons.

            a. When a mother adopts or fosters a baby (or child of any age) and desires to breastfeed (sometimes referred to as adoptive breastfeeding)

            b. When a relation/friend stimulates lactation to nourish an infant if the biological mother is unable (for example, in the case of maternal human immunodeficiency virus, maternal death or absence, the maternal inability to breastfeed because of a physical abnormality) (Hormann et al., 1998; Slome, 1956)

    c. When emergency situations exist following a natural disaster, warfare, or civil strife (Brown, 1978; Gribble, 2005b; Hormann et al., 1998; WHO, 2009)

    d. When an adoptive child seeks the comfort of the breast, or the mother or grandmother finds nursing at the breast calms an emotionally labile child (Gribble, 2005a, 2005c, 2006; Slome, 1956)

3. Relactation has been practiced:

    a. When the mother wishes to recommence breastfeeding after weaning, to enhance maternal-infant bonding

    b. To ameliorate an infant health problem that followed weaning, such as:

       i. Proven or suspected intolerance or allergy to artificial baby milks (Agarwal et al., 2010; Avery, 1973; Hormann et al., 1998)

       ii. Constipation

4. The situation that led to weaning, or to failure to initiate breastfeeding, has been overcome or ameliorated.

    a. Maternal breast or nipple conditions (Kesaree et al., 1993; Seema et al., 1997), illness, or maternal-infant separation (Agarwal et al., 2010; Brown, 1978).

    b. Unsupportive hospital practices that have prevented the initiation of breastfeeding in the postnatal period (De, 2003).

    c. Infant conditions such as prematurity (Thompson, 1996), oral-facial anomalies (Menon et al., 2002), malnutrition (WHO, 2009), severe dehydration (Sofer et al., 1993), or hospitalization (Auerbach et al., 1979b, 1979c).

5. The child initiates breastfeeding following weaning (Phillips, 1993; Thorley, 1997).

6. Emergency or disaster situations exist following a natural disaster, warfare, or civil strife (Brown, 1977; Gribble, 2005b; Hormann et al., 1998; WHO, 2009).

III. Induced Lactation: Clinical Practice

A. Assessment of the adoptive mother or wet nurse

1. History

    a. Previous pregnancies and endocrine history:

       i. How many?

       ii. Duration of pregnancies?

       iii. How long ago?

    b. Does she have a history suggestive of hormonal imbalance or anomalies?

       i. Reason for adoption (for instance, related to obstetrical or hormonal difficulties)

       ii. History of infertility (for example, hormonal, polycystic ovary syndrome)

       iii. Other hormonal abnormalities (such as thyroid or pituitary disorders)

2. Previous breastfeeding experience

    a. Has the woman breastfed previous children, and if so, for how long?

    b. Did she have any breastfeeding difficulties? If so, what, and were they resolved?

      c. What were her reason(s) for weaning and the age of the child?

      d. How long is the lactation gap (length of time from last breastfeeding to commencing induction of lactation)?

         i. A longer lactation gap has been associated with a longer time to achieve a milk flow (Agarwal et al., 2010; De et al., 2002; Lakhkar et al., 1999).

         ii. A long lactation gap, even years, has not been an obstacle in other case series (Banapurmath et al., 1993b; Lakhkar, 2000; Nemba, 1994; Slome, 1956).

         iii. Women who had never previously lactated experienced more difficulty in inducing a milk flow in some studies (Auerbach et al., 1979a); in others, there was no disadvantage (Marieskind, 1973; Nemba, 1994).

      e. Was the previous breastfeeding experience with an adopted baby? The experience with a different adopted baby may be different (Mobbs et al., 1971).

      f. Assess the mother's education on breastfeeding in general (Auerbach et al., 1979a), such as reading, classes, and videos, irrespective of presence or absence of previous breastfeeding experience.

  B. Cultural influences

    1. Assess the mother's support system.

    2. Determine her expectations about her ability to make breastmilk.

    3. Determine her expectations about her ability to introduce her baby to the breast.

    4. Assess her concerns regarding modesty.

    5. Does she hold religious beliefs regarding breastmilk and breastfeeding that affect family relationships, including relationships of this baby with other children?

    6. In an indigenous culture, is this a traditional adoption where the baby will go from the birth mother to the adoptive mother at or soon after birth? If so, the baby may be able to be breastfed by the biological mother while the adoptive mother is establishing lactation (Nemba, 1994).

    7. In cases of surrogacy, if the birth mother agrees, the baby may be breastfed by her while the adoptive mother is establishing lactation, thus accustoming the child to breastfeeding and providing optimum nutrition.

  C. Reasons for wanting to breastfeed an adopted baby

    1. To normalize the arrival of a child and to simulate the experience of biological motherhood

    2. To enhance attachment and develop a close mother–infant relationship

    3. To optimize the baby's health

    4. To ensure that the baby will not miss out on the experience

    5. To give a debilitated infant a chance at survival (e.g., during a natural disaster)

IV. Prior to Receiving the Infant

  A. Requirements, essential (Brown, 1977)

    1. A healthy woman, with intact pituitary, motivated to establish lactation

    2. A baby willing to suckle, or a mother willing to do milk expression (manual or mechanical) for breast stimulation

  3. A support network that may consist of:
   a. Family and friends
   b. Mother-support group (breastfeeding specific)
   c. Internet websites supportive of adoptive breastfeeding (Gribble, 2001; see **Table 35-2**)
   d. Professional support (Szucs et al., 2010)
  4. Confidence, or confidence-building (Banapurmath et al., 2003; Nemba, 1994)
  5. Rehydration therapy, if induced lactation is undertaken for a dehydrated or ill infant (Brown, 1977)

B. Requirements, desirable
  1. Preparation by reading or other education on induction of lactation (Auerbach et al., 1979a; Nemba, 1994; Thearle et al., 1984)
  2. Reading and videos for education on the normal management of breastfeeding if the mother has limited experience of observing others breastfeeding (Auerbach et al., 1979a; Szucs et al., 2010)

C. Questions to be addressed
  1. How long will it be until the mother receives the adopted child she plans to breastfeed?
   a. The mother should be warned of difficulty in predicting the date when she will receive her adopted baby, especially with overseas adoptions.
   b. She may receive her baby on short notice, reducing the expected preparation time, or
   c. She may have a longer wait than anticipated.
   d. Few mothers today will receive their adoptive babies at or soon after birth. Exceptions include:
     i. Following the birth of the baby to a surrogate mother
     ii. Traditional adoptions; for instance, in some indigenous cultures or within a family
  2. Approximately how old does she expect the child to be (for example, newborn, older than 6 months, older than 12 months)?
  3. What type of milk is the child being fed at present and is it an appropriate choice?
  4. How is the child currently being fed (for example, wet nursed, fed by bottle, fed by cup)?

D. Infant's age
  1. Newborns and babies younger than 8 weeks are most likely to suckle willingly (Auerbach et al., 1981); this may be because suck is initially reflexive and changes to a voluntary action by about 3 months (Walker, 2006).
  2. Adopted infants older than 2 months of age may either resist or respond when put to the breast (Auerbach et al., 1980), and some may require similar techniques to resolve breast refusal as for an infant born to the mother.
  3. Early rejection of the breast need not mean the baby will always refuse (Auerbach et al., 1979a; Seema et al., 1997; Thearle et al., 1984).

Table 35-2 Selected Internet Resources on Adoptive Breastfeeding for Professionals and Clients*

Source and Description	Web Site
Protocols	
Academy of Breastfeeding Medicine	*http://www.bfmed.org/Media/Files/Protocols/Protocol 9 - English 1st Rev. Jan 2011.pdf*
Protocol #9: Use of galactogogues in initiating or augmenting maternal milk supply.	
Goldfarb L, Newman J	*http://www.asklenore.info/breastfeeding/induced_lactation/ gn_protocols.shtml*
The Newman-Goldfarb protocols for induced lactation.	
Breastfeeding Aids	
Lact-Aid	*http://www.lact-aid.com/facts-about-lact-aid*
A tube-type feeding system that permits the baby to learn to breastfeed safely by supplementing at the breast.	
Supplemental Nursing System	*http://www.medelabreastfeedingus.com/products/51/ supplemental-nursing-system-sns*
Long-term supplemental tube feeding system enabling the baby to stay on the breast.	
Support	
La Leche League International	*http://www.lalecheleague.org/NB/NBadoptive.html*
Frequently asked questions; Online articles from LLLI publications, New Beginnings, and Leaven.	
Adoption Media LLC	*http://breast-feeding.adoption.com*
Resources, articles, forums, Chat line, community outreach. Adoption procedures for US, Canada, UK.	
Yahoo Groups	*http://groups.yahoo.com/group/adoptivebreastfeeding*
Adoptive Breastfeeding; an online chat group and links to other supports.	
The Adoptive Breastfeeding Resource Website	*http://www.fourfriends.com/abrw*
Naomi B. Duane Resources, milk calculator, articles, news, message boards, support.	

Compiled by Virginia Thorley

*_Note_: Web sites change over time. These URLs were valid as of May 13, 2012.

4. Babies who are older than 6 months are likely to require patience in the gradual process of introducing the breast.

5. The older the child is when introduced to the breast, the less willing he or she may be to suckle (Auerbach et al., 1979a), unless he or she is being breastfed by the biological mother or a foster mother at the time of the adoption or has previously been breastfed.

6. For a baby older than 9 months, factors influencing willingness to accept breast-feeding attempts include high-quality foster care prior to adoption (vs. negative care with little physical contact) and the child's personality (ABA, 2004).

7. Children, including toddlers, who have breastfed previously, may seek the breast of their own accord (Gribble, 2005c; Phillips, 1993).

E. Breasts and nipples

1. Assess physical characteristics of the breasts that may make inducing a milk supply a greater challenge.

a. Anomalies, scars, history of any surgical procedures

b. Breast size and shape; for example, signs of underdevelopment, such as tubular, asymmetrical, or pendulous breasts (Huggins et al., 2000)

2. Assess the size and shape of the nipples and areola.

a. Normal, inverted, flat, and retracted nipples

b. Nipple or areola anomalies and the existence of supernumerary nipples

c. The direction the nipple points; this will influence how best to position the baby

V. Planning

A. Expected outcome

1. Counseling:

a. Explain to the mother that two partners are involved, mother and baby.

b. Ascertain her expectations and how she defines breastfeeding success.

c. Emphasize the breastfeeding relationship and realistic levels of achievement (Szucs et al., 2010).

i. Success is best defined as how the individual mother feels about the experience (Auerbach et al., 1981).

ii. Focus on the baby's willingness to go to the breast.

iii. Some mothers will achieve exclusive breastfeeding or breastmilk feeding (Szucs et al., 2010); others may not.

d. Build on her confidence because low confidence, lack of support, and infrequent suckling have been associated with poorer outcomes in adoptive mothers (Lakhkar, 2000); thus confidence, a factor in lactation success following a pregnancy (Blyth et al., 2002; Dennis, 1999; Meedya et al., 2010; Persad et al., 2008), is also an important factor in inducing lactation nonpuerperally.

e. Encourage her to build the trust of her baby, especially with an older baby, before attempting to offer the breast (ABA, 2004).

f. Reassure the mother that, although full lactation/exclusive breastfeeding might never be achieved by some mothers, many mothers and their adopted babies have continued supplemented breastfeeding for extended periods.

 i. The breast can become a place of comfort, where the baby feels safe.

 ii. The mother can offer breastmilk as a drink or mixed in other food, even if the child never accepts nursing at the breast.

2. The first drops of milk in the absence of a baby can be expected after a few days to a few weeks of preparation.

3. If the baby is suckling effectively, breastmilk may be evident earlier, but there is wide individual variation. Consequently, it is advisable not to give the mother a number value for how long this will take.

B. Support for the mother

1. Support from family and friends (Avery, 1973; Hormann, 1977; Lakhkar et al., 1999), including psychological support and household assistance.

2. Support, encouragement, and appropriate information from the lactation consultant or other healthcare professional, with an emphasis on confidence-building (Banapurmath et al., 2003; De et al., 2002; Szucs et al., 2010).

3. Access to an online support group for adoptive breastfeeding mothers, to normalize the experience (Gribble, 2001; see Table 35-2).

4. Mothers may receive little support or outright discouragement from adoption agencies, family, and friends. Mothers need to be prepared for addressing this issue.

VI. Establishing Lactation: Inducing Milk Production

A. Stimulation to induce breastmilk production

1. Nipple stimulation (through nipple exercises or stroking, suckling, or expressing) for development and maturation of breast tissue prior to breastfeeding (Auerbach et al., 1979a; WHO, 2009).

2. Many women have induced lactation solely by expressing and/or by putting the baby to the breast, or combining this with nipple stimulation (Auerbach et al., 1979a; Banapurmath et al., 1993b; Cohen, 1971; Kleinman et al., 1980; Lakhkar, 2000).

a. Milk expression sessions may start with only a few minutes, according to comfort, building up to a maximum of 15 to 25 minutes.

b. Simultaneous expression of both breasts was believed to enhance prolactin secretion (Hill et al., 1999; Zinaman et al., 1992), but a Cochrane Review found no difference in serum prolactin or milk yield when postnatal mothers pumped both breasts simultaneously (Becker et al., 2009).

c. Simultaneous expression of both breasts does, however, save time (Becker et al., 2009).

d. Listening to a relaxation tape may enhance milk expression (Becker et al., 2009), though this has not been studied in women inducing lactation or relactating.

     e. Attention to optimal latch and breastfeeding technique when the child is placed at the breast (Academy of Breastfeeding Medicine [ABM] Protocol Committee, 2011).

3. Breast and nipple stimulation has included the following:

     a. Nipple exercises for about 4 weeks prior to receiving the baby, every three to four hours (Auerbach et al., 1979a).

     b. Breast massage or application of warmth (Auerbach et al., 1979a; Phillips, 1969).

     c. The baby suckling at the breast, as the sole or main stimulus (ABA, 2004; Lakhkar, 2000; WHO, 2009).

     d. Manual expression has been shown to extract colostrum more effectively than use of a hospital-grade breast pump in postnatal women (ABM Protocol Committee, 2011; Ohyama et al., 2010); this is likely to be applicable to the low volume of fluid in the early stages of inducing lactation.

     e. A tube feeding device that delivers milk while the baby is simultaneously suckling at the breast (ABA, 2004; Auerbach et al., 1979a; Hormann et al., 1998; Kulski et al., 1981; WHO, 2009).

          i. Whether a commercial device or a homemade one is used, this provides stimulation of the breasts and a breastfeeding experience for the baby, while at the same time eliminating the use of bottle nipples.

          ii. The mother is taught to raise or lower the milk receptacle to adjust the rate of flow.

4. Some mothers may not have breast secretions prior to putting the baby to the breast.

     a. Mothers who have previously breastfed are more likely to have milk after manual or mechanical stimulation prior to putting the adopted baby to the breast, although the difference is not always significant.

     b. Tandem breastfeeding (continuing to breastfeed an older baby along with the new baby) means there is already milk available.

5. Galactagogues (medications or other substances believed to increase milk yield):

     a. Priming medications:

          i. Estrogen and progesterone in the oral contraceptive pill (OCP), begun as many weeks as possible before the adoption (Auerbach et al., 1979a; Kramer, 1995; Nemba, 1994; Szucs et al., 2010; see Table 35-2 for induced lactation protocols available online). Breastfeeding or expressing has been begun on cessation of the OCP.

          ii. Caution is advised because of the risk of deep vein thrombosis associated with high doses and older age.

b. Prolactin secretion, necessary for lactogenesis, is set in motion by stimulation of sensory nerves in the breast, via neural pathways. This is why physical stimulation, as described earlier, is recommended (ABM Protocol Committee, 2011). Additional stimulation of prolactin release, in addition to breastfeeding or expressing, is believed to be provided by the use of drugs that are dopamine antagonists (Gabay, 2002; Hale, 2010; McNeilly et al., 1974).

   i. The Academy of Breastfeeding Medicine's revised protocol of galactogogues provides levels of evidence for four substances commonly used as galactogogues (ABM Protocol Committee, 2011). (See Table 35-2.)

   ii. Use of the following pharmaceuticals as galactogogues is an off-label use (ABM Protocol Committee, 2011).

   iii. Metoclopramide (ABM Protocol Committee, 2011; Auerbach et al., 1980; Banapurmath et al., 1993a; Bose et al., 1981; Brown, 1973; Budd et al., 1993; Hale, 2010; Kauppila et al., 1983). Level of Evidence: III (ABM Protocol Committee, 2011). The effects on lactation appear to be dose related (Hale, 2010). Reducing the dose gradually before discontinuing metaclopramide is advised to prevent the reduction in supply experienced by some women (Hale, 2010). Side effects make this medication less desirable than domperidone (Hale, 2010).

   iv. Domperidone (Brown, 1978; Hale, 2010; Hofmeyr et al., 1983; Hofmeyr et al., 1985); available outside the United States, but may sometimes be obtained from compounding pharmacies in the United States. Optimal time for commencing dose is after milk has appeared (Lawrence et al., 2011). Level of Evidence: I (ABM Protocol Committee, 2011).

   v. Sulpiride, an antidepressant and antipsychotic, in low doses, because it is not dose dependent (Aono et al., 1982; Cheales-Siebenaler, 1999; Hale, 2010; Ylikorkala et al., 1982, 1984); used in South Africa, but unavailable in some countries. It is not recommended because of pyramidal side effects and maternal weight gain (ABM Protocol Committee, 2011; Gabay, 2002).

c. Less-used pharmaceutical galactagogues:

   i. Thyrotropin-releasing hormone (Emery, 1996; Hill et al., 1999; Peters et al., 1991); not advised for general use (ABM Protocol Committee, 2011; Hormann et al., 1998)

   ii. Chlorpromazine, a tranquilizer with a long half-life (Ehrenkranz et al., 1986); has side effects such as sedation and should be avoided (Hale, 2010; Sousa et al., 1975)

   iii. Human growth hormone (Hale, 2010; Hofmeyr et al., 1985; Milsom et al., 1992), for which there is a lack of clinical experience of this off-label use (Gabay, 2002).

6. The hormone oxytocin stimulates the milk ejection reflex through acting on receptors in the breast; it stimulates the contraction of the myoepithelial cells surrounding the alveoli, forcing out the milk (Lawrence et al., 2011).
   a. Suckling or other nipple stimulation causes the release of oxytocin from the hypothalamus without recourse to pharmaceuticals (Lawrence et al., 2011).
   b. Other senses can trigger oxytocin release and the milk ejection reflex (Lawrence et al., 2011), for example, touch (such as skin-to-skin contact) and visual, auditory, and olfactory stimuli.
   c. Because oxytocin release can become a conditioned response (Hill et al., 1999), the mother may find that developing a ritual or routine, including breast stimulation, just prior to breastfeeding or expressing will trigger this response (Szucs et al., 2010), without recourse to pharmaceuticals.
   d. Synthetic forms of this hormone should be used only after there is milk present to be ejected and the mother's milk ejection reflex is ineffective.
   e. Oxytocin is usually administered as an intranasal spray (Syntocinon); not available in some countries, though in the United States it can be mixed at a compounding pharmacy (Walker, 2006).
   f. Hale (2010) suggests the intranasal spray be limited to the first week post-partum. In induced lactation, it would be reasonable to extrapolate this to the first week after milk is present beyond a few drops, although this has not been studied (Lawrence et al., 2011).
   g. The oxytocin nasal spray (Lawrence et al., 2011) and buccal oxytocin (Ylikorkala et al., 1984) are unlikely to have any effect on actual milk yield (Fewtrell et al., 2006).

7. Herbal medications, dietary supplements, and alternative medicine have been used in most cultures as galactagogues.
   a. Most information is anecdotal and, in the absence of randomized controlled trials, the placebo effect cannot be ruled out.
   b. It is common for mothers who are inducing lactation to improve their own diets and increase fluid intake (similarly to women who are lactating following childbirth) (Auerbach et al., 1979a; De et al., 2002).
   c. Many mothers believe that dietary supplements or increasing fluid intake will stimulate milk production, but evidence that special foods or herbal products enhance milk synthesis is lacking. Those that have been used traditionally include:
      i. Brewer's yeast (may cause fussiness in some infants).
      ii. Beer. Alcohol may, however, both inhibit the milk ejection reflex and reduce the baby's suckling behavior and sleep and thus may be counterproductive (Mennella, 2001; Mennella et al., 1993; Mennella et al., 2005).

    d. Herbal drugs, such as fenugreek, fennel, and anise (not star anise), have a long history of use as herbal galactagogues; they may be allergenic in susceptible individuals (Humphrey, 2003; Lawrence et al., 2011).

        i. *Fenugreek*: Generally regarded as safe, but may have a hypoglycemic effect on the mother (Bryant, 2006; Hale, 2010). Evidence is from observational studies only (Hale, 2010), and randomized controlled trials are as yet lacking. Level of Evidence: II-3 (ABM Protocol Committee, 2011).

        ii. *Fennel*: Considered safe, but no documentation of galactogogue effects (Hale, 2010).

        iii. *Milk thistle (Silybum marianum)*: Taken as a tea, milk thistle significantly increased milk yield in one study, compared with placebo (Di Pierro et al., 2008; Lawrence et al., 2011). Level of Evidence: II-1 (ABM Protocol Committee, 2011).

        iv. So-called natural treatments should be used with caution, especially in blended products, because some herbal products have been found to be detrimental to infant health (Rosti et al., 1994) and products may not be free of contamination (ABM Protocol Committee, 2011).

        v. Although never claimed to be a galactogogue, the herb comfrey, banned in some countries, should be avoided absolutely because of the danger of hepatotoxicity (Lawrence et al., 2011); this includes topical use as well as orally (Hale, 2010).

    e. Acupuncture, through enhancing prolactin secretion (Clavey, 1996; Jenner et al., 2002; Sheng et al., 1989).

B. Expressing

    1. Assess the mother's comfort with manual or mechanical expressing.

    2. Teach and assess her ability to hand express the breasts.

    3. Discuss the types of manual and electric breast pumps available and the mother's ability to access them. (See Chapter 34: Breastfeeding Devices and Equipment.)

        a. Simultaneous bilateral (double) pumping with a portable, hospital-grade electric pump is more efficient in use of time than other pumping options (Siebenaler, 2002).

    4. Assess the mother's ability to use these technologies correctly. If she is using a mechanical or electronic pump, ensure that it is effective and not causing pain. Pumps are sometimes ineffective or cause pain (Dwyer, 2008; Lawrence et al., 2011).

    5. Assess the mother's ability to achieve expression frequency.

        a. Ideally, as frequently as a newborn would breastfeed (8–12 times per 24 hours; Hormann & Savage, 1998), or

        b. Two-hourly (Lakhkar, 2000), with one or more expressions at night, or

        c. At least six times per 24 hours, at 15 minutes per breast (Szucs et al., 2010)

      6. Discuss expression strategies while traveling, if the mother is required to travel to another country in the case of an overseas adoption.

         a. Manual expression is always available and requires no equipment other than a collecting container.

         b. Mechanical pumping: Does the electric pump have a manual mode and does the mother know how to use it?

         c. Power adapters are necessary for countries with incompatible power.

         d. Can the pump run on batteries, and will the mother have sufficient batteries with her?

C. The most common challenges adoptive mothers might encounter (Auerbach et al., 1979a)

    1. Lack of preparation time

    2. Maintaining the newly stimulated breastmilk supply while traveling to collect the baby

    3. Getting the baby to nurse, or experiencing breast refusal through infant frustration

       a. Rewarding the baby with supplemental milk through the drop and drip technique (dripping donor breastmilk or artificial baby milk [ABM] onto the areola) or through a supplemental feeding tube device can reduce frustration (Lakhkar et al., 1999).

    4. Worry about the baby getting enough milk (Auerbach et al., 1979a) or self-doubt leading to stress (Bose et al., 1981)

    5. Fatigue

    6. Uncertainty about decreasing supplements

       a. Regular contact with relevant members of the healthcare team (International Board Certified Lactation Consultant [IBCLC], physician, child health nurse) for guidance

       b. Emotional support/reassurance

    7. Expressing/feeding equipment difficulties

    8. Finding the time to initiate lactation as a result of competing demands of other children or employment

D. Physiological responses to induced lactation and related discomforts (Auerbach et al., 1979a)

    1. Nipple pain (Seema et al., 1997), which should be addressed by:

       a. Reassurance and attention to the baby's attachment and positioning (Banapurmath et al., 2003)

       b. Selection of appropriate diameter of the breast pump flange and correct use of it

    2. Breast pain

    3. Nipple and breast changes, including fullness (ABA, 2004; Riordan, 2010)

    4. Signs of milk ejection

    5. Menstrual cessation or irregularities (Hormann, 1977; Riordan, 2010)

6. Increased appetite (Auerbach et al., 1979a)

7. Maternal weight changes; Auerbach et al. (1979a) reported either gain or loss

E. Infant suckling

1. Skin-to-skin contact:

   a. Begin skin contact when the baby is not showing hunger cues and is still sleepy.

   b. Older babies not used to being held close may at first find skin-to-skin threatening, so patience and respect for the baby's feelings are needed.

2. Establish breastfeeding.

   a. Facilitate good attachment and positioning.

   b. Encourage the mother to begin to nurse the infant on the side on which he or she is used to being fed (for example, if bottle-fed on the left side, begin breastfeeding on the left breast).

   c. Facilitate short, frequent breastfeeds (8–12 each 24 hours).

   d. The infant should not be forced to the breast or to breastfeed.

      i. Early refusal is not predictive; infants who reject the breast initially may later learn to accept it (Auerbach et al., 1980).

   e. To encourage a reluctant baby, teach the mother to:

      i. Assuage hunger with partial feeding before breastfeeds, using a cup, syringe, or bottle, or finger feeding with a feeding tube.

      ii. Use the drop and drip method to encourage suckling; that is, dribble milk onto the areola while the baby is attached (Kesaree, 1993; Lakhkar, 2000). The milk can be dropped from a spoon, dropper, syringe, or bottle.

      iii. Breastfeed when the baby is drowsy.

      iv. Breastfeed in a darkened, quiet room.

      v. Use a supplemental feeding tube device to deliver milk while the baby is suckling at the breast (Auerbach et al., 1980; Bryant, 2006); placing the device's milk container higher will initially allow for a faster flow.

      vi. Some babies will take the breast without the supplement at night.

      vii. Some babies will latch and stay attached if the mother walks around; wearing the baby in a sling may facilitate breastfeeding.

   f. Teach the mother to recognize milk transfer.

   g. Do not allow the infant to cry at the breast; the breastfeeding experience should be pleasurable.

      i. Remove a crying baby from the breast and soothe or divert her or him in other ways.

      ii. Talk or sing to the baby while at the breast.

   h. Begin with short, frequent breastfeeding attempts, extending the time as the child indicates willingness.

   i. Once the child accepts the breast, expressing can be gradually discontinued and replaced with frequent suckling.

3. Supplementation (for induced lactation or relactation):
  a. Supplementation is essential for the baby's well-being while the mother's milk supply is being established.
  b. If banked human milk is unavailable, the ABM that the baby was already drinking should be continued, unless there is good reason to change it.
  c. Eliminate/decrease the use of bottles and artificial nipples, including pacifiers, by putting the child to the breast frequently and providing whatever additional nourishment is needed via feeding tube device at the breast, or by cup or syringe after breastfeeding. A combination of methods has been used (de Aquino et al., 2009).
  d. If a supplemental feeding tube device is not being used and milk has been observed:
    i. Offer the supplement only after the baby has nursed at the breast.
    ii. Offer the ABM after every second feed, provided breastfeeds are approximately two-hourly.
    iii. Feed the baby exclusively on the breast at night, if the mother and baby are sleeping in close proximity and able to breastfeed ad lib.
  e. If a cup is used for supplements, teach the mother to cup-feed the baby in an upright position. (See Chapter 33.)
  f. If supplements are given by bottle, bottle-feed on both the left and right sides to avoid a one-sided preference.
  g. If the baby is accustomed to being fed by bottle with a fast flow, introduce bottle nipples with a slower flow to accustom the baby to receiving milk more slowly; pace the feeds, pausing several times.
  h. Gradually decrease ABMs and other foods as appropriate, using infant output and growth as guides. However,
    i. Do not keep the baby hungry in an attempt to encourage suckling at the breast; this is counterproductive because the baby becomes weak and less effective at nursing (Avery, 1973).
    ii. Do not dilute the supplementary milk, for similar reasons.
    iii. Do not restrict the amounts of supplements.
    iv. If the baby's output lessens or growth falters, temporarily increase the supplement.
  i. Replace milk expression/pumping with additional breastfeeds; however, expression after some feeds may be necessary for additional stimulation if the baby is weak and suckles poorly.
  j. Gradually reduce any galactogogue being used.
  k. Some babies will require supplementation for as long as the mother nurses.
F. Evaluation
  1. Mother–infant relationship.
    a. Skin-to-skin contact is facilitating bonding.
    b. A harmonious mother–infant relationship is developing, with mother–infant dyad happy and contented.

2. Infant breastfeeding.
   a. Infant suckling at the mother's breast.
   b. The infant is contented to suckle at the breast for increasing periods.
3. Mother is producing breastmilk.
   a. Mother is producing breastmilk in increasing quantities.
   b. Milk secretion observed on expression.
4. Infant indicators of breastmilk intake.
   a. Evidence of milk transfer/swallowing.
   b. Changes in stools, which may vary through the day.
   c. Milk/food intake from other sources diminishing, while the urinary output (diaper count) remains normal.
   d. Pre- and postfeed weights to assess amounts of milk obtained directly from the breasts, if necessary.
   e. Weight checks every 3 to 5 days and then weekly, to assess that adequate growth continues.

G. Infant taking all nutrition from breast
1. Infant receiving only breastmilk
   a. Cessation of supplementary ABM/foods
   b. Cessation of use of feeding tubes, bottles, cups, or other devices
   c. Other stimulation (expressing, galactagogues) no longer needed
   d. Milk production maintained by infant's breastfeeding
2. Infant receiving only breastmilk and age-appropriate complementary (solid) foods
   a. As stated previously, except for the inclusion of solid foods

VII. Relactation

A. Definition:
1. Relactation, or the reestablishment of lactation, is similar in many aspects to induced lactation and to lactation generally.
2. Information in this section applies in situations where relactation is initiated by the mother.
3. In the less usual situation where relactation is initiated by an older baby or child who is an experienced breastfeeder (Phillips, 1993), and who is eating semi-solid complementary foods daily, little assistance may be required other than reassurance.

B. Assessment:
1. History
   a. Questions that apply when a mother is relactating for her biological child:
      i. Did the mother breastfeed this child at all?
      ii. If so, for how long?
      iii. What was the reason for weaning/not breastfeeding (Phillips, 1992)?
      iv. Were there any maternal breastfeeding difficulties, such as inverted nipples, illness, breast hypoplasia (underdevelopment), hormonal conditions?

     v. Have maternal difficulties been adequately addressed?

     vi. How and what is the infant currently being fed?

     vii. Does the mother understand basic breastfeeding techniques, such as effective latch?

C. Infant's current health status:

    1. Birth details (for example, normal vaginal, forceps, vacuum extraction, cesarean, birth asphyxia).

    2. Infant's health history, and current growth and developmental status.

    3. Is the infant strong enough to suckle?

    4. Were previous feeding difficulties caused by infant factors, for instance, prematurity, tongue tie, other oral anomalies, hypertonic bite, developmental lag, neurological issues? If so, have these factors resolved themselves or been adequately addressed (Phillips, 1992)?

    5. Age of infant.

      a. Babies who are younger than 2 or 3 months old may be more willing to accept the breast because at this stage suckling is reflexive.

      b. Babies older than this may respond to measures appropriate to breast refusal.

      c. Children who are older than 12 months and who have a long history of breastfeeding may remember how to breastfeed effectively (Phillips, 1993).

D. Cultural influences:

    1. Assess the mother's support system.

    2. Identify any cultural or community barriers to her resuming breastfeeding, such as beliefs about modesty and ability to breastfeed away from home.

E. Breast and nipple assessment:

    1. Refer to the "Breasts and nipples" subsection in the section titled "IV. Prior to Receiving the Infant" earlier in this chapter.

    2. Breastmilk production:

      a. Is the mother producing any breastmilk at present?

      b. How long has it been since the last breastfeeding or expression of milk?

      c. A very short lactation gap may mean a short time to achieving a flow of milk (De et al., 2002).

F. Planning:

    1. Expected outcome:

      a. Encourage the mother to define her success as the reestablishment of the breastfeeding relationship, rather than milk yield.

      b. Determine her expectations about her ability to make breastmilk.

      c. Determine her expectations about her ability to reintroduce her baby to the breast.

      d. Encourage realistic levels of achievement.

    2. Counseling:

      a. Emphasize the breastfeeding relationship, facilitated by skin-to-skin contact.

    b. Focus on having the baby learn to accept and actively suckle the mother's breast.

    c. Provide additional support to the mother who is relactating for a child with an intolerance to other milks because she may be under considerable stress (Riordan, 2010). This support should include:

       i. Stress management.

       ii. Ascertaining what replacement feeding is being used and whether the child is tolerating it. If not, advise the mother to consult her baby's pediatrician.

       iii. Information about the availability of a human milk bank, if applicable.

3. Ascertain the mother's level of breastfeeding confidence, which is important for relactation, just as it is for lactation immediately following a delivery (Blyth et al., 2002; Dennis, 1999; Meedya et al., 2010; Persad et al., 2008).

4. Provide appropriate and intensive support because confidence-building support from a knowledgeable health worker has been recommended by various authors (Agarwal et al., 2010; Banapurmath et al., 2003; De et al., 2002; Gribble, 2001; Seema et al., 1997).

5. Remind the mother that two parties are involved in relactation: the mother and her baby (Riordan, 2010).

6. Ask if the mother is employed and working at the moment.

    a. If so, is she able to reduce her hours temporarily?

    b. What are her goals? For some mothers, mixed feeding may be an achievable goal while employed; that is, giving the baby breastmilk with some ABM or age-appropriate complementary foods.

7. Provide regular telephone contact, which may be an appropriate form of professional support.

8. Avoid suggesting a specific time frame because of individual variation and the numerous mother and baby factors involved (Agarwal et al., 2010).

    a. If the baby is suckling at very frequent intervals, a flow of breastmilk can appear in a few days to a few weeks.

    b. Although some mothers fully relactate, some mothers may never achieve full lactation but are able to breastfeed, with supplementation, for an extended period.

G. Support from family and others:

    1. Psychological support and household assistance

    2. Appropriate information, support, and encouragement from a knowledgeable health worker (Seema et al., 1997)

    3. Ongoing support from a mother's support group or breastfeeding counselor

H. Reestablishing lactation/reversal of weaning:

    1. Stimulation to induce breastmilk production

       a. Many women have achieved relactation simply by nursing the baby intensively at the breast, usually with but sometimes without manual stimulation of the breast and nipples (Agarwal et al., 2010; Banapurmath et al., 2003; Kesaree et al., 1993; Marquis et al., 1998; Scantlebury, 1923; Seema et al., 1997; Taylor, 1995).

    b. Banapurmath et al. (1993a) and Lakhkar et al. (1999) found no difference in relactation outcomes between mothers who used breast/nipple hyperstimulation (very frequent suckling) and those who used metoclopramide as well.

    c. Encourage optimal latch and breastfeeding technique to maximize stimulation and milk removal (ABM Protocol Committee, 2011).

    d. Back massage, up and down both sides of the spinal column, has been used to enhance oxytocin release in conjunction with stimulation of the breasts and nipples (Agarwal et al., 2010).

I. Infant suckling at the breast is desirable. To encourage the infant, do the following:

    1. Provide a flow of milk through a feeding tube supplementer while at breast, or use the drop and drip method, with a drop of milk by tube or syringe to reward each suck (Agarwal et al., 2010).

    2. Put the baby to the breast while sleepy and not fully awake, and use other techniques associated with breast refusal.

J. Expressing:

    1. Discuss expression of the breasts by hand or with an electric or manual pump, if mother and baby are separated or the baby is reluctant to suckle.

        a. Provides stimulus to the breasts

        b. Allows milk production to be initiated or increased, which, in turn, increases the infant's willingness to nurse

    2. Teach and assess the skill of hand expression.

    3. Assess the effectiveness of the breast pump of the mother's choice, if she is using one, and her ability to use it. A pump that is ineffective, faulty, or that causes pain undermines the mother's efforts (Dwyer, 2008; Lawrence et al., 2011).

    4. Assess the mother's ability to achieve expression frequency in the case of a nonnursing baby (minimum six times in 24 hours/15 minutes each expression; twohourly if possible).

K. Galactagogues. See subsections 5, 6, and 7 in the section titled "VI. Establishing Lactation: Inducing Milk Production" earlier in the chapter.

L. Evaluation. Refer to subsection F in "VI. Establishing Lactation: Inducing Milk Production" earlier in the chapter.

M. Challenges:

    1. Relactation is not always easy, nor is it necessarily easier than induced lactation.

    2. Although for some mother–baby dyads a flow of milk is soon established, for others it may take weeks to increase the milk yield.

    3. Nonacceptance of the breast, or refusing out of frustration before there is a milk flow.

    4. Unreliable milk ejection reflex.

    5. Insufficient milk for the baby's needs, necessitating supplementation.

    6. Fatigue.

N. Supplementation. See subsection E(3) in "VI. Establishing Lactation: Inducing Milk Production" earlier in the chapter.

VIII. Milk Composition Following Induced Lactation and Relactation

A. Milk composition following induced lactation has been shown in other species (for example, bovine and rat) to be similar to breastmilk produced after a pregnancy and delivery (Lawrence et al., 2011.

B. Case series and case studies have repeatedly noted normal growth on human milk produced after induced lactation/relactation (Abejide et al., 1997; Banapurmath et al., 1993b; De et al., 2002; Mobbs et al., 1971; Nemba, 1994; Scantlebury, 1923; Seema et al., 1997).

C. Relactation has been used to correct poor growth in weaned infants (Marquis et al., 1998).

D. Few papers have been published specifically on the nutritional and immunological composition of milk produced in induced lactation or relactation.

   1. Investigations of the milk composition of adoptive mothers involve only a handful of cases.

   2. Breastmilk composition following relactation or unweaning of a biological child has yet to be investigated; literature searches do not find any published sources.

   3. Research on breastmilk after induced lactation is still very limited and contradictory because methodology differs.

     a. Kulski et al. (1981) included two adoptive mothers who had induced lactation in their case series of nonpuerperal lactation, with other cases involving galactorrhea resulting from pathologies.

       i. Total protein concentrations in the first milk of the adoptive mothers approximated those of transitional milk following a pregnancy, with no colostral phase.

       ii. The proportions of proteins differed from that of the biological mothers, with lower IgA and higher a-lactalbumin than colostrum, though the values were between those of transitional and mature milk.

       iii. Concentrations of lactose, potassium, and chloride in the first milk of nonbiological mothers approximated those of the transitional or mature milk of the biological mothers.

     b. Kleinman et al. (1980) compared the breast secretions of five adoptive mothers who had induced lactation with those of five biological mothers.

       i. A colostral phase was absent in the milk of the nonbiological mothers.

       ii. The total protein values of the first milk resembled that of the transitional and mature milk of biological mothers.

References

Abejide, O. R., Tadese, M. A., Babajide, D. E., et al. (1997). Non-puerperal induced lactation in a Nigerian community: Case reports. *Annals of Tropical Paediatrics, 17*, 109–114.

Academy of Breastfeeding Medicine Protocol Committee. (2011). ABM clinical protocol no. 9: Use of galactogogues in initiating or augmenting the rate of maternal milk secretion (first revision January 2011). *Breastfeeding Medicine, 6*, 41–49.

Agarwal, S., & Jain, A. (2010). Early successful relactation in a case of prolonged lactation failure. *Indian Journal of Pediatrics, 77*(2), 214.

Anonymous. (1845). Chemistry, pharmacy, and material medica: Analysis of milk taken from a he-goat. *Lancet, 45*(1115), 38.

Aono, T., Aki, T., Koike, K., & Kurachi, K. (1982). Effect of sulpiride on poor puerperal lactation. *American Journal of Obstetrics and Gynecology, 143*, 927–932.

Archer, M. (1990). Coming to grips with male nipples. *Australian Natural History, 23*, 494–495.

Auerbach, K. G., & Avery, J. L. (1979a). *Nursing the adopted infant: Report from a survey* [Monograph]. Denver, CO: Resources in Human Nurturing International.

Auerbach, K. G., & Avery, J. L. (1979b). *Relactation after a hospital-induced separation: Report from a survey* [Monograph]. Denver, CO: Resources in Human Nurturing International.

Auerbach, K. G., & Avery, J. L. (1979c). *Relactation after an untimely weaning: Report from a survey* [Monograph]. Denver, CO: Resources in Human Nurturing International.

Auerbach, K. G., & Avery, J. (1980). Relactation: A study of 366 cases. *Pediatrics, 65*, 236–242.

Auerbach, K. G., & Avery, J. (1981). Induced lactation: A study of adoptive nursing and counseling in 240 women. *American Journal of Diseases of Children, 135*, 340–334.

Australian Breastfeeding Association. (2004). *Relactation and adoptive breastfeeding* (2nd ed.). East Malvern, Australia: Author.

Avery, J. L. (1973). *Induced lactation: A guide for counseling and management.* Denver, CO: J. J. Avery.

Banapurmath, C. R., Banapurmath, S. C., & Kesaree, N. (1993a). Initiation of relactation. *Indian Pediatrics, 30*, 1329–1332.

Banapurmath, C. R., Banapurmath, S. C., & Kesaree, N. (1993b). Successful induced non-puerperal lactation in surrogate mothers. *Indian Journal of Pediatrics, 60*, 639–643.

Banapurmath, S., Banapurmath, C. R., & Kesaree, N. (2003). Initiation of lactation and establishing relactation in outpatients. *Indian Pediatrics, 40*, 343–347.

Basedow, H. (1925). *The Australian aboriginal.* Adelaide, South Australia: F. W. Preece & Sons.

Becker, G. E., McCormick, F. M., & Renfrew, M. J. (2009). Methods of milk expression for lactating women [Review]. Cochrane Collaboration. *Cochrane Library, 3*, 1–40.

Blyth, R., Creedy, D. K., Dennis, C. L., et al. (2002). Effect of maternal confidence on breastfeeding duration: An application of breastfeeding self-efficacy theory. *Birth, 29*, 278–284.

Bose, C. L., D'Ercole, J., Lester, A. G., et al. (1981). Relactation by mothers of sick and premature infants. *Pediatrics, 67*, 565–569.

Boyle, D. (1993, January–February). Adoptive nursing. *Leaven*, 3–5, 10.

Brown, R. (1973). Breastfeeding in modern times. *American Journal of Clinical Nutrition, 26*, 556–562.

Brown, R. (1977). Relactation: An overview. *Pediatrics, 60*, 116–120.

Brown, R. E. (1978). Relactation with reference to application in developing countries. *Clinical Pediatrics, 17*, 333–337.

Bryant, C. A. (2006). Nursing the adopted infant. *Journal of the American Board of Family Medicine*, *19*, 374–379.

Budd, S., Erdman, S., Long, D., et al. (1993). Improved lactation with metoclopramide. *Clinical Pediatrics*, *32*, 53–57.

Cheales-Siebenaler, N. J. (1999). Induced lactation in an adoptive mother. *Journal of Human Lactation*, *15*, 41–43.

Clavey, S. (1996). The use of acupuncture for the treatment of insufficient lactation (Que Ru). *American Journal of Acupuncture*, *24*, 35–46.

Cohen, R. (1971). Breast feeding without pregnancy. *Pediatrics*, *48*, 996–997.

Creel, S. R., Monfort, S. L., Wildt, D. E., et al. (1991). Spontaneous lactation is an adaptive result of pseudopregnancy. *Nature*, *351*, 660–662.

Datta, P., Embree, J. E., Kreiss, J. K., et al. (1993). Resumption of breast-feeding in later childhood: A risk factor for mother to mother immunodeficiency virus type 1 transmission. *Pediatric Infectious Disease Journal*, *11*, 974–976.

De, N. C. (2003). Baby friendly hospitals: How friendly are they? *Indian Pediatrics*, *40*, 378–379.

De, N. C., Pandit, B., Mishra, S. K., et al. (2002). Initiating the process of relactation: An institute based study. *Indian Pediatrics*, *39*, 173–178.

de Aquino, R. R., & Osório, M. M. (2009). Relactation, translactation, and breast-orogastric tube as transition methods in feeding preterm babies. *Journal of Human Lactation*, *25*(4), 420–426.

Dennis, C. L. (1999). Theoretical underpinnings of breastfeeding confidence: A self-efficacy framework. *Journal of Human Lactation, 15*, 195–2001.

Di Pierro, F., Callegari, A., Carotenuto, D., et al. (2008). Clinical efficacy, safety and tolerability of Bio-CÒ (micronized silymarin) as a galactogogue. *Acta Biomedica, 79*, 205–210.

Dwyer, D. (2008). Coping with breast pump problems. *Nursing, 25*.

Ehrenkranz, R. A., & Ackerman, B. A. (1986). Metoclopramide effect on faltering milk production by mothers of premature infants. *Pediatrics*, *78*, 614–620.

Emery, M. M. (1996). Galactagogues: Drugs to induce lactation. *Journal of Human Lactation, 12*, 55–57.

Fewtrell, M. S., Loh, K. L., Blake, A., et al. (2006). Randomised double blind trial of oxytocin nasal spray in mothers expressing breast milk for preterm infants. *Archives of Disease in Childhood*, *91*, F169–F174.

Gabay, M. P. (2002). Galactogogues: Medications that induce lactation. *Journal of Human Lactation*, *18*, 274–279.

Gribble, K. D. (2001). Mother-to-mother support for women breastfeeding in unusual circumstances: A new method for an old model. *Breastfeed Review*, *9*, 13–19.

Gribble, K. D. (2005a). Breastfeeding a medically fragile foster child. *Journal of Human Lactation*, *21*, 42–46.

Gribble, K. D. (2005b). Infant feeding in the post Indian ocean tsunami context: Reports, theory and action. *Birth Issues*, *14*, 121–127.

Gribble, K. D. (2005c). Post-institutionalized adopted children who seek breastfeeding from their new mothers. *Journal of Prenatal and Perinatal Psychology and Health*, *19*, 217–235.

Gribble, K. D. (2006). Mental health, attachment and breastfeeding: Implications for adopted children and their mothers. *International Breastfeeding Journal*, *1*, 5.

Hale, T. (2010). *Medications and mothers' milk: A manual of lactational pharmacology* (14th ed.). Amarillo, TX: Hale Publishing.

Hill, P. D., Aldag, J. C., & Chatterton, R. T. (1996). The effect of sequential and simultaneous breast pumping on milk volume and prolactin levels: A pilot study. *Journal of Human Lactation, 12*, 193–199.

Hill, P. D., Chatterton, R. T., & Aldag, J. C. (1999). Serum prolactin in breastfeeding: State of the science. *Biological Research for Nursing, 1*, 65–75.

Hofmeyr, G., & van Iddekinge, B. (1983). Domperidone and lactation. *Lancet, 1*, 647.

Hofmeyr, G., van Iddekinge, B., & Blott, J. A. (1985). Domperidone: Secretion in breast milk and effect on puerperal prolactin levels. *British Journal of Obstetrics and Gynaecology, 92*, 141–144.

Hormann, E. (1977). Breastfeeding the adopted baby. *Birth and the Family Journal, 4*, 165–172.

Hormann, E., & Savage, F. (1998). *Relactation: Review of experience and recommendations for practice.* Geneva, Switzerland: World Health Organization.

Huggins, K. E., Petok, E. S., & Mireles, O. (2000). Markers of lactation insufficiency: A study of 34 mothers. In K. Auerbach (Ed.), *Current issues in clinical lactation 2000* (pp. 25–35). Sudbury, MA: Jones and Bartlett.

Humphrey, S. (2003). *The nursing mother's herbal.* Minneapolis, MN: Fairview Press.

International Lactation Consultant Association (2011). ILCA encourages breastfeeding support in emergencies. Press release. Available from from http://www.ilca.org/files/in_the_news/Emergencies/2011-03_PressRelease_JapanEarthquake.pdf Retrieved March 9, 2012.

Jenner, C., & Filshie, J. (2002). Galactorrhoea following acupuncture. *Acupuncture in Medicine, 20*, 107–108.

Kauppila, A., Kivinen, S., & Ylikorkala, O. (1981). A dose response relation between improved lactation and metoclopramide. *Lancet, 1*, 1175–1177.

Kauppila, A., Kivinen, S., & Ylikorkala, O. (1983). Metoclopramide and breastfeeding: Transfer into milk and the newborn. *European Journal of Clinical Pharmacology, 25*, 819–823.

Kesaree, N. (1993). Drop and drip method. *Indian Pediatrics, 30*, 277–278.

Kesaree, N., Banapurmath, C. R., Banapurmath, S., & Shamanur, K. (1993). Treatment of inverted nipples using a disposable syringe. *Journal of Human Lactation, 9*, 27–29.

Kleinman, R., Jacobson, L., Hormann, E., & Walker, W. (1980). Protein values of milk samples from mothers without biologic pregnancies. *Journal of Pediatrics, 97*, 612–615.

Kramer, P. (1995). Breastfeeding of adopted infants [Letter]. *British Medical Journal, 311*, 188–189.

Kulski, J., Hartmann, P., Saint, W., et al. (1981). Changes in milk composition of nonpuerperal women. *American Journal of Obstetrics and Gynecology, 139*, 597–604.

Lakhkar, B. B. (2000). Breastfeeding in adopted babies. *Indian Pediatrics, 37*, 1114–1116.

Lakhkar, B. B., Shenoy, V. D., & Bhaskaranand, N. (1999). Relactation—Manipal experience. *Indian Pediatrics, 36*, 700–703.

Lawrence, R. A., & Lawrence, R. M. (2011). *Breastfeeding: A guide for the medical profession* (7th ed.). Maryland Heights, MO: Elsevier.

Marieskind, H. (1973). Abnormal lactation. *Journal of Tropical Pediatrics and Environmental Child Health, 19*, 123–128.

Marquis, G. S., Diaz, J., Bartolini, R., et al. (1998). Recognizing the reversible nature of child-feeding decisions: Breastfeeding, weaning and relactation patterns in a shanty town community of Lima, Peru. *Social Science and Medicine, 47*, 645–656.

McNeilly, A., Thorner, M., Volans, G., & Besser, G. M. (1974). Metoclopramide and prolactin. *British Medical Journal, 2*, 729.

Meedya, S., Fahy, K., & Kable, A. (2010). Factors that positively influence breastfeeding duration to 6 months: A literature review. *Women and Birth*, *23*(4), 135–145.

Mennella, J. A. (2001). Sleep disturbances after acute exposure to alcohol in mother's milk. *Alcohol*, *25*, 153–158.

Mennella, J., A. & Beauchamp, G. (1993). Beer, breastfeeding and folklore. *Developmental Psychobiology*, *26*, 459–466.

Mennella, J. A., Pepino, M. Y., & Teff, K. L. (2005). Acute alcohol consumption disrupts the hormonal milieu of lactating women. *Journal of Endocrinology and Metabolism*, *90*, 1970–1985.

Menon, J., & Mathews, L. (2002). Relactation in mothers of high-risk infants. *Indian Pediatrics*, *39*, 983–984.

Milsom, S., Breier, B., Gallaher, B., et al. (1992). Growth hormone stimulates galactopoesis in healthy lactating women. *Acta Endocrinologica*, *127*, 337–343.

Mobbs, G. A, & Babbage, N. F. (1971). Breast feeding adopted children. *Medical Journal of Australia*, *2*, 436–437.

Nemba, K. (1994). Induced lactation: A study of 37 non-puerperal mothers. *Journal of Tropical Pediatrics*, *40*, 240–242.

Ohyama, M., Watabe, H., & Hayasaka, Y. (2010). Manual expression and electric pumping in the first 48h after delivery. *Pediatrics International*, *52*, 39–43.

Persad, M. D., & Mensinger, J. L. (2008). Maternal breastfeeding attitudes: Association with breastfeeding intent and socio-demographics among urban primiparas. *Journal of Community Health*, *33*(2), 53–60.

Peters, F., Schulaze-Tollert, J., & Schuth, W. (1991). Thyrotrophin-releasing hormone: A lactation promoting agent? *British Journal of Obstetrics and Gynaecology*, *98*, 880–985.

Phillips, V. (1969). Non-puerperal lactation among Australian Aboriginal women. Part I. *Nursing Mothers' Association of Australia News*, *5*(4). Reprinted as NMAA Research Bulletin No. 1.

Phillips, V. (1992). Relactation and high needs infants. *Journal of Human Lactation, 8*, 64.

Phillips, V. (1993). Relactation in mothers of children over 12 months. *Journal of Tropical Pediatrics*, *39*, 45–47.

Raphael, D. (1973). Breastfeeding the adopted baby. In *The tender gift: Breastfeeding* (pp. 89–96, 105–115, Chap. 9). Englewood Cliffs, NJ: Prentice Hall.

Riordan, J. (2010). Women's health and breastfeeding. In J. Riordan & K. Wambach (Eds.), *Breastfeeding and human lactation* (4th ed., pp. 530–533). Sudbury, MA: Jones and Bartlett.

Rosti, L., Nardini, A., Bettinelli, M. E., & Rosti, D. (1994). Toxic effects of a herbal tea mixture in two newborns. *Acta Paediatrica*, *83*, 683.

Scantlebury, V. (1923). The establishment and maintenance of breastfeeding. *Transactions of 1923 Australasian Medical Congress*, 190–191.

Seema, Patwari, A. K., & Satyanarayana, L. (1997). Relactation: An effective intervention to promote exclusive breastfeeding. *Journal of Tropical Pediatrics*, *43*, 213–216.

Sheng, P. L., & Xie, Q. W. (1989). Relationship between effect of acupuncture on prolactin secretion and central catecholamine and R-aminobutyric acid. *Zeng Ci Yan Jiu*, *14*, 446–451. (Abstract in English)

Siebenaler, N. (2002). Adoptive mothers and breastfeeding. In M. Walker (Ed.), *Core curriculum for lactation consultant practice* (pp. 416–421). Sudbury, MA: Jones and Bartlett Publishers.

Slome, C. (1956). Non-puerperal lactation in grandmothers. *Journal of Pediatrics*, *49*, 550–552.

Sofer, S., Ben-Ezer, D., & Dagan, R. (1993). Early severe dehydration in young breast-fed newborn infants. *Israel Journal of Medical Science, 29*, 85–89.

Sousa, P. L. R., Barros, F. C., Pinheiro, G. N. M., & Gazalle, R. V. (1975). Re-establishment of lactation with metoclopramide. *Journal of Tropical Pediatrics, 321*, 214–215.

Szucs, K. A., Axline, S. E., & Rosenman, M. B. (2010). Induced lactation and exclusive breast milk feeding of adopted premature twins. *Journal of Human Lactation, 26*(3), 309–313.

Taylor, R. (1995). Relactation on the Peloponnese. *Midwives, 108*, 152.

Thearle, M. J., & Weissenberger, R. (1984). Induced lactation in adoptive mothers. *Australian and New Zealand Journal of Obstetrics and Gynaecology, 24*, 283–286.

Thompson, N. M. (1996). Relactation in a newborn intensive care setting. *Journal of Human Lactation, 12*, 233–235.

Thorley, V. (1997). Relactation: What the exceptions can tell us. *Birth Issues, 6*, 24–29.

Thorley, V. (2010). *Relactation and induced lactation: Bibliography and resources* (Rev. ed.). Brisbane, Australia: Thorley.

Waletzky, L., & Herman, E. (1976). Relactation. *American Family Practitioner, 14*, 69–74.

Walker, M. (2006). *Breastfeeding management for the clinician: Using the evidence.* Sudbury, MA: Jones and Bartlett.

Wieschhoff, H. A. (1940). Artificial stimulation of lactation in primitive cultures. *Bulletin of the History of Medicine, 8*, 1403–1415.

World Health Organization. (2009). *Infant and young child feeding: Model chapter for textbooks for medical students and allied health professionals.* Geneva, Switzerland: Author.

Ylikorkala, O., Kauppila, A., Kivinen, S., et al. (1982). Sulpiride improves inadequate lactation. *British Medical Journal, 285*, 249–251.

Ylikorkala, O., Kauppila, A., Kivinen, S., et al. (1984). Treatment of inadequate lactation with oral sulpiride and buccal oxytocin. *Obstetrics and Gynecology, 63*, 57–60.

Zinaman, M. J., Hughes, V., Oueenan, J. Y., et al. (1992). Acute prolactin and oxytocin response and milk yield to infant suckling and artificial methods of expressing in lactating women. *Pediatrics, 89*, 437–440.

CHAPTER 36
Donor Human Milk Banking

Mary Rose Tully, MPH, IBCLC
Revised by Frances Jones, MSN, RN, IBCLC

OBJECTIVES

- List appropriate uses of donor human milk.
- Describe similarities and differences between donor milk banking operations in different countries.
- List benefits and costs of using donor milk for at-risk infants.
- Discuss the risks of informal milk sharing.
- Discuss the history of donor milk banking.

INTRODUCTION

Donor human milk banking is the process of providing human milk to a recipient other than the donor's own child. It involves recruiting and screening donors; storing, treating, and screening donated milk; and distributing the milk on physician order (Human Milk Banking Association of North America [HMBANA], 2011; National Institute for Health and Clinical Excellence, 2010; Springer, 1997). Donor milk banking should not be confused with storage and handling of mother's own milk for her own child in any setting (HMBANA, 2011).

Support for and emphasis on the importance of mother's own milk for her own infant should not be overlooked. Donor milk cannot duplicate the benefits of mother's own milk but is the second choice when mother's own milk is unavailable (World Health Organization [WHO], 2003).

In hospitals where donor milk is used, it is often prescribed as a supplement to a mother's own supply until she has sufficient milk for her baby's or babies' needs, to feed the baby whose mother cannot lactate, to feed the baby whose mother's milk cannot be used temporarily, or to feed an adopted baby (HMBANA, 2011; see **Table 36-1**). It is also used for feeding an infant who is not being breastfed and is not thriving on human milk substitutes, as a short-term therapy after gastrointestinal surgery (Rangecroft et al., 1978), to provide a source of immunoglobulin A (IgA) for an infant

(continues)

who is not being breastfed, or for an older child or adult suffering from IgA deficiency (Merhav et al., 1995; Tully, 1990).

Table 36-1

Donor milk can be prescribed for the treatment of various medical conditions, including, but not limited to:

1. Prematurity

2. Malabsorption

3. Feeding intolerance

4. Immunologic deficiencies

5. Congenital anomalies

6. Postoperative nutrition

7. Trophic feeds/gut priming

8. Any medically indicated need for infant supplemention

If supplies of banked milk are sufficient, milk may be dispensed by prescription for a large variety of situations, including but not limited to:

1. Absent or insufficient lactation

2. Adoption or surrogacy

3. Illness in the mother requiring temporary interruption of breastfeeding

4. Health risk to the infant from the milk of the biological mother

5. Death of the mother

6. When human milk is required for medical indications, and mother's own milk is insufficient or unavailable.

Source: Used with permission HMBANA Guidelines, 2011.

Donor milk is never intended to replace mother's own, but is meant to provide human milk where there is a medical need (Kim et al., 2010). In the United States and Canada, donor milk is occasionally used for infants whose mothers cannot provide it when the parents desire to use human milk and can afford the processing fee. Health insurance does not cover the fee if the baby does not have a medical need. An order from the infant's physician is still required. Donor milk is recommended by the World Health Organization (WHO, 2003), the American Academy of Pediatrics (Gartner et al., 2005), and in the Surgeon General's Call to Action (U.S. Department of Health and Human Services, 2011) as an alternative when mother's own milk is not available.

A compelling argument can be made to support the investment necessary to make donor milk available to every preterm or sick infant as a result of the body of evidence citing sufficient risks to not feeding human milk (Arslanoglu et al., 2010; Bertino et al., 2009; Gartner et al., 2005). The Convention on the Rights of the Child, Article 24 (UNICEF, 2011), recognizes the right of every child to "the enjoyment of the highest attainable standard of health and to facilities for the treatment of illness and rehabilitation to health." Ethically, the question becomes one of offering the highest standard of care to all infants, regardless of the individual mother's ability to provide her own milk.

I. Research Findings

A. Research and clinical practice have shown that preterm infants fed human milk, including banked donor milk, have improved outcomes related to the nutritional qualities, ease of digestibility, and immunological components of human milk (Wight, 2001). Wight (2001) estimates that because of the reduction in length of stay and decreased rates of necrotizing enterocolitis (NEC) and sepsis, there is a relative savings of approximately $11 to the hospital or healthcare plan for each $1 spent for donor milk obtained from a nonprofit bank.

   1. A multicenter study in the United Kingdom found that infants fed at least some human milk in the first month of life (donor or mother's own, all by gavage) had higher IQs at 7.5 to 8 years of age, even when controlling for psychosocial influences (Lucas et al., 1992).

   2. Further studies of this cohort as they reached adolescence showed that the children who were fed donor human milk had lower cholesterol and better high-density lipoprotein to low-density lipoprotein ratios than those children fed preterm formula (Singhal et al., 2001).

B. A meta-analysis of randomized controlled trials comparing incidence of NEC, a devastating bowel disease that is frequently fatal for preterm infants, showed that use of donor human milk compared to human milk substitutes (formula) was protective.

   1. A recent study indicated that use of human milk–based fortifier versus bovine milk–based fortifier in human milk resulted in significantly lower rates of NEC for extremely premature infants (Sullivan et al., 2010). None of the earlier individual studies show a significant risk to using formula, although in aggregate the studies showed that infants who were fed donor milk when mother's own was not available were four times less likely to develop confirmed NEC (McGuire et al., 2003). A Cochrane review of five randomized clinical trials with premature and low-birth-weight infants indicated a significantly higher incidence of NEC in formula-fed babies ((Quigley et al., 2007). A systematic review and meta-analysis of formula versus donor milk found that donor milk as the sole diet reduced the risk of NEC by almost 80% (Boyd et al., 2007).

   2. A paper by Schanler et al. (2005) reported that donor milk "offered little observed short-term advantage over [preterm formula] for feeding extremely premature infants" (p. 400).

   3. However, as Wight (2005) pointed out, this study did show a significantly lower incidence of chronic lung disease among the babies fed mother's own and donor milk compared to those fed preterm formula as well as a trend toward fewer days on a ventilator.

C. Boyd's systematic review (Boyd et al., 2007) indicated that, like mother's own milk, enhanced feeding tolerance occurred with donor milk. Other researchers have postulated that donor milk may play a key role in priming the immune system through its immune-active properties such as oligosaccharides and long-chained polyunsaturated fatty acids (LCPUFAs), which remain after pasteurization (Arslanoglu et al., 2010).

D. Several case reports in the literature describe the use of donor milk for treatment of a variety of conditions or to provide immunologic support and appropriate nutrition to full-term infants and older children (Tully et al., 2004) as well as some adults.

   1. Infants with chronic renal failure (Anderson et al., 1993), metabolic disorders (Arnold, 1995), IgA deficiency, and allergy (Tully, 1990) have been fed donor milk as adjunct to other treatments.

   2. Milk banks report many cases of feeding intolerance and allergy that have been treated with donor milk but not reported in the literature, including infants who have failed to thrive on anything but human milk. Donor milk is typically a treatment of last resort in these cases, primarily because of the expense.

   3. Some adult conditions respond to human milk, including hemorrhagic conjunctivitis (Centers for Disease Control and Prevention, 1982), IgA deficiency in liver transplant recipients (Merhav et al., 1995), and gastrointestinal problems, such as severe reflux (Wiggins et al., 1998).

II. Therapeutic Components of Human Milk for Adults

A. Certain proteins unique to human milk are being investigated for their therapeutic value for adults.

   1. Human milk contains a unique protein, multimeric alpha-lactalbumin, which induces apoptosis (programmed cell death) in certain cancer cells (Gustafsson et al., 2005; Hakansson et al., 1995).

   2. Human alpha-lactalbumin made lethal to tumor cells by treating human milk has been confirmed in a rat model as a very specific treatment for human glioblastomas (brain tumors) (Gustafsson et al., 2005).

   3. Alpha-lactalbumin-oleic acid isolated from human milk has been found to be successful as a topical treatment for skin papillomas resistant to traditional treatment (Gustafsson et al., 2004).

B. With publication of this research, interest in donor milk for treatment of cancer has increased (Hallgren et al., 2008; Rough et al., 2009). For cancer patients the improved quality of life that results from use of human milk in combination with more traditional therapies may be the most important factor (Rough et al., 2009).

III. Acceptance of Donor Milk

A. Generally, donor milk is acceptable to the families of the recipient babies. Parents need to understand how the donors are screened and the milk is processed and tested (Ighogboja et al., 1995; Kim et al., 2010).

   1. Some families request donor milk for an adopted baby or a baby whose mother cannot lactate simply because of the advantages of human milk feeding for all infants. Cost can be a factor in the decision, and there may be limited availability of milk if there are no medical reasons for needing the donor milk. In some countries, donor milk is dispensed only to infants in the hospital.

   2. Milk donors are anonymous except in special circumstances.

      a. Few milk banks are set up to do directed donations.

      b. However, among Muslims, it is important that the recipient mother and donor mother meet, because the Koran decrees that all babies who receive milk from the same mother are siblings and it would be an act of incest for the two women's children to marry when they are older (al-Naqeeb et al., 2000). Specific suggestions have been developed after consultation with Islamic religious leaders (Ramli et al., 2010).

IV. Donor Milk Banking Worldwide

A. Donor human milk banks are found in most parts of the world and are typically associated with a neonatal intensive care unit (NICU).

B. The use of donor milk is more common in some countries than in others.

   1. Central and South America

      a. With 299 active donor milk banks, Brazil has the most extensive national network of donor milk banks in the Americas and possibly in the world (Rede Nacional de Bancos de Leite Humano, 2005).

         i. These milk banks all operate under quality control from the national standard bank at Fiocruz University in Rio de Janeiro, and all milk bank personnel go through a 40-hour training course established by the national standard bank.

         ii. Donor milk is the feeding of choice for all infants who do not have mother's own milk to meet their needs in Brazilian hospitals (Gutiérrez et al., 1998).

         iii. The national network of donor milk banks is also the organization charged with promoting breastfeeding and offering clinical care and services to breastfeeding mothers and babies.

         iv. In 2003, with the assistance of the Pan American Health Organization, a structured process was developed to expand the Brazilian Network of Milk Banks internationally, particularly to Portuguese- and Spanish-speaking countries. In 2005, the Latin American Network of Human Milk Banks was formed. Many countries in South and Central America as well as a few African and European countries have established donor milk bank networks, or at least individual banks, based on the Brazilian model and have relied on the Brazilian central bank to provide training for personnel (Rede Nacional de Bancos de Leite Humano, 2005).

2. North America: In 2012, the Human Milk Banking Association of North America had 12 distributing banks and 5 developing banks as members.

   a. The United States has ten nonprofit donor milk banks and five developing banks with more hospitals considering opening banks. These ten milk banks serve both inpatients and outpatients across the country and accept donations from mothers across the country. Milk can be shipped frozen by overnight express.

   b. Canada has two active donor milk banks and two other centers actively pursuing establishment of milk banks.

3. Europe: In 2010, the European Milk Banking Association (EMBA) was formed. In 2012, EMBA had 26 member countries with 166 distributing milk banks and 12 planned banks (European Milk Bank Association, n.d.).

   a. The United Kingdom has 17 donor milk banks, located in hospitals in England, Scotland, Ireland, and Wales.

   b. The Scandinavian countries—Denmark, Norway, Sweden, and Finland—have a total of 59 donor milk banks. Norway is unique because the majority of donor milk for premature infants is used raw after careful screening (Grovslien et al., 2009).

   c. Germany has 10 milk banks and one additional planned bank, with most of them situated in former East Germany (Springer et al., 2008).

   d. In France, there are 18 donor milk banks and milk is shipped as needed. Some of the milk banks lyophilize (freeze dry) milk after pasteurization (Voyer et al., 2000).

   e. Italy has 26 donor milk banks with three more planned banks, all associated with neonatal intensive care units (NICUs).

   f. Switzerland has six milk banks.

   g. The remaining 30 European EMBA member countries have one to six milk banks and the number is growing annually.

4. Asia and Africa

   a. India has seven milk banks for NICU infants, with the first established in 1987 (Women's Feature Service, 2009).

   b. Although China has a history of donor milk banks (Arnold, 1996), plans to open the first current milk bank were canceled because of low breastfeeding rates (Li, 2008).

   c. Kuwait has one donor milk bank (al-Naqeeb et al., 2000).

    d. Donor milk banking is growing in Africa.

       i. In South Africa, there are three main milk banks, which belong to an umbrella body, the Human Milk Banking Association of South Africa (HMBASA) and have other smaller banks associated with them. They provide milk to infants in hospital as well as AIDS orphans.

       ii. In Cameroon, a retired British physician, Peter McCormick, has supported the development of five donor milk banks all operating on very limited budgets and in a manner that is sustainable in Cameroon.

       iii. Several other countries in Africa are working to establish milk banks.

    e. In Australia, there are four milk banks currently operating (B. Hartmann, personal communication, June 26, 2011).

    f. New Zealand is working on establishing a milk bank (Bartle, n.d.).

V. Donor Compensation

Typically, donors are not paid for their milk; however, in some countries, donors are compensated for expenses incurred at the end of their donation (Grovslien & Gronn, 2009). Most donors have altruistic motives of helping others and sharing with babies who are not as healthy as their own (Osbaldiston et al., 2007; Pimenteira et al., 2008). Donating milk also can be an important and therapeutic part of the grieving process for mothers whose babies have died (Miracle et al., 2010).

    A. The HMBANA guidelines, which are used in the United States and Canada, prohibit compensation to donors, as do the Brazilian government guidelines (Gutiérrez et al., 1998; HMBANA, 2011).

    B. A few European banks do compensate donors nominally.

      1. Usually the compensation is sufficient to cover expenses directly incurred to donate milk, for example, breast pump rental (Grovslien et al., 2009).

      2. Some milk banks loan breast pumps to donors during the period of donation (Voyer et al., 2000).

    C. Buying and selling donor milk as a commodity is discouraged for several reasons.

      1. The mother may feel economic pressure to sell her milk rather than feeding her own baby.

      2. It is difficult to ensure quality of screening of the potential donor.

      3. It is difficult to ensure the quality of the milk purchased (that is, has it been diluted or contaminated?).

      4. There is no long-term follow-up of recipients or donors or valid recordkeeping.

VI. Milk Bank Operation

A. In developed countries, donors typically use electric breast pumps at home; however, in developing countries, milk is often hand expressed, or the donor goes to the milk bank daily to pump.

B. Donor milk banks are located in hospitals or are freestanding in the community (Wilson-Clay, 2006).

   1. In hospital, the milk bank may be within the NICU, the food service department, or the blood or tissue banking department (HMBANA, 2011; Omarsdottir et al., 2008; Springer et al., 2008).

   2. In some countries, milk banks are regulated by the government (Putet, 2008).

C. Milk banks are staffed by a milk bank director/coordinator who oversees day-to-day operations and supervises donor recruiting and screening and milk processing and dispensing and a medical director who supervises medical decisions and may or may not do a physical exam on each donor and her infant. In some banks, rather than having a medical director, there is an advisory committee consisting of experts in key fields including medical representation that takes responsibility for overseeing the milk bank operations (HMBANA, 2011).

   1. The milk bank director/coordinator may be an International Board Certified Lactation Consultant, nurse, physician, or a trained milk bank coordinator.

   2. Frequently, a trained technician does the milk processing.

   3. The medical director, who is often (but not always) a neonatologist, or the advisory committee is responsible for clinical decisions and oversight of the milk banking operations.

   4. In Brazil, a 40-hour training course is required for milk bank personnel, and many countries in Central and South America use this same course for training milk bank personnel (Giugliani et al., 2005; Rede Nacional de Bancos de Leite Humano, 2005).

   5. Most donor milk banks are also sources of breastfeeding support and counseling. In many developing countries, they are a part of implementation of the Baby-Friendly Hospital Initiative (Giugliani et al., 2005).

D. Some countries, including Brazil (Giugliani et al., 2005), France (Putet, 2008), Norway (Grovslien et al., 2009), and the United Kingdom (National Institute for Health and Clinical Excellence, 2010), have national milk banking regulations through the Ministry of Health or other recognized national body. However, others, including the United States, Canada, and Italy, are regulated through professional organizations or general tissue banking guidelines (Arslanoglu et al., 2010; HMBANA, 2011).

   1. Cost to recipient varies by country and by service setting. With nonprofit banks, if there is·a charge, it is to cover the expense of screening the donors and processing the milk, not for the milk itself. For example, in France the cost is set by the Ministry of Health at 80 euros per liter (about $3.50/ounce) to institutions (G. Putet, personal communication, May 5, 2011). In the United States, nonprofit milk banks charge from $3–5 per ounce and $1.25 per ounce in Canada.

Most donor milk in the United States is dispensed to hospitals, and typically there is no charge to the patient. In Central and South America, the milk is used only with hospitalized patients and is a part of the care, so there is no charge to the patient.

VII. Screening and Storage

A. Milk donors and the donor milk are carefully screened, just as with other donor human tissues.

  1. In developed countries, donors are serum screened for such communicable diseases as human immunodeficiency virus (HIV), human T-lymphoma virus (HTLV), hepatitis B and C, and syphilis (Arslanoglu et al., 2010; HMBANA, 2011; Putet, 2008).

    a. Because blood banks screen for all of these diseases, so do donor milk banks even though HIV and HTLV are the only diseases known to be potentially transmitted via human milk.

B. The cost of serum screening is borne by the milk bank or the national health system, not the donor.

C. Some milk banks require a form to be completed by the donor's physician and her infant's physician.

D. Some milk banks have physicians on staff who perform a physical examination of each mother and infant.

E. Because cost is prohibitive in developing countries and the donor milk is so vital, some banks do a verbal/written screening to eliminate high-risk donors and rely on heat treatment to kill viruses and other pathogens (Giugliani et al., 2005)

F. All donor milk is screened for bacteria before it is dispensed.

  1. In Norway and in parts of Germany, after donor screening, milk is screened for bacteria and dispensed raw (Grovslien et al., 2009; Springer et al., 2008).

  2. It may be stored refrigerated or frozen until it is dispensed, depending on the length of time it is stored.

  3. HMBANA guidelines (HMBANA, 2011) allow for dispensing of milk raw in rare circumstances in North America; however, since 1988 no bank has reported a request for raw milk in the United States or Canada.

G. In most other countries, the donor milk is stored frozen at –20°C until it is heat processed and used, and it is refrozen after processing until it is distributed.

  1. Although freezing preserves most of the nutritional, immunologic, hormonal, and other unique properties of the milk, it does not destroy many pathogens.

  2. Careful heat treatment with Holder pasteurization (62.5°C timed for 30 minutes after the center container reaches temperature) preserves as many of the properties of the milk as possible (Tully et al., 2001). See **Table 36-2**.

H. Either a commercial human milk pasteurizer (HMBANA, 2011; National Institute for Health and Clinical Excellence, 2010) or a standard laboratory shaking water bath is used (HMBANA, 2011).

Table 36-2 Selected Components of Human Milk After Freezing and Pasteurization

	Function	Percentage Activity	References
IgA and sIgA*	Binds microbes in the baby's digestive tract to prevent their passage into other tissues	67–100	19,27,30
IgM*	Antibodies specifically targeted against pathogens to which the mother has been exposed	0	30,33
IgG*	Antibodies specifically targeted against pathogens to which the mother has been exposed	66–70	30,34
Lactoferrin (iron-binding capacity)*	Binds iron required by many bacteria and thus retards bacterial growth	27–43	19,33,34
Lysozyme*	Attacks bacterial cell walls and thus destroys many bacteria	75	33,34
Lipoprotein lipase*	Partly responsible for lipolysis of milk triglycerides to release monoglycerides and free fatty acids	0	23,38
Bile salt activated lipase*	Partly responsible for lipolysis of milk triglycerides to release monoglycerides and free fatty acids	0	23,38
Monoglycerides produced by lipolysis of milk triglycerides*	Disrupts the membrane coating of many viruses and protozoans, destroying them	100	37,38,39
Free fatty acids produced by lipolysis of milk triglycerides**	Disrupts the membrane coating of many viruses and protozoans, destroying them	100	37,38,39
Linoleic acid (18:2n6)**	Essential fatty acid; metabolic precursor for prostaglandins and leukotrienes	100	37,38,39
α-linolenic acid (18:3n3)**	Essential fatty acid; metabolic precursor for docosahexaenoic acid; important for eye and brain development	100	37,38,39

*These biologically active components do not occur in commercial formula.

**Some manufacturers are now adding docosahexaenoic acid and other supplemental fats to selected infant formula preparations.

Source: Used with permission from Tully, D. B., Jones, F., & Tully, M. R.(2001). Donor human milk: What's in it and what's not. *Journal of Human Lactation, 17,* 152.

1. The shaking water bath is considerably less expensive but more time intensive because the milk containers must be physically moved to a vat containing an ice slurry for quick chilling after heat treatment (Tully, 2000).
2. In Brazil, the central standards bank has developed a chart for processing time based on container volume, which minimizes even further the damage to the milk components (Almeida et al., 2006).

   I. Milk banks use a wide variety of containers for processing and storing milk. Some decisions have been based on scientific investigation and others are based on convenience (Goes et al., 2002; HMBANA, 2011; Portal Brazil, 2011).
   J. Most milk banks accept initial donations in whatever container the donor has been using but will then provide containers for future donations.

VIII. Records

A. Donor milk bank records allow tracking of milk from donor to recipient. They also include each donor's screening profile and data on each batch of milk screened, processed, and dispensed.
1. Just as with other donor human tissue, it is important to be able to track milk from the time it arrives at the bank through the batch in which it is processed, screened, and dispensed.
B. Records on each individual batch of milk are maintained, including the processing and bacterial screening results.
C. Once a batch of milk is dispensed to a hospital, it is the hospital's responsibility to maintain accurate records of which patients received donor milk, from which bank, and from which batch(es).
D. In most countries, such records must be maintained until all recipients would have reached age of majority plus 3 years.
E. There are no adverse outcome reports on donor milk in the published literature in English. In addition, a review of legal torts by a law student in 2009 resulted in no cases being identified (Pauline Sakamoto, personal communication, August 31, 2011).

References

Almeida, S. G., & Dorea, J. G. (2006). Quality control of banked milk in Brasilia, Brazil. *Journal of Human Lactation, 22*(3), 335–339.

al-Naqeeb, N. A., Azab, A., Eliwa, M. S., & Mohammed, B. Y. (2000). The introduction of breast milk donation in a Muslim country. *Journal of Human Lactation, 16*, 346–350.

Anderson, A., & Arnold, L. D. (1993). Use of donor breast milk in the nutrition management of chronic renal failure: Three case histories. *Journal of Human Lactation, 9*, 263–264.

Arnold, L. D. (1995). Use of donor milk in the treatment of metabolic disorders: Glycolytic pathway defects. *Journal of Human Lactation, 11*, 51–53.

Arnold, L. D. (1996). Donor milk banking in China: The ultimate step in becoming baby friendly. *Journal of Human Lactation, 12*(4), 319–321.

Arslanoglu, S., Ziegler, E. E., & Moro, G. E. (2010). Donor human milk in preterm infant feeding: Evidence and recommendations. *Journal of Perinatal Medicine, 38*(4), 347–351.

Bartle, C. (n.d.). Donor human milk—what human milk banks do and what they don't do. Retrieved from http://www.nzno.org.nz/LinkClick.aspx?fileticket=LL9hJe41BXE%3D&tabid=605

Bertino, E., Giuliani, F., Occhi, L., Coscia, A., Tonetto, P., Marchino, F., & Fabris, C. (2009). Benefits of donor human milk for preterm infants: Current evidence. *Early Human Development*, *85*(10 Suppl.), S9–10.

Boyd, C. A., Quigley, M. A., & Brocklehurst, P. (2007). Donor breast milk versus infant formula for preterm infants: Systematic review and meta-analysis. *Archives of Disease in Childhood: Fetal and Neonatal Edition*, *92*, F169–175.

Centers for Disease Control and Prevention. (1982). Acute hemorrhagic conjunctivitis—American Samoa. *Morbidity and Mortality Weekly Report*, *31*(3), 21–22.

European Milk Bank Association. (n.d.). Home page. Retrieved from http://www.europeanmilkbanking.com.

Fernandez, A., Mondkar, J., & Nanavati, R. (1993). The establishment of a human milk bank in India. *Journal of Human Lactation,9*, 189–190.

Flatau, G., & Brady, S. (2006). *Starting a donor human milk bank: A practical guide*. Raleigh, NC: Human Milk Banking Association of North America.

Gartner, L. M., Morton, J., Lawrence, R. A., et al. (2005). Breastfeeding and the use of human milk. *Pediatrics*, *115*, 496–506.

Giugliani, E., & de Almeida, J. (2005, October 17–18). *The role of donor milk banking in breastfeeding promotion: Brazil's experience*. Presentation at Human Milk Banking: A Global Perspective on Best Practice, sponsored by HMBANA, Alexandria, VA.

Goes, H. C., Torres, A. G., Donangelo, C. M., & Trugo, N. M. (2002). Nutrient composition of banked human milk in Brazil and influence of processing on zinc distribution in milk fractions. *Nutrition*, *18*(7), 590–594.

Grovslien, A., & Gronn, M. (2009). Donor milk banking and breastfeeding in Norway. *Journal of Human Lactation*, *25*(2), 206–210.

Gustafsson, L., Hallgren, O., Mossberg, A. K., et al. (2005). HAMLET kills tumor cells by apoptosis: Structure, cellular mechanisms, and therapy. *Journal of Nutrition*, *135*, 1299–1303.

Gustafsson, L., Leijonhufvud, I., Aronsson, A., et al. (2004). Treatment of skin papillomas with topical alpha-lactalbumin-oleic acid. *New England Journal of Medicine*, *350*, 2663–2672.

Gutiérrez, D., & de Almeida, J. A. (1998). Human milk banks in Brazil. *Journal of Human Lactation*, *14*, 333–335.

Hakansson, A., Zhivotovsky, B., Orrenius, S., et al. (1995). Apoptosis induced by a human milk protein. *Proceedings of the National Academy of Sciences USA*, *92*, 8064–8068.

Hallgren, O., Aits, S., Brest, P., Gustafsson, L., Mossberg, A. K., Wulit, B., & Svanborg, C. (2008). Apoptosis and tumor cell death in response to HAMLET (human alpha-lactalbumin made lethal to tumor cells). *Advances in Experimental Medicine and Biology*, *606*, 217–240.

Human Milk Banking Association of North America. (2011). *Guidelines for the establishment and operation of a donor human milk bank*. Raleigh, NC: Author.

Ighogboja, I. S., Olarewaju, R. S., Odumodu, C. U., & Okuonghae, H. O. (1995). Mothers' attitudes towards donated breastmilk in Jos, Nigeria. *Journal of Human Lactation*, *11*, 93–96.

Kim, J. H., & Unger, S. (2010). Human milk banking. Canadian Pediatric Society. *Paediatrics and Child Health*, *15*(9), 595–598.

Li, C. (2008). Plans dry up for breast milk bank. *China Daily*, November 9. Retrieved March 15, 2012 from http://www.chinadaily.com.cn/cndy/2008-10/09/content_7088914.htm.

Lucas, A., Morley, R., Cole, T. J., Lister, G., & Leeson, P. C. (1992). Breast milk and subsequent intelligence quotient in children born preterm [see comments]. *Lancet, 339*, 261–264.

McGuire, W., & Anthony, M. Y. (2003). Donor human milk versus formula for preventing necrotising enterocolitis in preterm infants: Systematic review. *Archives of Disease in Childhood: Fetal and Neonatal Edition, 88*, F11–F14.

Merhav, H. J., Wright, H. I., Mieles, L. A., & Van Thiel, D. H. (1995). Treatment of IgA deficiency in liver transplant recipients with human breast milk. *Transplant International, 8*, 327–329.

Miracle, D., & Wellborn, J. (2010, April 13). *Bereavement and milk donation.* Presentation at 100 Years of Milk Banking: Looking Back and Reaching Forward, Boston, MA.

National Institute for Health and Clinical Excellence. (2010). *NICE clinical guideline 93. Donor breast milk banks: The operation of donor milk bank services.* London, England: Author.

Omarsdottir, S., Casper, C., Akerman, A., Polberger, S., & Vanpee, M. (2008). Breastmilk handling routines for preterm infants in Sweden: a national cross-sectional study. *Breastfeeding Medicine, 3*(3), 165–170.

Osbaldiston, R., & Mingle, L. A. (2007). Characterization of human milk donors. *Journal of Human Lactation, 23*(4), 350–357.

Pimenteira, T., Maia, L., da Silva, O. T., Furtadoi, M. N. C., Dantas, A. J. E., Fernando, R. S. C., & Calado, C. J. (2008). The human milk donation experience: Motives, influencing factors, and regular donation. *Journal of Human Lactation, 1*, 69–76.

Portal Brazil. (2011). Milk banks.Found at http://www.brasil.gov.br/sobre/health/programs-and-campaigns/milk-banks-1/br_video?set_language=en. Accessed on August 31, 2011.

Putet, G. (2008, October 17). *New French law on human milk bank's good practices.* Presentation at the 2nd International Human Milk Banking Meeting: Donor Breastmilk: So Precious That We Keep It in a Bank, Milan, Italy.

Quigley, M. A., Henderson, G., Anthony, M. Y., & McQuire, W. (2007). Formula milk versus donor breast milk for feeding preterm or low birth weight infants. *Cochrane Database of Systematic Reviews, 4*, CD002971.

Ramli, N., Ibrahim, N. R., & Hans, V. R. (2010). Human milk banks—the benefits and issues in an Islamic setting. *Eastern Journal of Medicine, 15*, 163–167.

Rangecroft, L., de San Lazaro, C., & Scott, J. E. (1978). A comparison of the feeding of the postoperative newborn with banked breast-milk or cow's-milk feeds. *Journal of Pediatric Surgery, 13*, 11–12.

Rede Nacional de Bancos de Leite Humano. (2005). Bancos de Leite Humano no Brasil. Retrieved from http://www.redeblh.fiocruz.br

Rough, S., Sakamoto, P., Fee, C., & Hollenbeck, C. B. (2009). Qualitative analysis of cancer patients' experiences using donated human milk. *Journal of Human Lactation, 25*(2), 211–219.

Schanler, R. J., Lau, C., Hurst, N. M., & Smith, E. O. (2005). Randomized trial of donor human milk versus preterm formula as substitutes for mothers' own milk in the feeding of extremely premature infants. *Pediatrics, 116*, 400–406.

Singhal, A., Cole, T. J., & Lucas, A. (2001). Early nutrition in preterm infants and later blood pressure: Two cohorts after randomised trials. *Lancet, 357*, 413–419.

Springer, S., & Gebauer, C. (2008, October 17). *Trends in human milk banking in Germany.* Presentation at the 2nd International Human Milk Banking Meeting: Donor Breastmilk: So Precious That We Keep It in a Bank, Milan, Italy.

Sullivan, S., Schanler, R. J., Kim, J. H., Patel, A. L., Trawoger, R., Kiechl-Kohlendorfer, U., Chan, G. M., Blanco, C. L., Abrams, S., Cotton, C. M., Laroia, N., Ehrenkranz, R. A., Dudell, G., Cristifalo, E. A., Meier, P., Lee, M. L., Rechtman, D. J., & Lucas, A. (2010). An exclusively human milk-based diet is associated with a lower rate of necrotizing enterocolitis than a diet of human milk and bovine milk-based products. *Journal of Pediatrics, 156*(4), 562–567.

Tully, D. B., Jones, F., & Tully, M. R. (2001). Donor milk: What's in it and what's not. *Journal of Human Lactation, 17*, 152–155.

Tully, M. R. (1990). Banked human milk in treatment of IgA deficiency and allergy symptoms. *Journal of Human Lactation, 6*, 75–76.

Tully, M. R. (2000). Cost of establishing and operating a donor human milk bank. *Journal of Human Lactation, 16*, 57–59.

Tully, M. R., Lockhart-Borman, L., & Updegrove, K. (2004). Stories of success: The use of donor milk is increasing in North America. *Journal of Human Lactation, 20*, 75–77.

UNICEF. (2011). Convention on the Rights of the Child: The human rights framework. Retrieved from http://www.unicef.org/crc/index_framework.html

U.S. Department of Health and Human Services. (2011). The Surgeon General's call to action to support breastfeeding. Washington, DC: U.S. Department of Health and Human Services, Office of the Surgeon General. Retrieved from http://www.surgeongeneral.gov/topics/breastfeeding/index.html.

Voyer, M., Nobre, R., & Magny, J. F. (2000). Human milk banks organization in France: Legal proceedings and their consequences on milk bank activities. In G. De Nisi (Ed.), *La Banca Del Latte Materno* (pp. 21–28). Trento, Italy: New Magazine.

Weaver, G. (1999). Every drop counts: News from the United Kingdom Association for Milk Banking. *Journal of Human Lactation, 15*, 251–253.

Wiggins, P. K., & Arnold, L. D. (1998). Clinical case history: Donor milk use for severe gastroesophageal reflux in an adult. *Journal of Human Lactation, 14*, 157–159.

Wight, N. E. (2001). Donor human milk for preterm infants. *Journal of Perinatology, 21*(4), 249–254.

Wight, N. E. (2005). Donor milk: Down but not out. *Pediatrics, 116*, 1610–1611.

Wilson-Clay, B. (2006). The milk of human kindness: The story of the Mothers Milk Bank at Austin. *International Breastfeeding Journal, 1*(1), 6.

Women's Feature Service. (2009). India: Banking on mother's milk. *News Blaze.* Retrieved April 16, 2012 from http://newsblaze.com/story/20090106052848iwfs.nb/topstory.html.

World Health Organization. (2003). *Global strategy for infant and young child feeding.* Geneva, Switzerland: Author.

CHAPTER 37
Pregnancy, Labor, and Birth Complications

Marsha Walker, RN, IBCLC
Revised by Suzanne Cox, AM, IBCLC, FILCA

OBJECTIVES

- Describe several maternal problems that can occur in the perinatal period.
- Plan for how breastfeeding can continue under adverse situations.
- Ascertain whether any of these conditions are present when working with a breastfeeding problem.
- Discuss how these situations can affect the baby and breastfeeding.

INTRODUCTION

Although pregnancy, labor, and birth are normal and natural processes, occasional problems arise that might have an impact on breastfeeding. These complications can change a mother's birth plan and might affect access to her infant after delivery. The lactation consultant can benefit from knowledge of the more common alterations in maternal health and strategies to circumvent any impediment to breastfeeding that might be present.

I. Hypertensive Disorders of Pregnancy

These include preeclampsia, severe preeclampsia, eclampsia (toxemia), and HELLP syndrome.

A. Preeclampsia
1. Determined by increased blood pressure after 20 weeks of gestation (pregnancy-induced hypertension) accompanied by proteinuria, edema, or both.
2. Occurs in 3% to 5% of otherwise normal pregnancies (Dietl, 2000; Higgins et al., 2001) and more frequently in women who have chronic renal or vascular diseases such as diabetes, collagen vascular disease, or chronic hypertension.
3. Preterm delivery usually occurs to improve the mother's condition and decrease infant morbidity associated with growth retardation and fetal asphyxia.

B. Severe preeclampsia

   1. A progression to higher blood pressure, increased proteinuria (protein in the urine), oliguria (decreased urine output), cerebral or visual changes, severe headaches, epigastric pain, pulmonary edema, or cyanosis.

C. Eclampsia

   1. If the baby is not delivered as severe preeclampsia continues, then the pre-eclampsia can progress to eclampsia (toxemia).

   2. Eclampsia denotes the occurrence of convulsions not caused by neurologic disease and usually occurs after 32 weeks gestation.

   3. Seizures can occur even after the baby is delivered.

   4. Women who have severe preeclampsia are usually hospitalized and placed on seizure precautions.

   5. The mother might be sedated and given antihypertensive medications and anticonvulsive medications, such as magnesium sulfate.

     a. Magnesium sulfate is compatible with breastfeeding (Hale, 2010).

     b. Magnesium sulfate given to the mother prior to delivery might lead to neonatal neuromuscular blockage with hypotonia and urine retention (Blackburn, 2007, p. 397).

   6. Breastfeeding depends on the condition of the mother and the baby.

   7. Because it is important to reduce stress and other noxious stimuli that could provoke a seizure, breastfeeding with mother and baby in skin-to-skin contact might actually be therapeutic as a result of the calming and sedating effects of prolactin and oxytocin (Light et al., 2000; Uvnäs Moberg et al., 2005).

   8. If the baby cannot go to the breast, arrangements need to be made for expressing breastmilk within hours of the birth.

   9. Antihypertensive medications are likely to continue after the baby is born.

D. HELLP syndrome

   1. H (intravascular hemolysis), EL (elevated liver enzymes: aspartate aminotransferase and alanine aminotransferase), LP (low platelets).

   2. A very small percentage (0.1%) of women who have preeclampsia develop HELLP syndrome (Abraham et al., 2001).

   3. It occurs most often early in the third trimester and is thought to result from a circulating immunologic component.

   4. Management is still controversial. To improve maternal and fetal prognosis, two approaches are usually considered.

     a. Immediate delivery after stabilization of the clinical condition (Haram et al., 2000) but with the risk of fetal complications related to prematurity. OR

     b. Conservative treatment using corticosteroids. The use of corticosteroids is only beneficial in increasing the rate of platelet recovery, but to date there is no evidence to support routine use (Gasem et al., 2009).

5. Women who develop HELLP might also experience disseminated intravascular coagulation (DIC) and require intensive medical care.

    a. DIC is caused by a process that consumes the plasma's clotting factors and platelets so that hemorrhage occurs.

    b. Severe hemorrhage associated with DIC can result in pituitary necrosis (Sheehan syndrome), a well-recognized cause of lactation failure (see the section titled "IV. Sheehan Syndrome") (Kelestimur, 2003).

6. During any intensive care period, the mother with HELPP is likely to need assistance to hand express or pump her milk regularly to ensure high levels of circulating prolactin and to increase prolactin receptor sites (De Carvalho et al., 1983). If the breasts are not drained regularly, then the alveoli become distended and the amount of prolactin released into the lactocyte decreases (Cregan et al., 2002).

II. Cesarean Delivery

A. The most frequently performed surgery in industrialized societies around the world.

    1. Usually performed under epidural or spinal anesthesia.

    2. Breastfeeding should not be delayed unless the conditions of the mother and/or baby preclude it.

B. Occasionally, a mother receives general anesthesia.

    1. Mother can breastfeed as soon as she is awake and able to respond.

    2. General anesthetic agents such as thiopental sodium and halothane are considered to be usually compatible with breastfeeding (Hale, 2010).

C. Compatible with skin-to-skin contact and breastfeeding.

    1. Mother can nurse her infant as soon as she feels ready, including in the recovery room (Cox, 2006).

    2. Most incisions are a lower uterine segment transverse, enabling the mother to more comfortably position her baby for breastfeeding across her lap.

    3. Vertical incisions are usually done when other surgery is indicated at the same time or in emergency deliveries.

D. Full-term healthy babies and mothers can and should recover together after cesarean delivery in skin-to-skin contact in the recovery room (Spear, 2006).

E. Medications:

    1. Mothers who are receiving pain relief intrathecally (around the spine) are usually quite comfortable and ready to breastfeed soon after surgery.

    2. Regular pain relief needs to be given to ensure that no breakthrough pain occurs, that the mother is comfortable to breastfeed whenever her baby requires, and to allow her to become ambulatory.

    3. Pain medication is usually required for 72 hours.

        a. Most common postoperative pain medications require no interruption or delay in breastfeeding, with morphine (Duramorph, Infumorph) being preferred because of absence of pediatric side effects.

    b. In comparison, meperidine (Demerol/pethidine) has been shown to cause neonatal sedation and poor sucking (Hale, 2010).

F. An unexpected cesarean delivery can be a significant disappointment to the mother, and time needs to be made for debriefing.

    1. Some mothers experience anger, resentment, remorse, grief, or relief at this point.

    2. Skin-to-skin contact and the concomitant release of extra oxytocin may alleviate both her pain and disappointment (Uvnäs-Moberg et al., 2005) and need to be instituted as soon as possible after the surgery.

G. An urgent cesarean may result in delayed secretory activation (Pang et al., 2007). Lactogenesis II (Dewey, 2001) and skin-to-skin contact following surgery (Uvnäs-Moberg et al., 2005) and/or frequent hand expressing (Morton et al., 2009) may assist in overcoming this early delay.

    1. Pang et al., (2007) suggest the use of the term *secretory activation* to replace the term *lactogenesis II* because it is more explanatory of what is occurring in the breast as the milk supply is commenced or initiated.

H. Some babies might be lethargic at first, especially if the mother has labored, the labor was protracted, and it involved long exposure to analgesia or anesthesia (Kuhnert et al., 1998; Rosenblatt et al., 1991; Scherer et al., 1995; Sepkoski et al., 1994; Volikas et al., 2005).

I. Suctioning of the mouth and throat might cause breastfeeding problems because it may temporarily cause infant oral defensiveness (Widstrom et al., 1987).

J. Finding a comfortable position in which to breastfeed can be worrisome to mothers.

    1. Placing the baby between the mother's breasts as she lies on her back, with a pillow behind her head, allows the baby time to follow prefeeding cues and self-latch (Matthiessen et al., 2001) as the mother watches.

    2. If the mother lies on her side, it is often easier for the baby to be placed so that the baby's nose is opposite the top breast. The mother can draw the baby forward behind the shoulders with her free top arm so that the baby's chin touches the breast and feeding reflexes and responses are elicited and he or she can self-latch.

    3. When the mother is sitting up, a pillow can be used to cover her cesarean incision area and to rest the baby on once he or she has latched.

    4. Fathers and other helpers should be encouraged to lift and change the baby and help position the baby at the breast.

K. The mother should breastfeed her baby 8 to 12 times each 24 hours including at night, when the infant demonstrates readiness to feed, and refrain from sending her baby to the nursery for long periods of time. Separation of mother and baby decreases opportunities for frequent breastfeeding and increases the likelihood of supplemental feedings, both of which adversely affect maternal milk production and the baby's interest in feeding at the breast.

L. In the early days, mothers who have had a cesarean need their rest; visitors are best limited to allow for napping and breastfeeding during the day.

M. Low-grade maternal fever (above 99°F [37°C] but below 100°F [37.8°C]) can occur. In the absence of other symptoms such as tachycardia, tachypnea, and wound redness/oozing, low-grade fever should not interrupt breastfeeding.

1. Even with antibiotic therapy breastfeeding should continue because antibiotics are "usually compatible with breastfeeding" (Hale, 2010).

N. If the baby is born preterm or is unable to breastfeed for some time, using a hospital-grade breast pump, preferably with a double collection kit, combined with hand expression (Morton et al., 2009) stimulates optimal milk production. (See Chapter 30.)

O. If the baby is temporarily unable to latch on to the breast, the mother can hand express colostrum into a spoon or cup and feed it to the baby (Collins et al., 2004; Dowling et al., 2002).

P. Mothers who receive antibiotics might be placed at a higher risk for *Candida* overgrowth.

III. Postpartum Hemorrhage

A. The most common obstetric emergency (5% of deliveries) and is life threatening (Reynders et al., 2006).

B. Considerable blood volume can be lost and intravenous fluids, including blood transfusion, might be necessary.

C. Oxytocic agents such as ergonovine maleate (Ergotrate, Ergometrine) or pitocin (Syntocinon or Syntometrine) are given intravenously, and if use is prolonged, they can affect milk production (Hale, 2010).

D. The mother will need assistance with positioning her baby for easy latch while she has an intravenous infusion and her blood pressure is low.

E. The mother will be exhausted and needs to be told that she will have low energy levels for between 6 and 12 weeks while she is replacing her red blood cells.

1. During this period, breastfeeding is an excellent time for her to rest.

2. She will need assistance with her baby's care.

IV. Sheehan Syndrome

A. Caused by a severe postpartum hemorrhage and hypotension often associated with disseminated intravascular coagulation (Kelestimur, 2003).

1. The decreased blood flow to the pituitary gland leads to an infarction and necrosis or other complications.

B. At the end of pregnancy, the pituitary is very sensitive to decreased blood flow because of its vascularity and increased size.

C. With no prolactin secretion, the alveoli can involute and lactation might be suppressed.

D. Prolactin-stimulating drugs such as metoclopramide (Reglan, Maxolon), supleride (Lawrence et al., 1999), and domperidone (Motilium; not available in the United States as a galactogogue) have been used to treat this condition (Hale, 2010).

E. Mild cases of pituitary disruption can occur with a delay in secretory activation (lactogenesis II). During this period, as well as frequent breastfeeding or pumping, there may be a need to offer supplementary fluid to the infant, preferably donor milk if available.

V. Episiotomy

A. A surgical incision of the perineum made to facilitate birth as the fetal head distends the perineum.
   1. A midline episiotomy, which is a straight line incision toward the rectum OR
   2. A mediolateral episiotomy, which is angled down and off to one side, usually the right
B. This procedure is often done routinely in industrialized countries.
C. Current research does not support routine episiotomies (Hartmann et al., 2005).
D. Usually done therapeutically for shoulder dystocia to allow more room for manual maneuvers to free the impacted shoulders of the infant.
E. Also used with forceps to provide more room for their application.
F. Naturally occurring lacerations involve less tissue and muscle impairment than do episiotomies, are less painful, and heal well without suturing (Lundquist et al., 2000).
G. Complications include excessive blood loss, infection of the incision, necrotizing fasciitis, extension of the midline episiotomy into a third-degree tear (into the rectal sphincter), and further extension into a fourth-degree perineal laceration (into the anterior rectal wall).
H. Can be extremely painful, and if pain is not controlled, it could interfere with the milk ejection reflex, impeding milk flow to the baby.
   1. To lessen the need for medications, ice therapy is frequently used.
   2. Cold packs are usually applied immediately following delivery, and iced sitz baths are also used for pain and to hasten healing; these are more effective for pain relief than warm sitz baths (Ramler et al., 1986).
   3. Extreme pain may require analgesic rectal suppositories such as diclofenac (Voltaren) that transfers in extremely low levels into breastmilk (Hale, 2010).
   4. Topical preparations have not been shown to hasten healing or decrease pain (Minassian et al., 2002).
I. Positioning to alleviate pain:
   1. Mothers who have episiotomies may have pain lasting up to 2 weeks or longer and often find it very hard to assume a comfortable position, especially when sitting upright.
   2. Therefore, these mothers may need assistance to position themselves and their babies in a laidback or side-lying position , or with a soft cushion under their buttocks if sitting up.
J. Mothers can be counseled during the prenatal period to request that an episiotomy not be done unless absolutely necessary.

VI. Assisted Birth or Operative Vaginal Delivery

A. Forceps use has declined in many countries.

  1. They can cause trauma to the baby, such as bruising to the face where the blades are applied, facial nerve paralysis, or cephalhematoma (hemorrhage into the subperiosteum that does not cross a suture line) that can be associated with intracranial bleeding or skull fracture.

B. Vacuum extraction does not need more room in the vagina than forceps do for application and therefore episiotomies are rarely done.

  1. Some babies who undergo this procedure have marked hematomas or contusions on the face, with associated increased bilirubin levels, and poor feeding (Hall et al., 2002; Johnson et al., 2004).

VII. Retained Placenta

A. Subinvolution of the uterus caused by retained placental fragments is typically diagnosed after the mother has been discharged from the hospital.

B. It might present itself as bleeding that is uncharacteristic for the length of time post delivery: normal change from rubra (red) loss on day 3, to serosa (serous) loss until day 9, and then alba (pale creamy-brownish loss).

C. Placental retention can inhibit secretory activation (lactogenesis II) by keeping inhibitory hormones at levels that are representative of pregnancy (Anderson, 2001; Neifert et al., 1981).

  1. Mothers might experience little to no breast fullness by days 3 to 5 and might still be producing colostrum when transitional milk should be seen.

  2. Failure to see breast fullness might occur prior to excessive bleeding or hemorrhage (Anderson, 2001).

  3. Curettage might be required, after which spontaneous milk flow should commence (Anderson, 2001; Neifert et al., 1981).

D. Retained placenta can be suspected (Anderson, 2001) if the mother complains of one of the following:

  1. Little to no breast fullness by day 5

  2. A colostrum stage of milk that persists beyond day 4

  3. Continued bright-red vaginal bleeding that continues to be heavy after 3 days

  4. A uterus that might be painful to palpation and larger than expected

  5. With an infant who:

    a. Is not satisfied at the breast

    b. Has less than the normal amount of wet and soiled diapers per day

    c. Is possibly showing visible signs of jaundice

VIII. Venous Thrombosis

A. Defined as the formation of a blood clot inside a blood vessel.

B. A reduction in this complication has been seen because of:

1. Early ambulation following delivery

2. Fewer operative deliveries using general anesthesia

3. Better health of women during pregnancy

4. Routine use of subcutaneous enoxoprin (Clexane, Lovenox) anticoagulant therapy daily for 3 days after cesarean section; enoxoprin is compatible with breastfeeding (Hale, 2010)

C. Deep vein thrombosis is serious because pulmonary embolism can result if thrombi formed in the legs migrate to the lungs.

D. A pulmonary embolism can be fatal.

E. Procedures to establish a diagnosis and systemic medications involved in treatment are considerations during lactation.

1. Scans using radiocontrast media might be necessary to confirm a diagnosis.

   a. Interruption or delay in breastfeeding is not necessary if radio-opaque or radiocontrast agents are used (Hale, 2010).

2. Radioactive materials vary in their half-lives, with some requiring little disruption to breastfeeding and others requiring pumping and discarding milk for up to 2 weeks; the lactation consultant should ascertain the contrast medium being used, its half-life if radioactive, and when breastfeeding can recommence.

3. Anticoagulant treatment can involve heparin, warfarin, or a newer, lower-molecular-weight fraction of heparin, enoxoprin (Clexane, Lovenox), all of which are considered compatible with breastfeeding (Hale, 2010).

4. If long-term anticoagulant therapy is initiated, prothrombin (clotting) time in the infant is usually monitored monthly and the infant might be given extra vitamin K if necessary.

F. Some mothers can experience a lengthy hospital stay or readmission and possible separation from their baby.

1. Plans must be made for continued breastfeeding and/or for the expressing of breastmilk.

G. Some hospital units enable babies to room with their mothers if an adult caretaker is available to be responsible for the infant.

1. Because the mother might be on bed rest and pain medication, a helper is usually needed for baby care and to provide infant access to the mother.

IX. Postpartum Infection

A. Infection processes might remain localized in the reproductive or genital area, urinary tract, or breasts, or it might progress, resulting in metritis, endometritis, peritonitis, or parametritis.

B. Prenatal risk factors associated with postpartum infections include preexisting infections, chronic diseases, anemia, diabetes, obesity, and poor nutritional status.

C. Intrapartum risk factors include prolonged rupture of the membranes, frequent vaginal examinations, intrauterine fetal monitoring, intrauterine manipulation, lacerations in the reproductive tract, operative delivery, retained placental fragments, manual removal of the placenta, hematomas, postpartum hemorrhage, and improper aseptic technique.

D. Portals for bacterial entry include the placental site, the episiotomy, cesarean incision, the vagina, the urinary tract, the breasts, and the lymphatic system along the uterine veins.

E. Perineal, vaginal, and cesarean incision infections are usually easily treated with antibiotics that are compatible with breastfeeding; these infections, however, are a source of significant discomfort for the mother (making positioning for breastfeeding cumbersome; see the section titled "II. Cesarean Delivery").

F. Endometritis, an infection of the lining of the uterus, is the most frequent cause of postpartum infection.
   1. Early endometritis occurs within 48 hours of the delivery.
   2. Mothers usually experience elevated temperatures, considerable pain, malaise, and often foul-smelling lochia.
      a. *Note:* Early temperature rises are also seen with epidural anesthesia/analgesia (Philip et al., 1999).
   3. The most important risk factor is premature rupture of the membranes or non-elective cesarean section after the onset of labor with rupture of the membranes.
   4. Treatment is usually with broad-spectrum antibiotics that are compatible with breastfeeding.
   5. The mother's condition will determine how breastfeeding proceeds.

G. Parametritis (also known as pelvic cellulitis) is an extension of the infectious process beyond the endometrium into the broad ligaments.
   1. Typically occurs during the second week postpartum.
   2. Mothers usually experience a persistent high fever, malaise, chills, lethargy, and marked pain over the affected area.
   3. The lactation consultant must remember to ask whether pain is present in areas other than the breasts because some of these infections present with symptoms similar to mastitis.
   4. Intravenous antibiotics are used; needle aspiration or surgery might be required to drain an abscess.
      a. The baby needs to feed or the mother pump just before surgery so that breastfeeding/pumping can resume as soon as the mother is conscious after the surgery.
      b. Antibiotics and anesthetic agents are compatible with breastfeeding (Hale, 2010).
   5. Separation and interrupted breastfeeding might occur.
      a. Arrangements for access to the baby and/or a breast pump need to be made.

H. Urinary tract infections (UTIs) caused by urine retention after childbirth are common.

1. Causes include trauma to the base of the bladder, use of regional anesthesia, increased capacity and decreased sensitivity of the puerperal bladder, and the use of oxytocin infusion after birth, which induces potent antidiuretic effects. Once the oxytocin is discontinued, rapid diuresis follows.

2. Catheterization is a frequent cause of UTIs because the insertion of the catheter introduces residual urine and bacteria into the bladder.

3. Mothers can experience fever and considerable pain.

4. Treatment includes antibiotic therapy that is compatible with breastfeeding, urinary alkalinizers, increased fluid intakes, and good nutrition.

I. Cesarean incision infections occur in 10% of mothers following cesarean section (Johnson et al., 2006) even with the use of prophylactic antibiotics (Bagratree et al., 2002).

1. The most common symptom is fever occurring on about the fourth day.

2. Treatment is with antibiotics usually compatible with breastfeeding (Hale, 2010) and less frequently with surgical drainage.

X. Side Effects of Intrapartum Medications That Can Affect Breastfeeding

A. In optimal birth settings, mothers are encouraged to have uninterrupted skin-to-skin contact and rooming-in options, which minimize effects of labor medications on lactation success (Halpern et al., 1999; Righard et al., 1990).

B. Both mothers and babies are affected by intrapartum medications in the early postpartum period.

1. The use of large amounts of intravenous oxytocin to induce labor combined with an epidural affects the pulsatile release of oxytocin during breastfeeds on the second postpartum day (Jonas et al., 2009), and cortisol levels differ significantly among mothers who receive epidurals whether or not this is combined with oxytocics for labor induction (Handlin et al., 2009).

2. Some mothers feel drugged or "hung over" or may be immobilized by the epidural.

3. Neonates may show poor feeding abilities during the early postpartum period (Nissen et al., 1997; Righard et al., 1990; Riordan et al., 2000).

4. Mothers may need assistance to position and latch their babies.

5. Mothers who are affected by analgesia/anesthesia and whose babies are in skin-to-skin contact should be under constant supervision until the medications are no longer effective.

C. Epidural medications are measurable in the fetal circulation within 10 minutes of administration (Hale, 2010). Following birth:

1. Neonates who are separated from their mothers after medicated labors show a delayed and depressed sucking and rooting behavior (Righard et al., 1990).

2. Neonates' feeding abilities may be affected by the metabolite of meperidine (normeperidine) for 63 hours after administration (Quinn, cited in Hale, 2010).

3. Following the use of epidural, neonates:
   a. Have a delay in normal prefeeding behaviors, increased crying, and a higher temperature (Ransjo-Arvidson et al., 2001)
   b. Are less likely to initiate breastfeeding in the first 4 hours after birth; more often given artificial milk during their hospital stay; are less likely to be fully breastfed at hospital discharge (Wiklund et al., 2009)
   c. Are less likely to have more than two successful breastfeeds in the first 24 hours (Baumgarder et al., 2003)
4. Babies are likely to have a shorter breastfeeding duration (Henderson et al., 2003).
5. Neonates have poor neonatal alertness and orientation when their mothers have postnatal intravenous patient-controlled analgesia with meperidine (Wittels, cited in Hale, 2010).

D. Metabolites of some medications, particularly meperidine (Demerol, pethidine; regardless of route of administration) and intrathecal fentanyl, can affect the baby until they are excreted (Scherer et al., 1995).
   1. *Fentanyl:* Has a short half-life and is found in very low concentrations in colostrum (Hale, 2010). High-dose fentanyl epidurals (>150 micrograms) have been shown to impede the establishment of breastfeeding (Jordan et al., 2005) or lead to early cessation in breastfeeding in women who have breastfed previous babies (Beilin et al., 2005). Supportive breastfeeding practices postnatally can overcome the effect of fentanyl doses (<150 micrograms) (Wieczorek et al., 2010).
   2. *Bupivicaine (Marcaine):* Because of its lack of effect on neonates and low levels of detection in breastmilk (Naulty, cited in Hale, 2010), it has become the most commonly used epidural and local anesthetic in labor (Hale, 2010).

E. Prenatal education needs to include advice to women that epidurals increase the length of labor and lead to higher levels of instrumental delivery (Rosenblatt et al., 1991).

References

Abraham, K. A., Connolly, G., Farrell, J., & Walshe, J. J. (2001). The HELLP syndrome, a prospective study. *Renal Failure, 23,* 705–713.

Anderson, A. M. (2001). Disruption of lactogenesis by retained placental fragments. *Journal of Human Lactation, 17,* 142–144.

Bagratee, J. S., Moodley, J., Kleinschmidt, I., & Zawilski, W. (2002). A randomized controlled trial of antibiotic prophylaxis in elective caesarean delivery. *BJOG, 109,* 1423–1424.

Baumgarder, D. J., Muehl, P., Fischer, M., et al. (2003). Effect of labor epidural anesthesia on breast-feeding of healthy full-term newborns delivered vaginally. *Journal of the American Board of Family Practitioners, 16*(1), 7–13.

Beilin, Y., Bodian, C. A., Weiser, J., et al. (2005). Effect of labor epidural analgesia with and without fentanyl on infant breast-feeding: A prospective, randomized, double-blind study. *Anesthesiology, 103,* 1111–1112.

Blackburn, S. T. (2003). *Maternal, fetal and neonatal physiology: A clinical perspective* (2nd ed.). Basel, Switzerland: Elsevier Science.

Collins, C. T., Ryan, P., Crowther, C. A., et al. (2004). Effect of bottles, cups, and dummies on breast feeding in preterm infants: A randomised controlled trial. *British Medical Journal, 329,* 193–198.

Cox, S. G. (2006). *Breastfeeding with confidence.* New York, NY: Meadowbook Press, Simon & Schuster.

Cregan, M. D., Mitoulas, L. R., & Hartmann, P. E. (2002). Milk prolactin, feed volume and duration between feeds in women breastfeeding their full-term infants over a 24 hour period. *Experimental Physiology, 87*(2), 207–214.

Curtin, W. M., & Weinstein, L. (1999). A review of HELLP syndrome. *Journal of Perinatology, 19,* 138–143.

De Carvalho M., Robertson, S., Friedman, A., & Klaus, M. (1983). Effect of frequent breast-feeding on early milk production and infant weight gain. *Pediatrics, 72*(3), 307–311.

Dewey, K. G. (2001). Maternal and fetal stress are associated with impaired lactogenesis in humans. *Journal of Nutrition, 131,* 3012S–3015S.

Dietl, J. (2000). Pathogenesis of pre-eclampsia—new aspects. *Journal of Perinatal Medicine, 28,* 464.

Dowling, D. A., Meier, P. P., DiFiore, J. M., et al. (2002). Cup-feeding for preterm infants: Mechanics and safety. *Journal of Human Lactation, 8,* 13–20.

Gasem, T., Al Jama, F. E., Burshaid, S., et al. (2009). Maternal and fetal outcome of pregnancy complicated by HELLP syndrome. *Journal of Maternal-Fetal and Neonatal Medicine, 12,* 1140–1143.

Hale, T. W. (2010). *Medications and mothers' milk* (13th ed.). Amarillo, TX: Hale Publishing.

Hall, R. T., Mercer, A. M., Teasley, S. L., et al. (2002). A breastfeeding assessment score to evaluate the risk for cessation of breastfeeding by 7 to 10 days of age. *Journal of Pediatrics, 141,* 659–664.

Halpern, S. H., Levine, T., Wilson, D. B., et al. (1999). Effect of labor analgesia on breastfeeding success. *Birth, 26,* 83–88, 275–276.

Handlin, L., Jonas, W., Petersson, M., et al. (2009). Effects of sucking and skin-to-skin contact on maternal ACTH and cortisol levels during the second day postpartum—influence of epidural analgesia and oxytocin in the perinatal period. *Breastfeeding Medicine, 4*(4), 207–220.

Haram, K., Svendsenm E., & Abildgaard, U. (2009). The HELLP syndrome: Clinical issues and management. A Review. *Biomed Central Pregnancy & Childbirth, 9,* 8.Published online 2009 February 26. doi: 10.1186/1471-2393-9-8 PMCID: PMC2654858

Hartmann, K., Visawanthan, M., Palmieri, R., et al. (2005). Outcomes of routine episiotomies: A systematic review. *Journal of the American Medical Association, 293,* 2141–2148.

Henderson, J. J., Dickinson, J. E., Evans, S. F., et al. (2003). Impact of intrapartum epidural analgesia on breast-feeding duration. *Australian and New Zealand Journal of Obstetrics and Gynaecology, 43*(5), 372–377.

Higgins, J. R., & de Swiet, M. (2001). Blood pressure measurement and classification in pregnancy. *Lancet, 357,* 131–135.

Johnson, A., Young, D., & Reilly, J. (2006). Caesarean section surgical site infection surveillance. *Journal of Hospital Infection, 64*(1), 30–35.

Johnson, J. H., Figueroa, R., Garry, D., Elimian, A., & Maulik, D. (2004). Immediate maternal and neonatal effects of forceps and vacuum-assisted deliveries. *Obstetrics and Gynecology, 103*(3), 513–518.

Jonas, K., Johansson, L. M., Nissen, E., et al. (2009). Effects of intrapartum oxytocin administration and epidural analgesia on the concentration of plasma oxytocin and prolactin, in response to suckling during the second day postpartum. *Breastfeeding Medicine, 4*(2), 71–82.

Jordan, S., Emery, S., Bradshaw, C., et al. (2005). The impact of intrapartum analgesia on infant feeding. *BJOG, 112,* 927–934.

Kelestimur, F. (2003). Sheehan's syndrome. *Pituitary, 6,* 181–188.

Kuhnert, B. R., Kennard, M. J., & Linn, P. L. (1998). Neonatal behaviour after epidural anesthesia for caesarean section: A comparison of bupivacaine and chloroprocaine. *Anesthesia and Analgesia*, *67*, 64–68.

Lawrence, R. A., & Lawrence, R. M. (1999). *Breastfeeding: A guide for the medical profession* (5th ed.). St. Louis, MO: Mosby.

Light, K. T., Smith, T. E., Johns, J. M., et al. (2000). Oxytocin responsivity in mothers and infants: A preliminary study of relationships with blood pressure during laboratory stress and normal ambulatory activity. *Health Psychology*, *90*, 560–567.

Lundquist, M., Olsson, A., Nissen, E., & Norman, M. (2000). Is it necessary to suture all lacerations after a vaginal delivery. *Birth*, *27*, 79–85.

Matthiessen, A.-S., Ransjo-Arvidsson, A.-B., Nissen, E., & Uvnäs-Moberg, K. (2001). Postpartum maternal oxytocin release by newborns: Effects of infant hand massage and sucking. *Birth*, *28*, 13–19.

Minnassian, V. A., Jazayeri, A., Prien, S. D., et al. (2002). Randomized trial of lidocaine ointment versus placebo for the treatment of postpartum perineal pain. *Obstetrics and Gynecology*, *100*, 1239–1243.

Morton, J., Hall, J. Y., Wong, R. J., et al. (2009). Combining hand techniques with electric pumping increases milk production in mothers of preterm infants. *Journal of Perinatology*, *29*(11), 757–764.

Neifert, M., McDonough, S. L., & Neville, M. C. (1981). Failure of lactogenesis associated with placental retention. *American Journal of Obstetrics and Gynecology*, *140*, 477–478.

Nissen, E., Widstrom, A., Lilja, G., et al. (1997). Effects of routinely given pethidine during labour on infants' developing breastfeeding behaviour. Effects of dose-delivery time interval and various concentrations of pethidine/norpethidine in cord plasma. *Acta Paediatrica*, *86*(2), 201–208.

Pang, W. W., & Hartmann, P. E. (2007). Initiation of human lactation: Secretory differentiation and secretory activation. *Journal of Mammary Gland Biology and Neoplasia*, *12*(4), 211–221.

Philip, J., Alexander, J. M., Sharma, S. K., et al. (1999). Epidural analgesia during labor and maternal fever. *Anaesthesiology*, *90*(3), 1250-1252.

Ramler, D., & Roberts, J. (1986). A comparison of cold and warm sitz baths for relief of postpartum perineal pain. *Journal of Obstetric, Gynecologic, and Neonatal Nursing*, *15*, 471–474.

Ransjo-Arvidson, A. B., Matthiessen, A. S., Lilja, G., et al. (2001). Maternal analgesia during labor disturbs newborn behavior: Effects on breastfeeding temperature: Effects on breastfeeding, temperature and crying. *Birth*, *28*(1), 5–12.

Reynders, F. C., Senten, L., Tjalma, W., & Jacquemyn, Y. (2006). Postpartum hemorrhage: Practical approach to a life threatening complication. *Clinical and Experimental Obstetrics and Gynecology*, *33*, 81–84.

Righard, L., & Alade, M. O. (1990). Effect of delivery room routines on success of first breast-feed. *Lancet*, *336*, 1105–1107.

Riordan, J., Gross, A., Angeron, J., et al. (2000). The effect of labor pain relief medication on neonatal suckling and breastfeeding duration. *Journal of Human Lactation*, *16*(1), 7–12.

Rosenblatt, D., Belsey, E., Lieberman, B. A., et al. (1991). The influence of maternal analgesia on neonatal behaviour. II. Epidural bupivacaine. *British Journal of Obstetrics and Gynaecology*, *88*, 407–413.

Scherer, R., & Holzgreve, W. (1995). Influence of epidural analgesia on fetal and neonatal well-being. *European Journal of Obstetrics and Gynecology and Reproductive Biology*, *59*(Suppl.), S17–S19.

Sepkoski, C. M., Lester, B. M., Ostheimer, G. W., & Brazelton, T. B. (1994). The effects of maternal epidural anaesthesia on neonatal behaviour during the first month. *Developmental Medicine and Child Neurology, 36*, 91–92.

Spear, H. J. (2006). Policies and practices for maternal support options during childbirth and breastfeeding initiation after caesarean in south-eastern hospitals. *Journal of Obstetric, Gynecologic, and Neonatal Nursing, 35*(5), 634–643.

Uvnäs-Moberg, K., & Petersson, M. (2005). Oxytocin, a mediator of anti-stress, well-being, social interaction, growth and healing. *Zeitschrift für Psychosomatische Medizin und Psychotherapie , 51*, 51–80. (In German; abstract in English)

Visser, W., & Wallenburg, H. C. (1995). Maternal and perinatal outcome of temporizing management in 254 consecutive patients with severe preeclampsia remote from term. *European Journal of Obstetrics and Gynecology and Reproductive Biology, 63*, 147–154.

Volikas, I., Butwick, A., Wilkinson, C., et al. (2005). Maternal and neonatal side-effects of remifentanil patient controlled analgesia in labour. *British Journal of Anaesthesia, 95*, 504–509.

Widstrom, A. M., Ransjo-Arvidson, A. B., Christensson, K., et al. (1987). Gastric suction in healthy newborn infants. Effects on circulation and developing feeding behaviour. *Acta Paediatrica Scandinavica, 76*, 566–572.

Wieczorek, P. M., Guest, S., Balki, M., et al. (2010). Breastfeeding success rate after vaginal delivery can be high despite the use of epidural fentanyl: An observational cohort study. *International Journal of Obstetric Anesthesia, 19*(3), 273–277.

Wiklund, I., Norman, M., & Uvnäs-Moberg, K. (2009). Epidural analgesia: Breast-feeding success and related factors. *Midwifery, 25*(2), e31–e38.

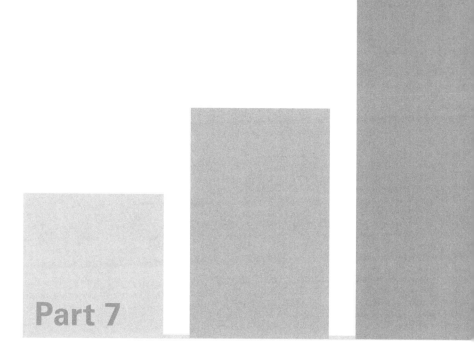

Part 7

Breastfeeding Problem Solving: Maternal and Infant Issues

CHAPTER 38
Congenital Anomalies, Neurologic Involvement, and Birth Trauma

Catherine Watson Genna, BS, IBCLC

OBJECTIVES

- Discuss how congenital anomalies, neurologic impairments, and birth trauma can affect early breastfeeding.
- List strategies for assisting these babies with initiating breastfeeding.

INTRODUCTION

A number of conditions presenting at birth or shortly thereafter can have a significant impact on the initiation and duration of breastfeeding. Some of these conditions are temporary whereas others remain for a lifetime. Compromised babies especially benefit from the provision of breastmilk and/or breastfeeding. A few babies cannot feed at the breast, but provision of breastmilk for them can and should continue as long as possible. Some of these conditions are first be brought to the attention of a healthcare provider because of poor feeding, with the inability to breastfeed being a marker or symptom of the problem. Mothers of these babies can experience an enormous range of emotions. They might be frightened, frustrated, anxious, fatigued, angry, or depressed. Their emotional well-being should not be neglected in the flurry of activity surrounding the baby.

I. Postmature Infants, Those Born at the Onset of Week 42 of Gestation

A. Fully mature infants who have remained in utero beyond the time of optimal placental function.

B. Aging of the placenta and reduced placental function impair nutrient and oxygen transport to the fetus, placing the fetus at risk for a lower tolerance to the stresses of labor and delivery, including hypoxia.

1. In response to hypoxia, meconium might be passed, increasing the risk for meconium aspiration.

2. Amniotic fluid might be decreased, increasing the risk for meconium aspiration and umbilical cord compression.

C. If the placenta continues to function well, the baby might become large for gestational age (LGA) and thereby increase the risk for shoulder dystocia and possible fractured clavicle.

D. Postmature infants are characterized by the following:

    1. Loss of weight in utero

    2. Dry, peeling skin that appears to hang as a result of the loss of subcutaneous fat and muscle mass

    3. A wrinkled, wide-eyed appearance

    4. Lack of vernix caseosa (the waxy or cheese-like substance coating the newborn's skin; composed of sebum and skin sloughed in utero)

    5. Reduced glycogen stores in the liver

E. These babies might be at higher risk for hypoglycemia as a result of low glycogen reserves.

    1. Skin-to-skin contact from birth, and early, frequent breastfeeding, or feeding of colostrum if not latching can help maintain blood glucose levels.

F. These babies might feed poorly, appear lethargic, and require considerable incentives to sustain suckling, including alternate massage/breast compression, expressed colostrum incentives, skin-to-skin contact (because their body temperature is quite labile), and avoidance of crying episodes, which can further drop their blood glucose levels.

II. Birth Trauma

A. Forceps use might result in small areas of ecchymosis (bruising) on the sides of the face where the blades were placed.

B. Neurological injuries:

    1. Trauma to the facial nerves can occur; any muscles innervated by these nerves might be temporarily hypotonic, making latching and sucking difficult; observe for an asymmetric movement of the mouth, a drooping mouth, or a drooping eyelid.

    2. Forceps, vacuum, and especially failure of one followed by use of the other can result in shoulder dystocia and brachial plexus injury, causing paralysis or weakness of the hand or arm (Brimacombe et al., 2008). These injuries can interfere with stable positioning and normal manual breast seeking, stimulating and shaping behaviors at breast.

C. Vacuum-assisted deliveries can pose an increased risk of cranial hemorrhage (Ng, 1995; U.S. Food and Drug Administration [FDA], 1998) as can vacuum or forceps use during labor or cesarean birth during labor. (Towner et al., 1999).

    1. Extracranial hemorrhage (bleeding between the skin and cranial bone):

        a. Caput succedaneum, hemorrhagic edema of the soft tissues of the scalp, usually resolves within the first week of life.

        b. Cephalhematoma, bleeding that is contained within the subperiosteal space, preventing it from crossing suture lines (see **Figure 38-1**).

   c. Subgaleal hemorrhage can represent a significant blood loss to the infant.

      i. It presents as a fluctuant area of the scalp, sometimes increasing in size to the point of blood dissecting into the subcutaneous tissue of the back of the neck (Cavlovich, 1994).

      ii. These babies need special help in positioning to keep pressure off the hemorrhagic area.

      iii. Some infants feed poorly or not at all until some of the hemorrhage has resolved, a condition that presents an increased risk for high bilirubin levels as the body breaks down the red blood cells and recycles the hemoglobin.

2. Intracranial hemorrhage (not visible externally):

   a. The baby might present with common signs such as sleepiness, feeding intolerance, and decreased muscle tone.

   b. Subdural (cerebral) hemorrhage is the most common intracranial hemorrhage resulting from a traumatic delivery (Steinbach, 1999). Subarachnoid hemorrhage incidence increased more after vacuum than forceps births, and both were higher compared with unassisted vaginal deliveries (Wen et al., 2001). Intraventricular hemorrhages were more likely after forceps birth but were also increased in vacuum deliveries (Wen et al., 2001).

   c. Some of the signs and symptoms become evident following discharge; babies who have a history of vacuum extraction that demonstrate lethargy, feeding problems, hypotonia, increased irritability, diffuse swelling of the head, and pallor need an immediate follow-up (Davis, 2001).

   d. Ability to suck, swallow, and root are sensitive to neurologic insults (Katz-Salamon, 1997), and feeding difficulties are more likely in infants born by vacuum or forceps (Wen et al., 2001).

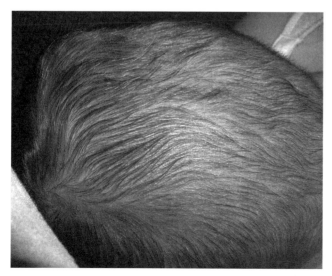

Figure 38-1 Cephalhematoma in newborn.

D. Fractured clavicle:

1. Can occur with an LGA infant or with malpresentations of the baby.

2. The baby might display a decreased movement of the arm or distress with arm movements; the arm and shoulder are immobilized and special positioning might be needed to breastfeed the baby.

3. Some babies are not diagnosed until after discharge when certain positions are noted to cause crying in the baby; the clutch hold or placing the baby on the unaffected side at each breast might be helpful.

III. Inborn Errors of Metabolism

A. Galactosemia

1. Caused by a deficiency of the enzyme galactose-1-phosphate uridyltransferase (GALT), causing an inability in the infant to metabolize galactose.

2. Infant can have severe and persistent jaundice, vomiting, diarrhea, electrolyte imbalance, cerebral involvement, and weight loss.

3. These babies are weaned from the breast to a lactose- and galactose-free formula.

4. Duarte Galactosemia: Low but functional levels of GALT allow breastfeeding to continue. Despite slightly elevated levels of galactose breakdown products in blood and urine, developmental outcomes are not improved by restricting lactose intake during the first year of life (Ficicioglu et al., 2010; Ficicioglu et al., 2008).

B. Phenylketonuria (PKU)

1. The most common of the amino acid metabolic disorders.

2. An autosomal recessive, inherited disorder where the amino acid phenylalanine accumulates because of the absence of the enzyme phenylalanine hydroxylase, which converts phenylalanine to tyrosine for further breakdown.

3. Newborn screening for PKU is done in all 50 states in the United States and in more than 30 other countries.

4. Babies need some phenylalanine.

5. Infants who have PKU can continue to breastfeed when a balance is maintained between the use of a phenylalanine-free formula and breastmilk (van Rijn et al., 2003).

6. Human milk has lower levels of phenylalanine than standard commercial formulas do (Duncan et al., 1997).

7. The amount of phenylalanine-free formula and breastmilk can be calculated by weight, age, blood levels, and the need for growth.

8. Another approach is to feed the baby 10 to 30 milliliters of the special formula followed by breastfeeding.

   a. As long as phenylalanine levels are properly maintained, the exact calculations of breastmilk and formula might not need to be made.

   b. Breastmilk might be more than half of the diet, improving the baby's exposure to the trophic (tissue building), immune, and immunomodulating functions of human milk.

9. Breastfeeding before diagnosis and dietary intervention has been shown to produce a 14-point higher IQ than babies who are artificially fed prediagnosis (Riva et al., 1996).

IV. Other Genetic Disorders

A. Cystic fibrosis (CF)

1. A congenital disease involving a generalized dysfunction of exocrine glands resulting from a mutation in the transmembrane conductance regulatory protein.

2. The glands produce abnormally thick and sticky secretions that block the flow of pancreatic digestive enzymes, clog hepatic ducts, and affect the movement of the cilia in the lungs.

3. Increased sodium chloride in the child's sweat is frequently the first indicator of the condition; the baby tastes salty when nuzzled.

4. Another early indicator of CF is intestinal obstruction or ileus.

   a. The meconium blocks the small intestine, resulting in abdominal distension, vomiting, and failure to pass stools (resulting in the failure to gain weight).

5. Babies who have CF produce normal amounts of gastric lipase, which combined with the milk lipase in breastmilk enhances fat absorption.

6. Breastfed infants with CF are less likely to need intravenous antibiotics (Parker et al., 2004).

7. Breastfed infants with CF can present with protein malnutrition (edema) and reduced weight gain but may escape the characteristic infections, confounding diagnosis.

   a. Pancreatic enzymes can be given to the baby to improve protein metabolism (Cannella et al., 1993).

8. There is no need to interrupt breastfeeding (Luder et al., 1990).

B. Neurologic disorders

1. Infants who have neurologic impairments often have extremely complex needs.

2. The infant's nervous system can be damaged, abnormally developed, immature, or temporarily incapacitated from insults such as asphyxia, sepsis, trauma, or drugs.

3. Infants can have an absent or depressed rooting response, gag reflex, sucking reflex, and/or may have difficulty swallowing (dysphagia).

4. Giving a bottle to a baby who is to be breastfed provides inconsistent sensory input that additionally disorganizes the nervous system.

5. A depressed or absent suck reflex, where infants might exhibit a limited response to stimulation to the palate and tongue; these babies might have decreased muscle tone.

6. A weak or poorly sustained sucking reflex.

   a. Denotes an oral musculature weakened to the point of an inability to sustain a rhythmic suck.

   b. The rhythm is interrupted by irregular pauses and sometimes a lack of the 1:1 suck:swallow ratio.

       c. Adequate negative intraoral pressure is not generated, causing the nipple to fall out of the mouth.

       d. Lips do not form a complete seal.

       e. The hypotonic tongue might remain flat, not cupping around the breast.

   7. Uncoordinated sucking includes a mistiming of the component muscle movements of the suck–swallow cycle.

       a. The lactation consultant might see extraneous movements of the mouth, head, or neck.

       b. The infant might have difficulty organizing feeding behaviors and initiating sucking.

       c. Hypersensitivity or hyposensitivity might be seen in other areas of the body.

       d. Infant might have dysfunctional tongue movements and uncoordinated swallowing, increasing risk of aspiration.

C. Down syndrome

   1. Results from an extra chromosome 21 (trisomy 21)

       a. Common characteristics that relate to feeding include the following:

          i. A flaccid tongue that appears too large for the mouth as a result of reduced growth of the mandible (lower jaw). (see **Figure 38-2**)

          ii. Generalized hypotonia, including the oral musculature.

          iii. Heart defects that decrease aerobic capacity for feeding and might require surgery.

          iv. Incomplete development of the gastrointestinal (GI) tract.

          v. Hyperbilirubinemia is common.

          vi. Infant is especially prone to infection.

          vii. Might have a depressed sucking reflex or a weak suck, or both.

       b. Some babies have no problem sucking while others might exhibit initial sucking difficulties.

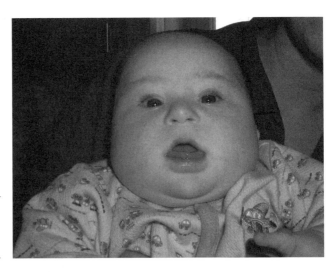

Figure 38-2 Infant with Down Syndrome. Note hypotonia and small mandible that increase tongue protrusion.

    c. The dancer hand position (Danner, 1992) may stabilize the jaw and support the masseter muscles, which decreases the intraoral space and enhances the generation of negative pressure.

        i. The breast is supported by the third, fourth, and fifth fingers so that the webbing between the thumb and index finger forms a U-shaped cup on which the baby's chin rests.

        ii. The thumb and index finger support the cheeks with gentle traction toward the corner of the lips.

        iii. The baby should be in a quiet-alert state to feed.

        iv. The infant might need hindmilk supplementation to gain weight and may benefit from the use of a supplementer at breast to deliver it.

D. Fetal distress and hypoxia (decreased levels of oxygen)

  1. Infants can be compromised in utero or during delivery from low levels of oxygen caused by the following:

    a. Insufficient placental reserve

    b. Umbilical cord compression

    c. Umbilical cord prolapse

  2. Newborns are vulnerable to brain cell death from hypoxia.

    a. *Neonatal encephalopathy* is the current term for altered level of consciousness, seizures, apnea, and reduced brain stem function, including feeding ability.

    b. Recovery begins after 3 to 4 days; some infants remain compromised and may develop cerebral palsy or other neurologic deficits.

    c. Low Apgar scores combined with inability to suck requiring tube feeding is the most sensitive indicator of later disability, followed by seizures and need for mechanical ventilation (Moster et al., 2002).

    d. Colostrum is very important to these babies because their GI tract might have suffered hypoxic damage; colostrum should be expressed and used as soon as the baby can tolerate feedings by mouth; mothers should frequently hand express or pump during this time.

    e. Hypoxia decreases the motility of the gut and reduces the gut-stimulating hormones.

    f. These infants might have a depressed suck that is not well coordinated with the swallow, and they may have difficulty bottle-feeding.

    g. A supplementer device, cup, or other feeding device might be needed initially until the infant's feeding skills recover. Mothers need to express milk when their infant is unable to remove milk (Academy of Breastfeeding Medicine [ABM], 2005).

    h. The hypotonic (low muscle tone) baby might breastfeed better in a clutch hold with the trunk stabilized against the mother's side (McBride et al., 1987) or prone on a semireclined mother.

    i. The hypertonic (high muscle tone) baby should be held in a flexed, well-supported position to reduce the overall extensor patterning.

    j. Breastfeeding interventions are similar to those for the baby who has Down syndrome, including cheek and jaw support (dancer hand position).

    k. These infants have increased effort of feeding, fatigue easily, and may require very short, frequent feedings.

    l. Recovery usually proceeds for many months, and infants who cannot breastfeed at birth may develop the skills later, especially if oral motor therapy is provided.

E. GI tract disorders

  1. Esophageal atresia (EA)

    a. A congenital defect of the esophagus. In most cases, the upper esophagus does not connect with the lower esophagus and stomach. May be associated with other birth defects.

    b. Tracheoesophageal fistula (TEF) occurs when the esophagus communicates with the trachea and is a common variation of EA. Occurs in 1 of every 3,000–5,000 live births.

    c. Usually detected in the first few hours of life and is considered a surgical emergency.

    d. Symptoms can include excess amniotic fluid during pregnancy and difficulties with feeding such as coughing, spilling fluid from the lips, gagging, choking, and cyanosis.

    e. There is no research to justify test feeds of sterile or glucose water to diagnose TEF or EA. Water or low-chloride fluids in the neonatal airway have the potential to cause prolonged apnea (Thach, 1997).

  2. Gastroesophageal reflux (GER)

    a. A persistent, nonprojectile regurgitation (spitting up) seen after feeds.

    b. Can be mild and self-limiting, requiring no modification or interventions.

    c. Can be more severe, with worsening regurgitation and weight gain or loss problems.

    d. Can present as follows:

      i. Fussiness at the breast as stomach contents contact the lower section of the esophagus.

      ii. Might be more apparent in certain side-lying positions at the breast.

      iii. Mothers might report increased fussing at the breast, a baby who arches off or pulls away from the breast, or a baby who cries until placed upright.

      iv. Baby mouths refluxed milk between feedings ("cud chewing").

      v. Upper respiratory infections and congestion may occur from chronic aspiration of refluxing fluid (ascending aspiration).

      vi. Feeding refusal.

      vii. Micro- and macroaspiration may manifest as nasal congestion that increases throughout the feeding, coughing, or wheezing during or between feeds (Catto-Smith, 1998). Aspiration can also be caused by high milk flow or infant inability to properly coordinate sucking, swallowing, and breathing.

e. Mothers are encouraged to keep providing breastmilk, nurse the baby in an upright position (in clutch hold or straddled across her lap or diagonal with mother reclining), nurse on one breast at each feeding to keep from overdistending the stomach, feed frequently, and keep the baby upright for 10–20 minutes after feedings (Boekel, 2000).

f. Reflux needs to be differentiated from hyperlactation with overfeeding or lactose overload.

   i. Generally, if the infant is gaining rapidly, has signs of gut irritation and rapid intestinal transit time (green, mucousy stools), and is fussy, maternal hyperlactation might be responsible.

   ii. Reducing milk production by gradually increasing the amount of time before changing breasts is generally successful (block feeding) (van Veldhuizen-Staas, 2007).

g. If the reflux is severe, the baby might undergo diagnostic tests and be placed on medication.

3. Pyloric stenosis

   a. A stricture or narrowing of the pylorus (muscular tissue controlling the outlet of the stomach) caused by muscular hypertrophy, more common in nonbreastfed infants (Osarumwese Osifo et al., 2009; Pisacane et al., 1996).

   b. It usually occurs between the 2nd and 6th week of life, although it can occur any time after birth.

   c. Vomiting is characteristic, intermittent at first, progressing to after every feeding, and projectile in nature. Baby usually begins to refuse feeds.

   d. Dehydration, electrolyte imbalance, and weight loss can occur in extreme situations.

   e. If the baby does not outgrow the condition or if it is severe, surgery can be performed after rehydration and correction of electrolyte balance.

   i. A breastfed baby can resume breastfeeding earlier than a formula-fed baby because of the faster stomach emptying time and zero curd tension of human milk.

   ii. Mothers should feed with one breast initially after surgery to prevent overfilling the baby's stomach; these limited feedings gradually expand the stomach and can be advanced as the baby tolerates it.

   iii. Mothers can position the baby upright in a straddle position to avoid stress on the incision.

F. Congenital heart defects

1. Seen along a continuum of mild with no symptoms to severe with cyanosis, rapid breathing, shortness of breath, and lowered oxygen levels (desaturation) that requires surgical correction.

2. Cardiac disease is not a medical indication to interrupt or cease breastfeeding (Barbas et al., 2004).

3. Feeding at the breast presents less work for the baby, keeps oxygen levels higher than with bottle-feeding, and keeps heart and respiratory rates stable when the baby is at the breast (Marino et al., 1995).

4. A baby who has more serious heart involvement might be either unable to sustain sucking at the breast or might need to pause frequently to rest; if intake is inadequate, the baby will not gain weight or will exhibit weight loss.

5. Infants with cardiac disease often have increased caloric requirements.

6. Mothers might describe these babies in any number of ways, including the following:
   a. Able to sustain sucking for only short periods of time
   b. Pulling off the breast frequently
   c. Turning blue around the lips (circumoral cyanosis)
   d. Rapid breathing or panting; rapid heart rate
   e. Sweating while at the breast
   f. Requiring very frequent feedings

7. If surgery is planned, it is typically scheduled after the baby reaches a predetermined weight and/or age.
   a. Small, frequent feeds might be necessary.
   b. If additional calories are needed, consider hindmilk supplementation at the breast with a supplementer device.

G. Sudden infant death syndrome (SIDS) or sudden unexplained infant death (SUID)

1. Also known as crib death or cot death; the leading cause of death in infants in developed countries who are older than 1 month; rates vary worldwide.

2. The etiology seems to be related to brain stem serotonin abnormalities (Kinney, 2005; Kinney et al., 2003; Paterson et al., 2006) that interfere with gasping for breath while anoxic during sleep (Tryba et al., 2006). Parental smoking is the greatest risk factor.

3. The sleeping position dramatically affects the rates; babies placed on their backs (supine) are less prone to SIDS.

4. The majority of deaths occur between 2 and 6 months of age with a peak at about 10 weeks of age.

5. Artificially fed infants have higher risk of SIDS than do breastfed infants. A recent meta-analysis (Hauck et al., 2011) found a .27 odds ratio (OR) for exclusively breastfed infants and .4 OR for infants who receive some breastmilk.
   a. Breastfeeding offers dose-response protection across race and socioeconomic levels; it is associated with a 50% reduction in risk on meta-analysis, but the quality of the included studies was deficient (McVea et al., 2000).
   b. The exact protective mechanism is not well understood.
      i. Breastfeeding reduces minor infections such as acute upper-respiratory infections and diarrheal infections that are frequently associated with SIDS.
      ii. Breastfeeding and breastmilk enhance the development of the central nervous system and the brain stem, which might also provide protection.

6. The American Academy of Pediatrics (AAP Task Force on Sudden Infant Death Syndrome, 2005) statement on SIDS recommends against bedsharing and for pacifier use during sleep for infants older than 1 month of age.

   a. Lactation consultants can help ensure that pacifier use is delayed and does not unduly affect breastfeeding while continuing to call for higher quality studies that recognize mother–baby togetherness and breastfeeding as the human norm.

H. Respiratory disorders

  1. Common features

   a. Increased effort of breathing leaves less energy for feeding.

   b. Increased baseline respiratory rate reduces the amount of swallowing that can be done because swallowing inhibits breathing (Glass et al., 1994).

   c. Short sucking bursts are typical signs of respiratory disorders.

   d. Very careful pacing of the feed (making sure the infant can control the speed of milk flow), head extension to reduce airway resistance to air flow (Ardran et al., 1968; Wolf et al., 1992), prone feeding positions (with mother reclined), and more frequent feedings are generally helpful.

   e. Growth should be monitored closely, and expressed milk provided by slow-flow methods if the infant is unable to meet needs at breast.

  2. Laryngomalacia

   a. Epiglottis lacks normal stiffness and collapses into airway on inspiration, causing inspiratory stridor, suprasternal retractions, and increased work of breathing, particularly during crying, feeding, and supine positioning.

   b. Strongly associated with GER because of increased pressure on the lower esophageal sphincter.

   c. Head extension and prone positioning during feeding reduce airway resistance; short frequent feeds may be necessary to prevent failure to thrive (Wolf et al., 1992).

   d. Generally outgrown by 6 to 18 months as the neck elongates and structures become anatomically separated.

  3. Tracheomalacia

   a. Cartilage rings in trachea may be malformed and are insufficiently stiff so that rapid air flow during expiration (and inspiration as well in newborns) causes partial collapse of trachea (Wiatrak, 2000).

   b. Can be seen as sternal retraction and heard as stridor. See **Figure 38-3**.

   c. Increases work of respiration.

   d. Same strategies are helpful as for laryngomalacia; also is outgrown in the first year or two of life.

  4. Laryngeal webs

   a. Persistence of tissue in the lumen of the airway that can cause significant respiratory distress.

   b. Infant may have great difficulty feeding; very careful pacing of feeding is necessary to prevent hypoxia.

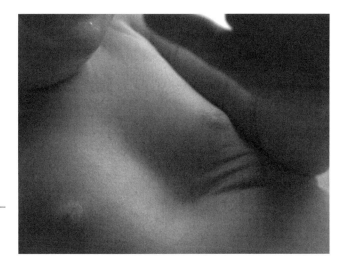

Figure 38-3 Sternal and substernal retraction due to tracheomalacia.

5. Laryngeal clefts
    a. Opening between the larynx and esophagus of variable size and position
    b. Cause stridor and/or aspiration during feeding (Chien et al., 2006)
    c. Usually require repair to allow the infant to feed safely
    d. Might be comorbid with tracheobronchomalacia or tracheoesophageal fistula (Rahbar et al., 2006)
6. Vocal fold paresis
    a. Usually unilateral from injury to fold or nerve.
    b. Hoarse cry.
    c. Reduces airway protection on the affected side.
    d. Infant will usually coordinate swallowing and breathing better if the weak or paralyzed cord is oriented upward.
7. Velopharyngeal insufficiency/incompetence
    a. Hypoplasia or dysfunction of the soft palate and pharyngeal constrictor muscles that prevent milk from entering the nasopharynx, sometimes resulting from submucosal cleft palate.
    b. Nasal regurgitation, harsh respiration in feeding pauses, apnea from milk in the nasopharynx, feeding resistance.
    c. Careful pacing and upright positioning (straddle) may help.
    d. See Chapter 27: Assessment of Infant Oral Anatomy, for information about clefts of the lip and palate.

References

Academy of Breastfeeding Medicine Protocol Committee. (2008). ABM Clinical Protocol #6: Guideline on Co-Sleeping and Breastfeeding. Retrieved March 11, 2012 from http://www.bfmed.org/Media/Files/Protocols/Protocol_6.pdf.

Academy of Breastfeeding Medicine Protocol Committee. (2007). *ABM clinical protocol no. 3: Hospital guidelines for the use of supplementary feedings in the healthy term breastfed neonate, revised 2009.* Retrieved from http://www.bfmed.org/Media/Files/Protocols/ABMProtocol_3%20Revised.pdf

American Academy of Pediatrics Task Force on Sudden Infant Death Syndrome. (2005). The changing concept of sudden infant death syndrome: Diagnostic coding shifts, controversies regarding sleeping environment, and new variables to consider in reducing risk. *Pediatrics, 116*, 1245–1255.

Ardran, G., & Kemp, F. (1968). The mechanism of changes in form of the cervical airway in infancy. *Medical Radiography and Photography, 44*, 26–38, 54.

Barbas, K. H., & Kelleher, D. K. (2004). Breastfeeding success among infants with congenital heart disease. *Pediatric Nursing, 30*, 285–289.

Boekel, S. (2000). *Gastroesophageal reflux disease (GERD) and the breastfeeding baby.* Independent Study Module. Raleigh, NC: International Lactation Consultant Association.

Brimacombe, M., Iffy, L., Apuzzio, J. J., Varadi, V., Nagy, B., Raju, V., & Portuondo, N. (2008). Shoulder dystocia related fetal neurological injuries: The predisposing roles of forceps and ventouse extractions. *Archives of Gynecology and Obstetrics, 277*, 415–422.

Cannella, P. C., Bowser, E. K., Guyer, L. K., et al. (1993). Feeding practices and nutrition recommendations for infants with cystic fibrosis. *Journal of the American Dietetic Association, 93*, 297–300.

Catto-Smith, A. G. (1998). Gastroesophageal reflux in children. *Australian Family Physician, 27*, 465–473.

Cavlovich, F. E. (1994). Subgaleal hemorrhage in the neonate. *Journal of Obstetric, Gynecologic, and Neonatal Nursing, 24*, 397–404.

Chien, W., Ashland, J., & Haver K. (2006). Type 1 laryngeal cleft: Establishing a functional diagnostic and management algorithm. *International Journal of Pediatric Otorhinolaryngology, 70*, 2073–2079.

Danner, S. C. (1992). Breastfeeding the neurologically impaired infant. *NAACOG's Clinical Issues in Perinatal and Women's Health Nursing, 3*, 640–646.

Davis, D. J. (2001). Neonatal subgaleal hemorrhage: Diagnosis and management. *Canadian Medical Association Journal, 164*(10), 1452–1453.

Duncan, L. L., & Elder, S. B. (1997). Breastfeeding the infant with PKU. *Journal of Human Lactation, 13*, 231–235.

Ficicioglu, C., Hussa, C., Gallagher, P. R., Thomas, N., & Yager, C. (2010). Monitoring of biochemical status in children with Duarte galactosemia: Utility of galactose, galactitol, galactonate, and galactose 1-phosphate. *Clinical Chemistry, 56*, 1177–1182.

Ficicioglu, C., Thomas, N., Yager, C., et al. (2008). Duarte (DG) galactosemia: A pilot study of biochemical and neurodevelopmental assessment in children detected by newborn screening. *Molecular Genetics and Metabolism, 95*, 206–212.

Glass, R. P., & Wolf, L. S. (1994). Incoordination of sucking, swallowing and breathing as an etiology for breastfeeding difficulty. *Journal of Human Lactation, 10*,185–189.

Hauck, F., Thompson, J. M. D., Tanabe, K. O., et al. (2011, June 13). Breastfeeding and reduced risk of sudden infant death syndrome: A meta-analysis. *Pediatrics*, doi:10.1542/peds.2010-3000 [Advance online publication]

Katz-Salamon, M. (1997). Perinatal risk factors and neuromotor behaviour during the neonatal period. *Acta Paediatrica, 419*(Suppl.), 27–36.

Kinney, H. C. (2005). Abnormalities of the brainstem serotonergic system in the sudden infant death syndrome: A review. *Pediatric and Developmental Pathology, 8*, 507–524.

Kinney, H. C., Randall, L. L., Sleeper, L. A., et al. (2003). Serotonergic brainstem abnormalities in Northern Plains Indians with the sudden infant death syndrome. *Journal of Neuropathology and Experimental Neurology, 62*, 1178–1191.

Luder, E., Kattan, M., Tanzer-Torres, G., et al. (1990). Current recommendations for breastfeeding in cystic fibrosis centers. *American Journal of Diseases of Children, 144*, 1153–1156.

Marino, B. L., O'Brien, P., & LoRe, H. (1995). Oxygen saturations during breast and bottle feedings in infants with congenital heart disease. *Journal of Pediatric Nursing, 10*, 360–364.

McBride, M. C., & Danner, S. C. (1987). Sucking disorders in neurologically impaired infants. *Clinical Perinatology, 14*, 109–130.

McVea, K. L. S. P., Turner, P. D., & Peppler, D. K. (2000). The role of breastfeeding in sudden infant death syndrome. *Journal of Human Lactation, 16*, 13–20.

Moster, D., Lie, R. T., & Markestad, T. (2002). Joint association of Apgar scores and early neonatal symptoms with minor disabilities at school age. *Archives of Disease in Childhood: Fetal and Neonatal Edition, 86*, F16–F21.

Ng, P. C. (1995). Subaponeurotic haemorrhage in the 1990s: A 3-year surveillance. *Acta Paediatrica, 84*, 1065–1069.

Osarumwese Osifo, D., & Evbuomwan, I. (2009). Does exclusive breastfeeding confer protection against infantile hypertrophic pyloric stenosis? A 30-year experience in Benin City, Nigeria. *Journal of Tropical Pediatrics, 55*(2), 132–134.

Parker, E. M., O'Sullivan, B. P., Shea, J. C., Regan, M. M., & Freedman, S. D. (2004). Survey of breast-feeding practices and outcomes in the cystic fibrosis population. *Pediatric Pulmonology, 37*, 362–367.

Paterson, D. S., Trachtenberg, F. L., Thompson, E. G., et al. (2006). Multiple serotonergic brainstem abnormalities in sudden infant death syndrome. *Journal of the American Medical Association, 296*, 2124–2132.

Pisacane, A., de Luca, U., & Criscuolo, L. (1996). Breast feeding and hypertrophic pyloric stenosis: Population based case-control study. *British Medical Journal, 312*, 745–746.

Rahbar, R., Rouillon, I., & Roger G. (2006). The presentation and management of laryngeal cleft: A 10-year experience. *Archives of Otolaryngology—Head and Neck Surgery, 132*, 1335–1341.

Riva, E., Agostoni, C., Biasucci, G., et al. (1996). Early breastfeeding is linked to higher intelligence quotient scores in dietary treated phenylketonuric children. *Acta Paediatrica, 85*, 56–58.

Steinbach, M. T. (1999). Traumatic birth injury—intracranial hemorrhage. *Mother and Baby Journal, 4*, 5–14.

Thach, B. T. (1997). Reflux associated apnea in infants: Evidence for a laryngeal chemoreflex. *American Journal of Medicine, 103*(5A), 120–124.

Towner, D., Castro, M. A., Eby-Wilkens, E., & Gilbert, W. M. (1999). Effect of mode of delivery in nulliparous women on neonatal intracranial injury. *New England Journal of Medicine, 341*(23), 1709–1714.

Tryba, A. K., Peña, F., & Ramirez, J. (2006). 5-HT2A activity is required for fictive gasping. *Journal of Neuroscience, 26*(10), 2623–2634.

U.S. Food and Drug Administration. (1998, May 21). *Public health advisory: Need for caution when using vacuum assisted delivery devices*. Washington, DC: Author.

van Rijn, M., Bekhof, J., Dijkstra, T., et al. (2003). A different approach to breast-feeding of the infant with phenylketonuria. *European Journal of Pediatrics, 162*, 323–326.

van Veldhuizen-Staas, C. G. (2007). Overabundant milk supply: An alternative way to intervene by full drainage and block feeding. *International Breastfeeding Journal, 2*, 11.

Wen, S. W., Liu, S., Kramer, M. S., Marcoux, S., Ohlsson, A., Sauve, R., & Liston, R. (2001). Comparison of maternal and infant outcomes between vacuum extraction and forceps deliveries. *American Journal of Epidemiology*, 153, 103–107.

Wiatrak, B. (2000). Congenital anomalies of the larynx and trachea. *Otolaryngology Clinics of North America*, *33*, 91–110.

Wolf, L. S., & Glass, R. P. (1992). *Feeding and swallowing disorders in infancy: Assessment and management*. Tucson, AZ: Therapy Skill Builders.

Wolf, L. S., & Glass, R. P. (1993). Feeding and oral motor skills. In J. Case Smith (Ed.), *Pediatric occupational therapy and early intervention*. Los Angeles, CA: Butterworth-Heinemann.

CHAPTER 39
Breast Pathology

Angela Smith, RM, BA, IBCLC, and Joy Heads, RM, MHPEd, IBCLC

OBJECTIVES

- Describe common breastfeeding problems related to the lactating breast.
- Describe preventative and prophylactic measures for these problems.
- Differentiate between common presenting signs and symptoms.
- Identify appropriate interventions by the lactation consultant.
- Identify relevant educational issues for the mother with a breastfeeding problem.

INTRODUCTION

A number of common problems relate to the lactating breast. Although most can either be prevented or improved, early recognition, prompt treatment and/or referral, and close follow-up are required to preserve breastfeeding. Some of these problems can be painful and extend over a period of time, which can be disappointing and frustrating to the new mother. Many lactation consultants use a number of therapeutic interventions that are based on long years of clinical experience rather than on randomized, controlled trials, which often are not available. These strategies likely vary from region to region and country to country. Some strategies are commonly seen in daily practice and others are used more rarely. All solutions to problems depend on careful assessment and management plans developed in conjunction with the mother using any available evidence-based recommendations.

I. Differentiation Between Normal and Engorged Breasts

A. Normal fullness:

1. Many women experience normal fullness when the milk increases during lactogenesis II.
2. The increase in blood flow to the breast, triggered by the prolactin surge, is accompanied by an increase in milk volume and interstitial tissue edema; this results in normal fullness in most women.

    3. Normal fullness can be differentiated from problematic engorgement.

       a. The normally full breast will be larger, warmer, and uncomfortable; milk flow will be normal.

       b. The engorged breast will look tight and shiny and feel painful; milk flow may be compromised.

    4. Pathologic engorgement is generally a preventable postpartum complication. Restrictive feeding practices, suboptimal attachment, and/or ineffective sucking compromise milk removal and result in pathologic engorgement as identified by Woolridge in 1986.

B. Engorgement. In 2010, a Cochrane review was conducted on treatments for breast engorgement during lactation by Mangesi et al.

    1. When milk production increases rapidly, the volume of milk in the breast can exceed the capacity of the alveoli to store it.

    2. If milk is not removed, overdistention of the alveoli can cause the lactocytes to become flattened and drawn out; the alveoli's integrity relies on the junctions between each lactocyte being tightly closed. When these junctions are not tight, as might occur with increased pressure, a paracellular pathway may occur that allows components of breastmilk, for example, lactose, to leak into the interstitial tissue, resulting in inflammation and then possibly infection (Fetherston et al., 2005; Humenick et al., 1994; Nguyen et al., 1998).

    3. The distention can partly or completely occlude the capillary blood circulation surrounding the alveolar cells, further decreasing cellular activity. This distention can partly or completely occlude the oxytocin-rich capillary blood reaching the myoepithelial complex.

    4. Congested blood vessels leak fluid into the surrounding tissue space, contributing to interstitial edema, which further compresses and impedes the milk flow. A cycle of congestion/edema/poor flow/congestion can occur easily.

    5. Pressure and congestion obstruct the lymphatic drainage of the breasts, stagnating the system that rids the breasts of toxins, bacteria, and cast-off cell parts, thereby predisposing the breast to mastitis (both inflammatory and infectious).

    6. It is also thought that a protein called the feedback inhibitor of lactation (FIL) accumulates in the mammary gland during milk stasis, further reducing milk production (Daly et al., 1995; Peaker et al., 1996).

    7. Accumulation of milk and the resulting engorgement are a major trigger of apoptosis, or programmed cell death, that causes involution of the lactocytes, milk reabsorption, collapse of the alveolar structures, and the cessation of milk production (Marti et al., 1997).

    8. Engorgement has also been classified as involving only the areola, only the body of the breast, or both.

    9. Areolar engorgement in its simple form can occur more frequently with large pendulous breasts or women with generalized edema from large amounts of intravenous fluids or hypertension.

C. Prevention of engorgement requires efficient, thorough, and frequent milk removal.

1. Approaches to prevention:
   a. Optimal attachment/latch.
   b. Early and frequent feedings.
   c. Feeding according to cue of baby.
   d. Not restricting frequency or length of feeds.
   e. Finishing the first breast before offering the second. This directive is sometimes confusing; therefore, the lactation consultant should give examples of how to determine this to the mother.
2. The degree/duration of engorgement that poses an unrecoverable situation is unknown. The breast compensates to a point as milk production in the unaffected areas continues normally.
3. Predicting an individual mother's risk for engorgement might not be possible, but some general principles can help the lactation consultant anticipate situations that predispose women to a higher risk.
   a. Failure to prevent or resolve milk stasis resulting from infrequent or inadequate drainage of the breasts
   b. Women who have small breasts (other than hypoplastic and tubular) causing lack of room for expansion
   c. Mothers with high rates of milk synthesis (hyperlactation) because milk stasis magnifies whenever milk volume significantly exceeds milk removal

II. Treatment Modalities

A. Common treatment modalities.
   1. Warmth: Where a milk ejection reflex is thought to be compromised or slow, warmth has been shown to improve oxytocin uptake.
   2. Softening the areola prior to attachment helps achieve optimal attachment.
   3. If areolar edema is apparent, gentle massage of the interstitial fluid away from the nipple helps shape the areola, reveal the nipple, and improve milk flow.
      a. Originally referred to as *feathering* by British midwives, this technique has been redefined and described by Miller et al. (2004) as areolar compression and by Cotterman (2004) as reverse pressure softening.
   4. Cold therapy (cryotherapy):
      a. There is wide variation in the clinical use of cryotherapy (ice packs, gel packs, frozen bags of vegetables, frozen wet towels) and guidelines continue to be made on an empirical basis (Bleakley et al., 2004).
      b. Clinical and physiological evidence suggests that cryotherapy lowers tissue temperature by the withdrawal of heat from the body to achieve a therapeutic objective.
      c. Resultant vasoconstriction and suppressed cellular metabolic rate reduce the inflammatory response and lessen pain and edema.
      d. After removal of the cryotherapy, the mean skin temperature rises but does not return to the pretest level (Kanlayanaphotporn et al., 2005). This indicates a hemodynamic exchange between superficial and deep tissue and

offers an explanation of the reduction of pain, muscle spasm, and edema observed (Emwemeka et al., 2002).

5. Chilled cabbage leaves:
   a. Chilled cabbage leaves are commonly used because they appear to have a rapid effect on reducing edema and increasing milk flow.
   b. Roberts (1995) and Arora et al. (2009) compared chilled cabbage leaves and gel packs, both showing similar significant reduction in pain. The Roberts group found that two-thirds of the mothers preferred the cabbage because of a stronger, more immediate effect.
   c. Roberts et al., (1998) studied the use of cabbage extract cream applied to the breasts, which had no more effect than the placebo cream.

6. Expressing milk: Hand expressing or pumping to comfort reduces the buildup of FIL, decreases the mechanical stress on the alveoli (preventing the cell death process), prevents blood circulation changes, alleviates the impedance to lymph and fluid drainage, decreases the risk of mastitis and compromised milk production, and reduces maternal pain (Peaker et al., 1996; Prentice et al., 1989).

III. Plugged Ducts, Blocked Ducts, Caked Breast, Milk Stasis

A. Contributing factors
   1. Presents as localized tenderness and/or a firm red area in the breast usually as a result of inadequate milk removal from one duct.
   2. Compromised milk drainage from the breast can occur from external pressure to the breast. For example, a tight-fitting bra, baby carrier straps, mother's fingers, or baby's fist.
   3. Ineffective drainage of the breast by factors such as ineffective or inefficient sucking, suboptimal attachment, disorganized or dysfunctional sucking, skipped or irregular feeds, or hyperlactation.
   4. The section of the breast behind this blockage might experience a focal area of engorgement; an older name for this was *caked breast*.
   5. The mother might complain of tenderness, heat, or possibly redness over a palpable lump; the lump has well-defined margins and no fever is present.
   6. Management is by hot compresses and gentle massage before the feed. During the breastfeed, gentle pressure behind the blockage may improve milk flow. Alternating the baby's position at the breast can assist in milk removal; however, optimal attachment is still the most crucial component.
   7. Bleb: A blocked nipple pore is another potential cause of milk stasis.
      a. Frequently described as a solitary bleb/white dot or pressure cyst on the tip of the nipple (Day, 2001; Spencer, 2008).
      b. It is shiny, smooth, and less than 1 millimeter in diameter and causes pinpoint pain.
      c. The bleb blocks the terminal opening for drainage of one of the lobes of the breast and as such could contribute to milk stasis in a larger area of the breast.
      d. Warm soaks and optimal attachment sometimes resolve the problem.

e. After removal, the initial flow of milk is often "cheesy" followed by normal milk.

f. The bleb may require a health professional to open it with a sterile needle; it often reforms and requires repeated opening; the mother may need to be shown how to remove it herself.

8. Other descriptions of milk expressed from blocked areas of the breast include strings that look like spaghetti or lengths of fatty-looking material.

a. This type of blockage might account for the ropy texture of an obstructed area and the thought that thickened milk could be responsible for the blockage.

b. Lawrence et al. (2010) describe improvement in this condition when the mother's diet contains only polyunsaturated fats and a lecithin supplement is added to meals.

IV. Mastitis and Abscess

A. The role of bacterial pathogens in lactational mastitis remains unclear (Kvist et al., 2008).

B. A preventable but common lactation complication (Amir et al., 2007; Fetherston, 1998; Foxman et al., 2002).

C. Approximately 10% of women with mastitis wean because of the debilitating nature of the condition (Fetherston, 1997; Wambach et al., 2005).

D. Onset is usually in the first 3 to 4 weeks postpartum or with abrupt weaning or sudden changes in breast usage (Foxman et al., 2002).

E. An inflammatory process that may or may not progress to a breast infection.

1. The initial cause of mastitis is thought to be an unresolved increase in the intra-ductal pressure, first causing a flattening of the lactocytes and an increase in permeability of the tight junctions.

2. A paracellular pathway may then occur between the cells, which allows some of the components in breastmilk to leak into the interstitial tissue, resulting in an inflammatory response.

3. This inflammatory response and resultant tissue damage can be precursors to infective mastitis.

4. Studies have suggested that an elevated sodium/potassium ratio, an increase in sodium chloride, increased immunoglobulins, and a decrease in lactose with consequent decrease in milk volume are early signs of mastitis, which is often demonstrated by infant breast refusal (Fetherston, 2001). This is commonly referred to as subclinical mastitis (Hale et al., 2007; Kvist, 2010; Michie et al., 2003; Willumsen et al., 2000).

F. Usually associated with lactation, can be acute or chronic, and often occurs as a result of poor breastfeeding techniques.

G. Can progress to an infection and provoke serious sequelae, such as an abscess and early unnecessary weaning if it is treated inappropriately (World Health Organization [WHO], 2000).

H. Incidence varies among studies; it is estimated to occur in 24–33% of lactating women (Fetherston, 2001).

I. Mastitis has a variety of definitions that usually describe different aspects of the problem and are often based on the symptoms or ultimate treatment approach (Academy of Breastfeeding Medicine Protocol Committee, 2008).

J. Most clinicians simply use a cluster of signs and symptoms to diagnose mastitis (the infection).

1. Fever. 38°C (100.4°F)
2. Chills/headache
3. Increased pulse
4. Flu-like body aches
5. Pain/swelling at the site
6. Red, tender, hot area
7. Increased sodium levels in the milk (the baby might reject the breast because of the salty taste of the milk)
8. Red streaks extending toward the axilla
9. Thomsen et al. (1983) microscopically examined the milk itself to differentiate between milk stasis, inflammation, and infection; all of the mothers in their study complained of tender, red, hot, and swollen breasts.
10. Diagnosis of a breast infection was made by counting (not culturing) leukocytes and bacteria in milk samples taken from the affected breast and studied under a microscope (Thomsen et al., 1983).
11. Three clinical states were identified.
    a. Milk stasis: less than 10(6) leukocytes and 10(3) bacteria/milliliter of milk Symptoms persisted for 2.1 days
    b. Noninfectious inflammation: Greater than 10(6) leukocytes, milliliter of milk. The milk was sterile or contaminated by skin flora bacteria. Average duration of symptoms was 5.3 days
    c. Infectious mastitis: Greater than 10(6) leukocytes and bacteria greater than 10(3)/milliliter of milk
    d. Kvist (2010) suggests that although this classification is often cited, it might be questionable because cultivation can take up to 48 hours and the inflammation may have progressed.

K. The highest occurrence is generally at 2 to 3 weeks postpartum (WHO, 2000).

L. There seems to be a fairly equal distribution of cases between the right and left breasts. Bilateral mastitis occurs much less frequently (usual organism, Streptococcus).

M. Breastmilk is not sterile.

1. The vast majority of confirmed cases of mastitis show S. aureus as the causative organism.
2. Although lactating women potentially have pathogenic bacteria on their skin or in their milk, most do not go on to develop infectious mastitis (Kvist et al., 2008).
3. Conversely, in many women who actually develop an infection, pathogenic bacteria cannot be cultured in their milk.

N. Buescher et al. (2001) found that milk from a woman with mastitis has the same anti-inflammatory components and characteristics of normal milk, with elevations in selected components that may help protect the infant from developing clinical illness resulting from feeding from the affected mastitis breast.

O. Contributing factors:

1. Milk stasis

   a. If the pressure rises high enough, as with severe, unrelieved, and prolonged engorgement, small amounts of milk components are forced out from the tight junctions between the epithelial cells that line the ductal system and into the surrounding breast tissue.

   b. This triggers a localized inflammatory response, which involves pain, local swelling, redness, and heat over the affected area and/or a general response of a rise in body temperature and pulse rate.

   c. The disruption of the tight junction integrity can also provide a partial explanation for why women develop recurrent mastitis within a particular lactation.

   d. If milk components also leak into the vascular channels, capillaries, and bloodstream, this situation can account for the systemic/autoimmune response of fever, aches, fatigue, and general malaise that accompany mastitis.

   e. The body's response to both the inflammatory agents in the milk (interleukin-1) and the antigenic response to the milk proteins (which are recognized as foreign) are thought to contribute to the flu-like symptoms described.

2. Inefficient milk removal

P. Conditions and situations contributing to inefficient emptying of the breast and hence milk stasis:

1. Scheduled, interrupted, or erratic feeding patterns
2. A sudden change in the number of feeds
3. Mother's or baby's illness
4. Baby sleeping longer at night
5. Overabundant milk supply (hyperlactation)
6. Sucking at breast displaced by pacifiers or bottles
7. Separation of mother and baby
8. Breastfeeding technique (switching too soon from the first breast to the second before the baby has adequately drained the first side)
9. Abrupt weaning
10. Baby's oral anatomy that leads to inefficient emptying of the breast (for example, short frenulum, cleft palate, Pierre Robin syndrome)
11. Baby with a neurological impairment
12. Cracked or damaged nipples indicating ineffective latch (Foxman et al., 2002)
13. Breast pump use (Foxman et al., 2002)

Q. Hyperlactation:

1. van Veldhuizen-Staas (2007) describes several factors of maternal hyperlactation consisting of a high rate of milk synthesis and an abundant milk supply. This is an often underdiagnosed condition in well, healthy, lactating women.

R. Cracked or damaged nipples:

    1. Research suggests the possibility of an ascending infection (Miltenburg et al., 2008).

    2. However, studies by Kawada et al. (2003) found that methicillin-resistant S. aureus (MRSA) or methicillin-sensitive S. aureus may be transmitted between healthy lactating mothers without mastitis and their infants by breastfeeding.

S. Maternal stress and/or fatigue:

    1. Stress and sleep deprivation can lower a woman's immune response and are thought to be contributing factors (Michie et al., 2003).

    2. Wambach (2003) also identified the burden mastitis places on women. Women reported that mastitis had a greater impact on their daily living than on their breastfeeding outcome.

T. Use of nipple creams and/or gel pads:

    1. It has been hypothesized that the use of creams and lotions alters the pH of the nipple and areolar epithelium and blocks the glands of Montgomery or alters their secretions, thus reducing the natural protective factors of the areola.

    2. Use also may indicate the presence of damaged nipples and could appear as one of a cluster of situations or conditions simply associated with mastitis.

    3. Jonsson et al. (1994) found that the use of a nipple cream several times a day was associated with an increased incidence of mastitis.

U. Recurrent mastitis:

    1. Usually caused by delayed or inadequate treatment of the initial mastitis.

    2. Condition most frequently recurs when:

        a. Bacteria are resistant or not sensitive to the prescribed antibiotic.

        b. Antibiotics are not continued long enough.

        c. Mother stopped nursing on the affected side.

        d. The initial cause of the mastitis was not addressed (such as milk stasis).

    3. Clinicians can recommend that the mother continues to feed (or pump) on the affected side, that she take a full 10- to 14-day course of antibiotics, and that the cause or precipitating factors be identified and remedied (Hale et al., 2010).

    4. At the first recurrence, Lawrence et al. (2010) recommend milk cultures as well as cultures of the infant's nasopharynx and oropharynx.

        a. Other family members can be cultured as necessary to identify the source of the bacteria to keep it from reinfecting the mother.

        b. Culture and sensitivity testing is important to determine that the proper antibiotic is given.

        c. Nasal carriers of S. *aureus* should be identified and can be treated with mupirocin 2% (Bactroban nasal ointment) (Amir, 2002).

        d. Lawrence et al. (2010) also state that if the infection is chronic, low-dose antibiotics can be instituted for the duration of the lactation (erythromycin 500 mg/day).

e. Mothers with a history of mastitis in previous lactations need to be especially vigilant in preventing milk stasis and in ensuring optimal positioning and latch-on of the baby.

f. Ultrasound examination of the breast is used when either a cyst or an abscess is suspected. If the breast shows a fluid-filled cavity, an abscess is likely to be present.

g. "Because inflammatory breast cancer can resemble mastitis, this condition should be considered when the presentation is atypical or when the response to treatment is not as expected" (Spencer, 2008).

V. Prevention of mastitis:

1. Begins with accurate breastfeeding education and information.

   a. The lactation consultant needs to enable the mother to be able to confidently feed her infant and to recognize and implement management of problems such as mastitis.

2. Such education should include:

   a. Importance of early, frequent, unrestricted access to the breast

   b. Optimal positioning of the baby at the breast

   c. Individual mother's unique breast storage capacity and feeding pattern

   d. Early signs and symptoms of mastitis

   e. Common predisposing factors

3. Twenty-four-hour rooming in and increased skin-to-skin contact promotes the prompt recognition of infant feeding cues, reduces skipped feedings (especially at night), and leads to more frequent breast drainage during the early days.

4. Avoiding the use of pacifiers, which displaces sucking from the breast; this situation causes the breasts to remain full of milk as the time between breastfeeds increases.

5. Recognition and prompt attention of early warning signs that lead to milk stasis.

6. Plugged milk ducts can be massaged during the feed/expression to encourage the removal of the plug and enhance milk flow.

7. If a baby remains an inefficient feeder for whatever reason, the mother may need to hand express or pump following feeds to ensure adequate breast drainage and to provide additional milk for the baby. The mother can also use alternate massage/breast compression to improve milk drainage if the infant is unable to drain the breast adequately.

8. Adequate rest, help around the house and with other children, good nutrition, and hand washing before manual expression are common guidelines that can contribute to better overall health of the mother.

9. Limited milk expression might be needed if the baby abruptly starts sleeping for longer periods at night or if there is a substantial decrease in the number of breastfeedings for any reason.

10. Mothers who have a history of mastitis in previous lactations or women who have undergone breast surgery need to be especially vigilant in preventing milk stasis and in ensuring proper positioning and latch-on of the baby.

W. Management of mastitis:
1. Although antibiotics treat the infection, they do not treat the underlying cause of mastitis.
   a. If a mother develops infectious mastitis, then symptomatic treatments and antibiotic therapy must be joined by the third part of the intervention plan: identification and treatment of the underlying cause.
   b. Failure to do so can lead to recurrent mastitis.
2. Clinical assessment:
   a. Because milk stasis is the primary contributor to both inflammation and infection in the lactating breast, a lactation history is crucial in determining the underlying cause.
   b. Feeding assessment should ensure optimal attachment and milk transfer.
3. Management plan:
   a. Supportive counseling.
   b. Bed rest as much as can be managed.
   c. Increase fluid intake.
   d. Analgesic/antipyretic (acetaminophen, paracetamol).
   e. A more rapid reduction of inflammation may be seen by treatment with a nonsteroidal anti-inflammatory drug such as ibuprofen.
   f. Warm compresses prior to feeds if milk release appears to be delayed.
   g. Continue feeding on both breasts, including MRSA mastitis (Lawrence et al., 2010).
      i. Begin the feed on the affected side unless the breast is so painful that latch is impossible.
      ii. The rationale for this is that most babies will suck more vigorously and effectively on the first side.
   h. Use warm moist packs or cold/cabbage compresses between feeds, whichever gives greatest comfort (WHO, 2000).
   i. If there is no improvement within 12 to 24 hours, if her symptoms worsen, or the woman has multiple risk factors such as bilateral nipple damage, previous mastitis history, or unwell baby, then the mother needs immediate referral to her physician for antibiotic therapy.
   j. Other comfort measures:
      i. Immersing the affected breast in warm water before feeding.
      ii. Utilizing gravity by lying in a bath of hot water with the affected breast hanging.
      iii. Feeding in a hands-and-knees body position.
      iv. Ultrasound's efficacy is thought to be more likely from the radiant heat or massage than from the ultrawave emitting crystal.

X. Microbiology:

1. Breastmilk is seldom obtained for routine culture and sensitivity testing for appropriate antibiotic prescribing.

2. Culture and sensitivity testing should be undertaken if the following situations occur:

   a. There is no response to antibiotics within 2 days.

   b. If the mastitis recurs more than twice.

   c. If it occurs while the mother is still in hospital. Globally, MRSA and ORSA are becoming more common both in the hospital setting and in the community.

3. Severe or unusual cases:

   a. Because *S. aureus* is most commonly associated with breast infections, choices of antibiotics are generally penicillinase-resistant penicillins or cephalosporins, which are effective against *S. aureus*.

   b. Common drugs of choice are dicloxacillin and flucloxacillin; other antibiotics that may be used include erythromycin, nafcillin, and clindamycin.

   c. In streptococcal infections (often bilateral mastitis), penicillin might be preferable.

   d. In the case of a penicillin allergy, erythromycin would be the drug of choice.

4. Mothers who are treated with antibiotics for mastitis may subsequently develop candidiasis (Amir et al., 2002).

Y. Breast abscess:

1. Can be a complication of mastitis—incidence 2–11% of women who have mastitis (Amir et al., 2004; Foxman et al., 2002).

2. Almost always follows inappropriate/ineffective management of mastitis (Brodribb, 2004; WHO, 2000).

3. An abscess is a localized collection of pus that the body walls off; once encapsulated, it must be surgically drained/aspirated.

4. Risk factors:

   a. Prior mastitis

   b. A delay in therapy

   c. Noncompliance with antibiotic therapy

   d. Inappropriate choice of antibiotics or insufficient length of treatment

   e. Antibiotic resistance

   f. Failure to drain the affected breast

   g. Avoiding breastfeeding on the affected side

   h. Abrupt weaning

5. The most common offending organism is S. aureus, although other organisms are occasionally cultured from an abscess.

6. Prevention of an abscess resides on a continuum.

   a. Efficient milk transfer from breast to baby

   b. Avoidance and/or intervention for milk stasis

    c. Quick relief of breast inflammation

    d. The prompt treatment of breast infection, which includes continued and frequent nursing or pumping on the affected side

    e. Maternal education regarding gradual rather than abrupt weaning

    f. Health professional and maternal education regarding type, duration, and compliance with antibiotic prescribing

7. It is not always possible to confirm or exclude the presence of an abscess by clinical examination alone.

8. Mammography might not reveal an abscess because of extreme tenderness of the breast and very dense tissue.

9. Ultrasound (diagnostic):

    a. Can exclude the presence of an abscess and thereby avoid unnecessary surgery (Christensen et al., 2005).

    b. Ultrasound-guided aspiration is less invasive than traditional surgery and has a high rate of success (Christensen et al., 2005; Karstrup et al., 1993).

    c. Mothers can breastfeed throughout the course of ultrasound-guided needle aspiration drainage and possibly avoid surgery, admission to the hospital, and separation from their baby and families.

10. Surgical drainage of a breast abscess in some cases may be the necessary method of management.

11. Weaning or inhibiting lactation might hinder the rapid resolution of the abscess by producing increasingly viscid fluid that tends to promote rather than reduce breast engorgement.

12. The baby is not affected with continued breastfeeding unless the surgical site prevents optimal attachment/latch; pumping may be initially necessary.

    a. Some babies, however, might refuse to feed from the affected side because of a change in the taste of the milk.

    b. Following the onset of mastitis, changes in protein, carbohydrate, and electrolyte concentrations of milk from the affected breast have been observed.

    c. In particular, there is a decreased level of lactose and a marked rise in the concentrations of sodium and chloride; this situation has the temporary effect of causing the milk to taste salty.

    d. The decreased level of lactose also causes a decrease in volume of breastmilk produced (Neville et al., 1983).

V. Other Breast Conditions

A. Galactocele

1. A benign cyst in the ducts of the breast that contains a milky fluid; often called a milk retention cyst.

2. Presence of a galactocele should not interrupt breastfeeding (Merewood et al., 2001).

3. Contents of the cyst at first are pure milk but change to a thickened cheesy or oily consistency.

4. Cyst is smooth and rounded and might cause milk to ooze from the nipple when it is pressed.

5. Thought to be caused by the blockage of a milk duct.

6. Cyst can be aspirated but usually refills with milk.

7. If deemed necessary, it can be surgically removed under local anesthesia without interfering or interrupting breastfeeding; some spontaneously resolve.

8. Diagnosis can be made with ultrasound (Sabate et al., 2007).

B. Duct ectasia

1. Also known as periductal mastitis.

2. Most common cause of a bilateral, multiduct, multicolored, intermittent sticky nipple discharge (Brodribb, 2006).

3. Presenting symptoms, in addition to nipple discharge, are noncyclical mastalgia, nipple retraction, or a subareola abscess (Guray et al., 2006).

4. Result of dilatation of the terminal ducts (within 2–3 cm of the nipple); can occur in pregnancy, but is most commonly seen between 35 and 40 years of age. Risk increases with smoking.

5. An irritating lipid forms in the ducts, producing an inflammatory reaction and nipple discharge.

6. Women complain of burning, itching, pain, and swelling of the nipple and areola, which must be differentiated from symptoms of *Candida*.

7. A palpable, wormlike mass might develop as the condition progresses that mimics cancer, with chronic inflammation leading to fibrosis.

8. Surgery is not indicated unless the condition becomes severe and bleeding commences from the nipple.

9. Lactation can aggravate this condition but is not contraindicated.

10. Idiopathic granulomatous mastitis (IGM) a rare benign, chronic inflammatory condition of the breast can mimic duct ectasia and inflammatory breast cancer (Al-Khaffaf et al., 2008).

    a. It usually appears during lactation or within 5 years of childbirth as a firm discrete unilateral mass.

    b. Management ranges from conservative measurers to the use of corticosteroids and, rarely, excision (Nzegwu et al., 2007).

C. Fibrocystic breast condition (FCC)

1. Also known over the years as benign breast disease, chronic cystic mastopathy, mammary dysplasia, fibrocystic mastopathy, and chronic cystic mastopathy (Guray et al., 2006).

2. The term *fibrocystic changes* (FCC) is now the preferred terminology because the condition is observed clinically in up to 50% of women and histologically in 90% of women (Guray et al., 2006).

3. FCC may be multifocal and bilateral.

4. Palpable irregularities in breast tissue can be felt in varying degrees in response to the normal menstrual cycle.

a. These occur as proliferations of the alveolar system under hormonal influence.

5. Women might experience pain, tenderness, palpable thickenings, and nodules of varying sizes.

6. This condition might regress during pregnancy and does not contraindicate breastfeeding.

7. Some women describe varying degrees of relief from the condition when they eliminate caffeine from their diet and take vitamin E supplements. However, there is no evidence to support this.

D. Fibroadenoma

1. The most common benign lesion of the breast; occurs in 25% of asymptomatic women.

2. Peak incidence is 20–40 years (Miltenburg et al., 2008).

3. Lumps are nontender, mobile, firm, oval/almond shaped with well-defined borders.

4. Are hormone-dependent neoplasms that lactate during pregnancy (Guray et al., 2006).

5. Breastfeeding is not contraindicated.

6. Management is conservative with emphasis on educating the woman to ensure adequate milk removal to prevent the increased risk of milk stasis caused by the placement of the fibroadenoma.

E. Other lumps, cysts, and discharges

1. Nipple discharge is usually benign. Women with discharge can be divided into risk groups by a combination of clinical and radiological findings. Gray et al. (2007) developed a management algorithm.

2. Intraductal papilloma is a benign tumor or wart-like growth on the epithelium of mammary ducts that bleeds as it erodes.

3. The discharge is usually spontaneous from a single duct, and a nontender lump might be felt under the areola.

4. After serious disease has been ruled out, breastfeeding can continue.

a. Mothers are usually advised to pump the affected breast until the milk is clear of blood and continue breastfeeding on the other side.

b. If the baby tolerates the milk, many can simply continue breastfeeding.

c. The baby's stools might contain black flecks or temporarily become discolored and tarry.

5. If the discharge does not stop, the affected duct can be surgically removed.

6. Sometimes the first sign of this condition is when the baby spits up blood or when a mother who is pumping sees blood or pink-tinged milk.

7. This condition is extremely upsetting to the mother; infant disease can be ruled out by checking the regurgitated blood for fetal or adult hemoglobin (Apt test) to determine from whom the blood came.

F. Breast cancer

1. Inflammatory breast cancer must be differentiated from mastitis and plugged ducts.

2. Lumps that do not disappear in a couple of days, that are fixed with no clearly defined margins, and a pink slightly swollen breast that does not resolve with frequent breastfeeding or anti-inflammatory/antibiotic medications should be evaluated by a physician.

3. The majority of nipple discharge in women of childbearing age is not clinically concerning and requires no specific treatment.

4. Serous or blood-stained spontaneous discharge, especially if the discharge is coming from one duct only and is persistent, needs prompt referral and evaluation.

5. Approximately 1–3% of masses diagnosed during pregnancy and lactation are malignant.

6. Ductal carcinoma in situ (DCIS) may present as bloodstained nipple discharge with abnormal cells identified on cytology.

7. Paget disease of the nipple is a superficial manifestation of an underlying breast malignancy and is 1–3% of all breast cancers.

   a. The first symptom is usually a unilateral eczema-like rash. It appears as a well-demarcated, red, scaly plaque involving the nipple, areola, or both.

   b. The woman might also complain of a serous or blood-tinged discharge, pain, crusting, itching, burning, skin thickening, redness, ulceration, or nipple retraction.

   c. There is an underlying breast mass about 60% of the time.

   d. Lesion tends to appear on the nipple first and then spread to the areola.

8. Prominent masses need prompt evaluation; mammography might be difficult to interpret; fine needle biopsy can be performed with minimal problems during lactation; ultrasound or magnetic resonance imagery can be used to confirm a solid mass.

9. Treatment might include surgery, chemotherapy, and radiation therapy.

10. Infants are usually weaned from the breast if chemotherapy is necessary.

11. Young women who are treated with breast-conserving therapy and radiation for early stage cancer can experience subsequent full-term pregnancies and successful breastfeeding on the untreated breast and some women may successfully breastfeed on the treated breast.

12. The milk volume of the treated breast might be diminished.

13. Sometimes a baby will refuse to nurse from a cancerous breast, which is the first clue that a problem exists.

14. There is compelling evidence that breastfeeding is protective against developing premenopausal and probably postmenopausal breast cancer (Martin et al., 2005; Zheng et al., 2000).

    a. There is convincing evidence of a dose-response effect, with longer duration and more exclusive breastfeeding being more protective.

b. A review of 47 studies carried out in 30 countries indicated that the relative risk of breast cancer decreased by 4.3% for every 12 months of breastfeeding (Beral, 2002).

VI. Breast Surgery

A. Augmentation mammoplasty

1. Implants for breast augmentation are done for a variety of reasons, such as asymmetric breasts, hypoplastic breasts, breast reconstruction from surgery, or more commonly for purely cosmetic reasons.

2. Breasts undergoing augmentation might lack functional breast tissue, so the reason for the augmentation affects breastfeeding management.

3. Some augmentation procedures are done on adolescents.

4. Submuscular implants seldom cause interruption of ducts, nerves, or blood supply.

5. Surgical techniques vary, with the milk glands being most affected by periareolar incisions, which can damage ducts, nerves, and blood supply.

6. Subglandular and large-sized implants can compress the milk ducts and impede milk flow.

7. All women who have had augmentation surgery face the possibility of compromising maximum milk volume not only from the site of the incision but also from nerve disruption and pressure from the implant on breast structures.

8. Since 2008, hyaluronic acid injections (Macrolane), directly into breast tissue, have been used as a noninvasive option to enhance breast size.

a. Hyaluronic acid injections are not a contraindication to breastfeeding. The oral bioavailability of hyaluronic acid is nil and therefore even if it were to transfer into milk, it would not be readily absorbed by the baby's GI tract (Hale, 2010; infantrisk.com, March 2011)

9. Women need antenatal assessment and planning. Skin-to-skin contact at birth and early frequent, unrestricted breastfeeds are essential. Follow-up should include monitoring of engorgement and infant weight gain.

10. Women who received silicone implants are usually concerned about the leakage of silicone into breastmilk.

a. For the most part, silicone implants seem to pose little hazard to the breast-fed baby (Hale, 2010).

b. Silicone measurements of infant formula show vastly higher amounts in artificial baby milks than in breastmilk from women who have implants.

c. Most implants used currently are saline filled, but silicone implants will reappear because the U.S. Food and Drug Administration has cleared them for use again.

B. Breast reduction mammoplasty

1. Women may have breast reduction for aesthetic or health reasons. Large pendulous breasts (macromastia) may cause chronic pain of the head, neck, back, and shoulders, plus circulation and breathing problems. Brassiere straps may abrade or irritate the skin.

2. Full breastfeeding might not always be possible after reduction surgery. The outcome depends on the surgical technique used, the amount of glandular tissue removed, and the resultant integrity of blood supply and nerve pathways (Ramsay et al., 2005; Suto et al., 2003).

3. Techniques common for breast-reduction surgery are:

   a. The pedicle technique leaves the nipple and areola attached to the breast gland on a stalk of tissue. A wedge is removed from the undersides of the breast; for the most part, the breast tissue, blood supply, and some nerves remain intact, and breastfeeding will have varying degrees of success (Baumeister, 2003; Cruz-Korchin et al., 2007).

   b. The free nipple technique (auto transplantation of the nipple) involves removing the nipple/areola entirely so that larger amounts of breast tissue can be removed; the blood supply to the nipple/areola is severed and nerve damage occurs; this situation might result in diminished sensations in the nipple/areola.

   c. More recently, liposuction, which removes fatty tissue only and is almost scarless.

4. Women who have breast reduction surgery should be encouraged to breastfeed early and frequently to stimulate the breasts to provide as much breastmilk as possible. Monitoring of infant output is essential. The infant might need to be supplemented post breastfeeds.

   a. Supplementation can often be done at the breast with a supply line/lactation aid so that the mother and baby can enjoy each other and the breastfeeding experience.

   b. It is important that the mother–child relationship be as positive as possible.

   c. Some women may find this relationship is maintained if they supplement with the breast post bottle-feeds.

5. Nommsen-Rivers (2003) identifies the alternatives to reduction surgery, such as supportive bras and physical therapy resources for large-breasted women experiencing neck and shoulder pain, as well as clothing styles for breastfeeding.

VII. Other Infections

A. Dermatitis

1. Dermatitis may affect any area of skin on the body including the breasts (Whitaker-Worth et al., 2000).

2. Dermatitis may be caused by contact with an allergen, viral dermatitis may be caused by herpes simplex infection, and bacterial dermatitis may occur with impetigo (Thorley, 2000) or staphylococcus infection.

3. There is also a case report of a mother developing dermatitis on the nipple and areola after having developed an allergy to her infant's saliva (Kirkman, 1997).

4. Nipple eczema:

   a. Tends to present with redness, crusting, oozing, scales, fissures, blisters, excoriations (slits), or lichenification.

     b. Mothers might complain of burning and itching, and the eczema can extend onto and beyond the areola.

     c. This condition can occur on both nipples and is usually treated with topical corticosteroids applied sparingly post breastfeeds (Hale, 2010, pp. 1198–2000).

     d. If the eczema appears to be infected, indicated by a yellowish discharge, then topical antibiotic treatment may be necessary in addition to the corticosteroid.

     e. When eczema appears on just one nipple, referral to a physician should be considered to rule out Paget's disease, a superficial manifestation of underlying breast malignancy.

5. Allergic contact dermatitis

     a. Can present in a similar manner.

     b. Arises from the use of lanolin, emollients, or ointments containing beeswax or chamomile.

     c. The lactation consultant should ask what is being applied to the nipples that might be causing this problem.

6. Psoriasis, a chronic autoimmune disease, can affect any area of the breast and can present as a pink plaque that appears moist with minimal or no scale.

7. Seborrheic dermatitis can occur on the breast, most commonly in the mammary folds.

     a. It exhibits a greasy white or yellow scale on a reddened base and can be treated topically with ketoconazole, zinc, or selenium sulfide preparations.

8. Herpes simplex virus type 1 (HSV-1) with active oozing lesions on the nipple or areola requires a culture of the lesions and immediate treatment.

     a. Breastfeeding on that side should be interrupted until the lesions heal.

B. Mammary candidiasis

1. Recent research studies have questioned the diagnosis of mammary/ductal candidiasis (Eglash et al., 2006; Hale et al., 2009). Humans have an active cellular immune system that prevents fungal growth, and lactoferrin in breastmilk has been demonstrated to inhibit growth of *C. albicans* (Hale et al, 2009; Morrill et al., 2003).

2. Diagnosis is frequently based on a cluster of symptoms, the most common being persistent nipple and/or breast pain despite optimal position and latch of baby, rather than on laboratory evidence or a standard technique. May begin after a period of pain-free nursing (Newman, 2003).

3. The offending organism *C. albicans* is a commensal organism until a change in pH disrupts the balance between the fungus and its host, the human body.

     a. An example of this disruption is the use of antibiotics and the often-resultant vaginal overgrowth of *Candida* (Amir et al., 2002).

     b. Thrush in the oral cavity of a baby.

     c. The organism *C. albicans*, found frequently in the vagina and gastrointestinal tract, is the most frequent cause of thrush in the oral cavity of a baby. Women with vaginal thrush during pregnancy are considered at greater risk.

4. Intact dry skin is protective against *C. albicans*, while the warm, moist nipple possibly damaged or eroded from suboptimal latch may be a perfect host for colonization and infection.

5. *C. albicans* can exist in a number of forms, from the spherical cells on the surface of the nipple to the invasive form that is capable of penetrating cell walls.

6. Infant symptoms of oral thrush range from no visible symptoms to a white plaque coating the tongue to cottage cheese-like fungal colonies on the tongue, buccal mucosa, soft palate, gums, or tonsils.

   a. These plaques, if wiped, might reveal a reddened or bleeding base.

7. A fiery red diaper/nappy rash with glistening red patches, clear margins, and pustules that enlarge, appear outside the rash, and rupture, resulting in scaly and peeling skin, might be present on the baby.

8. An infected nipple might appear red, shiny, and have sloughing skin or be merely pink; the areola might have irregular shiny confluences.

9. Women complain of burning, itching, and stinging pain in the nipples that persists between feedings for many days and that is unresponsive to position changes or sucking corrections. Observation of a breastfeed, to rule out any nipple compression on detachment, should be part of the initial assessment.

10. Some mothers also complain of burning and shooting pain in the breasts or pain with milk release, which needs to be differentiated from a bacterial infection or nipple vasospasm that can cause the same symptoms (Anderson et al., 2004).

11. The value of skin swabs of the nipple/areola has been questioned (Hale et al., 2009; Spencer, 2008).

12. Examination of the nipple/areola under a microscope in a potassium hydroxide wet mount for the presence of superficial candidiasis may enable the proper use of antifungals. Excessive use has produced resistant strains.

    a. Culturing may confirm the *Candida* species (Amir et al., 2002).

    b. Milk cultures are difficult because lactoferrin inhibits fungal growth (Hale et al., 2009; Morrill et al., 2003). Using the laboratory technique that adds iron to counteract the action of lactoferrin was shown to reduce the likelihood of false-negative results and improve the accuracy of detecting Candida in human milk (Morrill et al., 2003). Hale et al. (2009), however, found no growth of *C. albicans* in the samples used which "strongly" suggested that there was no *C. albicans* present.

    c. A few small studies have demonstrated that the milk cultures among women with chronic breast pain are more likely to reveal bacterial pathogens rather than candidiasis (Eglash et al., 2006).

13. If mammary candidiasis is confirmed, both mother and baby should be treated simultaneously, even if the baby shows no signs in his or her mouth (Amir et al., 2002).

14. More than 40% of *Candida* strains are resistant to topical nystatin (usually the first medication prescribed); other topical treatments recommended are clotrimazole and miconazole (Amir et al., 2002).

    a. Gentian violet (methylrosanilinium chloride): Gentian violet is classified as an antifungal/antimicrobial agent. The previously used common practice of painting the baby's mouth and the mother's nipple with methylrosanilinium chloride (gentian violet) has been discontinued in some countries (e.g., Australia, United Kingdom). In the United States and Canada, some authors continue to recommend 0.5–1.0% solutions applied once daily for 3–5 days as a simple, effective treatment for both the baby and the mother (Hale, 2010; Newman, 2003).

15. Pacifiers are a continuous source of reinfection, so all items coming into contact with the baby's mouth need to be boiled, bleached, or washed daily (Amir et al., 2002).

16. Iatrogenic factors increase the risk of *Candida*, including the use of antibiotics, oral contraceptives, and steroids.

17. Fatigue and stress have been linked to increased risk of *Candida* (Abou-Dakin et al., 2009; Amir et al., 2002).

18. If all topical medications fail to bring relief, systemic oral fluconazole has been prescribed for 14 to 28 days.

C. Nipple pain and damage

1. In late pregnancy and early breastfeeding, there is normal tenderness because nipple sensitivity is heightened. This peaks on days 3 to 6 postpartum and is relieved as the volume of milk increases.

2. Women feel nipple discomfort as the collagen fibers are stretched with early sucking. This discomfort decreases as nipple flexibility increases.

3. Increased vascularity of the nipple and normal epithelial denudement can occur with optimal latch but increase initial tenderness.

4. Transient latch-on pain may occur from lack of established keratin layer on the nipple epithelium.

5. Prior to milk ejection, unrelieved negative pressure increases nipple tenderness. This is relieved with milk ejection.

6. Any severe nipple pain is not normal. Discomfort that lasts longer than a week and that is felt throughout a feed is not normal and requires intervention.

7. Skin color, hair color, prenatal preparation, or limiting sucking time at the breast are not related to the discomfort experienced (Dyson et al., 2006). Pain during a feed is most commonly a result of incorrect latch.

8. Nipple pain/protractility and baby's oral anatomy and functional suck require assessment, review, and/or correct positioning.

9. Eliminate diagnosis of impetigo, eczema, *C. albicans* overgrowth, nipple vasospasm.

10. Observance of nipple shape as the baby detaches is diagnostic and may present as:

    a. Horizontal or vertical red or white stripes

     b. Asymmetrical stretching

     c. Blisters

     d. Fissures, cracks, or bleeding

     e. Sharp pain experienced in one or both nipples post feed

     f. Blanching (vasospasm)

11. Nipple pain is aggravated by engorgement and the level of existing nipple damage.

12. The individual pain response of the mother mediates nipple pain.

13. Some mothers present with a long history of acutely sensitive nipples prior to pregnancy.

14. Sexual abuse and domestic violence can be complicating factors (Kendall-Tackett, 1998; Klingelhafer, 2007).

15. Nipple shields should not be considered as a part of routine management for nipple damage. They may be indicated if maternal and infant anatomy prevent optimal latch or if the history of acute sensitivity and/or sexual abuse is a complicating factor in degree of nipple pain experienced.

16. Vasospasm of the nipple (a Raynaud-like condition of the nipple):

     a. Described as causing extreme pain, stinging, and burning of the nipple during and/or between feeds.

     b. Emotional stress and cold are classic triggers of the phenomenon (Anderson et al., 2004).

     c. The shape of the nipple post feed indicates proper latch, but pain is evident.

     d. Nipple appears blanched post feed, and then the classic triphasic color change of white to blue to red is apparent.

     e. Babies who bite at the breast, clench their jaw, or chew on the nipple can cause nipple spasms (spasms of the blood vessels within the nipple).

     f. Symptomatic management of vasospasm that has shown to be of benefit (Anderson et al., 2004; Holmen et al.., 2009; Lawlor-Smith et al., 1997) includes the following techniques:

          i. Initiate the milk ejection reflex or express drops of colostrum before putting the baby to the breast.

          ii. Feed on the less tender side first.

          iii. Ensure correct positioning.

          iv. Use warm compresses.

          v. Avoid cold air.

          vi. Avoid substances that induce vasoconstriction such as some nasal sprays, nicotine, and caffeine.

          vii. Use pain relief.

          viii. Ensure adequate vitamin B6 intake.

          ix. Supplement calcium.

          x. Supplement magnesium.

     g. Medical management with nifedipine has been shown to be effective long term (Anderson et al., 2004; Hale, 2010; Holmen et al., 2009; Page et al., 2006).

References

Abou-Dakn, M., Schafer-Graf, U., & Wockkel, A. (2009). Psychological stress and breast diseases during lactation. *Breastfeeding Review, 17*(3), 19–26 .

Academy of Breastfeeding Medicine Protocol Committee. (2008). ABM clinical protocol no. 4: Mastitis. Revision, May 2008. *Breastfeeding Medicine, 3*(3). doi:10.1089/bfm.2008.999

Al-Khaffaf, B., Knox, F., & Bungred, N. J. (2008). Idiopathic granulomatous mastitis. *Journal of the American College of Surgeons, 206*(2), 269–273. doi:101016/j/jamcollsiurg.2007.07.041

Amir, L. H. (2002). Breastfeeding and *Staphylococcus aureus*: Three case reports. *Breastfeeding Review,10*, 15–18.

Amir, L. H., Forster, D. A., Lumley, J., & McLaughlin, H. (2007). A descriptive study of mastitis in Australian breastfeeding women: Incidence and determinants. *BMC Public Health , 7,* 62.

Amir, L. H., Forster, D., McLachlan, H., & Lumley, J. (2004). Incidence of breast abscess in lactating women: Report from an Australian cohort. *British Journal of Obstetrics and Gynaecology, 111*, 1378–1381.

Amir, L. H., & Hoover, K. (2002). Candidiasis and breastfeeding. In *Lactation Consultant Series Two*, Unit 6. Schaumburg, IL: La Leche League International.

Anderson, J. E., Held, N., & Wright, K. (2004). Raynaud's phenomenon of the nipple: A treatable cause of painful breastfeeding. *Pediatrics, 113*, 360–364.

Arora, S., Vatsa, M., & Dadhwal, V. (2009). Cabbage leaves vs hot and cold compresses in the treatment of breast engorgement. *Nursing Journal of India, 100*(3), 52.

Baumeister, R. G. H. (2003). Curtain type combined pedicled reduction mammoplasty with internal suspension for extensive hypertrophic and ptotic breasts, *British Journal of Plastic Surgery*, 56(2), 114–119.

Beral, V. (2002). Breast cancer and breastfeeding: Collaborative reanalysis of individual data of 47 epidemiological studies in 30 countries, including 50,302 women with breast cancer and 96,973 women without the disease. *Lancet, 360*, 187–195, 202–210.

Beral, V. (2003). Breast cancer and breastfeeding: Collaborative reanalysis of individual data of 47 epidemiological studies in 30 countries, including 50,302 women with breast cancer and 96,973 women without the disease [Comments]. *Lancet, 361*, 176–177.

Bertzold, C. M. (2005). Infections of mammary ducts in the breastfeeding mothers. *Journal of Nurse Practitioners, 1*(1), 15–21.

Bleakley, C., McDonough, S., & MacAuley, D. (2004). The use of ice in the treatment of acute soft-injury: Systematic review of randomized controlled trials. *American Journal of Sports Medicine, 32*, 251–261. doi:10.1177/0363546503260757

Brent, N., Rudy, S .J., Redd, B., Rudy, T. E., & Roth, L. A. (1998). Sore nipples in breast-feeding women: A clinical trial of wound dressings vs conventional care. *Archives of Pediatric and Adolescent Medicine, 152*, 1077–1082.

Brodribb, W. (Ed.). (2004). *Breastfeeding management in Australia* (3rd ed.). Malvern, Victoria, Australia: Australian Breastfeeding Association.

Brodribb, W. (2006). *Nipple discharge*. Malvern, Victoria, Australia: Australian Breastfeeding Association, Lactation Resource Centre. Retrieved from http://www.lrc.asn.au/publications.html

Buescher, E. S., & Hair, P. S. (2001). Human milk anti-inflammatory component contents during acute mastitis. *Cell Immunology, 21*(2), 87–95.

Christensen, A. F., Al-Suliman, N., Nielsen, K. R., et al. (2005). Ultrasound-guided drainage of breast abscesses: Results in 51 patients. *British Journal of Radiology, 78*, 186–188.

Cotterman, J. K. (2004). Reverse pressure softening: A simple tool to prepare areola for easier latching during engorgement. *Journal of Human Lactation, 2,* 227–237.

Cruz, N. I., & Korchin, L. (2007). Lactational performance after breast reduction with different pedicles. *Plastic and Reconstructive Surgery, 120*(1), 35-40.

Cruz-Korchin, N., & Korchin, L. (2004). Breast-feeding after vertical mammaplasty with medial pedicle. *Plastic and Reconstructive Surgery,* 114(4), 890–894. doi:10.1097/01. PRS.0000133174.64330.CC

Daly, S. E. J., & Hartmann, P. E. (1995). Infant demand and milk supply. Part 2: The short-term control of milk synthesis in lactating women. *Journal of Human Lactation, 11,* 27–37.

Day, J. (2001). Report of Australian Breastfeeding Association White Spot study. LRC *Topics in Breastfeeding,* Set 13. Retrieved from http://www.lrc.asn.au/publications.html

Dyson, L., Renfrew, M., McFadden, A., McCormick, F., Herbert, G., & Thomas, J. (2006). *Promotion of breastfeeding initiation and duration. Evidence into practice briefing.* England: National Institute for Health and Clinical Excellence.

Eglash, M. D., Plane, M. B., & Mundt, M. S. (2006). History, physical and laboratory findings, and clinical outcomes of lactating women treated with antibiotics for chronic breast and/or nipple pain, *Journal of Human Lactation, 22*(4). doi:10.1177/0890334406293431

Enwemeka, C. S., Allen, C., Avilla, P., Bina, J., Konrade, J., & Munns, S. (2002). Soft tissue thermodynamics before, during and after cold pack therapy. *Medicine and Science in Sports and Exercise, 34,* 45–50.

Fetherston, C. (1997). Characteristics of lactation mastitis in a Western Australian cohort. *Breastfeeding Review, 5,* 5–11.

Fetherston, C. (1998). Risk factors for lactation mastitis. *Journal of Human Lactation, 14,* 101–109.

Fetherston, C. (2001). Mastitis in lactating women: Physiology or pathology? *Breastfeeding Review, 9,* 5–12.

Fetherston, C. M., Lai, C. T., Mitsoulas, L. R., & Hartmann, P. E. (2005). Excretion of lactose in urine as a measure of increased permeability of the lactating breast during lactation. *Acta Obstetricia et Gynecologica Scandinavica, 85,* 20–25.

Foxman, B., D'Arcy, H., Gillespie, B., et al. (2002). Lactation mastitis: Occurrence and medical management among 946 breastfeeding women in the United States. *American Journal of Epidemiology, 155,* 103–114.

Foxman, B., Schwartz, K., & Looman, S. J. (1994). Breastfeeding practices and lactation mastitis. *Social Science and Medicine, 38,* 755–761.

Gray, R. J., Pockaj, M. D., & Karstaedt, M. D. (2007). Navigating murky waters: A modern treatment algorithm for nipple discharge. *American Journal of Surgery, 194,* 850–855. doi:10.1016/j.amjsurg.2007.08.027

Guray, M., & Sahin, A. A. (2006). Benign breast disease: Classifications, diagnosis, and management. *Oncologist, 11*(5), 435–449. doi:10.1634/theoncologist.11-5-435

Hale, T. W. (2010). *Medications and mothers' milk* (14th ed.). Amarillo, TX: Hale Publishing.

Hale, T. W., Bateman, T. L., Finkelman, M. A., & Berens, P. D. (2009). The absence of *Candida albicans* in milk samples of women with clinical symptoms of ductal candidiasis. *Breastfeeding Medicine, 4*(2), 57–61.

Hale, T. W., & Berens, P. (2010). *Clinical therapies in breastfeeding patients* (2nd ed.). Amarillo, TX: Pharmasoft Publishing.

Hale, T. W., & Hartmann, P. E. (2007). *Textbook of human lactation.* Amarillo, TX: Hale Publishing.

Hanson, L. A. (2007). The role of breastfeeding in the defense of the infant. In T. W. Hale & P. E. Hartmann (Eds.), *Textbook of human lactation* (p. 180). Amarillo, TX: Hale Publishing.

Holeman, O. L., & Backe, B. (2009). An underdiagnosed cause of nipple pain presented on a camera phone. *British Medical Journal*, *339*, b2553.

Humenick, S. S., Hill, P. D., & Anderson, M. A. (1994). Breast engorgement: Patterns and selected outcomes. *Journal of Human Lactation*, *10*, 87–93.

Jonsson. S., & Pulkkinen, M. O. (1994). Mastitis today: Incidence, prevention and treatment. *Annales Chirurgiae et Gynaecologiae*, *208*, 84–87.

Kanlayanaphotporn, R., & Janwantanakul, P. (2005). Comparison of skin surface temperature during the application of various cryotherapy modalities. *Archives of Physical Medicine and Rehabilitation*, *86*, 1411–1415.

Karstrup, S., Solvig, J., Nolsoe, C. P., et al. (1993). Acute puerperal breast abscess: US-guided drainage. *Radiology*, *188*, 807–809.

Kawada, M., Okuzumi, K., Hitomi, S., & Sugishita, C. (2003). Transmission of *Staphylococcus aureus* between healthy, lactating mothers and their infants by breastfeeding. *Journal of Human Lactation*, *19*, 411–417.

Kendall-Tackett, K. (1998). Breastfeeding and the sexual abuse survivor. *Journal of Human Lactation*, *14*, 125–130.

Kirkman, W. (1997). Breast dermatitis. *La Leche League News*, *97*, 6–7.

Klingelhafer, S. K. (2007). Sexual abuse and breastfeeding. *Journal of Human Lactation*, *23*, 194–197.

Kvist, L. J. (2010). Review: Towards a classification of the concept of mastitis as used in empirical studies of breast inflammation during lactation. *Journal of Human Lactation*, *26*, 53–59.

Kvist, L. J., Larsson, B. W., Hall-Lord, M. L., Steen, A., & Schalen, C. (2008). The role of bacteria in lactational mastitis and some considerations of the use of antibiotic treatment. *International Breastfeeding Journal*, *3*, 6. doi:10.1186-1746-4358-3-6

Lawlor-Smith, L. S., & Lawlor-Smith, C. L. (1997). Vasospasm of the nipple: A manifestation of Raynaud's phenomenon; case reports. *British Medical Journal*, *314*, 644–645.

Lawrence, R. A., & Lawrence, R. M. (2010). *Breastfeeding: A guide for the medical profession* (7th ed.). St. Louis, MO: Elsevier/Mosby.

Mangesi, L., & Dowswell, T. (2010). Treatments for breast engorgement during lactation. *Cochrane Database of Systematic Reviews*, *9*, CD006946. doi:10.1002/14651858.CD006946.pub2

Marti, A., Feng, Z., Altermatt, H. J., & Jaggi, R. (1997). Milk accumulation triggers apoptosis of mammary epithelial cells. *European Journal of Cell Biology*, *73*, 158–165.

Martin, R. M., Middleton, N., Gunnell, D., Owen, C. G., & Smith, G. D. (2005). Breast-feeding and cancer: The Boyd Orr cohort and a systemic review with meta-analysis. *Journal of the National Cancer Institute*, *97*, 1446–1457.

Merewood, A., & Philipp, B. L. (2001). *Breastfeeding conditions and disease: A reference guide*. Amarillo, TX: Pharmasoft Publishing.

Michie, C., Lockie, F., & Lynn, W. (2003). The challenge of mastitis. *Archives of Disease in Childhood*, *88*(9), 818–821.

Miller, V., & Riordan, J. (2004). Treating postpartum breast edema with areolar compression. *Journal of Human Lactation*, *20*, 223–226.

Miltenburg, D. M., & Speights, V. O., Jr. (2008). Benign breast disease. *Obstetrics and Gynecology Clinics of North America*, *35*, 285–300.

Morrill, J. M., Pappagianis, D., Heinig, M. J., et al. (2003). Detecting *Candida albicans* in human milk. *Journal of Clinical Microbiology, 41*, 475–478.

Neville, M., Allen, J., & Watters, C. (1993). The mechanism of milk secretion. In M. C. Neville & M. R. Neifert (Eds.), *Lactation: Physiology, nutrition and breastfeeding*. New York, NY: Plenum Press.

Newman, J. (2003). *Using gentian violet*. Handout no. 6. Retrieved from http://www.breastfeedingonline.com/6pdf.pdf

Nguyen, D. D., & Neville, M. C. (1998). Tight junction regulation in the mammary gland. *Journal of Mammary Gland Biology and Neoplasia, 3*, 233–246.

Nommsen-Rivers, L. (2003). Cosmetic breast surgery—is breastfeeding at risk? *Journal of Human Lactation, 19*(1), 7–8. doi:10.1177/0890334402239729

Nzegwu, M. A., Agu, K. A., & Amaraegbulam, P. I. (2007). Idiopathic granulomatous mastitis lesion mimicking inflammatory breast cancer. *Canadian Medical Association Journal, 176*, 13. doi:10.1503/cmaj.061110

Page, S., & McKenna, D. S. (2006). Vasospasm of the nipple presenting as painful lactation. *Obstetrics and Gynecology, 108* (3, pt. 2), 806–808. doi:1097/01.AOG.0000214671.19023.68

Peaker, M., & Wilde, C. J. (1996). Feedback control of milk secretion from milk. *Journal of Mammary Gland Biology and Neoplasia, 1*, 307–314.

Prentice, A., Addey, C. V. P., & Wilde, C. J. (1989). Evidence for local feedback control of human milk secretion. *Biochemical Society Transactions, 15*, 122.

Ramsay, D. T., Kent, J. C., Hartmann, R. A., & Hartmann, P. E. (2005). Anatomy of the lactating human breast redefined with ultrasound imaging. *Journal of Anatomy, 206*(6), 525–534. doi:10.1111/j.1469-7580.2005.00417

Roberts, K. L. (1995). A comparison of chilled cabbage leaves and chilled gelpaks in reducing breast engorgement. *Journal of Human Lactation, 11*, 17–20.

Roberts, K. L., Reiter, M., & Schuster, D. (1998). Effects of cabbage leaf extract on breast engorgement. *Journal of Human Lactation, 14*, 231–236.

Sabate, J. M., Clotet, M., Torrubia, S., et al. (2007). Radiologic evaluation of breast disorders related to pregnancy and lactation. *Radiographics, 27*(Suppl. 1), 101–124. doi:10.1148/rg.27si075505

Spencer, J. P. (2008). Management of mastitis in breastfeeding women. *American Family Physician, 78*(6), 727–731.

Suto, G. C., Giugliani, E. R., Giugliani, C., & Schneider, M. A. (2003). The impact of breast reduction surgery on breastfeeding performance. *Journal of Human Lactation, 19*(1), 43–49.

Thomsen, A. C., Housen, K. B., & Moller, B. R. (1983). Leukocyte counts and microbiologic cultivation in the diagnosis of puerperal mastitis. *American Journal of Obstetrics and Gynecology, 146*, 938–941.

Thorley, V. (2000). Impetigo on the areola and nipple. *Breastfeeding Review, 8*, 25–26.

van Veldhuizen-Staas, C. G. A. (2007). Overabundant milk supply: An alternative way to intervene by full drainage and block feeding. *International Breastfeeding Journal, 2*, 11. doi:10.1186/1746-4358-2-11

Wambach, K., Campbell, S. H., Gill, S. L., et al. (2005). Clinical lactation practice: 20 years of evidence. *Journal of Human Lactation, 21*, 245–258.

Wambach, K. A. (2003). Lactation mastitis: A descriptive study of the experience. *Journal of Human Lactation, 19*(1), 24–34.

Whitaker-Worth, D. L., Carlone, V., Susser, W. S., et al. (2000). Dermatologic diseases of the breast and nipple. *Journal of the American Academy of Dermatology, 43*, 733–754.

Willumsen, J. F., Filteau, S. M., Coutsoudis, A., Uebel, K. E., Newell, M. L., & Tomkins, A. M. (2000). Subclinical mastitis as a risk factor for mother–infant HIV transmission. *Advances in Experimental Medicine and Biology, 478*, 211–223.

Woolridge, M. W. (1986a). Aetiology of sore nipples. *Midwifery, 2*, 172–176.

Woolridge, M. W. (1986b). The "anatomy" of infant sucking. *Midwifery, 2*, 164–171.

World Health Organization. (2000). *Mastitis: Causes and management.* Geneva, Switzerland: Author.

Zheng, T., Duan, L., Lui, Y., et al. (2000). Lactation reduces breast cancer risk in Shandong Province, China. *American Journal of Epidemiology, 152*, 1129–1135.

CHAPTER 40
Hyperbilirubinemia and Hypoglycemia

Sallie Page-Goertz, MN, CPNP, IBCLC

OBJECTIVES

- Define and differentiate the characteristics of physiologic jaundice, breastfeeding-associated jaundice, pathologic jaundice, and breastmilk jaundice.
- Describe the breastfeeding management of the infant who is experiencing jaundice.
- List strategies for the prevention of breastfeeding-associated jaundice.
- List the criteria for referral for medical evaluation.
- List the risk factors for the development of hypoglycemia.
- Describe breastfeeding management of the infant who has hypoglycemia.
- List measures for preventing hypoglycemia in a newborn infant.

INTRODUCTION

During the immediate newborn period, two problems affect and are affected by breast-feeding management: hyperbilirubinemia and hypoglycemia. Appropriate breastfeeding routines, awareness of the risk factors, and continuous assessment of the newborn are critical elements in preventing or reducing morbidity from these two concerns.

Part 1: Hyperbilirubinemia: Background Information

Hyperbilirubinemia is the presence of elevated bilirubin. Jaundice describes yellow staining of the skin and sclera caused by abnormally high blood levels of the bile pigment bilirubin, irrespective of the cause. Sections I through VI in this part discuss issues related to indirect (unconjugated) hyperbilirubinemia, where increased bilirubin is secondary to either increased bilirubin production, or decreased bilirubin metabolism/excretion. The terms *bilirubin* and *hyperbilirubinemia* refer to indirect/unconjugated bilirubin, unless indicated otherwise. Direct (conjugated) hyperbilirubinemia is caused by hepatocellular disorders such as hepatitis and biliary tree abnormalities such as biliary atresia. These disorders are considered if an infant or child has persistent hyperbilirubinemia, with an elevation of the direct bilirubin component, and are outside the scope of this discussion.

High bilirubin levels can lead to a spectrum of bilirubin-induced neurologic dysfunction (BIND) evidenced by damage primarily to the basal ganglia, central and peripheral neurologic pathways, hippocampus, brain stem nuclei for oculomotor function, and the cerebellum. Damage can be minimal to severe. Extremely high levels of bilirubin can lead to kernicterus, which is chronic, irreversible brain damage. Clinical sequelae include movement disorders (dystonia and athetosis), abnormalities of gaze and other visual difficulties, auditory disorders (hearing loss, processing disorders), and dysplasia of the enamel of deciduous teeth (Bhutani et al., 2005). Johnson et al. (2009) report that each infant with a total serum bilirubin (TSB) greater than 35 mg/dL in the United States Pilot Kernicterus Registry evidenced moderate to severe posticteric neurodevelopmental deficits consistent with permanent BIND. Further, the case reviews reveal that providers did not monitor these newborns per current standards of care.

Fortunately, for many children who experience marked hyperbilirubinemia, sequelae might resolve over time (Harris et al., 2001). Newman et al. (2006) report neurodevelopmental outcome of 140 infants who had bilirubin ≥ 25 mg/dL and were treated with either phototherapy (n = 136) or exchange transfusion (n = 5). Neurologic and developmental testing demonstrated that adverse outcomes at ages 2 and 5 years were not statistically different from those in the random control group of 419 infants who did not experience hyperbilirubinemia. The nine children who had bilirubin over 30 mg/dL did have slightly lower IQ scores. Kernicterus and BIND are rare but nonetheless should be "never events" because they are preventable when evidence-based newborn care is provided.

Reports of infants experiencing complications from hyperbilirubinemia as well as concurrent dehydration and excessive weight loss show that the majority were breastfeeding, apparently ineffectively, and as in the Registry group, did not receive recommended monitoring (Salas et al., 2009). Cases are also reported, although with less frequency, from other countries including Canada, Denmark, Holland, New Zealand, and Nigeria (Kaplan et al., 2004; Udoma et al., 2001).

The American Academy of Pediatrics (American Academy of Pediatrics [AAP] Subcommittee on Neonatal Hyperbilirubinemia, 2004) guideline for prevention and treatment of hyperbilirubinemia recommends that all newborns have either a formal risk assessment performed or a bilirubin level obtained prior to hospital dismissal. The 2004 AAP guideline includes risk stratification and treatment recommendation nomograms to guide care. The risk nomogram requires a TSB result along with the exact hour of age of the infant at the time of obtaining the sample. If transcutaneous bilirubin (TcB) levels are used, an adjustment must be made to account for the difference in TcB as compared to TSB to avoid inaccurate risk assessment (El-Beshbishi et al., 2009). At the BiliTool website (www.bilitool.org), practitioners can enter an infant's weight, date and time of birth, and the bilirubin result with date and time of sampling to obtain a risk assessment and treatment recommendation based on the nomograms (see **Figures 40-1** and **40-2**) used in the AAP guideline. Screening with TcB or TSB leads to more appropriate treatment of infants with decreased frequency of readmission for hyperbilirubinemia, decreased incidence of high bilirubin levels, and more use of phototherapy for infants who met treatment guidelines as opposed to those who did not (Kuzniewicz et al., 2009; Petersen et al., 2005).

Maisels et al. (2009) published a commentary including updated screening recommendations and clarifications of the AAP 2004 guideline, particularly related to thinking about the effect of risk on decisions for treatment and follow-up. Maisels et al. (2009) recommend universal testing with either TSB or TcB and do not endorse the AAP 2004 option of doing risk assessment only.

The Academy of Breastfeeding Medicine's (Academy of Breastfeeding Medicine [ABM] Protocol Committee, 2010) protocol 22 addresses breastfeeding management for prevention of problematic hyperbilirubinemia. These ABM recommendations are congruent with the International Lactation Consultant Association's *Clinical Guidelines for Establishment of Exclusive Breastfeeding* (International Lactation Consultant Association [ILCA], 2005). The ABM protocol also addresses breastfeeding management for the infant with hyperbilirubinemia. The lactation consultant should review each of these documents for the best understanding of prevention and management of hyperbilirubinemia.

It is not known at this time if the AAP guidelines and the more recently published clarification commentary (Maisels, Bhutani et al., 2009) are appropriate for populations or systems of care dissimilar to that in the United States (Kaplan et al., 2005; Manning, 2005). Furthermore, performing a TcB on every newborn leads to a cost of $9,191,352 for prevention of one case of kernicterus in the United States (Suresh et al., 2004). If clinical guidelines for appropriate policies and practices of newborn care were in fact implemented, this type of expense could be avoided.

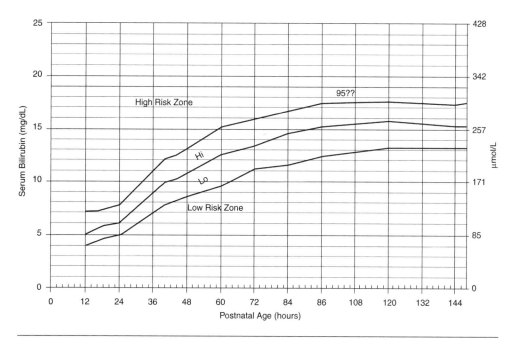

Figure 40-1 Risk Nomogram for Infants > 35 Weeks Gestation

Source: Reproduced with permission from American Academy of Pediatrics Subcommittee on Neonatal Hyperbilirubinemia. (2004). Management of hyperbilirubinemia in the newborn infant 35 or more completed weeks of gestation. *Pediatrics 114*, 301.

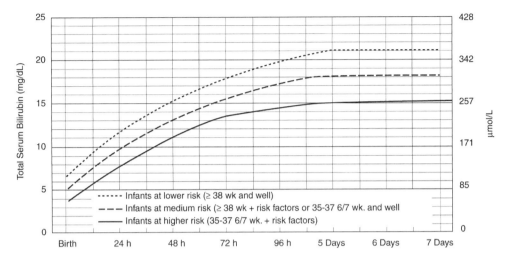

• Risk factors: isoimmune hemolytic disease, G6PD deficiency, asphyxia, significant lethargy, temperature instability, sepsis, acidosis, or albumin <3.0 gd:
• For well infants 35-37 6.7 wk can adjust TSB levels for interfvention around the medium risk line. It is an option to intervene at lower TSB leveles for infants closer to 35 wks, and at higher TSB levels for those closer to 37 6;7wk.
• It is an option to provide conventional phototherapy in hospital or at home at TSB levels 2-3 mg/dl (35-50mmol/L_ below those shown but home phototherapy should not be used in any infant with risk factors

Figure 40-2 Guidelines for Phototherapy in Hospitalized Infants of 35 or More Weeks' Gestation

Source: Reproduced with permission from American Academy of Pediatrics Subcommittee on Neonatal Hyperbilirubinemia. (2004). Management of hyperbilirubinemia in the newborn infant 35 or more completed weeks of gestation. *Pediatrics, 114*, 304.

Often, the lactation consultant is asked to evaluate and manage the breastfeeding of an infant who has hyperbilirubinemia. **Table 40-1** describes the most common causes of hyperbilirubinemia in the newborn. Jaundiced infants might present to the consultant's practice with family members who are unaware of the significance of jaundice. In certain situations, a jaundiced infant might also have excessive weight loss as well as other underlying health problems contributing to ineffective feeding. There might even be life-threatening situations caused by associated dehydration and hypernatremia. The lactation consultant must work in collaboration with the infant's primary healthcare provider (PCP) in the medical management of the infant with hyperbilirubinemia.

Persistent hyperbilirubinemia in the breastmilk-fed infant is a vexing problem. There is a growing list of factors that might contribute to persistent jaundice in newborns. Preer et al., (2011) published an excellent review of this clinical problem, including an algorithm suggesting a step-by-step approach to the evaluation of the infant with persistently elevated bilirubin so that practitioners can more confidently distinguish among breastmilk jaundice and other pathologic conditions (see Figure 40-4).

Table 40-1 Comparison of Common Causes of Indirect Hyperbilirubinemia in the Term Newborn Infant

	Physiologic Jaundice	Breastfeeding-Associated Jaundice	Breastmilk Jaundice
Onset of clinical jaundice	48–72 hours	48–72 hours	5–10 days of age
Peak	Day 3–5	Day 3–5+	Day 15
Rate of rise	2 mg/dL/day	5 mg/dL/day	1–2 mg/dL/day
Cause	RBC breakdown	Starvation/delayed defecation	Unknown
Condition of infant	Thriving; normal weight loss; normal output; clinically jaundiced	Lethargic/fussy; excessive weight loss; ineffective feeding; scant urine/stool output; signs of dehydration	Thriving; clinically jaundiced
Breastfeeding management	Monitor in order to ensure effective breastfeeding and initiation of normal weight gain	Increase caloric intake; intervene to establish effective breastfeeding; assist with supplementation; stimulate milk supply	No intervention needed
Medical management	Monitor; return visit at 72 hours of age; phototherapy per guidelines (seldom needed)	Phototherapy per guidelines; supplementation if indicated	Monitor bilirubin until stable; consider brief interruption of mother's milk feedings (preferable to avoid this strategy)

Source: Page-Goertz, S., & McCamman, S. (1996). *Hyperbilirubinemia in the breastfed infant, lectures to go.* Overland Park, KS: Best Beginnings Productions. Used with permission from Best Beginnings Productions.

I. Bilirubin Physiology in the Normal Newborn

A. Red blood cells (RBCs) break down after birth with the transition to a higher-oxygen environment.

B. Bilirubin is one of the breakdown products of these RBCs; it is released into the bloodstream.

C. Bilirubin is then bound to albumin in the bloodstream and is carried to the liver, where it is conjugated with the aid of a hepatic enzyme UDGT 1A1 (uridine diphosphate glucorosyltransferase 1A1).

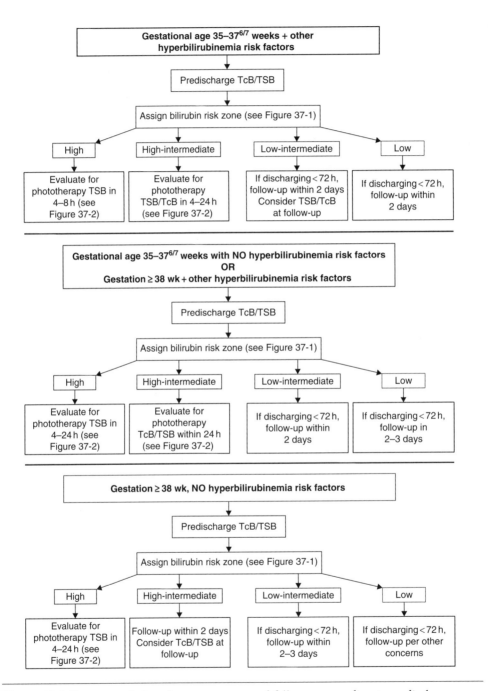

Figure 40-3 Recommendations for management and follow-up according to predischarge bilirubin measurements, gestation, and risk factors for subsequent hypebilirubinemia.

Source: Reproduced with permission from *Pediatrics, 127,* 575, Copyright 2009 by the AAP

D. Conjugated bilirubin is then excreted via the bile duct into the small intestine.

E. Intestinal flora convert it to stercobilin for excretion into the stool.

F. If stooling is delayed, conjugated bilirubin can be deconjugated by an enzyme in the brush border of the gut, be absorbed by the gut mucosa, and returned to the liver via the portal circulation. This is known as enterohepatic circulation.

II. Screening/Testing for Hyperbilirubinemia

A. Who/when to screen/test?

1. Current recommendation (AAP Subcommittee on Neonatal Hyperbilirubinemia, 2004) is that predischarge risk appraisal should be done on all infants via bilirubin screening (TcB or TSB and/or risk assessment questionnaire), with TSB to be obtained on those noted to be at high risk.

2. Maisels et al. (2009) note that combining TcB with just two risk factors, gestational age and exclusive breastfeeding, improves prediction of later hyperbilirubinemia.

3. Keren et al. (2008) found that the combination of TcB with gestational age was a simple and accurate approach to risk assessment.

B. How to test?

1. Risk assessment using TcB:

a. TcB levels may be lower or higher than TSB, and correlation should be made between TCB levels and TSB levels in the laboratory being used.

b. Risk nomograms currently in use are based on TSB levels and require that the infant's exact age in hours be noted to use the nomogram (AAP Subcommittee on Neonatal Hyperbilirubinemia, 2004; De Luca et al., 2008).

2. Visual appraisal is shown to be inaccurate, both underestimating and overestimating predicted bilirubin (Kaplan et al., 2008; Szabo et al., 2004).

III. Physiologic and Pathologic Hyperbilirubinemia

A. Physiologic jaundice is the normal increase in bilirubin associated with RBC breakdown after birth and immaturity of bilirubin metabolism systems. It is unusual for bilirubin levels in purely physiologic jaundice to reach the high-risk zones (Herschel et al., 2005). All newborns experience physiologic rises in bilirubin, but the level may not rise high enough to result in visible jaundice.

1. Age and bilirubin

a. Bilirubin levels in normal newborns of at least 35 weeks gestation increase most rapidly in the first 6 to 18 hours of life and less rapidly from 18 to 42 hours of life, followed by a slower increase until the peak is reached at 3 to 5 days of age.

b. Decreased gestational age and exclusive breastfeeding were associated with higher bilirubin levels at 24, 48, 72, and 96 hours of age (Maisels et al., 2006).

c. Late-preterm infants (35–37 completed weeks) may have bilirubin levels that peak later, on days 5 to 7, and are more likely to develop significant hyperbilirubinemia compared to those of 38 to 42 weeks (Sarici et al., 2004).

2. Race and bilirubin
   a. Babies of Caucasian and Asian descent have higher physiologic bilirubin levels than do babies of African descent (Newman et al., 1999).
   b. Despite low incidence of hyperbilirubinemia, babies of African descent comprise 25% of reported kernicterus and BIND cases in the United States, Ireland, and the United Kingdom (Watchko, 2010). This may be because of the difficulty of detecting clinical jaundice, in addition to the higher risk for G6PD deficiency.
   c. Huang et al. (2009) report Chinese ethnic origin as an independent risk for hyperbilirubinemia as compared to babies of Malay or Indian descent.
   d. Research demonstrates a genetic difference in Asians that may account for the increased propensity of about 20% of Asian infants for severe neonatal indirect hyperbilirubinemia (Akakba et al., 1998).
   e. Johnson et al. (1986) reported that Navajo infants had exaggerated levels of bilirubin as well.
   f. Many babies are of mixed racial background, and both the clinical observation and the parents' report may not reflect the child's actual racial background (Beal et al., 2006).
B. Neonatal pathologic hyperbilirubinemia:
   1. Overproduction or lack of effective excretion of bilirubin, or both, results in bilirubin levels requiring active intervention to prevent complications.
   2. Infants with pathologic jaundice must be under the care of a PCP in addition to receiving assistance from a lactation consultant.
   3. Suspect pathologic jaundice if:
      a. Infant has onset of jaundice within the first 24 hours of life.
      b. Bilirubin levels are rising rapidly; or the infant is jaundiced beyond 3 weeks of life *and* not thriving (AAP Subcommittee on Neonatal Hyperbilirubinemia, 2004).
   4. Causes of increased production/presence of circulating bilirubin beyond the liver's capability to metabolize it include:
      a. Hemolysis resulting from pathologic causes such as ABO or Rh incompatibility, congenital RBC disorders such as spherocytosis and G6PD deficiency
      b. Polycythemia (placenta-to-infant or twin-to-twin transfusion)
      c. Birth trauma with resultant bruising (AAP Subcommittee on Neonatal Hyperbilirubinemia, 2004), such as cephalohematoma or bruising elsewhere, seen especially with vacuum- or forceps-assisted vaginal deliveries
   5. Interference with the liver's capability to metabolize bilirubin:
      a. Genetic variants/disorders of conjugation such as Gilbert syndrome, Crigler-Najjar syndrome
      b. Hypothyroidism
      c. Genetic mutations

6. Interference with the body's ability to excrete bilirubin via stooling:
   a. Inadequate intake resulting from ineffective feeding (for example, breast-feeding-associated jaundice) and resultant delayed stooling
   b. Intestinal obstruction such as meconium ileus, other congenital intestinal anomalies

IV. Risk Factors for Hyperbilirubinemia

A. Maternal factors
   1. Factors that may result in insufficient milk production or ineffective feeding
   2. Diabetes and other endocrinopathies (Neubauer et al., 1993)
   3. Anatomic breast abnormality (Huggins et al., 2000)
   4. Breast surgery, especially breast reduction/periareolar incision (Neifert et al., 1990)
   5. Retained placenta (Anderson, 2001)
   6. Hypertension/eclampsia
   7. Mother–infant separation (Yamauchi et al., 1990b)
   8. Delayed first feeding (Yamauchi et al., 1990b)

B. Labor and delivery factors that may result in increased RBC hemolysis
   1. Epidural analgesia because of the associated increased risk of interventional delivery using forceps or vacuum extraction (Thorp et al., 1996) and associated bruising of the infant
   2. Birth trauma and associated bruising

C. Infant risk factors
   1. Family history of RBC disorders such as spherocytosis, G6PD deficiency, or Gilbert syndrome
   2. Factors associated with ineffective feeding/inadequate intake
      a. Sleepy infant/infrequent feedings (Yamauchi et al., 1990a)
      b. Congenital oral-facial anomalies, such as cleft palate, ankyloglossia, or Pierre Robin syndrome (Marques et al., 2001)
      c. Congenital heart disease/neurologic impairment, such as an infant with trisomy 21 or large ventricular septal defect
      d. Oral motor difficulties, such as difficulties with attachment or effective suckling
   3. Small for gestational age or prematurity

V. Assessing the Jaundiced Infant

A. Quick appraisal to determine the immediate need for a medical evaluation:
   1. Lethargic, unable to arouse
   2. Refusal to feed
   3. Excessive weight loss (≥ 10%; AAP Subcommittee on Neonatal Hyperbilirubinemia, 2004)
   4. Vomiting
   5. Inadequate urine or stool output for the infant's age

6. Visible jaundice in the first 24 hours, or jaundice extending below the shoulders/upper chest at any time (AAP Subcommittee on Neonatal Hyperbilirubinemia, 2004)

B. History:

1. Infant history

   a. Assess for presence of the risk factors (see the section titled "IV. Risk Factors for Hyperbilirubinemia" in this part).

   b. Know the child's risk level based on the use of the AAP risk nomogram (Figure 40-1) or as obtained at www.bilitool.org if bilirubin levels are available. Confer with the medical provider if the child is in an elevated risk category.

   c. Assess color of urine; it should be yellow and not orange.

   d. Assess for presence of uric acid crystals in the urine (brick dust appearance in the diaper); this can indicate dehydration but is also common in the first 1–2 days of life.

   e. Assess stool color—expect transitional stools days 2 to 3 and breastmilk stools (yellow, runny) by days 4–5. An infant with white/clay color stools needs immediate referral because this might indicate biliary atresia, a medical emergency (direct bilirubin will be elevated in this case).

   f. Assess infant's behavior over the past 24 to 48 hours.

      i. Waking to feed?

      ii. Content after feedings?

      iii. Fussy or unsatisfied with feedings?

2. Maternal history

   a. Health history; underlying risk factors (see the section titled "IV. Maternal Factors" in this part)

   b. Breast health history; underlying risk factors (see the section titled "IV. Maternal Factors")

   c. Mother's perception of breast fullness by days 3–4 (evidence of lactogenesis II)

   d. Breast/nipple pain or discomfort

   e. Evidence of milk ejection reflex

3. Feeding history

   a. Frequency of feeds

   b. Length of active feeding

   c. Swallows present

   d. Number of voids and stools per 24 hours:

      i. First 24 hours: 1 wet diaper and 1 meconium stool(s)

      ii. Day 2: 2 to 3 wet diapers and 1 meconium stool(s)

      iii. Day 3: 4 to 6 wet diapers and transitional stools

      iv. Day 4: 4 to 6 wet diapers and transitional stools

      v. Day 5: 6+ wet diapers and 3 to 4 yellow stools

C. Assessment:
  1. Infant
    a. General appearance
    b. Level of vigor: alert/active versus difficult to arouse/lethargic
    c. Evidence of dehydration
      i. Check capillary refill. Press the infant's finger or toe to blanch it, and observe how quickly it becomes pink again (this should take 2 seconds or less). Capillary refill longer than 2 seconds is the most sensitive indicator of dehydration other than weight loss (Gorelick et al., 1997).
      ii. Check skin turgor. Pull up on the skin and observe the elasticity. Skin should immediately recoil with no tenting.
      iii. Check mucous membranes for moistness.
    d. Presence of any congenital oral-facial anomalies or other syndromes that might interfere with effective breastfeeding
    e. Current weight and the percentage of weight loss since birth
    f. The extent of jaundice:
      i. When jaundice extends beyond the upper chest, visual inspection is *not* accurate for judging degree of jaundice at the upper extremes (Szabo et al., 2004).
      ii. Refer to the PCP for evaluation.
  2. Feeding assessment
    a. Latch-on technique.
    b. Presence/frequency and length of bursts of swallows.
    c. Impact of change of feeding positions on the quality of feeding.
    d. Consider pre- and postfeeding test weighing if weight loss more than 8% has occurred.
      i. Test weight documents intake for a single feeding; one cannot be sure if it represents the best or worst feeding effort the infant is capable of.
      ii. Whether or not test weighing is done, a follow-up weight check within 24 hours must be obtained to ensure the infant's safety.
  3. Maternal breast assessment
    a. Scars, marked asymmetry, inverted/flat nipples, tubular breasts, or widely spaced breasts
    b. Nipple trauma
    c. Engorgement
D. Table 40-1 summarizes and compares the findings in causes of jaundice related to breastfeeding.
E. Breastfeeding management:
  1. Infant with hyperbilirubinemia who demonstrates appropriate weight for age:
    a. No interruption of breastfeeding (with the exception of galactosemia)
    b. Continued exclusive breastfeeding
    c. No supplementation

2. Infant who has excessive weight loss or inadequate weight gain (See Chapter 43, Slow Weight Gain and Failure to Thrive):

   a. Establish effective breastfeeding techniques and routines.

   b. Provide supplemental fluid/calories at the breast or by other methods as indicated. Use expressed mother's milk or a human milk substitute.

   c. Initiate additional stimulation of milk supply.

   d. Monitor bilirubin per primary care provider's instruction.

   e. Weight check within 24 hours, with repeat checks until appropriate weight gain established.

   f. If supplement is used, reduce or increase the amount based on weight gain, hydration status, and the infant's breastfeeding capabilities.

   g. The child's PCP decides on the need for phototherapy or other medical intervention.

   h. Although medical therapy might be effective in reducing the bilirubin levels, the infant still needs careful feeding evaluation to ensure adequate hydration, weight gain, and restoration of effective breastfeeding as well as sufficient maternal milk supply.

F. Medical management of hyperbilirubinemia:

   1. Establish a definitive cause. (see Table 40-1)

   2. Treat based on the definitive cause.

   3. Intervene to decrease bilirubin level if it is at potentially dangerous or high level.

      a. Phototherapy

         i. Under the influence of phototherapy lights, photoisomers of bilirubin are formed that are more easily excreted by the liver.

         ii. Phototherapy lights or fiber-optic blankets are used.

         iii. Phototherapy lights are preferred for efficient management of significant hyperbilirubinemia.

         iv. Certain high-risk infants (≤ 37 weeks gestation, positive Coombs, and short treatment) are at risk for significant rebound after phototherapy and need close follow-up (Kaplan et al., 2006).

      b. Exchange transfusion

         i. Rarely needed

         ii. Used only in the case of extremely high bilirubin level

         iii. Used when not responding to intensive phototherapy

         iv. iv. More likely to be needed for the preterm infant and with severe hemolytic disease

   4. New treatments being researched:

      a. Tin-mesoporphyrin

         i. A metal that inhibits bilirubin formation.

         ii. One or two injections are administered to the infant, usually resulting in a rapid fall in bilirubin levels without the need for phototherapy. Research trials to establish safety and efficacy are in process (Hansen, 2010).

           iii. Not approved by the U.S. Food and Drug Administration at this time but may be available under compassionate use protocol for Jehovah's Witnesses whose child would otherwise require exchange transfusion.

      b. L-aspartic acid

           i. Being studied for its ability to prevent the occurrence of high bilirubin levels without disrupting breastfeeding.

           ii. Infants receiving six oral doses of this beta glucuronidase inhibitor had significantly lower peak bilirubin levels (Gourley et al., 2005).

G. Danger signs that indicate an immediate need for referral to the PCP:

    1. Excessive weight loss of 10% or more of birth weight

    2. History of inadequate urine output for the age of the infant

    3. Vomiting

    4. Refusal to feed

    5. Excessive sleeping or continued fretfulness

    6. Jaundiced color below the upper chest

    7. White or clay-colored stool indicative of biliary atresia

H. Education and counseling:

    1. Remember that families view hyperbilirubinemia and its treatment as a threat to their infant (Hannon et al., 2001; Willis et al., 2002).

    2. Expect parents to have ongoing feelings of concern that they caused the baby's illness. They will need continued support to continue exclusive breastfeeding.

    3. Explain the reason for the jaundiced color and the implications related to breastfeeding

    4. Teach how to determine whether the infant is feeding effectively.

    5. Provide written information regarding the clinical indicators of sufficient intake and infant danger signals.

    6. Assist the mother with techniques for the stimulation of milk supply if supplement is required.

      a. Frequent, effective feeding or

      b. Hand or mechanical milk expression as an adjunct if supplementation has been recommended

    7. Advocate for the avoidance of mother–infant separation if phototherapy is required.

    8. Work with the PCP to develop a feeding plan that is individualized to the mother–infant dyad's particular need.

    9. Provide a feeding diary to record feedings, supplement amounts, and the infant output.

    10. Ensure understanding of the importance of close follow-up.

I. Evaluation:

    1. Normal infant weight gain, with 20 to 28 grams weight gain per day after day 4 of life (Lawrence et al., 2011).

2. Bilirubin level will decrease with the onset of effective feeding and resultant stooling for the baby with breastfeeding-associated jaundice (see the section titled "VI. Breastfeeding-Associated Jaundice" that follows). There may be a rapid fall in the bilirubin level if effective feeding is established within 12 to 24 hours, which might eliminate the need for medical therapy.

3. Maternal milk supply will develop normally, or improve if it had been insufficient, as evidenced by infant weight/hydration/stool patterns and the ability to decrease or eliminate supplement.

4. The breastfeeding relationship will be maintained and strengthened based on the previous parameters.

5. Failure of the infant to improve within 12 to 24 hours indicates other underlying problems and a need for reappraisal of the infant by the PCP. Further exploration of reasons for insufficient milk supply may also be indicated.

VI. Breastfeeding-Associated Jaundice (Also Called Starvation Jaundice, Lack of Breastfeeding Jaundice, Nonbreastfeeding Jaundice)

A. One of the significant causes of hyperbilirubinemia
   1. Lack of intake leads to delayed stooling and recirculation of bilirubin.
   2. One of the most common complications the lactation consultant will encounter.
   3. Neither breastfeeding nor breastmilk causes the jaundice; rather, a lack of effective breastfeeding causes the problem.
   4. Infants who have hyperbilirubinemia caused by lack of appropriate intake may be significantly dehydrated as well, occasionally presenting to the practitioner in a life-threatening state.
   5. Quick appraisal and timely referral to the PCP is a critical component of the lactation consultant's responsibility.

B. Pathophysiology
   1. An infant who is not feeding effectively may experience jaundice in part related to the delay in passing meconium and in part because of dehydration.
   2. Meconium contains conjugated bilirubin.
   3. If the meconium is not passed in a timely manner, bilirubin is deconjugated, reabsorbed from the intestine back into the bloodstream, and transported to the liver via portal circulation where it must be conjugated again for excretion (enterohepatic circulation).

C. Health implications for the infant
   1. Ineffective feeding is associated with inadequate fluid intake and resultant dehydration. Unal et al. (2008) report that 47% of infants with hypernatremic dehydration also had elevated bilirubin.
   2. Severe hypernatremic dehydration results from lack of fluid intake and from the increased sodium content noted in breastmilk of women whose babies are feeding ineffectively (so-called weaning milk). *This is potentially life threatening.*
   3. Rarely kernicterus or BIND can occur if bilirubin levels remain greater than 25 to 30 milligrams per deciliter in the term infant.

D. Typical infant with breastfeeding-associated jaundice
  1. History
    a. Onset of jaundiced appearance at 48 to 72 hours of age
    b. Delayed or scant meconium output
    c. Scant urine output; may have uric acid crystals present in the urine (brick dust urine)
    d. Either infrequent, ineffective feeds or frequent, ineffective feedings
    e. Either lethargic with few requests for feedings or very fussy and not content after feedings
  2. Physical assessment
    a. Thin, jaundiced infant
    b. Lethargic, difficult to arouse or fussy, and difficult to console
    c. Excessive weight loss or lack of appropriate interval weight gain for age
  3. Feeding assessment
    a. Problems with latch-on
    b. Scant swallows noted during the feeding
    c. Maternal engorgement possible
E. Feeding management (see item E, section V, Assessing the Jaundiced Infant" earlier)
F. Prevention
  1. Implement *Clinical Guidelines for the Establishment of Exclusive Breastfeeding* (ILCA, 2005) that enumerate practices that prevent breastfeeding-associated jaundice, among other breastfeeding complications
  2. Timely initiation of breastfeeding
  3. Frequent breastfeeding (de Carvalho et al., 1982; Yamauchi et al., 1990a)
  4. Avoidance of water supplement/complement (de Carvalho et al., 1981)
  5. Effective breastfeeding
  6. Early follow-up with the PCP (within 48–72 hours of birth or sooner if high risk) for an assessment of the weight, hydration, breastfeeding effectiveness, and cardiovascular assessment (AAP Subcommittee on Neonatal Hyperbilirubinemia, 2004)
G. Education and counseling (see item H in the section titled "V. Assessing the Jaundiced Infant")
H. Evaluation (see item I in "V. Assessing the Jaundiced Infant")

VII. Breastmilk Jaundice

A. Overview
  1. Infants who have breastmilk jaundice are healthy breastfed infants who have no pathologic cause for indirect hyperbilirubinemia. They are breastfeeding effectively, have good weight gain, and have no other signs or symptoms of illness.
  2. Diagnosis is made by excluding other causes of delayed-onset, persistent hyperbilirubinemia either by history or laboratory testing before assuming that breastmilk jaundice is the cause of the persistent hyperbilirubinemia

(Preer et al., 2011). Preer et al. recommend diagnostic evaluation for infants who have TSB of ≥ 12 mg/dL (see **Figure 40-4**). The infant with breastmilk jaundice may have clinically perceptible jaundice for up to 3 months.

B. Introduction

1. Physiology

 a. Not well understood.

 b. Elevated levels of epidermal growth factor in both the breastmilk and serum of affected infants were seen in one case-control study (Kumral et al., 2009).

2. Tends to recur in subsequent infants in the family

3. No other health implications/risks for the infant

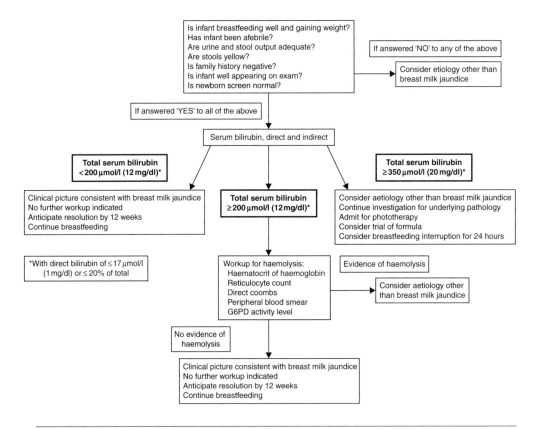

Figure 40-4 Algorithm for assessment and management of suspected breast milk jaundice.

Source: Preer GL, Philipp BL. Understanding and managing breast milk jaundice. *Arch Dis Child Fetal Neonatal Ed* (2010;doi10.1136/adc.2010.184416) Includes correction of published erratum

C. History
    1. Breastmilk jaundice may appear between 5 and 10 days of age after physiologic jaundice has peaked and declined.
    2. Positive family history of late-onset jaundice.
    3. Infant is vigorous, feeding well, and gaining weight appropriately.

D. Physical assessment
    1. Assess level of jaundice.
    2. Assess alertness.
    3. Assess the weight status.

E. Breastfeeding assessment
    1. Expect effective breastfeeding.

F. Management
    1. Ensure continued, effective breastfeeding.
    2. The healthcare provider will decide on the frequency of bilirubin monitoring and need for further diagnostic testing for other causes of persistent jaundice.
        a. Typically, bilirubin levels are monitored until the level plateaus.
        b. An infant who has additional risk factors, such as prematurity or race, might experience levels high enough to require phototherapy.
        c. Some healthcare providers advise interruption of breastfeeding for 12 to 24 hours, although this is not the preferred approach.
            i. Bilirubin levels drop precipitously with formula feeding.
            ii. This strategy serves as a diagnostic method; if the bilirubin level drops, then one does not have to look further for the cause of jaundice.
            iii. It is not thought to be necessary by most experts (Preer et al., 2011).
            iv. Interruption of breastfeeding might jeopardize the breastfeeding relationship between the mother and her infant.
            v. Risks and benefits of breastfeeding interruption need to be carefully assessed.
        d. If phototherapy is required, advocate for the avoidance of mother–infant separation.

G. Education and counseling
    1. Reassure the family that the infant is not seriously ill.
    2. Work with the PCP to develop a breastfeeding plan.
    3. If breastfeeding is interrupted, teach the mother how to maintain her milk supply and safely store expressed milk for later use.

H. Evaluation
    1. Maintenance of the breastfeeding relationship
    2. Continued normal weight gain
    3. A gradual decrease in jaundiced appearance in the infant over 3 to 12 weeks of age

Part 2: Hypoglycemia

Sustained hypoglycemia can lead to abnormal neurologic or developmental outcomes. However, it still is uncertain just how low the blood glucose must be or how long an episode is necessary to incur neurologic sequelae. It is likely that the absolute glucose level that leads to damage is different for different risk situations, further complicating the question of screening and management. Additionally, there is still no specific glucose value which defines hypoglycemia (Hawdon, 2010; Hay et al., 2009). Cornblath et al. (2000) offer operational thresholds below which intervention should be considered; many healthcare providers use these values. These have not been updated in the interim 11 years.

Adamkin and the Committee for the Fetus and Newborn (2011) published a clinical report (as opposed to a policy or practice guideline) with a recommended guide for screening and treatment of infants who are high risk for hypoglycemia (**Figure 40-5**). The authors present a practical approach based on Cornblath's operational threshold levels of glucose. Operational thresholds as recommended by Cornblath et al. might not be applicable to breastfed infants because of differences in metabolism. Despite their lower caloric intake, they have higher concentrations of ketone bodies than formula-fed babies (Cornblath et al., 2000). Ketone bodies serve as an effective alternate fuel source for newborns.

Rozance et al. (2010) summarize the state of the science:

> Plasma glucose concentration is the only practical measure of glucose sufficiency, but by itself is a very limited guide. Key to preventing complications from glucose deficiency is to identify infants at risk, promote early and frequent feedings, normalize glucose homeostasis, measure glucose concentrations early and frequently in infants at risk, and treat promptly when glucose deficiency is marked and symptomatic. (p. 275)

Effective breastfeeding provides the normal newborn infant with sufficient calories to prevent hypoglycemia (Diwakar et al., 2002). Healthy, large-for-gestational-age infants do not appear to be harmed by transient mild hypoglycemia (Brand et al., 2005). Certain infants have a higher risk for experiencing hypoglycemia. If risk factors are present, effective breastfeeding with intake of normal amounts of colostrum might not be sufficient to support unusual metabolic demands. In these cases, a supplement might be required. The baby's PCP can determine whether calories are best supplied as an oral supplement or by using intravenous glucose infusion.

Hypoglycemia is most likely to occur after the first 2 to 3 hours of birth, before fat metabolism has begun, and particularly if any other risk factors are present (Hoseth et al., 2000). Infants who are born prior to 38 completed weeks have limited glycogen reserves. Infants who are intrauterine growth retarded or who are small for gestational age have limited fat reserves. Infants of diabetic mothers quickly deplete their glycogen stores after birth as a result of hyperinsulinism, which is caused by producing large amounts of insulin in response to maternal hyperglycemia while in utero (de Rooy et al., 2010). Newborns who have persistent hypoglycemia in the first days of life require further evaluation to determine the cause.

Incidence of hypoglycemia in healthy term infants is difficult to determine because a standard definition of hypoglycemia has not been used across studies. Reported rates using 1.8 mmol/L (32 mg/dL) range from 0.4% to 34%. Rates using 2.2 mmol/L (40 mg/dL) range from 4% to 40% (Hoseth et al., 2000). Reports of readmission of 280 newborns to a regional hospital in Kenya noted that 23% were hypoglycemic. Eighty-one percent of the hypoglycemic infants were younger than 7 days of age (English et al., 2003). Hypoglycemia was correlated with weight of < 2,500 grams and inability to breastfeed effectively. Infants with hypoglycemia (blood glucose less than 2.2 mmol [40 mg/dL]) had much higher mortality as well. A Nepalese study looked at incidence of hypoglycemia in nearly 600 infants born at the largest maternity hospital. In this hospital, maintaining a neutral thermic environment was problematic. Forty-one percent of newborn infants had mild hypoglycemia (< 2.6 mmol/L) and 11% had moderate hypoglycemia (< 2 mmol/L). Risk factors included delayed initiation of breastfeeding and cold ambient temperatures. Feeding delay increased the risk of hypoglycemia at age 12 to 24 hours of age (Pal et al., 2000).

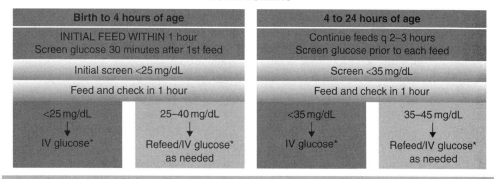

Figure 40-5 Screening and management of postnatal glucose homeostasis in late preterm and term SGA, IDM/LGA infants.

Source: Reproduced with permission from *Pediatrics*, *127*, 575, Copyright 2011 by the AAP.

I. Glucose Regulation in the Fetus and Newborn

A. The fetus receives energy continuously via the placenta.

B. Glycogen reserves that are available for conversion to glucose during the immediate neonatal period are laid down during the later part of the third trimester.

C. Newborns have a greater demand for glucose than children and adults because of their large brain-to-body weight.

D. Preterm infants have an even greater demand for glucose and have limited to absent glycogen reserves.

E. Glucose is the primary nutrient for brain metabolism, and the placentally derived supply terminates at birth.

F. Neonatal physiology:

1. At birth, there is a transition period as glucose homeostasis is established by the infant.

2. Change in glucoregulatory hormones are as follows:
   a. Increased epinephrine.
   b. Increased norepinephrine.
   c. Increased glucagon.
   d. The net effect is mobilization of glycogen and fatty acids.

G. The collective activities that maintain glucose homeostasis are called *counterregulation* and consist of the following:

1. *Glycogenolysis:* Mobilization and release of glycogen from body stores to form glucose

2. *Gluconeogenesis:* Production of glucose by the liver and kidneys from noncarbohydrate substrates such as fatty acids and amino acids

H. The rate of glucose production is 4 to 6 mg/kg/minute (Eidelman, 2001).

1. To meet the requirements of the brain 3.7 mg/kg per minute are needed.

2. About 70% is provided by glucose oxidation with the rest being provided from alternative fuels.

3. Alternative brain fuels are also produced, such as ketone bodies.

I. Dietary intake and gluconeogenesis:

1. After 12 hours, the baby is dependent on glucose made from dietary intake of milk components (20–50%) and gluconeogenesis to maintain blood glucose (galactose, amino acids, glucerol, lactate) as well as free fatty acids from fat stores and milk.

2. Breastmilk is more ketogenic than formula, enabling the breastfed baby to create high levels of alternative fuels until the milk supply increases sufficiently to draw on milk components for glucose synthesis (de Rooy et al., 2002).

3. High levels of ketone bodies enable breastfed babies to demonstrate lower measured blood glucose levels but still maintain the optimal production of brain fuels (de Rooy et al., 2002).

4. Glycogen stores are converted to glucose (glycogenolysis), rapidly depleting glycogen stores over the first hours of life; liver glycogen stores are 90% depleted by 3 hours and gone by 12 hours.

5. Fat metabolism provides glucose substrate beginning at 2 to 3 days of age.

II. Definition of Hypoglycemia

A. No consensus on the definition of hypoglycemia in a full-term infant; hypoglycemia is a continuum of falling blood glucose levels, not an arbitrary number (Cornblath et al., 2000).

B. Serum glucose below 36 to 45 mg/dL (2.0–2.5 mmol/L) in the newborn is considered the threshold for intervention (operational threshold) (Cornblath et al., 2000).

III. Testing for Hypoglycemia

A. Recommendations for glucose screening (AAP Section on Breastfeeding, 2005; Adamkin & Committee on the Fetus and Newborn, 2011 (See Figure 40-5); Wight, Marinelli, & ABM, 2006):

1. Universal screening is not recommended (Adamkin & Committee on the Fetus and Newborn, 2011; Hoops et al., 2010).

2. Screen infants who are at risk.

   a. Any infant who is symptomatic (Perrson, 2009): Weak cry, apnea, cyanosis, temperature instability, hypothermia, feeding problems, irritability, tremors or seizures, lethargy, hypotonia.

   b. Infants with high-risk criteria: Large or small for gestational age, intrauterine growth retardation, infant of a diabetic mother, late-preterm, asphyxiation, sepsis, cold stress, Rh disease, congestive heart failure.

   c. Jitteriness is a very common, nonspecific finding. Linder et al. (1989) suggest that if jitteriness ceases with suckling, there is no need to be concerned about hypoglycemia or hypocalcemia (another cause of newborn tremor).

B. Which screening method?

1. Bedside screening devices (point-of-care [POC]) are in general not designed to be accurate in the lower ranges, but rather in the normal and higher ranges (Beardsall, 2010).

   a. For newborns, the greatest need is for accuracy in the hypoglycemia ranges.

   b. A comparison of three different POC devices found that none was satisfactory as the *only* measuring device (Roth-Kleiner et al., 2010).

2. Reagent strips are of limited accuracy in newborns. Visual interpretation of test strip results in highly inaccurate results and is not recommended.

3. Accuracy depends on following the directions precisely.

4. Significant variability of the results has been noted.

5. Results from most POC devices are affected by the infant's hemoglobin status. Low hemoglobin (anemia) results in falsely elevated glucose measurement, while high hemoglobin (polycythemia) depresses glucometer readings (Ho et al., 2006).

C. Confirm abnormal screening results with a serum glucose level sent to a laboratory.
D. If an infant has galactosemia, some screening tests will give falsely high glucose results.
E. If screening glucoses are abnormally high, confirm these with serum glucose level because the infant may in fact be profoundly hypoglycemic (Newman et al., 2002).
F. Do not delay treatment while waiting for the serum glucose results (AAP Subcommittee on Neonatal Hyperbilirubinemia, 2004).

IV. Health Implications for a Breastfed Infant

A. Neonatal hypoglycemia is linked to later developmental difficulties.
B. Delay in first feeding and ineffective breastfeeding can contribute to the development of hypoglycemia, even in low-risk infants (Moore et al., 1999).

V. Risk Factors for Hypoglycemia in a Full-Term Newborn

A. Maternal risk factors
 1. Gestational diabetes; women are not always aware of their glycemic status (Simmons et al., 2000)
 2. Diabetes, type 1 or 2 (insulin- or noninsulin-dependent) (Hartmann et al., 2001)
 3. Anatomic or physiologic disorders affecting lactogenesis including maternal obesity (Nommsen-Rivers et al., 2010)
 4. Hypertension (pregnancy-induced or essential)
B. Labor and delivery management factors
 1. Maternal intravenous fluids using dextrose and water solutions
 2. Cool room temperature
 3. Infant separation from mother
 4. Delayed feeding
 5. Crying that is not quickly attended to
C. Infant risk factors
 1. Large for gestational age (LGA) (> 4,000 g)
 2. Small for gestational age (SGA) (< 2,500 g)
  a. LGA and SGA infants may develop hypoglycemia as late as 10 days of age (Hume et al., 1999).
 3. Intrauterine growth retardation
 4. Preterm (≤ 37 completed weeks of gestation)

VI. Prevention of Hypoglycemia in Newborns

A. Implementation of the *Clinical Guidelines for the Establishment of Exclusive Breastfeeding* (ILCA, 2005) provides conditions that prevent hypoglycemia as well as other newborn complications.
B. Labor and delivery management:

1. If intravenous fluids are used for the laboring woman, choose balanced electrolyte solutions rather than dextrose and water to reduce the risk of hyperinsulinism in the infant.
2. Provide a neutral thermal environment.
3. Avoid cold stress in the infant.
   a. Towel dry.
   b. Place baby in skin-to-skin contact with the mother and cover the dyad (Moore et al., 1999; Moore et al., 2007).
   c. Babies separated from their mother have lower body temperatures, cry more, and have lower blood glucose levels (Christensson et al., 1992; Williams, 1997).
4. Prevent infant crying because crying rapidly depletes glycogen stores.
   C. Feeding routine:
   1. Early first feeding:
      a. Hypoglycemia is *not* associated with lack of feeding in the first 6 hours of life in healthy infants who are appropriate for gestational age (Diwakar et al., 2002).
      b. However, this finding does not negate the importance of early first feeding for the establishment of exclusive breastfeeding.
      c. Feeding within the first hour of birth is associated with higher glucose levels than first feed occurring later (Chertok et al., 2009).
   2. Frequent feeding (Hawdon et al., 1992). After the first few hours, the major determinant of blood glucose concentration is the interval between feeds.
   3. Ensure effective feedings.
   4. Avoid dextrose water complement or supplemental feedings because this leads to rebound hypoglycemia (AAP Subcommittee on Neonatal Hyperbilirubinemia, 2004).

VII. Postdischarge Follow-up

A. Perform an early follow-up at 48 hours of age to ensure infant well-being and establishment of effective breastfeeding.
B. Teach families the early symptoms of hypoglycemia.

VIII. Implementation and Planning

A. Monitor the infant closely to assess for signs of hypoglycemia.
B. Notify the PCP if the infant is symptomatic.
C. Ensure effective breastfeeding.
D. If breastfeeding has been effective and infant's glucose level is still low, provide an appropriate supplement per order of the healthcare provider.
E. If breastfeeding is ineffective and the infant's glucose levels are low, initiate supplementation according to the PCP recommendation (expressed mother's milk or human milk substitute is preferred to glucose water for the prevention of rebound hypoglycemia).

F. If supplementation is required, supplement at the breast if the infant can breastfeed effectively.

G. If the infant is unable to sustain suckling at the breast, feed away from the breast using a method that is best suited to the infant's capabilities and the parents' and provider's preference.

1. The mother can hand express colostrum into a spoon and spoon feed it frequently to her baby.

2. The protein and fat in colostrum provide substrates for gluconeogenesis, enhance ketogenesis, and increase gut motility and gastric emptying time, which causes a rapid absorption of nutrients.

3. The healthcare provider might use intravenous glucose if the initial feedings are not sufficient to increase the infant's serum glucose level.

H. All infants require close monitoring after discharge by either home or office visits with a healthcare provider at 48 to 72 hours of age to assess well-being.

1. Case reports describe breastfed infants who had no other risk factors yet became symptomatic of hypoglycemia on the third day of life, presenting with seizures at home (Moore et al., 1999). Each of these infants was experiencing feeding difficulties.

2. Hume et al. (1999) reported on preterm infants (gestation of ≤ 37 weeks) who were at risk for hypoglycemia at the time of discharge. Their findings stressed the importance of timely feedings to avoid hypoglycemia at home.

IX. Education and Counseling

A. Explain to the family the short-term feeding implications for an infant who has low blood sugar.

1. Need for short-term supplementation; importance of frequent feedings

2. Need for blood tests to monitor glucose levels until normoglycemia is established

B. If supplementation is needed, assist the mother with initiating milk expression.

C. Assist family in administering oral supplementation if ordered.

D. Ensure that the family understands the importance of a timely return visit to the healthcare provider.

E. Teach the family the indicators of effective breastfeeding.

F. Teach the family the symptoms of hypoglycemia.

X. Evaluation

A. The infant will be able to maintain blood glucose without the need for supplementation.

B. A breastfeeding plan will be established prior to discharge from the birthing site.

References

Academy of Breastfeeding Medicine Protocol Committee. (2010). Clinical protocol no. 22: Guidelines for management of jaundice in the breastfeeding infant equal to or greater than 35 weeks' gestation. *Breastfeeding Medicine, 5*(2), 87–93.

Adamkin, D. H., & Committee on the Fetus and Newborn. (2011). Clinical report—postnatal glucose homeostasis in late-preterm and term infants. *Pediatrics, 127*(3), 576.

Akakba, K., Kimura, T., Sasaki, A., et al. (1998). Neonatal hyperbilirubinemia and mutation of the bilirubin uridine diphosphate-glucorosyltransferase gene: A common missense mutation among Japanese, Koreans, and Chinese. *Biochemistry and Molecular Biology International, 46*, 21–26.

American Academy of Pediatrics Section on Breastfeeding. (2005). Breastfeeding and the use of human milk. *Pediatrics, 115*, 496–506. Retrieved from http://aappolicy.aappublications.org/cgi/content/full/pediatrics;115/2/496

American Academy of Pediatrics Subcommittee on Neonatal Hyperbilirubinemia. (2004). Management of hyperbilirubinemia in the newborn infant 35 or more completed weeks of gestation. *Pediatrics, 114*, 297–316.

Anderson, A. M. (2001). Disruption of lactogenesis by retained placental fragments. *Journal of Human Lactation, 17*, 142–144.

Beal, A. C., Chou, S.-C., Palmer, R. H., Testa, M. A., Newman, C., & Ezhuthachan, S. (2006). The changing face of race: Risk factors for neonatal hyperbilirubinemia. *Pediatrics, 117*(5), 1618–1625.

Beardsall, K. (2010). Measurement of glucose levels in the newborn. *Early Human Development, 86*, 263–267.

Bhutani, V. K., Johnson, L. H., & Keren, R. (2005). Treating acute bilirubin encephalopathy before it is too late. *Contemporary Pediatrics, 22*, 57–74.

Brand, P. L. P., Molenaar, N. L. D., Kaaijk, C., & Wierenga, W. S. (2005). Neurodevelopmental outcome of hypoglycaemia in healthy, large for gestational age, term newborns. *Archives of Disease in Childhood, 90*, 78–81.

Chertok, I. R. A., Raz, I., Shoham, I., Haddad, H., & Wiznitzer, A. (2009). Effects of early breastfeeding on neonatal glucose levels of term infants born to women with gestational diabetes. *Journal of Human Nutrition and Dietetics, 22*(2), 166–169.

Christensson, K., Siles, C., Moreno, L., et al. (1992). Temperature, metabolic adaptation and crying in healthy full-term newborns cared for skin-to-skin or in a cot. *Acta Paediatrica, 81*, 488–493.

Cornblath, M., Hawdon, J. M., Williams, A. F., et al. (2000). Controversies regarding definition of neonatal hypoglycemia: Suggested operational thresholds. *Pediatrics, 105*, 1141–1145.

de Carvalho, M., Hall, M., & Havey, D. (1981). Effects of water supplementation on physiological jaundice in breastfed babies. *Archives of Disease in Childhood, 56*, 568–569.

de Carvalho, M., Klaus, M. H., & Merkatz, R. B. (1982). Frequency of breastfeeding and serum bilirubin concentration. *American Journal of Diseases of Children, 136*, 737–738.

De Luca, D., Romagnoli, C., Tiberi, E., Zuppa, A. A., & Zecca, E. (2008). Skin bilirubin nomogram for the first 96 h of life in a European normal healthy newborn population, obtained with multiwavelength transcutaneous bilirubinometry. *Acta Paediatrica, 97*(2), 146–150.

de Rooy, L., & Hawdon, J. (2002). Nutritional factors that affect the postnatal metabolic adaptation of full-term small- and large-for-gestational-age infants. *Pediatrics, 109*, E42.

de Rooy, L., & Johns, A. (2010). Management of the vulnerable baby on the postnatal ward and transitional care unit. *Early Human Development, 86*, 281–285.

Diwakar, K. K., & Sasidhar, M. V. (2002). Plasma glucose levels in term infants who are appropriate size for gestation and exclusively breast fed. *Archives of Disease in Childhood: Fetal and Neonatal Edition*, *87*, F46–F48.

Eidelman, A. I. (2001). Hypoglycemia and the breastfed neonate. *Pediatric Clinics of North America*, *48*, 377–387.

El-Beshbishi, S. N., Shattuck, K. E., Mohammad, A. A., & Petersen, J. R. (2009). Hyperbilirubinemia and transcutaneous bilirubinometry. *Clinical Chemistry*, *55*(7), 1280–1287.

English, M., Ngama, M., Musumba, C., et al. (2003). Causes and outcome of young infant admissions to a Kenyan district hospital. *Archives of Disease in Childhood*, *88*, 438–443.

Gartner, L. (2010). Jaundice and the breastfed baby. In J. Riordan & K. Wambach (Eds.), *Breastfeeding and human lactation* (4th ed., pp. 365–378). Sudbury, MA: Jones and Bartlett.

Gorelick, M. H., Shaw, K. N., & Murphy, K. O. (1997). Validity and reliability of clinical signs in the diagnosis of dehydration in children. *Pediatrics*, *99*(5), E6.

Gourley, G. R., Zhanhai, K., Kreamer, B. L., & Kosorok, M. R. (2005). A controlled, randomized, double blind trial of prophylaxis against jaundice among breastfed newborns. *Pediatrics*, *116*, 385–391.

Hannon, P. R., Willis, S. K., & Scrimshaw, S. C. (2001). Persistence of maternal concerns surrounding neonatal jaundice: An exploratory study. *Archives of Pediatric and Adolescent Medicine*, *155*, 1357–1363.

Hansen, T. W. R. (2010). Core concepts: Bilirubin metabolism. *NeoReviews*, *11*(6), e316–e322.

Harris, M. C., Bernbaum, J. C., Polin, J. R., et al. (2001). Developmental follow-up of breastfed term and near-term infants with marked hyperbilirubinemia. *Pediatrics*, *107*, 1075–1080.

Hartmann, P., & Cregan, M. (2001). Lactogenesis and the effects of insulin-dependent diabetes mellitus and prematurity. *Journal of Nutrition*, *131*(11), 3016S–3020S.

Hawdon, J. M. (2008). Investigation and management of impaired metabolic adaptation presenting as neonatal hypoglycaemia. *Paediatrics and Child Health*, *18*, 161–165.

Hawdon, M. J., Ward Platt, M. P, & Annsley-Green, A. (1992). Patterns of metabolic adaptation for term and preterm infants in the first neonatal week. *Archives of Disease in Childhood*, *67*, 357–365.

Hawdon, M. J. (2010). Best practice guidelines: Neonatal hypoglycaemia. *Early Human Development*, *86*, 261.

Hay, W., Jr., Raju, T. K., Higgins, R. D., Klahan, S. C., & Devaskar, S. U. (2009). Knowledge gaps and research needs for understanding and treating neonatal hypoglycemia: Workshop report from Eunice Kennedy Shriver National Institute of Child Health and Human Development. *Journal of Pediatrics*, *155*(5), 612–617.

Ho, H. T., Yeung, W. K. Y., & Young, B. W. Y. (2004). Evaluation of "point of care" devices in the measurement of low blood glucose in neonatal practice. *Archives of Disease in Childhood: Fetal and Neonatal Edition*, *89*, F356–359.

Hoops, D., Roberts, P., Van Winkle, E., Trauschke, K., Mauton, N., DeGhelder, S., Scalise, A., Jackson, S., Cato, D., Roth, C., Jones, A., Kautz, M., & Whaley, L. (2010). Should routine peripheral blood glucose testing be done for all newborns at birth? *MCN American Journal of Maternal and Child Nursing*, *35*(5), 264–270.

Hoseth, E., Joergensen, A., Ebbesen, J., & Moeller, M. (2000). Blood glucose levels in a population of healthy, breast fed, term infants of appropriate size for gestational age. *Archives of Disease in Childhood: Fetal and Neonatal Edition*, *83*, F117–F119.

Herschel, M., & Gartner, L. (2005). Jaundice and the breastfed baby. In J. Riordan (Ed.), *Breastfeeding and human lactation* (pp. 311–321). Sudbury, MA: Jones and Bartlett.

Huang, A., Tai, B. C., Wong, L. Y., Lee, J., & Yong, E. L. (2009). Differential risk for early breastfeeding jaundice in a multi-ethnic Asian cohort. *Annals Academy of Medicine Singapore, 38*, 217–224.

Huggins, K. E., Petok, E. S., & Mreles, O. (2000). Markers of lactation insufficiency: A study of 34 mothers. *Current Issues in Clinical Lactation*, 25–35.

Hume, R., McGeechan, A., & Burchell, A. (1999). Failure to detect preterm infants at risk of hypoglycemia before discharge. *Journal of Pediatrics, 134*, 499–502.

International Lactation Consultant Association. (2005). *Clinical guidelines for the establishment of exclusive breastfeeding.* Raleigh, NC: Author.

Jain, A., Aggarwal, R., Jeevasanker, M., Agarwal, R., Deorari, A. K., & Paul, V. K. (2008). Hypoglycemia in the newborn. *Indian Journal of Pediatrics, 75*, 63–67.

Jangaard, K. A., Fell, D. B., Dodds, L.. & Alledn, A. C. (2008). Outcomes in a population of healthy term and near-term infants with serum bilirubin levels of ≥325 μmol/L (≥19 mg/dL) who were born in Nova Scotia, Canada, between 1994 and 2000. *Pediatrics, 122*(1), 119–124.

Johnson, J. D., Angelus, P., Aldrich, M., & Skipper, B. J. (1986). Exaggerated jaundice in Navajo neonates. *American Journal of Diseases of Children, 140*, 889–890.

Johnson, L., Bhutani, V. K., Karp, K., Sivieri, E. M., & Shapiro, S. M. (2009). Clinical report from the pilot USA Kernicterus Registry (1992 to 2004). *Journal of Perinatology, 29*, S25–S45. doi:10.1038/jp.2008.211

Kaplan, M., & Hammerman, C. (2004). Understanding and preventing severe hyperbilirubinemia: Is bilirubin neurotoxicity really a problem in the developed world? *Clinical Perinatology, 31*, 555–575.

Kaplan, M., & Hammerman, C. (2005). American Academy of Pediatrics guidelines for detecting neonatal hyperbilirubinemia and preventing kernicterus: Are there worldwide implications? *Archives of Disease in Childhood: Fetal and Neonatal Edition, 90*, F448–F449.

Kaplan, M., & Hammerman, C. (2010). Glucose-6-phosphate deyhdrogenase deficiency and severe neonatal hyperbilirubinemia: A complexity of interactions between genes and environment. *Seminars in Fetal and Neonatal Medicine, 15*, 148–156.

Kaplan, M., Kaplan, E., Hammerman, C., Algur, N., Bromiker, R., Schimmel, M. S., & Eidelman, A. I. (2006). Post-phototherapy neonatal bilirubin rebound: A potential cause of significant hyperbilirubinaemia. *Archives of Disease in Childhood, 91*(1), 31–34.

Kappas, A. (2004). A method for interdicting the development of severe jaundice in newborns by inhibiting the production of bilirubin. *Pediatrics, 113*, 119–123.

Keren, R., Luan, X., Friedman, S., Saddlemire, S., Cnaan, A., & Bhutani, V. K. (2008). A comparison of alternative risk-assessment strategies for predicting significant neonatal hyperbilirubinemia in term and near-term infants. *Pediatrics, 121*(1), e170–179.

Kumral, A., Ozkan, H., Duman, N., Yesilirmak, D. C., Islekel, H., & Ozalp, Y. (2009). Breast milk jaundice correlates with high levels of epidermal growth factor. *Pediatric Research, 66*(2), 218–221.

Kuzniewicz, M. W., Escobar, G. J., & Newman, T. B. (2009). Impact of universal bilirubin screening on severe hyperbilirubinemia and phototherapy use. *Pediatrics, 124*(4), 1031–1039.

Laptook, A. R., & Watkinson, M. (2008). Temperature management in the delivery room. *Seminars in Fetal and Neonatal Medicine, 13*, 383–391.

Lawrence, R. A., & Lawrence, R. M. (2011). *Breastfeeding: A guide for the medical profession* (7th ed.). St. Louis, MO: Mosby.

Linder, N., Moser, A. M., Asli, I., et al. (1989). Suckling stimulation test for neonatal tremor. *Archives of Disease in Childhood, 64*, 44–46.

Maisels, M. J., Bhutani, V. K., Bogen, D., Newman, T. B., Stark, A. R., & Watchko, J. F. (2009). Hyperbilirubinemia in the newborn infant > or =35 weeks' gestation: An update with clarifications. *Pediatrics*, *124*(4), 1193–1198.

Maisels, M. J., DeRidder, J. M., Kring, E. A., & Balasubramaniam, M. (2009). Routine transcutaneous bilirubin measurements combined with clinical risk factors improve the prediction of subsequent hyperbilirubinemia. *Journal of Perinatology*, *29*, 612–617.

Maisels, M. J., & Kring, E. (2006). Transcutaneous bilirubin levels in the first 96 hours in a normal newborn population of ≥ 35 weeks gestation. *Pediatrics*, *117*, 1169–1173.

Manning, D. (2005). American Academy of Pediatrics guidelines for detecting neonatal hyperbilirubinemia and preventing kernicterus: Are they applicable in Britain? *Archives of Disease in Childhood: Fetal and Neonatal Edition*, *90*, F450–F451.

Marques, I. L., de Sousa, T. V., Carneiro, A. F., et al. (2001). Clinical experience with infants with Robin sequence: A prospective study. *Cleft Palate-Craniofacial Journal*, *38*, 171–178.

Moore, A. M., & Perlman, M. (1999). Symptomatic hypoglycemia in otherwise healthy, breastfed term newborns. *Pediatrics*, *103*, 837–839.

Moore, E. R., Anderson, G. C., & Bergman, N. (2007). Early skin-to-skin contact for mothers and their healthy newborn infants. *Cochrane Database of Systematic Reviews*, CD003519.

Neifert, M., De Marzo, S., Seacat, J., et al. (1990). The influence of breast surgery, breast appearance, and pregnancy-induced breast changes on lactation sufficiency as measured by infant weight gain. *Birth*, *17*, 31–38.

Neubauer, S. H., Ferris, A. M., Chase, C. G., et al. (1993). Delayed lactogenesis in women with insulin-dependent diabetes mellitus. *American Journal of Clinical Nutrition*, *58*, 54–60.

Newman, J. D., Ramsden, C. A., & Balazs, N. D. H. (2002). Monitoring neonatal hypoglycemia with the Accu-chek Advantage II glucose meter: The cautionary tale of galactosemia. *Clinical Chemistry*, *48*, 2071.

Newman, T. B., Easterling, J., Goldman, E. S., et al. (1999). Frequency of neonatal bilirubin testing and hyperbilirubinemia in a large health maintenance organization. *American Journal of Diseases of Children*, *144*(3), 364–368.

Newman, T. B., Liljestrand, P., Jeremy, R. J., Ferriero, D. M., Wu, Y. W., Hudes, E. S., & Escobar, G. J., for the Jaundice and Infant Feeding Study Team. (2006). Outcomes among newborns with total serum bilirubin levels of 25 mg per deciliter or more *New England Journal of Medicine*, *354*, 1889–1900.

Nommsen-Rivers, L. A., Chantry, C. J., Peerson, J. M., Cohen, R. J., & Dewey, K. G. (2010). Delayed onset of lactogenesis among first-time mothers is related to maternal obesity and factors associated with ineffective breastfeeding. *American Journal of Clinical Nutrition*, *92*(3), 574–584.

Pal, D. K., Manandhar, D. S., Rajbhandari, S., et al. (2000). Neonatal hypoglycaemia in Nepal 1. Prevalence and risk factors. *Archives of Disease in Childhood: Fetal and Neonatal Edition*, *82*, F46–F51.

Persson, B. (2009). Neonatal glucose metabolism in offspring of mothers with varying degrees of hyperglycemia during pregnancy. *Seminars in Fetal and Neonatal Medicine*, *14*, 106–110.

Petersen, J. R., Okorodudu, A. O., Mohammad, A. A., et al. (2005). Association of transcutaneous bilirubin testing in hospital with decreased readmission rate for hyperbilirubinemia. *Clinical Chemistry*, *51*, 540–544.

Preer, G. L., & Philipp, B. L. (2011). Understanding and managing breast milk jaundice. *Archives of Disease in Childhood: Fetal and Neonatal Edition*, *96*(6), F461–466. doi:10.1136/adc.2010.184416 (Advance online publication)

Roth-Kleiner, M., Diaw, C. S., Urfer, J., & Ruffieux, C. (2010). Evaluation of different POCT devices for glucose measurement in a clinical neonatal setting. *Early Human Development, 169*, 1387–1395.

Rozance, P. J., & Whay, W. W. (2010). Describing hypoglycemia—definition or operational threshold? *Early Human Development, 86*, 275–280.

Salas, A. A., Salazar, J., Burgoa, C. V., De-Villegas, C. A., Quevedo, V., & Soliz, A. (2009). Significant weight loss in breastfed term infants readmitted for hyperbilirubinemia. *BMC Pediatrics, 9*(82), 1–6.

Sarici, S. U., Sedar, M. A., Korkmaz, A., et al. (2004). Incidence, course, and prediction of hyperbilirubinemia in near-term and term newborns. *Pediatrics, 113*, 775–780.

Simmons, D., Thompson, C. F., & Conroy, C. (2000). Incidence and risk factors for neonatal hypoglycaemia among women with gestational diabetes mellitus in South Auckland. *Diabetic Medicine, 17*, 830–834.

Suresh, G. K., & Clark, R. E. (2004). Cost-effectiveness of strategies that are intended to prevent kernicterus in newborn infants. *Pediatrics, 114*, 917–924.

Szabo, P., Wolf, M., Bucher, H. U., et al. (2004). Detection of hyperbilirubinemia in jaundiced full-term neonates by eye or by bilirubinometer? *European Journal of Pediatrics, 163*, 722–727.

Thorp, J. A., & Breedlove, G. (1996). Epidural analgesia in labor: An evaluation of risks and benefits. *Birth, 23*, 63–83.

Udoma, E. J., Udo, J. J., Etuk, S. J., & Duke, E. S. (2001). Morbidity and mortality among infants with normal birth weight in a new born baby unit. *Nigerian Journal of Paediatrics, 28*, 13.

Unal, S., Arhan, E., Kara, N., Uncu, N., & Aliefendioglu, D. (2008). Breast-feeding-associated hypernatremia: Retrospective analysis of 169 newborns. *Pediatrics International, 50*, 29–34.

Watchko, J. F. (2010). Hyperbilirubinemia in African American neonates: Clinical issues and current challenges. *Seminars in Fetal and Neonatal Medicine, 15*, 176–182.

Wight, N., Marinelli, K. A., & Academy of Breastfeeding Medicine Protocol Committee. (2006). Clinical protocol no. 1: Guidelines for glucose monitoring and treatment of hypoglycemia in breastfed neonates. *Breastfeeding Medicine, 1*(3), 178–184. Retrieved from http://www.bfmed.org/Media/Files/Protocols/hypoglycemia.pdf

Williams, A. (1997). *Hypoglycaemia of the newborn*. Geneva, Switzerland: World Health Organization.

Willis, S. K., Hannon, P. R., & Scrimshaw, S. C. (2002). The impact of the maternal experience with a jaundiced newborn on the breastfeeding relationship [Abstract]. *Journal of Family Practice, 51*, 465.

Yamauchi, Y., & Yamanouchi, I. (1990a). Breastfeeding frequency during the first 24 hours after birth in full-term neonates. *Pediatrics, 86*, 171–175.

Yamauchi, Y., & Yamanouchi, I. (1990b). The relationship between rooming-in/not rooming-in and breast-feeding. *Acta Paediatrica Scandinavica, 79*, 1017–1022.

Suggested Reading

Canadian Paediatric Society. (2007). Guidelines for detection, management and prevention of hyperbilirubinemia in term and later preterm newborn infants (35 or more weeks' gestation). *Paediatrics and Child Health, 12*(5), 1B–12B.

Duvanel, C., Fawer, C. L., Cotting, J., et al. (1999). Long-term effects of neonatal hypoglycemia on brain growth and psychomotor development in small-for-gestational-age preterm infants. *Journal of Pediatrics, 134*, 492–498.

McDonagh, A. F. (2010). Controversies in bilirubin biochemistry and their clinical relevance. *Seminars in Fetal and Neonatal Medicine, 15,* 141–147.

NAAN Board of Directors. (2010). Prevention of acute bilirubin encephalopathy and kernicterus in newborns; position statement no. 3049. *Advances in Neonatal Care, 10*(3), 112–118.

Nylander, G., Lindemann, R., Helsing, E., & Bendvold, R. (1991). Unsupplemented breastfeeding in the maternity ward. *Acta Obstetricia et Gynecologica Scandinavica, 70,* 205–209.

Smith, J. R, Donze, A., & Schuller, L. (2007). An evidence-based review of hyperbilirubinemia in the late preterm infant with implications for practice: Management, follow-up and breastfeeding support. *Neonatal Network, 26*(6), 395–405.

Stevenson, D. K., Dennery, P. A., & Hintz, S. R. (2001). Understanding newborn jaundice. *Journal of Perinatology, 21*(Suppl. 1), S21–S24.

Watchko, J. F., & Lin, Z. (2010). Exploring the genetic architecture of neonatal hyperbilirubinemia. *Seminars in Fetal and Neonatal Medicine, 15,* 169–175.

Wight, N., Marinelli, K. A., & Academy of Breastfeeding Medicine Protocol Committee. (2006). ABM clinical protocol no. 1: Guidelines for glucose monitoring and treatment of hypoglycemia in breastfed neonates. *Breastfeeding Medicine, 1*(3), 178–184.

CHAPTER 41
Maternal Acute and Chronic Illness

Marsha Walker, RN, IBCLC
Revised by Susan W. Hatcher, RN, BSN, IBCLC

OBJECTIVES

- Describe the influence of acute and chronic maternal illness on breastfeeding and lactation.
- Identify breastfeeding management strategies to preserve breastfeeding under adverse situations.
- Discuss contraindications to breastfeeding.

INTRODUCTION

Not only has there been an increase in the number of women choosing to breastfeed, but more women now than ever have been able to conceive and carry a pregnancy to term or near term under a variety of acute and chronic health conditions. Almost all of these mothers can breastfeed partially or totally, even if they are taking medications or are experiencing viral or bacterial infections. The lactation consultant should gain familiarity with a number of the more common health challenges to better provide lactation care and services when confronted with maternal health problems.

I. Pituitary Disorders

A. Sheehan's syndrome (panhypopituitarism)

1. Caused by severe postpartum hemorrhage and hypotension; this can lead to the failure of the pituitary gland to produce gonadotropins.

2. Symptoms of severe Sheehan's syndrome include weight gain and then loss postpartum, loss of pubic and axillary hair, intolerance to cold, low blood pressure, and vaginal and breast tissue atrophy.

3. Milder cases might see a delay in milk synthesis; frequent breastfeeding or pumping would be required to stimulate the number and sensitivity of breast prolactin receptors and to take advantage of what little prolactin might be available.

    4. The role of the pituitary gland might be permissive rather than completely responsible for the success of lactation; women who have varying levels of pro-lactin have been shown to produce adequate amounts of milk for their infants (Cox et al., 1996).

    5. The breast and body have compensatory mechanisms that make lactation a robust activity; autocrine control of milk production can fill in for a less-than-optimal hormonal environment (Cregan et al., 2000).

B. Prolactinomas; prolactin-secreting adenomas

    1. Prolactin-secreting tumors that can produce amenorrhea and galactorrhea do not show a correlation with milk production (DeCoopman, 1993).

    2. Women can breastfeed with this condition (Verma et al., 2006).

    3. Chronic, high levels of prolactin also can be caused by certain medications (such as oral estrogens, medications for hypothyroidism, or medications for the treat-ment of psychiatric conditions), excessive breast manipulation, hypothyroid states, hyperthyroid disease, chronic renal failure, and several less-frequently seen syndromes (Verhelst et al., 2003).

II. Diabetes

A. Diabetes is a chronic disease of impaired carbohydrate metabolism.

    1. Type 1 diabetes, also termed insulin-dependent diabetes mellitus (insufficient insulin).

    2. Type 2 diabetes, also termed late-onset or nnoninsulin-dependent diabetes that is usually not insulin dependent (inefficient use of insulin).

      a. There are some incidences where type 2 diabetics are prescribed insulin to better manage their insulin levels.

      b. Reduced by breastfeeding.

    3. Gestational diabetes is a glucose intolerance that is seen in about 2% of preg-nancies in previously healthy women.

      a. Women who have gestational diabetes during a pregnancy are 30–40% more likely to develop type 2 diabetes within 10 years.

      b. Based on epidemiologic studies, there is a relationship between the duration of lactation and the risk of subsequent development of type 2 diabetes. For every year of lactation, the risk decreases by an average of 15% (Steube et al., 2005; Taylor et al., 2005).

B. The breast has insulin-sensitive tissue and requires insulin to initiate milk production.

    1. There can be a 15- to 28-hour delay in lactogenesis II as the mother's body competes with the breasts for the available insulin (Arthur et al., 1994; Hartmann et al., 2001).

C. Lactation has an insulin-sparing effect on the mother.
1. This can cause lower insulin requirements during lactation.
2. The constant conversion of glucose to galactose and lactose during milk synthesis lowers the insulin requirement.
3. The diabetic mother also needs extra calories while lactating.
D. Diabetic mothers should be encouraged to breastfeed.
1. Their infants might be large and are prone to hypoglycemia, so very frequent feedings of colostrum are necessary; if mother and baby are separated, pumping should be initiated as soon as possible (California Diabetes and Pregnancy Program, 2002; Wight, Marinelli, & Academy of Breastfeeding Medicine Protocol Committee, 2006).
2. Some babies of diabetic mothers are observed in a nursery for a number of hours following birth.
   a. Separation increases the chances for supplemental feeding and delayed initiation of breastfeeding.
   b. Hand-expressed colostrum can stabilize blood glucose levels; colostrum (donor milk or breastmilk substitutes in the absence of colostrum) can be offered to the baby by cup, spoon, dropper, or tube feeding device.
   c. Mothers can hand express colostrum into a spoon and spoon feed it to the baby.
   d. Mothers with diabetes can express colostrum during the prenatal period, freeze it, and bring it to the hospital for use if necessary instead of infant formula (Cox, 2006).
3. Insulin is a large molecule that does not pass into the milk of a mother on insulin replacement therapy.
E. Mothers who have diabetes might be more prone to infection, mastitis, and overgrowth of *Candida albicans*.
1. Hypoglycemia in the mother might increase the release of epinephrine, reducing milk production and interfering with the milk ejection reflex (Asselin et al., 1987).
2. The presence of acetone signals the need for more calories and carbohydrates; acetone can be transferred to the milk and stress the newborn's liver (Lawrence et al., 2011).

III. Thyroid Disease

A. The thyroid gland controls the body's metabolism and is involved with the hormones of pregnancy and lactation.
B. Because untreated hypothyroidism has a low probability for the maintenance of a pregnancy, most mothers who have this condition are already receiving thyroid replacement therapy (which is compatible with breastfeeding) (Braverman et al., 2008).
C. Low thyroid levels have been associated with low milk production and insufficient weight gain in some babies and should be examined in these situations.
D. Hypothyroidism has also been identified in postpartum mothers who have prolonged "baby blues," a new onset of depression, or extended fatigue.

    E. Hyperthyroidism is an excess amount of thyroid hormone that can result in rapid weight loss, increased appetite, nervousness, heart palpitations, and a rapid pulse at rest.

      1. The ability to lactate is not compromised by this condition.

      2. Hyperthyroidism with bulging eyes is called Graves' disease.

      3. Laboratory examination of a blood sample can usually diagnose this condition; sometimes radioiodine studies are recommended. The lactation consultant should identify the compound being used and its compatibility with breastfeeding.

      4. Treatment is usually an antithyroid drug that is safe for the infant.

      5. Sometimes the baby's thyroid function is measured periodically.

IV. Cystic Fibrosis (CF)

    A. Cystic fibrosis (CF) is characterized by the dysfunction of the exocrine glands and includes chronic pulmonary disease, obstruction of the pancreatic ducts, and pancreatic enzyme deficiency.

    B. Formerly, life expectancy was short with few women reaching adulthood. The life expectancy of patients with CF largely depends on the severity of the manifestations (Buescher et al., 2008).

    C. More sophisticated treatments in early stages are now enabling women to live into adulthood, reproduce, and breastfeed.

    D. Concerns center on the mother maintaining her own weight and her health status, rather than quality or quantity of her breastmilk.

      1. Mothers who have CF usually need plenty of extra calories and supplements to their own diet to maintain their weight.

      2. Mothers with mild pulmonary disease are able to maintain their own weight during breastfeeding, and their milk can support the health needs of an infant for growth and development (Michel et al., 1994).

    E. Individuals who have CF are chronic carriers of pathologic bacteria such as *Staphylococcus aureus* and *Pseudomonas*.

      1. Breastmilk lymphocytes are sensitized to these pathogens carried by the mother and are passed to the baby in breastmilk, protecting him or her from infections by these agents (Larson, 2004).

V. Phenylketonuria (PKU)

    A. Phenylketonuria (PKU) is an inborn error of metabolism whereby the body lacks the enzyme to break down the amino acid phenylalanine, which can result in lowered intelligence.

    B. Because of widespread newborn screening for this condition and early treatment, many women with PKU are reaching their childbearing years with normal intelligence.

    C. Dietary restrictions should not be discontinued at any age, especially in women (Lee et al., 2005).

        1. Blood phenylalanine levels should be 4 milligrams in women (Matalon et al., 1986).

        2. Breastfeeding is compatible with the condition (Matalon et al., 1986).

        3. The milk of mothers who have PKU is of normal composition (Fox-Bacon et al., 1997).

VI. Systemic Lupus Erythematosus (SLE)

    A. Systemic lupus erythematosus (SLE) is an autoimmune disease of the connective tissue primarily affecting women of childbearing age.

    B. Symptoms are diverse, exacerbated by pregnancy, and include the following: fatigue, fibromyalgia, joint redness and swelling, and a butterfly rash on the cheeks and nose.

    C. Women who have SLE experience higher rates of miscarriage and delivery of pre-term infants.

    D. Raynaud's phenomenon is present in about 30% of cases.

    E. Insufficient milk supply is the most frequent complaint during lactation.

        1. Infant weight gain must be carefully watched, and babies might need supplementation.

        2. Fatigue and some medications can contribute to faltering milk production.

    F. Nonsteroidal anti-inflammatory medications and corticosteroids are frequent medications that are given to handle symptoms and are usually compatible with breast-feeding (Hale, 2010).

    G. Breastfeeding is especially beneficial to mothers who have SLE because it enables them to rest while feeding the baby and helps space out pregnancies.

VII. Osteoporosis

    A. Osteoporosis is a condition of bone thinning that is generally associated with older, postmenopausal women.

    B. Normal lactation-associated bone mineral mobilization takes place and does not require drug therapy or nutritional supplements.

    C. Bone loss can be measurable during lactation but returns to normal baseline following weaning (Eisman, 1998).

    D. Because a lactating woman's body is more efficient in energy use and nutrient uptake, lumbar bone density actually increases the longer a woman breastfeeds and the more infants she nurses (Kalkwarf et al., 1995; Kalkwarf et al., 1996).

    E. Age, diet, body frame size, and weight-bearing exercise all contribute to good (or poor) bone health.

VIII. Seizure Disorders (Epilepsy)

A. Mothers who have epilepsy can successfully breastfeed and should be encouraged to do so.

B. The major concern is the sedating effect on the baby of maternal medications.

C. Antiepileptic drugs tend to make a baby sleepy and depress his or her sucking in the early days following birth until he or she is better able to handle drug clearance (Hale, 2010).

    1. It is important that mothers pump milk following feedings or if the baby feeds poorly to provide breast stimulation in the absence of adequate sucking by the baby during the early days.

D. Some mothers have been advised not to breastfeed because they might drop the baby if they have a seizure while breastfeeding; this situation is no more likely to occur during breastfeeding than during bottle-feeding.

IX. Migraine Headaches

A. These severe episodic headaches tend to be worse during the first trimester of pregnancy and are sensitive to hormones and other triggers.

B. Many remedies, both pharmacologic and of a biofeedback nature, are used to help this condition.

C. Pharmacologic treatment does not preclude breastfeeding. Medications such as Fioricet (butalbital, acetaminophen, and caffeine), Percocet (oxycodone and acetaminophen), codeine, and sumatriptan are all considered compatible with breastfeeding (Hale, 2010).

D. When a mother experiences this type of headache and if it is severe enough, she might not feel well enough to breastfeed (although pumping may not be much of a relief).

E. Mothers can store extra milk in the freezer in case others need to feed the baby.

X. Raynaud's Phenomenon of the Nipple

A. Raynaud's phenomenon is an intermittent ischemia (narrowing of the blood vessels) usually affecting the fingers and toes, especially when exposed to cold and more commonly seen in women.

B. In some women, this condition shows indications of blanching of the nipple before, during, or after breastfeedings.

C. These nipple spasms also have been seen clinically as a result of babies biting at the breast, jaw clenching, and in the presence of severe nipple damage; such sucking variations need to be corrected to help eliminate the trigger to the spasms (Lawlor-Smith et al., 1997).

D. The mother feels extreme pain during this nipple spasm, which might continue to spasm and relax for up to 30 minutes after a feeding.

E. Exposure to cold and/or ingestion of caffeine can exacerbate this problem.

F. Some maternal medications, such as fluconazole and oral contraceptives, might be associated with vasospasm.

G. Mothers usually feel relief by applying warm compresses to the breasts or a heating pad.

H. Mothers may also get relief from using a nipple compression technique (using thumb and index finger) to "trap" any remaining blood in the end of the nipple. This compression may also interrupt the spasm itself.

I. Other anecdotal remedies for this condition that have not been thoroughly studied include the following:

1. Ibuprofen

2. Nifedipine (minimum 5 mg 3 times per day, or up to one daily 30 mg slow release tablet; both up to 2 week treatment time; Anderson et al., 2004)

3. Supplemental calcium (2,000 mg/day)

4. Supplemental magnesium (1,000 mg/day)

XI. Surgery

A. Breastfeeding can continue through almost all situations that require surgery.

B. Mothers can usually breastfeed upon arousal from anesthesia (Hale, 2010).

C. Concern is over anesthetic and pain medications, the mother's ability to hold and feed the baby, access to the baby, access to a breast pump, and the ability to pump on a regular basis.

D. Babies might be able to room with the mother during her hospital stay as long as an assistant is present to care for the baby.

1. Otherwise, the baby can be brought to the hospital for feedings.

2. If this situation is not possible, the mother should have access to a hospital-grade electric breast pump with a double collection kit.

3. If she is physically unable to pump, then the nurse, family member, or caregiver can pump the breasts for her.

E. With elective surgery, the mother has time to arrange for access to the baby, a private room, and perhaps express extra milk and freeze it for use any time she is unavailable to feed.

XII. Viral Infections (Pickering, 2006)

A. Breastfeeding is rarely contraindicated in maternal infection.

B. Exceptions relate to specific infectious agents with strong evidence of transmission and to the association of increased morbidity and mortality in the infant.

C. Cytomegalovirus (CMV; one of the human herpes viruses):

1. Congenital infections are usually asymptomatic but can result in later hearing loss or learning disability.

2. Infections in full-term infants acquired at birth from maternal cervical secretions or breastmilk are usually not associated with symptoms (Lawrence et al., 2011).

3. Infants who have congenital or acquired CMV do better if they are breastfed because of the antibody protection delivered through breastmilk.

4. Nonbreastfed infants can be infected through other secretions, including saliva, and receive no protective antibodies or other host resistance factors that are present in breastmilk.
   a. They can have significant health effects from the disease, including microcephaly and mental retardation.
   b. High rates of transmission occur in child care centers.
5. Term infants can be fed breastmilk when the mother is shedding virus in her milk because of the passively transferred maternal antibodies (Lawrence, 2006).
6. Preterm infants can develop the disease, even from breastmilk; recommendations include scalding the breastmilk for 3 to 7 days at 220°C, which decreases infectivity but does not totally eliminate the virus (Lawrence, 2006).

D. Herpes simplex virus:
   1. Infection in the early neonatal period is serious and can be fatal.
   2. The infection is most frequently transmitted to the baby through the birth canal.
   3. Only lesions on the breast would require a temporary interruption of breast-feeding on that breast until the lesions have completely cleared (American Academy of Pediatrics [AAP] Section on Breastfeeding, 2005).
   4. Active lesions elsewhere on the body should be covered, and the mother should be instructed to wash her hands before handling the infant; breastfeeding is not affected.
   5. A mother who has cold sores on her lips should refrain from kissing and nuzzling the baby until the lesions have crusted and dried.

E. Herpes varicella zoster (chickenpox):
   1. Perinatal exposure can be problematic. If a mother develops varicella during a period of 5 days prior to delivery to 2 days after delivery, the infant is a candidate to receive varicella immune globulin (AAP, 2009). It is presumed that infants in this time period face an infectious challenge for which they have not received any transplacental antibody from the mother prior to birth. Birth during this time frame can be deadly to the infant.
   2. If a mother develops varicella prior to 5 days before delivery, her body has time to develop an antibody response, which is passed on to the unborn baby.
   3. Babies born to mothers with varicella, regardless of when the lesions presented, are still encouraged to breastfeed. The infant has already been exposed because of the timing of the delivery and may or may not have received transplacental antibody. There are no current indications to separate mothers and infants in these cases.

F. Respiratory syncytial virus (RSV):
   1. RSV is a common cause of respiratory illness in children.
   2. Mortality can be high in neonates, especially preterm babies or ill full-term babies.
   3. There is no reason to stop breastfeeding during maternal RSV infection; in fact, breastmilk might be protective against severe RSV (Lawrence & Lawrence, 2011).

4. If a mother develops RSV during lactation, she would need to practice good hand washing techniques, avoid coughing on her infant, and be diligent in the management of her respiratory secretions (Buescher et al., 2008).

5. Infants who have RSV should breastfeed.

G. Human immunodeficiency virus 1 (HIV-1):

1. HIV-1 can be transmitted through breastmilk, but the risk is relative to other factors, such as onset, access to medications, and other illnesses common to underdeveloped countries (U.S. Department of Health and Human Services [USDHHS], 2011).

2. HIV-1 antibodies also occur in the breastmilk of infected women.

3. A major dilemma in estimating the risk from breastfeeding is in the difficulty of determining when the HIV infection actually occurs in the infant.

4. Current research from the National Institutes of Health (NIH) shows evidence that breastfeeding is acceptable in infants, if their mothers are receiving antiretroviral treatment throughout the breastfeeding experience. However, the U.S. Department of Health and Human Services continues to recommend that HIV-infected mothers in the United States use infant formula (USDHHS, 2011).

5. Current standards of the Occupational Safety and Health Administration do not require gloves for the routine handling of expressed human milk.

   a. Health workers should wear gloves in situations where exposure to expressed breastmilk would be frequent or prolonged, such as in milk banking (Nommsen-Rivers, 1997).

6. Expressed breastmilk from HIV-positive mothers can be made safe for infant consumption via pasteurization or by maternal antiretroviral treatment and should be carefully considered for use, especially in areas of the world where breastmilk substitute use would pose a grave threat to the life of the infant.

   a. Refer to Chapter 23.

H. Hepatitis:

1. The varying types of hepatitis carry different risks of contagion, pathways of exposure, treatments, and preventive measures.

2. Hepatitis A is an acute illness and is usually transmitted through food-borne and water-borne routes as well as commonly in child care settings through fecal contamination.

   a. A newborn can be infected by vertical transmission from an infected mother during delivery.

   b. The baby should be isolated from other babies in the nursery (such as rooming-in).

   c. Gamma globulin is given to the baby if the mother developed the disease within 2 weeks of the delivery.

   d. The mother also receives gamma globulin.

   e. Hepatitis A is not transmitted via breastmilk. Breastfeeding should proceed as usual. Mothers should exercise good hand washing and personal hygiene to prevent transmission.

3. Hepatitis B can cause a wide variety of infections, from asymptomatic conversion to fulminant fatal hepatitis.
   a. Prenatal testing reveals the mother's status prior to delivery.
   b. Infants who are born to mothers who have the active disease or who are active carriers receive hepatitis B specific immunoglobulin (HBIG) at birth or soon after, followed by an immunization program.
   c. As soon as HBIG is given, breastfeeding should begin (Lawrence et al., 2011).
   d. Although hepatitis B virus has been detected in human milk from infected mothers, current data show that breastfeeding does not significantly increase the risk of infant infection.
   e. Breastfeeding is not contraindicated, and appropriate care should be taken to prevent any infant contact with maternal blood (Buescher et al., 2008).
4. Hepatitis C infection has an insidious onset, with many people not aware that they are affected.
   a. The risk of infection via breastmilk has not been documented (AAP Section on Breastfeeding, 2005). Antibodies against hepatitis C have been detected in milk of infected mothers, thus leaving some question theoretically of whether it could be passed via human milk.
   b. Concern arises if a mother has a coinfection, such as HIV.
   c. The virus might be inactivated in the infant's gastrointestinal tract or neutralized in colostrum; mothers who have hepatitis C can and should breastfeed.
   d. The current AAP policy on breastfeeding states that maternal hepatitis C infection is not a contraindication for breastfeeding (AAP Section on Breastfeeding, 2005).
5. Hepatitis D, E, and G:
   a. Not much is known about transmission of these forms of hepatitis through breastfeeding.
   b. Hepatitis D is usually a coinfection or superimposed on a hepatitis B infection.
   c. Once immunoglobin has been given and the vaccine has begun, breastfeeding should proceed as usual.
   d. Hepatitis E is self-limited and is not a chronic disease (usually associated with water contamination).
   e. Breastfeeding has not been shown to transmit this disease and should proceed as usual.
   f. Hepatitis G seems associated with blood transfusions but has not been shown to be transmitted through breastmilk.
   g. Reports of infected mothers breastfeeding infants are few, but no clinical infections have been reported.

XIII. Tuberculosis

A. Breastfeeding is not contraindicated in women who have previously positive skin tests and no evidence of disease.

   1. A mother who has had a recent conversion to a positive skin test should be evaluated for the disease, and if there is no sign of disease, breastfeeding should begin or continue (AAP, 2006).

   2. If a mother has suspicious symptoms, she might need to express milk and have it fed to the baby until a diagnosis is made. The mother's milk is safe to feed to baby because tuberculosis is usually spread via respiratory droplets.

   3. In developing countries where nonbreastfed infants have a high mortality rate, breastfeeding is not interrupted. In developed countries where there are safe alternatives to direct breastfeeding, mothers might need to express milk during the time they are being evaluated.

   4. If there is confirmation of the disease, the mother needs to be treated and breastfeeding can begin or resume after 2 weeks of maternal therapy (AAP, 2006).

   5. Current medications used in treatment of tuberculosis, such as rifampin, isoniazid, ethambutol, and streptomycin, are considered compatible with breastfeeding (Hale, 2010).

   6. If it is safe for the mother to be in contact with her baby, then it is safe to breastfeed.

References

American Academy of Pediatrics Section on Breastfeeding. (2005). Breastfeeding and the use of human milk. *Pediatrics, 115*(2), 496–506.

American Academy of Pediatrics. (2006). Tuberculosis. In L. K. Pickering (Ed.), *Red book: 2006 report of the Committee on Infectious Diseases* (27th ed.). Elk Grove Village, IL: American Academy of Pediatrics.

American Academy of Pediatrics. (2009). Varicella-zoster infections. In *Red book: 2009: Transmission of infectious agents via human milk* (pp. 714–727). Elk Grove Village, IL: American Academy of Pediatrics.

Anderson, J. E., Held, N., & Wright, K. (2004). Raynaud's phenomenon of the nipple: A treatable cause of painful breastfeeding. *Pediatrics, 113*, e360–e364.

Arthur, P. G., Kent, J. C., & Hartmann, P. E. (1994). Metabolites of lactose synthesis in milk from diabetic and non-diabetic women during lactogenesis II. *Journal of Pediatric Gastroenterology and Nutrition, 19*, 100–108.

Asselin, B. L., & Lawrence, R. A. (1987). Maternal disease as a consideration in lactation management. *Clinical Perinatology, 14*, 71–87.

Braverman, L., & Barbour, L. (2008). Pregnancy and thyroid disease. National Endocrine and Metabolic Diseases Information Service. Retrieved from http://endocrine.niddk.nih.gov/pubs/pregnancy

Buescher, E. S., & Hatcher, S. W. (2008). *Breastfeeding and diseases: A reference guide.* Amarillo, TX: Hale Publishing.

California Diabetes and Pregnancy Program. (2002). *Guidelines for care: Sweet success express.* Sacramento, CA: Maternal and Health Branch, Department of Health Services.

Cox, D. B., Owens, R. A., & Hartmann, P. E. (1996). Blood and milk prolactin and the rate of milk synthesis in women. *Experimental Physiology, 81*, 1007–1020.

Cox, S. G. (2006). Expressing and storing colostrum antenatally for use in the newborn period. *Breastfeeding Review, 14*, 11–16.

Cregan, M. D., DeMello, T. R., & Hartmann, P. E. (2000). Pre-term delivery and breast expression: Consequences for initiating lactation. *Advances in Experimental Medicine and Biology, 478*, 427–428.

DeCoopman, J. (1993). Breastfeeding after pituitary resection: Support for a theory of autocrine control of milk supply? *Journal of Human Lactation, 9*, 35–40.

Eisman, J. (1998). Relevance of pregnancy and lactation to osteoporosis? *Lancet, 352*, 504–505.

Fox-Bacon, C., McCamman, S., Therou, L., et al. (1997). Maternal PKU and breastfeeding: Case report of identical twin mothers. *Clinical Pediatrics, 36*, 539–542.

Hale, T. W. (2010). *Medications and mothers' milk.* Amarillo, TX: Hale Publishing.

Hartmann, P. E., & Cregan, M. (2001). Lactogenesis and the effects of insulin-dependent diabetes mellitus and prematurity. *Journal of Nutrition, 131*(11), 3016S–3020S. Retrieved from http://jn.nutrition.org/cgi/content/full/131/11/3016S

Kalkwarf, H. J., & Specker, B. L. (1995). Bone mineral loss during lactation and recovery after weaning. *Obstetrics and Gynecology, 86*, 26–32.

Kalkwarf, H. J., Specker, B. L., Heubi, J. E., et al. (1996). Intestinal calcium absorption of women during lactation and after weaning. *American Journal of Clinical Nutrition, 63*, 526–531.

Larson, L. A. (2004). *Immunobiology of human milk: How breastfeeding protects babies.* Amarillo, TX: Pharmasoft Publishing.

Lawlor-Smith, L., & Lawlor-Smith , C. (1997). Vasospasm of the nipple—a manifestation of Raynaud's phenomenon: Case reports. *British Medical Journal, 314*, 844–845.

Lawrence, R. A., & Lawrence, R. M. (2011). *Breastfeeding: A guide for the medical profession* (7th ed.). St. Louis, MO: Mosby.

Lawrence, R. M. (2006). Cytomegalovirus in human breast milk: Risk to the premature infant. *Breastfeeding Medicine, 1*, 99–107.

Lee, P. J., Ridout, D., Walter, J. H., & Cockburn, F. (2005). Maternal phenylketonuria: Report from the United Kingdom Registry 1978–97. *Archives of Disease in Childhood, 90*, 143–146.

Matalon, R., Michals, K., & Gleason, L. (1986). PKU: Strategies for dietary treatment and monitoring compliance. *Annals of the New York Academy of Science, 477*, 223–230.

Michel, S. H., & Mueller, D. H. (1994). Impact of lactation on women with cystic fibrosis and their infants: A review of five cases. *Journal of the American Dietetic Association, 94*, 159–165.

Montgomery, A., Hale, T. W., and Academy of Breastfeeding Medicine Protocol Committee. (2006). ABM clinical protocol no. 15: Analgesia and anesthesia for the breastfeeding mother. *Breastfeeding Medicine, 1*(4), 271–277.

Nommsen-Rivers, L. (1997). Universal precautions are not needed for health care workers handling breast milk. *Journal of Human Lactation, 13*, 267–268.

Pickering, L. K. (Ed.). (2006). *Red book: Report of the Commission on Infectious Diseases* (27th ed.). Elk Grove Village, IL: American Academy of Pediatrics.

Stuebe, A. M., Rich-Edwards, J. W., Willett, W. C., Manson, J. E., & Michels, K. B. (2005). Duration of lactation and the incidence of type 2 diabetes. *Journal of the American Medical Association, 294*, 2601–2610.

Taylor, J. S., Kacmar, J. E., Nothnagle, M., & Lawrence, R. A. (2005). A systematic review of the literature associating breastfeeding with type 2 diabetes and gestational diabetes. *Journal of the American College of Nutrition*, *24*, 320–326.

U.S. Department of Health and Human Services. (2011, March 3). Six-month drug regimen cuts HIV risk for breastfeeding infants, NIH study finds. *NIH News*. Retrieved from http://www.nih.gov/news/health/mar2011/niaid-03.htm

Verhelst, J., & Abs, R. (2003). Hyperprolactinemia: Pathophysiology and management. *Treatments in Endocrinology*, *2*, 23–32.

Verma, S., Shah, D., & Faridi, M. M. (2006). Breastfeeding a baby with mother on Bromocriptine. *Indian Journal of Pediatrics*, *73*, 435–436.

Wight, N., Marinelli, K. A., & Academy of Breastfeeding Medicine Protocol Committee. (2006). ABM clinical protocol no. 1: Guidelines for glucose monitoring and treatment of hypoglycemia in breastfed neonates. Revision June, 2006. *Breastfeeding Medicine*, *1*(3), 178–184.

CHAPTER 42
Insufficient Milk Production

Kay Hoover, MEd, IBCLC, FILCA, and Lisa Marasco, MA, IBCLC, FILCA

OBJECTIVES

- Explain normal milk production.
- Delineate between real and perceived insufficient milk production.
- Discuss the etiology of insufficient milk.
- Describe potential indicators of insufficient milk.
- List options for improvement of insufficient milk production.

INTRODUCTION

Insufficient milk is diagnosed when a mother is not making enough milk to fuel sufficient growth for her baby. *Insufficient milk production* specifically refers to the inadequate rate of milk synthesis over time, while *insufficient milk supply* reflects the amount of available stored milk at a given moment. Although these terms are often used interchangeably, it is the rate of production that ultimately results in low milk supply.

Inadequate milk production continues to be the major reason given by mothers worldwide for the discontinuation of breastfeeding. Whether the problem is real or perceived is addressed by a careful history and breastfeeding assessment. True low milk production can be caused by a number of factors and is often a combination of these factors (termed overlapping etiologies). Perceived insufficient milk production is a mother's misinterpretation of infant behaviors such as frequent feedings or apparent unsettledness after a feed. Many mothers reporting infant fussiness after breastfeeding give the baby a bottle of formula to "satisfy" the infant. Supplementing the baby usually begins a downward spiral to real insufficient milk unless interrupted. The percentage of mothers reporting insufficient milk in the literature varies, with many reports not differentiating between real and perceived insufficiency.

I. Normal Milk Production

    A. Normal milk production begins with successful mammogenesis.

        1. Three important periods of mammary gland development: embryo/fetal, puberty, and pregnancy (Knight et al., 2001).

        2. Whereas growth hormone is essential for puberty, estrogen has primary influence on the breast gland, causing ductal growth into the mammary fat pad. Progesterone, the second major hormone of mammary gland development, stimulates development of alveoli along the ducts and ductules (Lawrence et al., 2011, p. 43).

        3. With each successive menstrual cycle, estrogen rises during the first half while progesterone dominates the second half of the cycle, continuing on a minute level to stimulate glandular growth until approximately age 30–35 (Hale et al., 2007; Hartmann et al., 1996; Lawrence et al., 2011).

        4. During pregnancy, the major hormones that stimulate mammary growth and differentiation include (but are not limited to) estrogen, progesterone, human placental lactogen, prolactin, and chorionic gonadotropin (Lawrence et al., 2011).

        5. Change in breast volume is most closely associated with concentration of human placental lactogen (Cox et al., 1999). The additional placenta present in multiple pregnancies stimulates greater mammogenesis (Knight et al., 2001).

        6. Generally speaking, lactation capability is reached approximately halfway through pregnancy. At this time, colostrum begins to be made and the substrates for milk production are laid down (lactogenesis I).

    B. Initiation of lactogenesis II is hormonally (endocrine) controlled.

        1. Onset is triggered by separation of placenta from uterus, removing progesterone interference with prolactin receptors and allowing lactogenesis II to begin.

        2. Key hormones necessary for initiation of lactation are prolactin, insulin, and cortisol (Lawrence et al., 2011).

        3. Under normal circumstances, change to more copious milk production usually begins in 30 to 40 hours (Chapman et al., 1999) and is usually noticed by Western mothers between days 2 and 4.

        4. Milk production at 5 days is highly variable, with mothers producing between 200 and 900 grams per 24 hours (Kent et al., 1999; Woolridge, 1996).

        5. Early milk removal (within first 48 hours) is associated with higher milk output (Hill et al., 2001; Hill et al., 2005; Neville et al., 2001). Milk production begins to shut down if milk removal does not begin at the onset of copious milk production (typically 3–4 days).

    C. Maintenance of milk production (lactogenesis III) is locally (autocrine) controlled.

        1. Transition from endocrine to autocrine control occurs in the first couple of weeks postpartum as milk output is progressively calibrated to the baby's needs, increasing in most cases but sometimes decreasing (Woolridge, 1996). Milk removal is the key factor to calibration of milk production. If milk production is to be sustained, milk must be consistently and effectively removed.

a. The emptier the breast, the faster the rate of milk synthesis. The fuller the breast, the slower the rate of synthesis (production).

b. Unremoved milk exerts an inhibitory effect on milk production, downregulating the amount produced through the accumulation of a whey protein known as the feedback inhibitor of lactation, or the FIL factor (Hale et al., 2007; Wilde et al., 1995).

c. Inhibition of oxytocin/milk ejection can affect ability to remove milk.

2. The average infant consumes approximately 750–800 milliliters per 24 hours from 1 month to 6 months of age (Kent, 2007; Kent et al., 1999; Kent et al., 2006).

a. Total milk required is a function of a combination of baby's sex, baby's metabolic needs, and caloric content of the milk.

b. Boys take in more than girls on average; thus, mothers of boys make more milk than mothers of girls on average (Kent et al., 2006).

c. After 1 month and again around 6 months, a baby's energy requirements per kilogram of body weight decrease (Butte, 2005).

3. Milk output is not constrained at 750–800 milliliters per 24 hours because mothers of twins are quite capable of outputs of 1,500 milliliters per 24 hours (Saint et al., 1986).

4. It is normal for one breast to make more milk, even significantly more, than the other; this effect has been found to be independent of the infant (Engstrom et al., 2007; Kent et al., 2006).

5. Prolactin receptor theory: Successful transition to autocrine control might rely in part on continued development of prolactin receptors, which appears to be influenced by frequency of feeding (Woolridge, 1996).

6. Interference with the calibration of the breasts during the early days can cause the breasts to calibrate at an inappropriate level.

D. Weaning is the end of the lactation cycle. As milk demand declines, involution of the breast occurs as unneeded lactocytes are destroyed via apoptosis (programmed cell death) and the remaining stroma is remodelled. "The amount of breast tissue remains constant from 1 to 6 months of lactation, but decreases significantly between 6 and 9 months, when there is only a small decrease in milk production." The breasts return to their preconception size by 15 months of lactation (Kent, 2007, p. 568).

II. Unsubstantiated Low Milk Production (Perceived Insufficiency)

A. Mothers might misjudge their milk production based on infant behavior or personal experiences such that they perceive insufficiency when in reality they have plenty of milk (Gatti, 2008).

1. Some newborns desire to nurse very frequently until the milk increases with lactogenesis II. Mothers can interpret this as "not enough milk" and "starving the baby" and initiate supplemental feeds prior to full lactogenesis II.

2. Mothers often describe an unsettled baby who fusses after feedings; a baby who feeds for long periods at the breast; or a baby who feeds constantly at the breast

and fusses when put down. Although this can be the result of low supply, it also can be the result of infant discomfort or high sucking needs. This behavior can also be seen when the baby is sucking at the breast and not transferring milk (i.e., impaired milk ejection reflex, infant suckling problem, etc.).

3. Sometimes the symptoms of oversupply (baby pulling away from the breast and crying, fussy baby who still wants to nurse) can be mistaken for insufficient milk production.

4. Normal newborn patterns of wakefulness and feeding more often at night can be misinterpreted as low production.

5. Perceptions by the mother that her production is low because of softer breasts, normal decrease in size of the breasts, breasts feeling less full, cessation of leakage, or a change in the sensation of the milk ejection.

6. Mothers doubt their ability to make sufficient milk.

B. Psychosocial concerns (Williams, 2002).

1. Social support:

a. Importance of mother feeling supported for her desire to breastfeed.

b. Motivation to breastfeed is higher when mother feels it is her choice and not something forced on her.

2. Postpartum depression (O'Brien et al., 2004).

3. Emotional problems: How a mother feels about her new role of motherhood and the experience of breastfeeding can affect breastfeeding management and milk production.

4. Severe psychological issues can affect oxytocin release and impair milk ejection, which can lead to low production if chronic (rare).

a. Posttraumatic stress syndrome: Nursing can awaken unwanted memories or fears (Seng, 2010; Williams, 1997).

b. History of sexual abuse (Beck, 2004).

III. Secondary Milk Production Problems: Interferences That Can Cause Inappropriate Calibration of the Breasts

A. Iatrogenic:

a. Supplemental feeds of water or formula.

b. Interrupted or delayed breastfeeding without compensatory removal of milk (milk expression), often caused by the following conditions: (*Note:* These conditions can be managed so that breastfeeding is maintained):

i. Hyperbilirubinemia

ii. Hypoglycemia

iii. Maternal medications

iv. Maternal illness

v. Infant illness

c. Unrelieved engorgement. A mother might have been engorged and mistakenly told not to pump milk because she would just make more milk, resulting in prolonged fullness that signals the breasts to reduce production.

      d. A mother might have been encouraged to send her baby to the nursery at night, leading to undermining situations such as mother–baby separation, infant introduction to artificial nipples, or infant dissatisfaction with colostrum after larger boluses of formula. This in turn can start a downward spiral of supplementation and downregulation of milk production.

B. Maternal mismanagement/misunderstanding of the process:

  1. Potential risk factors:

      a. Mothers who are less informed about breastfeeding.

      b. Only making the decision to breastfeed in late pregnancy or just after birth, resulting in potential lack of information.

      c. Intending to breastfeed for a short or limited period of time.

      d. Planning to "do both" (mixed feeding) (Holmes et al., 2011).

      e. Planning to "sleep train" baby, resulting in ignoring feeding cues by infant (Marasco et al., 1998).

      f. Initiation of milk removal greater than 48 hours and/or low frequency of milk removal when baby is unable to feed (Hill et al., 2001).

      g. Being less confident about her ability to breastfeed; mothers who are tentative and say that they are going to "try" to breastfeed.

      h. Breastfeeding in front of others and being sensitive to a lack of privacy.

      i. Receiving little encouragement from partner, mother, and/or mother-in-law.

      j. Having a poorer health status and more problems with illness while breastfeeding.

      k. Nipple pain.

      l. Breast pain (engorgement, mastitis).

      m. Discomfort in positioning from cesarean surgery or episiotomy.

      n. After 6 weeks, this condition might be more difficult to reverse (Woolridge, 1996).

  2. Common management problems that undermine breastfeeding:

      a. Limited number of feedings.

      b. Mother who is not breastfeeding enough:

        i. Unusual stress or fatigue

        ii. Logistics of returning to work or school and maintaining adequate milk removal and stimulation

        iii. Following an infant feeding schedule instead of feeding on cue (Marasco et al., 1998)

      c. Feedings that are not long enough to drain the breasts adequately.

      d. An infant sucking on pacifiers, fingers, thumbs, or nipple shield (Auerbach, 1990; Woolridge et al., 1980).

      e. Preterm baby: Mother might not express her milk to her peak yield, but just to the transient limited needs of the small baby at the time, causing a lowered calibration of milk yield.

3. Medications and foods:
    a. Reports of sage, parsley, and mint reducing milk supply (anecdotal; no formal research).
    b. Cigarette smoking:
        i. Interpretations of research are conflicting (Amir, 2001; Amir et al., 2003; de Mello et al., 2001).
        ii. Reduces the length of breastfeeding (Amir, 2001).
        iii. Believed to reduce prolactin secretion (Andersen et al., 1982).
        iv. Lower milk yield (Hopkinson et al., 1992; Vio et al., 1991).
        v. Lower total lipid levels and docosahexaenoic acid content of milk (Agostoni et al., 2003; Hopkinson et al., 1992).
    c. Some over-the-counter and prescription medicines reduce milk supply.
        i. Pseudoephedrine: Nasal decongestant for colds and allergies (Aljazaf et al., 2003; Hale et al., 2004).
        ii. Bromocriptine, cabergoline, ergotamine.
        iii. Hormonal birth control (oral, injectable, implants, transdermal patch, vaginal ring, or emergency contraceptives), especially before 6 weeks postpartum (Academy of Breastfeeding Medicine [ABM] Protocol Committee, 2006; Betzold et al., 2010; Kennedy et al., 1997; Smith et al., 2006).
            (a) Progesterone may reduce milk supply in early weeks/months (Betzold et al., 2010; Kennedy et al.,1997).
            (b) Estrogen reduces the milk supply (Ball et al., 1999; Hale et al., 2007).
        iv. Estrogen patch for postpartum depression.
        v. Bupropion: Antidepressant; smoking deterrent (Hale, 2010, p. 141).
        vi. Parkinson's disease treatments such as levodopa or dopamine agonists may decrease prolactin and milk production.
        vii. Blood pressure medicine: Methyldopa suppresses prolactin (Lawrence et al., 2011, p. 580).
        viii. Marijuana may reduce milk supply (Djulus et al., 2005).
        ix. Overdoses of vitamin B_6 may reduce milk for some women (conflicting research).
        x. Alcohol consumption:
            (a) Prolactin response to suckling after ingestion of alcohol is greater.
            (b) Oxytocin response to suckling is lower after ingestion of alcohol, with slowed milk ejection (Cobo, 1973; Mennella, 2001b; Mennella et al., 2005).
            (c) Babies transfer less milk during the immediate hours after maternal ingestion of alcohol, though they are able to make up for it later when the effects of the alcohol have worn off (Mennella, 2001b).
            (d) Frequent ingestion of alcohol can cause lowered milk production (de Araújo Burgos et al., 2004; Mennella, 2001a).
C. Teach mothers about normal physiologic breastfeeding.

D. Infant problems: Baby is not capable of sufficient milk removal to maintain adequate supply.
1. Take a thorough infant history.
    a. Gestational age (Wight, 2003).
    b. Late preterm infants may not suckle well enough for adequate milk removal.
2. Consider normal variants of growth.
    a. Small parents, so baby is growing to his or her genetic potential.
    b. Premature babies do not grow at the same rate as age-matched peers.
    c. Large-at-birth baby may have postnatal "catch down" growth.
3. Assess the baby. See Chapters 16 and 18.
    a. Check the baby's oral and facial anatomy (Abadie et al., 2001).
    b. Infant health:
        i. Any infant medical condition that can affect weight gain
        ii. Inadequate caloric intake
        iii. Inability to utilize ingested nutrients due to reduced absorption/excessive loss of nutrients, metabolic problems, obstructions, disease process, etc.
        iv. Excessive utilization of energy as a result of metabolic problems, disease process, and so forth
4. Observe a feeding (Yurdakök et al., 1997).
    a. Positioning.
    b. Good latch.
    c. Audible swallowing, one per suck at the start of the feeding.
    d. Rhythmic sucking; a baby should be able to sustain 10 to 30 suck:swallow:breathe patterns in a row at the start of the feeding (McMillan, 2006, p. 382; Taki et al., 2010).
    e. Satisfied baby at the end of the feeding.
    f. Test feed weights (on electronic scale accurate to 2 grams).
5. Infant conditions that can affect milk removal and milk production:
    a. Preterm or late preterm baby may have difficulty with sucking or feeding stamina.
    b. Tongue mobility restriction:
        i. Tongue-tie (ABM Protocol Committee, 2005; Amir, 2006; Ballard et al., 2002; Fernando, 1999; Forlenza et al., 2010; Geddes et al., 2008; Hazelbaker, 2010; Knox, 2010; Manfro et al., 2010; Miranda et al., 2010; Wilson-Clay et al., 2008).
        ii. Tight maxillary frenum (lip of upper jaw) can restrict lip flexibility and affect seal (Kotlow, 2010).
    c. Airway problems (Genna, 2013):
        i. Check that nostrils are not too narrow or obstructed for comfortable breathing.
        ii. Laryngomalacia: Floppy laryngeal structures are pulled into the airway upon inspiration (stridor is heard with inspiration).

      iii. Tracheomalacia: Softening of the cartilaginous ring surrounding the trachea (stridor is heard with expiration).

      iv. Position baby to optimize breathing.

  d. Palatal problems:

      i. High, bubble, channel (Burke-Snyder, 1997).

      ii. Partial or complete cleft of soft or hard palate (Glenny et al., 2005; Wilton, 1998).

      iii. Submucosal cleft can interfere with ability to create proper oral vacuum (velopharyngeal insufficiency) for removing milk (Genna, 2013).

  e. Infant pain:

      i. Fractured clavicle; repeated heel sticks

      ii. Scalp or brain bleeds from vacuum extraction

  f. Hyper- or hypotonia (high or low muscle tone).

  g. Sensory integration problems. Affected infants may not feed well, leading to poor breast stimulation, milk removal, and decreased milk production (Genna, 2001; Weiss-Salinas et al., 2001).

IV. Primary (Pathophysiology) Lactation Problems

  A. Delayed lactogenesis II: onset of lactation longer than 72 hours (Dewey et al., 2003)

    1. Temporary problem, usually self-resolving if managed well.

    2. Risk factors (Hurst, 2007):

      a. Stress during labor (Chen et al., 1998)

      b. Second stage of labor longer than 1 hour (Dewey et al., 2003)

      c. Significant edema of extremities, such as swollen legs and ankles, especially when pregnancy edema worsens after delivery or the edema develops for the first time after birth (Chantry et al., 2011; Nommsen-Rivers et al., 2010)

      d. Cesarean birth, especially when urgent (Chapman et al., 1999; Leung et al., 2002)

      e. Forceps or vacuum delivery (Leung et al., 2002)

      f. Epidural analgesia affects duration of breastfeeding (Henderson et al., 2003; Jordan et al., 2009)

      g. Augmentation of labor with Pitocin (intravenous oxytocin; Dewey et al., 2003)

      h. Flat or inverted nipples (Dewey et al., 2003)

      i. Hypertension (Hall et al., 2002)

      j. Type 1 diabetes (average 24-hour delay) (Hartmann et al., 2001; Miyake et al., 1989; 1989; Neubauer et al., 1993; Ostrom et al., 1993)

        i. Poorly controlled may affect pregnancy mammary growth, prolactin (Marasco, 2009).

        ii. Fluctuations in maternal glucose can cause fluctuations in milk production (Ferris et al., 1988).

      k. Obesity (Chapman et al., 1999); maternal body mass index (BMI) greater than 27 kilograms per meter squared (Baker et al.,2004; Dewey et al., 2003;

Elliott et al., 1997; Hilson et al., 1997, 2004, 2006; Kugyelka et al., 2004; Lovelady, 2005; Nommsen-Rivers et al., 2010; Nommsen-Rivers, Chantry, Peerson, Cohen, & Dewey, 2011; Rasmussen, 2007; Rasmussen et al., 2001; Raamussen et al., 2006)

    i. Can blunt prolactin response in some women (Rasmussen et al., 2004)

    ii. May cause a delay of 0.5 hours for every one unit of BMI over normal at the time of conception (Hilson et al., 2004)

    iii. May also be related to underlying metabolic cause of obesity

  l. Selective serotonin reuptake inhibitor (SSRI) antidepressant use during pregnancy (Marshall et al., 2010)

  m. Preterm birth (Cregan, 2007; Cregan et al., 2002)

  n. Corticosteroid treatment for premature labor (i.e., betamethasone) (Henderson et al., 2008; Henderson et al., 2009)

  o. Maternal age older than 30 years (Escobar et al., 2002; Nommsen-Rivers et al., 2010)

3. Other causes of delayed lactation:

  a. Retained placental tissue

    i. May continue to issue progesterone and interfere with full milk production until passed or removed (Anderson, 2001; Neifert et al., 1981).

    ii. Placenta accreta/increta/percreta; the more severe forms are more difficult to resolve.

    iii. Medications such as Methergine (methylergonovine maleate) used to treat these conditions may suppress lactation (Arabin et al., 1986; Hale, 2010).

  b. Gestational ovarian theca lutein cysts—a condition that causes high testosterone levels during pregnancy

    i. In some cases, it may also cause virilization (balding, deepening of the voice, facial or abdominal hair growth, pimples on the face or back, or enlargement of the clitoris).

    ii. High testosterone gradually resolves days to weeks after birth on its own. With continued breast stimulation some women eventually have produced a full milk supply, though it has taken as long as 30 days before milk dramatically increased in volume (Betztold et al., 2004; Dahl et al., 2008; Hoover et al., 2002).

B. Impaired lactation (chronic)

  1. Structural

    a. Maternal nipple anomalies (Wilson-Clay et al., 2008)

      i. Large (Caglar et al., 2006)

      ii. Long

      iii. Meaty/nonpliable

      iv. Flat or inverted (Caglar et al., 2006; Cooper et al., 1995; Dewey et al., 2003; Livingstone et al., 2000; Neifert et al., 1990; Wilson-Clay et al., 2002; Yaseen et al., 2004)

      v. Few or no patent ducts through nipple

      vi. Pierced nipples—scarring may obstruct milk flow (Garbin et al., 2009)

  b. Maternal breast anatomy

      i. Surgery (Andrade et al., 2010; Michalopoulos, 2007)

        (a) Breastmilk insufficiency has been particularly noted when periareolar incisions are used (Hurst, 1996; Neifert et al., 1990; Souto et al., 2003).

        (b) Augmentation (Andrade et al., 2010; Michalopoulos, 2007).

        (c) Reduction (Chiummariello et al., 2008; Harris et al., 1992).

        (d) Cyst removal.

        (e) Surgical drainage of abscess or galactocele, especially if incision not radial.

        (f) Biopsy.

        (g) Cancer:

          (i) Lumpectomy

          (ii) Mastectomy

        (h) Nipple surgery.

      ii. Other damaging events

        (a) Chest tube as preterm baby (Rainer et al., 2003).

        (b) Destruction of glandular tissue by abscess.

        (c) Pathologic engorgement.

        (d) Trauma, burns, radiation (Dow et al., 1994; McCullough et al., 2010; Rosenfield et al., 1989).

        (e) Spinal cord injuries:

          (i) Breast innervated T4–T6; if damage occurs T6 or above, lactation may be affected (Halbert, 1998).

          (ii) Lactation often falters after 3 months, but a report of three cases suggests that aiding milk ejection via visualization or synthetic oxytocin spray may help sustain lactation (Cowley, 2005).

        (f) Environmental disruptor theory implicates environmental contaminants such as TCDD, BPA, PCBs, and PCAHs (Fenton et al., 2002; Guillette et al., 2006; Hond et al., 2002; Lewis et al., 2001; Markey et al., 2003; Moral et al., 2008; Roy et al., 2009; University of Rochester Medical Center, 2009; Vorderstrasse et al., 2004; Weldon et al., 2010; Wolff et al., 2008).

2. Pregnancy-related mammary development problems

  a. Placental insufficiencies can negatively affect mammary development during pregnancy (O'Dowd et al., 2008).

   b. With premature deliveries between 22 and 34 weeks, mammogenesis may or may not be sufficiently complete for full lactation (Cregan, 2007). If progesterone drops as a result of threatened premature labor, rat studies suggest that immediate progesterone supplementation may help rescue mammary gland development and lactation (Wlodek et al., 2009).

   c. Inappropriate hormonal exposure to environmental contaminants during critical windows can affect mammary development (Lew et al., 2009).

   d. Low progesterone could affect breast development.

3. Primary hypoplasia: Insufficient glandular tissue (IGT) (Wilson-Clay & Hoover, 2008)

   a. Defined as insufficient lactation tissue to produce enough milk to support adequate infant growth and development (Neifert et al., 1987; Neifert et al., 1985).

   b. IGT is not always evident visually, but more evident on palpation. Some breasts present with normal dimensions, but their appearance suggests a failure to respond normally to pregnancy hormones.

   c. Assessing breast tissue:

      i. Degree of changes during pregnancy (growth, sensitivity, areolar enlargement, darkening).

      ii. Enlargement postpartum.

      iii. Palpate for granular versus smooth tissue.

   d. Presentations of IGT vary.

      i. "Classic" or more obvious IGT:

         (a) Frequent asymmetry in size and/or shape of breasts.

         (b) One or both breasts may be conical/tubular in shape.

      ii. Breasts may be completely underdeveloped.

         (a) "Hypoplasia: Underdevelopment of breast" (Lawrence et al., 2011, p. 45)

         (b) "Amastia: Congenital absence of the breast and nipple" (Lawrence et al., 2011, p. 45)

         (c) An endocrine disorder resulting in faulty development or lack of development of secondary sex characteristics

      iii. Breasts may be large, even pendulous, while palpating as soft fatty tissue.

   e. Risk factors for IGT/poor lactation (Huggins et al., 2000)

      i. Little or no breast enlargement either during pregnancy or early postpartum

      ii. Greater than 1.5 inches (3.8 cm) between breasts

      iii. Lack of significant visible veining on breasts

      iv. Stretch marks (striae) on breast in the absence of breast growth

      v. Higher risk for poor lactation, but may produce more milk over time with sustained effort, and may produce more milk with subsequent pregnancies

      vi. Diet-induced obesity caused aberrant mammary development in rats (Kamikawa et al., 2009)

4. Maternal conditions
   a. Illness of mother
      i. Infection (including mastitis)
      ii. Anemia (Henly et al., 1995)
   b. Chronic conditions
      i. Thyroid dysfunction—may affect both oxytocin and prolactin (Marasco, 2006).
         (a) Hypothyroidism (Hapon et al., 2003, 2005; Stein, 2002).
         (b) Thyroid surgery.
         (c) Hyperthyroid: Rat studies show problems with impaired oxytocin and milk ejection as well as lipid metabolism (Rosato et al., 1992).
         (d) Thyroid dysfunction—risk higher with PCOS, type 1 diabetes, and smoking (de Mello et al., 2001; Janssen et al., 2004).
         (e) Subclinical and/or borderline thyroid dysfunction may present through lactation problems; laboratory values may not always be clear (Marasco, 2006).
      ii. Lupus erythematosus (Ferris et al., 1994)
      iii. Parkinson's disease (some Parkinson's medications are dopamine agonists, which can inhibit prolactin)
      iv. Autoimmune disease
      v. Connective tissue disease
      vi. Renal failure
      vii. Hypertension
      viii. Hypopituitarism
         (a) Prior radiation to the brain may damage the pituitary gland.
         (b) Sheehan's syndrome (described later).
      ix. Diabetes, especially when poorly controlled (Ferris et al., 1994; Lau et al., 1993; Miyake et al., 1989)
         (a) Decreases prolactin and placental lactogen in rats (Botta et al., 1984).
         (b) Thyroid dysfunction may occur concomitantly with diabetes (Gallas et al., 2002).
         (c) Rapid weight gain during pregnancy and gestational diabetes.
         (d) Mothers with gestational diabetes breastfeed for shorter time (Hummel et al., 2008).
         (e) Pituitary necrosis and lactation failure a rare but possible complication (Park et al., 2010).
         (f) Lactation duration decreases as severity of diabetes increases (Hummel et al., 2008; Soltani et al., 2009).

   c. Pregnancy- or birth-related complications

      i. Hemorrhage after birth, especially causing large sudden drop in blood pressure and/or requiring blood transfusion (500 milliliter loss is normal) (Thompson et al., 2010; Willis et al., 1995) May cause damage to pituitary, ranging from mild insult to major infarction.

       (a) Sheehan's syndrome: Severe hemorrhage and drop in blood pressure may result in necrosis of the anterior pituitary. Onset is typically in the weeks after birth but may also show up months later (Dökmetas et al., 2006; Gei-Guardia et al., 2010; Sheehan et al., 1938).

      ii. Hypertension; pregnancy-induced hypertension; hemolysis, elevated liver, low platelets (HELLP) syndrome (Leeners et al., 2005)

      iii. Pregnancy during lactation (Marquis et al., 2002)

5. Other hormonal problems

   a. Something may go wrong internally when the system switches from endocrine to autocrine control.

   b. Might have seen evidence of higher milk output at an earlier stage, but output has inexplicably dropped despite good management.

   c. Hormone receptor problems—not well researched for lactation, but if there are not enough receptors (downregulated) or they are resistant to binding, then even if there is a normal amount of hormone, the hormone cannot have an effect (Collier et al., 1984).

   d. Hormonal problems may or may not be easily pinpointed (West et al., 2009).

   e. Risk factors for hormonal milk production problems:

      i. History of irregular menses or very late menarche.

      ii. Infertility with underlying hormonal imbalance or deficiency.

      iii. Required fertility medications to achieve pregnancy.

      iv. In vitro fertilization pregnancy.

      v. Obesity-related problems may be chronic and not just delayed lactogenesis.

      vi. Postpartum thyroiditis (Stagnaro-Green, 2002).

       (a) Onset anywhere in first year after birth, occurs in 5–7% of all pregnancies

       (b) Risk higher with history of diabetes or tobacco use

       (c) Frequently starts with hyperthyroidism (high thyroid) and then eventually burns out and becomes hypothyroidism (low thyroid), but may also occur as low to high, or just low or just high thyroid

       (d) May or may not be recognized, diagnosed, or treated

       (e) Typically resolves within 12 months

   f. Hyperandrogenism (Carlsen et al., 2010)

      i. Male hormones such as testosterone, dihydrotestosterone, dehydroepinandrosterone (DHEA), dehydroepinandrosterone sulfate (DHEAS), androstenedione.

      ii. Origin may be ovarian or adrenal.

iii. May occur independently or the result of a condition: polycystic ovary syndrome, Cushing's syndrome, congenital adrenal hyperplasia, or androgen-secreting tumors may potentially cause lactation problems.

iv. Effects include downregulation of estrogen and prolactin receptors.

v. Can affect mammary development and/or milk synthesis.

g. Polycystic ovary syndrome (PCOS) with its possible hormonal aberrations include low progesterone levels, insulin resistance, elevated estrogen levels, and hyperandrogenism (high levels of androgens such as testosterone and androstenedione with their possible effect of downregulating estrogen and prolactin receptors) (Marasco et al., 2000; Vanky et al., 2008).

h. Prolactin problems

i. Prolactin deficiency

(a) Cases of familial deficiencies reported (Powe et al., 2010; Zargar et al., 1997)

(b) May develop as the result of poor prolactin surges secondary to other conditions such as obesity

ii. Prolactin resistance theory (Zargar et al., 2000)

i. Sjögren's syndrome

i. "Women with Sjögren's Syndrome may have poor milk supply partially responsive to hydroxychloroquine" (Revai et al., 2010, p. 332).

ii. "Primary Sjögren's Syndrome, which involves the glands of secretion (sweat, salivary), is known to be associated with hyperprolactinemia, but because of the characteristic abnormalities of secreting glands, lactation may not be successful" (Lawrence et al., 2011, p. 580).

j. Women with a family history of alcoholism exhibit lower prolactin surges during breastfeeding and a pattern of more frequent feedings than mothers without the same family history (Mennella et al., 2008, 2010).

6. Nutrition-related issues

a. Deposits of fat during pregnancy subsidize lactation.

b. Breastfeeding women need at least 1,500 calories per day.

c. Lesser intakes have been related to reductions in milk production (Institute of Medicine, 1991).

i. Minimum caloric requirements vary according to individual metabolism and level of activity (Picciano, 2003).

ii. Generally speaking, an extra 500 kilocalories per day over normal are needed the first 6 months; this drops to 400 kilocalories per day from 7 to 9 months (Picciano, 2003).

d. History of an eating disorder is rarely a problem unless the disorder is active. Active binge/purge of bulimia can cause lower prolactin levels; implications are unknown (Bowles et al., 1990; Monteleone et al., 1998; Weltzin et al., 1991).

e. Severe restriction of food intake during pregnancy or lactation may cause milk supply problems (Motil et al., 1994; Paul et al., 1979).

   f. Gastric bypass surgery (Grange et al., 1994; Martens et al., 1990; Wardinsky et al., 1995).
      i. Must also consider underlying cause of obesity leading to gastric bypass surgery.
      ii. If mother still in high caloric restriction phase, risk for problems is higher (Stefanski, 2006).
      iii. High risk of poor absorption of nutrients essential to milk composition, most especially vitamin B_{12} (Grange et al., 1994; Martens et al., 1990; Stefanski, 2006; Wardinsky et al., 1995).
      iv. Recommend at least 65 grams of protein daily (Stefanski, 2006).

V. Management of Milk Insufficiency

   A. Therapeutic interventions depend on the cause of the problem.
      1. Mothers should be taught how to position their baby at the breast, what constitutes an effective latch-on, and how to know when the baby is swallowing milk.
      2. Nipple pain during a feeding can indicate that the baby is not positioned correctly or is not suckling correctly; each increases the likelihood of poor milk transfer, less milk removed from the breast, and less milk synthesized (Geddes et al., 2010; Geddes et al., 2008; McClellan et al., 2008).
      3. Mothers should be taught infant behavioral feeding cues, be encouraged to eliminate watching the clock, and to feed the baby when he or she demonstrates feeding readiness.
         a. Feeding cues include rapid eye movements under the eyelids, sucking movements of the mouth and tongue, hand-to-mouth movements, body movements, and small sounds; these indicate a light sleep state moving to alertness when the baby is more likely to feed efficiently. Babies who are in a deep sleep state do not breastfeed; feeding at prescribed intervals might catch the baby repeatedly at times when he or she is not "available" to feed.
         b. Babies should be fed at least 8–12 times each 24 hours; feedings should not be skipped, complemented, or supplemented unless medically indicated; mothers should manually express or pump milk if the baby cannot go to the breast.
         c. Mothers should demonstrate an awareness of the normalcy of cluster or bunched feedings that typically occur in the late afternoon or early evening but that could also occur at other times.
         d. Alternate massage or breast compressions can be used to initiate and sustain suckling at the breast; some babies require the presence of milk flow to regulate their sucking (Stutte et al., 1988).
         e. A mother should know how to gauge whether her baby is getting enough milk; bowel movements can be an indicator (size and color change are important) (Nommsen-Rivers et al., 2008; Shrago, 2006), but ultimately weight gain is the best indicator (regain birth weight before 2 weeks and thereafter at least 5 to 8 ounces per week during the first 3 months).

    f. Larger than normal weight loss during the first 3 days in a baby whose mother had Pitocin and/or large amounts of intravenous fluids during labor should not be confused with insufficient milk intake (Dahlenburg et al., 1980; Nommsen-Rivers, 2010).

   4. Express milk after breastfeeding starting on the third day postpartum.

   5. Increase number of feedings/expressions. When expressing, try to express as often as baby feeds, with at least one pumping session between midnight and 5 a.m. (Mohrbacher, 2011).

   6. Massage the breast while breastfeeding/expressing.

   7. Compress the breast while feeding or pumping (hand express while breastfeeding).

   8. Hand express after pumping to drain residual milk and stimulate production further (ABM Protocol Committee, 2011; Morton et al., 2009).

   9. Hold the baby skin to skin for as many hours a day as possible.

  10. Supplement the baby with a tube feeding device while the baby is breastfeeding.

  11. Switch nursing: Move baby back and forth between breasts several times whenever he or she slows down.

B. Make sure the baby is getting enough milk by assessing weight gain. See **Table 42-1**.

C. Protect the mother's milk supply with compensatory milk removal.

D. Provide as close to a breastfeeding relationship as possible.
   1. Supplementer at the breast if the baby has the ability to transfer milk
   2. Alternative feeding (bottle, finger, etc.) while holding baby against the bare breast

E. If necessary, a woman's 24-hour milk production can be estimated by having her express every hour for four sessions:
   1. The first two expressions will yield more milk than the third and fourth.
   2. Take the third and fourth expressions and add them together. Multiply by 12 to obtain her 24-hour milk production (Lai et al., 2004).

F. In the first week, supplement a newborn as needed with colostrum/donor human milk/formula, per expected intake based on baby's age and weight. See **Table 42-2**.

G. Needs of young babies from 1 week to 3 months:
   1. American/British system, up to 10 pounds: Multiply 2.5 (2 to 3) by the baby's body weight in pounds to obtain the approximate number of ounces needed for 24 hours. Divide by number of feedings.
   2. Metric system, up to 4.5 kilograms: 165 (150 to 200) milliliters times baby's weight in kilograms for number of milliliters needed in 24 hours (Riordan et al., 2010, p. 355).

H. After the first week, infant intake begins to stabilize. By 1 month, most babies are taking in approximately 750–800 milliliters per 24 hours.

Table 42-1 Average weight gain per week for a full–term infant WHO 2006

Age of infant (months)	Grams per week	Ounces per week	WHO boys	WHO girls
0–3	149–243	5–8	208–250–300g 7–8–10 oz	183–216–266 6–7–9 oz
3–6	80.5–143.5	2.5–4.5	140–160–180g 4.6–5.3–6 oz	120–140–180g 4–4.7–6 oz
6–9	44–96	1.5–3.5	80–90–110 2.7–3–3.6 oz	80–100–120g 2.7–3.3–4 oz
9–12	31–81	1–3	60–70–90 2–2.3–3 oz	60–80–100 2–2.7–3.3 oz

VI. Additional Therapies for Increasing Milk Production

    A. Pharmacologic galactogogues

        1. No drug is manufactured specifically for the purpose of increasing milk production; all galactogogue drugs are off-label uses (in United States, not reviewed or approved by the Food and Drug Administration for this application).

        2. Medications in common use (ABM Protocol Committee, 2011):

            a. Metoclopramide (Reglan and Maxeran) is used quite successfully to increase a faltering milk supply, especially in preterm birth situations; some mothers experience depression as a side effect; mothers who have a history of depression might not be good candidates for use of this medication; other mothers find significant benefits from its use.

            b. Domperidone (Motilium) is used for the treatment of certain gastrointestinal disorders; it is quite effective at increasing milk production without the side effects of metoclopramide (de Silva et al., 2001; Gabay, 2002). "Domperidone is the only galactogogue available that has been scientifically evaluated through a randomized, double-blind, placebo-controlled study" (ABM Protocol Committee, 2011). Typical dosage is 10 to 20 milligrams, three to four times daily (Hale, 2010, p. 326). Domperidone is not always available in the United States but may sometimes be available from compounding pharmacies.

        3. Medications not commonly used:

            a. Major tranquilizers such as chlorpromazine (Largactil and Thorazine) and haloperidol (Haldol) typically increase milk production as a side effect; however, significant side effects of sedation, fatigue, and neurologic aberrations preclude their use for insufficient milk supply; sulpiride is used as an antipsychotic in some countries and also increases milk production, but its side effects are similar to tranquilizers, and it is used only in emergency or disaster situations.

Table 42-2 Hospital Guidelines for the Use of Supplementary Feedings

Newborn's age (in hours from birth)	Normal Volume per feed, assuming 8 feeds per 24 hours (in ml. per feed)
1–24	2–10
24–48	5–15
48–72	15–30
72–96	30–60

  b. Thyrotropin-releasing hormone has been used successfully to increase prolactin levels and milk production; in larger doses, side effects can include
  hyperthyroidism.
  c. Human growth hormone has been shown to significantly increase milk production in both term and preterm mothers; adverse effects have not been
  reported in either mothers or babies (Breier et al., 1993; Milsom et al., 1992;
  Milsom et al., 1998).
B. Other medicinal therapies
 1. Oxytocin nasal spray to increase milk flow
  a. Has been used successfully in past (Renfrew et al., 2000; Ruis et al., 1981).
  b. Some conflicting research (Fewtrell et al., 2006). This therapy is likely
  more effective when milk ejection is a real problem than if used as a general
  galactogogue.
 2. Metformin
  a. Normally used to treat type 2 diabetes and PCOS
  b. Has helped increase milk production in some PCOS women (Gabbay et al.,
  2003)
  c. May work by improving insulin resistance, which in turn reduces hyperandrogenism interference with lactation
 3. Recombinant human prolactin (Powe et al., 2010; Welt et al., 2006)
C. Herbal galactogogues (ABM Protocol Committee, 2011; Ayers, 2000; Marasco, 2008).
 1. Have been used for millennia to support and increase a mother's milk supply,
  but more controversial in Western world.
 2. Limited formal research to validate effectiveness.
 3. When effective, galactogogues work best in conjunction with good management (that is, frequent and effective milk removal).
 4. Quality can vary between manufacturers.
 5. Dosage is largely anecdotal due to lack of formal testing.

6. Mothers considering using herbal galactogogues should be provided with available evidence-based resources regarding their impact on milk production and any potential effect on baby. International Board Certified Lactation Consultants (IBCLCs) should record all relevant information, refer to other experts as needed, and work collaboratively with mother's other healthcare providers (International Board of Lactation Consultant Examiners, 2008).
7. Common reputed herbal galactogogues (Abascal et al., 2008; Bruckner, 1993; Humphrey, 2003; Low-Dog, 2009; Whitten, 2010):
   a. Alfalfa (*Medicago sativa*)
   b. Anise seed (*Pimpinella anisum*)
   c. Black seed (*Nigella sativa*)
   d. Blessed thistle (*Cnicus benedictus*)
   e. Caraway seed (*Carum carvi*)
   f. Coriander seed (*Coriandrum sativum*)
   g. Dill seed (*Anethum graveolens*)
   h. Fennel seed (*Foeniculum volgare*)
   i. Fenugreek seed (*Trigonella foenum-graecum*)
   j. Goat's rue (*Galega officinalis*)
   k. Malunggay or Drumstick (*Moringa oleifera*; Briton-Medrano et al., 2002; Estrella et al., 2000)
   l. Marshmallow root (*Althaea officinalis*)
   m. Milk thistle (*Silybum marianum*; Di Pierro et al., 2008)
   n. Nettle (*Urtica urens* or *Urtica dioica*)
   o. Shatavari (*Asparagus racemosus*)
D. Complementary therapies
   1. Imagery/relaxation/hypnosis audiotapes (Becker et al.., 2008; Feder et al., 1989; Pincus, 1996)
   2. Acupuncture/acupressure (Clavey, 1996)
      a. Acupuncture has been used in China for low milk production since A.D. 256 (Clavey, 1996).
      b. Reports indicate that acupuncture is most effective if started within 20 days post delivery; little to no results will be obtained if started after 6 months (Clavey, 1996).
      c. Milk production can start to increase as soon as 2 to 4 hours following treatment or as late as 72 hours; the faster the response, the better the outcome (Clavey, 1996).
      d. There seem to be few (if any) side effects.
   3. Reflexology (Tipping et al., 2000)
   4. Chiropractics to correct subluxations interfering with lactation nerve pathways (Vallone, 2007)

References

Abadie, V., André, A., Zaouche, A., et al. (2001). Early feeding resistance: A possible consequence of neonatal oro-oesophageal dyskinesia. *Acta Paediatrica. 90*, 738–745.

Abascal, K., & Yarnell, E. (2008). Botanical galactagogues. *Alternative and Complementary Therapies, 14*(6), 288–294.

Academy of Breastfeeding Medicine Protocol Committee. (2005). Clinical protocol no. 11: Guidelines for the evaluation and management of neonatal ankyloglossia and its complications in the breastfeeding dyad. *ABM News and Views, 11*, 6–8. Retrieved from http://www.bfmed.org

Academy of Breastfeeding Medicine Protocol Committee. (2006). Clinical protocol no. 13: Contraception during breastfeeding. *Breastfeeding Medicine, 1*, 43–51.

Academy of Breastfeeding Medicine Protocol Committee. (2009). Clinical protocol no. 3: Hospital guidelines for the use of supplementary feedings in the healthy term breastfed neonate. *Breastfeeding Medicine, 4*, 175–182.

Academy of Breastfeeding Medicine Protocol Committee. (2011). Clinical protocol no. 9: Use of galactogogues in initiating or augmenting the ate of maternal milk secretion. *Breastfeeding Medicine, 6*, 41–49.

Agostoni, C., Marangoni, F., Grandi, F., Lammardo, A. M., Giovannini, M., Riva, E., & Galli, C. (2003). Earlier smoking habits are associated with higher serum lipids and lower milk fat and polyunsaturated fatty acid content in the first 6 months of lactation. *European Journal of Clinical Nutrition, 57*, 1466–1472.

Aljazaf, K., Hale, T. W., Ilett, K. F., et al. (2003). Pseudoephedrine: Effects on milk production in women and estimation of infant exposure via breastmilk. *British Journal of Clinical Pharmacology, 56*, 18–24.

Amir, L. (2001). Maternal smoking and reduced duration of breastfeeding: A review of possible mechanisms. *Early Human Development, 64*, 45–67.

Amir, L. H. (2006). Breastfeeding—managing "supply" difficulties. *Australian Family Physician, 35*, 686–689.

Amir, L. H., & Donath, S. M. (2003). Does maternal smoking have a negative physiological effect on breastfeeding? The epidemiological evidence. *Breastfeeding Review, 11*, 19–29.

Andersen, A., Lund-Andersen, C., Larsen, J., et al. (1982). Suppressed prolactin but normal neurophysin levels in cigarette smoking breast-feeding women. *Clinical Endocrinology* (Oxf), *17*, 363–368.

Anderson, A. M. (2001). Disruption of lactogenesis by retained placental fragments. *Journal of Human Lactation, 17*, 142–144.

Andrade, R. A., Coca, K. P., & Abrao, A. C. (2010). Breastfeeding pattern in the first month of life in women submitted to breast reduction and augmentation. *Jornal de pediatria, 86*, 239–244.

Arabin, B., Ruttgers, H., & Kubli, F. (1986). Effects of routine administration of methylergometrin during puerperium on involution, maternal morbidity and lactation. *Geburtshilfe Frauenheilkd, 46*, 215–220.

Araújo Burgos, M. G., Bion, F. M., & Campos, F. (2004). Lactation and alcohol: Clinical and nutritional effects. *Archivos Latinoamericanos de Nutrición, 54*, 25–35.

Auerbach, K. (1990). The effect of nipple shields on maternal milk volume. *Journal of Obstetric, Gynecologic, and Neonatal Nursing, 19*, 419–427.

Ayers, J. F. (2000). The use of alternative therapies in the support of breastfeeding. *Journal of Human Lactation, 16*, 52–56.

Baker, J. L., Michaelsen, K. F., Rasmussen, K. M., & Sorensen, T. I. (2004). Maternal prepregnant body mass index, duration of breastfeeding, and timing of complementary food introduction are associated with infant weight gain. *American Journal of Clinical Nutrition, 80*, 1579–1588.

Ball, D. E., & Morrison, P. (1999). Oestrogen transdermal patches for postpartum depression in lactating mothers—a case report. *Central Africa Journal of Medicine, 45*, 68–70.

Ballard, J. L., Auer, C. E., & Khoury, J. C. (2002). Ankyloglossia: Assessment, incidence, and effect of frenuloplasty on the breastfeeding dyad. *Pediatrics, 110*, e63.

Beck, C. T. (2004). Post-traumatic stress disorder due to childbirth: The aftermath. *Nursing Research, 53*(4), 216–224.

Becker, G. E., McCormick, F. M., & Renfrew, M. J. (2008). Methods of milk expression for lactating women. *Cochrane Database of Systematic Reviews, 4*, CD006170.

Betzold, C., & DeNicola, G. (2010). Progestin-only contraception during lactation: A re-analysis. *Breastfeeding Medicine, 5*, 339.

Betzold, C. M., Hoover, K. L., & Snyder, C. L. (2004). Delayed lactogenesis II: A comparison of four cases. *Journal of Midwifery and Women's Health, 49*, 132–137.

Botta, R., Donatelli, M., Bucalo, M., et al. (1984). Placental lactogen, progesterone, total estriol and prolactin plasma levels in pregnant women with insulin-dependent diabetes mellitus. *European Journal of Obstetrics and Gynecology and Reproductive Biology, 16*, 393–401.

Bowles, B. C., & Williamson, B. P. (1990). Pregnancy and lactation following anorexia and bulimia. *Journal of Obstetric, Gynecologic, and Neonatal Nursing, 19*, 243–248.

Breier, B. H., Milsom, S. R., Blum, W. F., et al. (1993). Insulin-like growth factors and their binding proteins in plasma and milk after growth hormone-stimulated galactopoiesis in normally lactating women. *Acta Endocrinologica, 129*, 427–435.

Briton-Medrano, G., & Perez, L. (2002). The efficacy of malunggay (*Moringa oleifera*) given to near term pregnant women in inducing early postpartum breast milk production—a double blind randomized clinical trial. Unpublished manuscript.

Bruckner, C. (1993). A survey on herbal galactogogues used in Europe. *Medicaments et Aliments: L'Approche Ethnopharmacologique*, 140–145. Retrieved from http://horizon.documentation.ird.fr/exl-doc/pleins_textes/pleins_textes_6/colloques2/010005528.pdf

Burke-Snyder, J. (1997). Bubble palate and failure to thrive: A case report. *Journal of Human Lactation, 13*, 139–143.

Butte, N. F. (2005). Energy requirements of infants. *Public Health and Nutrition, 8*, 953–967.

Caglar, M. K., Ozer, I., & Altugan, F. S. (2006). Risk factors for excess weight loss and hypernatremia in exclusively breast-fed infants. *Brazilian Journal of Medical and Biological Research, 39*, 539–544.

Carlsen, S. M., Jacobsen, G., & Vanky, E. (2010). Mid-pregnancy androgen levels are negatively associated with breastfeeding. *Acta Obstetricia et Gynecologica Scandinavica, 89*, 87–94.

Chantry, C. J., Nommsen-Rivers, L. A., Peerson, J. M., et al. (2011). Excess weight loss in first-born breastfed newborns relates to maternal intrapartum fluid balance. *Pediatrics, 127*, e171–e179.

Chapman, D., & Perez-Escamilla, R. (1999). Does delayed perception of the onset of lactation shorten breastfeeding duration? *Journal of Human Lactation, 15*, 107–110.

Chen, D. C., Nommsen-Rivers, L., Dewey, K. G., & Lonnerdal, B. (1998). Stress during labor and delivery and early lactation performance. *American Journal of Clinical Nutrition, 68*, 335–344.

Chiummariello, S., Cigna, E., Buccheri, E., et al. (2008). Breastfeeding after reduction mammaplasty using different techniques. *Aesthetic Plastic Surgery, 32*, 294–297.

Clavey, S. (1996). The use of acupuncture for the treatment of insufficient lactation (QueRu). *American Journal of Acupuncture, 24*, 35–46.

Cobo, E. (1973). Effect of different doses of ethanol on the milk-ejecting reflex in lactating women. *American Journal of Obstetrics and Gynecology, 115*, 817–821.

Collier, R. J., McNamara, J. P., Wallace, C. R., & Dehoff, M. H. (1984). A review of endocrine regulation of metabolism during lactation. *Journal of Animal Science, 59*(2), 498–510.

Cooper, W., Atherton, H., Kahana, M., & Kotagal, U. (1995). Increased incidence of severe breastfeeding malnutrition and hypernatremia in a metropolitan area. *Pediatrics, 96*, 957–960.

Cowley, K. (2005). Psychogenic and pharmacologic induction of the let-down reflex can facilitate breastfeeding by tetraplegic women: A report of 3 cases. *Archives of Physical Medicine and Rehabilitation, 86*, 1261–1264.

Cox, D., Kent, J., Casey, T., et al. (1999). Breast growth and the urinary excretion of lactose during human pregnancy and early lactation: Endocrine relationships. *Experimental Physiology, 84*, 421–434.

Cregan, M. D. (2007). Complicating influences upon the initiation of lactation following premature birth (abstract A14). *Journal of Human Lactation, 23*, 77.

Cregan, M. D., De Mello, T. R., Kershaw, D., McDougall, K., & Hartmann, P. E. (2002). Initiation of lactation in women after preterm delivery. *Acta Obstetricia et Gynecologica Scandinavica, 81*, 870–877.

Dahl, S. K., Thomas, M. A., Williams, D. B., & Robins, J. C. (2008). Maternal virilization due to luteoma associated with delayed lactation. *Fertility and Sterility, 90*(5), e17–19.

Dahlenburg, G. W., Burnell, R. H., & Braybrook, R. (1980). The relationship between cord serum sodium levels in newborn infants and maternal intravenous therapy during labour. *British Journal of Obstetrics and Gynaecology, 87*, 519–522.

De Araujo Burgos, M.G., Bion, F.M., Campos, F. (2004). Lactation and alcohol: clinical and nutritional effects. *Archivos Latinoamericanos de Nutrición, 54*(1), 25–35.

de Carvalho, M., Robertson, S., Merkatz, R., & Klaus, M. (1982). Milk intake and frequency of feeding in breastfed infants. *Early Human Development, 7*, 155–163.

de Mello, P. R., Pinto, G. R., & Botelho, C. (2001). The influence of smoking on fertility, pregnancy and lactation. *Journal of Pediatrics (Rio J), 77*, 257–264.

de Silva, O. P., Knoppert, D. C., Angeline, M. M., & Forret, P. A. (2001). Effect of domperidone on milk production in mothers of premature newborns: A randomized, double blind, placebo-controlled trial. *Canadian Medical Association Journal, 164*, 17–21.

Dewey, K., Nommsen-Rivers, L., Heinig, M., et al. (2003). Risk factors for suboptimal infant breastfeeding behavior, delayed onset of lactation, and excess neonatal weight loss. *Pediatrics, 112*, 607–619.

Di Pierro, F., Callegari, A., Carotenuto, D., & Tapia, M. M. (2008). Clinical efficacy, safety and tolerability of BIO-C (micronized Silymarin) as a galactagogue. *Acta BioMedica, 79*, 205–210.

Djulus, J., Moretti, M., & Koren, G. (2005). Marijuana use and breastfeeding. *Canadian Family Physician, 51*, 349–350.

Dökmetas, H. S., Kilicli, F., Korkmaz, S., & Yonem, O. (2006). Characteristic features of 20 patients with Sheehan's syndrome. *Gynecological Endocrinology, 22*, 279–283.

Dow, K. H., Harris, J. R., & Roy, C. (1994). Pregnancy after breast-conserving surgery and radiation therapy for breast cancer. *Journal of the National Cancer Institute—Monographs, 16*, 131–137.

Elliott, K. G., Kjolhede, C. L., Gournis, E., & Rasmussen, K. M. (1997). Duration of breastfeeding associated with obesity during adolescence. *Obesity Research, 5*, 538–541.

Engstrom, J. L., Meier, P. P., & Jegier, B. J. (2007). Factors associated with milk output differences from the right and left breasts. *Journal of Human Lactation, 23*, 80.

Escobar, G. J., Gonzales, V. M., Armstrong, M. A., et al. (2002). Rehospitalization for neonatal dehydration. *Archives of Pediatric and Adolescent Medicine, 156*, 155–161.

Estrella, M., Mantaring, J., & David, G. (2000). A double blind, randomised controlled trial on the use of malunggay (*Moringa oleifera*) for augmentation of the volume of breastmilk among non-nursing mothers of preterm infants. *Philippine Journal of Pediatrics, 49*, 3–6.

Feder, S. D., Berger, L. R., Johnson, J. D., & Wilde, J. B. (1989). Increasing breast milk production for premature infants with a relaxation/imagery audiotape. *Pediatrics, 83*, 57–60.

Fenton, S. E., Hamm, J. T., Birnbaum, L. S., & Youngblood, G. L. (2002). Persistent abnormalities in the rat mammary gland following gestational and lactational exposure to 2,3,7,8-Tetrachlorodibenzo-p-dioxin (TCDD). *Toxicological Sciences, 67*, 63–74.

Fernando, C. (1999). *Tongue-tie: From confusion to clarity.* Sydney, Australia: Tandem Publications.

Ferris, A. M., Dalidowitz, C. K., Ingardia, C. M., et al. (1988). Lactation outcome in insulin-dependent diabetic women. *Journal of the American Dietetic Association, 88*(3), 317–322.

Ferris, A. M., & Reece, E. A. (1994). Nutritional consequences of chronic maternal conditions during pregnancy and lactation: Lupus and diabetes. *American Journal of Clinical Nutrition, 59*(Suppl.), 465S–473S.

Fewtrell, M. S., Loh, K. L., Blake, A., et al. (2006). Randomised, double blind trial of oxytocin nasal spray in mothers expressing breast milk for preterm infants. *Archives of Disease in Childhood: Fetal and Neonatal Edition, 91*, F169–F174.

Forlenza, G. P., Paradise Black, N. M., McNamara, E. G., et al. (2010). Ankyloglossia, exclusive breastfeeding, and failure to thrive. *Pediatrics, 125*, e1500–e1504.

Gabay, M. P. (2002). Galactogogues: Medications that induce lactation. *Journal of Human Lactation, 18*, 274–279.

Gabbay, M., & Kelly, H. (2003). Use of metformin to increase breastmilk production in women with insulin resistance: A case series. *ABM News and Views, 9*, 20–21.

Gallas, P. R., Stolk, R. P., Bakker, K., et al. (2002). Thyroid dysfunction in pregnancy and the first postpartum year in women with diabetes mellitus type 1. *European Journal of Endocrinology, 147*, 443–451.

Garbin, C. P., Deacon, J. P., Rowan, M. K., et al. (2009). Association of nipple piercing with abnormal milk production and breastfeeding. *Journal of the American Medical Association, 301*, 2550–2551.

Gatti, L. (2008). Maternal perceptions of insufficient milk supply in breastfeeding. *Image: Journal of Nursing Scholarship, 40*, 355–363.

Geddes, D. T., Kent, J. C., McClellan, H. L., et al. (2010). Sucking characteristics of successfully breastfeeding infants with ankyloglossia: A case series. *Acta Paediatrica, 99*, 301–303.

Geddes, D. T., Langton, D. B., Gollow, I., et al. (2008). Frenulotomy for breastfeeding infants with ankyloglossia: Effect on milk removal and sucking mechanism as imaged by ultrasound. *Pediatrics, 122*, e188–e194.

Gei-Guardia, O., Soto-Herrera, E., Gei-Brealey, A., & Chen-Ku, C. H. (2010). Sheehan's syndrome in Costa Rica: Clinical experience on 60 cases. *Endocrine Practice. 1*, 1–27.

Genna, C. W. (2001). Tactile defensiveness and other sensory modulation difficulties. *Leaven, 37*(3), 51–53.

Genna, C. W. (2013). *Supporting sucking skills in breastfeeding infants.* Burlington, MA: Jones and Bartlett Learning.

Glenny, A. M., Hooper, L., Shaw, W. C., et al. (2005). Feeding interventions for growth and development in infants with cleft lip, cleft palate or cleft lip and palate. *Cochrane Database of Systemic Reviews, 3*, CD003315.

Grange, D. K., & Finlay, J. L. (1994). Nutritional vitamin B$_{12}$ deficiency in a breastfed infant following maternal gastric bypass. *Pediatric Hematology and Oncology, 11*, 311–318.

Guillette, E. A., Conrad, C., Lares, F., et al. (2006). Altered breast development in young girls from an agricultural environment. *Environmental Health Perspectives, 114*, 471–475.

Halbert, L. (1998). Breastfeeding in the woman with a compromised nervous system. *Journal of Human Lactation, 14*, 327–331.

Hale, T., Ilett, K., Hartmann, P., et al. (2004). Pseudoephedrine effects on milk production in women and estimation of infant exposure via human milk. *Advances in Experimental Medicine and Biology, 554*, 437–438.

Hale, T. W. (2010). *Medications and mothers' milk* (14th ed.). Amarillo, TX: Hale Publishing.

Hale, T. W., & Hartmann, P. (2007). *Textbook of human lactation.* Amarillo, TX: Hale Publishing.

Hall, R. T., Mercer, A. M., Teasley, S. L., et al. (2002). A breastfeeding assessment score to evaluate the risk for cessation of breastfeeding by 7 to 10 days. *Journal of Pediatrics, 141*, 659–664.

Hapon, M., Simoncini, M., Via, G., et al. (2003). Effect of hypothyroidism on hormone profiles in virgin, pregnant and lactating rats, and on lactation. *Reproduction, 126*, 371–382.

Hapon, M., Varas, S., Jahn, G., & Gimenez, M. (2005). Effects of hypothyroidism on mammary and liver lipid metabolism in virgin and late-pregnant rats. *Journal of Lipid Research, 46*, 1320–1330.

Harris, L., Morris, S. F., & Freiberg, A. (1992). Is breastfeeding possible after reduction mammaplasty? *Plastic and Reconstructive Surgery, 89*(5), 836–839.

Hartmann, P., & Cregan, M. (2001). Lactogenesis and the effects of insulin-dependent diabetes mellitus and prematurity. *Journal of Nutrition, 131*, 3016S–3020S.

Hartmann, P. E., Owens, R. A., Cox, D. B., & Kent, J. C. (1996). Establishing lactation: Breast development and control of milk synthesis. *Food and Nutrition Bulletin, 17*. Retrieved from http://archive.unu.edu/unupress/food/8F174e/8F174E02.htm

Hazelbaker, A. K. (2010). *Tongue-tie: Morphogenesis, impact, assessment and treatment.* Columbus, OH: Aidan and Eva Press.

Heinig, M. J., Nommsen, L. A., Peerson, J. M., Lonnerdal, B., & Dewey, K. G. (1993). Energy and protein intakes of breast-fed and formula-fed infants during the first year of life and their association with growth velocity: The DARLING study. *American Journal of Clinical Nutrition, 58,* 152–161.

Henderson, J. J., Dickinson, J. E., Evans, S. F., et al. (2003). Impact of intrapartum epidural analgesia on breastfeeding duration. *Australian and New Zealand Journal of Obstetrics and Gynaecology, 43*, 372–377.

Henderson, J. J., Hartmann, P., Newnham, J., & Simmer, K. (2008). Effect of preterm birth and antenatal corticosteroid treatment on lactogenesis II in women. *Pediatrics, 121*, e92–e100.

Henderson, J. J., Newnham, J. P., Simmer, K., & Hartmann, P. E. (2009). Effects of antenatal corticosteroids on urinary markers of the initiation of lactation in pregnant women. *Breastfeeding Medicine, 4*, 201–206.

Henly, S. J., Anderson, C. M., Avery, M. D., et al. (1995). Anemia and insufficient milk in first-time mothers. *Birth, 22*, 87–92.

Hill, P. D., Aldag, J. C., & Chatterton, R. T. (2001). Initiation and frequency of pumping and milk production in mothers of nonnursing preterm infants. *Journal of Human Lactation, 17*, 9–13.

Hill, P. D., Aldag, J. C., Chatterton, R. T., & Zinaman, M. (2005). Comparison of milk output between mothers of preterm and term infants: The first 6 weeks after birth. *Journal of Human Lactation, 21*, 22–30.

Hilson, J. A., Rasmussen, K. M., & Kjolhede, C. L. (1997). Maternal obesity and breastfeeding success in a rural population of white women. *American Journal of Clinical Nutrition, 66*, 1371–1378.

Hilson, J. A., Rasmussen, K. M., & Kjolhede, C. L. (2004). High prepregnant body mass index is associated with poor lactation outcomes among white, rural women independent of psychosocial and demographic correlates. *Journal of Human Lactation, 20*, 18–29.

Hilson, J. A., Rasmussen, K. M., & Kjolhede, C. L. (2006). Excessive weight gain during pregnancy is associated with earlier termination of breast-feeding among white women. *Journal of Nutrition, 136*, 140–146.

Holmes, A. V., Auinger, P., & Howard, C. R. (2011). Combination feeding of breast milk and formula: Evidence for shorter breastfeeding duration from the national health and nutrition examination survey. *Journal of Pediatrics, 159*(2), 186–191.

Hond, E. D., Roels, H. A., Hoppenbrouwers, K., et al. (2002). Sexual maturation in relation to polychlorinated aromatic hydrocarbons: Sharpe and Skakkebaek's hypothesis revisited. *Environmental Health Perspectives, 8*, 771–776.

Hoover, K. L., Barbalinardo, L. H., & Platia, M. P. (2002). Delayed lactogenesis II secondary to gestational ovarian theca lutein cysts in two normal singleton pregnancies. *Journal of Human Lactation, 18*, 264–268.

Hopkinson, J., Schanler, R., Fraley, J., et al. (1992). Milk production by mothers of premature infants: Influence of cigarette smoking. *Pediatrics, 90*, 934–938.

Huggins, K. E., Petok, E. S., & Mireles, O. (2000). Markers of lactation insufficiency: A study of 34 mothers. In K. Auerbach (Ed.), *Current issues in clinical lactation 2000* (pp. 25–35). Sudbury, MA: Jones and Bartlett.

Hummel, S., Hummel, M., Knopff, A., Bonifacio, E., & Ziegler, A. G. (2008). Breastfeeding in women with gestational diabetes. *Deutsche Medizinische Wochenschrift, 133*, 180–184.

Humphrey, S. (2003). *The nursing mother's herbal*. Minneapolis, MN: Fairview Press.

Hurst, N. M. (1996). Lactation after augmentation mammoplasty. *Obstetrics and Gynecology, 87*, 30–34.

Hurst, N. M. (2007). Recognizing and treating delayed or failed lactogenesis II. *Journal of Midwifery and Women's Health, 52*, 588–594.

Institute of Medicine. (1991). *Nutrition during lactation*. Washington, DC: National Academy Press.

International Board of Lactation Consultant Examiners. (2008). *Scope of practice for International Board certified lactation consultants*. Retrieved from http://www.iblce.org/upload/downloads/ScopeOfPractice.pdf

Janssen, O., Mehlmauer, N., Hahn, S., et al. (2004). High prevalence of autoimmune thyroiditis in patients with polycystic ovary syndrome. *European Journal of Endocrinology, 150*, 363–369.

Jordan, S., Emery, S., Watkins, A., et al. (2009). Associations of drugs routinely given in labour with breastfeeding at 48 hours: Analysis of the Cardiff Births Survey. *BJOG, 116*(12), 1622–1632. doi:10.1111/j.1471-0528.2009.02256x

Kamikawa, A., Ichii, O., Yamaji, D., et al. (2009). Diet-induced obesity disrupts ductal development in the mammary glands of nonpregnant mice. *Developmental Dynamics, 238*, 1092–1099.

Kennedy, K. I., Short, R. V., & Tully, M. R. (1997). Premature introduction of progestin-only contraceptive methods during lactation. *Contraception, 55*, 347–350.

Kent, J. (2007). How breastfeeding works. *Journal of Midwifery and Women's Health, 52*, 564–570.

Kent, J., Mitoulas, L., Cox, D., et al. (1999). Breast volume and milk production during extended lactation in women. *Experimental Physiology, 84*, 435–447.

Kent, J. C., Mitoulas, L. R., Cregan, M. D., et al. (2006). Volume and frequency of breastfeedings and fat content of breast milk throughout the day. *Pediatrics, 117*, 387–395.

Knight, C. H., & Sorenson, A. (2001). Windows in early mammary development: Critical or not? *Reproduction, 122*, 337–345.

Knox, J. (2010). Tongue tie and frenotomy in the breastfeeding newborn. *NeoReviews, 11*, e513–e519.

Kotlow, L. A. (2010). The influence of the maxillary frenum on the development and pattern of dental caries on anterior teeth in breastfeeding infants: Prevention, diagnosis, and treatment. *Journal of Human Lactation, 26*(3), 304–308.

Kugyelka, J. G., Rasmussen, K. M., & Frongillo, E. A. (2004). Maternal obesity is negatively associated with breastfeeding success among Hispanic but not black women. *Journal of Nutrition, 134*, 1746–1753.

Lai, C. T., Hale, T., Kent, J., et al. (2004). *Hourly rate of milk synthesis in women*. Cambridge, England: International Society for Research into Human Milk and Lactation.

Lau, C., Sullivan, M., & Hazelwood, R. (1993). Effects of diabetes mellitus on lactation in the rat. *Proceedings of the Society for Experimental Biology and Medicine, 204*, 81–89.

Lawrence, R. A., & Lawrence, R. M. (2011). *Breastfeeding: A guide for the medical profession* (7th ed.). Maryland Heights, MO: Elsevier Mosby.

Leeners, B., Rath, W., Kuse, S., & Neumaier-Wagner, P. (2005). Breast-feeding in women with hypertensive disorders in pregnancy. *Journal of Perinatal Medicine, 33*, 553–560.

Leung, G. M., Lam, T.-H., & Ho, L.-M. (2002). Breastfeeding and its relation to smoking and mode of delivery. *American College of Obstetrics and Gynecology, 99*, 785–794.

Lew, B. J., Collins, L. L., O'Reilly, M. A., & Lawrence, B. P. (2009). Activation of the aryl hydrocarbon receptor (AhR) during different critical windows in pregnancy alters mammary epithelial cell proliferation and differentiation. *Toxicological Sciences, 111*(1), 151–162.

Lewis, B. C., Hudgins, S., Lewis, A., et al. (2001). In utero and lactation treatment with 2,3,7,8-tetrachlorodibenzo-p-dioxin impairs mammary gland differentiation but does not block the response to exogenous estrogen in the postpubertal female rat. *Toxicological Sciences, 62*, 46–53.

Livingstone, V. H., Willis, C. E., Abdel-Wareth, L. O., et al. (2000). Neonatal hypernatremic dehydration associated with breast-feeding malnutrition: A retrospective survey. *Canadian Medical Association Journal, 162*, 647–652.

Loveclady, C. A. (2005). Is maternal obesity a cause of poor lactation performance. *Nutrition Reviews, 63*, 352–355.

Low Dog, T. (2009). The use of botanicals during pregnancy and lactation. *Alternative Therapies in Health and Medicine, 15*, 54–58.

Manfro, A. R., Manfro, R., & Bortoluzzi, M. C. (2010). Surgical treatment of ankyloglossia in babies—case report. *International Journal of Oral and Maxillofacial Surgery, 39*, 1130–1132.

Marasco, L. (2006). The impact of thyroid dysfunction on lactation. *Breastfeeding Abstracts, 25*, 9–12.

Marasco, L. (2008). Inside track. Increasing your milk supply with galactogogues. *Journal of Human Lactation, 24*(4), 455.

Marasco, L. (2009). Lactation. In L. Jovanovic (Ed.), *Medical management of pregnancy complicated by diabetes* (4th ed., pp. 83–86). Alexandria, VA: American Diabetes Association.

Marasco, L., & Barger, J. (1998). Cue vs scheduled feeding: Revisiting the controversy. *Mother–Baby Journal, 3*(4), 39–42.

Marasco, L., Marmet, C., & Shell, E. (2000). Polycystic ovary syndrome: A connection to insufficient milk supply? *Journal of Human Lactation, 16*, 143–148.

Markey, C., Rubin, B., Soto, A., & Sonnenschein, C. (2003). Endocrine disruptors: From Wingspread to environmental developmental biology. *Journal of Steroid Biochemistry and Molecular Biology, 83*, 235–244.

Marquis, G. S., Penny, M. E., Diaz, J. M., & Marin, R. M. (2002). Postpartum consequences of an overlap of breastfeeding and pregnancy: Reduced breast milk intake and growth during early infancy. *Pediatrics, 109*, e56.

Marshall, A. M., Nommsen-Rivers, L. A., Hernandez, L. L., et al. (2010). Serotonin transport and metabolism in the mammary gland modulates secretory activation and involution. *Journal of Clinical Endocrinology and Metabolism, 95*, 837–846.

Martens, W. S., 2nd, Martin, L. F., Berlin, C. M., Jr. (1990). Failure of a nursing infant to thrive after the mother's gastric bypass for morbid obesity. *Pediatrics, 86*, 777–778.

McClellan, H., Geddes, D., Kent, J., et al. (2008). Infants of mothers with persistent nipple pain exert strong sucking vacuums. *Acta Paediatrica, 97*, 1205–1209.

McCullough, L., Ng, A., Najita, J., et al. (2010). Breastfeeding in survivors of Hodgkin lymphoma treated with chest radiotherapy. *Cancer, 116*, 4866–4871.

McMillan, J. A. (Ed.). (2006). *Oski's pediatrics: Principles and practice* (4th ed., p. 382). Philadelphia, PA: Lippincott Williams & Wilkins.

Mennella, J. A. (2001a). Alcohol's effect on lactation. *Alcohol Research and Health, 25*, 230–234.

Mennella, J. A. (2001b). Regulation of milk intake after exposure to alcohol in mothers' milk. *Alcoholism: Clinical and Experimental Research, 25*, 590–593.

Mennella, J. A., & Pepino, M. Y. (2008). Biphasic effects of moderate drinking on prolactin during lactation. *Alcoholism: Clinical and Experimental Research, 32*, 1899–1908.

Mennella, J. A., & Pepino, M. Y. (2010). Breastfeeding and prolactin levels in lactating women with a family history of alcoholism. *Pediatrics, 125*, e1162–e1170.

Mennella, J. A., Pepino, M. Y., & Teff, K. L. (2005). Acute alcohol consumption disrupts the hormonal milieu of lactating women. *Journal of Clinical Endocrinology and Metabolism, 90*, 1979–1985.

Michalopoulos, K. (2007). The effects of breast augmentation surgery on future ability to lactate. *Breast Journal, 13*, 62–67.

Milsom, S. R., Breier, B. H., Gallaher, B. W, et al. (1992). Growth hormone stimulates galactopoiesis in healthy lactating women. *Acta Endocrinologica, 127*, 337–343.

Milsom, S. R., Rabone, D. L., Gunn, A. J., & Gluckman, P. D. (1998). Potential role for growth hormone in human lactation insufficiency. *Hormonal Research, 50*, 147–150.

Miranda, B. H., & Milroy, C. J. (2010). A quick snip: A study of the impact of outpatient tongue tie release on neonatal growth and breastfeeding. *Journal of Plastic Reconstructive Aesthetic Surgery, 63*, e683–e685.

Miyake, A., Tahara, M., Koike, K., & Tanizawa, O. (1989). Decrease in neonatal suckled milk volume in diabetic women. *European Journal of Obstetrics and Gynecology and Reproductive Biology, 33*, 49–53.

Mohrbacher, N. (2011). The magic number and long-term milk production. *Clinical Lactation, 2*, 15–18.

Monteleone, P., Brambilla, F., Bortolotti, F., et al. (1998). Plasma prolactin response to D-fenfluramine is blunted in bulimic patients with frequent binge episodes. *Psychological Medicine, 28*, 975–983.

Moral, R., Wang, R., Russo, I. H., et al. (2008). Effect of prenatal exposure to the endocrine disruptor bisphenol A on mammary gland morphology and gene expression signature. *Journal of Endocrinology, 196*, 101–112.

Morton, J., Hall, J. Y., Wong, R. J., et al. (2009). Combining hand techniques with electric pumping increases milk production in mothers of preterm infants. *Journal of Perinatology, 29*, 757–764.

Motil, K. J., Sheng, H.-P., & Montandon, C. M. (1994). Case report: Failure to thrive in a breastfed infant is associated with maternal dietary protein and energy restriction. *Journal of the American College of Nutrition, 13*, 203–208.

Neifert, M., DeMarzo, S., Seacat, J., et al. (1990). The influence of breast surgery, breast appearance, and pregnancy-induced breast changes on lactation sufficiency as measured by infant weight gain. *Birth, 17*, 31–38.

Neifert, M. R., McDonough, S. L., & Neville, M. C. (1981). Failure of lactogenesis associated with placental retention. *American Journal of Obstetrics and Gynecology, 140*, 477–478.

Neifert, M. R., & Seacat, J. M. (1987). Lactation insufficiency; a rational approach. *Birth, 14*, 182–190.

Neifert, M. R., Seacat, J. M., & Jobe, W. E. (1985). Lactation failure due to insufficient glandular development of the breast. *Pediatrics, 76*, 823–828.

Neubauer, S. H., Ferris, A. M., Chase, C. G., et al. (1993). Delayed lactogenesis in women with insulin-dependent diabetes mellitus. *American Journal of Clinical Nutrition, 58*, 54–60.

Neville, M., & Morton, J. (2001). Physiology and endocrine changes underlying human lactogenesis II. *Journal of Nutrition, 131*, 3005S–3008S.

Nommsen-Rivers, L. A., Chantry, C. J., Peerson, J. M., Cohen, R. J., & Dewey, K. G. (2010). Delayed onset of lactogenesis among first-time mothers is related to maternal obesity and factors associated with ineffective breastfeeding. *American Journal of Clinical Nutrition, 92*, 574–584.

Nommsen-Rivers, L. A., Dolan, L. M., & Huang, B. (2011). Timing of stage II lactogenesis is predicted by antenatal metabolic health in a cohort of primiparas. *Breastfeeding Medicine, 7*, 43–49.

Nommsen-Rivers, L. A., Heinig, M. J., Cohen, R. J., & Dewey, K. G. (2008). Newborn wet and soiled diaper counts and timing of onset of lactation as indicators of breastfeeding inadequacy. *Journal of Human Lactation, 24*, 27–33.

O'Brien, L. M., Heycock, E. G., Hanna, M., et al. (2004). Postnatal depression and faltering growth: A community study. *Pediatrics, 113*, 1242–1247.

O'Dowd, R., Wlodek, M. E., & Nicholas, K. R. (2008). Uteroplacental insufficiency alters the mammary gland response to lactogenic hormones in vitro. *Reproduction, Fertility, and Development, 20*, 460–465.

Ostrom, K. M., & Ferris, A. M. (1993). Prolactin concentrations in serum and milk of mothers with and without insulin-dependent diabetes mellitus. *American Journal of Clinical Nutrition, 58*, 49–53.

Park, H. J., Kim, J., Rhee, Y., Park, Y. W., & Kwon, J. Y. (2010). Antepartum pituitary necrosis occurring in pregnancy with uncontrolled gestational diabetes mellitus: A case report. *Journal of Korean Medical Science, 25*, 794.

Paul, A. A., Muller, E. M., & Whitehead, R. G. (1979). The quantitative effects of maternal dietary energy intake on pregnancy and lactation in rural Gambian women. *Transactions of the Royal Society of Tropical Medicine and Hygiene, 73*, 686–692.

Picciano, M. F. (2003). Pregnancy and lactation: Physiological adjustments, nutritional requirements and the role of dietary supplements. *Journal of Nutrition, 133*, 1997S–2002S.

Pincus, L. (1996). How hypnosis can help increase breast milk production. *Medela Round-Up, 13*, 5.

Powe, C. E., Allen, M., Puopolo, K. M., et al. (2010). Recombinant human prolactin for the treatment of lactation insufficiency. *Clinical Endocrinology, 73*, 645–653.

Rainer, C., Gardetto, A., Frühwirth, M., et al. (2003). Breast deformity in adolescence as a result of pneumothorax drainage during neonatal intensive care. *Pediatrics, 111*, 80–86.

Rasmussen, K. (2007). Association of maternal obesity before conception with poor lactation performance. *Annual Review of Nutrition, 27*, 103–121.

Rasmussen, K. M., Hilson, J. A., & Kjolhede, C. L. (2001). Obesity may impair lactogenesis II. *Journal of Nutrition, 131*, 3009S–3011S.

Rasmussen, K. M., & Kjolhede, C. L. (2004). Prepregnant overweight and obesity diminish the prolactin response to suckling in the first week postpartum. *Pediatrics, 113*, e465–e471.

Rasmussen, K. M., Lee, V. E., Ledkovsky, T. B., & Kjolhede, C. L. (2006). A description of lactation counseling practices that are used with obese mothers. *Journal of Human Lactation, 22*, 322–327.

Renfrew, M. J., Lang, S., & Woolridge, M. (2000). Oxytocin for promoting successful lactation. *Cochrane Database of Systematic Reviews, 2*, CD000156.

Revai, K., Briars, L., & Cochran, K. (2010). Case series of Sjögren's syndrome and poor milk supply. *Breastfeeding Medicine, 5*, 332. doi:10.1089/bfm.2010.9982

Riordan, J., & Wambach, K. (2010). *Breastfeeding and human lactation* (4th ed.). Sudbury, MA: Jones and Bartlett.

Rosato, R., Gimenez, M., & Jahn, G. (1992). Effects of chronic thyroid hormone administration on pregnancy, lactogenesis, and lactation in the rat. *Acta Endocrinologica* (Copenh), *127*, 547–554.

Rosenfield, N. S., Haller, J. O., & Berdon, W. E. (1989). Failure of development of the growing breast after radiation therapy. *Pediatric Radiology, 19*, 124–127.

Roy, J. R., Chakraborty, S., & Chakraborty, T. R. (2009). Estrogen-like endocrine disrupting chemicals affecting puberty in humans—a review. *Medical Science Monitor, 15*, RA137–145.

Ruis, H., Rolland, R., Doesburg, W., et al. (1981). Oxytocin enhances onset of lactation among mothers delivering prematurely. *British Medical Journal (Clinical Research Edition), 283*, 340–342.

Saint, L., Maggiore, P., & Hartmann, P. E. (1986). Yield and nutrient content of milk in eight women breastfeeding twins and one woman breastfeeding triplets. *British Journal of Nutrition, 56*, 49–58.

Seng, J. (2010). Posttraumatic oxytocin dysregulation: Is it a link among posttraumatic self-disorder, posttraumatic stress disorder, and pelvic visceral dysregulation conditions in women? *Journal of Trauma and Dissociation, 11*, 387–406.

Sheehan, H. L., & Murdoch, R. (1938). Post-partum necrosis of the anterior pituitary: Pathological and clinical aspects. *Journal of Obstetrics and Gynaecology of the British Empire, 45*, 456–489.

Shrago, L. C. (2006). The neonatal bowel output study: Indicators of adequate breast milk intake in neonates. *Pediatric Nursing, 32*, 195–201.

Smith, C., & Valentine, C. (2006). Early hormonal contraception associated with increased galactogogue use. *Journal of Human Lactation, 22*, 469–470.

Soltani, H., & Arden, M. (2009). Factors associated with breastfeeding up to 6 months postpartum in mothers with diabetes. *Journal of Obstetric, Gynecologic, and Neonatal Nursing, 38*, 586–594.

Souto, G. C., Giugliani, E. R. J., Giugliani, C., & Schneider, M. A. (2003). The impact of breast reduction surgery on breastfeeding performance. *Journal of Human Lactation, 19*, 43–49.

Stagnaro-Green, A. (2002). Postpartum thyroiditis. *Journal of Clinical Endocrinology and Metabolism, 87*, 4042–4047.

Stefanski, J. (2006). Breastfeeding after bariatric surgery. *Today's Dietitian, 8*, 47–50.

Stein, M. (2002). Failure to thrive in a four-month-old nursing infant. *Journal of Developmental and Behavioral Pediatr*ics, *23*, S69–S73.

Stutte, P., Bowles, B., & Morman, G. (1988). The effects of breast massage on volume and fat content of human milk. *Genesis, 10*, 22–25.

Taki, M., Mizuno, K., Murase, M., et al. (2010). Maturational changes in the feeding behaviour of infants—a comparison between breast-feeding and bottle-feeding. *Acta Paediatrica, 99*, 61–67.

Thompson, J. F., Heal, L. J., Roberts, C. L., & Ellwood, D. A. (2010). Women's breastfeeding experiences following a significant primary postpartum haemorrhage: A multicentre cohort study. *International Breastfeeding Journal, 5*, 5.

Tipping, L., & Mackereth, P. A. (2000). A concept analysis: The effect of reflexology on homeostasis to establish and maintain lactation. *Complementary Therapies in Nursing and Midwifery, 6*, 189–198.

University of Rochester Medical Center. (2009, June 9). Dioxins in food chain linked to breastfeeding ills. *Science Daily.*

Vallone, S. A. (2007). The role of subluxation and chiropractic care in hypolactation. *Journal of Clinical Chiropractic Pediatrics, 8*, 518–524.

Vanky, E., Isaksen, H., Moen, M. H., & Carlsen, S. M. (2008). Breastfeeding in polycystic ovary syndrome. *Acta Obstetricia et Gynecologica Scandinavica, 87*, 531–535.

Vio, F., Salazar, G., & Infante, C. (1991). Smoking during pregnancy and lactation and its effects on breast-milk volume. *American Journal of Clinical Nutrition, 54*, 1011–1016.

Vorderstrasse, B., Fenton, S., Bohn, A., et al. (2004). A novel effect of dioxin: Exposure during pregnancy severely impairs mammary gland differentiation. *Toxicological Sciences, 78*, 248–257.

Wall, V., & Glass, R. (2006). Mandibular asymmetry and breastfeeding problems: Experience from 11 cases. *Journal of Human Lactation, 22*, 328–334.

Wardinsky, T. D., Montes, R. G., Friederich, R. L., et al. (1995). Vitamin B_{12} deficiency associated with low breast-milk vitamin B_{12} concentration in an infant following maternal gastric bypass surgery. *Archives of Pediatric and Adolescent Medicine, 149*, 1281–1284.

Weiss-Salinas, D., & Williams, N. (2001). Sensory defensiveness: A theory of its effect on breastfeeding. *Journal of Human Lactation, 17*(2), 145–151.

Weldon, R. H., Webster, M., Harley, K. G., et al. (2010). Serum persistent organic pollutants and duration of lactation among Mexican-American women. *Journal of Environmental and Public Health, 2010*, 861757.

Welt, C., Page-Wilson, G., & Smith, P. (2006, November 4–6). *Recombinant human prolactin is biologically active: Potential treatment for lactation insufficiency.* Paper presented at American Public Health Association annual meeting, Boston, MA.

Weltzin, T., McConaha, C., MeKee, M., et al. (1991). Circadian patterns of cortisol, prolactin, and growth hormone secretion during bingeing and vomiting in normal weight bulimic patients. *Biological Psychiatry, 30*, 37–48.

West, D., & Marasco, L. (2009). *The breastfeeding mother's guide to making more milk.* New York, NY: McGraw-Hill.

Whitten, D. (2010). Expert opinion: Addressing concerns about breastmilk supply: Simple steps to prevent premature cessation of breastfeeding. *Global Natural Medicine,* November 2010*;* Retrieved March 23, 2012: http://www.globalnaturalmedicine.com/expert-opinion-003/

Wight, N. E. (2003). Breastfeeding the borderline (near-term) preterm infant. *Pediatric Annals, 32*, 329–336.

Wilde, C. J., Addey, C. V., Boddy, L. M., & Peaker, M. (1995). Autocrine regulation of milk secretion by a protein in milk. *Biochemistry Journal, 305*, 51–58.

Williams, N. (1997). Maternal psychological issues in the experience of breastfeeding. *Journal of Human Lactation, 13*(1), 57–60.

Williams, N. (2002). Supporting the mother coming to terms with persistent insufficient milk supply: The role of the lactation consultant. *Journal of Human Lactation, 18*, 262–263.

Willis, C., & Livingstone, V. (1995). Infant insufficient milk syndrome associated with maternal postpartum hemorrhage. *Journal of Human Lactation, 11*, 123–126.

Wilson-Clay, B., & Hoover, K. (2008). *The breastfeeding atlas* (4th ed.). Austin, TX: LactNews Press.

Wilson-Clay, B., & Maloney, B. M. (2002). A reporting tool to facilitate community-based follow-up for at-risk breastfeeding dyads at hospital discharge. In K. G. Auerbach (Ed.), *Current issues in clinical lactation* (pp. 59–67). Sudbury, MA: Jones and Bartlett.

Wilton, J. M. (1998). Cleft palates and breastfeeding. *AWHONN Lifelines, 2*, 11.

Wlodek, M. E., Ceranic, V., O'Dowd, R., et al. (2009). Maternal progesterone treatment rescues the mammary impairment following uteroplacental insufficiency and improves postnatal pup growth in the rat. *Reproductive Sciences, 16*, 380–390.

Wolff, M. S., Britton, J. A., Boguski, L., et al. (2008). Environmental exposures and puberty in inner-city girls. *Environmental Research, 107*, 393–400.

Woolridge, M. (1996). Problems of establishing lactation. *Food and Nutrition Bulletin, 17*, 316–323. Available: http://archive.unu.edu/unupress/food/8F174e/8F174E06.htm

Woolridge, M. W., Baum, J. D., & Drewett, R. F. (1980). Effect of a traditional and of a new nipple shield on sucking patterns and milk flow. *Early Human Development, 4*, 357–364.

WHO Working Group on the Growth Reference Protocol and WHO Task Force on Methods for the Natural Regulation of Fertility. (2000). Growth patterns of breastfed infants in seven countries. *Acta Paediatrica, 89*, 215–222.

World Health Organization. (n.d.). WHO child growth standards. Retrieved from http://www.who.int/childgrowth/standards/chts_boys_p.pdf and http://www.who.int/childgrowth/standards/chts_girls_p.pdf

World Health Organization. (n.d.). WHO growth charts from the Centers for Disease Control. Retrieved March 2012; Boys: *http://www.cdc.gov/growthcharts/data/who/grchrt_boys_24lw_9210.pdf* Girls: http://www.cdc.gov/growthcharts/data/who/grchrt_girls_24lw_9210.pdf

Yaseen, H., Salem, M., & Darwich, M. (2004). Clinical presentation of hypernatremic dehydration in exclusively breast-fed neonates. *Indian Journal of Pediatrics, 71*, 1059–1062.

Yurdakök, K., Özmert, E., & Yalçin, S. S. (1997). Physical examination of breast-fed infants. *Archives of Pediatric and Adolescent Medicine, 151*, 429–430.

Zargar, A. H., Masoodl, S. R., Laway, B. A., et al. (1997). Familial puerperal alactogenesis: Possibility of a genetically transmitted isolated prolactin deficiency. *British Journal of Obstetrics and Gynaecology, 104*, 629–631.

Zargar, A. H., Salahuddin, M., Laway, B. A., et al. (2000). Puerperal alactogenesis with normal prolactin dynamics: Is prolactin resistance the cause? *Fertility and Sterility, 74*, 598–600.

CHAPTER 43
Slow Weight Gain and Failure to Thrive

Roberto Mario Silveira Issler, PhD, MD, IBCLC; and
Barbara Wilson-Clay, BS, IBCLC, FILCA

OBJECTIVES

- Distinguish between slow weight gain and failure to thrive.
- List the main causes of slow weight gain and failure to thrive.
- Discuss and assess parameters for an infant who is slow to gain weight.
- Develop appropriate management strategies according to the etiology of the slow weight gain.
- Develop appropriate management strategies to manage the infant with failure to thrive, including feeding for recovery weight gain, test weighing, and augmented breast stimulation.

INTRODUCTION

Inadequate weight gain in the breastfed infant is a condition that occurs mainly in infants younger than 6 months of age. Growth faltering is generally reversible once identified. True failure to thrive (FTT) is potentially dangerous, requiring early recognition and corrective action. FTT beyond 1 month of age is often associated with organic illness of the mother or baby (Emond et al., 2007; Lawrence et al., 2011; Lukefahr, 1990). Once identified, clinicians have a responsibility to provide effective lactation support and to document the recovery of infants who have lost excessive weight or who gain at a rate below the 10th percentile beyond 1 month of age (Iver et al., 2008).

I. Definitions

    A. Slow weight gain (Powers, 2001)

        1. Breastfed infants grow robustly in the first few months following birth (Dewey et al., 1992). Deviations from this normal pattern merit evaluation. When infants and children gain weight consistently, although slowly, this condition may be familial or genetic.

2. Slow weight gain can become problematic in the following situations:
   a. An infant is small for gestational age (SGA) (Lawrence et al., 2011).
      i. SGA infants often have feeding difficulty and their caloric needs match the requirements of an infant of appropriate weight for gestation.
      ii. Their intake should be calculated at a higher level than their birth weight suggests.
   b. A newborn infant who is less than 2 weeks of age is more than 10% below birth weight.
      i. Clinicians should be aware that once infants lose an excess percentage of their birth weight, their sucking often becomes weak and ineffective.
      ii. Such infants may be at the breast continuously without being able to remove enough milk to recover lost weight.
      iii. Mothers should be instructed to augment breast emptying with hand expression or a breast pump to bring in a full milk supply and to collect milk for supplementation until the infant recovers birth weight.
   c. An infant's weight at 2 weeks is less than birth weight.
   d. An infant has no urine and stool output in any given 24-hour period during the first month of life (Lawrence & Lawrence, 2011). (See the subsection "Infant Aspects" in "VI. Taking a History.")
   e. An infant has stools that have not changed to a yellow color by the end of the first week.
   f. An infant has clinical signs of dehydration.
B. Failure to thrive
   1. Rate of weight gain is less than the −2 SD (standard deviation) value during an interval of 2 months or longer for infants less than 6 months of age, or 3 months or longer for infants older than 6 months of age, and the weight for length is less than the 5th percentile (Fomon et al., 1993).
   2. Definition of FTT according to Lawrence et al. (2011) is as follows:
      a. Infant continues to lose weight after 10 days of life.
      b. Does not regain birth weight by 3 weeks of age.
      c. Gains at a rate below the 10th percentile for weight beyond 1 month of age.

II. Growth of Breastfed Children Is Normally Robust

A. The World Health Organization (WHO, 2007) Child Growth Standards establish the breastfed infant as the standard for measuring healthy growth. The International Growth Reference from the U.S. National Center for Health Statistics, which is based on predominantly formula-fed infants, is inadequate for the breastfed infant.
B. A key characteristic of the new standard is that it shows how children should grow when their health and housing needs are properly met and they are exclusively breastfed for 6 months. It is recommended by the WHO that children breastfeed (along with receiving complementary solid foods) until the end of the second year (WHO, 2007).

1. According to the WHO references, a fully breastfed girl gains an average of 1,000 grams in the first month, 900 grams in the second month, 700 grams in the third month, and 600 grams in the fourth month of life.
2. A fully breastfed boy gains an average of 1,200 grams in the first month, 1,100 grams in the second month, 800 grams in the third month, and 600 grams in the fourth month.

III. Distinction Between Slow Weight Gain and Failure to Thrive

A. Slow weight gain
   1. Alert, responsive, and a healthy appearance
   2. Normal muscle tone and skin turgor
   3. Dilute urine, six or more times per day
   4. Frequent stools (or infrequent, but large amount)
   5. Good suck with swallowing heard for the majority of the feeding
   6. Eight or more breastfeeds per day with infant determining length of feeding (Lawrence et al., 2011)
   7. Efficient milk ejection reflex
   8. Weight gain slow, but consistent
B. Failure to thrive
   1. Apathetic or weakly crying infant
   2. Poor muscle tone and skin turgor
   3. Concentrated urine, a few times per day
   4. Infrequent, scanty stools
   5. Fewer than eight breastfeeds per day, usually brief, or constant feeding with poor intake
   6. No or erratic signs of milk ejection reflex
   7. Poor and erratic weight gain or no weight gain
   8. Swallowing only with the milk ejection reflex or sporadic swallowing

IV. Conditions Associated with Infant Weight Gain Problems (Table 43-1)

A. Poor intake
   1. Poor latch, poor sucking
   2. Physical and/or structural factors
      a. Cleft lip/palate
      b. Short frenulum
      c. Micrognathia
      d. Macroglossia
      e. Choanal atresia
      f. Tracheomalacia or laryngomalacia
   3. Preterm (Lucas et al., 1997), near-term, postterm, small for gestational age (SGA), intrauterine growth restriction (IUGR), large for gestational age (LGA) (may lack mature feeding skills)

Table 43-1 Infant Factors That May Contribute to Slow Weight Gain

Factor	Effect
Gestational age and growth	Preterm, near-term, postterm, SGA, IUGR, and LGA infants may lack mature feeding skills. Provision of breastmilk is especially important for SGA infants because it promotes better catch-up growth in head circumference (brain growth) than supplementing with a standard formula (Lucas et al., 1997).
Alterations in oral anatomy	Alterations such as ankyloglossia, cleft lip, cleft of hard or soft palate, bubble palate, facial growth anomalies such as micrognathia, or congenital syndromes that affect the oral structure may contribute to poor milk intake.
Alterations in oral functioning	Hypotonia, hypertonia, neurologic pathology or physiology that may interfere with the performance, strength, or stamina of the structures involved in the suck, swallow, breathe cycling.
High energy requirements	Cardiac disease, respiratory involvement (bronchopulmonary dysplasia—BPD), metabolic disorders that create a need for increased caloric intake or volume restriction that place limits on intake.
Known illness	Infection, trisomy 21, cystic fibrosis, or cardiac defects often put the infant at risk for poor growth because of the combination of a low endurance for feeding and high metabolic demands. Growth faltering may be apparent in the early months due to atopic dermatitis (Agostoni et al., 2000).
Maternal medications	Certain prenatal prescription medications or recreational drugs may interfere with normal sucking physiology.
Intrapartum factors	Cesarean delivery, hypoxia, anoxia, labor medications, state control difficulties, epidural analgesia, forceps, and vacuum extraction that affect brain function, anatomical structures, and nerves, contributing to ineffective milk transfer.
Iatrogenic factors	Hospital routines that separate mothers and infants, provide inappropriate supplementation, offer pacifiers, or provide conflicting or poor breastfeeding instruction leave both mothers and infants lacking needed feeding skills.
Gastrointestinal or metabolic/ malabsorption problems	Gastroesophageal reflux or other conditions that limit nutrient intake or metabolism.

   B. Peripartum factors
      1. Meperidine and bupivacaine given to mothers during labor were associated with short-term infant neurological depression and resultant poor feeding (Lawrence et al., 2011).

    2. Poor feeding frequency: Initiation of lactation does not depend on suckling until the third or fourth day; subsequently, secretion of milk declines if milk is not regularly removed from the breast (Daly et al., 1996; Lawrence et al., 2011).

    3. Vacuum extraction, urgent cesarean, separation (Hall et al., 2002).

    4. Mismanagement of early breastfeeding (for example, prolonged breast engorgement).

    5. Cesarean delivery (Evans et al., 2003).

C. Infant medical conditions (Lawrence et al., 2011)

    1. Anoxia/hypoxia

    2. Preterm

    3. Neonatal jaundice

    4. Trisomy 13, 18, or 21

    5. Hypothyroidism

    6. Neuromuscular dysfunction

    7. Central nervous system impairment

    8. Abnormal suckling patterns—*feeding skills disorder* (terminology proposed by Ramsay et al., 1993)

        a. Abnormal feeding-related symptoms that appear shortly after birth that suggest that the infant may be minimally neurologically abnormal and require closer evaluation to prevent difficulties in mother–infant interaction

    9. Allergies (Agostoni et al., 2000)

    10. Infection/sepsis (Collet et al., 2009 ; Vilavona Juanola et al., 1989)

    11. Inborn errors of metabolism (Ficicioghi et al., 2009)

D. Infrequent/fewer feeds (Walker, 2006)

    1. Mother–infant separation

    2. Overuse of pacifiers

    3. Water/juice supplementation

    4. Early solids

    5. Baby "training" programs that inhibit ability to breastfeed on cue

E. Low net milk intake

    1. Vomiting (pyloric stenosis, severe reflux)

    2. Diarrhea

    3. Malabsorption (such as in the following conditions: neonatal hypothyroidism, galactosemia) (Lawrence et al., 2011)

F. Infants with high energy requirements

    1. SGA infant

    2. Stimulants in the milk

    3. Neurologic disorders

    4. Severe congenital heart disease

V. Maternal Factors (Table 43-2)

   A. Inadequate milk production

      1. Severe postpartum hemorrhage (Willis et al., 1995)

      2. Mismanagement

         a. Improper positioning

         b. Low frequency/duration of feedings. Use of pacifiers to delay feeding

         c. Rigid feeding schedules

         d. Absence of night feedings

         e. Rigid adherence to "switch nurse" technique (sometimes leading to short duration of feedings or decreased intake of hindmilk)

         f. Unsupervised or inappropriate use of nipple shields (especially in the absence of efforts to protect the milk supply with hand expression or pumping)

         g. Prolonged, unrelieved breast engorgement (Daly et al., 1996)

         h. Nongraspable nipples (flat, inverted, large, or long) (Geddes, 2007; Hall et al., 2002)

         i. Lack of adequate assessment

      3. Insufficient glandular development (Neifert et al., 1985)

         a. No or minimal breast changes during pregnancy and no postpartum breast fullness

         b. Maternal breast variation. Marked differences in the shape and size of the breasts Vazininejad et al., 2009)

      4. Other maternal physical factors (Chapman et al., 1999; Dewey et al., 2003; Hall et al., 2002; Lawrence et al., 2011)

         a. Illness/infection

         b. Hypothyroidism

         c. Untreated or inadequately managed diabetes

         d. Sheehan's syndrome

         e. Pituitary tumors

         f. Mental illness

         g. Retained placenta

         h. History of infertility or polycystic ovary syndrome

         i. Fatigue

         j. Emotional disturbance (postdelivery "blues," postpartum depression, chronic mental illness)

         k. Obesity (Nommsen-Rivers et al., 2010)

         l. Other or rare conditions such as gestational ovarian theca lutein cysts (Hoover et al., 2002)

Table 43-2 Maternal Factors That May Contribute to Slow Infant Weight Gain

Factor	Effect
Breast abnormalities	Previous breast surgery, insufficient glandular development, augmentation, reduction, and trauma may influence the ultimate volume of milk that the breasts will produce but do not preclude breastfeeding.
Nipple anomalies	Flat, retracted, inverted, oddly shaped, or dimpled nipples may make latching more difficult and reduce milk intake. Improper suckling on nipples may also damage them, further reducing infant milk intake.
Ineffective or insufficient milk removal	Improperly positioned/latched infant, ineffective suckling, unresolved engorgement leaves residual milk and reduces supply, making less milk available to the infant.
Delayed lactogenesis II	Mother who is overweight, obese, or diabetic may experience an initial delay in lactogenesis II. With copious milk production delayed, frequency of feedings must increase to offset volume deficit.
Poor breastfeeding management	Delayed or disrupted early feeding opportunities, separation, too few feedings, and illness reduce feeding opportunities at breast. Failure to pump milk in the absence of an infant suckling at breast may interfere with proliferation and sensitivity of prolactin receptors.
Medications/drugs	Prescription or recreational drugs, labor medications, and IV fluids may delay lactogenesis II or interfere with infant suckling. Oral contraceptives can reduce lactose content and overall milk volume (Hale, 2006). Smoking may also decrease volume (Vio et al., 1991) and fat content of milk (Hopkinson et al., 1992).
Hormonal alterations	Hypothyroid, retained placenta, superimposed pregnancy, pituitary disorders, polycystic ovarian syndrome, theca lutein cysts (Hoover et al., 2002), oral contraceptives, diabetes insipidus, assisted reproduction/difficulty conceiving, or other endocrine-related problems may interfere with the normal progression of milk production.
Milk ejection problems	Drugs, alcohol, smoking, stress, pain, or other factors that inhibit the let-down reflex reduce the amount of milk available to the infant.
Miscellaneous factors	Lack of vitamin B_{12} in a vegetarian diet, parenting programs that limit feedings, ineffective breast pump or pumping schedule, inadequate weight gain during pregnancy, postpartum hemorrhage, anemia, cesarean delivery (Evans et al., 2003).

5. Drugs (Hale, 2010)
   a. Estrogen
   b. Antihistamine
   c. Pseudoephedrine
   d. Sedatives
   e. Diuretics
   f. Large doses of vitamin B_6
   g. Prenatal administration of corticosteroids to the mother within 3 to 9 days of birth (Henderson et al., 2008)
   h. Alcohol
   i. Nicotine (smoking can decrease fat content of milk and inhibit the milk ejection reflex) (Hopkinson et al., 1992; Vio et al., 1991)
6. Severe maternal diet restriction
7. Breast reduction and other breast surgeries
8. Pregnancy
9. Impaired milk ejection reflex
   a. Psychological inhibition
   b. Stress
   c. Pain
10. Abnormal milk composition
    a. Very low fat diet.
    b. Strict vegan vegetarian without vitamin B_{12} supplementation.
    c. Gastric bypass (mothers need dietary counseling).
    d. Stimulants in the milk (coffee, tea, cola) may increase infant metabolic rate (Lawrence et al., 2011).

VI. Taking a History (Powers, 2001, 2010)

A. Details of the breastfeeds/feedings
   1. Frequency of breastfeeds
      a. Usually an exclusively breastfed baby feeds *at least* eight times per 24 hours. Before 12 weeks of life, most babies do not sleep for more than 4 to 5 hours at a stretch. Infants who sleep one 6-hour stretch may make up for missed feedings by increasing their frequency of feeding at other times of the day (American Academy of Pediatrics [AAP] Section on Breastfeeding, 2005; Lawrence & Lawrence, 2011).
   2. Duration
      a. Normally, infant should breastfeed on one breast until he or she comes off spontaneously; then the baby can be placed on the other side. "The duration of the feeding is normally determined by the infant's response and not by time. Enough time must be spent on a single breast to assure getting the fat-rich, calorie-rich hindmilk" (Lawrence et al., 2011).

   b. Preterm, weak, ill, or lethargic infants may become exhausted after only a few minutes of effective sucking, during which they primarily consume lower-calorie foremilk. They may spend the rest of the time asleep at breast. Once effective sucking stops, the milk supply is better stimulated by emptying the breast with hand expression or a pump so that expressed hindmilk is available for supplementation.

      i. Other strategies to improve milk intake may include teaching the mother signs of effective feeding, supervised use of an appropriately sized nipple shield (Meier et al., 2000), test weights, teaching mothers to separate foremilk from hindmilk for supplementation, skin-to-skin holding, and peer support (Meier, 2003; Spatz, 2004).

3. Signs of the milk ejection reflex

   a. Leaking or spraying of milk

   b. Tingling or burning sensations within the breast

   c. Does the baby consistently swallow, or is swallowing seen only when the milk release occurs?

4. History of the use of supplements

   a. Is there a history of supplementation of other liquids and foods? Was medical necessity documented?

   b. If supplementation was initiated, was complementary milk expression begun?

   c. What feeding method was used to supplement?

      i. Is the supplementation method effective? Efficient? Well tolerated by the infant?

B. Infant history

1. General health (including information about the birth, including history of birth trauma)

2. Birth weight/adequacy for gestational age

3. Lowest weight after birth and the age at that time

4. Sleep pattern

5. Fussiness

6. Frequency of urine and stool output

   a. An infant is usually getting enough milk if there are at least six soaking wet diapers a day after day 4, and three or more bowels movements per day in infants younger than 6 weeks of age (Lawrence et al., 2011). See **Table 43-3**.

   b. An infant can be well hydrated enough to urinate but may be calorically deprived.

      i. Stool frequency may be a better marker for adequate caloric intake.

      ii. Parents may need specific education to help them distinguish between a normal size bowel movement and one too small to be counted.

7. Replacement of breast stimulation resulting from overuse of pacifiers

Table 43-3 Signs of Sufficient Breastmilk Intake

Age	Wet Diapers	Color	Urates	Stools	Color	Volume	Consistency	Weight Gain
Day 1	1	pale	possible	1	black	≥15 gm	tarry/sticky	<5% loss
Day 2	2–3	pale	possible	1–2	greenish/black	≥15 gm	changing	<5% loss
Day 3	3–4	pale	possible	3–4	greenish/yellow	≥15 gm	soft	≤8–10% loss
Day 4	≥4–6 disposable ≥6–8 cloth	pale	none	4 large 10 small	yellow/seedy	≥15 gm	soft/liquidy	15–30 gm/day

Sources: Adapted from Powers, N. G., & Slusser, W. (1997). Breastfeeding update 2: Clinical lactation management. *Pediatrics in Review, 18,* 147–161; Black, L. S. (2001). Incorporating breastfeeding care into daily newborn rounds and pediatric office practice. *Pediatric Clinics of North America, 48,* 299–319; Neifert, M. R. (2001). Prevention of breastfeeding tragedies. *Pediatric Clinics of North America, 48,* 273–297.

C. Maternal assessment
  1. General health
  2. Psychological aspects
  3. The mother's social support for breastfeeding (Scott et al., 2001; Sheeshka et al., 2001)
  4. Dietary habits including herbal use
    a. Excessive caffeine intake may increase infant metabolic rate.
  5. Workload
    a. Overload of maternal daily activities or stress
    b. Constraints on milk expression in the workplace
  6. Sleep patterns
  7. Smoking
  8. Alcohol consumption
  9. Medications

VII. Physical Assessment of the Infant Relative to Breastfeeding

A. Assess the infant's hydration status and passage of meconium (Lawrence et al., 2011).
  1. Assess the number of wet diapers each 24 hours.
    a. Day 1: At least 1 void of urine
    b. Day 2: At least 2 voids of urine
    c. Day 3: At least 3 voids of urine
    d. First 30 days: At least 6 to 8 daily voids of urine
  2. Assess the number of stools each 24 hours.
    a. Day 1: At least 1 stool
    b. Day 2: At least 2 stools
    c. Day 3: Meconium should be passed and lightening stool color observed
    d. First 30 days: Minimum of 3 sizable stools daily
  3. Moist mucous membranes should be observed.
  4. The anterior fontanelle should not appear sunken.
  5. Skin turgor should be observed without signs of tenting.
B. Compare the infant's weight, length, and head circumference with previous measurements and determine the baby's pattern of weight gain.
C. Observe anatomic abnormalities of the mouth and major neurologic disturbances.
  1. Observe the ability to root, suck, and swallow.
  2. Observe muscle tone and mouth, tongue, and facial movements.

VIII. Assessment of the Maternal Breast

A. Condition and size of breast/nipples/areolae
B. Presence of scars and history of previous breast surgery
C. Symmetry
D. History of pattern of early breast engorgement

    E. Signs of mastitis
        1. Decreased milk production is a symptom of mastitis.
        2. Decreased milk production can occur with subclinical mastitis (Filteau et al., 1999).

IX. Observation of the Feeding

    A. Typical breast fullness-to-softness changes during feeding.
    B. Positioning.
    C. Latch-on.
    D. Infant suck.
        1. Degree of vigor
        2. Coordination
        3. Rhythmic sucking and swallowing
    E. Signs of adequate milk "release."
        1. Milk flows from the opposite breast.
        2. Milk flows when feeding is interrupted abruptly.
        3. Baby's sucking pattern changes from shallow, rapid sucking to a slower pattern with deep jaw excursions.
    F. Interaction between mother and baby.
    G. Observation of a feeding on the breast including history taking about the pattern of breast usage. Does the mother offer both breasts? Does the infant feed from both breasts?
    H. Test weighing with a sensitive electronic scale provides a more accurate assessment of infant intake than does observation alone, permits targeted supplementation, and prevents overfeeding (Hurst et al., 2004; Meier et al., 1996).

X. Laboratory Tests (Lawrence et al., 2011)

    A. In specific situations, specialized laboratory tests might be of help.
        1. Prolactin levels
            a. Used to rule out inadequate glandular tissue or a primary prolactin secretion defect.
            b. Intrafeeding (after 15 minutes of breastfeeding) prolactin value should be at least twice that of the baseline (Lawrence et al., 2011).
        2. Sodium, chloride, potassium, pH, blood urea, nitrogen, and hematocrit when the infant is dehydrated
            a. When electrolyte levels are abnormal, sodium, chloride, and potassium should be measured in the mother's milk (Lawrence et al., 2011).

XI. Management

    A. All infants who experience failure to thrive should be seen by their primary medical care providers.
    B. If an underlying medical condition is suspected, the lactation consultant will refer the mother and/or baby for medical/surgical assessment.

C. The management of slow weight gain and failure to thrive is based on etiology (see related chapters).

D. When the mother's milk supply is low:

1. Be sure that the baby is correctly positioned and latched on.

2. Suggest to the mother the following actions:

   a. Increase the number of breastfeeds, but verify that the infant is removing milk. If the infant is not transferring milk, use a combination of hand expression and pumping to remove milk to protect the milk supply (Morton et al., 2009).

   b. If the mother has been offering only one breast at a feeding, offer both breasts at each feeding.

   c. Ensure that the infant receives the hindmilk.

   d. Use breast compression when the baby is on the breast but no longer seems to be getting milk, if the baby is sleepy or not sucking actively (Powers, 2001).

   e. Avoid bottles, pacifiers, and nipple shields unless clinically indicated. Supervise their use and devise a plan to withdraw these interventions when no longer necessary.

   f. Ideally give only mother's milk in the first 6 months; however, formula supplements may be required if the milk supply is deficient and a safe source of donor human milk is unavailable.

   g. Weaning foods may be introduced earlier than 6 months in addition to breastfeeding as an alternative to formula in some cases (AAP Section on Breastfeeding, 2005).

   h. Provide counseling for the mother to eat a well-balanced diet, drink enough fluids, and rest.

E. Supplementary feeding might be necessary (Academy of Breastfeeding Medicine [ABM] Protocol Committee, 2009).

1. Temporary or permanent supplementation:

   a. Recovery from malnutrition is ideally achieved with human milk feeds (Graham et al., 1996). Pumped own mother's milk, human donor milk from a safe source or accredited human donor milk bank, or formula may be required if the mother's milk supply is temporarily or permanently insufficient to meet the infant's growth needs.

2. Recommendations on the type and method of supplemental feedings depend on motivation and conditions (physical and emotional) of the mother, as well as availability of donor human milk banks (ABM Protocol Committee, 2009).

   a. There is little evidence regarding safety or efficacy of various feeding methods.

3. Select method of feeding based on cost and availability, ease of use and cleaning, stress to the infant, whether the adequate milk volume can be fed in 20–30 minutes, and maternal preference.

4. When cleanliness is suboptimal, cup feeding is recommended (WHO, 2003).

5. When the mother's supply is adequate, the first choice is to supplement the child with her own fresh milk.

    a. Maternal milk volume is greater when electric breast pumps are used to stimulate production. Although hand expression may be used, for best results combine techniques (Curtis, 2010).

    b. Expressed hindmilk can be used as a high-calorie supplement (Meier, 2003).

    c. Mothers can skim off the cream layer of milk that has sat in a refrigerator for 24 hours.

    d. In many circumstances, when the infant has neuromuscular or central nervous system disorders, consultation with an occupational therapist (OT) may be necessary to assist in the selection of optimal feeding method to facilitate full feedings.

6. In some selected cases, when routine methods fail, and maternal prolactin levels are documented to be low, maternal medications (metoclopramide, domperidone, sulpiride) may be considered by the physician (ABM Protocol Committee, 2011; Hale, 2010; Zuppa et al., 2010).

    a. Because of the risk of side effects, these medications should be used with caution.

    b. Galactagogues should be prescribed at the lowest possible doses for the shortest period of time.

    c. Counsel mothers not to exceed therapeutic doses.

    d. Counsel mothers to taper off galactagogue use under physician supervision in accordance with the ABM guidelines.

    e. Inquire about any herbs the mother may also be taking and alert the physician to monitor for potential drug–herb interactions.

7. When no obvious cause for low milk supply is identified, a positive attitude toward supplemented breastfeeding is helpful: Develop a written plan describing optimal number and length of feedings, amount of required supplementation, and recommend attention to diet and rest for the mother. If possible, counsel the family or friend support systems in ways to assist the mother.

F. Evaluation. Follow-up is an important aspect of management of the infant with FTT/SGA. An early contact by phone within 48 hours is optimal, and reevaluation and a reweigh should take place within 1 week to ensure that interventions are successful in promoting catch-up growth.

1. After a period of catch-up growth, assess whether the infant is now gaining weight within the normal limits.

2. Is the infant now correctly positioned and latched on?

3. Have possible causes of failure to thrive been removed?

4. Has the infant had all necessary medical/surgical assessments?

References

Academy of Breastfeeding Medicine Protocol Committee. (2009). ABM clinical protocol no. 3: Hospital guidelines for the use of complementary feeding in the healthy breastfed neonate. *Breastfeeding Medicine, 4*(3), 175–183. Retrieved from http://www.bfmed.org/Media/Files/Protocols/ABMProtocol_3%20Revised.pdf

Academy of Breastfeeding Medicine Protocol Committee. (2011). ABM clinical protocol no. 9: Use of galactogogues in initiating or augmenting the rate of maternal milk secretion. *Breastfeeding Medicine, 6*(1), 41–49. Retrieved from http://www.bfmed.org/Media/Files/Protocols/Protocol%209%20-%20English%201st%20Rev.%20Jan%202011.pdf

Agostoni, C., Grandi, F., Scaglioni, S., et al. (2000). Growth pattern of breastfed and nonbreastfed infants with atopic dermatitis in the first year of life. *Pediatrics, 106*, e73.

American Academy of Pediatrics Section on Breastfeeding. (2005). Policy statement: Breastfeeding and the use of human milk. *Pediatrics, 115*(2), 496–506.

Chapman, D., & Perez-Escamilla, R. (1999). Identification of risk factors for delayed onset of lactation. *Journal of the American Dietetic Association, 99*(4), 450–454.

Collet, E., Diebold, P., & Paccaud, D. (2009). A 6-week old infant with failure to thrive: Insidious presentation of group B streptococcal ventriculitis. *Archives of Pediatrics, 16*(4), 360–363.

Curtis, B. (2010, July). *Comparison of Ugandan mother's milk expression technique for infants in special care nurseries.* Oral research presented at the International Lactation Consultant Association Annual Conference, San Antonio, TX.

Daly, S., Kent, J., Owens, R., et al. (1996). Frequency and degree of milk removal and the short-term control of human milk synthesis. *Experimental Physiology, 81*(5), 861–875.

Dewey, K., Heinig, M. J., Nommsen, L. A., et al. (1992). Growth of breastfed and formula fed infants from 0 to 18 months: The DARLING study. *Pediatrics, 89*(6, Pt. 1), 1035–1041.

Dewey, K., Nommsen-Rivers, L., & Heinig, M. (2003). Risk factors for suboptimal infant breastfeeding, delayed onset of lactation, and excess neonatal weight loss. *Pediatrics, 112*(3, Pt. 1), 607–619.

Emond, A., Drewett, R., Blair, P., et al. (2007). Postnatal factors associated with failure to thrive in term infants in the Avon Longitudinal Study of parents and children. *Archives of Disease in Childhood, 92*(2), 115–119.

Evans, K. C., Evans, R. G., Royal, R., et al. (2003). Effect of cesarean section on breast milk transfer to the normal term newborn over the first week of life. *Archives of Disease in Childhood: Fetal and Neonatal Edition, 88*, F380–F382.

Ficicioghi, C., & Haack, K. (2009). Failure to thrive: When to suspect inborn errors of metabolism. *Pediatrics, 124*(3), 972–979.

Filteau, S., Rice, A., Ball, J., et al. (1999). Breast milk immune factors in Bangladeshi women supplemented   postpartum with retinol or beta-carotene. *American Journal of Clinical Nutrition, 69*(5), 953–958.

Fomon, S. J., & Nelson, S. E. (1993). Size and growth. In S. J. Fomon (Ed.), *Nutrition of normal infants* (pp. 36–84). St. Louis, MO: Mosby Yearbook.

Garza, C., Frongillo, E., Dewey, K. G., et al. (1994). Implications of growth patterns of breastfed infants for growth references. *Acta Paediatrica, 402*(2, Suppl.), 4–10.

Geddes, D. (2007). Gross anatomy of the lactating breast. In T. Hale & P. Hartmann (Eds.), *Hale and Hartmann's textbook of human lactation*. Amarillo, TX: Hale Publishing.

Graham, G., MacLean, W. C., Jr., & Brown, K. H. (1996). Protein requirements of infants and children: Growth during recovery from malnutrition. *Pediatrics, 97*(4), 499–505.

Hale, T. W. (2010). *Medications and mother's milk* (14th ed.). Amarillo, TX: Hale Publishing.

Hall, R., Mercer, A., Teasley, S., et al. (2002). A breast-feeding assessment score to evaluate the risk for cessation of breast-feeding by 7 to 10 days of age. *Journal of Pediatrics, 141*(5), 659–664.

Henderson, J., Hartmann, P., Newnham, J. P., et al. (2008). Effect of preterm birth and antenatal corticosteroid treatment on lactogenesis II in women. *Pediatrics, 121*(1), e92–e100.

Hoover, K. L., Barbalinardo, L. H., & Platia, M. P. (2002). Delayed lactogenesis II secondary to gestational ovarian theca lutein cysts in two normal singleton pregnancies. *Journal of Human Lactation, 18*, 264–268.

Hopkinson, J. M., Schanler, R. J., Fraley, J. K., & Garza, C. (1992). Milk production by mothers of premature infants: Influence of cigarette smoking. *Pediatrics, 90*, 934–938.

Hurst, N., Meier, P., Engstrom, J., et al. (2004). Mothers performing in-home measurement of milk intake during breastfeeding of their preterm infants: Maternal reactions and feeding outcomes. *Journal of Human Lactation, 20*(2), 178–187.

Iver, N. P., Srinivasan, R., & Evans, K. (2008). Impact of an early weighing policy on neonatal hypernatremic dehydration and breast feeding. *Archives of Disease in Childhood, 93*(4), 297–299.

Lawrence, R. A., & Lawrence, R. M. (2011). *Breastfeeding: A guide for the medical profession* (7th ed.). Maryland Heights, MO: Elsevier Mosby.

Lucas, A., Fewtrell, M. S., Davies, P. S. W., et al. (1997). Breastfeeding and catch-up growth in infants born small for gestational age. *Acta Paediatrica, 86*, 564–569.

Lukefahr, J. (1990). Underlying illness associated with failure to thrive in breastfed infants. *Clinical Pediatrics, 29*(8), 468–470.

Meier, P. (2003). Supporting lactation in mothers with very low birth weight infants. *Pediatric Annals, 32*(5), 317–325.

Meier, P., Brown, L., Hurst, N., et al. (2000). Nipple shields for preterm infants: Effect on milk transfer and duration of breastfeeding. *Journal of Human Lactation, 16*(2), 106–114.

Meier, P., & Engstrom, J. (2007). Test weighing for term and premature infants is an accurate procedure [Letter]. *Archives of Disease in Childhood: Fetal and Neonatal Edition, 92*(2), F155–F156.

Meier, P., Engstrom, J., Fleming, B., et al. (1996). Estimating milk intake of hospitalized preterm infants who breastfeed. *Journal of Human Lactation, 12*(1), 21–26.

Morton, J., Hall, J. Y., Wong, R. J., et al. (2009). Combining hand techniques with electric pumping increases milk production in mothers of preterm infants. *Journal of Perinatology, 87*, 1–8.

Neifert, M., Seacat, J., & Jobe, W. (1985). Lactation failure due to insufficient glandular development of the breast. *Pediatrics, 76*(5), 823–827.

Nommsen-Rivers, L., Chantry, C., & Peerson, J. M., et al. (2010). Delayed onset of lactogenesis among first-time mothers is related to maternal obesity and factors associated with ineffective breastfeeding. *American Journal of Clinical Nutrition, 92*(3), 574–584.

Powers, N. G. (2001). How to assess slow growth in the breastfed infant. Birth to 3 months. *Pediatric Clinics of North America, 48*, 345–363.

Powers, N. G. (2010). Low intake in the breastfed infant: Maternal and infant considerations. In J. Riordan & K. Wambach (Ed.), *Breastfeeding and human lactation* (4th ed., pp. 277–309). Sudbury, MA: Jones and Bartlett.

Ramsay, M., Gisel, E., Boutry, M., et al. (1993). Non-organic failure to thrive: Growth failure secondary to feeding skills disorder. *Developmental Medicine and Child Neurology, 35*(4), 285–297.

Scott, J., Landers, M., Hughes, R., et al. (2001). Psychosocial factors associated with abandonment of breastfeeding prior to hospital discharge. *Journal of Human Lactation, 17*(1), 24–30.

Sheeshka, J., Potter, B., Valaitis, R., et al. (2001). Women's experiences breastfeeding in public places. *Journal of Human Lactation*, *17*(1), 31–38.

Spatz, D. (2004). Ten steps for promoting and protecting breastfeeding for vulnerable infants. *Journal of Perinatology and Neonatal Nursing*, *18*(4), 385–396.

Vazirinejad, R., Darakhshan, S., Esmaelli, A., & Hadadian, S. (2009). The effect of maternal breast variations on neonatal weight gain in the first seven days of life. *International Breastfeeding Journal*, *4*(13). doi:10.1186/1746-4358-4-13

Vilavona Juanola, J. M., Juanola, J. M., Canos Molinos, J., & Rosell Arnold, E. (1989). Urinary tract infection in the newborn infant. *Anales Españoles de Pediatría*, *31*(2), 105–109.

Vio, F., Salazar, G., & Infante, C. (1991). Smoking during pregnancy and lactation and its effects on breast milk volume. *American Journal of Clinical Nutrition*, *54*, 1011–1016.

Walker, M. (2006). *Breastfeeding management for the clinician: Using the evidence.* Sudbury, MA: Jones and Bartlett.

Willis, C., & Livingstone, V. (1995). Infant insufficient milk syndrome associated with maternal postpartum hemorrhage. *Journal of Human Lactation*, *11*(2), 123–126.

World Health Organization. (2007). The WHO child growth standards. Retrieved from http://www.who.int/childgrowth

World Health Organization Multicenter Growth Reference Study Group. (2006). Assessment of differences in linear growth among populations in the WHO Multicenter Reference Study. *Acta Paediatrica*, *450*(Suppl.), 86–95.

Zuppa, A. A., Sindico, P., Orchi, C., Carducci, C., Cardiello, V., & Romagnoli, C. (2010). Safety and efficacy of galactogogues: Substances that induce, maintain and increase breast milk production. *Journal of Pharmacy and Pharmaceutical Sciences*, *13*(2), 162–174.

APPENDIX A

Summary of the *International Code of Marketing of Breast-milk Substitutes* and Subsequent World Health Assembly Resolutions

Summary

Inappropriate feeding practices lead to infant malnutrition, morbidity, and mortality in all countries, and improper practices in the marketing of breast milk substitutes and related products can contribute to these major public health problems. (*International Code* Preamble)

The *International Code* was adopted by the World Health Assembly on May 21, 1981. The *International Code* is intended to be adopted as a minimum requirement by all governments and aims to protect infant health by preventing the inappropriate marketing of breastmilk substitutes.

Scope

The *International Code* covers the marketing of all breastmilk substitutes (Article 2) and breastfeeding-related items, including the following:

- Infant formula (including so-called hypoallergenic formula, preterm milks, and other "special" baby milks)
- Follow-up milks
- Complementary foods such as cereals, teas and juices, water, and other baby foods that are marketed for use before the baby is 6 months old
- Feeding bottles and teats

Provision of Clear Information

Informational and educational materials dealing with the feeding of infants that are intended to reach health professionals, pregnant women, and mothers of infants and young children should include clear information about all of the following points:

- The benefits and superiority of breastfeeding
- Maternal nutrition and the preparation for and maintenance of breastfeeding
- The negative effect on breastfeeding of introducing partial bottle-feeding
- The difficulty of reversing the decision not to breastfeed
- Where needed, the proper use of infant formula

When such materials contain information about the use of infant formula, they should include the following points:

- Social and financial implications of its use.
- Health hazards of inappropriate foods or feeding methods.
- Health hazards of unnecessary or improper use of infant formula and other breastmilk substitutes.
- Such materials should not use pictures or text that might idealize the use of breastmilk substitutes (Articles 4.2, 7.2).

No Promotion to the Public

There should be no advertising or other form of promotion to the general public of products that are within the scope of the *International Code*. There should be no point-of-sale advertising, giving of samples, or giving any other promotional device to induce sales directly to the consumer at the retail level, such as special displays, discount coupons, premiums, special sales, loss-leaders, and tie-in sales. Marketing personnel should not seek direct or indirect contact with pregnant women or with mothers of infants and young children (Article 5).

No Gifts to Mothers or Health Workers

Manufacturers and distributors should not distribute to pregnant women or mothers of infants and young children any gifts of articles or utensils that might promote the use of breast-milk substitutes or bottle-feeding. No financial or material inducements to promote products within the scope of the *International Code* should be offered to healthcare workers or members of their families. Financial support for professionals who are working in infant and young child health professions should not create conflicts of interest (Articles 5.4 and 7.3, WHA 49.15 [1996]).

No Promotion to Healthcare Facilities

Facilities of healthcare systems should not be used to promote infant formula or other products within the scope of the *International Code*, nor should they be used for the display of products, placards, or posters concerning such products, or for the distribution of material bearing the brand name of products covered by the *International Code* (Articles 6.2, 6.3, and 4.3).

No Promotion to Health Workers

Information provided to health professionals by manufacturers and distributors regarding products covered by the *International Code* should be restricted to scientific and factual matters and should not imply or create a belief that bottle-feeding is equivalent or superior to breastfeeding. Samples of products covered by the *International Code*, or equipment or utensils for their preparation or use, should not be provided to healthcare workers except where necessary for the professional evaluation or research at the institutional level (Articles 7.2 and 7.4).

No Free Samples or Supplies

Neither manufacturers nor healthcare workers should give pregnant women or mothers of infants and young children samples of products covered by the *International Code*. Free or low-cost supplies of breastmilk substitutes should not be given to any part of the healthcare system (which includes maternity wards, hospitals, nurseries, and child care institutions). Donated supplies in support of emergency relief operations should be given only for infants who have to be fed on breastmilk substitutes and should continue for as long as the infants who are concerned need them. Supplies should not be used as a sales inducement (Articles 5.2 and 7.4). *Note:* Articles 6.6 and 6.7 of the *International Code* have been superseded (WHA Resolutions 39.28; 1986, WHA 45.34; 1992, and WHA 47.5; 1994).

No Promotion of Complementary Foods Before They Are Needed

It is important for infants to receive appropriate complementary foods at about 6 months of age. Every effort should be made to use locally available foods. Any food or drink given before complementary feeding is nutritionally required might interfere with the initiation or maintenance of breastfeeding and therefore should not be promoted for use by infants during this period. Complementary foods should not be marketed in ways that undermine exclusive and sustained breastfeeding (*International Code* Preamble; WHA Resolution 39.28, 1986; WHA 45.34, 1992; WHA 47.5, 1994; and WHA 49.15, 1996).

Adequate Labels: Clear Information, No Promotion, and No Baby Pictures

Labels should provide the necessary information about the appropriate use of the product and should not discourage breastfeeding. Infant formula manufacturers should ensure that each container has a clear, conspicuous, and easily readable message in an appropriate language that includes all of the following points:

- The words "Important Notice" or their equivalent
- A statement about the superiority of breastfeeding
- A statement that the product should be used only on the advice of a healthcare worker as to the need for its use and the proper method of use
- Instructions for appropriate preparation and a warning of the health hazards of inappropriate preparation

Neither the container nor the label should have pictures of infants or other pictures or text that might idealize the use of infant formula. The terms *humanized*, *maternalized*, or similar terms should not be used (Articles 9.1 and 9.2).

Companies Must Comply with the *International Code*

Monitoring the application of the *International Code* and subsequent resolutions should be carried out in a transparent, independent manner, free from commercial influence (WHA 49.15, 1996).

Independently of any other measures taken for implementation of the *International Code*, manufacturers and distributors of products covered by the *International Code* should regard themselves as responsible for monitoring their marketing practices according to the principles and aim of the *International Code*.

Manufacturers should take steps to ensure that their conduct at every level conforms to all the preceding provisions (Article 11.3).

APPENDIX B
Universal Precautions and Breastmilk

The Centers for Disease Control and Prevention (CDC) maintains a detailed database on the topic of breastfeeding. The following is reprinted with permission from a section in a monograph titled "Frequently Asked Questions (FAQs)" (www.cdc.gov/breastfeeding/faq/index.htm).

Are special precautions needed for handling breast milk?

CDC does not list human breast milk as a body fluid for which most health care personnel should use special handling precautions. Occupational exposure to human breast milk has not been shown to lead to transmission of HIV or HBV infection. However, because human breast milk has been implicated in transmitting HIV from mother to infant, gloves may be worn as a precaution by health care workers who are frequently exposed to breast milk (e.g., persons working in human milk banks).

For additional information regarding universal precautions as they apply to breast milk in the transmission of HIV and hepatitis B infections, visit the following resources:

- Perspectives in disease prevention and health promotion update: Universal precautions for prevention of transmission of human immunodeficiency virus, hepatitis B virus, and other bloodborne pathogens in health-care settings. (1998). *Morbidity and Mortality Weekly Report*, *37*(24), 377–388.
- CDC. (1987). Recommendations for prevention of HIV transmission in health-care settings. *Morbidity and Mortality Weekly Report*, *36*(Suppl. 2S), 1S–18S.

In regard to Standard Number 1910.1030, "Breast milk does not constitute occupational exposure as defined by standard," the following letter is reprinted from the Department of Labor, Occupational Safety and Health Administration and is available on the Internet:

www.osha.gov/pls/oshaweb/owadisp.show_document?p_table
=INTERPRETATIONS&p_id=20952

December 14, 1992

Ms. Marjorie P. Alloy
Reed, Smith, Shaw & McClay
8251 Greensboro Drive
Suite 1100
McLean, Virginia 22102-3844

Dear Ms. Alloy:

This is in response to your letter of November 23, addressed to the Acting Assistant Secretary, Dorothy L. Strunk. You wrote on behalf of the International Lactation Consultants Association and inquired into the applicability of the Occupational Safety and Health Administration (OSHA) regulation 29 CFR 1910.1030, "Occupational Exposure to Bloodborne Pathogens," to breast milk.

Breast milk is not included in the standard's definition of "other potentially infectious materials." Therefore contact with breast milk does not constitute occupational exposure, as defined by the standard. This determination was based on the Centers for Disease Control's findings that human breast milk has not been implicated in the transmission of the human immunodeficiency virus (HIV) or the hepatitis B virus (HBV) to workers although it has been implicated in perinatal transmission of HIV and the hepatitis surface antigen has been found in the milk of mothers infected with HBV. For this reason, gloves should be worn by health-care workers in situations where exposures to breast milk might be frequent, for example, in milk banking.

We hope this information is responsive to your concerns and thank you for your interest in worker safety and health.

Sincerely,

Roger A. Clark,
Director
Directorate of Compliance Programs

INDEX

A

AA. *See* arachidonic acid
AAP. *See* American Academy of Pediatrics
abandonment of LC-client relationship, 217, 218
abscess of breast, 757–758
accountability, professional, 6, 13, 17, 27
acquisition of parental role, 66–67
active alert, infant behavioral state, 86
active listening, 59, 139
active participation, in adult learning, 54, 55
active sleep, 86, 89
acupuncture to increase milk production, 835
adaptive oral reflexes, 284–285, 303
administrators, hospital lactation service, 244–247
adolescence
    breast development, 262
    consent, 220–221
    maternal nutrition, 322, 325, 327
    support for adolescent mothers, 74–75
adoptive lactation. *See* induced lactation
adult learning principles, 54–55
adult sleep cycles, 89
adult use of donor human milk, 704
adverse child experiences (ACEs) as stressor, 101–102
advertising and marketing. *See also* International Code of Marketing of Breast-milk Substitutes (International Code)
    formula, 9, 41–42
    lactation consultant services, 26–27, 230–231
Africa, donor human milk use, 706–707
age of child
    and bilirubin, 779
    breastfeeding expectations, 594
    gestational, slow weight gain, 852
    induced lactation, 680
    weaning, 596–597
air pollution exposure, 452–453
airway. *See* breathing, infant
alcohol consumption, 332, 464–465, 822
alertness, infant, 86, 91, 540

allergies
    allergy medications, 428, 437–440
    breastmilk protective effects, 348, 400, 402–404, 412
    food sensitivities, 402–403, 414
    lactating women, 331
alpha-lactalbumin, 358, 363, 704
alternate hypothesis, 183, 185
altitude (height) as communication component, 57
aluminum exposure, 456
alveoli, breast, 264–266
ambivalently attached infants, 67
amenorrhea, 70–71
American Academy of Pediatrics (AAP)
    breastfeeding duration, 596
    hyperbilirubinemia, 774–775
    pacifier use and SIDS, 305–306, 741
amino acids in breastmilk, 358. *See also* protein
amniotic fluid, swallowing, 303
amphetamines, 466–467
analgesics
    in breastmilk, 365
    cesarean delivery, 717–718
    labor intervention, 498–499
    lactational pharmacology, 428, 435–436
anatomy
    basic terminology, 275–277
    breasts, 261–272
    infant oral and feeding, 275–285, 302, 475–492
anemia, 325, 344, 565, 828
anklyloglossia, 30, 283, 284, 482–483
anonymity in qualitative research, 211
anorexia, 328
ANOVA (analysis of variance), 186, 187
antacids, 428, 442–443
antepartum secretion. *See* colostrum
anthrax *(Bacillus anthracis)* exposure, 462–463
anthropology, qualitative research, 204
anti-diarrheal medications, 428, 444
anti-infection protections, 365, 394–395, 411–416

fibroadenoma, 760
fibrocystic breast condition (FBC), 759–760
FIL. *See* feedback inhibitor of lactation
financial vulnerability, 141
first contact, neonates, 499–504
Fisher's Exact Test, 187
fit between infant oral anatomy and maternal
       breast/nipple, 492
flat nipples, 271
flavor of breastmilk, 365
flexible work programs, 123
fluids and beverages, 323, 341, 385–386
fluoride, 345–346
folate, 326, 342
follow-on formula, 379
follow-up counseling, 59, 62, 140, 519, 795
fontanels, 278
food
    additives in, 332–333
    allergies to, 402–403, 414
    exclusive *vs.* partial breastfeeding, 383–386
    inadequate, for lactating women, 322
    inappropriate, 385–386
    infant intake effects, 330–333
    for newborns, resistance to change, 155
    solid foods, 414, 578–579, 596
Food and Drug Administration (FDA) on
       formula, 372, 375
food handling, 348
football hold, 73, 508, 510, 540, 548, 573, 574
forceps, 720, 721, 732
foremilk, 292–293
formal stage, parental role acquisition, 66–67
formaldehyde exposure, 453–454
forms, legal, 215
formula, 371–386
    acceptable medical reasons for use of
       (BFHI), 49
    vs. breastmilk, 365–366, 373–376, 404–405
    components of, 371–373
    costs, 383
    exclusive *vs.* partial breastfeeding, 383–386
    forms of, 372–373
    guidelines for nutrient content, 372
    hazards, 378–383, 405
    immune system effects, 376–378, 404–405
    infant growth curves, 590–595
    and infant sleep, 91–92
    labels, 42, 373
    low-income families, 136

    microorganisms in, 43–44
    nervous system development effects, 376–378,
       405
    nutrients in, 373–376
    recalls, 373
    silicone in, 462
    types of, 372
fortified breastmilk, 529, 533–534, 575
fortifiers, liquid and powder, 534
fractured clavicle, neonate, 734
frankness, in adult learning, 54
frenotomy (tongue-tie), 283, 284, 483, 485,
      486, 823
frequency of breastfeeding
    breastmilk expression, 627–628
    cesarean delivery, 717
    infant growth and development, 590, 591,
      595–596
    slow weight gain, 853
    weight gain problems, 856
FTT. *See* failure to thrive
funsters personality, 159

G

GAD. *See* generalized anxiety disorder
gag reflex, 285, 303, 491
galactagogues, 684–687, 694, 833–836
galactocele, 758–759
galactopoesis. *See* lactogenesis II
galactosemia, 734
gastric bypass surgery, 831
gastroesophageal reflux (GER), 738–739
gastrointestinal (GI) disorders
    breastmilk protective effects, 405, 412–416
    esophageal atresia, 738
    gastroesophageal reflux (GER), 738–739
    infant, 738–739
    nutrition for lactating women, 322–323, 328
    pyloric stenosis, 739
    slow weight gain, 852
gatekeepers, employers, 125
gel dressings, 650–651, 754
gender differences, infant growth, 591–593,
      831–834
generalist education level, 168
generalized anxiety disorder (GAD), 104
genetic disorders. *See* infant genetic and
      congenital disorders